This book is sent to you on permanent
loan but is still Library property

To keep our computer records up to date,
it is essential that you inform Library Staff
Sue Storey/Morag Stanley, if you transfer this
book to another person.

The Library
ZENECA Central Toxicology Laboratory
Alderley Park
Macclesfield
Cheshire SK10 4TJ

The Metabolism of Drugs and Other Xenobiotics

THE METABOLISM OF DRUGS AND OTHER XENOBIOTICS

Edited by Bernard Testa and John Caldwell

The Metabolism of Drugs and Other Xenobiotics:
Biochemistry of Redox Reactions
Bernard Testa

The Metabolism of Drugs and Other Xenobiotics:
Biochemistry of Hydration and Dehydration Reactions (in preparation)
Bernard Testa and Joachim M. Mayer

The Metabolism of Drugs and Other Xenobiotics:
Biochemistry of Conjugation Reactions (in preparation)
Bernard Testa, Joachim M. Mayer and John Caldwell

The Metabolism of Drugs and Other Xenobiotics:
Biological Regulation and Consequences (in preparation)
John Caldwell and Bernard Testa

THE METABOLISM OF DRUGS AND OTHER XENOBIOTICS

BIOCHEMISTRY OF REDOX REACTIONS

Bernard Testa
School of Pharmacy
University of Lausanne
CH-1015 Lausanne, Switzerland

ACADEMIC PRESS
Harcourt Brace and Company, Publishers
London   San Diego   New York
Boston   Sydney   Tokyo   Toronto

ACADEMIC PRESS LIMITED
24–28 Oval Road
London, NW1 7DX

United States Edition published by
ACADEMIC PRESS INC.
San Diego, CA 92101

A catalogue record for this book
is available from the British Library

ISBN 0-12-685391-6

Typeset by Keyset Composition, Colchester, Essex
Printed and bound in Great Britain by The Bath Press, Avon

This book is dedicated to the loving memory of my parents,

Humbert Guido Testa (1909–1991)

and

Lina Klara Testa-Grau (1911–1993),

whose main goal in life
was the education and happiness of their children.

FOREWORD

Mammals have only a limited ability to pick and choose among the molecules in their diet. Therefore, these animals take on board a vast range of substances, which at best serve no nutritional role, and at worst can produce acute or chronic tissue damage. Ultimately, the biological defences against this chemical invasion are the physiological pathways of molecular elimination via the liver and kidneys. However, these animals have also developed a first-line defensive apparatus, an extensive ensemble of enzymes which oxidize or reduce, hydrolyze or conjugate these foreign, xenobiotic molecules. The essential design principle of these enzymes is non-selectivity: they recognize common, general, chemical features of organic molecules, not the molecules themselves. This system of xenobiotic metabolism, which is adapted to molecular invasion, is as vital to mammalian survival as the immunological apparatus which has been adapted to deal with invasion by organisms. At the molecular level, they share the same design principles of non-selectivity. Built-in non-discriminatory activity has, however, got a down side: the immunological system sometimes sees self as foreign and becomes self-destructive; the xenobiotic metabolic system sometimes generates products more reactive and biologically destructive than the original substrate.

The extensive apparatus for cellular communication, the system of hormones and their conjugate receptors, involves an entirely different design principle. Hormone receptors have evolved with a high degree of molecular discrimination. Medicinal chemists have been incredibly successful in making specific ligands for these receptors which often show remarkable, even unique, selectivity for a specific receptor. However, almost invariably, these selective ligands or drugs are substrates for one or more of the xenobiotic enzyme systems. Quite often, this blind metabolism produces a highly reactive product which can be the basis of a drug's toxicity.

Evidently, xenobiotic metabolism is a subject of great physiological, pathological and pharmacological importance. Professor Bernard Testa is now preparing a several-volume survey of xenobiotic metabolism. He is uniquely qualified to do so. Not only has he spent his life intensely researching this area, but he also has the experience of co-authoring a previous review published in 1976. More important, however, is Professor Testa's philosophical objective of a search for underlying principles so that newcomers will be attracted to pursuing new ideas. The first volume is a one man's view, a highly expert view, of redox reactions. Each chapter comprehensively covers, *inter alia*, reaction mechanisms and catalytic cycle, regio- and stereoselectivities, types of substrates, reactivity of intermediates and drug–enzyme interactions. Testa's deep comprehension of his subject and his scholarly commitment make sure that this volume is not only comprehensive but eminently readable as well.

Sir James Black
Nobel Laureate

PREFACE

The 17th of January 1991 is a day many will remember. In the middle of the night, I was as usual busy writing this book when the barely audible background music on the radio was interrupted by a broadcast announcing that "Operation Desert Storm" had begun. During the next few hours, I continued to alternate typing and listening to the news until sleep could no longer be resisted. But then the telephone rang, announcing that my father had just died. It is to his memory, first, that this book is dedicated, he who was a living example of modesty, kindness, altruism and rectitude—an example that remains with us undiminished.

Two years later, while I had much advanced in this work, misfortune came again with the sudden death of my mother. She was a woman of penetrating intelligence and creativity who had worked hard and against trying odds to ensure well-being to her family. The second dedication is to her memory, so that the names of my parents, who were united in life for more than a half-century, appear together at the beginning of this book.

The genesis of *The Metabolism of Drugs and Other Xenobiotics* (code name "MEDOX") can be traced back to 1976, in other words to the publication of the book on drug metabolism I wrote with Peter Jenner (Testa and Jenner, 1976). This book presented drug metabolism from two vantage points, chemical and biological. Its presentation was based on functional groups, metabolic pathways and biological factors rather than on classes of substrates, giving it a clear heuristic value. The book commanded attention as soon as it was published, and it continued to be used and cited for well over a decade (Testa and Jenner, 1990). But the science of xenobiotic metabolism has progressed enormously since 1976, both in terms of accumulation of data and creation of powerful concepts. The 1976 book is now severely outdated, both in content and in structure.

Ten years ago, I began to consider seriously the writing of a new book on drug metabolism. At this stage, three things became rapidly apparent. First, Professor Peter Jenner had by then moved to molecular pharmacology and felt his interests to be too remote from drug metabolism to enable him to participate in this new endeavour. However, Peter provided much needed guidance at the first stages of the conception of MEDOX. Since then, he has kept a benevolent eye on the project, and he deserves much gratitude for his help and encouragement. The second thing that became clear when conceiving the work was the futility of simply updating the 1976 book, or preparing a new edition of it. Indeed, only an entirely new book, or rather several volumes, could allow the clear presentation and synthesis of the many recent data and concepts that have added so much to our knowledge. I cannot stress too strongly that *The Metabolism of Drugs and Other Xenobiotics* is not a second edition of the 1976 book, but an entirely newly written work. In fact, not a single sentence has been transferred from the 1976 book to the present work.

But there was a third problem with MEDOX that arose from the sheer size of the project. Clearly, a one-man operation was impossible, and I had to find one or two colleagues whom I could trust as partners in the endeavour. This is why I have been fortunate to team up with Professor John Caldwell and Dr Joachim M. Mayer. The former is the senior editor of the volume on *Biological Regulation and Consequences*, but he is also the co-editor of the Series, and as such has provided essential help in the preparation of this volume, not only in terms of ideas and advice, but also in carefully and critically reading and correcting the entire text. What this volume owes to John is beyond evaluation, and it must be stressed that I alone must be blamed for any errors and ambiguities that remain. As for Joachim Mayer, he has been indispensable in two ways, first because he is the co-author of a volume now being written, and second because as explained below he was the technical coordinator in the preparation of the artwork of this volume.

The actual writing of this volume took five years, including an extensive updating to integrate the many recent findings published while the work was in progress. As a result, all chapters of this volume have been updated with material published up to the end of 1993. The nomenclature of cytochrome P450 enzymes used here is entirely based on the review on the CYP superfamily published in January 1993 by Nelson and colleagues. Professor Daniel W. Nebert was kind enough to send a preprint of this essential work early enough for it being smoothly taken into account.

One person who deserves special gratitude is Professor William F. Trager, who read part of the book in its first version and made most useful suggestions to improve clarity and readability. And then, we should not forget the many colleagues who during symposia or at other occasions encouraged me to update the 1976 book and who, upon learning of MEDOX, wholeheartedly supported the idea.

A particular mention must be made of a number of persons who were instrumental editorially or technically to make this book possible. Peter Brown has known and trusted me for more than a decade, giving advice with distinction and understanding. I owe him much not only for this book, but also more generally for other opportunities he has offered.

The writing of this book would have proved outright impossible had word processing and graphics processing not existed. Like many others, I learned to bypass the pen-and-paper step of text writing, saving myself a lot of time and avoiding the need for secretarial assistance. In contrast, help was needed for the artwork. Joachim Mayer proved invaluable in directing two of our graduate students, Marieke Roy-de Vos and Christian Audergon, who enthusiastically took it upon them to draw all chemical formulae and figures using graphics processing. Marieke and Christian were patient enough to modify and correct the drawings time and again until I was satisfied. Needless to say, any error that remains in the artwork is entirely my fault.

The last, but by no means the least, two persons to deserve my warmest gratitude are the writer of the Foreword and my wife Jacqueline. That Sir James, despite innumerable commitments, has accepted and found time to write a Foreword is an honour for the Series and a resonant recognition of the significance of xenobiotic metabolism in drug research and molecular toxicology. As for Jacqueline, she gave precious help with the bibliography, but above all provided unfailing understanding and good-humoured support while having to bear with her husband's absent-mindedness. By simply being who she is, she has given meaning and purpose to my efforts and has allowed them to bear fruits. Anything else that can be said does not need to be made public.

Bernard Testa
February 1994

REFERENCES

Testa B. and Jenner P. (1976). *Drug Metabolism: Chemical and Biochemical Aspects*. Dekker, New York.

Testa B. and Jenner P. (1990). The coming of age of drug metabolism. A "Citation Classic" commentary. *Current Contents Life Sciences* **33**(33), 17.

CONTENTS

Chapter 2: *Dehydrogenation of Alcohols and Aldehydes, Carbonyl Reduction*　41

Chapter 3: *The Nature and Functioning of Cytochromes P450 and Flavin-containing-monooxygenases*　70

Chapter 4: Carbon Oxidations Catalyzed by Cytochromes P450   122

Chapter 7: Monooxygenase-catalyzed Oxidation of Oxygen- and Sulfur-Containing Compounds   235

Chapter 8: Oxidative Dehalogenation, and Dealkylation of Organometallics   284

introduction

XENOBIOTIC METABOLISM: THE GLOBAL VIEW
(A General Introduction to the Series)

by Bernard Testa and John Caldwell

Contents

i.1 INTERACTIONS OF FOREIGN CHEMICALS WITH LIVING SYSTEMS

We live in an environment which abounds in natural and synthetic chemicals lacking nutritional value or the function of vitaminics (Albert, 1987). These anutrient chemicals are often called **xenobiotics**, as they are foreign to the energy-yielding metabolism and other physiological functions of the body. The major categories of xenobiotics are listed in Table i.1. It is virtually impossible to estimate the number of these xenobiotics to which living organisms might be exposed, but some idea of the scale of the problem can be seen from the probably more than ten million compounds synthesized in the last 150 years or so by the ingenuity of chemists, the many tens of thousands of natural compounds responsible for the flavour and fragrance of our foods, and so on.

TABLE i.1 *Major categories of xenobiotics* (modified from Testa, 1984)

- Drugs
- Food constituents devoid of physiological roles
- Food additives (preservatives, colouring and flavouring agents, antioxidants, etc)
- Chemicals of "leisure and pleasure" and of abuse (ethanol, coffee and tobacco constituents, hallucinogens, etc)
- Agrochemicals (fertilizers, insecticides, herbicides, etc)
- Industrial and technical chemicals (solvents, dyes, monomers, polymers, etc)
- Pollutants of natural origin (radon, sulfur dioxide, hydrocarbons, etc)
- Pollutants produced by microbial contamination (aflatoxins, etc)
- Pollutants produced by physical or chemical transformation of natural compounds (polycyclic aromatic hydrocarbons by burning, Maillard reaction products by heating, etc)

TABLE i.2 *Major phases of drug action* (Ariëns, 1970; Ariëns and Simonis, 1977)

Phase	Processes
Pharmaceutical phase	• Desaggregation of the pharmaceutical form
	• Liberation and dissolution of active ingredients (drugs)
Pharmacokinetic phase	• Absorption
	• Distribution
	• Binding and storage
	• Biotransformation (Metabolism)*
	• Excretion
Pharmacodynamic phase	• Interaction between the drug and its site(s) of action (receptors, enzymes, membranes, nucleic acids, etc)

*This is the narrow meaning of the word "metabolism", and the one usually used in this book.

accidental or coincidental upon their use in other circumstances (in industry, agriculture, etc), it is very important indeed to consider the *consequences of such exposures*. This clearly includes the interaction of such compounds with specific sites in the body, dealt with by the science of pharmacology, and the specific and non-specific unwanted effects which are the realm of the toxicologist. However, as well as considering the wanted or unwanted effects, we must have an understanding of how xenobiotics behave in the organism. The study of the disposition—or fate—of xenobiotics in living systems thus includes the consideration of their absorption into the organism; how and where they are distributed and stored; the chemical and biochemical transformations they may undergo; and how and by what route(s) they are finally excreted and returned to the environment. Note that nowhere in the above list is the word "metabolism" to be found. As a matter of fact, in this context the word has acquired two meanings, being synonymous with disposition (i.e. the sum of the processes affecting the fate of a chemical substance in the body) and with biotransformation (Di Carlo, 1982). Only by considering the context can the meaning be clarified, but let us make it very clear here that in this book, metabolism is often equated with biotransformation. In particular, this is the meaning of the word in the book's title. As for the word "elimination", which is also absent from the above list and from Table i.2, it designates biotransformation plus excretion.

We have thus characterized above two aspects of the behaviour of xenobiotics, which may be simplified to "what the compound does to the body" and "what the body does to the compound". In pharmacology, one speaks of "**pharmacodynamic effects**" to indicate what a drug does to the body, and "**pharmacokinetic effects**" to indicate what the body does to the drug (Table i.2). Already at this stage of the discussion, it is critical to appreciate that these two aspects of the behaviour of xenobiotics are inextricably interdependent. Pharmacokinetic effects will obviously have a decisive influence on the intensity and duration of pharmacodynamic effects, and metabolism will generate new chemical entities (metabolites) which may have distinct pharmacodynamic effects properties of their own. Conversely, by its own pharmacodynamic effects, a compound may affect the state of the organism (e.g. hemodynamic changes, enzyme activities, etc) and hence its capacity to handle xenobiotics. Only a systemic approach (i.e. an approach based on systems theory) is capable of appreciating the global nature of this interdependence (Testa, 1987).

i.2 A First Glance at the Fate of Xenobiotics

i.2.1 Absorption

In general, xenobiotics enter by passive diffusion across lipidic membranes unless deliberately injected into the organism (Austel and Kutter, 1980). The most common "portals of entry" are the gastrointestinal tract, the respiratory tract and the skin. A good deal is known about absorption from the **gut**, where ionization and lipophilicity both play major roles. Other influences include gut motility and transit time and the presence of food and other possible sequestering agents in the gut lumen. A small number of xenobiotics are absorbed by active processes but these are generally drugs which mimic nutrients and are taken up by the same me‹   s, e.g. α-methyl-DOPA and 5-fluorouracil. In such cases, the mechanism is generally of low capacity and is highly restrictive in terms of the substrates it recognizes (high substrate specificity).

Entry from the **respiratory tract** is open to volatile compounds and aerosols in the atmosphere. The absorption of volatiles is a function of respiratory rate and tidal volume, and of the lipid solubility and partial pressure of the compound. The disposition of inhaled aerosols depends on the same physiological factors and on particle size. The vast majority of an inhaled aerosol actually leaves the respiratory tract at the back of the nose and is swallowed. The distribution of the remainder is determined by particle size, with smaller particles travelling further into the smaller airways and ultimately reaching the alveoli. Particle size may increase as a result of hydration so that predicting the disposition of an inhaled aerosol is extremely difficult. Absorption across the membranes of the respiratory tract appears to follow the same principles as for the gut, with lipophilicity playing a significant role.

The **skin** encounters an enormous number of xenobiotics and may represent an important barrier to their penetration. The outermost layer of the skin, the stratum corneum, comprises collapsed, keratinized cells which effectively divide the inside from the outside. However, many compounds applied to the skin built up a slowly mobilized depot in the stratum corneum which cannot be removed by washing. Entry to the systemic circulation after dermal application occurs by two routes, either through the cells of the epidermis (the transcellular route) or through gaps between them (the paracellular route). The experimental distinction of these two options is difficult but available evidence indicates that the transcellular route is the more important by far.

i.2.2 Distribution

Once a compound has been absorbed into the general circulation, its distribution throughout the body will be a function of physicochemical and structural properties (e.g. ionization and lipophilicity) due to the balance of factors retaining it in the blood (**binding to blood**

macromolecules) and those forcing the equilibrium in favour of the tissues (**binding to tissue macromolecules, storage into adipose tissues**, etc) (Austel and Kutter, 1983; Fichtl *et al.*, 1991; Tillement *et al.*, 1984). These are processes of **retention** of the xenobiotic or its metabolites. Specific uptake mechanisms into particular cell types will also play a role: examples include uptake of large molecules into Kupffer cells, the uptake of amines in the lung, and drugs stored in adrenergic neurones. There are at least two apparent barriers to drug distribution in the body, the blood–brain barrier and the placental barrier which prevent access of a range of xenobiotics to the brain and the fetus, respectively.

i.2.3 Elimination

Molecules circulating in the blood may undergo one of three distinct fates, which all contribute to the elimination of a given xenobiotic compound:

- excretion unchanged
- non-enzymatic chemical transformation
- enzymatic metabolism.

There are important examples of each of these possibilities but, in quantitative terms, enzymic metabolism greatly predominates over non-enzymic transformation while the fraction excreted unchanged decreases with increasing lipophilicity of the xenobiotic (Austel and Kutter, 1980; Testa, 1982). The **metabolism of drugs and other xenobiotics** is typically a biphasic process in which the compound first undergoes a functionalization reaction (Phase I reaction) of oxidation, reduction or hydrolysis, which introduces or unveils within its structure a functional group (e.g. $-OH$, $-NH_2$) suitable for linkage with an endogenous moiety in the second step of conjugation (Phase II reaction). In some cases, compounds possessing a suitable functionality do undergo conjugation directly, while Phase I metabolites may be excreted prior to conjugation. Also well documented are the reactions of functionalization which a number of conjugates undergo prior to their excretion.

The possible products in the excreta thus include Phase I metabolites and their conjugates, together with the unchanged compound and its own conjugates. But what are the routes of **excretion**? **Urine** is obviously the major and most common route of excretion of xenobiotics and their metabolites. Three processes are involved in the urinary excretion of chemicals, namely glomerular filtration, passive reabsorption, and for some compounds active tubular transport. As a rule, the renal excretion of chemicals decreases with increasing extent of protein binding, and with their increasing lipophilicity (due to increased tubular reabsorption). **Faecal excretion** is also of significance and results from three sources, namely: limited gastrointestinal absorption; biliary excretion; and passive diffusion from blood to intestinal lumen (Dayton *et al.*, 1983). Like urinary excretion, biliary excretion depends on certain physicochemical properties of the compound, in particular an amphipathic character and a molecular weight of sufficient magnitude, itself dependent upon the animal species in question.

Other routes of excretion also exist that are often overlooked, e.g.:

- the **cutaneous route** (perspiration), which involves compounds of good hydrophilicity and/or volatility;
- the **pulmonary route** (breath), which is restricted to highly volatile compounds such as aliphatic halides and some sulphides of low molecular weight;
- the **mammary route** (passage into milk), of potential significance when cows are fed contaminated food, or when lactating mothers are administered lipophilic drugs (Begg and Atkinson, 1993; Gallenberg and Vodicnik, 1989; Wilson, 1983).

i.3 ENDOGENOUS BIOCHEMISTRY VS. XENOBIOTIC METABOLISM: THE EVOLUTIONARY VIEW

i.3.1 Introduction

Section i.1 above has defined xenobiotics by listing them (Table i.1) and by contrasting them with environmental compounds of physiological value (e.g. nutrients, vitamins, minerals, water and oxygen). The latter compounds, after their entry into the body, are metabolized to endogenous substances (the so-called **endobiotics**) which are substrates and/or products of endobiotic-metabolizing enzymes. Xenobiotics can therefore also be contrasted with endobiotics, leading to speculation as to whether and by how much endogenous biochemistry and xenobiotic metabolism involve the same, exclusive, or overlapping metabolic pathways and enzymes (Jenner *et al.*, 1981). This question is intimately related to the intriguing fact that most of the xenobiotic-metabolizing enzymes made their appearance early in evolution, billions of years ago, while their human-made substrates are only decades old (Testa *et al.*, 1981).

Schematically, two answers can be proposed to account for this puzzle. The first explanation would be that enzymes have evolved solely to metabolize endobiotics of ever increasing variety and complexity, and that xenobiotics are fortuitous substrates due to their structural similarities with the physiological substrates. The second solution would be that specialized xenobiotic-metabolizing enzymes have evolved to protect organisms from natural xenobiotics produced by, for example, combustion and plants, artificial xenobiotics of contemporary appearance being substrates simply because they resemble these natural xenobiotics. As will be seen, both explanations apply depending on the enzymes and substrates in question.

i.3.2 The evolution of xenobiotic-metabolizing enzymes

The so-called xenobiotic-metabolizing enzymes (Table i.3) share to a variable extent a number of characteristics that apparently contrast them with the enzymes of endogenous biochemistry (Jakoby and Ziegler, 1990; Jenner *et al.*, 1981; Ziegler, 1990):

(a) They have low orders of substrate specificities, being promiscuous for large varieties of structurally diverse substrates.
(b) In some cases, they may even display low chemospecificity and/or product specificities, being able to catalyze the formation of more than one type of functional group.
(c) They tend to have low catalytic rates, which are sometimes compensated for by the presence of very large amounts of the enzyme.
(d) They have a distinct preference for lipophilic substrates which they convert to more polar products which may be more easily excreted so that loss of water is minimal.
(e) They are inducible by many xenobiotics, particularly by some of their substrates. How much this property is shared by the enzymes of endogenous metabolism remains to be better understood.

As a consequence of the above, the major function of xenobiotic-metabolizing enzymes can be seen as the **elimination of physiologically useless compounds**. Some of these compounds are harmless, but others are harmful: witness the tens of thousands of toxins produced by plants to protect themselves against fungi, insects, and animal predators (Ames and Profet, 1992). The function of **toxin inactivation** thus justifies the designation of "**enzymes of detoxication**", although it is a sad irony, as discussed in Section i.4, that in a significant number of cases

TABLE i.3 *A compilation of enzymes acting on xenobiotics* (In such a list, the discrimination between the so-called xenobiotic-metabolizing enzymes and the enzymes of endogenous biochemistry is not easily made)

Oxidoreductases	*Transferases*
Alcohol dehydrogenases	Catechol O-methyltransferase
Aldo-keto reductases	N-Methyltransferases
Quinone reductase	S-Methyltransferases
Aldehyde dehydrogenases	Phenol sulfotransferases
Dihydrodiol dehydrogenases	Alcohol sulfotransferases
Cytochromes P450	Steroid sulfotransferases
FAD-containing monooxygenases	Amine sulfotransferases
Hemoglobin	Glucuronyltransferases
Dopamine β-mono-oxygenase	Glucosyltransferases
Monoamine oxidase	N-Acetyltransferases
Xanthine oxidase	O-Acetyltransferases
Aldehyde oxidase	Arylformamidase
Copper-containing amine oxidases	Cholesterol ester synthase
Prostaglandin-endoperoxide synthase	Acyl-coenzyme A synthetases
Myeloperoxidase and other peroxidases	N-Acyltransferases
	O-Acyltransferases
Hydrolases	Glutathione S-transferases
Carboxylesterases	Phosphotransferases
Arylesterases	
Cholinesterase	*Lyases*
Glucuronidases	Cysteine-S-conjugate β-lyase
Thiolester hydrolases	Dehydrochorinases
Endo- and exo-peptidases	
Arylsulfatases	
Phosphatases	
Epoxide hydrolases	

"detoxication reactions" actually generate one or more highly reactive/toxic metabolites that may cause damage at the molecular, cellular and organismic levels. Nevertheless, the detoxication function of these enzymes remains genuine and could well be more far-reaching than believed hitherto. The recent characterization of a unique multifunctional protein from rat liver which links enzymatic and immunological detoxication systems raises fascinating perspectives (Blocki *et al.*, 1992).

It is probably the function of detoxication that accounts for the prodigious evolution of the genes of xenobiotic-metabolizing enzymes during the last 0.5 billion years, a continuous molecularly driven co-evolution of plants producing phytotoxins and animals responding with new (iso)enzymes to detoxify these chemicals—the so-called "**animal-plant warfare**" (Gonzalez and Nebert, 1990). The evolution of the P450 gene superfamily is exemplary in this respect, with an ancestral gene appearing more than 3.5 billion years ago (see Section i.3.3), and many contemporary genes and their products (enzymes) in the various families and subfamilies having emerged during the past 0.4 billion years.

Because animals and plants may have begun to diverge approximately 1.2 billion years ago, the "animal-plant warfare" cannot account for the much earlier appearance of some ancestral enzymes. This has led some scientists to present thought-provoking speculations about their possible functions. For example, the ancestral form of cytochrome P450 appeared before the advent of free oxygen in the atmosphere, its low redox potential allowing it to function under reducing conditions. It may then have provided an early line of defence against the progressively appearing molecular oxygen. And when this protective role in detoxifying oxygen was superseded by the development of aerobic organisms, its other activities retained their usefulness in the transformation of endogenous and exogenous compounds (Wickramasinghe and Villee, 1975).

Another enzymatic activity in prokaryotes and early eukaryotes may have been the **metabolic control of the steady-state levels** of various ligands modulating cell division, growth, homeostasis, differentiation and morphogenesis, and neuroendocrine functions (Nebert, 1991). Such functions, of course, remain operative today and have lost nothing of their significance, but they seem no longer to be mediated by the same (iso)enzymes that metabolize xenobiotics (see below).

i.3.3 Endogenous biochemistry and xenobiotic metabolism

Because Nature is at the same time both prodigious and thrifty, the coexistence in organisms of endogenous biochemistry and xenobiotic metabolism takes many forms, and may involve the same, exclusive, or overlapping metabolic pathways and enzymes.

A simple form of overlap is the sharing of common cofactors (e.g. NADPH) or common electron transfer enzymes (e.g. cytochrome b_5) (Estabrook and Werringloer, 1979). A more complex form of overlap occurs when xenobiotics and endobiotics are substrates of the same enzymes, as documented in a number of cases.

The previous section clearly suggests that xenobiotic-metabolizing enzymes have evolved precisely to fulfil such a function. However, this does not imply the inadequacy of the first explanation offered at the end of Section i.3.1, namely that xenobiotics may also be **fortuitous substrates** of the enzymes of endogenous biochemistry. Indeed, it seems that most enzymes in Table i.3 (e.g. dopamine β-monooxygenase, monoamine oxidase, xanthine oxidase, prostaglandin-endoperoxide synthase, myeloperoxidase, catechol O-methyltransferase) have not, to the best of our knowledge, evolved to metabolize xenobiotics. Nevertheless, they do metabolize a very large number of xenobiotics, but only because these display some structural resemblance to the physiological substrates.

The situation is more complex when it comes to large superfamilies of enzymes, e.g. the cytochromes P450. Here, it appears that some families, subfamilies, or individual enzymes have evolved to metabolize xenobiotics, and others to mediate the anabolism and/or catabolism of endogenous compounds. Thus, those cytochromes P450 responsible for the oxidation of xenobiotics are found principally in the endoplasmic reticulum, whereas the steroid-generating enzymes are found in the mitochondria of endocrine organs. However, overlaps do exist and may even be more common than believed.

i.4 IMPACT OF METABOLISM ON PHARMACODYNAMICS AND ON THE ACTIONS OF XENOBIOTICS

The kinetics of absorption, distribution and elimination of a drug (its pharmacokinetics) or a toxin (its toxicokinetics) are bound to have a major influence on the pharmacodynamic or toxicodynamic effects of this xenobiotic. In other words, the disposition of a xenobiotic will influence the intensity and duration of its biological effects, an obvious cause-and-effect relationship. In the case of metabolism (i.e. biotransformation) however, the situation is far more complex since metabolites may have biological effects of their own.

In the simple case of a xenobiotic having a single metabolite, four possibilities exist:

(a)   Both the xenobiotic and its metabolite are devoid of biological effects (at least in the concentration or dose range investigated).
(b)   Only the xenobiotic elicits biological effects.
(c)   Both the xenobiotic and its metabolite are biologically active.
(d)   The observed biological activity is due exclusively to the metabolite.

Case (a) represents an ideal situation characteristic of a number of innocuous xenobiotics. In contrast, it is irrelevant to therapeutic agents, which by definition are bound to elicit a pharmacological response. Case (b) is interesting and corresponds to the **deactivation** of a drug or the **detoxication** of a toxin. Here, the duration and intensity of a xenobiotic's actions will also be influenced, sometimes predominantly, by its rate and extent of metabolism.

Cases (c) and (d) account for the increased complexity mentioned above, and this is particularly true for case (c) (Drayer, 1982). Here, a metabolite may prolong a drug's action (if it has a comparable activity) or expand the range of observed effects (if its activity is different). The production of an active metabolite may therefore be beneficial, or it may be detrimental when it is at the origin of unwanted or downright toxic effects. Case (d) is of particular significance in drug research and toxicology. "Inactive" drugs that yield active metabolites are well known as **prodrugs** (Section 1.8). More is to be said here about xenobiotics that are inactive *per se* but yield reactive metabolites.

When a drug or another xenobiotic is transformed into a toxic metabolite, the reaction is one of **toxication** (Neumann, 1986). Such a metabolite may act or react in a number of ways to elicit a variety of toxic responses at different biological levels (Timbrell, 1991). However, it is essential to stress here, as will be done again in Section 1.8, that the occurrence of a reaction of toxication (i.e. toxicity at the molecular level) does **not** necessarily imply toxicity at the levels of organs and organisms. In other words, the occurrence of a reaction of toxication is by no means a sufficient condition for toxicity. Several factors account for this sobering and often underemphasized fact:

(a)   Metabolic reactions of toxication are always accompanied by competitive and/or sequential reactions of detoxication that compete with the formation of the toxic metabolite and/or inactivate it. A profusion of biological factors control the relative effectiveness of these competitive and sequential pathways.

(b)   The reactivity and half-life of a reactive metabolite condition its sites of action and determine whether it will reach sensitive sites (Gillette, 1983).

(c)   Dose, rate and route of entry into the organism are all factors of known significance.

(d)   Above all, there exist mechanisms of essential survival value which operate to repair molecular lesions, remove them immunologically, and/or regenerate the lesioned sites.

i.5 FACTORS AFFECTING XENOBIOTIC METABOLISM

Xenobiotic metabolism occurs in a biological environment that profoundly affects it in qualitative, quantitative and kinetic terms. A great number of physiological and pathological factors have been characterized which are of importance in drug research and toxicology. It is customary to distinguish between inter-individual and intra-individual factors depending on whether they vary between or within given organisms or individuals, respectively (Table i.4).

The **inter-individual factors** as a rule remain constant during the life span of an organism or individual. Species differences in xenobiotic metabolism are a well-known issue of significance to the extrapolation to humans of metabolic, pharmacological, and toxicological data obtained in animals (Boxenbaum and D'Souza, 1990; Caldwell *et al.*, 1989; Chappell and Mordenti, 1991; Smith, 1991). Genetic differences result from the fact that some xenobiotic-metabolizing enzymes (e.g. the CYP2D6 enzyme) are deficient in a number of individuals. The consequences of this genetic polymorphism are a greatly impaired metabolism of the drugs (or prodrugs) which are substrates of such enzymes, and a marked risk of adverse effects through overdose (or therapeutic failure) in affected individuals. **Pharmacogenetics** has thus become in recent years a major issue in clinical pharmacology and pharmacotherapy (Daly *et al.*, 1993; Meyer *et al.*, 1990). Sex is also

TABLE i.4 *Factors affecting xenobiotic metabolism*

Inter-individual factors	Intra-individual factors
• Animal species • Genetic factors • Sex	• Age • Biological rhythms • Pregnancy • Stress • Diseases • Nutritional factors • Enzyme induction • Enzyme inhibition

a factor of significance in a number of cases, being related, like some intra-individual factors, to hormonal influences on enzyme activities.

Intra-individual factors are related to physiological changes or pathological states affecting for example the hormonal balance and immunological mechanisms of individuals. Thus, the age of a person may markedly influence his or her ability to metabolize xenobiotics, especially at the extremes of life. Biological rhythms are of the utmost but not always recognized importance; their study is the realm of **chronopharmacology** (Bélanger, 1993). Pregnancy affects xenobiotic metabolism for several reasons, one being the activity of the placenta and another the profound hormonal and physiological changes in the mother (Pasanen and Pelkonen, 1990). Human data are scarce for obvious reasons, while animal data are of limited extrapolative value. The influence of stress is connected with hormonal and haemodynamic changes but is not well documented. In contrast, a wealth of information is available on the influence of disease, although only partial rationalizations and explanatory mechanisms have been proposed (Jenner and Testa, 1981).

The **influence of chemicals** on xenobiotic metabolism is intimately connected with intra-individual factors. Here, we encounter the influence of nutritional factors, namely diet, nutrients and starvation. As far as drug therapy and toxicology are concerned, factors of even greater significance are **enzyme induction** and **enzyme inhibition** (Barry and Feely, 1990; Conney, 1967; Greim, 1981; Murray and Reidy, 1990; Okey, 1990; Testa and Jenner, 1981). Enzyme inducers act by increasing the concentration and hence activity of some enzymes or isozymes, while inhibitors decrease the activity of some enzymes or isozymes by reversible inhibition or irreversible inactivation. A given xenobiotic may induce and/or inhibit its own metabolism, thus acting respectively as an auto-inducer and/or auto-inhibitor, but the vast majority of available data document the influence of xenobiotics on metabolic reactions affecting other xenobiotics.

Enzyme induction and enzyme inhibition by co-administered drugs is one of the major causes of **drug–drug interactions**. Other causes of a pharmacokinetic nature include interactions at the level of absorption, protein binding, active transport and excretion. Pharmacodynamic interactions also occur but are relatively predictable and fall outside the realm of the present work (Ariëns and Simonis, 1977). A very large number of examples are known of drugs inhibiting the metabolism of other drugs and thus intensifying and prolonging their effects. In contrast, enzyme induction is frequently accompanied by a decrease in efficacy (Ariëns, 1970; Greim, 1981). An in-depth knowledge of the biochemistry, enzymology and physiology of drug metabolism is indispensable for a proper understanding of drug–drug interactions.

i.6 XENOBIOTIC METABOLISM: ITS HISTORY, AND IMPORTANCE IN DRUG RESEARCH AND XENOBIOTIC RESEARCH

Given all the evidence outlined in the previous sections, it is easy to understand why xenobiotic metabolism has evolved in the last decades to become a mature science whose multidisciplinary nature is particularly noteworthy (Testa, 1976). But the **history of xenobiotic metabolism** is much older than just the past few decades. Xenobiotic metabolism was born in 1841 with the discovery of the biotransformation of benzoic acid into hippuric acid, and the major pathways were discovered in the 19th Century (Conti and Bickel, 1977). The first half of the 20th Century saw an accumulation of data on many xenobiotics, recognized the role of enzymes, and bathed in the belief that metabolism means detoxication (Bachmann and Bickel, 1986). The state of knowledge in the middle of the 20th Century was summarized in a most comprehensive and authoritative manner by R.T. Williams (Williams, 1947 and 1959).

The second half of the 20th Century has seen the maturation of xenobiotic metabolism. From the many examples available, it became possible to deduce generalizations and rules and to use them as guides for future advances (Testa and Jenner, 1976 and 1990). As a modern science, xenobiotic metabolism draws from many other disciplines and progresses by way of a permanent interplay between methodology, findings and concepts. In recent years, the contributions of molecular biology and computational chemistry have been particularly impressive.

But what fuels the explosive growth of xenobiotic metabolism as a science? Of course it affords one path to increasing our understanding of life and ourselves, but this reason alone, however essential and noble, is not sufficient to explain the utilization of so many resources and the involvement of so many scientists. What explains the current and still growing interest in xenobiotic metabolism, we believe, resides in the central position it has acquired in the investigation of drugs and xenobiotics of all kinds, fundamental and applied research alike.

In **drug research and development**, metabolism is of pivotal importance due to the interconnectedness between pharmacokinetic and pharmacodynamic processes. Very early in the testing of a newly synthesized promising compound metabolic studies must be initiated to identify the metabolites; the pathways by which they are formed; and the possible intermediates. Based on these findings, the metabolites can be synthesized and tested for their own pharmacological and toxicological effects. In preclinical and early clinical studies, much pharmacokinetic data must be obtained and relevant criteria must be satisfied before a drug candidate can enter large-scale clinical trials (Balant *et al.*, 1990). As a result of these demands, the metabolic and pharmacokinetic registration files of a new drug may well be larger than the pharmacological and toxicological registration files.

The products of **xenobiotic research and development** are monomers, oligomers and polymers, dyes, agrochemicals, food additives, and innumerable other types of compounds. Here again, a major aim is the marketing of safe and useful products, with metabolic studies being central in the safety evaluation of new chemicals (Ariëns, 1984; Parke and Ioannides, 1990).

i.7 METABOLISM AND ECOTOXICOLOGY

In recent years, the environmental implications of xenobiotic metabolism have been recognized as an issue of world-wide proportions. In nature, chemicals undergo processes of passive distribution, active transport, storage, and elimination by transformation, that differ in scale but not in essence from the pharmacokinetic processes in the animal body (Zakrzewski, 1991).

The **transformation** of xenobiotics in the environment occurs both abiotically (e.g. photochemical and surface-catalyzed reactions) and biotically. In the latter case, particular mention must be made of soil and water microorganisms and plants, fishes, birds and reptiles, and ruminants (James, 1989; Lamoureux, 1989; Miyamoto, 1989). Our appreciation of the capacities of nature (or, perhaps, of Gaia as a living organism; Lovelock, 1987 and 1989) in handling chemicals (natural and artificial) is still rudimentary. In contrast, much knowledge has accumulated on mammalian metabolism. Yet here again, it appears that Gaia and some of the higher organisms that are part of her display essential similarities in their handling of chemicals despite obvious differences in scale and level of complexity.

In such a perspective, the mammalian metabolism of xenobiotics which constitutes the focus of this series of volumes is just a particular case of the planetary (Gaian) handling of chemicals both natural and artificial. And just as unphysiological compounds may accumulate in our bodies and elicit deleterious effects, so Earth may be poisoned by "unnatural" chemicals which affect her subsystems and equilibria.

i.8 PHILOSOPHY, SCOPE AND LAYOUT OF MEDOX

The above sections set the stage for the chapters and volumes to follow. How this treatise came to be conceived and brought to existence has been described in the Preface. What remains to be explained now is the philosophy of *The Metabolism of Drugs and Other Xenobiotics* (MEDOX), as implicit in its scope and layout.

Given the explosive development of the science of xenobiotic metabolism in the last decades, a coverage aiming at completeness would be outright impossible—and most likely would be useless and unusable even if it could be assembled. What is needed, we believe, is a work that brings *order and structure* to an extravagantly abundant body of information which may well appear chaotic even to experienced investigators. To achieve this goal, we aim at *comprehensiveness*. In other words, we try in these volumes to cover as many aspects of xenobiotic metabolism as possible and to illustrate them with a limited number of selected examples of particular didactic value and pharmacological relevance.

The logic we have followed in conceiving and preparing *The Metabolism of Drugs and Other Xenobiotics* is to go from the relatively simple to the more complex, from the molecular level to the whole organism, yet restricting the presentation to a two-tier approach. The first tier is the **molecular level** and covers the **biochemistry of xenobiotic metabolism**, i.e. enzymes and their properties; catalytic reactions and their mechanisms, structure–metabolism relationships and related aspects. The second tier is the **systemic level** and covers the **physiology of xenobiotic metabolism**, i.e. the enzymes and their regulation, the many inter-individual and intra-individual factors affecting xenobiotic metabolism, its pharmacological and toxicological consequences, and related aspects.

To attempt the creation of order out of chaos as mentioned above may be a most timely and fashionable concept, but the reader must realize that such an act of creation is not the exclusive privilege (or should we say the duty?) of authors. To benefit fully from the study of this work, our readers are invited to be active partners rather than passive onlookers. We have done our modest best to make MEDOX inviting and profitable in the service of human and Gaian health and evolution.

i.9 REFERENCES

Albert A. (1987). The behaviour of foreign substances in the human body. *Trends Pharmacol. Sci.* **8**, 258–261.

Ames B.N. and Profet M. (1992). Nature's pesticides. *Natural Toxins* 1, 2–3.

Ariëns E.J. (1970). Reduction of drug action by drug combination. In *Progress in Drug Research*, Vol. 14 (ed. Jucker E.) pp. 11–58. Birkhäuser, Basel.

Ariëns E.J. (1984). Domestication of chemistry by design

of safer chemicals: structure–activity relationships. *Drug Metab. Rev.* **15**, 425–504.

Ariëns E.J. and Simonis A.M. (1977). Pharmacodynamic aspects of drug interactions. *Naunyn-Schmied Arch. Pharmacol.* **297**, S37–S41.

Austel V. and Kutter E. (1980). Practical procedures in drug design. In *Drug Design*, Vol. 10 (ed. Ariëns E.J.). pp. 1–69. Academic Press, New York.

Austel V. and Kutter E. (1983). Absorption, distribution, and metabolism of drugs. In *Quantitative Structure–Activity Relationships of Drugs*, Vol. 19 (ed. Topliss J.G.). pp. 437–496. Academic Press, New York.

Bachmann C. and Bickel M.H. (1986). History of drug metabolism: the first half of the 20th Century. *Drug Metab. Rev.* **16**, 185–253.

Balant L.P., Roseboom H. and Gundert-Remy U.M. (1990). Pharmacokinetic criteria for drug research and development. In *Advances in Drug Research*, Vol. 19 (ed. Testa B.). pp. 1–138. Academic Press, London.

Barry M. and Feely J. (1990). Enzyme induction and inhibition. *Pharmacol. Therap.* **48**, 71–94.

Begg E.J. and Atkinson H.C. (1993). Modelling the passage of drugs into milk. *Pharmacol. Therap.* **59**, 301–310.

Bélanger P.M. (1993). Chronopharmacology in drug research and therapy. In *Advances in Drug Research*, Vol. 24 (ed. Testa B.). pp. 1–80. Academic Press, London.

Blocki F.A., Schlievert P.M. and Wackett L.P. (1992). Rat liver protein linking chemical and immunological detoxification systems. *Nature* **360**, 269–270.

Boxenbaum H. and D'Souza R.W. (1990). Interspecies pharmacokinetic scaling, biological design and neoteny. In *Advances in Drug Research*, Vol. 19 (ed. Testa B.). pp. 139–196. Academic Press, London.

Caldwell J., Weil A. and Tanaka Y. (1989). Species differences in xenobiotic conjugation. In *Xenobiotic Metabolism and Disposition* (eds. Kato R., Estabrook R.W. and Cayen M.N.). pp. 217–224. Taylor & Francis, London.

Chappell W.R. and Mordenti J. (1991). Extrapolation of toxicological and pharmacological data from animals to humans. In *Advances in Drug Research*, Vol. 20 (ed. Testa B.). pp. 1–116. Academic Press, London.

Conney A.H. (1967). Pharmacological implications of microsomal enzyme induction. *Pharmacol. Rev.* **19**, 317–366.

Conti A. and Bickel M.H. (1977). History of drug metabolism: discoveries of the major pathways in the 19th Century. *Drug Metab. Rev.* **6**, 1–50.

Daly A.K., Cholerton S., Gregory W. and Idle J.R. (1993). Metabolic polymorphisms. *Pharmacol. Therap.* **57**, 129–160.

Dayton P.G., Israili Z.H. and Henderson J.D. (1983). Elimination of drugs by passive diffusion from blood to intestinal lumen: factors influencing nonbiliary excretion by the intestinal tract. *Drug Metab. Rev.* **14**, 1193–1206.

Di Carlo F.J. (1982). Metabolism, pharmacokinetics, and toxicokinetics defined. *Drug Metab. Rev.* **13**, 1–4.

Drayer D.E. (1982). Pharmacologically active metabolites of drugs and other foreign compounds. Clinical, pharmacological, therapeutic and toxicological considerations. *Drugs* **24**, 519–542.

Estabrook R.W. and Werringloer J. (1979). The microsomal enzyme system responsible for the oxidative metabolism of many drugs. In *The Induction of Drug Metabolism* (eds. Estabrook R.W. and Lindenlaub E.). pp. 187–199. Schattauer Verlag, Stuttgart.

Fichtl B., v. Nieciecki A. and Walter K. (1991). Tissue binding versus plasma binding of drugs: General principles and pharmacokinetic consequences. In *Advances in Drug Research*, Vol. 20 (ed. Testa B.). pp. 117–166. Academic Press, London.

Gallenberg L.A. and Vodicnik M.J. (1989). Transfer of persistent chemicals in milk. *Drug Metab. Rev.* **21**, 277–317.

Gillette J.R. (1983). The use of theoretical pharmacokinetic concepts in studies of the mechanisms of formation of chemically reactive metabolites *in vitro* and *in vivo*. *Drug Metab. Rev.* **14**, 9–33.

Gonzalez F.J. and Nebert D.W. (1990). Evolution of the P450 gene superfamily: animal-plant "warfare", molecular drive and human genetic differences in drug oxidation. *Trends Genet.* **6**, 182–186.

Greim H.A. (1981). An overview of the phenomena of enzyme induction and inhibition: Their relevance to drug action and drug interactions. In *Concepts in Drug Metabolism*, Part B (eds. Jenner P. and Testa B.). pp. 219–263. Dekker, New York.

Jakoby W.B. and Ziegler D.M. (1990). The enzymes of detoxication. *J. Biol. Chem.* **265**, 20,715–20,718.

James M.O. (1989). Conjugation and excretion of xenobiotics by fish and aquatic invertebrates. In *Xenobiotic Metabolism and Disposition* (eds. Kato R., Estabrook R.W. and Cayen M.N.). pp. 283–290. Taylor & Francis, London.

Jenner P. and Testa B. (1981). Altered drug disposition in disease states: The first pieces of the jigsaw. In *Concepts in Drug Metabolism*, Part B (eds. Jenner P. and Testa B.). pp. 423–513. Dekker, New York.

Jenner P., Testa B. and Di Carlo F.J. (1981). Xenobiotic and endobiotic metabolizing enzymes: an overstretched discrimination? *Trends Pharmacol. Sci.* **2**, 135–137.

Lamoureux G.L. (1989). Plant metabolism of herbicides in relation to detoxification, selectivity, antidoting, and synergism. In *Xenobiotic Metabolism and Disposition* (eds. Kato R., Estabrook R.W. and Cayen M.N.). pp. 267–274. Taylor & Francis, London.

Lovelock J.E. (1987). *Gaia—A New Look at Life on Earth*. Oxford University Press, Oxford, UK.

Lovelock J.E. (1989). *The Ages of Gaia—A Biography of Our Living Earth*. Oxford University Press, Oxford, UK.

Meyer U.A., Zanger U.M., Grant D. and Blum M. (1990). Genetic polymorphisms of drug metabolism. In *Advances in Drug Research*, Vol. 19 (ed. Testa B.). pp. 197–241. Academic Press, London.

Miyamoto J. (1989). Comparative metabolism of xenobiotics in the environment; fundamentals for risk assessment. In *Xenobiotic Metabolism and Disposition* (eds. Kato R., Estabrook R.W. and Cayen M.N.). pp. 257–265. Taylor & Francis, London.

Murray M. and Reidy G.F. (1990). Selectivity in the inhibition of mammalian cytochromes P-450 by chemical agents. *Pharmacol. Rev.* **42**, 85–101.

Nebert D.W. (1991). Proposed role of drug-metabolizing enzymes: Regulation of steady state levels of the ligands that effect growth, homeostasis, differentiation, and neuroendocrine functions. *Molec. Endocrinol.* **5**, 1203–1214.

Neumann H.G. (1986). Toxication mechanisms in drug metabolism. In *Advances in Drug Research*, Vol. 15 (ed. Testa B.). pp. 1–28. Academic Press, London.

Okey A.B. (1990). Enzyme induction in the cytochrome P-450 system. *Pharmacol. Therap.* **45**, 241–298.

Parke D.V. and Ioannides C. (1990). The role of metabolism studies in the safety evaluation of new chemicals. *Acta Pharm. Jugosl.* **40**, 363–382.

Pasanen M. and Pelkonen O. (1990). Human placental xenobiotic and steroid biotransformations catalyzed by cytochrome P450, epoxide hydrolase, and glutathione S-transferase activities and their relationships to maternal cigarette smoking. *Drug Metab. Rev.* **21**, 427–461.

Smith D.A. (1991). Species differences in metabolism and pharmacokinetics: are we close to an understanding? *Drug Metab. Rev.* **23**, 355–373.

Testa B. (1976). Preface. Drug metabolism as a mutation—Drug metabolism in mutation. *Drug Metab. Rev.* **5**(2), i–ii.

Testa B. (1982). Nonenzymatic contributions to xenobiotic metabolism. *Drug Metab. Rev.* **13**, 25–50.

Testa B. (1984). Drugs? Drug research? Advances in drug research? Musings of a medicinal chemist. In *Advances in Drug Research*, Vol. 13 (ed. Testa B.). pp. 1–58. Academic Press, London.

Testa B. (1987). Pharmacokinetic and pharmacodynamic events: can they always be distinguished? *Trends Pharmacol. Sci.* **8**, 381–383.

Testa B. and Jenner P. (1976). *Drug Metabolism: Chemical and Biochemical Aspects*. Dekker, New York.

Testa B. and Jenner P. (1981). Inhibitors of cytochrome P-450s and their mechanisms of action. *Drug Metab. Rev.* **12**, 1–117.

Testa B. and Jenner P. (1990). The coming of age of drug metabolism. *Current Contents Life Sci.* **33**(33), 17.

Testa B., Di Carlo F.J. and Jenner P. (1981). Xenobiotic metabolism: Necessity, chance, mishap, or none of the above? In *Concepts in Drug Metabolism*, Part B (eds. Jenner P. and Testa B.). pp. 515–535. Dekker, New York.

Tillement J.P., Houin G., Zini R., Urien S., Albengres E., Barré J., Lecomte M., D'Athis P. and Sébille B. (1984). The binding of drugs to blood plasma macromolecules: Recent advances and therapeutic significance. In *Advances in Drug Research*, Vol. 13 (ed. Testa B.). pp. 59–94. Academic Press, London.

Timbrell J.A. (1991). *Principles of Biochemical Toxicology*, 2nd edition. Taylor & Francis, London.

Wickramasinghe R.H. and Villee C.A. (1975). Early role during chemical evolution for cytochrome P450 in oxygen detoxification. *Nature* **256**, 509–511.

Williams R.T. (1947). *Detoxication Mechanisms*. Chapman & Hall, London.

Williams R.T. (1959). *Detoxication Mechanisms*, 2nd edition. Chapman & Hall, London.

Wilson J.T. (1983). Determinants and consequences of drug excretion in breast milk. *Drug Metab. Rev.* **14**, 619–652.

Zakrzewski S.F. (1991). *Principles of Environmental Toxicology*. American Chemical Society, Washington, DC.

Ziegler D.M. (1990). Flavin-containing monooxygenases: enzymes adapted for multisubstrate specificity. *Trends Pharmacol. Sci.* **11**, 321–324.

chapter 1

XENOBIOTIC METABOLISM: THE BIOCHEMICAL VIEW

Contents

1.1 INTRODUCTION

The present volume of the *Metabolism of Drugs and Other Xenobiotics* is the first of the volumes dealing with the **molecular and biochemical levels of xenobiotic metabolism** (see Section i.8). This suggests a broad coverage and a variety of viewpoints. Briefly explained, each chapter will cover as many of the following aspects as possible and as appropriate:

- Various biochemical properties of the enzymes/isozymes;
- Drug–enzyme interactions;
- The various chemical reactions catalyzed by the enzyme(s);
- Reaction mechanisms and catalytic cycle;
- Regio- and stereoselectivities;
- Types of moieties and molecules being metabolized;
- Structure–metabolism relationships;
- Reactivity of metabolic intermediates, molecular aspects of toxication and detoxication;
- Molecular mechanisms of direct and indirect enzyme inhibition.

To avoid an impossibly encyclopaedic treatment of the subject, selective coverage of the above aspects characterizes each chapter. Choices have been made on the basis of the availability of data and their interest.

Concisely stated, the goal is to offer both *information* and *knowledge*. In other words, we intend the reader to find in these volumes, at first a large body of factual information, and upon deeper and creative study a network of rationalizations and concepts that should be truly formative. Remember the poet:

> *"Where is the wisdom we have lost in knowledge?*
> *Where is the knowledge we have lost in information?"*
> (T.S. Eliot).

1.2 THE REDUCTIONISTIC APPROACH

In a first approximation, the approach taken in the volumes covering the biochemistry of xenobiotic metabolism is clearly a reductionistic one, meaning that it is based on the study of parts (reactions, enzymes, etc) taken in isolation. With such an approach, information is supplied, but knowledge demands a more global and integrated view. For this reason, it should be clear that any fragmentary approach can only be futile in the long-term, as eloquently demonstrated by Briggs and Peat (1985). However, discovering, collecting and presenting pieces of the jigsaw is the unavoidable and indispensable foundation of any scientific construction. Only in this way can systems of knowledge be synthesized in the various scientific disciplines.

In the biochemical volumes, the fragmentary approach is mainly twofold. First, the various **metabolic reactions** or **sequences of reactions** are considered separately. In other words, each major reaction and relevant enzyme(s) are treated in turn. This simplification, however necessary, may be misleading to the reader who is not aware of the complexity of the metabolic fate of most xenobiotics. To illustrate the point, let us consider **propranolol**, a β-blocker whose metabolism in humans has been quantitatively established in a study of exemplary but all too rare comprehensiveness (Walle *et al.*, 1985). As shown in Fig. 1.1, the metabolism of propranolol involves a relatively complex pattern of competitive and sequential reactions. Two unidentified metabolites were also seen which together accounted for 7% of the dose. Globally, over 90% of the dose

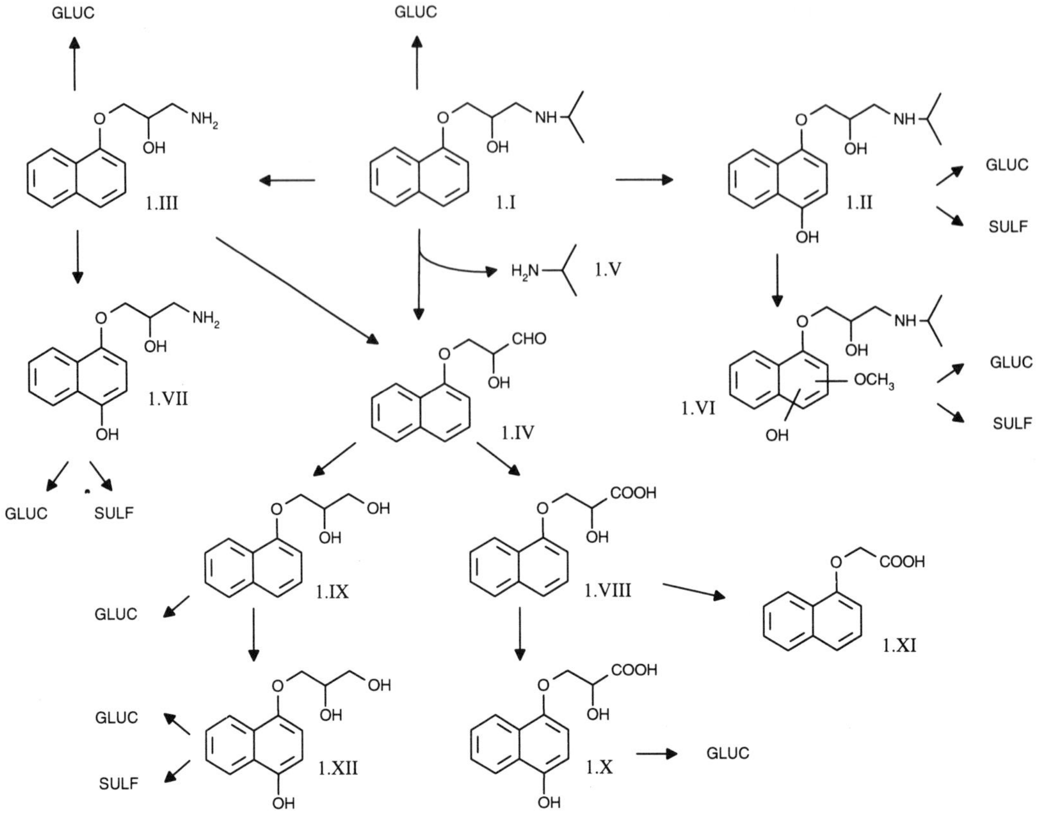

FIGURE 1.1 The metabolism of propranolol (**1.I**) in humans, accounting for more than 90% of the dose (Walle *et al.*, 1985). The metabolites are (approximate percent of dose in 24 h urine):
- propranolol (**1.I**) (its glucuronide = 14%);
- ring[mainly 4]-hydroxylated propranolol (**1.II**) (its glucuronide = 9%, its sulfate = 18%);
- N-desisopropylpropranolol (**1.III**) (its glucuronide = 1%);
- propranolol aldehyde (**1.IV**);
- isopropylamine (**1.V**);
- hydroxymethoxypropranolol (**1.VI**);
- ring-hydroxylated N-desisopropylpropranolol (**1.VII**) (its glucuronide = 1.5%, its sulfate = 5%);
- α-naphthoxylactic acid (**1.VIII** = 17%);
- propranolol glycol (**1.IX**) (its glucuronide = 1.5%);
- ring-hydroxylated α-naphthoxylactic acid (**1.X**) (its glucuronide = 1%);
- α-naphthoxyacetic acid (**1.XI**) (1%);
- ring-hydroxylated propranolol glycol (**1.XII**) (its glucuronide = 2%, its sulfate = 3%);

GLUC = glucuronide conjugate(s); SULF = sulfate conjugate(s).

were accounted for in the 0–96 h urine collections, indicating that the scheme shown in Fig. 1.1 offers a fair view of the metabolic behaviour of propranolol in humans. The missing 10% of the dose may be accounted for by other, minor and presumably quite numerous metabolites, e.g. those resulting from ring hydroxylation at other positions or from the progressive breakdown of glutathione conjugates.

Rather than discussing reactions separately and more or less independently, we could have selected a large variety of xenobiotics and for each one in turn present the totality of its known metabolic fate in a manner analogous to Fig. 1.1. This format, also found in pharmacopoeias and compilations, is useful as a depository of information but has low didactic and extrapolative value; it is therefore alien to the purpose and scope of this book. In contrast, the fragmentary approach followed here allows for rationalizations, generalizations and extrapolations, but only with an active participation of the reader. Indeed, the greatest benefit will be derived from this book if it is first *studied and understood*, followed by *creative action* to build an individual synthetic and integrated view. In this dynamic perspective, with both writer and reader active participants, the reductionistic approach will be transcended and the book will gain a heuristic value which will differ from one reader to another.

The second fragmentary approach adopted in the biochemical volumes concerns **enzymes and enzyme systems**, which are presented independently from biological regulations, and without consideration for the possible influence of biological organization. As explained in the Introduction, it is precisely the scope of the volume on physiology and regulations to discuss regulatory factors that influence xenobiotic metabolism. But what about biological organization and its influence on enzyme activities? Indeed, organelles, cells, tissues, organs, organisms and populations display an extremely high and poorly understood degree of organization and integration characteristic of all **biological systems**. Consider for example the direct transfer of metabolites from one enzyme site to the next by means of enzyme–enzyme complex formation (Srivastava and Bernhard, 1986). Such a phenomenon dispenses with random diffusion and may markedly affect reaction rates, yet its occurrence and significance in xenobiotic metabolism remains to be investigated. In this case, a fragmentary approach is unavoidable due to our ignorance.

1.3   ENZYMATIC VS. NON-ENZYMATIC VS. POSTENZYMATIC REACTIONS

As a rule, biochemical reactions are catalyzed by enzymes, which as cogently discussed by Knowles (1991) are catalytic devices built on essentially definable principles. In thermodynamic terms, the effect of enzymes in particular, and catalysts in general, is to decrease the free energy of the reaction transition state (in other words, to stabilize it), thereby increasing the rate constant of the reaction by several orders of magnitude (Fig. 1.2). Enzymes can thus be defined as the catalytic operators of the biosphere.

Reactions of xenobiotic metabolism are not different from other biochemical reactions and are also catalyzed by enzymes. In fact, the outline of the biochemical volumes is based on enzymes as much as on metabolic reactions. However, a number of xenobiotics are labile enough

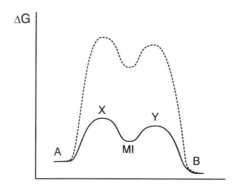

FIGURE 1.2 Reaction coordinates of a hypothetical metabolic reaction: absence of enzymatic catalysis (----); enzymatic catalysis (———). A: substrate; B: product; X and Y: transition states; MI: metabolic intermediate.

TABLE 1.1 *Enzymatic, non-enzymatic, and postenzymatic contributions to xenobiotic metabolism* (modified from Testa, 1982)*

	Reaction with:	
	a xenobiotic	a metabolic intermediate
Reaction of:		
• An enzyme	Enzymatic	Enzymatic
• A macromolecule	Borderline case (A)	Postenzymatic (B)
• An endogenous compound	Non-enzymatic (C)	Postenzymatic (D)
• A xenobiotic	Non-enzymatic (E)	Postenzymatic (F)
• H_2O, H_3O^+, HO^-, etc (G)	Non-enzymatic	Postenzymatic

*Cases A–G are discussed in the text.

to react non-enzymatically under biological conditions of pH and temperature (Hathway, 1980; Testa, 1982 and 1983). The major cases of **non-enzymatic reactions** are summarized in Table 1.1.

In a normal enzymatic reaction, metabolic intermediates (MI in Fig. 1.2) exist *en route* to the product(s) and do not leave the catalytic site. However, many exceptions to this rule are known, the metabolic intermediate leaving the active site and reacting with water, with an endogenous molecule or macromolecule, or with a xenobiotic. Such reactions are also of a non-enzymatic nature but are better designated as **postenzymatic reactions** (Fig. 1.3 and Table 1.1) (Testa, 1982 and 1983).

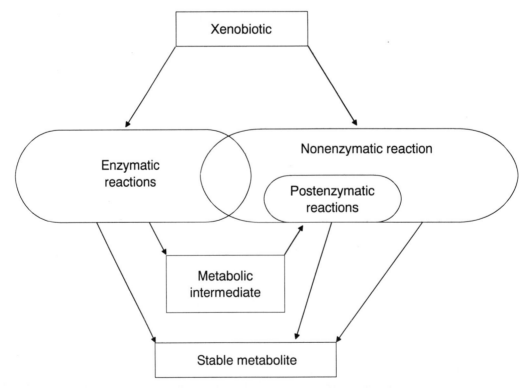

FIGURE 1.3 Enzymatic and non-enzymatic modes of xenobiotic metabolism.

The present section is just meant to offer a rapid overview and a conceptual framework of enzymatic versus non-enzymatic and postenzymatic reactions. However, some of the cases presented in Table 1.1 deserve a brief comment:

- *Case A* is exemplified by the capacity of serum albumin to catalyze (albeit not as efficiently as esterases) the hydrolysis of a number of esters. Other enzyme-like activities of serum albumin are known. The capacity of this protein to accelerate a number of reactions can be viewed as enzymatic or not depending on the definition given to enzymes.
- *Case B* is represented by the many known examples of covalent binding of reactive metabolites to macromolecules such as albumin or membranal proteins, forming adducts which are drug–macromolecule conjugates (Section 1.4). Metabolic intermediates can also react postenzymatically with endogenous compounds such as lipids, fatty acids or glutathione (Case D).
- *Case C* is particularly interesting and will be discussed in a number of chapters. The endogenous compounds able to react non-enzymatically with xenobiotics are nucleophiles such as NADH and NADPH (Chapter 13), glutathione and other thiols and electrophiles such as carbonyl compounds (Ketterer, 1982; O'Donnell, 1982) (cf. volume on conjugation reactions).
- A few xenobiotics (e.g. acetylsalicylic acid) are unstable enough to react with other xenobiotics (*Case E*).
- The reaction of a metabolic intermediate with an identical molecule or the parent compound leads for example to the formation of dimers (*Case F*). However, the most important cases of this type involve the reactions of reactive metabolites of molecular oxygen (e.g. $O_2^{\bullet -}$ H_2O_2, $HO^{\bullet}$, see Section 1.4) with a xenobiotic (Trager, 1982). Such postenzymatic reactions of oxidation have a major significance in xenobiotic metabolism (as discussed in this volume) and in pathophysiological processes.
- *Case G* represents for example various proton- or hydroxyl-catalyzed reactions of hydrolysis, ring opening, cyclization, or rearrangement. These can affect metabolic intermediates as well as a number of xenobiotics sufficiently labile to react under biological conditions. The volume on hydration reactions will examine cases of this type.

1.4 THE THREE TYPES OF METABOLITES: FUNCTIONALIZATION PRODUCTS, CONJUGATES, AND MACROMOLECULAR ADDUCTS

Biotransformation reactions affecting xenobiotics are traditionally separated into Phase I and Phase II reactions. The former involve the **creation or modification of functional groups** in a substrate molecule. For example, a $-CH_3$ moiety can be functionalized to become a $-CH_2OH$ group, or an $-NO_2$ group can be modified by reduction to $-NH_2$. In contrast, Phase II reactions involve the **conjugation of an endogenous molecule or fragment** to the substrate, yielding a metabolite known as a conjugate. Thus, an $-NH_2$ group can become $-NHCOCH_3$ upon conjugation with an acetyl moiety. While it is regularly observed that Phase II reactions follow Phase I reactions (e.g. $RNO_2 \rightarrow RNH_2 \rightarrow RNHCOCH_3$; see also Fig. 1.1), reversed situations are just as likely, for example the long sequence of Phase I reactions able to transform glutathione conjugates (cf. the volume of conjugation reactions).

The Phase I/Phase II nomenclature is therefore misleading inasmuch as it conveys the sometimes false idea that the former reactions must precede the latter. In this book, preference will be given to the more explicit terms of **functionalization** and **conjugation** to designate Phase I and Phase II processes, respectively (Testa and Jenner, 1978). To clarify further the meaning of these terms, Table 1.2 lists the chemical species being transferred during functionalization or

TABLE 1.2 *A classification of reactions of xenobiotic metabolism*
(Chemical entity being transferred to, and in some cases from, the substrate)[*]

Reactions of functionalization (Phase I)		Reactions of conjugation (Phase II)
Redox reactions	Reactions of hydration	
First volume	Second volume	Third volume
O	H_2O	methyl group
O_2	HO^-	acetyl and other acyl moieties
e^- (electron)		glucuronic acid, some sugars
$2e^-$		sulfate and phosphate moieties
H^- (hydride)		glycine and other amino acids
		two-carbon chain
		diglycerides
		cholesterol and other sterols
		glutathione and other sulfides
		CO_2
		carbonyl compounds
		S, etc

[*]The sequence in each column has no particular meaning.

conjugation reactions. This Table also has the advantage of presenting the content of the biochemical volumes in a schematic manner, neglecting a few exceptions that will become apparent in the relevant chapters.

Up to this point, Sections 1.3 and 1.4 have discussed metabolic **reactions** (enzymatic, non-enzymatic, postenzymatic, functionalization, conjugation). But what about the **products**, i.e. the metabolites? Logically, one could conclude from the above that only two types of metabolites exist, namely **functionalization products** and **conjugates**. However, with the growth of our knowledge, biochemists and pharmacologists have progressively come to recognize the existence of a third class of metabolites, namely **xenobiotic-macromolecule adducts**, also called macromolecular conjugates (Caldwell, 1982). Such peculiar metabolites are formed when a xenobiotic binds covalently to a biological macromolecule. Let us discuss in turn the three parts of this definition.

(a) The xenobiotic does not usually bind directly (except sufficiently reactive compounds such as alkylating agents), but must undergo **metabolic activation** (by functionalization and/or conjugation) to a reactive intermediate (see Section 1.3). Thus, xenobiotic oxidation leads to the formation of electrophilic intermediates (often cations and/or radicals), while reduction leads to nucleophilic radicals (Fig. 1.4). Even the formation of a disulfide bond (RSD–SR') by reaction of a thiol-containing xenobiotic with a thiol group in a protein is not believed to occur directly but after oxidation of the xenobiotic thiol to an electrophilic oxide or to a radical (Chapter 7) (Mason, 1986; Nelson, 1982; Trush *et al.*, 1982).

The reduction of molecular oxygen to activated forms is also shown in Fig. 1.4 because it should not be separated from other reactions of toxication. Formation of radicals and reduction of molecular oxygen are of particular toxicological significance and will receive ample attention in later chapters (Neumann, 1986; Ross, 1989; Sies, 1991).

(b) The **covalent** nature of the bond is an important part of the definition since reversible

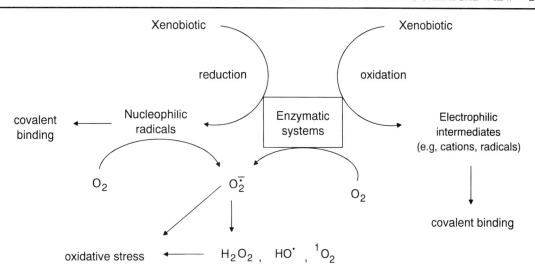

FIGURE 1.4 Schematic view of metabolic reactions of toxication. Note the formation of reactive metabolites of oxygen, namely the anion-radical superoxide ($O_2^{\bullet-}$), hydrogen peroxide (H_2O_2), the hydroxyl radical ($HO^{\bullet}$), or singlet oxygen ($^{1}O_2$). Formation of these metabolites produces oxidative stress in cells with progression to acute lethal cell injury. Oxidative stress is defined as a disturbance in the prooxidant–antioxidant balance in favour of the pro-oxidant state, and it elicits effects such as lipid peroxidation and changes in Ca^{2+} homeostasis (Nelson and Pearson, 1990; Sies, 1991).

binding by weak intermolecular forces does not lead to adduct formation. Covalent bonds are difficult to break, meaning that adduct formation is essentially irreversible. This is the case for adducts formed by **alkylation** of electrophilic or nucleophilic sites. **Acylation** of nucleophilic sites (e.g. $-NH_2$, $-OH$, $-SH$ or imidazole) forms adducts that might be slowly hydrolyzed, while **disulfides** may be cleaved slowly by reduction.

(c) The type of **biological macromolecule** involved will determine the nature of any toxicity that might result from covalent binding (Caldwell, 1982; Nelson and Pearson, 1990). Alkylation of nucleophilic sites in **nucleic acids** (DNA in particular) may result in scission at the molecular level, perhaps leading to mutagenesis or carcinogenesis at the cellular or tissular level (Hathway and Kolar, 1980; Latif *et al.*, 1988). Covalent binding to blood and cellular **proteins and glycoproteins** may have a variety of consequences, in particular immunological ones (Boelsterli, 1993; Park and Kitteringham, 1990). Thus, the xenobiotic–protein conjugate may be recognized as an immunogen (when capable of eliciting a specific immune response in the form of specific antibodies and/or lymphocytes) and an antigen (when capable of interacting with an antibody). Here, the xenobiotic behaves as an hapten, leading to hypersensitivity and tissue damage. Much information can be found in the excellent reviews by Park and Kitteringham (1990) and by Boelsterli (1993). Covalent binding to **carbohydrate macromolecules** is an additional possibility (Nelson and Pearson, 1990). **Lipids** can also bind covalently reactive intermediates (e.g. addition of nucleophilic radicals to unsaturated fatty acyl moieties).

In summary, the formation of macromolecular adducts resembles functionalization and conjugation, and differs from reversible protein binding, by the nature of the chemical bonds being formed (Fig. 1.5). However, macromolecular adducts cannot be classified together with "classical" conjugates, as there are too many differences existing in the underlying mechanisms and in the chemical properties and biological fate of the products. As always in biology, intermediate cases exist, e.g. the hydrid triglycerides to be discussed in the volume on conjugation reactions.

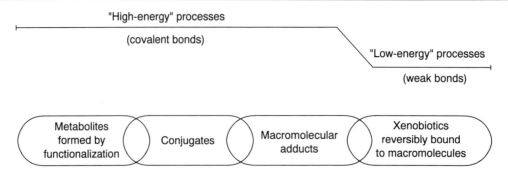

FIGURE 1.5 A comparison between chemical processes in xenobiotic metabolism and disposition: "High-energy" processes lead to the three types of metabolites, while weak bonds underlie reversible binding to macromolecules.

1.5 SPECIFICITY AND SELECTIVITY IN XENOBIOTIC METABOLISM

1.5.1 Specificity of enzymes vs. selectivity of metabolic reactions

Because the words "selectivity" and "specificity" will be used repeatedly in this work, their meaning should first be clarified. In **chemistry**, and more precisely in synthetic chemistry, the concepts of stereospecificity and stereoselectivity have well-defined meanings (Glossary of Terms, 1983). A reaction is termed stereospecific if stereoisomeric starting materials are converted into stereoisomeric products. This is different from stereoselectivity, which means the preferential formation of one stereoisomer over another. According to this definition, a stereospecific reaction is necessarily stereoselective, but not all stereoselective reactions are stereospecific. Another definition has recently been proposed (Davankov, 1991) which appears to contradict partly the established one.

In **biochemistry**, these two aspects of stereoreactivity are often intermingled, implying that it is seldom useful (if meaningful at all) to distinguish between stereoselectivity and stereospecificity as defined above (Alworth, 1972). To add to the confusion, some pharmacologists take stereospecific to mean "totally stereoselective" (Portoghese, 1970).

In this work, **the specificity of an enzyme** will be taken to mean an ensemble of properties, the description of which makes it possible to **specify** the enzyme's behaviour. For example, substrate specificity and stereospecificity belong to this ensemble of characteristic properties. In contrast, the present work will apply the term **selectivity** to **metabolic processes**, indicating that a given metabolic reaction or pathway is able to **select** some substrates or products from a larger set. In other words, **the selectivity of a metabolic reaction is the expression of the specificity of an enzyme.** Such definitions may not be universally accepted, but they have the merit of clarity. And since the emphasis given in this work is to metabolic reactions, selectivity will be discussed more often than specificity.

1.5.2 The discrimination of target groups, substrates, and enzymes

To understand the various enzyme specificities and reaction selectivities of significance in xenobiotic metabolism, we must first outline the three types of discrimination that underlie them. These are schematized in Fig. 1.6 together with a mechanistic interpretation based on the three

SPECIFICITY OF ENZYMES AND SELECTIVITY OF REACTIONS

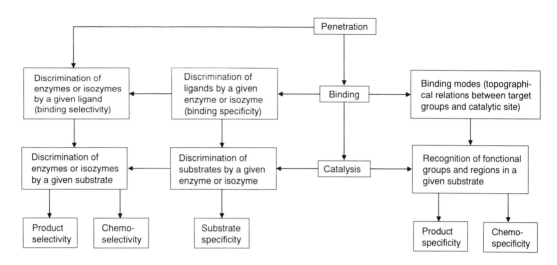

FIGURE 1.6 Scheme of the major types of specificity and selectivity characteristic of enzymes and metabolic reactions, respectively. Also shown is a mechanistic interpretation based on the three conceptual steps (penetration, binding and catalysis) underlying xenobiotic metabolism.

steps that exist in the interaction of a xenobiotic with a biological system. Indeed, it is useful when discussing pharmacodynamic and pharmacokinetic events to consider three conceptual steps, namely **penetration** (i.e. entry into the receptor or enzyme compartment), **binding** (e.g. to the receptor or the enzyme), and **activation** (e.g. receptor **activation** or enzymatic catalysis) (Testa, 1984).

When looking at the right-hand side of Fig. 1.6, we encounter the situation when a single substrate interacts with a single enzyme (or isozyme, see Section 1.6). Here, the only possible discrimination is that of target groups in the substrate, as influenced by binding (i.e. binding modes) and/or catalysis. This phenomenon accounts for the **chemospecificity** and **product specificity** of the enzyme.

When a single enzyme (or isozyme) reacts with several substrates, the former may discriminate between the latter, a property known as **substrate specificity** (Fig. 1.6, centre). Again binding (i.e. the binding specificity of the enzyme) and/or catalysis may cause this type of discrimination.

In contrast, a single substrate facing a number of enzymes (or isozymes) will be metabolized differently by each due to differences in penetration, binding, and/or catalysis. As a consequence, **chemoselectivity** and **product selectivity** may characterize the observed reactions (Fig. 1.6, left).

1.5.3 Chemospecificity, substrate selectivity, product selectivity, regioselectivity and stereoselectivity

What characterizes an enzyme from a catalytic viewpoint is first its **chemospecificity**, i.e. its specificity in terms of the type(s) of reaction it catalyzes (Fig. 1.6). Six main classes of enzymes are recognized based on the reactions being catalyzed (International Union of Biochemistry and Molecular Biology, 1992):

● Oxidoreductases (EC 1.), which catalyze oxidoreduction reactions;

- Transferases (EC 2.), which transfer a group from a donor to an acceptor;
- Hydrolases (EC 3.), which catalyze the hydrolytic cleavage of C–O, C–N, C–C and some other bonds;
- Lyases (EC 4.), which cleave C–C, C–O, C–N, C–S and other bonds by elimination, leaving double bonds or rings, or conversely add groups to double bonds;
- Isomerases (EC 5.), which catalyze geometric or structural changes within one molecule;
- Ligases (EC 6.), which catalyze the joining together of two molecules coupled with the hydrolysis of a pyrophosphate bond in ATP.

Note that the electron-transport proteins are not classified in these six classes. The vast majority of enzymes known to act on xenobiotics belong to oxidoreductases (this volume), hydrolases and transferases.

Besides chemospecificity, there exist a number of other components of enzyme specificity. These will be discussed here in terms of the observable selectivities that have been recognized in xenobiotic metabolism and are now receiving wide acceptance (Fig. 1.7) (Jenner and Testa, 1973; Testa and Jenner, 1980).

When two or more substrates are metabolized at different rates by a single enzyme under identical conditions, **substrate selectivity** is observed as schematized also in Fig. 1.6. In such a definition, and in contrast to definitions used by chemists (see above), the nature of the product(s) and their isomeric relationship are not considered. Substrate selectivity is distinct from **product selectivity**, which is observed when two or more metabolites are formed at different rates by a single enzyme from a single substrate. As shown in Fig. 1.6 and 1.7, substrate-selective reactions discriminate between different compounds, while product-selective reactions discriminate between different goups or positions in a given compound.

The substrates being metabolized at different rates may share various types of relationships. They may be chemically very or slightly different (e.g. analogues), in which case the term of substrate selectivity is used in a narrow sense. Alternatively, the substrates may be isomers such as positional isomers (regioisomers), stereoisomers (diastereomers or enantiomers), resulting in **substrate regioselectivity**, **substrate stereoselectivity**, **substrate diastereoselectivity** (seldom used) or **substrate enantioselectivity**, respectively.

Products formed at different rates in product-selective reactions may also share various types of relationships. Thus, they may be analogues, regioisomers, stereoisomers (diastereomers or enantiomers), resulting in product selectivity (narrow sense), **product regioselectivity**, **product stereoselectivity**, **product diastereoselectivity** (seldom used) or **product enantioselectivity**, respectively.

Note that the product selectivity displayed by two distinct substrates in a given metabolic reaction may be different, in other words the product selectivity may be substrate-selective. The term **substrate-product selectivity** can be used to describe such complex cases, which are conceivable for any type of selectivity but have been reported mainly for stereoselectivity (Fig. 1.7).

1.6 ISOZYMES AND THEIR SPECIFICITIES AS INTERFACE BETWEEN THE BIOCHEMISTRY AND THE PHYSIOLOGY OF XENOBIOTIC METABOLISM

1.6.1 Isozymes, orthologues and variants

One of the major paradigm shifts that occurred in recent years in xenobiotic metabolism has been the recognition of the significance of **isozymes** (isoenzymes) (Ogita and Markert, 1990). These are defined as multiple forms of enzymes, arising from genetically determined difference in the

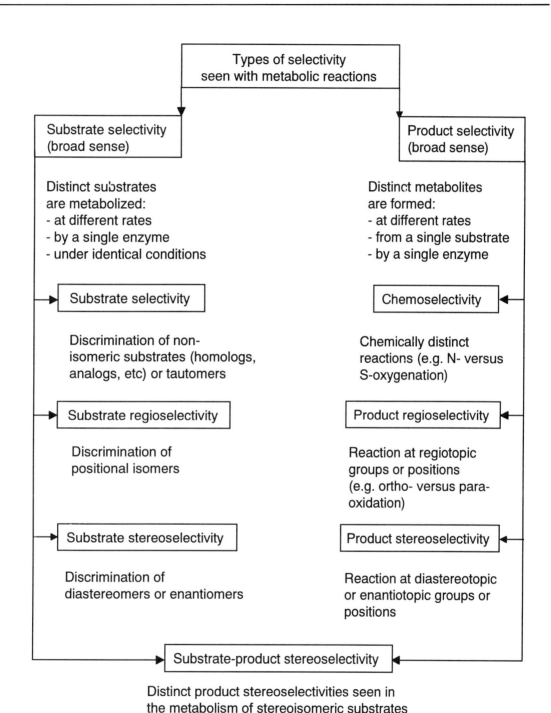

FIGURE 1.7 Scheme of the major types of substrate selectivity and product selectivity observed in metabolic reactions.

primary structure of their protein component, as distinct from multiple forms derived by post-translational modification of the same primary amino acid sequence. In other words, isozymes share comparable catalytic site, cofactor(s) and reaction mechanism(s), but they are almost always the products of distinct genes. While an enzyme such as monoamine oxidase (MAO, Chapter 9) exists as two isozymes known as MAO-A and MAO-B, cytochrome P450 (Chapter 3) has evolved into more than 200 gene products and is at present one of the most actively investigated enzyme systems.

Interestingly, the cytochrome P450 gene products are labelled by some authors as enzymes and by others as isozymes (Waterman and Johnson, 1991). They form a superfamily divided into families and subfamilies (Chapter 3). Within a single family, the P450 protein sequences have >40% resemblance, with a few exceptions; mammalian sequences within a subfamily always have >55% resemblance (Nebert *et al.*, 1991; Nelson *et al.*, 1993). These important aspects of the molecular biology of xenobiotic-metabolizing enzymes will be discussed in detail in the relevant volume.

The concept of **orthologous genes** is an important one in xenobiotic metabolism. According to Nebert *et al.* (1991), an orthologous gene in two species refers to a gene known with certainty to correspond to the ancestral gene which existed before the evolutionary divergence of the two species. Mutations occurring after the divergence have resulted in the two gene products differing not only in their primary amino acid sequence (the similarity between rat and human P450 orthologues is usually in the range 70–80%), but also in their substrate and product specificities (see below) (Nebert *et al.*, 1991; Soucek and Gut, 1992).

The existence of **alleles** (i.e. different forms of the same gene) results in the existence of gene products with slight differences in their protein sequence (microheterogeneity) but possibly large differences in specificities and catalytic activities. For cytochrome P450, proteins having less than 3% divergence (i.e. fewer than 15 amino acids in a 500-residue P450 protein) are arbitrarily considered as derived from alleles of the same gene, but there are several known exceptions (Nebert *et al.*, 1991). Such **allelic variants** of a given cytochrome P450 form may explain some catalytic differences between animal strains. For example, a Wistar-Munich strain of rats was found to have a functionally altered P450 2B1 variant resulting from a difference in a single residue (Kedzie *et al.*, 1991). Allelic variants can also underlie pharmacogenetic differences in drug metabolism seen between human individuals.

1.6.2 Aspects of the specificity of isozymes

The first important contributor to isozyme specificity is their **chemospecificity**. Some enzymes are able to catalyze only a single type of chemical reaction, a characteristic necessarily shared by their isozymes. In contrast, other enzymes catalyze several types of reactions, most notably cytochrome P450 which offers a particularly telling example (Chapters 3–8, 10–12). Much remains to be done to analyze the relative chemospecificities of individual forms of cytochrome P450 and their regulation by biological factors. The influence of biological factors is seen for example with a cytochrome P450 enzyme temporarily designated as P450 C_{21scc}. This single enzyme was found to have C-21 steroids as substrates and to catalyze two reactions, namely 17α-hydroxylation followed by C(17–20)-lyase activity (removal of the two-carbon side-chain) (Hall, 1991). The ratio of these two activities was markedly dependent on the availability of NADPH-cytochrome P450 reductase, the enzyme which delivers electrons to P450.

Substrate and product specificities also differ markedly among isozymes, as illustrated by innumerable studies with cytochrome P450 and other enzymes. An example is presented in Table 1.3, which compares the specificity of 11 rat liver isocytochromes P450 toward 13 substrates, and also documents differences in the regioselectivity of testosterone hydroxylation (Levin, 1990).

TABLE 1.3 *Substrate specificity and product regiospecificity of purified rat hepatic cytochromes P450* (Levin, 1990)

Isozyme*	Substrate and reaction (nmol min^{-1} [nmol P450]$^{-1}$)†												
	A	B	C	D	E	F	G	H	I	J	K	L	M
P450a	2.3	0.5	0.2	0.9	—	0.6	—	—	—	—	20.9	—	—
P450b	132.5	42.7	0.4	3.3	—	9.6	1.8	1.8	—	—	—	9.1	—
P450c	6.7	0.9	23.4	60.8	1.7	97.1	21.6	1.0	—	—	—	—	1.9
P450d	3.9	—	0.3	21.1	13.8	0.6	0.7	9.6	—	0.5	—	—	0.7
P450e	19.8	8.2	0.1	1.1	0.9	2.0	—	—	—	—	—	0.8	—
P450f	1.3	—	—	0.9	0.5	—	—	—	—	0.4	—	0.8	—
P450g	4.9	1.1	—	—	0.6	1.1	—	—	—	—	—	0.3	3.8
P450h	52.1	22.6	1.8	7.4	8.0	0.9	1.5	1.5	—	1.1	—	7.9	0.2
P450i	2.8	1.0	—	0.7	1.3	0.7	—	—	4.8	—	—	—	—
P450j	5.5	—	—	3.4	0.8	1.2	1.6	12.7	—	15.9	—	—	—
P450k	14.1	4.5	0.4	3.4	2.5	0.5	1.3	1.0	—	0.5	—	—	—

*See Table 3.2 in Chapter 3 for current nomenclature.
†Empty boxes indicate negligible values.

A: Benzphetamine N-demethylation
B: Hexobarbital 3-hydroxylation
C: Benzo[a]pyrene 3/9-hydroxylation
D: Zoxazolamine 6-hydroxylation
E: Estradiol-17β 2-hydroxylation
F: 7-Ethoxycoumarin O-dealkylation
G: p-Nitroanisole O-demethylation

H: Aniline p-hydroxylation
I: Androstane disulfate 15β-hydroxylation
J: N-Nitrosodimethylamine N-demethylation
K: Testosterone 7α-hydroxylation
L: Testosterone 16α-hydroxylation
M: Testosterone 6β-hydroxylation

Comparison of their substrate specificities reveals marked similarities between some isozymes (e.g. P450b and P450h), and considerable differences between others. And when the various substrates are compared, it becomes clear that each is oxidized by a distinct population of isozymes. Selectivity is also the rule in isozyme **induction** and **inhibition**, be it by competitive inhibitors, mechanism-based reversible inhibitors, or mechanism-based irreversible inhibitors (Murray and Reidy, 1990).

Biological factors controlling the function of enzymes (e.g. availability of and coupling to reductase; Chapter 3) may affect various aspects of the specificity of isozymes. However, such influences appear limited when compared to the importance of the tertiary structure of enzymes. Indeed, a number of differences between the specificities of isozymes can now be explained satisfactorily by subtle yet critical variations in their **substrate binding site**, i.e. the cavity in which substrates are bound and maintained more or less tightly or loosely, presenting one or more target sites for catalytic attack. Even small differences in the amino acid sequence may strongly affect specificity, witness mouse P450$_{15\alpha}$ (a steroid hydroxylase) and P450$_{coh}$ (a coumarin hydroxylase). In spite of their divergent catalytic activities, these two enzymes differ by only 11 amino acids within their 494 residues, with three positions being critical. Moreover, a single mutation is sufficient to convert the substrate specificity of P450$_{coh}$ from coumarin to steroid hydroxylation (Lindberg and Negishi, 1989). A telling example of regiospecificity is offered by the three mammalian lipoxygenases, which catalyze the oxygenation of arachidonic acid at position 5, 12 and 15, respectively. Substituting Met-418 with Val in 15-lipoxygenase afforded a mutant enzyme with an altered substrate binding pocket in which arachidonic acid could penetrate more deeply and be oxygenated equally well at positions 12 and 15 (Sloane *et al.*, 1991).

Investigations on the structure–function relationships of enzymes have become a fast advancing research front in biochemistry. In xenobiotic metabolism also, molecular biology techniques such as site-directed mutagenesis and the construction of chimeric proteins have led to innumerable discoveries and conceptual breakthroughs of the type outlined above (Johnson, 1992; Johnson *et al.*, 1992).

1.6.3 A connection between the biochemistry and the physiology of xenobiotic metabolism?

Large portions of the volume on physiology and regulations will be dedicated to the many biological factors influencing xenobiotic metabolism (see Introduction). The biochemical volumes for their part discuss metabolic reactions and, as often as possible and appropriate, mention the enzymes and isozymes involved. But is there a connection between the two approaches, namely between the physiology and the biochemistry of xenobiotic metabolism? A partial answer can now be found in the functional diversity of isozymes, whose differential distribution, turnover and regulation contribute to metabolic differences seen between tissues, animal species and strains, sexes, age groups, etc (Birkett *et al.*, 1993).

To give but an example, let us consider the carcinogenic compound N-nitrosodibutylamine (NDBA; **1.XIII**), which is metabolized mainly by hydroxylation of one butyl moiety at positions 3 and 4. While 3-hydroxylation appears as an innocuous reaction, 4-hydroxylation is believed to lead to metabolites accounting for the induction of urinary bladder cancers. NDBA is hydroxylated by cytochrome P450 2B and 4B, two isozymes which display regiospecificity for the 4- and 3-position, respectively. In addition, this substrate has high affinity for P450 2B and low affinity for P450 4B. The point to make here is that differences in regioselective hydroxylation of NDBA occurring as a function of tissue, species and substrate concentration were fully consistent with the differential distribution of P450 2B and P450 4B (Schulze *et al.*, 1990).

1.XIII

Such an example is particularly illustrative, but it should not mislead the reader into adopting the reductionistic belief that the differential distribution of enzymes and isozymes accounts for the totality of metabolic differences. Many other factors such as oxygen supply, redox state, availability of cofactors, and endogenous inhibitors will also be involved.

1.7 STRUCTURE–METABOLISM RELATIONSHIPS

Like all other biological responses, the biotransformation of drugs and other xenobiotics is markedly dependent upon their molecular structure (Testa, in press; Testa and Mayer, 1990). But unlike the passive processes of disposition in which solubility and lipophilicity properties often play a major role, biotransformation is influenced by all aspects of molecular structure, including steric and stereochemical features and stereoelectronic properties, in addition to lipophilicity. A further element of complexity is due to the existence of the two basic types of selectivity discussed in Section 1.5, namely substrate selectivity and product selectivity.

1.7.1 The concept of molecular structure in structure–activity and structure–metabolism relationships

Structure–activity relationships (SAR) are an important tool in current pharmacology, encompassing every type of biological response elicited by chemical compounds. When such responses pertain to biotransformation, disposition and even pharmacokinetics (i.e. metabolism in its broadest sense), structure–metabolism relationships (SMR) can be investigated. However, a realistic and informative description of molecular structure is an obligatory condition for conducting relevant SAR or SMR studies, for obtaining meaningful results, and for deducing reasonable interpretations and generalizations.

Molecular structure is conveniently approached by considering several conceptual levels of description (Testa and Kier, 1991). As presented in Table 1.4, the description starts at an elementary level, which offers very little information, and continues with levels of increasing complexity and information content. At the geometric levels, molecules are still considered as abstract entities, which however gain flesh and reality at the stereoelectronic level. At all these levels, the molecules are viewed in isolation, and it is only at the last level that interactions with the molecular environment are considered. This allows such significant properties as lipophilicity to enter into the picture.

Depending on the biological responses under consideration, some of the structural properties detailed in Table 1.4 will be found to play a predominant role in SMR. As schematized in Fig. 1.8, lipophilicity influences predominantly passive phenomena of penetration, while stereoelectronic properties control the binding and catalytic steps.

1.7.2 The unpredictable influence of configurational and conformational factors

The influence of **configurational factors** in xenobiotic metabolism is a well-known and abundantly documented phenomenon, resulting in substrate stereoselectivity and product stereoselectivity (enantio- and diastereoselectivity) as defined in Section 1.5.3 (Caldwell *et al.*, 1988; Jenner and Testa, 1973; Testa, 1988, 1990 and 1991; Testa and Jenner, 1980; Testa and Mayer, 1988). Thus, many relevant examples will be found in this and the following volumes, and the point does not need to be discussed further in this introductory chapter.

In contrast with configurational factors, the role of **conformational factors** in drug

TABLE 1.4 *The description of chemical structure* (simplified from Testa and Kier, 1991)

Conceptual levels	Properties
• Elementary	• Atomic composition, MW, . . .
• Geometric	• 2D structure (atom connectivity)
	• 3D structure (configuration, . . .)
• Stereoelectronic	• Volume, bulk, . . .
	• Spatio-temporal structure (flexibility, conformation, . . .)
	• Electronic properties (ionization, electron distribution, electrostatic field, . . .)
• Interactions with the environment	• Solvation, solubility, lipophilicity, . . .

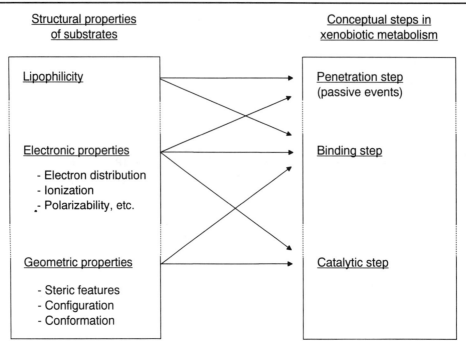

FIGURE 1.8 Conceptual steps in xenobiotic metabolism and their control by the structural properties of substrates.

metabolism has seldom been examined. Only a limited number of unambiguous cases are known to date, one of which is discussed here.

For a number of years, workers were intrigued by the paradox of the opposed substrate enantioselectivity and identical product regioselectivity seen in the hydroxylation of warfarin and phenprocoumon mediated by rat liver microsomes. Indeed, the reaction is selective for the 6- and 8-position of (R)-warfarin and (S)-phenprocoumon. This situation was finally explained by Heimark and Trager (1984), who showed that (R)-warfarin binds to cytochrome P450 as the cyclic hemiketal tautomer and with a conformation which renders it topographically equivalent to (S)-phenprocoumon despite opposite absolute configurations (Fig. 1.9).

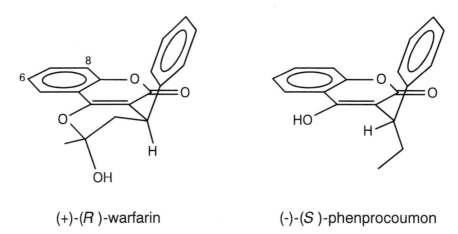

FIGURE 1.9 The topographical equivalent conformations of (R)-warfarin (left) and (S)-phenprocoumon (right) at the active site of cytochrome P450 (Heimark and Trager, 1984).

In short, both substrate stereoselectivity and product stereoselectivity are the rule in the metabolism of stereoisomeric and stereotopic drugs. But although these phenomena are to be expected *per se*, we are not able at present **to predict** either the stereoselectivities or conformational preferences of a given metabolic pathway. In other words, there is no way, except perhaps for closely related analogues, to predict which enantiomer will be the preferred substrate of a given metabolic reaction, which enantiomeric metabolite of a prochiral drug will predominate, or which conformer will be recognized by an enzyme or isozyme. This situation is due to the fact that the stereoselectivities depend as much on molecular factors of the substrate as on enzymatic factors (e.g. the stereoelectronic architecture of the catalytic site in the various isozymes involved). In fact, substrate and product stereoselectivities are determined by the binding mode(s) of the substrate and by the resulting topography of the enzyme–substrate complex (Fig. 1.6). No tool short of molecular modelling can help us in predicting stereo-selectivities (Korzekwa and Jones, 1993).

1.7.3 Interest and limitations of quantitative structure–metabolism relationships: the influence of electronic factors and lipophilicity

Besides qualitative SAR studies which seek trends and relations based on qualities, there exist numerico-statistical approaches termed as quantitative structure–activity relationships (QSAR), of which **quantitative structure–metabolism relationships** (QSMR) are a subset. Here, both the biological responses and the physicochemical and structural properties are expressed by numbers, and statistical methods based on various mathematical models are used to establish quantitative correlations. An impressive variety of physicochemical and structural parameters have found applications in QSAR and QSMR and can be classified according to the level of structural description to which they belong (Table 1.4) (van de Waterbeemd and Testa, 1987). Two groups of parameters of particular interest are those quantitating electronic properties and lipophilicity.

Stereoelectronic properties may influence the binding of substrates to enzymatic active sites in the same manner as they influence the binding of ligands to receptors. Of specific interest in the present context is the influence of electronic factors on the cleavage and formation of covalent bonds characteristic of a biotransformation reaction (i.e. the catalytic step). Correlations between **electronic parameters** and catalytic parameters obtained from *in vitro* studies (e.g. V_{max} or k_{cat}) allow a rationalization of substrate selectivity and some insight into reaction mechanisms.

Correlations between **lipophilicity** and metabolic parameters are interpreted to mean that binding and/or transport processes influence the reaction. Lipophilicity was shown to account for variations in metabolism in many series of compounds either *in vitro* or *in vivo*. For example, the type I spectral binding to cytochrome P450 and N-demethylation of 3-O-alkylmorphine homologues is controlled by their lipophilicity. For substrates with an O-alkyl group ranging from methyl to octyl, the spectral dissociation constant K_s and the kinetic affinity parameter K_m showed a comparable linear increase with lipophilicity (Eqs. 1.1 and 1.2, respectively) (Duquette *et al.*, 1983):

$$\log K_s = -0.370 \log P + 1.61 \tag{Eq. 1.1}$$
$$n = 8; r = 0.986$$

$$\log K_m = -0.552 \log P + 2.67 \tag{Eq. 1.2}$$
$$n = 8; r = 0.922$$

Eqs 1.1 and 1.2 are understandable in terms of the hydrophobic properties of the substrate binding site, but their limits are clearly set by the lack of fit of the lowest and highest homologues. In contrast to Eqs. 1.1 and 1.2, a relationship with lipophilicity was less apparent for V_{max}, the maximal velocity of the reaction, confirming that stereoelectronic and not lipophilic properties of substrates control the catalytic step. Many *in vivo* metabolic studies have also demonstrated a dependence of biotransformation on lipophilicity, suggesting a predominant role for transport and partitioning processes (Austel and Kutter, 1983). Quantitative relationships between structure and pharmacokinetics are also of great interest (Seydel and Schaper, 1982).

In such examples also, the extrapolative power of the correlations is doubtful, restricting their value to the chemical series investigated and to the range explored for each property (the so-called explored property space). However, recent statistical techniques such as PLS (partial least squares) analysis, cross-validation and CoMFA (comparative molecular field analysis) have done much to improve the analytical and extrapolative power of quantitative SMR studies (e.g. Altomare *et al.*, 1992). As a result, their contributions to drug design will certainly increase in the coming years.

1.8 METABOLISM AND DRUG DESIGN

1.8.1 Strategies in drug design

Drug design can be understood as the scientific discipline whose goal is the discovery of drugs with optimal therapeutic properties, i.e. the highest desired activities and the lowest possible occurrence of undesired effects. Such goals can be approached with the help of SAR, SMR, and also structure–toxicity relationships (Ariëns, 1984), all of which must be considered in the design of drugs with optimal therapeutic properties (Fig. 1.10).

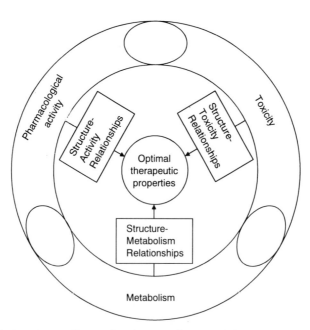

FIGURE 1.10 Drug design aims at discovering drugs with optimal therapeutic properties, i.e. high desired activities and lowest possible occurrence of unwanted effects. This must be achieved by giving attention not only to structure–activity relationships, but also to structure–toxicity relationships and structure–metabolism relationships (metabolism being taken here in its broadest sense).

Drug design is inseparable from the concept of **lead compounds**, which are defined as (Testa, 1984):

(a)   • either novel compounds displaying an interesting biological activity,
       • or known compounds with a newly discovered biological activity;
(b)   starting points for systematic or rational modifications aiming at:
       • increasing the desired activities and
       • decreasing the undesired activities.

With these definitions in mind, the two main strategies of drug design become easy to grasp (Testa, 1992):

• **Lead finding** aims at discovering compounds that fit one of the two definitions in (a);
• **Lead optimization** aims at improving lead compounds as defined in (b).

Drug metabolism can contribute to lead finding, for example when a metabolite is shown to display an activity far superior to, or qualitatively different from, that of the parent drug. The best known example is that of sulfanilamide, the lead compound of all antibacterial sulfonamides, which was discovered as a metabolite of Prontosil (see Section 12.4). However, only a few cases document the contribution of drug metabolism to lead finding. In sharp contrast, innumerable examples illustrate the major significance of drug metabolism in lead optimization, as outlined below.

1.8.2 Modulation of drug metabolism by structural variations: unmetabolized drugs, soft drugs, prodrugs, and chemical delivery systems

Much of the SMR discussed above involves overall molecular properties such as configuration, conformation, electronic distribution or lipophilicity. An alternative means of modulating metabolism is by structural modifications of the substrate at its **target moiety**, a direct approach whose outcome is often more predictable than that of altering molecular properties by structural changes not involving the reaction centre. Globally, structural variations at the reaction centre can aim either at decreasing or even suppressing biotransformation (metabolic stabilization), or at promoting it by introducing labile groups (metabolic promotion). Metabolic switching is a combination of the two goals, the aim being to block metabolism in one region of the molecule and to promote it in another.

Metabolic stabilization resulting in poorly or unmetabolized drugs can often be observed for highly hydrophilic or lipophilic compounds, a type of structural variation pertinent to the SMR discussed in Section 1.7.3. But high polarity and high lipophilicity tend to be avoided by drug designers because they often result in poor bioavailability and very slow excretion, respectively. Metabolic stabilization can be achieved more conveniently by replacing a labile group with another, less or non-reactive moiety. Classical examples include:

• Introducing an N-t-butyl group to prevent N-dealkylation;
• Inactivating aromatic rings toward oxidation by substituting them with strongly electron-withdrawing groups (e.g. CF_3, SO_2NH_2, SO_3^-);
• Replacing a labile ester linkage with an amide group;
• More generally protecting the labile moiety by steric shielding.

In addition, there have been hopes of decreasing or deflecting metabolism by specific deuteration of regioselectively oxidized positions. However, the scope of effectively using deuterium isotope effects in drug design is quite limited (Foster, 1985; Miwa and Lu, 1987).

Metabolic stabilization can present some conceivable advantages (Ariëns and Simonis, 1982), e.g.:

- Longer half-lives;
- Decreased possibilities of drug interactions;
- Decreased inter- and intra-patient variability;
- Decreased species differences;
- Decreased number and significance of active metabolites.

Nevertheless, drawbacks cannot be ignored, e.g. too long half-lives and a risk of accumulation, but the label of "hard" drugs is inadequate and polemical, and should be avoided. In contrast to metabolic stabilization, **metabolic switching** is a versatile means of deflecting metabolism away from toxic products to enhance the formation of therapeutically active metabolites and/or to obtain a suitable pharmacokinetic behaviour.

Metabolic promotion can be achieved by introducing into a lead compound a functional group of predictable metabolic reactivity, for example an ester linkage. This concept enjoys considerable success in the design of prodrugs, and is beginning to prove its therapeutic utility in the design of **soft drugs** as pioneered by Bodor and Collaborators (Bodor, 1982, 1984a and 1984b). The concept of soft drugs, which are defined as "biologically active compounds (drugs) characterized by a predictable *in vivo* metabolism to non-toxic moieties, after they have achieved their therapeutic role", has led to valuable and innovative drugs such a β-blockers with ultrashort duration of action (Quon and Gorczynski, 1986).

For the sake of fairness, it must also be mentioned that soft drugs are not without their limitations. While emphasis is placed on the predictability of their metabolism, we stress that this predictability is qualitative rather than quantitative. This is due to the many biological factors which influence biotransformation, among which inter-individual differences represent a most serious complication. Note that such a limitation also applies to prodrug design.

Prodrugs are defined as therapeutic agents which are inactive *per se* but are predictably transformed into active metabolites. As such, prodrugs must be contrasted with soft drugs, which as explained above are active *per se* and yield inactive metabolites. Prodrug design, which was earlier called drug latentiation (Harper, 1962; Riley, 1988), aims at overcoming a number of barriers to a drug's usefulness (Stella *et al.*, 1985) (Table 1.5). Based on these and other considerations, the major objectives of prodrug design can be listed as follows:

- Improved formulation (e.g. increased hydrosolubility);
- Improved chemical stability;
- Improved patient acceptance and compliance;
- Improved bioavailability;
- Prolonged duration of action;
- Improved organ selectivity;
- Decreased side-effects;
- Marketing considerations and "me-too" drugs.

The successes of prodrug design are many, and a large variety of such compounds have proved their therapeutic value (Waller and George, 1989). It is customary to distinguish between a number of (partly overlapping) classes of prodrugs (Bodor, 1984; Notari, 1981; Wermuth, 1984), i.e.:

- Carrier-linked prodrugs, i.e. drugs linked to a carrier moiety by a labile bridge;
- Bioprecursors, which do not contain a carrier group and are activated by the metabolic creation of a functional group;
- Site-specific chemical delivery systems;
- Macromolecular prodrugs;
- Drug–antibody conjugates.

Before briefly discussing these classes, a few generalizations must be made. Thus, it is always important to consider whether the activation occurs by an enzymatic and/or a non-enzymatic mechanism. The former implies biological variability and may result in difficult optimization and unpredictable behaviour, while a non-enzymatic activation is not subject to this limitation. Another essential aspect of prodrug design is the potential toxicity of the released carrier moiety or fragment. For example, some problems may be associated with formaldehyde-releasing prodrugs such as N- and O-acyloxymethyl derivatives or Mannich bases. And finally, the problem of tissue or organ selectivity is of significance even for prodrugs that are not site-specific chemical delivery systems.

Numerous **carrier-linked prodrugs** have been prepared from drugs containing a carboxylate, an amine or an amide group. Esters of carboxylic acids are quite popular, and their SMR are documented in many studies. But because of the large interspecies variability in enzymatic hydrolysis, non-enzymatic hydrolysis is often a goal of drug designers. This can occur for example with Mannich bases, (2-oxo-1,3-dioxol-4-yl)methyl esters, and oxazolidines (Chan and Li Wan Po, 1989). Under physiological conditions of pH and temperature, these compounds break down chemically. While most carrier-linked prodrugs are activated by hydrolysis, a number of other cases involve oxidation or reduction. Non-enzymatic cyclization reactions accompanied by loss of carrier moiety appear quite promising (Saari *et al.*, 1990). Carrier-linked prodrugs activated by hydrolysis or cyclization will be discussed in the next volume.

Bioprecursors are prodrugs that are activated by oxidation, reduction, or non-redox reactions (e.g. cyclization), without the release of a (non-existent) carrier group (Wermuth, 1984). Bioprecursors avoid potential toxicity problems caused by the carrier moiety, but here attention must be given to metabolic intermediates. Thus, arylacetylenes are toxic bioprecursors of anti-inflammatory arylacetic acids due to the formation of intermediate ketenes (Section 4.5). Differences in redox properties may also be used to reach tissue-selective activation, e.g. the preferential bioreduction of chemotherapeutic quinones in hypoxic tumour cells (Section 12.2).

TABLE 1.5 *Prodrugs: a concept to overcome barriers to drug's usefulness* (modified from Stella *et al.*, 1985)

Pharmaceutical barriers
- insufficient chemical stability
- poor solubility
- inacceptable taste or odour
- irritation or pain

Pharmacokinetic barriers
- insufficient oral absorption
- marked presystemic metabolism
- short duration of action
- unfavourable distribution in the body

Pharmacodynamic barriers
- toxicity

Site-specific chemical delivery systems, the "magic bullets" of drug design, are based on enzymatic or physicochemical characteristics of a given tissue or organ. For example, the selective presence of cysteine S-conjugate β-lyase in the kidney suggests that this enzyme might be exploited for delivery of sulfhydryl drugs to this organ (Section 7.7). To date, the most elaborate and versatile delivery systems are the brain-selective dihydropyridine carriers pioneered and developed by Bodor and collaborators (Bodor, 1984 and 1987) (Section 13.3). A large variety of drugs (e.g. neuropharmacological agents, steroidal hormones, chemotherapeutic agents) have been coupled to dihydropyridine carriers, resulting in improved and sustained brain delivery.

Macromolecular prodrugs and drug–antibody conjugates represent a vast field of investigation that is largely unexplored (Duncan, 1992; Franssen *et al.*, 1992; Kohn, 1991; Rajewski *et al.*, 1992).

1.8.3 The concept of toxophoric groups

Biotransformation to reactive metabolic intermediates is one of the major mechanisms by which drugs exert toxic effects, and particularly chronic toxicity (Hathway, 1984; Monks and Lau, 1988). As discussed in the Introduction, metabolic reactions of toxication as a rule are accompanied by reactions of detoxication occurring competitively or sequentially. For the reaction of toxication to occur at all, a proper moiety must be present, which has been termed a toxogenic, toxicophoric or toxophoric group, or a toxophore (e.g. Ariëns, 1984; Testa, 1984). Major **reactions of functionalization** by which toxophoric groups are activated are oxidation to electrophilic intermediates or reduction to nucleophilic radicals (Fig. 1.4). Note that the metabolic activation of xenobiotics may cause toxic effects by different mechanisms which may operate simultaneously, e.g. oxygen reduction leading to oxidative stress, and binding to bio(macro)-molecules producing critical or non-critical lesions (Section 1.4) (Kehrer, 1993; Neumann, 1986). Of more recent awareness is the fact that a number of **reactions of conjugation** may also lead to toxic metabolites, either reactive ones or long-retained residues, as discussed in the relevant volume.

A drug designer worthy of the name must be conversant with toxication reactions and toxophoric groups, which include:

- Some aromatic systems oxidizable to epoxides, quinones or quinone imines (Section 4.3);
- Ethynyl moieties activated by cytochrome P450 (Section 4.5);
- Some halogenated alkyl groups which can undergo reductive dehalogenation (Section 12.3);
- Nitroarenes which can be reduced to nitro anion-radicals, nitrosoarenes, nitroxides and hydroxylamines (Section 12.4);
- Aromatic amides activated to nitrenium ions (Section 5.6);
- Thiocarbonyl derivatives, particularly thioamides, which can be oxidized to S,S-dioxides (sulfenes) (Section 7.8).

In a comparable fashion, a list has been compiled of functional groups which would lead to a compound being classified as a potential carcinogen (Ashby and Tennant, 1988; Hay, 1988). The results have been presented in the form of a hypothetical compound containing these various groups, most of which are not reactive as such but must undergo bioactivation (Fig. 1.11).

However, it would be wrong to conclude from the above that the presence of a toxophore necessarily implies toxicity. Reality is far less gloomy, as only **potential toxicity** is indicated. Given the presence of a toxophoric group in a compound, a number of factors will operate to render the latter toxic or non-toxic, as discussed in the Introduction. In conclusion, the presence

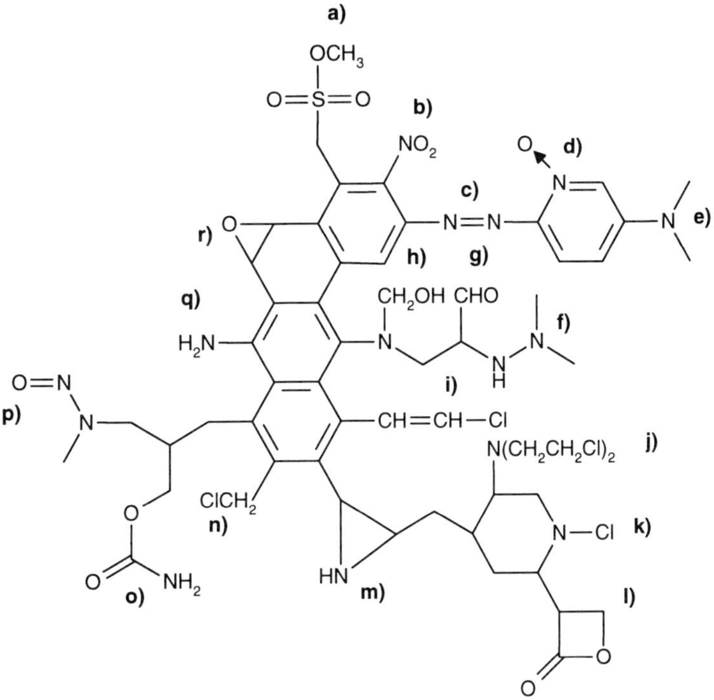

FIGURE 1.11 A hypothetical compound showing a number of functional groups (marked **a–r**) which would lead to a chemical being classed as a potential carcinogen (Ashby and Tennant, 1988; Hay, 1988). Most of these functional groups (i.e. **b–f, h, i, l–q**) display little or no carcinogenic potential prior to undergoing toxication reaction(s).

of a toxophoric group is by no means a sufficient condition for observable toxicity. And nor is it a necessary condition since other mechanisms of toxicity exist.

1.9 A CONCLUSION AND A TRANSITION

Following the general statements of Chapter i, the present chapter has presented an overview of significant concepts that are of value in clarifying our approach to and expanding our understanding of xenobiotic metabolism. Such fundamental concepts include the discrimination of enzymatic and non-enzymatic reactions, the three types of metabolic products, the many aspects of specificity and selectivity, the significance of isozymes, the interest of structure–metabolism relationships, and the role of metabolism in drug design.

With such concepts in mind, we are now ready to jump into the biochemistry of xenobiotic metabolism and examine in some detail the many reactions involved, first redox reactions (this volume), and then reactions of hydration and conjugation.

The classification of matters in this volume is based on both metabolic reactions and enzymes (International Union of Biochemistry and Molecular Biology, 1992). It can be outlined as follows:

- dehydrogenases and their reactions (Chapter 2);
- cytochrome P450, FAD-containing monooxygenase, and their reactions of mono-oxygenation (Chapters 3–8);

- various oxidases and monooxygenases and their reactions (Chapter 9);
- peroxidases and their reactions (Chapter 10);
- reductions (Chapter 12);
- various enzymatic and non-enzymatic reactions (Chapters 11 and 13).

A text, any text, necessarily follows a linear path in its presentation of matters, while the fragment of reality it aims at describing is multidimensional. To overcome to some extent the limitations of a linear presentation, cross-referencing has been generously used in this text, a technique that should help the reader in achieving a synthetic and integrated view, as stated in Section 1.2.

1.10 REFERENCES

Altomare C., Carrupt P.A., Gaillard P., El Tayar N., Testa B. and Carotti A. (1992). Quantitative structure-metabolism relationship analyses of MAO-mediated toxication of 1-methyl-4-phenyl-1,2,3,6-tetrahydropyridine and analogues. *Chem. Res. Toxicol.* **5**, 366–375.

Alworth W.L. (1972). *Stereochemistry and its Application in Biochemistry.* pp. 4–5. John Wiley, New York.

Ariëns E.J. (1984). Domestication of chemistry by design of safer chemicals: Structure-activity relationships. *Drug Metab. Rev.* **15**, 425–504.

Ariëns E.J. and Simonis A.M. (1982). Optimization of pharmacokinetics—an essential aspect of drug development—by "metabolic stabilization". In *Strategy in Drug Research* (ed. Keverling Buisman J.A.). pp. 165–178. Elsevier, Amsterdam.

Ashby J. and Tennant R.W. (1988). Chemical structure, Salmonella mutagenicity and extent of carcinogenicity as indicators of genotoxic carcinogens among 222 chemicals tested in rodents by the US NCI/NTP. *Mutat. Res.* **204**, 17–115.

Austel V. and Kutter E. (1983). Absorption, distribution, and metabolism of drugs. In *Quantitative Structure-Activity Relationships of Drugs* (ed. Topliss J.G.). pp. 437–496. Academic Press, New York.

Birkett D.J., Mackensie P.I., Veronese M.E. and Miners J.O. (1993). *In vitro* approaches can predict human drug metabolism. *Trends Pharmacol. Sci.* **14**, 292–294.

Bodor N. (1982). Designing safer drugs based on the soft drug approach. *Trends Pharmacol. Sci.* **3**, 53–56.

Bodor N. (1984a). Novel approaches to the design of safe drugs: Soft drugs and site-specific chemical delivery systems. In *Advances in Drug Research*, Vol. 13 (ed. Testa B.). pp. 255–331. Academic Press, London.

Bodor N. (1984b). Soft drugs: Principles and methods for the design of safe drugs. *Med. Res. Rev.* **4**, 449–469.

Bodor N. (1987). Redox drug delivery systems for targeting drugs to the brain. *Ann. NY Acad. Sci.* **507**, 289–306.

Boelsterli U.A. (1993). Specific targets of covalent drug-protein interactions in hepatocytes and their toxicological significance in drug-induced liver injury. *Drug Metab. Rev.* **25**, 395–451.

Briggs J.P. and Peat F.D. (1985). *Looking Glass Universe. The Emerging Science of Wholeness.* Fontana Paperbacks, London.

Caldwell J. (1982). Conjugation reactions in foreign-compound metabolism: definition, consequences, and species variations. *Drug Metab. Rev.* **13**, 745–777.

Caldwell J., Winter S.M. and Hutt A.J. (1988). The pharmacological and toxicological significance of the stereochemistry of drug disposition. *Xenobiotica* **18**, 59–70.

Chan S.Y. and Li Wan Po A. (1989). Prodrugs for dermal delivery. *Int. J. Pharmaceut.* **55**, 1–16.

Davankov V.A. (1991). Letter to the Editors: Should the terminology used in chirality be more precise. *Chirality* **3**, 442.

Duncan R. (1992). Drug-polymer conjugates: potential for improved chemotherapy. *Anti-Canc. Drugs* **3**, 175–210.

Duquette P.H., Erickson R.R. and Holtzman J.L. (1983). Role of substrate lipophilicity on the N-demethylation and type I binding of 3-O-alkylmorphine analogues. *J. Med. Chem.* **26**, 1343–1348.

Eliot T.S. (1974). *Collected Poems 1909-1962.* p. 161. Faber and Faber, London.

Foster A.B. (1985). Deuterium isotope effects in the metabolism of drugs and xenobiotics: Implications for drug design. In *Advances in Drug Research*, Vol. 14 (ed. Testa B.). pp. 1–40. Academic Press, London.

Franssen E.J.F., Koiter J., Kuipers C.A.M., Bruins A.P., Moolenaar F., de Zeeuw D., Kruizinga W.H., Kellogg R.M. and Meijer D.K.F. (1992). Low molecular weight proteins as carriers for renal drug targeting. Preparation of drug-protein conjugates and drug-spacer derivatives and their catabolism in renal cortex homogenates and lysosomal lysates. *J. Med. Chem.* **35**, 1246–1259.

Glossary of terms used in physical organic chemistry (1983). *Pure Appl. Chem* **55**, 1281–1371.

Hall P.F. (1991). Cytochrome P-450 C_{21scc}: One enzyme with two actions: hydroxylase and lyase. *J. Steroid. Biochem. Molec. Biol.* **40**, 527–532.

Harper N.J. (1962). Drug latentiation. In *Progress in Drug Research*, Vol. 4 (ed. Jucker E.). pp. 221–294. Birkhäuser, Basel.

Hathway D.E. (1980). The importance of (non-enzymic) chemical reaction processes to the fate of foreign compounds in mammals. *Chem. Soc. Rev.* **9**, 63–89.

Hathway D.E. (1984). *Molecular Aspects of Toxicology.* The Royal Society of Chemistry, London.

Hathway D.E. and Kolar G.F. (1980). Mechanisms of reaction between ultimate chemical carcinogens and nucleic acid. *Chem. Soc. Rev.* 9, 241–258.

Hay A. (1988). How to identify a carcinogen. *Nature* 332, 782–783.

Heimark L.D. and Trager W.F. (1984). The preferred solution conformation of warfarin at the active site of cytochrome P-450 based on the CD spectra in octanol/water model systems. *J. Med. Chem.* 27, 1092–1905.

International Union of Biochemistry and Molecular Biology (1992). *Enzyme Nomenclature 1992*. Academic Press, San Diego, USA.

Jenner P. and Testa B. (1973). The influence of stereochemical factors on drug disposition. *Drug Metab. Rev.* 2, 117–184.

Johnson E.F. (1992). Mapping determinants of the substrate selectivities of P450 enzymes by site-directed mutagenesis. *Trends Pharmacol. Sci.* 13, 122–126.

Johnson E.F., Kronbach T. and Hsu M.H. (1992). Analysis of the catalytic specificity of cytochrome P450 enzymes through site-directed mutagenesis. *FASEB J.* 6, 700–705.

Jones J.B. (1986). Enzymes in organic synthesis. *Tetrahedron* 42, 3351–3403.

Kedzie K.M., Balfour C.A., Escobar G.Y., Grimm S.W., He Y.A., Pepperl D.J., Regan J.W., Stevens J.C. and Halpert J.R. (1991). Molecular basis for a functionally unique cytochrome-P450IIB1 variant. *J. Biol. Chem.* 266, 22,515–22,521.

Kehrer J.P. (1993). Free radicals as mediators of tissue injury and disease. *Crit. Rev. Toxicol.* 23, 21–48.

Ketterer B. (1982). Xenobiotic metabolism by nonenzymatic reactions of glutathione. *Drug Metab. Rev.* 13, 161–187.

Knowles J.R. (1991). Enzyme catalysis: not different, just better. *Nature* 350, 121–124.

Kohn J. (1991). "Pseudo"-poly(amino acids). *Drug News Perspect.* 4, 289–294.

Korzekwa K.R. and Jones J.P. (1993). Predicting the cytochrome-P450 mediated metabolism of xenobiotics. *Pharmacogenetics* 3, 1–18.

Latif F., Moschel R.C., Hemminki K. and Dipple A. (1988). Styrene oxide as a stereochemical probe for the mechanism of aralkylation at different sites on guanosine. *Chem. Res. Toxicol.* 1, 364–369.

Levin W. (1990). Functional diversity of hepatic cytochromes P-450. *Drug Metab. Disposit.* 18, 824–830.

Lindberg R.L.P. and Negishi M. (1989). Alteration of mouse cytochrome P450COH substrate specificity by mutation of a single amino-acid residue. *Nature* 339, 632–634.

Mason R.P. (1986). Free radical metabolites of toxic chemicals. *Fed. Proc.* 45, 2464.

Miwa G.T. and Lu Y.H. (1987). Kinetic isotope effects and metabolic switching in cytochrome P-450-catalyzed reactions. *BioEssays* 7, 215–219.

Monks T.J. and Lau S.S. (1988). Reactive intermediates and their toxicological significance. *Toxicology* 52, 1–54.

Murray M. and Reidy G.F. (1990). Selectivity in the inhibition of mammalian cytochromes P-450 by chemical agents. *Pharmacol. Therap.* 42, 85–101.

Nebert D.W., Nelson D.R., Coon M.J., Estabrook R.W., Feyereisen R., Fujii-Kuriyama Y., Gonzales F.J., Guengerich F.P., Gunsalus I.C., Johnson E.F., Loper J.C., Sato R., Waterman M.R. and Waxman D.J. (1991). The P450 gene superfamily: Update on new sequences, gene mapping, and recommended nomenclature. *DNA Cell Biol.* 10, 1–14.

Nelson S.D. (1982). Metabolic activation and drug toxicity. *J. Med. Chem.* 25, 753–765.

Nelson S.D. and Pearson P.G. (1990). Covalent and non-covalent interactions in acute lethal cell injury caused by chemicals. *Ann. Rev. Pharmacol. Toxicol.* 30, 169–195.

Nelson D.R., Kamataki T., Waxman D.J., Guengerich F.P., Estabrook R.W., Feyereisen R., Gonzalez F.J., Coon M.J., Gunsalus I.C., Gotoh O., Okuda K. and Nebert D.W. (1993). The P450 superfamily: Update on new sequences, gene mapping, accession numbers, early trivial names of enzymes, and nomenclature. *DNA Cell Biol.* 12, 1–51.

Neumann H.G. (1986). Toxication mechanisms in drug metabolism. In *Advances in Drug Research*, Vol. 15 (ed. Testa B.). pp. 1–28. Academic Press, London.

Notari R.E. (1981). Prodrug design. *Pharmacol. Therap.* 14, 25–53.

O'Donnell J.P. (1982). The reaction of amines with carbonyls: Its significance in the nonenzymatic metabolism of xenobiotics. *Drug Metab. Rev.* 13, 123–159.

Ogita Z.I. and Markert C.L., eds. (1990). *Isozymes: Structure, Function, and Use in Biology and Medicine.* Wiley-Liss, New York.

Park B.K. and Kitteringham N.R. (1990). Drug-protein conjugation and its immunological consequences. *Drug Metab. Rev.* 22, 87–144.

Portoghese P.S. (1970). Relationships between stereostructure and pharmacological activities. *Ann. Rev. Pharmacol.* 10, 51–76.

Quon C.Y. and Gorczynski R.J. (1986). Pharmacodynamics and onset of action of esmolol in anesthetized dogs. *J. Pharmacol. Exp. Therap.* 237, 912–918.

Rajewski L.G., Stinnett A.A., Stella V.J. and Topp E.M. (1992). Enzymic and non-enzymic hydrolysis of a polymeric prodrug: hydrocortisone esters of hyaluronic acid. *Int. J. Pharmaceut.* 82, 205–213.

Riley T.N. (1988). The prodrug concept and new drug design and development. *J. Chem. Educ.* 65, 947–953.

Ross D. (1989). Mechanistic toxicology: a radical perspective. *J. Pharm. Pharmacol.* 41, 505–511.

Saari W.S., Schwering J.E., Lyle P.A., Smith S.J. and Engelhardt E.L. (1990). Cyclization-activated prodrugs. Basic esters of 5-bromo-2'-deoxyuridine. *J. Med. Chem.* 33, 2590–2595.

Schulze J., Richter E. and Philpot R.M. (1990). Tissue, species, and substrate concentration differences in the position-selective hydroxylation of N-nitrosodibutylamine. Relationship to the distribution of cytochrome P-450 isozymes 2 (IIB) and 5 (IVB). *Drug Metab. Disposit.* 18, 398–402.

Seydel J.K. and Schaper K.J. (1982). Quantitative structure-pharmacokinetic relationships and drug design.

Pharmacol. Therap. **15**, 131–182.

Sies H., ed. (1991). *Oxidative Stress: Oxidants and Antioxidants*. Academic Press, London.

Sloane D.L., Leung R., Craik C.S. and Sigal E. (1991). A primary determinant for lipoxygenase positional specificity. *Nature* **354**, 149–152.

Soucek P. and Gut I. (1992). Cytochromes P450 in rats: structures, functions, properties and relevant human forms. *Xenobiotica* **22**, 83–103.

Srivastava D.K. and Bernhard S.A. (1986). Metabolite transfer via enzyme-enzyme complexes. *Science* **234**, 1081–1086.

Stella V.J., Charman W.N.A. and Naringrekar V.H. (1985). Prodrugs: Do they have advantages in clinical practice? *Drugs* **29**, 455–473.

Testa B. (1982). Non-enzymatic contributions to xenobiotic metabolism. *Drug Metab. Rev.* **13**, 25–50.

Testa B. (1983). Non-enzymatic biotransformation. In *Biological Basis of Detoxication* (eds Caldwell J. and Jakoby W.B.). pp. 137–150. Academic Press, New York.

Testa B. (1984). Drugs? Drug research? Advances in drug research? Musings of a medicinal chemist. In *Advances in Drug Research*, Vol. 13 (ed. Testa B.). pp. 1–58. Academic Press, London.

Testa B. (1988). Substrate and product stereoselectivity in monooxygenase-mediated drug activation and inactivation. *Biochem. Pharmacol.* **37**, 85–92.

Testa B. (1990). Definitions and concepts in biochirality. In *Chirality and Biological Activity* (eds Holmstedt B., Frank H. and Testa B.). pp. 15–32. Liss, New York.

Testa B. (1991). Stereo-selectivity in drug disposition and metabolism: Concepts and mechanisms. In *New Trends in Pharmacokinetics* (eds Rescigno A. and Thakur A.K.). pp. 257–269. Plenum Press, New York.

Testa B. (1992). Medicinal chemistry: A teacher's and worker's perspective. *Chimia* **46**, 102–105.

Testa B. (in press). Drug Metabolism. In *Burger's Medicinal Chemistry and Drug Discovery*, 5th Edition, Volume 1 (ed. Wolff M.E.). Wiley, New York.

Testa B. and Jenner P. (1978). Novel drug metabolites produced by functionalization reactions: Chemistry and toxicology. *Drug Metab. Rev.* **7**, 325–369.

Testa B. and Jenner P. (1980). A structural approach to selectivity in drug metabolism and disposition. In *Concepts in Drug Metabolism*, Part A (eds Testa B. and Jenner P.). pp. 53–176. Dekker, New York.

Testa B. and Kier L.B. (1991). The concept of molecular structure in structure-activity relationship studies and drug design. *Med. Res. Rev.* **11**, 35–48.

Testa B. and Mayer J.M. (1988). Stereoselective drug metabolism and its significance in drug research. In *Progress in Drug Research*, Vol. 32 (ed. Jucker E.). pp. 249–303. Birkhäuser, Basel.

Testa B. and Mayer J.M. (1990). Drug metabolism and pharmacokinetics: Implications for drug design. *Acta Pharm. Jugosl.* **40**, 315–350.

Trager W.F. (1982). The non- and post-enzymatic chemistry of activated oxygen. *Drug Metab. Rev.* **13**, 51–70.

Trush M.A., Mimnaugh E.G. and Gram T.E. (1982). Activation of pharmacologic agents to radical intermediates. Implications for the role of free radicals in drug action and toxicity. *Biochem. Pharmacol.* **31**, 3335–3346.

van de Waterbeemd H. and Testa B. (1987). The parametrization of lipophilicity and other structural properties in drug design. In *Advances in Drug Research*, Vol. 16 (ed. Testa B.). pp. 85–225. Academic Press, London.

Walle T., Walle U.K. and Olanoff L.S. (1985). Quantitative account of propranolol metabolism in urine of normal man. *Drug Metab. Disposit.* **13**, 204–209.

Waller D.G. and George C.F. (1989). Prodrugs. *Brit. J. Clin. Pharmacol.* **28**, 497–507.

Waterman M.R. and Johnson E.F., eds (1991). *Cytochrome P450*. Methods in Enzymology, Volume 206. Academic Press, San Diego.

Wermuth C.G. (1984). Designing prodrugs and bioprecursors. In *Drug Design: Fact or Fantasy?* (eds Jolles G. and Woolridge K.R.H.). pp. 47–72. Academic Press, London.

chapter 2

DEHYDROGENATION OF ALCOHOLS AND ALDEHYDES, CARBONYL REDUCTION

Contents

2.1 INTRODUCTION

This chapter focuses on the carbonyl group and examines its pivotal role in reactions mediated by dehydrogenases. Specifically, it covers four major reactions, namely:

- dehydrogenation of primary and secondary alcohols to generate aldehydes and ketones, respectively;
- dehydrogenation of aldehydes to generate carboxylic acids;
- carbonyl reductions;
- dehydrogenation of dihydrodiols to generate catechols.

The reduction of quinones to hydroquinones has many analogies with carbonyl reduction and could be presented here. But as will be explained, its inclusion in Chapter 12 is preferable.

The oxidoreductases mediating the above reactions form a large and varied group of enzymes which use **nicotinamide adenine dinucleotide** (NAD$^+$/NADH) or **nicotinamide adenine dinucleotide phosphate** (NADP$^+$/NADPH) as cofactor (Weiner and Flynn, 1987 and 1989; Weiner et al., 1993). Enzymes of a different nature may also mediate some of the reactions discussed in this chapter, witness cytochrome P450 which can function as an alcohol oxidase (Section 7.6).

2.2 DEHYDROGENATION OF ALCOHOLS

Dehydrogenation plays a major role in the metabolism of alcohols, be they endogenous compounds, xenobiotics, or metabolites of the latter arising from hydroxylation reactions. A number of substrates will be presented below to illustrate the structural variety of alcohols (primary and secondary, aliphatic and alicyclic) undergoing dehydrogenation. Before so doing, however, essential enzymological aspects must be considered.

2.2.1 Alcohol dehydrogenases: biochemistry and reaction mechanism

Among the various enzymes mediating alcohol dehydrogenation, the best studied ones are certainly **alcohol dehydrogenases** [alcohol:NAD$^+$ oxidoreductase; EC 1.1.1.1; abbreviated ADH]. These zinc enzymes are found in the cytosol of the mammalian liver, in various extrahepatic tissues, and in yeast. Mammalian liver alcohol dehydrogenases (abbreviated LADHs) share many similarities in molecular weight, primary and tertiary structure, and zinc content. They are dimeric enzymes (in contrast to some tetrameric forms in microorganisms), each of the two subunits having a molecular weight of approximately 40,000 (number of amino acids in the range 365–412) and containing one structural and one catalytic zinc ion (Bosron and Li, 1980; Jörnvall et al., 1984; Pocker and De Roy, 1987; Vallee and Auld, 1990).

The **human enzymes** that have been well studied are the products of five separate genes (ADH_1–ADH_5) that encode the α, β, γ, π and χ subunits, respectively. Polymorphism has been demonstrated at ADH_2 (resulting in the three allelic variants β_1, β_2 and β_3) and ADH_3 (γ_1 and γ_2) (Chambers, 1990). The α, β and γ subunits share over 90% sequence identity and can form heterodimers as well as homodimers. In contrast, the π protein and the χ protein share only 50–60% sequence identity with the other subunits and can only form homodimers.

These combinations have led to the distinction of three or more different classes of human alcohol dehydrogenase enzymes (Bosron et al., 1979; Chambers, 1990; Eklund et al., 1990; Engeland and Maret, 1993; Hurley and Bosron, 1992; Jörnvall et al., 1984 and 1988; Smith, 1988; Weiner and Flynn, 1987):

- Class I, comprising the various isozymes that are homodimers or heterodimers of the α, β and γ subunits (e.g. the $\alpha\alpha$, $\beta_1\beta_1$, $\alpha\beta_2$ and $\beta_1\gamma$ isozymes);
- Class II, comprising the $\pi\pi$ enzyme;
- Class III, comprising the $\chi\chi$ enzyme.

Recently, a new alcohol dehydrogenase has been characterized from human stomach and named σ-ADH. Its properties suggest it to be a Class II isozyme (Moreno and Parés, 1991).

Other mammalian alcohol dehydrogenases are of interest, in particular the E and S isozymes of horse liver, the subunits of which differ only by 10 amino acid residues (Park and Plapp, 1992).

The **global reaction** of ADH-mediated alcohol oxidation is described by Eq. 2.1 (note that the reaction is a reversible one, carbonyl reduction being discussed in Section 2.4):

$$R'RCHOH + NAD^+ \rightleftarrows R'RC{=}O + NADH + H^+ \tag{Eq. 2.1}$$

Such an equation, however, is unrealistically simple and neglects the **ordered mechanism** leading to the obligatory formation of a ternary complex. Eqs. 2.2–2.4 depict such a mechanism, the thermodynamic and kinetic aspects of which have been examined (Pocker *et al.*, 1987; Sekhar and Plapp, 1990):

$$E + NAD^+ \rightleftarrows E{\cdot}NAD^+ \tag{Eq. 2.2}$$

$$E{\cdot}NAD^+ + R'RCHOH \rightleftarrows R'RC{=}O + E{\cdot}NADH + H^+ \tag{Eq. 2.3}$$

$$E{\cdot}NADH \rightleftarrows E + NADH \tag{Eq. 2.4}$$

The essential steps in the dehydrogenation reaction are first the deprotonation of the alcohol substrate to an alcoholate (R'RCHO$^-$), followed by removal of the hydrogen atom as a hydride anion (H$^-$) and its transfer to oxidized nicotinamide, as shown in Fig. 2.1. The reverse reaction, also shown in Fig. 2.1, will be discussed in Section 2.4.

The reaction of alcohol dehydrogenation is rendered possible by a complex mechanism of substrate activation which has been the object of considerable interest. An overall understanding of this **reaction mechanism** owes much to site-directed mutagenesis, X-ray crystallographic and molecular modelling studies of liver ADH complexed with substrates (e.g. Almarsson and Bruice, 1993; Bahnson *et al.*, 1993; Biellmann, 1986; Eklund *et al.*, 1982; Plapp *et al.*, 1978 and 1987a; Ramaswamy *et al.*, 1994). Fig. 2.2 shows the result of such a study, with benzyl alcohol bound to the active site of horse liver ADH. The catalytic zinc cation is coordinated to Cys-46, Cys-174, His-67, and the oxygen atom of the substrate. The latter additionally donates a hydrogen bond to Ser-48, and can be seen to bind (presumably by Van der Waals and hydrophobic forces) to a number of surrounding hydrophobic residues.

The deprotonation step can also be understood with the help of Fig. 2.2, since it is catalyzed by a proton relay system involving the hydroxyl group of Ser-48, the 2-hydroxyl of the ribosyl moiety, and the imidazolyl ring of His-51 (Eklund *et al.*, 1982).

Marked differences may exist between alcohol dehydrogenases in their substrate specificities, rates of reactions and sensitivity to inhibitors (see later). This can now be explained in terms of some amino acids in key positions being replaced by others playing an analogous but not

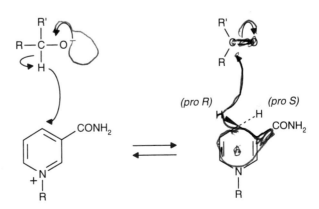

FIGURE 2.1 Hydride transfer in reactions catalyzed by oxidoreductases. Carbonyl reduction is arbitrarily depicted here as involving the *pro-R* hydrogen.

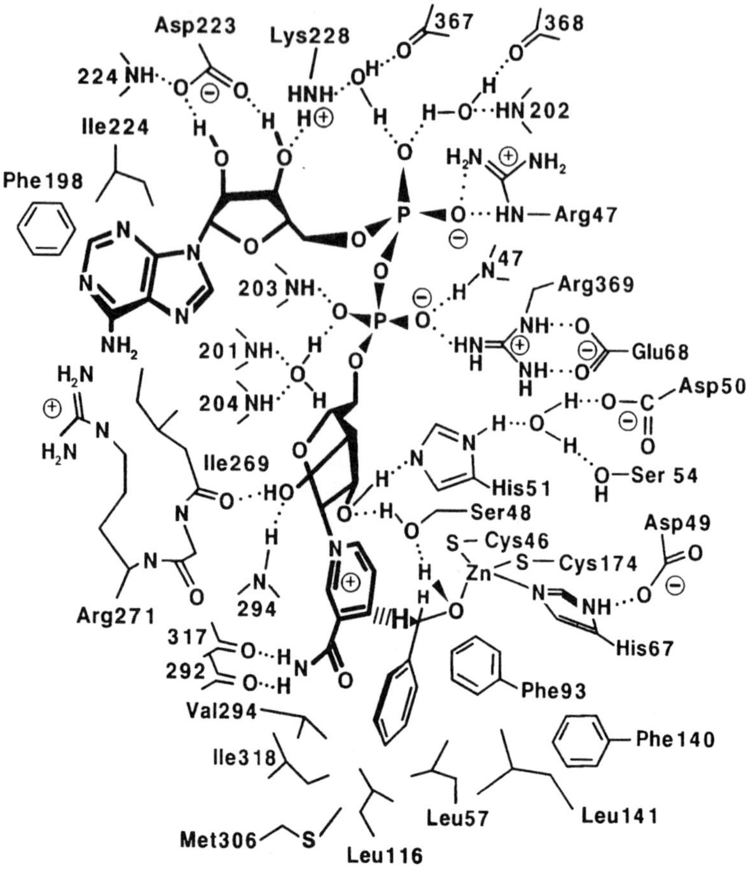

FIGURE 2.2 Active site of horse liver alcohol dehydrogenase with bound benzyl alcohol. This figure summarizes recent findings (Ramaswamy *et al.*, 1994) and was kindly made available by Dr Plapp, the copyright holder.

quantitatively identical role. Thus, Ser-48 in liver ADH is replaced by Thr-48 in yeast ADH. Similarly, some of the hydrophobic residues in the substrate binding pocket are replaced with larger residues such as Trp-93 and Trp-57, resulting in the narrower substrate specificity of yeast ADHs (Ganzhorn *et al.*, 1987; Plapp *et al.*, 1987a). The E and S isozymes of horse liver ADH also display marked differences in their substrate specificities and catalytic efficiency (Park and Plapp, 1992), as do the various human isozymes (e.g. Chambers, 1990; Eklund *et al.*, 1990; Hurley and Bosron, 1992; Jörnvall *et al.*, 1984; Light *et al.*, 1992).

2.2.2 Substrate selectivity in alcohol dehydrogenase-catalyzed oxidations

As shown in Eq. 2.1, the dehydrogenation of alcohols liberates one proton and this, among other causes, explains why reaction rates and selectivities are markedly pH-dependent. *In vitro*, higher or lower (neutral) pH values will shift the equilibrium toward dehydrogenation of alcohol or reduction of carbonyl, respectively, an informative example of **chemospecificity**. *In vitro* studies of liver ADHs have yielded pH optima in the range 10–11 for alcohol dehydrogenation, but the rather unphysiological character of these values prompts researchers to work closer to neutrality

(Bosron and Li, 1980). One interesting case of competition between oxidation and reduction was seen in the metabolism of 4-hydroxyalkenals (**2.I**, $n = 0$–10), which are natural cytotoxic products of lipid peroxidation (Section 10.5). The aldehydic group was reduced at pH 7.0 with marked substrate selectivities by various isozymes of human alcohol dehydrogenase. At pH 10, however, dehydrogenation of the 4-hydroxyl group occurred (Sellin *et al.*, 1991).

2.I

The high coenzyme specificity of mammalian ADHs for $NAD^+/NADH$ can be contrasted with their very broad **substrate specificity**. Most **primary and secondary aliphatic and aromatic alcohols** can be readily oxidized, while bulky secondary alcohols are poor substrates and **tertiary alcohols** cannot be dehydrogenated. A compilation of some representative data is given in Table 2.1. Interestingly, the maximal velocity of the reaction (V_{max}) ranges about one order of magnitude, whereas the Michaelis constant (K_m) spans four orders of magnitude. This is a clear indication, confirmed in numerous studies, that the affinity of substrates for ADHs is much more sensitive to structural effects than is their reactivity in the enzyme–substrate complex. As can be gathered from Table 2.1, lipophilic alcohols are better substrates than hydrophilic ones, and steric aspects also play a role. Indeed, quantitative structure–metabolism relationship (QSMR) studies have unravelled exquisite sensitivity to electronic and steric effects (e.g. Klinman, 1976).

TABLE 2.1 *Some kinetic parameters of alcohol dehydrogenation*

Substrate	Rat LADH[*]		Human LADH[†]		Human π-isozymes[#]	
	K_m	V_{max}	K_m	V_{max}	K_m	V_{max}
Methanol	[§]	—	7.0	0.09	no act.	
Ethanol	0.64	(1)	0.40	(1)	34	(1)
1-Propanol	0.22	0.95	0.10	0.9	3.0	0.8
1-Butanol	0.14	1.3	0.14	1.1	0.14	1.0
Isobutanol	0.19	0.80	—	—	—	—
1-Pentanol	—	—	—	—	0.036	1.0
1-Hexanol	—	—	0.06	0.9	—	—
2-Hexen-1-ol	—	—	0.003	1.4	—	—
Benzyl alcohol	0.036	0.47	—	—	—	—
Ethylene glycol	—	—	30	0.4	no act.	
1,4-Butanediol	9.5	1.5	—	—	—	—
1,6-Hexanediol	—	—	0.07	1.0	—	—
2-Butanol	12	0.48	—	—	—	—
Cyclohexanol	0.54	1.0	—	—	—	—

[*]pH 7.3, NAD^+ 0.5 mM, K_m in mM, V_{max} relative values (ethanol = 1.0) (data compiled by Plapp *et al.*, 1987b).
[†]pH 7.0, NAD^+ 0.5 mM, K_m in mM, V_{max} relative values (ethanol = 1.0) (data compiled by Bosron and Li, 1980).
[#]pH 7.5, NAD^+ 2.4 mM, K_m in mM, V_{max} relative values (ethanol = 1.0) (data compiled by Bosron and Li, 1980).
[§]Not investigated.

The oxidation of **diols and polyols** can be of physiological significance (e.g. glycerol, sugar alcohols), but in other cases it can have marked toxic consequences (e.g. ethylene glycol in Table 2.1, polyethylene glycols) (Herold *et al.*, 1989; Lenk *et al.*, 1989). **Unsaturated alcohols** are relatively good substrates as a rule, and the high affinity of retinol is worth noting in this context (Bosron and Li, 1980). Secondary alcohols are dehydrogenated to ketones, but an overall comparison between the reactivity of primary and secondary alcohols is difficult and may be misleading due to such factors as competitive reactions (see Sections 2.3 and 2.4), isozyme specificity, and the involvement of other dehydrogenases (see later). The sole comparison reported in Table 2.1 (1- versus 2-butanol) indicates lower affinity and reactivity of the latter substrate. This can be contrasted with the dehydrogenation of the two bicyclic alcohols **2.II** and **2.IV** by horse LADH. Under the conditions of the study, partial (ca. 30%) conversion of the primary alcohol **2.II** to the aldehyde **2.III** was observed, while dehydrogenation of the secondary alcohol **2.IV** to the ketone **2.V** was quantitative (MacInnes *et al.*, 1983). However, the major interest of this study lies in the particular reactivity of the substrates: the fact that the cyclopropane ring survived the reaction is proof that the transition state does not involve radical intermediates but a genuine hydride transfer.

2.II   2.III

2.IV   2.V

Liver ADH-catalyzed dehydrogenations (as well as reductions, see Section 2.4) are also characterized by their **stereoselectivity** as documented in a number of studies. **Substrate enantioselectivity** is seen for example in the dehydrogenation of 1,2-propanediol (**2.VI**) to lactaldehyde by horse liver ADH; the relative rates for (*R*)- and (*S*)-1,2-propanediol were 10:1. In contrast, no substrate enantioselectivity was seen in the dehydrogenation of the enantiomers of 1,3-butanediol (**2.VII**) and 3-methyl-1,2-butanediol (**2.VIII**) (Matos *et al.*, 1985). Note that compounds **2.VI–2.VIII** also demonstrate **product regioselectivity** in that dehydrogenation involves the primary but not the secondary alcohol group (see above). Marked differences in the substrate stereospecificity of human isozymes have also been reported and explained by computer graphics studies of the active sites (Stone *et al.*, 1989).

Liver ADH-catalyzed dehydrogenations can also display **product enantiospecificity** as seen in the preferential oxidation of the *pro-S* hydroxyl group in prochiral 1,5-pentanediols (**2.IX**) (Irwin and Jones, 1977). The stereospecificity of alcohol dehydrogenases corresponds to a stereochemical and mechanistic imperative as aptly discussed by Benner (1982). In addition, it is of major medicinal and synthetic significance, calling for versatile and reliable predictive rules. Jones and collaborators, for example, have refined an informative cubic-space active site model based on their innumerable results with alcohols and carbonyl derivatives of great structural variety (Jones and Jakovac, 1982).

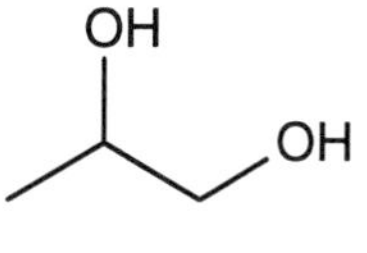

2.VI

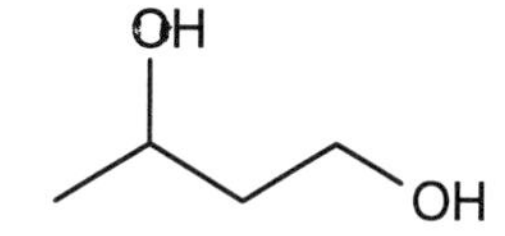

2.VII

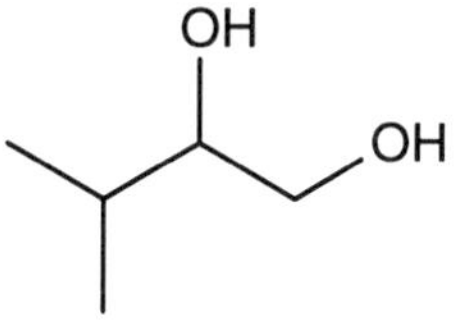

2.VIII

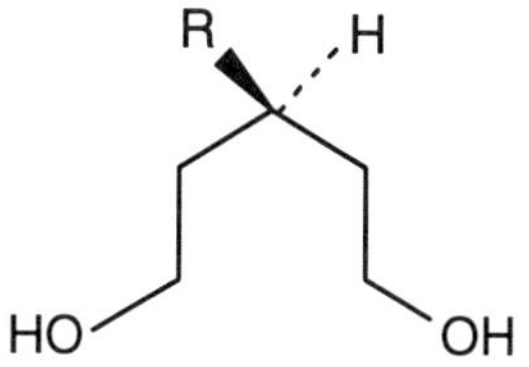

2.IX

2.2.3 Medicinal aspects of alcohol dehydrogenation

Mammalian ADHs have been shown to be operative in the dehydrogenation of various compounds having pharmacological or toxicological significance. For example, human liver ADH is an enzyme essential to the metabolism of **digitoxigenin (2.X)**, **digoxigenin** and **gitoxigenin**, the three active genins of the cardiac glycosides digoxin, digitoxin and gitoxin, respectively (Frey and Valle, 1979). The reaction involves the oxidation of the 3β-OH group to form the keto metabolite and is accompanied by a more than 90% loss in activity. This reaction is the first inactivation step in the metabolic sequence of digitalis glycosides and is thus of particular pharmacodynamic significance. Note that while ethanol, 5β-androstan-17β-ol-3-one and 5β-pregnan-3,20-dione were substrates of the same enzyme preparation, cortisone, corticosterone and 17α-methyltestosterone were not (Frey and Valle, 1979).

The dehydrogenation of some primary alcohols to aldehydes may be of potential toxicological significance due to the bioreactivity of the latter. However, in such cases the appearance of toxicity depends not only on the rate of formation of the aldehyde, but also on its further metabolism, as discussed in Section 2.3.

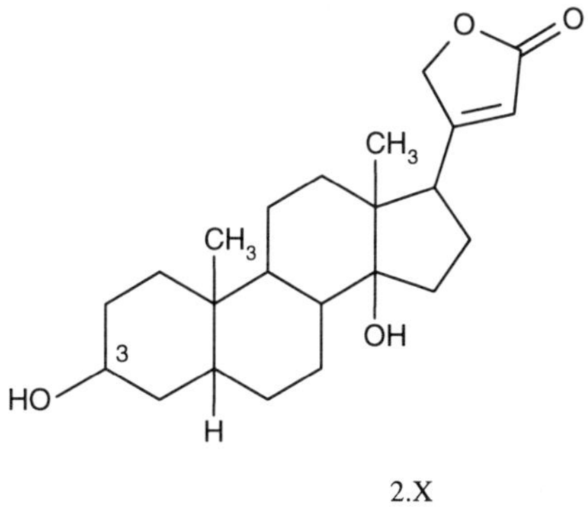

2.X

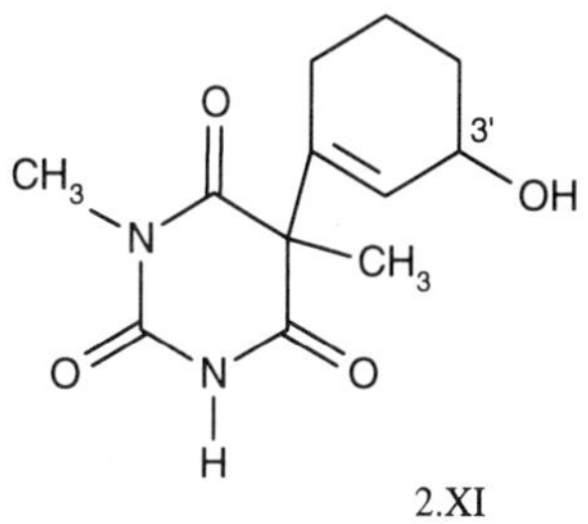

2.XI

All findings discussed above were obtained from *in vitro* studies using more or less purified enzyme preparations. **In vivo situations** are always much more complex, and the observed alcohol dehydrogenations may be mediated by various oxidoreductases among the considerable variety of such enzymes that exist in addition to ADH (Nakayama *et al.*, 1987). In particular, a number of **hydroxysteroid dehydrogenases** such as 3α- and 3β-hydroxysteroid dehydrogenases [EC 1.1.1.50 and EC 1.1.1.51, respectively] may well be involved more than currently believed. A case in point is that of **hexobarbital**, which like other barbiturates undergoes cytochrome P450-mediated side-chain hydroxylation. 3'-Hydroxyhexobarbital (**2.XI**), the resulting metabolite, is then dehydrogenated to 3'-oxohexobarbital, another major metabolite (Van der Graaff *et al.*, 1988). It was shown some years ago that in guinea-pigs the reversible oxidation of **2.XI** is catalyzed by an NADP$^+$-dependent oxidoreductase possessing a relatively narrow substrate specificity in comparison with the rabbit liver enzyme, and acting preferentially on 17β-hydroxysteroids (Kageura and Toki, 1975). We note also that 3α-hydroxyhexobarbital was oxidized four times faster by the guinea-pig enzyme than its 3β-diastereomer (Kageura and Toki, 1975).

It is a common case that *in vivo* dehydrogenations cannot be ascribed to a given enzyme. For example, (−)-menthol (**2.XII**) in rats yielded the diol **2.XIV** and the dihydroxy acid **2.XV** as its major urinary metabolites (Madyastha and Srivatsan, 1988). The postulated intermediate primary alcohol **2.XIII** was not detected, most likely due to its fast dehydrogenation to the aldehyde and then to the acid. No ketone arising from the dehydrogenation of the secondary alcohol group was reported. It is not possible with the data available to know which oxidoreductases were involved in the reaction and what factors account for the apparent inertness of the secondary alcohol group.

Fast dehydrogenation to the aldehyde and then to the acid (see Section 2.3) is a common fate for a number of drugs bearing a **primary alcohol group**. Such a metabolic reaction may be

2.XII

2.XIII

2.XIV

2.XV

unfavourable in terms of duration of action if the therapeutic effect is due to the alcohol, but it may be desirable and even so designed if the alcohol is a **prodrug** of an active acid. A classical illustration of such a situation is provided by β-pyridylcarbinol (**2.XVI**), a well-known prodrug of nicotinic acid. Oxidation of **2.XVI** to nicotinic acid is fast in rats. In humans dosed with labelled **2.XVI**, 80–90% of the circulating label was found to be nicotinic acid (Cohen, 1985; Fumagalli, 1971). Oxidation can also transform a directly active drug into an active metabolite, as seen in guinea-pigs with the *in vivo* formation of codeinone from codeine by dehydrogenation of its secondary alcohol group (Ishida *et al.*, 1991).

2.XVI

2.2.4 Inhibition of alcohol dehydrogenases

Inhibition of ADH is of interest from a biochemical and enzymological point of view. While earlier studies used ADH inhibitors to define better the involvement and functions of the enzyme, such inhibitors have in recent years become important tools in understanding stereo-electronic and mechanistic features of the active site.

Traditional and selective inhibitors of ADHs are **pyrazole** and **4-methylpyrazole** (**2.XVII**, R = H and R = CH$_3$, respectively) (Tolf *et al.*, 1985). These compounds bind tightly to the substrate binding site of the ADH–NAD$^+$ complex, with the N(2) atom forming an electrostatic interaction with the catalytic zinc cation (2.0–2.2 Å). The N(1) atom also contributes to the binding of pyrazoles; it is located 2.0 Å away from the C(4) atom of the nicotinamide ring, to which it can bind covalently (Becker and Roberts, 1984; Fries *et al.*, 1979; Hansch *et al.*, 1986). There is a hundredfold increase in the inhibitory potency of **2.XVII** when the 4-substituent X increases from methyl to *n*-hexyl, indicating that this substituent binds to a long hydrophobic channel, a molecular graphics representation of which has been published (Hansch *et al.*, 1986). Due to these precise topographical requirements, 3-substituted pyrazoles are far less active (Fries *et al.*, 1979).

2.XVII

2.XVIII

2.XIX

A large variety of ADH inhibitors are known, some of which were specifically designed and found to be highly effective (e.g. 4-substituted formylbenzylamines **2.XVIII**) (Biellmann, 1986). **Bifunctional active site-directed inactivators** of liver ADH have also added to our knowledge of this enzyme. Thus, in the ADH–NAD$^+$ complex 4-(*para*-bromoacetamidophenyl)butyric acid (**2.XIX**) binds with its carboxyl group to the catalytic zinc atom, while its bromoacetamido group alkylates Met-306 14 Å away in the substrate-binding pocket (Chen and Plapp, 1978). In the absence of a coenzyme, the carboxylate group forms an ionic bond with Arg-47 and Lys-228 while alkylation occurs at Cys-46 or Cys-174.

Alcohols of increased acidity (e.g. trifluoroethanol, propargyl alcohol, and 3-hydroxypropionitrile) were found to be informative inhibitors of ethanol dehydrogenation (Pocker and Page, 1990). There was a good correlation between pK_a and K_i (competitive inhibitory constant) such that greater acidity resulted in higher inhibitory activity. This indicated that inhibition is controlled by proton loss from these alcohols and formation of a Zn-bound alkoxide by direct ligation of the alcoholate oxygen to the catalytic zinc ion.

Unexpected inhibition of liver ADH occurs also with at least one drug, chloroprothixene, which bears none of the structural features of the above compounds (Kovar *et al.*, 1976). It appears that this tricyclic neuroleptic drug can fortuitously adopt a haptophoric structure allowing its binding in the active site pocket of liver ADH, but without participation of the zinc atom. This finding implies potential drug–drug and ascertained drug–ethanol interactions, and as such may have therapeutic consequences. It is also a warning that some quite unexpected drug–enzyme interactions may, and in fact do, occur.

2.3 DEHYDROGENATION OF ALDEHYDES

2.3.1 Aldehyde dehydrogenases and their substrates

Dehydrogenation of aldehydes is mediated by a large variety of enzymes, in particular (but not exclusively, see later) **aldehyde dehydrogenases** (ALDHs) [aldehyde:NAD(P)$^+$ oxidoreductases, EC 1.2.1.3 and EC 1.2.1.5]. Multiple forms of mammalian ALDHs exist in the cytosol, mitochondria and microsomes of various tissues. For example, four constitutive and four inducible ALDHs were isolated from rat liver and found to differ by a number of criteria (MW, coenzyme preference, quaternary structure, pI, etc) (Lindahl and Evces, 1984; Sladek *et al.*, 1989). It has been proposed that aldehyde dehydrogenases form a superfamily of related enzymes consisting of Class 1 enzymes (cytosolic), Class 2 enzymes (mitochondrial), and Class 3 enzymes (tumour-associated, and other isozymes) (Hempel *et al.*, 1989). Recently, a rat liver microsomal ALDH has been proposed to be a Class 4 enzyme (Miyauchi *et al.*, 1991). In all three major classes, constitutive and inducible isozymes exist (Lindahl, 1992). In general, the constitutive mammalian ALDHs function as tetramers of MW 220,000 to 250,000, being composed of identical subunits of MW approximately 55,000 (Guan and Weiner, 1987; Harrington *et al.*, 1987; Hempel and Jörnvall, 1987; Lindahl, 1992; Weiner, 1980). While considerable progress has been made in recent years to uncover the molecular biology of ALDHs (e.g. Dockham *et al.*, 1992; Lindahl, 1992), much more remains to be discovered in order to better understand the properties of these important enzymes.

The **global reaction** of the ALDH-mediated aldehyde dehydrogenase is described by Eq. 2.5:

$$RCHO + NAD(P)^+ + H_2O \rightleftarrows R-COOH + NAD(P)H + H^+ \qquad \text{(Eq. 2.5)}$$

In more detail, the reaction necessitates the formation of a ternary complex between enzyme, coenzyme and substrate. Within this complex, a covalent bond is formed between the substrate

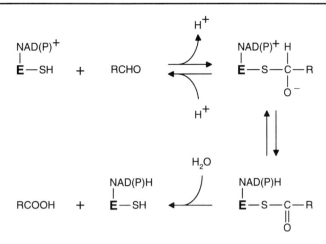

FIGURE 2.3 Mechanism of ALDH-mediated dehydrogenation of aldehydes. E-SH: enzyme with its nucleophilic thiol group.

and a nucleophilic group in the enzyme, as depicted in Fig. 2.3 (Abriola *et al.*, 1987; Dickinson and Haywood, 1987; Weiner, 1980). A hydride anion is then transferred to C(4) of the nicotinamide moiety, to become in all cases the *pro-R* hydrogen (Jones *et al.*, 1987). This hydride transfer effectively oxidizes the bound aldehyde to an acyl moiety, and the latter is finally liberated from the enzyme by a reaction of hydrolysis (see below).

The nature of the nucleophilic group in the active site of the enzyme was debated for years, but there is now compelling evidence that it is a reactive thiol group from a cysteinyl residue, in fact Cys-302 in human liver Class 1 and Class 2 ALDH and Cys-243 in Class 3 ALDH (Hempel *et al.*, 1991; Kitson *et al.*, 1991). Among other evidence, this is the only cysteinyl residue conserved in all aldehyde dehydrogenases sequenced so far (Blatter *et al.*, 1992).

It is of interest in the context of the above reaction mechanism, and particularly of its hydrolytic step, to note that ALDHs in fact display **two** enzymatic activities since they are also known to behave as **esterases** by hydrolyzing esters such as *para*-nitrophenyl acetate. A stimulating debate existed regarding the identity or non-identity of the dehydrogenase and esterase sites, with some evidence pointing to a two-site model and other to a single type of catalytic site (Blackwell *et al.*, 1983; Dickinson and Haywood, 1986; Duncan, 1985). The current belief is that Cys-302 is acylated during both aldehyde dehydrogenation and ester hydrolysis, in other words that ALDHs function with a single active site (Blatter *et al.*, 1992; Kitson *et al.*, 1991). This however does not exclude the possibility that other nucleophilic thiol groups in the protein react with electrophilic substrates such as reactive esters (and some inhibitors, see Section 2.3.3). The involvement of Cys-302 in both aldehyde dehydrogenation and ester hydrolysis has suggested that ALDHs and thiol proteases may have evolved from a common thiolesterase precursor (see next volume). Based on this concept, an informative molecular model of the active site of ALDH has been constructed using sequence alignments and computer graphics techniques (Hempel *et al.*, 1991).

The aldehyde dehydrogenases discussed in this section are enzymes with broad **substrate specificity**, as documented in a number of publications (e.g. Jones and Teng, 1983; Lindahl and Evces, 1984; Marselos and Lindahl, 1988; Sladek *et al.*, 1989; Weiner 1980). For example, three isozymes were purified from human liver, namely isozyme I (seemingly a Class 2 ALDH) and isozymes IIa and IIb (seemingly Class 1 ALDHs) (Jones and Teng, 1983); marked differences were seen in both affinities and maximal velocities of a variety of substrates (Table 2.2),

TABLE 2.2 *Some kinetic parameters for aldehydede hydrogenases isolated from human liver* (data from Jones and Teng, 1983)

Substrate	Isozyme I		Isozyme IIa		Isozyme IIb	
	K_m	V_{max}	K_m	V_{max}	K_m	V_{max}
Formaldehyde	27.0	3030	27.0	167	2.56	75
Acetaldehyde	5.0	5000	0.22	71	0.14	74
Propionaldehyde	1.0	3334	0.40	400	0.50	444
n-Butyraldehyde	0.106	820	0.019	200	0.035	118
Isobutyraldehyde	2.10	4000	0.25	333	0.40	500
Benzaldehyde	0.031	1026	0.0028	167	0.0056	125
para-Nitro-benzaldehyde	0.028	1695	*	—	0.0059	118
Phenylacetaldehyde	1.49	3334	—	—	—	—
Furfuraldehyde	0.027	455	0.057	218	0.063	166
Pyruvic aldehyde	0.38	333	0.33	100	0.14	81
(±)-Glyceraldehyde	1.30	2667	0.073	128	0.27	118
Glutaraldehyde	2.50	143	0.19	65	0.16	80

K_m values in mM, V_{max} values in $IU^{-3} mg^{-1}$.
*Not reported.

isoenzyme I being the most active. The high affinity of aromatic aldehydes in Table 2.2 contrasts with the lower affinity of aliphatic aldehydes. The dehydrogenation of acetaldehyde is of particular interest since it is the toxic metabolite of ethanol. The very high sensitivity of some individuals to ethanol is genetically based and results from the enhanced activity of an alcohol dehydrogenase (β_2) and/or the deficiency in ALDH isozyme I (Jones and Teng, 1983). More details can be found in some reviews (e.g. Chambers, 1990; Smith, 1988).

Table 2.2 contains both endogenous and exogenous substrates, and it must be stressed that ALDHs have may roles to play in the detoxication of **aldehyde metabolites of endogenous amines** such as monoamines, diamines and polyamines (Ambroziak and Pietruszko, 1991; Sladek

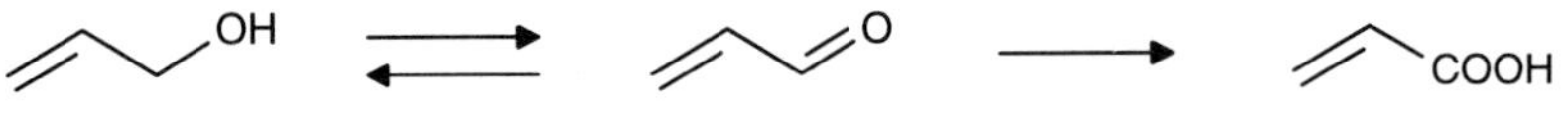

2.XX   2.XXI

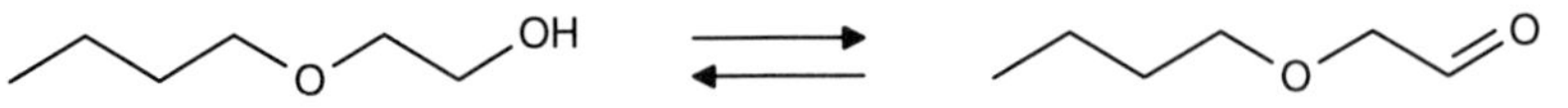

2.XXII

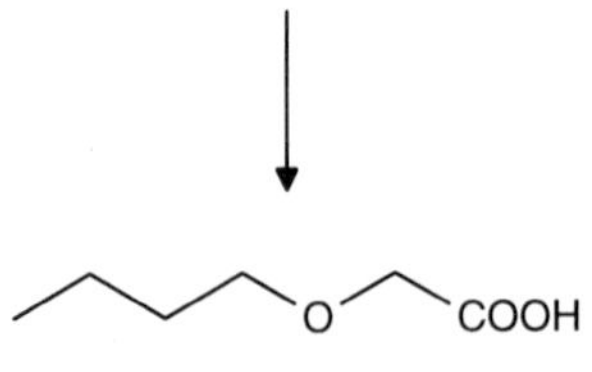

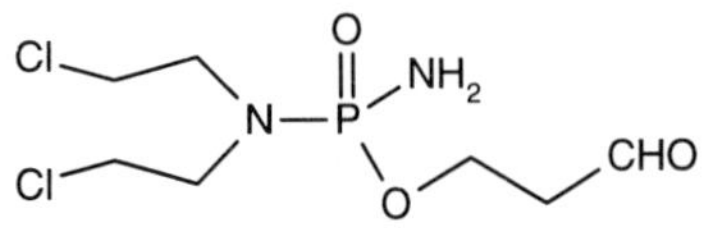

2.XXIV   2.XXIII

et al., 1989). Of particular significance may be the protective role of ALDHs against **aldehydic products of lipid peroxidation** (Lindahl, 1992; Lindahl and Petersen, 1991; Mitchell and Petersen, 1989).

A role has also been assigned to aldehyde dehydrogenase in detoxifying **acrolein (2.XXI)**, the hepatotoxic metabolite formed from allyl alcohol (**2.XX**) by alcohol dehydrogenase (Rikans and Moore, 1987). In contrast to these opposed effects, alcohol and aldehyde dehydrogenases act synergistically to transform **2-butoxyethanol (2.XXII)**, via the intermediate aldehyde, to the hematotoxin 2-butoxyacetic acid (**2.XXIII**) (Ghanayem *et al.*, 1987). Also worth mentioning is the oxidation of **aldophosphamide (2.XXIV)**, a metabolite of the anticancer prodrug cyclophosphamide, to the inactive metabolite carboxyphosphamide; this reaction is in competition with the formation of phosphoramide mustard, the actual cytotoxic agent (Lindahl, 1992; Sladek *et al.*, 1989).

2.3.2 Other enzymes

Beside the ALDHs of broad substrate specificity discussed in the previous section, there exist a number of **aldehyde dehydrogenases of narrow substrate specificity**, e.g. betaine-aldehyde dehydrogenase [EC 1.2.1.8], glyceraldehyde-3-phosphate dehydrogenase [EC 1.2.1.12], and succinate-semialdehyde dehydrogenase [EC 1.2.1.24] (Dockham *et al.*, 1992; Sladek *et al.*, 1989). Limited information is available on the capacity of these enzymes to metabolize xenobiotic aldehydes or aldehydes formed as metabolites of xenobiotics.

One enzyme however deserves a special mention, namely **formaldehyde dehydrogenase** [formaldehyde:NAD$^+$ oxidoreductase (glutathione-formylating); EC 1.2.1.1] which oxidizes formaldehyde to formic acid (Pourmotabbed and Creighton, 1986; Uotila and Koivusalo, 1987). The enzyme is of particular significance in detoxifying formaldehyde formed by metabolic reactions of demethylation (see Chapters 6 and 7) (Dicker and Cederbaum, 1986; Jones *et al.*, 1978; Waydhas *et al.*, 1978). Formaldehyde dehydrogenase is an NAD$^+$-dependent enzyme which requires but does not consume the tripeptide glutathione (GSH) and functions according to Eq. 2.6:

$$HCHO + GSH + NAD^+ \rightleftharpoons GS\text{--}CHO + NADH + H^+ \qquad \text{(Eq. 2.6)}$$

The intermediate S-formylglutathione (GS–CHO) is then rapidly broken down to formic acid and GSH by the specific S-formylglutathione hydrolase [EC 3.1.2.12]. Formaldehyde dehydrogenase has a wide distribution in human tissues and has a high affinity for formaldehyde ($K_m < 0.01$ mM). However, its true substrate is S-hydroxymethylglutathione (GS–CH$_2$OH) which is formed non-enzymatically from formaldehyde and GSH (high concentrations of which are present in most animal cells; also see the volume on conjugation reactions) (Pourmotabbed *et al.*, 1989). Multiple forms of the enzyme have been characterized, and there is evidence that formaldehyde dehydrogenase and mammalian Class III alcohol dehydrogenases (see Section 2.2.1) are identical enzymes (Holmquist and Vallee, 1991; Koivusalo *et al.*, 1989; Tsuboi *et al.*, 1992; Uotila and Koivusalo, 1987).

Other enzymes oxidizing aldehydes are the **molybdenum hydroxylases** aldehyde oxidase and xanthine oxidase (Section 9.5).

Finally, it must be stressed that liver **alcohol dehydrogenase** has also been proven capable of oxidizing aldehydes. For example, on incubation of horse liver ADH with *n*-octanol and NAD$^+$, the products were NADH as well as *n*-octanal and octanoic acid. It was found that during the reaction a portion of the octanal formed was not released from the enzyme but, in the presence of NAD$^+$, was oxidized to octanoic acid (Hinson and Neal, 1975). A similar sequence has been characterized in the ADH-catalyzed oxidation of *n*-heptanol (Battersby *et al.*, 1979). Furth-

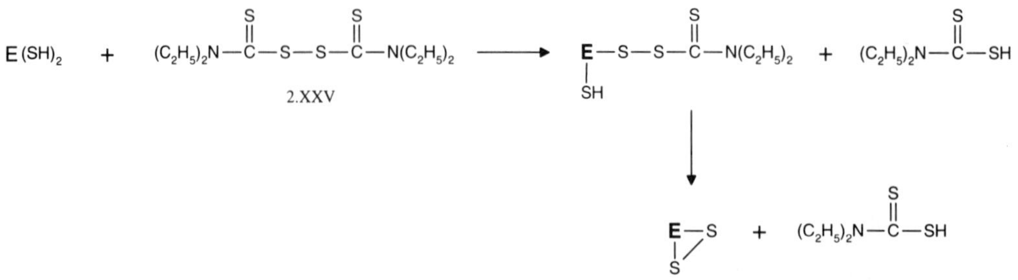

FIGURE 2.4 Mechanism of inhibition of aldehyde dehydrogenase by disulphiram (Vallari and Pietruszko, 1982). The enzyme is symbolized here by $E(SH)_2$ to indicate the involvement of two thiol groups.

ermore, the observation was made that under suitable conditions, the NAD^+ equivalent necessary for dehydrogenation of one molecule of heptanal was supplied by the ADH•NADH-catalyzed reduction of a second molecule of heptanal. In effect, liver ADH-catalyzed dismutation of heptanal was seen.

2.3.3 Inhibition of aldehyde dehydrogenases

Inhibition of ALDH is of interest not only from a fundamental and biochemical viewpoint, but also therapeutically in the treatment of alcoholism. The best known compound in this respect is **disulfiram (2.XXV** in Fig. 2.4), a substituted thiocarbamoyl disulfide which is thought to cause a disulfide interchange with a thiol group in ALDH, followed by the release of dithiocarbamic acid and concomitant formation of a cystine bridge (Fig. 2.4) (Vallari and Pietruszko, 1982). The various ALDH enzymes display marked differences in their sensitivity toward disulfiram (Zorzano and Herrera, 1990).

Inhibition of ALDH by disulfiram is mimicked by other **thiol reagents** such as iodoacetate and Hg^{2+} ions (Woenckhaus *et al.*, 1987). Interestingly, cyclopropanone hydrate (**2.XXVI**), the active metabolite of the natural product coprine isolated from the mushroom *Coprinus atramentarius*, is also an inhibitor of ALDHs and other thiol-containing enzymes: evidence indicates that it acts as a thiol reagent by forming a stable thiohemiketal (Wiseman and Abeles, 1979).

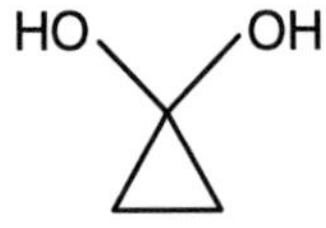

2.XXVI

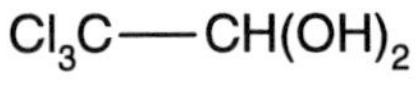

$$Cl_3C\!-\!CH(OH)_2$$

2.XXVII

A number of **aldehydes act as competitive inhibitors** of the enzyme, but the effects of some of them may be more complex at high concentrations. This is the case of chloral hydrate (**2.XXVII**), which at low concentrations elicits an inhibition that is competitive toward the aldehyde substrate, while at high concentrations it forms abortive ALDH•NADH•chloral and ALDH•NAD$^+$•chloral complexes (Dickinson and Haywood, 1987). In contrast, a reactive aldehyde such as acrolein (**2.XXI**) is a potent irreversible inhibitor of ALDHs (Mitchell and Petersen, 1988).

2.4 CARBONYL REDUCTION

2.4.1 Enzymes involved in carbonyl reduction

A vast array of enzymes are active in the reduction of aldehydes and ketones to primary and secondary alcohols, respectively. The role of **alcohol dehydrogenases** as carbonyl reductases has already been alluded to in Section 2.2, and indeed isolated human liver isozymes belonging to Class I, II and III (Section 2.2) proved capable of reducing a number of model aldehydes and ketones (Deetz *et al.*, 1984). In addition, a large variety of enzymes other than the alcohol dehydrogenases are active, namely aldehyde reductases and ketone reductases.

Enzymes categorized as **aldehyde reductases** include aldehyde reductase (NADPH) [alcohol:NADP$^+$ oxidoreductase; EC 1.1.1.2], glucuronate reductase [L-gulonate:NADP$^+$ 6-oxidoreductase; EC. 1.1.1.19], aldehyde reductase [alditol:NAD(P$^+$) 1-oxidoreductase; aldose reductase; polyol dehydrogenase (NADP$^+$); EC 1.1.1.21] and glycerol dehydrogenase (NADP$^+$) [glycerol:NADP$^+$ oxidoreductase; EC 1.1.1.72]. A number of other enzymes have been characterized, some of which such as lactaldehyde reductase (NADPH) [propane-1,2-diol:NADP$^+$ oxidoreductase; EC 1.1.1.55] must in fact be considered as different activities of aldehyde reductase (NADPH) (von Wartburg and Wermuth, 1980). A valuable compilation of enzymes and activities can be found in a review article by Felsted and Bachur (1980a). Aldehyde reductases are widely distributed in nature and occur in a considerable number of mammalian tissues. Their subcellular location is primarily cytosolic, and in some instances also mitochondrial. Their molecular weights seldom lie outside the range 29,000 to 44,000 in both native and denatured form, indicating a monomeric structure (von Wartburg and Wermuth, 1980; Felsted and Bachur, 1980a). The amino acid sequence of several aldehyde reductases has been established, with consequences for their classification to be discussed below (Bohren *et al.*, 1989; Wermuth *et al.*, 1987).

So-called **ketone reductases** are frequently mentioned but seldom well characterized. They include α- and β-hydroxysteroid dehydrogenases [e.g. EC 1.1.1.50 and EC 1.1.1.51], various prostaglandin ketoreductases [e.g. prostaglandin-F synthase, EC 1.1.1.188; prostaglandin-E$_2$ 9-reductase, EC 1.1.1.189], and many others which are comparable to aldehyde reductases in terms of distribution and range of molecular weights (Felsted and Bachur, 1980b; Oppermann *et al.*, 1991]. Most are NADPH-dependent, but a preference for NADH is also documented in some cases. A list of activities and enzymatic properties has been compiled by Felsted and Bachur (1980a).

Aldehydes are often good substrates for ketone reductases (see Section 2.4.3), which for this reason have come to be designated as **carbonyl reductases**, and form a group of enzymes collectively known as carbonyl reductase (NADPH) [secondary alcohol:NADP$^+$ oxidoreductase; EC 1.1.1.184]. Furthermore, the many similarities (including some marked overlap in substrate specificity) between monomeric, NADPH-dependent aldehyde reductase (AKR1), aldose reductase (AKR2), and carbonyl reductase (AKR3) have led to their designation as **aldo-keto reductases** (Davidson, 1987; Wermuth *et al.*, 1987; Wirth and Wermuth, 1985). It is for example quite revealing of the relatedness of aldo-keto reductases that four NADPH-dependent aldehyde reductases isolated from pig brain were identified with the high-K_m aldehyde reductase, aldose reductase (low-K_m aldehyde reductase), carbonyl reductase, and succinate-semialdehyde reductase, respectively (Cromlish and Flynn, 1985). Similarly, three reductases for carbonyl compounds purified to homogeneity from human liver cytosol were identified as alcohol dehydrogenase, aldehyde reductase, and carbonyl reductase (Nakayama *et al.*, 1985).

But while the grouping of all above enzymes as aldo-keto reductases is acceptable in terms of substrate specificities and physicochemical properties, it is not supported structurally. Indeed, aldehyde reductase, aldose reductase and carbonyl reductase from human tissues do not cross-react immunochemically, and even more importantly carbonyl reductase [EC 1.1.1.184] shows no sequence homology with other aldo-keto reductases, with which it appears very distantly related in an evolutionary perspective (Wermuth *et al.*, 1988; Wirth and Wermuth, 1985).

In short, aldo-keto reductases (AKR) are currently classified in three major groups of enzymes with closely related substrate specificities and physicochemical properties (Bohren *et al.*, 1989; Cromlish and Flynn, 1985; Wermuth *et al.*, 1988), i.e.:

- AKR1, aldehyde reductase, high-K_m aldehyde reductase, L-hexonate dehydrogenase;
- AKR2, aldose reductase, low-K_m aldehyde reductase;
- AKR3, carbonyl reductase, prostaglandin ketoreductases.

From a structural viewpoint, a different classification emerges. On the one hand, a superfamily exists comprising prostaglandin-F synthase, 3α-hydroxysteroid dehydrogenase, and aldehyde/aldose reductases (AKR1 and AKR2). On the other hand, carbonyl reductase remains practically alone being unrelated or too distantly related to this superfamily.

Enzyme preparations used in many studies are only partly purified and must therefore be viewed as mixes of enzymes and/or isozymes, often rendering any enzymatic assignment very difficult if not impossible.

2.4.2 Mechanism and stereoselectivity of carbonyl reduction

The major feature common to all reductases for carbonyl compounds [EC 1.1.1] is their pyridine nucleotide dependence. The mechanism of hydride transfer to and from the nicotinamide moiety (dehydrogenation and reduction, respectively) is that described in Fig. 2.1, and its **stereochemical consequences** deserve attention from the point of view of both the coenzyme and the substrate. As shown in Fig. 2.1, C(4) in reduced pyridine nucleotides is a prochiral centre with two attached diastereotopic hydrogen atoms (diastereotopic and not enantiotopic due to other chiral centres in NAD(P)H). The *pro-R* and *pro-S* hydrogens are commonly designated as H_A and H_B, respectively, and depending whether one or the other is transferred to the substrate the enzymes are said to be of the A- or B-type or, better, to be **pro-R** or **pro-S** specific (Fig. 2.5). Numerous studies have centred on the mechanism underlying this stereospecificity; these have been fruitful in terms of added knowledge, and promising as far as a profound understanding of stereo-electronic control in enzymes is concerned (Almarsson and Bruice, 1993; Donkersloot and Buck, 1981; Nambiar *et al.*, 1983; Oppenheimer, 1984).

Reduction by alcohol dehydrogenases leads to *pro-R* hydride transfer. This is also the case for the aldo-keto reductase superfamily discussed in Section 2.4.1, while carbonyl reductase transfers the *pro-S* hydrogen atom (Wermuth *et al.*, 1988). However, there are exceptions to this generalization (Felsted and Bachur, 1980a and 1980b; McMahon, 1982).

When the ketone group in the substrate is a centre of prochirality, its reduction leads to the creation of a new centre of chirality, and the enzymatic reaction has the potential of displaying **product stereoselectivity** in addition to substrate stereoselectivity. These stereochemical aspects, together with many interesting features of liver alcohol dehydrogenase, have made this enzyme a favourite tool of biostereochemists. Numerous studies have used purified ADH and an almost endless variety of ketones, especially cycloalkanones of restricted flexibility, to improve our insight of substrate–enzyme interactions and mechanistic intricacies. Representative publications of particular interest that have examined substrate and product stereoselectivity in liver ADH-mediated reduction used heteromonocyclic, heterobicyclic and cage-shaped ketones as

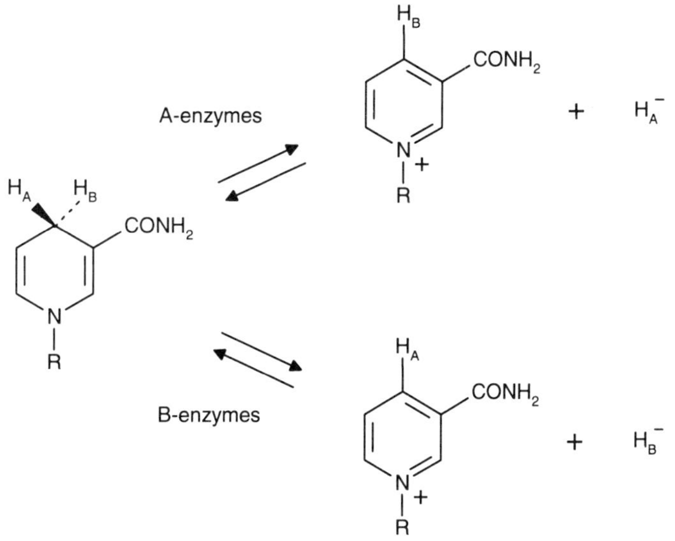

FIGURE 2.5 Transfer of *pro-R* and *pro-S* hydride (H_A and H_B, respectively) in NAD(P)H oxidoreductases.

substrates (Jones and Schwartz, 1981; Lam *et al.*, 1988; Nakazaki *et al.*, 1983). The role of critical amino acid residues in controlling *pro-R* hydrogen transfer is also being slowly uncovered (Weinhold *et al.*, 1991). Finally, the marked influence of organic solvents on the stereoselectivities of liver ADH-catalyzed oxidoreductions is particularly noteworthy and has raised great interest (Grunwald *et al.*, 1986).

A major goal of such enzymological studies is to rationalize structure–stereoselectivity relationships, and **topographical models** have proven most useful in this respect. The work of Prelog is epoch-making, and his "diamond lattice model" (Prelog, 1964) was refined by other workers who proposed the model shown in Fig. 2.6 (Lemière *et al.*, 1982) (see also Section 2.2.2). With the ketone group held in place by zinc ligation, an upper and a rear "wall" create strong steric hindrance, while interaction with a hydrophobic "barrel" increases affinity. This hydrophobic "barrel" must be identical with the hydrophobic channel discussed in Section 2.2.4 (Hansch *et al.*, 1986). A less comprehensive but more realistic model (i.e. based on the active site of liver ADH) has been presented by Dutler and Brändén (1981).

The **product stereospecificity** of carbonyl reductases was first rationalized by Prelog, who following pioneering work with microorganisms proposed the simple model shown in Fig. 2.7 (e.g. Baumann and Prelog, 1958). Of major interest in the context here, is the applicability of this model to mammalian ketone reductases. Thus, a *pro-S* specific, NADPH-dependent reductase partly purified from rabbit kidney cortex reduced acetophenone (Fig. 2.7, L = phenyl, S = methyl) to (−)-(*S*)-1-phenylethanol with 52% enantiomeric excess (Culp and McMahon, 1968). The same product enantioselectivity was observed during the *in vitro* and *in vivo* reduction of other aromatic ketones (e.g. propiophenone and phenylacetone) in rats and rabbits (Prelusky *et al.*, 1982). A case involving both substrate and product stereoselectivity is provided by the human metabolism of **amfepramone** (**2.XXVIII** in Fig. 2.8). This anorectic drug undergoes reactions of N-dealkylation and ketone reduction, resulting in the complex metabolic scheme shown in Fig. 2.8. Interestingly, the stereoselectivity of ketone reduction is again compatible with the model of Baumann and Prelog (Testa, 1973 and 1986).

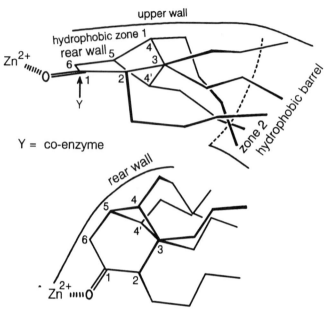

FIGURE 2.6 Lateral and upper view of a steric model accounting for the reduction of cyclic ketones by liver alcohol dehydrogenase. A rear and upper "wall" results in steric hindrance in positions 2β, 4β, 5 and 6. A hydrophobic "barrel" binds non-polar substituents in the 2α, 3 and 4' positions. Reproduced from Lemière *et al.* (1982) with the permission of the copyright holder.

Despite incomplete evidence, there may be reason to believe that the model of Baumann and Prelog is specifically applicable to *pro-S* specific ketone reductases. However, more studies with purified enzymes are necessary before the domain of applicability of this model can be delineated.

An intriguing aspect of several aldo-keto reductases is their capacity in some cases to catalyze **reactions of dehydrogenation** in addition to reductions, a phenomenon that has allowed mechanistic insights. Thus, human liver **aldehyde reductase** [EC 1.1.1.2] may also function as an alcohol dehydrogenase, as seen in its capacity to catalyze the reduction of the aldehydic group in D-glucuronate (forward reaction) and the oxidation of the alcoholic group in L-gulonate (reverse reaction) (Bhatnagar *et al.*, 1991). A histidinyl residue in the active site appears critical in controlling the direction of the reaction. When protonated, its imidazolyl moiety binds the aldehyde substrate by donating a hydrogen bond, thus facilitating hydride transfer from NADPH to the carbonyl carbon. In contrast, the non-protonated imidazolyl moiety binds the alcohol substrate by accepting a hydrogen bond and facilitating hydride transfer to $NADP^+$.

Carbonyl reductase [EC 1.1.1.184] has also been shown to be able to act as a dehydrogenase, more precisely as an aldehyde dehydrogenase. This was seen with guinea-pig pulmonary carbonyl reductase (an enzyme with specific properties) which irreversibly converted chloral hydrate (**2.XXVII**) into trichloroacetic acid and trichloroethanol (Hara *et al.*, 1991). Of significance in the present context is the fact that the ratio of the two metabolites was highly dependent on the cofactor used. Briefly stated, the enzyme oxidized the aldehyde in hydrated form to the acid with $NAD(P)^+$ as cofactor, and reduced the aldehyde in unhydrated form with NAD(P)H.

2.4.3 Substrate selectivity and inhibition of carbonyl reduction

A number of papers and reviews report the substrate selectivity of carbonyl reduction using various enzyme preparations such as human liver alcohol dehydrogenase isozymes, dog liver

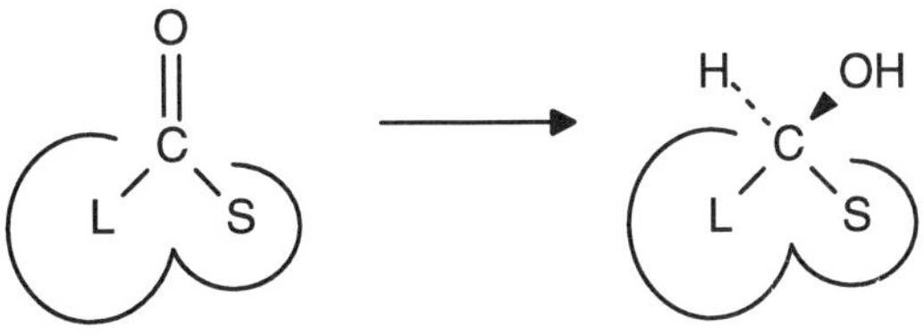

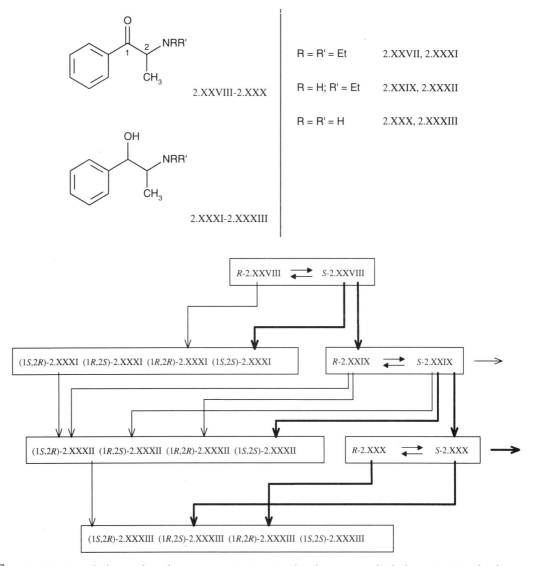

FIGURE 2.7 Model predicting the absolute configuration of secondary alcohols produced as metabolites of ketone reductases. L: larger substituent; S: smaller substituent (modified from Baumann and Prelog, 1958).

FIGURE 2.8 Metabolism of amfepramone (**2.XXVIII**, also known as diethylpropion) in the human, showing the substrate and product stereoselectivities of carbonyl reduction. The metabolites thus produced are the secondary and primary aminoketone (**2.XXIX** and **2.XXX**, respectively), and the corresponding ephedrine analogues (**2.XXXI**, **2.XXXII** and **2.XXXIII**) (modified from Testa, 1986). Thick and thin arrows represent major and minor pathways, respectively.

TABLE 2.3 *Some kinetic parameters for human NADPH-dependent aldo-keto reductase activities* (data from Nakayama *et al.*, 1985)

Substrate	High MW ALR*		Low MW ALR†		Carb. red.#	
	K_m	k_{cat}	K_m	k_{cat}	K_m	k_{cat}
Aldehydes						
Acetaldehyde	0.016	10.5	—		—	
n-Butyraldehyde	0.022	14.7	68.5	3.2	—	
Chloral hydrate	4.6	2.4	142	10.4	146	0.8
2-Nitrobenzaldehyde	0.024	8.7	—		2.3	16.1
3-Nitrobenzaldehyde	0.024	5.7	4.9	6.1	1.1	1.4
4-Nitrobenzaldehyde	0.021	8.1	0.96	7.3	1.2	3.2
Pyridine-3-aldehyde	0.36	4.2	1.2	9.8	15.6	4.9
Pyridine-4-aldehyde	0.036	6.8	2.6	10.5	3.7	12.9
Indole-3-acetaldehyde	0.033	8.5	2.9	5.4	2.2	1.1
(±)-Glyceraldehyde	4.0	0.85	2.9	1.5		—
Phenylglyoxal	0.85	6.9	0.92	10.4	7.0	7.6
Methylglyoxal	1.4	6.7	2.0	7.1	49.0	3.8
Ketones						
Acetone	—		—		—	
Cyclohexanone	1.2	2.9	—		—	
2,3-Butanedione	1.1	0.8	20.0	9.2	4.1	15.0
4-Nitroacetophenone	—		—		5.6	1.5
4-Benzoylpyridine	—		—		0.84	1.7
Benzoylacetone	—		—		0.94	0.8
Metyrapone (**2.XXXVIII**)	—		—		—	
Naloxone	—		—		—	
Toluquinone	—		—		0.091	11.3
Menadione	—		—		0.063	11.7

K_m values in mM, k_{cat} values in s^{-1}.
*High molecular weight (78,000) aldehyde reductase.
†Low molecular weight (32,000) aldehyde reductase.
#Carbonyl reductase (MW 31,000).
§Not detectable or very low activity.

carbonyl reductase, pig brain aldehyde reductases and human brain carbonyl reductase (Cromlish and Flynn, 1985; Deetz *et al.*, 1984; Hara *et al.*, 1986; Wermuth, 1981). To illustrate the **substrate specificity** of various human liver reductases, a coherent set of data is presented in Table 2.3 (Nakayama *et al.*, 1985). Clearly, aldehyde reductases are able to reduce some ketones, while carbonyl reductase is active towards ketones as well as aldehydes. The high activity of aldehyde reductase towards aromatic aldehydes with electron-withdrawing substituents is frequently reported; such is also the case for short-chain aliphatic aldehydes but not for higher homologues, as compiled extensively (Felsted and Bachur, 1980a; von Wartburg and Wermuth, 1980). Table 2.3 also lists a few drugs. Interestingly, a number of compounds such as metyrapone (see below) and naloxone are resistant to the three enzyme preparations. This of course does not imply that they will remain inert towards all reductases, and their reduction is indeed well characterized under other conditions (Felsted and Bachur, 1980a; Roerig *et al.*, 1976).

A variety of **drugs bearing a keto group** (drugs featuring an aldehydic group are exceedingly rare) are reduced *in vitro* and *in vivo* (Felsted and Bachur, 1980a). This applies to a few drugs containing an aliphatic keto group, e.g. warfarin (**2.XXXIV**), and mainly to aromatic ketones, e.g. acetohexamide (**2.XXXV**) and bunolol (**2.XXXVI**). The example of acetohexamide is intriguing because here, in contrast to other drugs, reduction of the aromatic keto group is reversible (Nagamine *et al.*, 1988). Reduction in humans of an aromatic group is documented for a number of drugs in addition to amfepramone discussed in Section 2.4.2. Thus, haloperidol (**2.XXXVII**) and metyrapone (**2.XXXVIII**) are efficiently reduced in human liver cytosol, the latter drug also in microsomes by a hydroxysteroid dehydrogenase (Inaba and Kovacs, 1989; Maser *et al.*, 1991). As a final example, let us mention the anticonvulsant agent nafimidone (**2.XXXIX**) which in dogs, primates and humans is extensively reduced to the secondary alcohol before undergoing a variety of other metabolic reactions such as ring oxidations (Section 4.3) and glucuronidation (Volume 2, this series) (Rush *et al.*, 1990).

2.XXXIV

2.XXXV

2.XXXVI

2.XXXVII

2.XXXVIII

2.XXXIX

Inhibition of aldo-keto reductases occurs with relative selectivity for the various groups of enzymes listed in Section 2.4.1. Quercitrin is the selective inhibitor of **ketone reductases**. In contrast, anticonvulsant drugs such as barbiturates, their open-chain analogues, glutarimides, succinimides, hydantoins and oxazolidinediones are potent *in vitro* inhibitors of **aldehyde reductase**. Their mechanism of inhibition is a non-competitive one, and activity requires an ionizable CO–NH–CO grouping as well as lipophilic substitution. The inhibition by phenobarbital and other compounds is directly related to the concentration of the anionic species, suggesting the involvement of an anion-binding group in the enzyme (Felsted and Bachur, 1980a; Schofield *et al.*, 1987). Valproate is similarly active. Furthermore, several neuroleptic phenothiazines (e.g. chlorpromazine and trifluoperazine) are moderate competitive inhibitors of aldehyde reductase.

Barbiturates and their analogues do not inhibit carbonyl reductase, and this selectivity is useful in discriminating the contribution of the two enzymes towards substrates of interest. Similarly, aldo-keto reductases are not inhibited by classical inhibitors of alcohol dehydrogenase (e.g. pyrazoles, disulfiram and metal chelators, see Section 2.2.4). Much interest has centred recently on selective, therapeutic inhibitors of **lens aldose reductase**, an enzyme involved in the pathogenesis of sugar-induced cataract. Such inhibitors include flavonoids and sorbinil, as well as an impressive number of compounds of novel structure, as extensively reviewed by Sarges (1989).

Contrasting with the selectivity of the above inhibitors, thiol-binding reagents like *para*-chloromercuribenzoate inhibit most aldehyde and aldose reductases, and some ketone reductases (Felsted and Bachur, 1980a; Nakayama *et al.*, 1985).

2.5 DEHYDROGENATION OF DIHYDRODIOLS

Dihydrodiols are metabolites produced by the attack of water on arene epoxides catalyzed by epoxide hydrolase (see next volume). The structure of benzene dihydrodiol is given here as an example (**2.XL** in Fig. 2.9; note the *trans*-configuration). These compounds can then be dehydrogenated by **dihydrodiol dehydrogenase** to the corresponding catechols (**2.XLI** in Fig. 2.9). As shown in Fig. 2.9, the **reaction mechanism** is a two-electron oxidation of one of the hydroxyl groups to yield an intermediate ketol which then enolizes to the catechol. Many catechol compounds, in particular the catechol derivatives of polycyclic aromatics, can easily form the corresponding *ortho*-quinone by autoxidation (Nohl *et al.*, 1986; Smithgall *et al.*, 1988) (see Section 7.6). Quinones being strong electrophilic compounds, tend to react readily with nucleophiles to form adducts, a phenomenon that often prevents their detection in biological media (e.g. Klein *et al.*, 1990).

Dihydrodiol dehydrogenases [*trans*-1,2-dihydrobenzene-1,2-diol:NADP$^+$ oxidoreductases; EC 1.3.1.20] are cytosolic enzymes several of which have been isolated, purified and characterized. Thus, four forms were isolated from mouse liver cytosol, two of which are monomers (MW 30,000 and 34,000) and two dimers (MW 64,000 and 65,000) (Bolcsak and Nerland, 1983). Although the isozymes were able to utilize NAD$^+$, the preferred cofactor was NADP$^+$. The dehydrogenation of benzene dihydrodiol exhibited K_m and V_{max} values in the range 0.32–5.3 mM and 1.6–3.9 μmol min^{-1} mg^{-1}, respectively. Similarly, a number of enzymes with dihydrodiol dehydrogenase activity were isolated from the liver of rabbits, monkeys and humans (Deyashiki *et al.*, 1992; Klein *et al.*, 1992; Nakagawa *et al.*, 1989).

Dihydrodiol dehydrogenases are not separate enzymes, but simply additional activities of some enzymes discussed earlier in this chapter. Indeed, the various forms isolated have been shown to be identical with isozymes of 3α-hydroxysteroid dehydrogenase [EC 1.1.1.50],

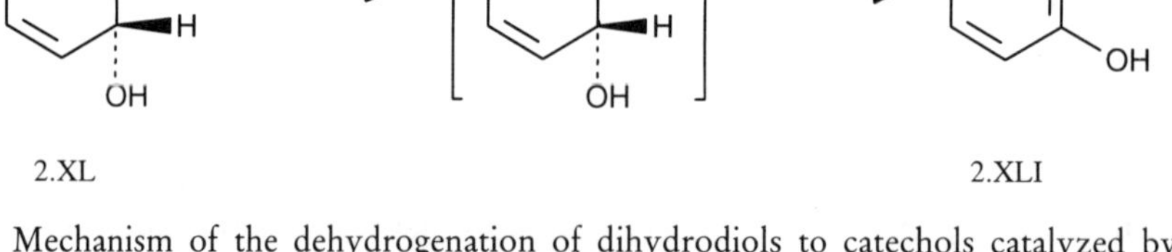

2.XL   2.XLI

FIGURE 2.9 Mechanism of the dehydrogenation of dihydrodiols to catechols catalyzed by dihydrodiol dehydrogenase. The reaction produces a ketol which then enolizes to the catechol. Benzene dihydrodiol is taken here as an example.

17β-hydroxysteroid dehydrogenase [EC 1.1.1.64], aldehyde reductase [EC 1.1.1.2], and carbonyl reductase [EC 1.1.1.184] e.g. Deyashiki *et al.*, 1992; Hara *et al.*, 1985; Klein *et al.*, 1992; Sawada *et al.*, 1988). For example, two dihydrodiol dehydrogenases isolated from human liver were found to be associated with 3α-hydroxysteroid dehydrogenase activity. Both forms (but one more than the other) were active towards benzene dihydrodiol, naphthalene dihydrodiol, alicyclic alcohols (tetralol and indan-1-ol), and a variety of 3α-hydroxylated steroids (Deyashiki *et al.*, 1992).

In addition to dihydrodiols, 17β-hydroxysteroid dehydrogenases can similarly dehydrogenate a large variety of *alicyclic alcohols* (e.g. 2-cyclohexen-1-ol) and particularly 17β-hydroxysteroids such as testosterone, testosterone analogues, and 17β-estradiol; they also reduce aldehydes, ketones and quinones (Sawada *et al.*, 1988; Vogel *et al.*, 1982).

2.XLII   2.XLIII   2.XLIV

An interesting structure–metabolism relationship study has been published on the dehydrogenation of dihydrodiols of polycyclic aromatic hydrocarbons (Klein *et al.*, 1991). Dihydrodiol dehydrogenase/3α-hydroxysteroid dehydrogenase isolated from rat liver cytosol was able to oxidize the dihydrodiols of a number of polycyclic aromatic hydrocarbons with high regio-selectivity. For example, the 1,2-dihydrodiol of chrysene (**2.XLII**) and the 1,2- and 3,4-dihydrodiol of benz[*a*]anthracene were good substrates, while the 5,6-dihydrodiol of **2.XLII** and the 5,6-, 8,9- and 10,11-dihydrodiol of **2.XLIII** were not accepted as substrates. Other convergent results were obtained which led to the 2D-topographical model of the binding/active site shown in Fig. 2.10. A lipophilic, largely planar binding region has been postulated; good substrates are those compounds which can bind with their target dihydrodiol moiety oriented towards Region 2 or (preferably) Region 1. Of particular relevance is the fact that a physiological substrate such as androsterone (**2.XLIV**) can fit very well to this model, thereby orienting the target 3α-hydroxyl towards Region 1.

Some dihydrodiol epoxides of polycyclic aromatic hydrocarbons are of high toxicological significance (Section 4.3), their potential for toxicity being strongly dependent on their subsequent detoxication by dehydrogenation or epoxide hydration (next volume in this series) (Glatt *et al.*, 1982). Thus studies such as the one discussed here are important for a proper understanding of the structure–toxicity relationships of polycyclic aromatic hydrocarbons.

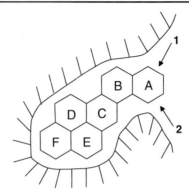

FIGURE 2.10 Two-dimensional topographical model of the binding/active site of dihydrodiol dehydrogenase/3α-hydroxysteroid dehydrogenase isolated from rat liver cytosol. Good substrates are those compounds which can bind with their target dihydrodiol moiety oriented towards Region 2 or 1. 3α-Hydroxysteroids are postulated to bind with their 3α-hydroxyl target group oriented towards Region 1 (modified from Klein *et al.*, 1991).

2.6 REFERENCES

Abriola D.P., Fields R., Stein S., MacKerell A.D. Jr and Pietruszko R. (1987). Active site of human liver aldehyde dehydrogenase. *Biochemistry* **26**, 5679–5684.

Almarsson O. and Bruice T.C. (1993). Evaluation of the factors influencing reactivity and stereospecificity in NAD(P)H dependent dehydrogenase enzymes. *J. Amer. Chem. Soc.* **115**, 2125–2138.

Ambroziak W. and Pietruszko R. (1991). Human aldehyde dehydrogenase. Activity with aldehyde metabolites of monoamines, diamines and polyamines. *J. Biol. Chem.* **266**, 13,011–13,018.

Bahnson B.J., Park D.H., Kim K., Plapp B.V. and Klinman J.P. (1993). Unmasking of hydrogen tunneling in the horse liver alcohol dehydrogenase reaction by site-directed mutagenesis. *Biochemistry* **32**, 5503–5507.

Battersby A.R., Buckley D.G. and Staunton J. (1979). Studies on enzyme-mediated reactions. Part 11. Experiments on the dismutation of aldehyde to alcohol and carboxylic acid by the complex of liver alcohol dehydrogenase and NAD⁺. *J. Chem. Soc. Perkin. Trans.* I, 2559–2562.

Baumann P. and Prelog V. (1958). Reaktionen mit Mikroorganismen. 5. Die stereospezifische Reduktion von stereoisomeren Dekalindionen-(1,4). *Helv. Chim. Acta* **41**, 2362–2379.

Becker N.N. and Roberts J.D. (1984). Structure of the liver alcohol dehydrogenase-NAD⁺-pyrazole complex as determined by ¹⁵N NMR spectroscopy. *Biochemistry* **23**, 3336–3340.

Benner S.A. (1982). The stereoselectivity of alcohol dehydrogenases—a stereochemical imperative. *Experientia* **38**, 633–637.

Bhatnagar A., Das B., Liu S.Q. and Srivastava S.K. (1991). Human liver aldehyde reductase: pH dependence of steady-state kinetic parameters. *Arch. Biochem. Biophys.* **287**, 329–336.

Biellmann J.F. (1986). Chemistry and structure of alcohol dehydrogenase: some general considerations on binding mode variability. *Acc. Chem. Res.* **19**, 321–328.

Blackwell L.F., Bennett A.F. and Buckley P.D. (1983). Relationship between the mechanisms of the esterase and dehydrogenase activities of the cytoplasmic aldehyde dehydrogenase from sheep liver. An alternative view. *Biochemistry* **22**, 3784–3791.

Blatter E.E., Abriola D.P. and Pietruszko R. (1992). Aldehyde dehydrogenase. Covalent intermediate in aldehyde dehydrogenation and ester hydrolysis. *Biochem. J.* **282**, 353–360.

Bohren K.M., Bullock B., Wermuth B. and Gabbay K.H. (1989). The aldo-keto reductase superfamily. *J. Biol. Chem.* **264**, 9547–9551.

Bolcsak L.E. and Nerland D.E. (1983). Purification of mouse liver benzene dihydrodiol dehydrogenases. *J. Biol. Chem.* **258**, 7252–7255.

Bosron W.F., Li T.K., Dafeldecker W.P. and Vallee B.L. (1979). Human liver π-alcohol dehydrogenase: kinetic and molecular properties. *Biochemistry* **18**, 1101–1105.

Bosron W.F. and Li T.K. (1980). Alcohol dehydrogenase. In *Enzymatic Basis of Detoxication*, vol. 1 (ed. Jakoby W.B.). pp. 231–248. Academic Press, New York.

Chambers G.K. (1990). The genetics of human alcohol metabolism. *Gen. Pharmacol.* **21**, 267–272.

Chen W.S. and Plapp B.V. (1978). Ambivalent active-site-directed inactivators of liver alcohol dehydrogenase. *Biochemistry* **17**, 4916–4922.

Cohen M. (1985). Antihyperlipidemic properties of β-pyridylcarbinol. A review of preclinical studies. *Life Sci.* **37**, 1949–1961.

Cromlish J.A. and Flynn T.G. (1985). Identification of pig brain aldehyde reductases with the high-K_m aldehyde reductase, the low-K_m aldehyde reductase and aldose reductase, carbonyl reductase, and succinic semialdehyde reductase. *J. Neurochem.* **44**, 1485–1493.

Culp H.W. and McMahon R.E. (1968). Reductase for aromatic aldehydes and ketones. The partial purification and properties of a reduced triphosphopyridine nucleotide-dependent reductase from rabbit kidney cortex. *J. Biol. Chem.* **243**, 848–852.

Davidson W.S. (1987). Comparison of the active sites of aldose reductase and aldehyde reductase from chicken. In *Enzymology and Molecular Biology of Carbonyl Metabolism* (eds Weiner H. and Flynn T.G.). pp. 275–285. Liss, New York.

Deetz J.S., Luehr C.A. and Vallee B.L. (1984). Human liver alcohol dehydrogenase isozymes: reduction of aldehydes and ketones. *Biochemistry* **23**, 6822–6828.

Deyashiki Y., Taniguchi H., Amano T., Nakayama T., Hara A. and Sawada H. (1992). Structural and functional comparison of two human liver dihydrodiol dehydrogenases associated with 3α-hydroxysteroid dehydrogenase activity. *Biochem. J.* **282**, 741–746.

Dicker E. and Cederbaum A.I. (1986). Inhibition of CO_2 production from aminopyrine or methanol by cyanamide or crotonaldehyde and the role of mitochondrial aldehyde dehydrogenase in formaldehyde oxidation. *Biochim. Biophys. Acta* **883**, 91–97.

Dickinson F.M. and Haywood G.W. (1986). The effects of Mg^{2+} on certain steps in the mechanisms of the dehydrogenase and esterase reactions catalysed by sheep liver aldehyde dehydrogenase. *Biochem. J.* **233**, 877–883.

Dickinson F.M. and Haywood G.W. (1987). Abortive complex formation and substrate activation and inhibition effects with sheep liver cytosolic aldehyde dehydrogenase. In *Enzymology and Molecular Biology of Carbonyl Metabolism* (eds Weiner H. and Flynn T.G.). pp. 25–35. Liss, New York.

Dockham P.A., Lee M.O. and Sladek N.E. (1992). Identification of human liver aldehyde dehydrogenases that catalyze the oxidation of aldophosphamide and retinaldehyde. *Biochem. Pharmacol.* **43**, 2453–2469.

Donkersloot M.C.A. and Buck H.M. (1981). The hydride-donation reaction of reduced nicotinamide adenine dinucleotide. 2. MINDO/3 and STO-3G calculations on the role of the CON_2 group in enzymatic reactions. *J. Amer. Chem. Soc.* **103**, 6554–6558.

Duncan R.J.S. (1985). Aldehyde dehydrogenase. An enzyme with two distinct catalytic activities at a single type of active site. *Biochem. J.* **230**, 261–267.

Dutler H. and Bränden C.I. (1981). Correlation studies based on enzyme structure and kinetic results: deduction of productive substrate orientation in the active-site pocket of horse liver alcohol dehydrogenase. *BioOrg. Chem.* **10**, 1–13.

Eklund H., Plapp B.V., Samama J.P. and Bränden C.I. (1982). Binding of substrate in a ternary complex of horse liver alcohol dehydrogenase. *J. Biol. Chem.* **257**, 14,349–14,358.

Eklund H., Müller-Wille P., Horjales E., Futer O., Holmquist B., Vallee B.L., Höög J.O., Kaiser R. and Jörnvall H. (1990). Comparison of three classes of human liver alcohol dehydrogenase. *Eur. J. Biochem.* **193**, 303–310.

Engeland K. and Maret W. (1993). Extrahepatic differential expression of 4 classes of human alcohol dehydrogenase. *Biochem. Biophys. Res. Commun.* **193**, 47–53.

Felsted R.L. and Bachur N.R. (1980a). Mammalian carbonyl reductases. *Drug Metab. Rev.* **11**, 1–60.

Felsted R.L. and Bachur N.R. (1980b). Ketone reductases. In *Enzymatic Basis of Detoxication*, vol. 1 (ed. Jakoby W.B.). pp. 281–293. Academic Press, New York.

Frey W.A. and Vallee B.L. (1979). Human liver alcohol dehydrogenase. An enzyme essential to the metabolism of digitalis. *Biochem. Biophys. Res. Commun.* **91**, 1543–1548.

Fries R.W., Bohlken D.P. and Plapp B.V. (1979). 3-Substituted pyrazole derivatives as inhibitors and inactivators of liver alcohol dehydrogenase. *J. Med. Chem.* **22**, 356–359.

Fumagalli R. (1971). Pharmacokinetics of nicotinic acid and some of its derivatives. In *Metabolic Effects of Nicotinic Acid and its Derivatives* (eds Gey K.F. and Carlson L.A.). pp. 33–49. Huber, Berne.

Ganzhorn A.J., Green D.W., Hershey A.D., Gould R.M. and Plapp B.V. (1987). Kinetic characterization of yeast alcohol dehydrogenase. *J. Biol. Chem.* **262**, 3754–3761.

Ghanayem B.I., Burka L.T. and Matthews H.B. (1987). Metabolic basis of ethylene glycol monobutyl ether (2-butoxyethanol) toxicity: role of alcohol and aldehyde dehydrogenases. *J. Pharmacol. Exp. Ther.* **242**, 223–231.

Glatt H.R., Cooper C.S., Grover P.L., Sims P., Bentley P., Merdes M., Waechter F., Vogel K., Guenthner T.M. and Oesch F. (1982). Inactivation of a diol epoxide by dihydrodiol dehydrogenase but not by two epoxide hydrolases. *Science* **215**, 1507–1509.

Grunwald J., Wirz B., Scollar M.P. and Klibanov A.M. (1986). Asymmetric oxidoreductions catalyzed by alcohol dehydrogenase in organic solvents. *J. Amer. Chem. Soc.* **108**, 6732–6734.

Guan K. and Weiner H. (1987). Molecular biology studies of beef liver aldehyde dehydrogenase. In *Enzymology and Molecular Biology of Carbonyl Metabolism* (eds Weiner H. and Flynn T.G.). pp. 15–24. Liss, New York.

Hansch C., Klein T., McClarin J., Langridge R. and Cornell N.W. (1986). A QSAR and molecular graphics analysis of hydrophobic effects in the interactions of inhibitors with alcohol dehydrogenase. *J. Med. Chem.* **29**, 615–620.

Hara A., Hayashibara M., Nakayama T., Hasebe K., Usui S. and Sawada H. (1985). Guinea-pig testosterone 17β-dehydrogenase (NADP+) and aldehyde reductase exhibit benzene dihydrodiol dehydrogenase activity. *Biochem. J.* **225**, 177–181.

Hara A., Nakayama T., Deyashiki Y., Kariya K. and Sawada H. (1986). Carbonyl reductase of dog liver: purification, properties, and kinetic mechanism. *Arch. Biochem. Biophys.* **244**, 238–247.

Hara A., Yamamoto H., Deyashiki Y., Nakayama T.,

Oritani H. and Sawada H. (1991). Aldehyde dismutation catalyzed by pulmonary carbonyl reductase: kinetic studies of chloral hydrate metabolism to trichloroacetic acid and trichloroethanol. *Biochim. Biophys. Acta* **1075**, 61–67.

Harrington M.C., Henehan G.T.M. and Tipton K.F. (1987). The roles of human aldehyde dehydrogenase isozymes in ethanol metabolism. In *Enzymology and Molecular Biology of Carbonyl Metabolism* (eds Weiner H. and Flynn T.G.). pp. 111–125. Liss, New York.

Hempel J. and Jörnvall H. (1987). Functional topology of aldehyde dehydrogenase structures. In *Enzymology and Molecular Biology of Carbonyl Metabolism* (eds Weiner H. and Flynn T.G.). pp. 1–14. Liss, New York.

Hempel J., Harper K. and Lindahl R. (1989). Inducible (class 3) aldehyde dehydrogenase from rat hepatocellular carcinoma and 2,3,7,8-tetrachlorodibenzo-*p*-dioxin-treated liver. Distant relationship to the class 1 and 2 enzymes from mammalian liver cytosol/mitochondria. *Biochemistry* **28**, 1160–1167.

Hempel J., Nicholas H. and Jörnvall H. (1991). Thiol proteases and aldehyde dehydrogenases: Evolution from a common thiolesterase precursor? *Proteins Struct. Funct. Genet.* **11**, 176–183.

Herold D.A., Keil K. and Bruns D.E. (1989). Oxidation of polyethylene glycols by alcohol dehydrogenase. *Biochem. Pharmacol.* **38**, 73–76.

Hinson J.A. and Neal R.A. (1975). An examination of octanol and octanal metabolism to octanoic acid by horse liver alcohol dehydrogenase. *Biochim. Biophys. Acta* **384**, 1–11.

Holmquist B. and Vallee B.L. (1991). Human liver class-III alcohol-dependent and glutathione-dependent formaldehyde dehydrogenase are the same enzyme. *Biochem. Biophys. Res. Commun.* **178**, 1371–1377.

Hurley T.D. and Bosron W.F. (1992). Human alcohol dehydrogenase: Dependence of secondary alcohol oxidation on the amino acids at positions 93 and 94. *Biochem. Biophys. Res. Commun.* **183**, 93–99.

Inaba T. and Kovacs J. (1989). Haloperidol reductase in human and guinea pig livers. *Drug Metab. Disposit.* **17**, 330–333.

Irwin A.J. and Jones J.B. (1977). Asymmetric syntheses via enantiotopically selective horse liver alcohol dehydrogenase catalyzed oxidations of diols containing a prochiral center. *J. Amer. Chem. Soc.* **99**, 556–561.

Ishida T., Yano M. and Toki S. (1991). *In vivo* formation of codeinone and morphinone from codeine. Isolation and identification from guinea pig bile. *Drug Metab. Disposit.* **19**, 895–899.

Jones J.B. and Jakovac I.J. (1982). A new cubic-space section model for predicting the specificity of horse liver alcohol dehydrogenase-catalyzed oxidoreductions. *Can. J. Chem.* **60**, 19–28.

Jones J.B. and Schwartz H.M. (1981). Enzymes in organic synthesis. 19. Evaluation of the stereoselectivities of horse liver alcohol dehydrogenase-catalyzed oxidoreductions of hydroxy- and ketothiolanes, -thianes, and -thiepanes. *Can. J. Chem.* **59**, 1574–1579.

Jones G.L. and Teng Y.S. (1983). A chemical and enzymological account of the multiple forms of human liver aldehyde dehydrogenase. *Biochim. Biophys. Acta* **745**, 162–174.

Jones K.H., Lindahl R., Baker D.C. and Timkovich R. (1987). Hydride transfer stereospecificity of rat liver aldehyde dehydrogenases. *J. Biol. Chem.* **262**, 10,911–10,913.

Jones D.P., Thor H., Andersson B. and Orrenius S. (1978). Detoxification reactions in isolated hepatocytes. Role of glutathione peroxidase, catalase and formaldehyde dehydrogenase in reactions relating to N-demethylation and the cytochrome P-450 system. *J. Biol. Chem.* **253**, 6031–6037.

Jörnvall H., Hempel J., Vallee B.L., Bosron W.F. and Li T.K. (1984). Human liver alcohol dehydrogenase: amino acid substitution in the $\beta_2\beta_2$ Oriental isozyme explains functional properties, establishes an active site structure, and parallels mutational exchanges in the yeast enzyme. *Proc. Natl. Acad. Sci. USA* **81**, 3024–3028.

Jörnvall H., Höög J.O., von Bahr-Lindström H., Johansson J., Kaiser R. and Persson B. (1988). Alcohol dehydrogenases and aldehyde dehydrogenases. *Biochem. Soc. Trans.* **16**, 223–227.

Kageura E. and Toki S. (1975). Guinea pig liver 3-hydroxyhexobarbital dehydrogenase. Purification and properties. *J. Biol. Chem.* **250**, 5015–5019.

Kitson T.M., Hill J.P. and Midwinter G.G. (1991). Identification of a catalytically essential nucleophilic residue in sheep liver cytoplasmic aldehyde dehydrogenase. *Biochem. J.* **275**, 207–210.

Klein J., Post K., Thomas H., Wörner W., Setiabudi F., Frank H., Oesch F. and Platt K.L. (1990). The oxidation of the highly tumorigenic benz[*a*]anthracene 3,4-dihydrodiol by rat liver dihydrodiol dehydrogenase. *Chem.-Biol. Interact.* **76**, 211–226.

Klein J., Seidel A., Frank H., Oesch F. and Platt K.L. (1991). Regiospecific oxidation of polycyclic aromatic dihydrodiols by rat liver dihydrodiol dehydrogenase. *Chem.-Biol. Interact.* **79**, 287–303.

Klein J., Thomas H., Post K., Worner W. and Oesch F. (1992). Dihydrodiol dehydrogenase activities of rabbit liver are associated with hydroxysteroid dehydrogenases and aldo-keto reductases. *Eur. J. Biochem.* **205**, 1155–1162.

Klinman J.P. (1976). Isotope effects and structure-activity correlations in the yeast alcohol dehydrogenase reaction. A study of the enzyme-catalyzed oxidation of aromatic alcohols. *Biochemistry* **15**, 2018–2026.

Koivusalo M., Baumann M. and Uotila L. (1989). Evidence for the identity of glutathione-dependent formaldehyde dehydrogenase and Class III alcohol dehydrogenase. *FEBS Lett.* **257**, 105–109.

Kovar J., Skursky L. and Blaha K. (1976). Chloroprothixene binding into the active site pocket of horse liver alcohol dehydrogenase. *Coll. Czech. Chem. Commun.* **41**, 928–940.

Lam L.K.P., Gair I.A. and Jones J.B. (1988). Enzymes in organic synthesis. 41. Stereoselective horse liver alcohol dehydrogenase catalysed reductions of heterocyclic bicyclic ketones. *J. Org. Chem.* **53**, 1611–1615.

Lemière G.L., Van Osselaer T.A., Lepoivre J.A. and Alderweireldt F.C. (1982). Enzymatic *in vitro* reduction of ketones. Part 8. A new model for the reduction of cyclic ketones by horse liver alcohol dehydrogenase (HLAD). *J. Chem. Soc. Parkin. Trans.* **II**, 1123–1128.

Lenk W., Löhr D. and Sonnenbichler J. (1989). Pharmacokinetics and biotransformation of diethylene glycol and ethylene glycol in the rat. *Xenobiotica* **19**, 961–979.

Light D.R., Dennis M.S., Forsythe I.J., Liu C.C., Green D.W., Kratzer D.A. and Plapp B.V. (1992). α-Isozyme of alcohol dehydrogenase from monkey liver—Cloning, expression, mechanism, coenzyme and substrate specificity. *J. Biol. Chem.* **267**, 12,592–12,599.

Lindahl R. (1992). Aldehyde dehydrogenases and their role in carcinogenesis. *Crit. Rev. Biochem. Molec. Biol.* **27**, 283–335.

Lindahl R. and Evces S. (1984). Rat liver aldehyde dehydrogenase. *J. Biol. Chem.* **259**, 11,986–11,996.

Lindahl R. and Petersen D.R. (1991). Lipid aldehyde oxidation as a physiological role for class 3 aldehyde dehydrogenases. *Biochem. Pharmacol.* **41**, 1583–1587.

MacInnes I., Nonhebel D.C., Orszulik S.T. and Suckling C.J. (1983). On the mechanism of hydrogen transfer by nicotinamide coenzymes and alcohol dehydrogenase. *J. Chem. Soc. Perkin. Trans.* **I**, 2777–2779.

Madyastha K.M. and Srivatsan V. (1988). Studies on the metabolism of *l*-menthol in rats. *Drug Metab. Disposit.* **16**, 765–772.

Marselos M. and Lindahl R. (1988). Substrate preference of a cytosolic aldehyde dehydrogenase inducible in rat liver by treatment with 3-methylcholanthrene. *Toxicol. Appl. Pharmacol.* **95**, 339–345.

Maser E., Gebel T. and Netter K.J. (1991). Carbonyl reduction of metyrapone in human liver. *Biochem. Pharmacol.* **42**, S93–S98.

Matos J.R., Smith M.B. and Wong C.H. (1985). Enantioselectivity of alcohol dehydrogenase-catalyzed oxidation of 1,2-diols and aminoalcohols. *BioOrg. Chem.* **13**, 121–130.

McMahon R.E. (1982). Alcohols, aldehydes, and ketones. In *Metabolic Basis of Detoxication* (eds Jakoby W.B., Bend J.R. and Caldwell J.). pp. 91–104. Academic Press, New York.

Mitchell D.Y. and Petersen D.R. (1988). Inhibition of rat liver aldehyde dehydrogenases by acrolein. *Drug Metab. Disposit.* **16**, 37–42.

Mitchell D.Y. and Petersen D.R. (1989). Oxidation of aldehydic products of lipid peroxidation by rat liver microsomal aldehyde dehydrogenase. *Arch Biochem. Biophys.* **269**, 11–17.

Miyauchi K., Masaki R., Taketani S., Yamamoto A., Akayama M. and Tashiro Y. (1991). Molecular cloning, sequencing and expression of cDNA for rat liver microsomal aldehyde dehydrogenase. *J. Biol. Chem.* **266**, 19,536–19,542.

Moreno A. and Parés X. (1991). Purification and characterization of a new alcohol dehydrogenase from human

stomach. *J. Biol. Chem.* **266**, 1128–1133.

Nagamine S., Otawa T., Nakae H. and Asada S. (1988). Estimation of the rates of available fraction for some 4-substituted acetophenone derivatives in the rat: reversible drug-metabolite pharmacokinetics. *Chem. Pharm. Bull.* **36**, 4612–4618.

Nakagawa M., Harada T., Hara A., Nakayama T. and Sawada H. (1989). Purification and properties of multiple forms of dihydrodiol dehydrogenase from monkey liver. *Chem. Pharm. Bull.* **37**, 2852–2854.

Nakayama T., Hara A., Yashiro K. and Sawada H. (1985). Reductases for carbonyl compounds in human liver. *Biochem. Pharmacol.* **34**, 107–117.

Nakayama T., Hara A., Kariya K., Hasebe K., Inoue Y., Matsuura K. and Sawada H. (1987). Hydrosteroids are physiological substrates of dehydogenases for alicyclic alcohols and benzene dihydrodiol in rodent and rabbit liver cytosol. In *Enzymology and Molecular Biology of Carbonyl Metabolism* (eds Weiner H. and Flynn T.G.). pp. 415–430. Liss, New York.

Nakazaki M., Chikamatsu H. and Sasaki Y. (1983). Stereochemistry of horse liver alcohol dehydrogenase (HLADH) mediated oxido reduction in cage-shaped carbonyl compounds. *J. Org. Chem.* **48**, 2506–2511.

Nambiar K.P., Stauffer D.M., Kolodziej P.A. and Benner S.A. (1983). A mechanistic basis for the stereoselectivity of enzymatic transfer of hydrogen from nicotinamide cofactors. *J. Amer. Chem. Soc.* **105**, 5886–5890.

Nohl H., Jordan W. and Youngman R.J. (1986). Quinones in biology: functions in electron transfer and oxygen activation. *Adv. Free Radic. Biol. Med.* **2**, 211–279.

Oppenheimer N.J. (1984). Stereoselectivity of enzymatic transfer of hydrogen from nicotinamide coenzymes: a stereochemical imperative? *J. Amer. Chem. Soc.* **106**, 3032–3033.

Oppermann U.C.T., Maser E., Mangoura S.A. and Netter K.J. (1991). Heterogeneity of carbonyl reduction in subcellular fractions and different organs in rodents. *Biochem. Pharmacol.* **42**, S189–S195.

Park D.H. and Plapp B.V. (1992). Interconversion of E and S isoenzymes of horse liver alcohol dehydrogenase. Several residues contribute indirectly to catalysis. *J. Biol. Chem.* **267**, 5527–5533.

Plapp B.V., Eklund H. and Brändén C.I. (1978). Crystallography of liver alcohol dehydrogenase complexed with substrates. *J. Mol. Biol.* **122**, 23–32.

Plapp B.V., Ganzhorn A.J., Gould R.M., Green D.W. and Hershey A.D. (1987a). Structure and function in yeast alcohol dehydrogenase. In *Enzymology and Molecular Biology of Carbonyl Metabolism* (eds Weiner H. and Flynn T.G.). pp. 227–236. Liss, New York.

Plapp B.V., Parsons M., Leidal K.G., Baggenstoss B.A., Ferm J.R.G. and Wear S.S. (1987b). Characterization of alcohol dehydrogenase from cultured rat hepatoma (HTC) cells. In *Enzymology and Molecular Biology of Carbonyl Metabolism* (eds Weiner H. and Flynn T.G.). pp. 203–215. Liss, New York.

Pocker Y. and De Roy S.C. (1987). The active site of liver alcohol dehydrogenase. Mechanistic inferences from the binding and turnover of 2-, 3-, and 4-pyridylcarbinols. In *Enzymology and Molecular Biology of Carbonyl Metabolism* (eds Weiner H. and Flynn T.G.). pp. 179–187. Liss, New York.

Pocker Y. and Page J.D. (1990). Zinc-activated alcohols in ternary complexes of liver alcohol dehydrogenase. *J. Biol. Chem.* **265**, 22,101–22,108.

Pocker Y., Li H. and Page J.D. (1987). Liver alcohol dehydrogenase: substrate orientation, metabolic activity and energetics of enzyme catalysis. In *Enzymology and Molecular Biology of Carbonyl Metabolism* (eds Weiner H. and Flynn T.G.). pp. 217–225. Liss, New York.

Pourmotabbed T. and Creighton D.J. (1986). Substrate specificity of bovine liver formaldehyde dehydrogenase. *J. Biol. Chem.* **261**, 14,240–14,245.

Pourmotabbed T., Shih M.J. and Creighton D.J. (1989). Bovine liver formaldehyde dehydrogenase. Kinetic and molecular properties. *J. Biol. Chem.* **264**, 17,384–17,388.

Prelog V. (1964). Specification of the stereospecificity of some oxido-reductases by diamond lattice sections. *Pure Appl. Chem.* **9**, 119–130.

Prelusky D.B., Coutts R.T. and Pasutto F.M. (1982). Stereospecific metabolic reduction of ketones. *J. Pharm. Sci.* **71**, 1390–1393.

Ramaswamy S., Eklund H. and Plapp B.V. (1994). Structures of horse liver alcohol dehydrogenase complexed with NAD$^+$ and substituted benzyl alcohols. *Biochemistry*, **33**, 230–5237.

Rikans L.E. and Moore D.R. (1987). Effect of age and sex on allyl alcohol hepatotoxicity in rats: role of liver alcohol and aldehyde dehydrogenase activities. *J. Pharmacol. Exp. Ther.* **243**, 20–26.

Roerig S., Fujimoto J.M., Wang R.I.H., Pollock S.H. and Lange D. (1976). Preliminary characterization of enzymes for reduction of naloxone and naltrexone in rabbit and chicken liver. *Drug Metab. Disposit.* **4**, 53–58.

Rush W.R., Alexander O.F., Hall D.J., Dow R.J., Tokes L., Kurz L. and Graham D.J.M. (1990). The metabolism of nafimidone hydrochloride in the dog, primates and man. *Xenobiotica* **20**, 123–132.

Sarges R. (1989). Aldose reductase inhibitors: Structure-activity relationships and therapeutic potential. In *Advances in Drug Research*, vol. 18 (ed. Testa B.). pp. 139–175. Academic Press, London.

Sawada H., Hara A., Nakayama T., Nakagawa M., Inoue Y., Hasebe K. and Zhang Y.P. (1988). Mouse liver dihydrodiol dehydrogenases. Identity of the predominant and a minor form with 17β-hydroxysteroid dehydrogenase and aldehyde reductase. *Biochem. Pharmacol.* **37**, 453–458.

Schofield P.J., De Jongh K.S., Smith M.M. and Edwards M.R. (1987). Inhibition of aldehyde reductases. In *Enzymology and Molecular Biology of Carbonyl Metabolism* (eds Weiner H. and Flynn T.G.). pp. 287–296. Liss, New York.

Sekhar V.C. and Plapp B.V. (1990). Rate constants for a mechanism including intermediates in the interconversion of ternary complexes by horse liver alcohol dehydrogenase. *Biochemistry* **29**, 4289–4295.

Sellin S., Holmquist B., Mannervik B. and Vallee B.L. (1991). Oxidation and reduction of 4-hydroxyalkenals catalyzed by isozymes of human alcohol dehydrogenase. *Biochemistry* **30**, 2514–2518.

Sladek N.E., Manthey C.L., Maki P.A., Zhang Z. and Landkamer G.J. (1989). Xenobiotic oxidation catalyzed by aldehyde dehydrogenases. *Drug Metab. Rev.* **20**, 697–720.

Smith M. (1988). Molecular genetic studies on alcohol and aldehyde dehydrogenase: individual variation, gene mapping and analysis of regulation. *Biochem. Soc. Trans.* **16**, 227–230.

Smithgall T.E., Harvey R.G. and Penning T.M. (1988). Spectroscopic identification of *ortho*-quinones as the products of polycyclic aromatic *trans*-dihydrodiol oxidation catalyzed by dihydrodiol dehydrogenase. *J. Biol. Chem.* **263**, 1814–1820.

Stone C.L., Li T.K. and Bosron W.F. (1989). Stereospecific oxidation of secondary alcohols by human alcohol dehydrogenases. *J. Biol. Chem.* **264**, 11,112–11,116.

Testa B. (1973). Some chemical and stereochemical aspects of diethylpropion metabolism in man. *Acta Pharm. Suec.* **10**, 441–454.

Testa B. (1986). Chiral aspects of drug metabolism. *Trends Pharmacol. Sci.* **7**, 60–64.

Tolf B.R., Dahlbom R., Åkeson Å. and Theorell H. (1985). Synthetic inhibitors of alcohol dehydrogenase. *Acta Pharm. Suec.* **22**, 147–156.

Tsuboi S., Kawase M., Takada A., Hiramatsu M., Wada Y., Kawakami Y., Ikeda M. and Ohmori S. (1992). Purification and characterization of formaldehyde dehydrogenase from rat liver cytosol. *J. Biochem.* **111**, 465–471.

Uotila L. and Koivusalo M. (1987). Formaldehyde dehydrogenase from human erythrocytes: purification, some properties and evidence for multiple forms. In *Enzymology and Molecular Biology of Carbonyl Metabolism* (eds Weiner H. and Flynn T.G.). pp. 165–177. Liss, New York.

Vallari R.C. and Pietruszko R. (1982). Human aldehyde dehydrogenase: mechanism of inhibition by disulfiram. *Science* **216**, 637–639.

Vallee B.L. and Auld D.S. (1990). Zinc coordination, function, and structure of zinc enzymes and other proteins. *Biochemistry* **29**, 5647–5659.

Van der Graaff M., Vermeulen N.P.E. and Breimer D.D. (1988). Disposition of hexobarbital: 15 years of an intriguing model substrate. *Drug Metab. Rev.* **19**, 109–164.

Vogel K., Platt K.L., Petrovic P., Seidel A. and Oesch F. (1982). Dihydrodiol dehydrogenase: Substrate specificity, inducibility and tissue distribution. *Arch. Toxicol. Suppl.* **5**, 360–364.

von Wartburg J.P. and Wermuth B. (1980). Aldehyde reductase. In *Enzymatic Basis of Detoxication*, Vol. 1 (ed. Jakoby W.B.). pp. 249–260. Academic Press, New York.

Waydhas C., Weigl K. and Sies H. (1978). The disposition of formaldehyde and formate arising from drug N-demethylations dependent on cytochrome P-450 in hepatocytes and in perfused rat liver. *Eur. J. Biochem.* **89**, 143–150.

Weiner H. (1980). Aldehyde oxidizing enzymes. In *Enzymatic Basis of Detoxication*, vol. 1 (ed. Jakoby W.B.). pp. 261–280. Academic Press, New York.

Weiner H. and Flynn T.G., eds (1987). *Enzymology and Molecular Biology of Carbonyl Metabolism*. Liss, New York.

Weiner H. and Flynn T.G., eds (1989). *Enzymology and Molecular Biology of Carbonyl Metabolism 2. Aldehyde Dehydrogenase, Alcohol Dehydrogenase, and Aldo-Keto Reductase*. Liss, New York.

Weiner H., Crabb D.W. and Flynn T.G., eds (1993). *Enzymology and Molecular Biology of Carbonyl Metabolism*, vol. 4. Plenum, New York.

Weinhold E.G., Glasfeld A., Ellington A.D. and Benner S.A. (1991). Structural determinants of stereospecificity in yeast alcohol dehydrogenase. *Proc. Natl. Acad. Sci. USA* **88**, 8420–8424.

Wermuth B. (1981). Purification and properties of an NADPH-dependent carbonyl reductase from human brain. Relationship to prostaglandin 9-ketoreductase and xenobiotic ketone reductase. *J. Biol. Chem.* **256**, 1206–1213.

Wermuth B., Omar A., Forster A., di Francesco Ch., Wolf M., von Wartburg J.P., Bullock B. and Gabbay K.H. (1987). Primary structure of aldehyde reductase from human liver. In *Enzymology and Molecular Biology of Carbonyl Metabolism* (eds Weiner H. and Flynn T.G.). pp. 297–307. Liss, New York.

Wermuth B., Bohren K.M., Heinemann G., von Wartburg J.P. and Gabbay K.H. (1988). Human carbonyl reductase. Nucleotide sequence analysis of a cDNA and amino acid sequence of the encoded protein. *J. Biol. Chem.* **263**, 16,185–16,188.

Wirth H.P. and Wermuth B. (1985). Immunochemical characterization of aldo-keto reductases from human tissues. *FEBS Lett.* **187**, 280–282.

Wiseman J.S. and Abeles R.H. (1979). Mechanism of inhibition of aldehyde dehydrogenase by cyclopropanone hydrate and the mushroom toxin coprine. *Biochemistry* **18**, 427–435.

Woenckhaus C., Bieber E. and Jeck R. (1987). Studies on the inactivation of aldehyde dehydrogenase. In *Enzymology and Molecular Biology of Carbonyl Metabolism* (eds Weiner H. and Flynn T.G.). pp. 53–65. Liss, New York.

Zorzano A. and Herrera E. (1990). Differences in the kinetic properties and sensitivity to inhibitors of human placental, erythrocyte, and major hepatic aldehyde dehydrogenase isoenzymes. *Biochem. Pharmacol.* **39**, 873–878.

chapter 3

THE NATURE AND FUNCTIONING OF CYTOCHROMES P450 AND FLAVIN-CONTAINING MONOOXYGENASES

Contents

3.1 INTRODUCTION

3.1.1 A first look at oxygenases

A wide variety of enzymes oxidize xenobiotic substrates, and in the previous chapter, oxidation by hydride abstraction (dehydrogenation) has been discussed. Oxidation by electron abstraction without oxygen incorporation is another mechanism characteristic of some oxidoreductases (Chapter 9) and also displayed by cytochrome P450 (e.g. Chapters 5 and 6). However, the most important reaction of oxidation in the metabolism of xenobiotics and endogenous compounds is incorporation of oxygen into the substrate, a reaction characterizing **oxygenases**. Depending whether one or both atoms of molecular oxygen are transferred to the substrate, the enzymes are categorized as **monooxygenases** and **dioxygenases**, respectively. In the present chapter and in those to follow, monooxygenases and monooxygenation reactions will be considered at length, although the pace of scientific progress is so fast at present that anything that can be written represents but a small fraction of the available knowledge. Dioxygenation reactions will be discussed in Chapter 10.

Monooxygenation reactions are mediated by various enzymes which differ markedly in their structure and properties. Among these, the most important as far as xenobiotic metabolism is concerned—and most likely also endobiotic metabolism—are the **cytochromes P450**, a very large group of enzymes encoded by the P450 gene superfamily and belonging to heme-coupled monooxygenases (Gonzalez, 1989 and 1990; Nebert and Gonzalez, 1987; Nebert *et al.*, 1987, 1989 and 1991). These cytochromes P450 are entered in the Enzyme Nomenclature mainly as **unspecific monooxygenase** [substrate, reduced-flavoprotein:oxygen oxidoreductase (RH-hydroxylating or -epoxidizing); microsomal P-450; EC 1.14.14.1] (International Union of Biochemistry and Molecular Biology, 1992). In addition, many other P450 activities are listed, e.g. cholesterol 7α-monooxygenase [EC 1.14.13.17], leukotriene-B_4 20-monooxygenase [EC 1.14.13.30], methyltetrahydroprotoberberine 14-monooxygenase [EC 1.14.13.37], tyrosine N-monooxygenase [EC 1.14.13.41], $(-)$-limonene 3-, 6- and 7-monooxygenases [EC 1.14.13.47, -.48 and -.49, respectively], camphor 5-monooxygenase [EC 1.14.15.1], steroid 11β-mono-oxygenase [EC 1.14.15.4], cortisone 18-monooxygenase [EC 1.14.15.5], cholesterol mono-oxygenase [EC 1.14.15.6], steroid 17α-monooxygenase [EC 1.14.99.9] and steroid 21-mono-oxygenase [EC 1.14.99.10].

Other monooxygenases whose role in xenobiotic metabolism is well recognized are the **flavin-containing monooxygenases** [EC 1.14.13.8] (Section 3.7), and **dopamine β-monooxygenase** [EC 1.14.17.1], a copper-dependent monooxygenase discussed in Section 9.3. In contrast to these enzymes, there exist other monooxygenases whose potential to metabolize xenobiotics is essentially unexplored, and which therefore will just be mentioned; these enzymes include the **copper-containing monooxygenases** collectively known as monophenol monooxygenase [monophenol, L-dopa:oxygen oxidoreductase; phenolase; tyrosinase; EC 1.14.18.1] (see also Section 9.6), and **pteridin-dependent monooxygenases** such as phenylalanine 4-monooxygenase [L-phenylalanine, tetrahydrobiopterin:oxygen oxidoreductase (4-hydroxylating); EC 1.14.16.1], tyrosine 3-monooxygenase [EC 1.14.16.2], and tryptophan 5-monooxygenase [EC 1.14.16.4] (Gunsalus *et al.*, 1975; Mesnil and Testa, 1984; Walsh, 1980a).

3.1.2 A first look at cytochrome P450

Cytochrome P450 is a hemoprotein of unusual properties found in almost all living organisms such as bacteria, yeast, plants, and animals (e.g. insects and vertebrates), but interestingly not in helminths (Holton *et al.*, 1993; Miners *et al.*, 1988; Ortiz de Montellano, 1986; Precious and Barrett, 1989; Ruckpaul and Rein, 1984). **Mammalian cytochromes P450** are found in almost all organs and tissues examined. These enzymes are membrane-bound, located mostly in the endoplasmic reticulum but also in mitochondria. In fact, they are present in almost all membranes and cells (Coon *et al.*, 1992; Guengerich, 1991; Kapke and Baron, 1980; LaBella, 1991; Soucek and Gut, 1992; Waterman and Johnson, 1991). It must also be noted, however, that soluble (i.e. cytosolic) cytochromes P450 are not unknown; besides the cytochrome P450cam discussed below, a mammalian soluble cytochrome P450 designated H450 has been reported (Hasegawa, 1983; Omura *et al.*, 1984).

The **appearance and evolution** of cytochrome P450 may be traced back to the early days of biological evolution (more than 3.5 billion years ago), before the advent of the oxygen atmosphere when its presence must have been associated with reductive reactions (Gonzalez, 1989 and 1990) (see Section i.3). Upon the gradual appearance of atmospheric oxygen, its main role is believed to have become that of a line of defence (Wickramasinghe and Villee, 1975), and only later evolving its manifold reactions of oxidation in (a) the anabolism and/or catabolism of endogenous compounds (e.g. steroids, fatty acids, leukotrienes, prostaglandins, biogenic amines, pheromones), and (b) in the detoxication of xenobiotics (in particular in the so-called animal–plant warfare). The long evolution of cytochrome P450 is certainly compatible with its present-day ubiquity, versatility and multiplicity (Estabrook *et al.*, 1982; Nebert and Gonzalez, 1985 and 1987; Nebert and Negishi, 1982; Nelson *et al.*, 1993).

The present chapter is centred on cytochrome P450 and examines first its structure (Section 3.2) and multiplicity (Section 3.3). The functioning of cytochrome P450 is next considered by breaking down its catalytic cycle into individual steps discussed successively in Sections 3.4 to 3.6. The chapter ends with an overview of the structure and functioning of another important enzyme system, the flavin-containing monooxygenase (Section 3.7). The reactions of monooxygenation catalyzed by cytochrome P450 and in some cases also by the flavin-containing monooxygenases are discussed in Chapters 4 to 8 and 11. That so many chapters are required to cover these topics gives the reader a first indication of the unique significance and position of cytochrome P450 biologically and as an object of scientific enquiry.

3.2 THE CHEMICAL STRUCTURE OF CYTOCHROME P450

Cytochrome P450, being a hemoprotein, consists of a **protein** (the apoprotein or apoenzyme) and a **heme moiety**, namely iron-protoporphyrin IX. This porphyrin is common not only to all cytochrome P450 enzymes, but also to other hemoproteins and enzymes such as hemoglobin, myoglobin, catalase and most peroxidases. In contrast to the constant porphyrin, the protein part of the enzyme varies markedly from one enzyme/isozyme to the other and accounts for the differences in their properties (see Section 3.3), e.g. molecular weight (approximate range 45 to 60 kDa), substrate and product specificities, and sensitivity to inhibitors.

3.2.1 Structure and electronic states of the prosthetic heme

The structure of the **prosthetic heme** of cytochrome P450 is shown in Fig. 3.1. The iron cation (which exists in the formal ferric and ferrous states, see below) is liganded to the four pyrrole nitrogens. Two additional non-porphyrin ligands in axial positions, the fifth ligand X and the sixth ligand Y, are also represented in Fig. 3.1; these will be discussed below, but at this stage we note that with X being the thiolate ligand, the chiral orientation of the haem shown in the figure is that found in cytochrome P450 (Ortiz de Montellano *et al.*, 1983). The detailed structure of

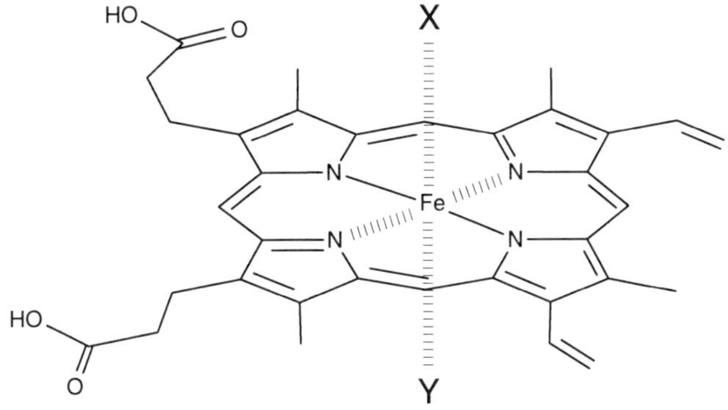

FIGURE 3.1 Structure of iron-protoporphyrin IX, the prosthetic heme of cytochrome P450. See text for further details.

protoporphyrin IX has been revealed by X-ray crystallographic studies (Caughey and Ibers, 1977). Extended X-ray absorption fine structure spectroscopy of cytochrome P450LM2 (ferric state, low spin) showed the Fe–N, Fe–C(α) and Fe–S distances to be 2.00, 3.07 and 2.19 Å, respectively (Cramer et al., 1978). Crystallographic studies of cytochrome P450cam, a soluble baterial enzyme, have yielded comparable results (Poulos, 1986, 1988 and 1991; Poulos and Raag, 1992).

The **fifth ligand** to the iron cation (i.e. X in Fig. 3.1) is a **thiolate group** (R–S⁻; note the anionic form) from an essential cysteine near the carboxyl end of the protein. The iron–sulfur bond is an unusually strong one, presumably due to other bonding forces, and it transfers considerable electron density to the iron (Black and Coon, 1985; Collman et al., 1976a; Poulos and Raag, 1992; Ruf et al., 1979; Silver and Lukas, 1984). These electronic features are indispensable for the catalytic activity of cytochrome P450, and formation of the inactive **cytochrome P420**, as induced for example by denaturation of the protein, involves displacement of the thiolate ligand (Fe–S rupture) or perhaps simply its protonation (thiol ligation).

The **sixth ligand** (Y in Fig. 3.1) has been the subject of lengthy debate. It became clear some years ago that this group, rather than being a stronger nitrogen-containing ligand, must be a weaker, oxygenated one (e.g. Dawson et al., 1982; White and Coon, 1982). A hydroxyl group, either from an adjacent amino acid residue or a water molecule, was postulated (Kumaki and Nebert, 1978). In some cases, the sixth ligand has now been shown to be a hydroxyl group belonging to a tyrosinyl residue located near the heme, while in cytochrome P450cam it appears to be a water molecule (Jänig et al., 1984; Poulos and Raag, 1992; Poulos et al., 1986).

The liganded heme can exist in a number of discrete electronic states which are responsible for many of the properties of cytochrome P450, most significantly for the binding of ligands and the activation of molecular oxygen. The iron atom formally exists in either ferric or ferrous **oxidation state** (although higher oxidation states also play a role in oxygen activation as discussed in Section 3.5). Two catalytically relevant **spin states** exist for both Fe(III) and Fe(II), i.e. low spin (abbreviated "ls") and high spin (abbreviated "hs"). The low spin states of Fe(III) ($S = 1/2$) and Fe(II) ($S = 0$) are hexacoordinated in hemoproteins; the iron atom is located in the plane of the four pyrrole nitrogens, and the six ligands occupy the vertices of an octahedron as suggested in Fig. 3.1. In contrast, the high spin states of Fe(III) ($S = 5/2$) and Fe(II) ($S = 2$) are too large in diameter to be coplanar with the four nitrogen ligands. The iron atom will therefore lie outside the plane of the porphyrin ring [0.3 Å for Fe(III) and 0.7 Å for Fe(II)] and as a result will be pentacoordinated (no sixth ligand Y) (e.g. Hahn et al., 1982; Hanson et al., 1977; Tang et al., 1976). The low spin/high spin equilibrium is depicted in Fig. 3.2 (see also Section 3.6). The

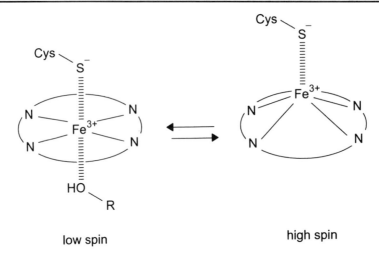

FIGURE 3.2 Low spin/high spin equilibrium in ferricytochrome P450 (the porphyrin is represented in simplified form).

interested reader may consult the comprehensive reviews by Scheidt and Reed (1981) and Lewis (1986) for further discussion of this topic.

3.2.2 The macromolecular structure of cytochrome P450

Cytochrome P450 exists in a considerable number of enzymic/isozymic forms (Section 3.3) differing in the structure of the apoprotein. As will be documented below, the primary structure (amino acid sequence) of many cytochromes P450 is now known, but to date the secondary and tertiary structures of only one form have been fully elucidated experimentally. Cytochrome P450 acts in monomeric form and thus has no quaternary structure, although its tendency to aggregate (a characteristic of membranal enzymes) will, in the absence of added detergents, give apparent molecular weights that are multiples of the genuine MW (Coon and Persson, 1980).

Peptide mapping has yielded much useful data on the **primary structure** of cytochrome P450 isozymes and has contributed to their characterization and differentiation, providing early evidence that they are not necessarily closely related peptides (e.g. Guengerich, 1978; Wang et al., 1983). There are about 400 to 500 amino acid residues, with high leucine content. The prokaryotic isozymes appear to have relatively fewer amino acids and lower hydrophobicity than do the eukaryotic ones.

A real breakthrough occurred when the first complete **amino acid sequences** of cytochrome P450 isozymes were established. Seemingly the first report is that of Haniu et al. (1982) on cytochrome P450cam (now known as cytochrome P450 101 or CYP101, see Section 3.3) isolated from *Pseudomonas putida*. This soluble enzyme was shown to be made of a single polypeptide chain of 412 amino acids, containing in particular eight cysteinyl residues. Since then, an increasing number of sequences have been determined, and the interested reader is referred to some excellent papers for compilations of the primary structure of many cytochrome P450 isozymes and for a critical evaluation of prominent features and homologies (Black and Coon, 1986; Lewis and Moereels, 1992). The short reviews by Guengerich et al. (1989) and Fuji-Kuriyama et al. (1989) also offer valuable information in condensed form.

For example, the sequencing of rabbit phenobarbital-induced, liver microsomal cytochrome

TABLE 3.1 *Invariant or highly conserved residues in cytochromes P450* (The residue numbering is that of cytochrome P450cam [P450 101]) (taken from Lewis and Moereels, 1992)

Residue	Type	Function
Pro-15	invariant	defines start of first turn into helix A
Gly-60	invariant	structural prerequisite
Arg-112	conserved	heme binding via propionate, and electron transfer ion-pair with cytochrome b_5 or redoxin
Gly-249	conserved	H-bonded pair defines substrate binding pocket
Thr-252	invariant	H-bonded pair defines substrate binding pocket
Glu-287	invariant	ion pair with Arg-290
Arg-290	invariant	ion pair with Glu-287
Arg-299	conserved	heme binding via propionate
Phe-350	invariant	possibly π–π stacking interactions with His-355 for electron conduction
Gly-353	invariant	defines heme binding pocket
His-355	conserved	charge relay from reductase to heme
Cys-357	invariant	heme ligation via thiolate (fifth ligand)
Gly-359	invariant	defines heme binding pocket
Ala-363	conserved	defines heme binding pocket
Leu-375	conserved	hydrophobic interaction with D helix

P450LM2 showed it to be a single chain made of 489 amino acids; homology with cytochrome P450cam is limited to a single eight-residue region, but it shows a high degree of homology with other mammalian isozymes (Heinemann and Ozols, 1983). A constitutive form of the rabbit liver microsomal cytochrome P450, namely isozyme 3b, is a single chain of 490 residues displaying 46% homology to cytochrome P450LM2 (Ozols *et al.*, 1985). Primary structure determination has even shown that an individual isozyme may in fact have a number of variants. Thus, the rabbit hepatic and pulmonary isozyme 2 could be separated into three variants B_0, B_1 and B_2; the lung contains only variants B_0 and B_1, while all three variants exist in the liver (Gasser *et al.*, 1988). These differences in amino acid sequence constitute the basis for a classification of the superfamily of cytochrome P450 enzymes into families, subfamilies and isozymes, as discussed in Section 3.3.

A number of **amino acid residues** are either invariant in all in cytochromes P450 or highly conserved (i.e. present in most forms), and their function is now understood (Table 3.1) (Gonzalez, 1989; Lewis and Moereels, 1992). The most important amino acid in the protein sequence is the thiolate-donating cysteine (i.e. the fifth ligand to the haem iron), which is used to align sequences. This critical, invariant residue is Cys-357 in cytochrome P450cam, Cys-422 in bovine cytochrome P450scc, Cys-436 in rabbit isozyme 2 and rat isozyme b, Cys-456 in rat isozyme d and mouse isozyme 3, Cys-458 in mouse isozyme 1, and Cys-461 in rat isozyme c (Black and Coon, 1985 and 1986). Other residues and their function are compiled in Table 3.1.

The secondary and tertiary structures of membrane cytochrome P450 isozymes are not yet known with certainty. Based on the primary structure, theoretical methods exist to predict the **secondary structure** of proteins. In a few cases, such approaches have been applied to cytochrome P450, for example rabbit liver isozyme 2 (Tarr *et al.*, 1983), the major phenobarbital-inducible isozyme of rat liver microsomes (cytochrome P450PB), and cytochrome P450cam (Gotoh *et al.*, 1983). Similarly, the predicted secondary structure of rat liver isozyme d yielded a maximum of 17 helices, four of which may be sufficiently hydrophobic to traverse the endoplasmic reticulum membrane (Haniu *et al.*, 1986). These approaches, although their degree of uncertainty cannot be neglected, have yielded coherent results that allow useful insights into function and membrane topology.

The only current method allowing the certain determination of the full three-dimensional structure of proteins is X-ray crystallography, which suffers the obvious and severe limitation that the protein must first be obtained in crystalline form. To date, this has been achieved only with **soluble cytochromes P450**, and the studies by Poulos and colleagues on both the camphor-bound and substrate-free cytochrome P450cam are true milestones (Poulos, 1986 and 1988; Poulos *et al.*, 1985 and 1986). For the first time, the crystalline **tertiary structure** of a cytochrome P450 isozyme is known beyond doubt. A schematic diagram of cytochrome P450cam is given in Fig. 3.3, showing the compact structure of the enzyme and the central and deeply buried position of the active site (Poulos *et al.*, 1985). A closer look at the active site in its substrate-free, low-spin form is given by Fig. 3.4. Further details will be given in Section 3.4.2 for the substrate-bound form. The structural and mechanistic understanding gained with this soluble isozyme is helping considerably in studying **membrane-bound cytochromes P450.** Thus, a secondary structure prediction of 52 membrane-bound cytochromes P450 was validated by its strong similarities with the tertiary structure of cytochrome P450cam (Nelson and Strobel, 1989). Even more powerful methods are the computational techniques of **sequence alignment and**

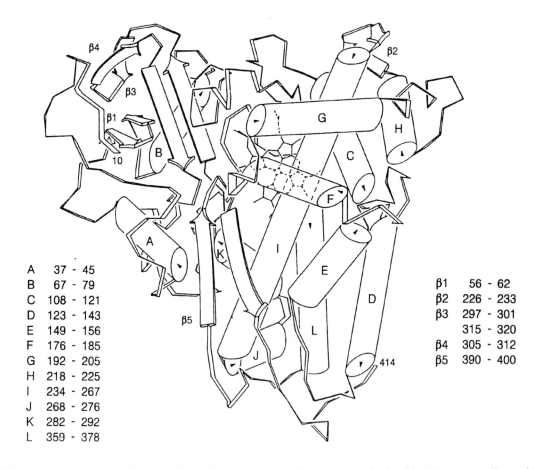

A	37 - 45				
B	67 - 79				
C	108 - 121		β1	56 - 62	
D	123 - 143		β2	226 - 233	
E	149 - 156		β3	297 - 301	
F	176 - 185			315 - 320	
G	192 - 205		β4	305 - 312	
H	218 - 225		β5	390 - 400	
I	234 - 267				
J	268 - 276				
K	282 - 292				
L	359 - 378				

FIGURE 3.3 Schematic diagram of cytochrome P450cam (P450 101) as obtained by X-ray crystallography. Helices are represented by rods and β-pleated sheets by flat arrows. The inset lists residues in helical segments and antiparallel β-sheet segments. The porphyrin ring is visible near the centre. Reproduced from Poulos *et al.* (1985) with the permission of the copyright holder.

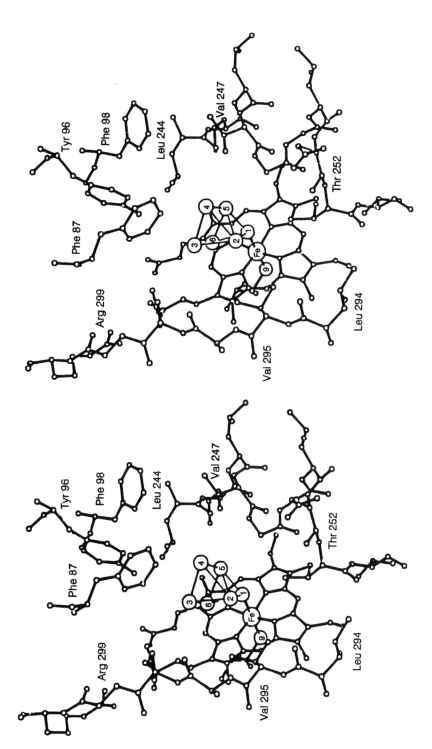

FIGURE 3.4 Model of active site environment in substrate-free, low-spin cytochrome P450cam. The sixth ligand is provided by a water molecule hydrogen-bonded to a number of companions (labelled 2–6 in the figure). To be visualized in 3D, this stereoscopic image must be altered in size by photocopying to reach a distance of about 6 cm between the same atoms. Reproduced from Poulos *et al.* (1986) with the permission of the copyright holder.

molecular modelling using the primary and tertiary structure of cytochrome P450cam as template. Such techniques have generated seemingly reliable models of the active sites of a number of mammalian cytochromes P450 (Korzekwa and Jones, 1993; Koymans *et al.*, 1992, 1993a and 1993b; Lewis and Moereels, 1992; Poulos, 1991; Vijayakumar and Salerno, 1992) (see Section 3.4.2). Mutations at specific positions offer one method to validate such models (Chen and Zhou, 1992; Tuck *et al.*, 1993).

In addition to differences in the protein structure, there is also the possibility that the molecular diversity of cytochrome P450 isozymes is further elaborated in the cells by **post-translational modifications** such as glycosylation and phosphorylation. **Glycosylation** has been shown for a few isozymes such as cytochrome P450scc isolated from bovine adrenocortical mitochondria (Ichikawa and Hiwatashi, 1982). Some cytochrome P450 isozymes of various origins must thus be considered as glycoproteins, although the extent of glycosylation is not extensive (7–9 mol mol^{-1} protein; 3–4% of total weight) (Armstrong *et al.*, 1983). In contrast, convincing proof exists that several other isozymes isolated from rat liver microsomes are not glycosylated in the native state (Armstrong *et al.*, 1983). **Phosphorylation** reactions appear of significance for the control of cytochrome P450 activity and perhaps also of degradation (Koch and Waxman, 1991).

3.3   THE MULTIPLICITY OF CYTOCHROMES P450

The concept of cytochrome P450 multiplicity had gained universal acceptance in the 1970s based on independent and converging lines of evidence, for example variations in substrate and product selectivities following induction and inhibition, and differences in these selectivities due to biological factors such as animal species and strain, age, sex, and others. The physical separation and characterization (see Section 3.2) of cytochrome P450 enzymes has given a direct proof of their existence, as thoroughly discussed in a number of excellent reviews (e.g. Aström and DePierre, 1986; Gelboin and Friedman, 1985; Guengerich, 1979; Ioannides and Parke, 1987; Lu, 1979; Mannering, 1981; Ullrich and Kremers, 1977).

3.3.1 A modern and powerful nomenclature system for the cytochrome P450 enzymes

Over the years, the number of cytochromes P450 that have been isolated and characterized by a variety of criteria has risen considerably. In particular, human cytochromes P450 have recently received increasing interest and a wealth of significant data can be found in the literature (e.g. Beaune *et al.*, 1986; Boobis and Davies, 1984; Wrighton *et al.*, 1986).

The result of this extraordinary international effort has been on the one hand the publication of innumerable data, and on the other hand much confusion about the identity or non-identity of the many forms reported, and about similarities or dissimilarities between them. Without the essential contributions of molecular biology, such a state of confusion would now have reached absurd proportions. Unravelling the sequence of P450 genes and isozymes has progressively led to a meaningful and robust classification, and a milestone paper was published in 1987 by Nebert and colleagues (Nebert *et al.*, 1987) who proposed a nomenclature for the *P450* **gene superfamily and gene products** based on evolution (Coon and Porter, 1988; Nebert *et al.*, 1989b; Puga and Nebert, 1990). In this nomenclature, genes and gene products are classified in families and subfamilies.

As outlined in Section 1.6, protein sequences within one family are defined as usually having >40% amino acid identity, but there are exceptions. For example, the CYP2D, CYP2J and CYP2K subfamilies include the most distant members of the CYP2 family. Similarly, two mitochondrial P450 proteins, scc and 11b, are included in the CYP11 family although the enzyme sequences are only 34% to 39% identical. Within the same subfamily, mammalian sequences are always >55% identical, but inclusion of non-mammalian vertebrates within the same subfamily drops this value to >46% (Nelson *et al.*, 1993).

The listing of *P450* genes, new protein sequences and recommended nomenclature is now updated every second year (Nebert *et al.*, 1989 and 1991; Nelson *et al.*, 1993). The latest available update of the P450 superfamily is presented in Table 3.2. Important reviews should also be consulted for detailed information (Gonzalez, 1989 and 1990; Guengerich, 1990; Koymans *et al.*, 1993a and 1993b; Nebert and Gonzalez, 1987; Nebert *et al.*, 1989; Porter and Coon, 1991; Soucek and Gut, 1992; Wrighton and Stevens, 1992). As of December 1992, 221 *P450* genes and 12 putative pseudogenes had been described in 31 eukaryotes (including eleven mammalian and three plant species) and in 11 prokaryotes (Nelson *et al.*, 1993).

The CYP1 family contains the enzymes that metabolize, and are induced by, polycyclic aromatic hydrocarbons such as 3-methylcholanthrene. In the CYP2 family, we find the phenobarbital-inducible enzymes that metabolize steroids and a large variety of xenobiotics. The CYP3 family also contains members that are highly active towards steroids and many different drugs. Essential physiological functions are fulfilled by members of the CYP4 family (which oxidize fatty acids) and of the CYP7 and CYP11 families (which metabolize cholesterol). The biosynthesis of steroids involves members of the CYP11, CYP17, CYP19, CYP21 and CYP27 families (Gonzalez, 1992). In humans, a number of cytochromes P450 are of particular significance in the metabolism of drugs and other xenobiotics, i.e. 1A1, 1A2, 2B6, 2C9, 2C10, 2C18, 2D6, 2E1, and 3A. The substrate specificity of most of them is illustrated in the next section.

3.3.2 Substrate specificity of cytochromes P450

As far as xenobiotic metabolism is concerned, a major consequence of cytochrome P450 multiplicity is the substrate specificity of these enzymes, a concept introduced and illustrated in Section 1.6. As apparent in Table 1.3, several isozymes can metabolize a given substrate by the same reaction, but one or a few isozymes are always much more active than the others. In practical terms, many xenobiotic substrates are metabolized mainly or exclusively of a single cytochrome P450. An illustrative list follows which features some important human cytochromes P450 and representative xenobiotic substrates (Cholerton *et al.*, 1992; Guengerich, 1990, 1992a and 1992b; Wrighton and Stevens, 1992):

- CYP1A1:   benzo[*a*]pyrene and other polycyclic aromatic hydrocarbons;
- CYP1A2:   caffeine, 2-naphthylamine and other arylamines, phenacetin, theophylline;
- CYP2C9/10:   hexobarbital, tolbutamide;
- CYP2C18:   cyclophosphamide, diazepam, hexobarbital, omeprazol, proguanil, propranolol;
- CYP2D6:   ajmaline, clomipramine, codeine, debrisoquine, dextromethorphan, encainide, haloperidol, imipramine, methadone, metoprolol, minaprine, perhexiline, phenformine, propafenone, propranolol, sparteine, thioridazine, timolol, tropisetrone;
- CYP2E1:   acetaminophen, acetone, aniline, benzene, carbon tetrachloride, chloroform, chlorzoxazone, diethyl ether, enflurane, ethanol and other alcohols, ethyl carbamate, ethylene dichloride, N-nitrosodimethylamine and other nitrosoamines, styrene, vinyl chloride and bromide;

- **CYP3A:** aflatoxins, bromocryptine, cyclosporine, diazepam, ergotamine, erythromycin, ethynylestradiol, lidocaine, methadone, midozolam, nifedipine and other dihydropyridines, quinidine, terfenadine, triazolam.

Such a list is obviously far from exhaustive, but it is sufficient to convey the concept of isozyme specificity. Interesting speculations on the relationships between substrate specificity of some cytochromes P450 and substrate structure have recently been presented (Smith and Jones, 1992). As often as possible in the chapters to follow, the cytochrome P450 isozymes involved will be mentioned when discussing metabolic reactions.

TABLE 3.2 *The P450 gene superfamily: A table of gene products*[*,†,#] (Nelson *et al.*, 1993; see also Gonzalez, 1990 and 1992; Nebert and Gonzalez, 1987; Soucek and Gut, 1992)

Family, Subfamily and Gene products	P450 isozymes (some of the trivial names in the literature)
P450 1 Family (*Mammalian aryl hydrocarbon hydroxylases; xenobiotic metabolism inducible by polycyclic aromatic hydrocarbons*)	
P450 1A Subfamily	
1A1	Dog (Dah1)
	Guinea-pig (GP 53K, GPc1)
	Hamster (IA1, HSc 1)
	Human (P_1, c, form 6)
	Monkey (MKah1)
	Mouse ($P_1$450)
	Rabbit (form 6)
	Rat (c, βNF-B)
	Trout (IA1)
1A2	Chicken (pP-450IA-61)
	Dog (P-450-D3, P-450-D2, Dah2)
	Hamster (MC4)
	Human (P_3, d, form 4)
	Monkey (MKah1)
	Mouse (P_3, P_2)
	Rabbit (LM_4)
	Rat (P-448, d, HCB)
P450 2 Family (*Mammalian; xenobiotic and steroid metabolism; constitutive and xenobiotic-inducible*)	
P450 2A Subfamily	
2A1	Rat (a1, a, 3, UT-F, RLM2b, IF-3)
2A2	Rat (a2, RLM2, UT-4)
2A3	Rat (a3)
2A4	Mouse (15αoh-1)
2A5	Mouse (15αoh-2)
2A6	Human (IIA3, P450(1), IIA4)
2A7	Human (IIA4)
2A8	Hamster (AFB, MC1)
2A9	Hamster (MC1-81)
2A10	Rabbit (NMa)
2A11	Rabbit (NMc)

TABLE 3.2 continued.

Family, Subfamily and Gene products	P450 isozymes (some of the trivial names in the literature)

P450 2B Subfamily (*Includes phenobarbital-inducible forms*)

2B1	Rat (b, PB-4, PB-B, PBRLM5, IIB1-WM [variant])
2B2	Rat (e, PB-5, PB-D, PBRLM6)
2B3	Rat
2B4	Rabbit (LM2, B0, B1, b14, b46, b54)
2B4P	Rabbit [pseudogene]
2B5	Rabbit (b52, HP1, B2)
2B6	Human (LM2, IIB1, hIIB)
2B7P	Human (IIB2 [pseudogene])
2B8	Rat [gene IV]
2B9	Mouse (pf26)
2B10	Mouse (pf3/46)
2B11	Dog (IIB)
2B12	Rat (IIB-gene 4)
2B13	Mouse (16αoh-b)
2B14	Rat (2By)
2B14P	Rat (2Bx)

P450 2C Subfamily (*Constitutive forms; includes sex-specific forms*)

2C1	Rabbit (PBc1)
2C2	Rabbit (PBc2, K, pHP2)
2C3	Rabbit (PBc3, 3b, 2C3v)
2C4	Rabbit (PBc4, 1-88)
2C5	Rabbit (form 1)
2C6	Rat (PB1, k, PB-C, pTF2, RLM5a, PB2, 2C6 [product of alternative splicing])
2C7	Rat (f, RLM5b, pTF1)
2C8	Human (form 1, IIC2, hP2-1, mp-12, mp-20, HPH, pB8)
2C9	Human (MP-1, MP-2, IIC1, human-2, mp-4, hPA22)
2C10	Human (mp, mp-8, [cloning artifact of 2C9?])
2C11	Rat (h, M-1, 16α, 2c, UT-A, RLM5, male, UT-2)
2C12	Rat (i, 15β, 2d, UT-I, female, F-2)
2C13	Rat (+g, −g, RLM3, UT-5)
2C14	Rabbit (pHP3)
2C15	Rabbit (b32-3)
2C16	Rabbit
2C17	Human (254c [splice variant of 2C18/2C19 ?])
2C18	Human (29c, 6b)
2C19	Human (11a)
2C20	Monkey (MKmp13)
2C21	Dog (DM 1-1)
2C22	Rat (Md)
2C23	Rat (cl17)
2C24	Rat
2C25	Hamster (hsm1)
2C26	Hamster (hsm2)
2C27	Hamster (hsm3)
2C28	Hamster (hsm4)

TABLE 3.2 continued.

Family, Subfamily and Gene products	P450 isozymes (some of the trivial names in the literature)
P450 2D Subfamily	
2D1	Rat (db1, UT-7, CMF1a)
2D2	Rat (db2, CMF2)
2D3	Rat (db3)
2D4	Rat (db4, CMF3)
2D5	Rat (db5, CMF1b)
2D6	Human (db1)
2D7P	Human (IID7 [pseudogene])
2D8P	Human (IID8 [pseudogene])
2D9	Mouse (16α, ca)
2D10	Mouse (cb)
2D11	Mouse (cc)
2D12	Mouse (cd)
2D13	Mouse (ce)
2D14	Cow (2D)
P450 2E Subfamily (*Ethanol-inducible*)	
2E1	Human (j)
	Monkey (MKj1)
	Mouse (j)
	Rabbit (3a)
	Rat (j, RLM6, DM)
2E2	Rabbit
P450 2F Subfamily	
2F1	Human
2F2	Mouse (Nah-2)
P450 2G Subfamily	
2G1	Rat (olf1)
	Rabbit (NMb)
P450 2H Subfamily (*Chicken P450*)	
2H1	Chicken (pCHP3, PB15)
2H2	Chicken (pCHP7)
P450 2J Subfamily	
2J1	Rabbit (ib)
P450 2K Subfamily	
2K1	Trout (LMC2)
P450 3 Family (*Mammalian; xenobiotic and steroid metabolism; steroid-inducible*)	
P450 3A Subfamily	
3A1	Rat (pcn1, PCNa, 6β-4, pIGC2)
3A2	Rat (pcn2, PCNb/c, 6β-1/3)
3A3	Human (HLp)
3A4	Human (nf-25, hPCN1, nf-10)
3A5	Human (hPCN3, HLp2)
3A5P	Human
3A6	Rabbit (3c)

TABLE 3.2 continued.

Family,
   Subfamily and
      Gene products
	P450 isozymes
	(some of the trivial
	names in the literature)

3A7	Human (HFLa, HFL33, HLp2)
3A8	Monkey (MKnf2)
3A9	Rat (olf2)
3A10	Hamster
3A11	Mouse (IIIAm1)
3A12	Dog (PBD-1)
3A13	Mouse (IIIAm2)

P450 4 Family (*Mammalian fatty acid ω- and (ω-1)-hydroxylases; peroxisome proliferator-inducible*)

P450 4A Subfamily

4A1	Rat (LAω)
4A2	Rat (IVA2, k-5, k-2)
4A3	Rat (IVA3, DM-2)
4A4	Rabbit (p-2, LPGw)
4A5	Rabbit (KDB3, kd)
4A6	Rabbit (ka-1, KDA6, LPGAw-1)
4A7	Rabbit (ka-2, R4, LPGAw-2)
4A8	Rat (PP1)
4A9	Human (HL14Acon)
4A10	Mouse (A14)
4A11	Human (HK$_w$)

P450 4B Subfamily

4B1	Human (lung P450, p-2-like, HLCF1) Rabbit (form 5) Rat (form 5, L-2)

P450 4C Subfamily

4C1	Cockroach (P-450)

P450 4D Subfamily

4D1	Fruit fly

P450 4E Subfamily

4E1	Fruit fly

P450 4F Subfamily

4F1	Rat (A3)
4F2	Human

P450 5 Family

5	Human (TXA synthase)

P450 6 Family (*In insects*)

P450 6A Subfamily

6A1	House fly (VIA1)
6A2	Fruit fly (DM P450-B1)

P450 6B Subfamily

6B1	Black swallowtail butterfly (CYP6B1v1, CYP6B1v2)

TABLE 3.2 continued.

Family, Subfamily and Gene products	P450 isozymes (some of the trivial names in the literature)
P450 7 Family (*Mammalian cholesterol 7α-hydroxylase*)	
7	Cow (7α)
	Human (7α)
	Rabbit (7α)
	Rat (7α)
P450 10 Family (*In snails*)	
10	Pond snail (P-450)
P450 11 Family (*Mammalian mitochondrial steroid hydroxylases*)	
P450 11A Subfamily (*Cholesterol side-chain cleavage*)	
11A1	Chicken (scc)
	Cow (scc)
	Human (scc)
	Pig (scc)
	Rat (scc)
P450 11B Subfamily (*Steroid 11β-hydroxylases*)	
11B1	Cow (CB11β-7, pcP-450(11β)-3, 11β-4)
	Human (11β)
	Mouse (11β)
	Rat (11β)
11B2	Cow
	Human (11β-2)
	Mouse (aldo synthase)
	Rat (11β, aldo 2, aldo)
11B3	Rat (B3)
11B4	Cow (CB11β-20)
11B5P	Cow (CB11β-1)
11B6P	Cow (CB11β-3)
11B7P	Cow (λB11β(15-1), (15-2), CB11β-21)
11B8P	Rat (B4)
P450 17 Family (*Mammalian steroid 17α-hydroxylase*)	
17	Chicken (17α)
	Cow (17α)
	Guinea-pig (17α)
	Human (17α)
	Mouse (17α)
	Pig (17α)
	Rat (17α)
	Trout (17α)
P450 19 Family (*Mammalian steroid aromatase*)	
19	Chicken (arom)
	Goldfish (arom)
	Human (arom)
	Mouse (gES-M10)

TABLE 3.2 continued.

Family, Subfamily and Gene products	P450 isozymes (some of the trivial names in the literature)
	Rat (arom)
	Trout (arom)

P450 21 Family (*Mammalian steroid 21-hydroxylases*)

   21A Subfamily

21A1	Cow (c21)
	Mouse (c21A)
	Pig (c21)
	Sheep (c21)
21A1P	Human (c21A [pseudogene])
21A2	Human (c21B)
21A2P	Mouse (c21B [pseudogene])

P450 24 Family

24	Rat (cc24)

P450 27 Family (*Mammalian steroid hydroxylase; mitochondrial*)

27	Human (27-hydroxylase)
	Rabbit (26-ohp)
	Rat (25-hydroxylase, P-450 26/25)

P450 51 Family (*Yeast 14-demethylase*)

51	*Saccharomyces cerevisiae* (14DM, ERG11)
	Candida tropicalis (14DM)
	C. albicans (14DM)

P450 52 Family (*In yeasts; alkane-inducible*)

   P450 52A Subfamily

52A1	*C. tropicalis* (alk1)
52A2	*C. tropicalis* (alk2)
52A3	*C. maltosa* (Cm1, ALK1-A, ALK1-B)
52A4	*C. maltosa* (Cm2, ALK3-A, ALK3-B)
52A5	*C. maltosa* (ALK2-A, ALK2-B)
52A6	*C. tropicalis* (alk3)
52A7	*C. tropicalis* (alk4)
52A8	*C. tropicalis* (alk5)
52A9	*C. maltosa* (ALK5-A)
52A10	*C. maltosa* (ALK7-A)
52A11	*C. maltosa* (ALK8-A)

   P450 52B Subfamily

52B1	*C. tropicalis* (alk6)

   P450 52C Subfamily

52C1	*C. tropicalis* (alk7)
52C2	*C. maltosa* (ALK6-A)

   P450 52D Subfamily

52D1	*C. maltosa* (ALK4-A)

TABLE 3.2 continued.

Family, Subfamily and Gene products	P450 isozymes (some of the trivial names in the literature)
P450 53 Family (*In yeasts*)	
53	*Aspergillus niger* (bphA)
P450 54 Family (*In yeasts*)	
54	*Neurospora crassa* (CI-1)
P450 55 Family (*In yeasts*)	
55	*Fusarium oxysporum* (dNIR)
P450 56 Family (*In yeasts*)	
56	*Saccharomyces cerevisiae* (DIT2)
P450 57 Family (*In yeasts*)	
57	*Nectria haematococca* (pdaT9)
P450 71 Family (*In plants*)	
71	Avocado
P450 72 Family (*In plants*)	
72	Madagascar periwinkle (P450)
P450 73 Family (*In plants*)	
73	Jerusalem artichoke (Ca4h)
P450 101 Family (*In prokaryotes*)	
101	*Pseudomonas putida* (cam)
P450 102 Family (*In prokaryotes*)	
102	*Bacillus megaterium* (BM-3)
P450 103 Family (*In prokaryotes*)	
103	*Agrobacterium tumefaciens* (pinF1)
P450 104 Family (*In prokaryotes*)	
104	*A. tumefaciens* (pinF2)
P450 105 Family (*In prokaryotes*)	
105A Subfamily	
105A1	*Streptococcus griseolus* (SU1)
105B Subfamily	
105B1	*S. griseolus* (SU2)
105C Subfamily	
105C1	*Streptococcus* species (choP)
105D Subfamily	
105D1	*S. griseys* (soy)

TABLE 3.2 continued.

Family, Subfamily and Gene products	P450 isozymes (some of the trivial names in the literature)
P450 106 Family (*In prokaryotes*)	
106	*Bacillus megaterium* (BM-1)
P450 107 Family (*In prokaryotes*)	
107A Subfamily	
107A1	*Saccharopolyspora erythraea* (eryF)
107B Subfamily	
107B1	*Sacc. erythraea* (orf405)
P450 108 Family (*In prokaryotes*)	
108	*Pseudomonas* species (terp)
P450 109 Family (*In prokaryotes*)	
109	*Bacillus subtilis* (ORF405)
P450 110 Family (*In prokaryotes*)	
110	*Anabaena* species (ORF3)
P450 111 Family (*In prokaryotes*)	
111	*Pseudomonas* species (lin)

*The author is deeply indebted to Prof. Daniel W. Nebert, University of Cincinnati Medical Center, for making available a preprint of the update paper by Nelson *et al.* (1993).

†Gene products (proteins) are designated here as, e.g. 1A1. Equally correct are the designation P450 1A1 or CYP1A1. In contrast, Greek letters, subscripts and superscripts must be avoided, and as examples $P450_{arom}$, $P450_{7\alpha}$ or $P450_{11\beta}$ should be referred to as P450arom, P450c7 or P450c11b, respectively (Nelson *et al.*, 1993).

#A pseudogene is a region of a chromosome with sequence similarity with a functional gene, but which contains deleterious mutations and is apparently not transcribed/translated (Guengerich, 1989).

3.4 BINDING OF DIATOMIC GASES, SUBSTRATES AND LIGANDS

A very large variety of chemicals bind to cytochrome P450, their affinity being characterized by several types of **binding selectivity**. First, isozyme specificity is of common occurrence but will not be considered here. Second, there is often a marked selectivity of ligands towards the various electronic states of cytochrome P450 (degree of oxidation and spin form), an aspect that will be given some attention below. Last and most important in the present context is a "selectivity" in terms of distinct modes of binding to the enzyme (Section 1.5).

3.4.1 Binding of diatomic gases

Some diatomic gases, i.e. molecular oxygen, carbon monoxide and nitric oxide, bind to cytochrome P450 (and other metalloporphyrins) as ligands of the iron cation. Molecular oxygen is the physiological ligand relevant to the present context (Section 3.5.2), while the latter two gases produce enzyme inhibition upon binding (reviewed in Testa and Jenner, 1981).

Molecular oxygen has a strong affinity for ferrous cytochrome P450, to which it is bound as a bent ligand; in other words, an angle exists between the line connecting the two oxygen atoms and that connecting the Fe–S ions. In addition, there is a marked electron transfer from Fe(II) to O_2 such that the latter is best viewed as bound superoxide $O_2^{\bullet -}$ (Fig. 3.5) (Collman et al., 1976b; Jung et al., 1979; Traylor et al., 1981). This electron transfer is of considerable biochemical significance in the catalytic cycle of cytochrome P450, as discussed in Section 3.5.

Carbon monoxide binds avidly to ferroporphyrins and is thus an inhibitor of hemoproteins. Quantum mechanical calculations (e.g. Jung et al., 1979) and experimental evidence indicate that the Fe(II)–C–O system is normally linear (Fig. 3.5) in contrast to the bent Fe(II)–O–O system. However, the presence of neighbouring amino acid residues in the active site of hemoproteins, including cytochrome P450, forces the FeCO system into an unfavourable bent conformation. As a result, CO affinity is considerably decreased and these enzymes are thus protected against massive poisoning by endogenous CO (Collman et al., 1976b). While all cytochrome P450 isozymes bind CO in their ferrous state, they nevertheless display different affinities most likely because of small differences in steric hindrance within the active site (Gray, 1982 and 1983).

Among other features, the **UV-visible spectra** of ferric cytochromes P450 have a typical Soret peak at approximately 417–419 nm in the low-spin form and at approximately 393 nm in the high-spin form; upon reduction, this band appears at 411–412 nm (e.g. White and Coon, 1982). The binding of CO to cytochrome P450 occurs with marked changes in the UV-visible spectrum of the enzyme, most remarkably a red-shift in the Soret peak, which appears at 448–452 nm (e.g. Wang et al., 1983). This shift in the Soret band is of historical significance since it allowed the first detection of cytochrome P450 as a pigment absorbing at 450 nm (Omura and Sato, 1964). Fig. 3.6 shows an example of the absolute spectra of total cytochrome P450 in liver microsomes from untreated male rats (Iba and Mannering, 1987; Iba et al., 1993; Nerland et al., 1981). In addition, crystallographic studies have revealed the precise 3-dimensional structure of the cytochrome P450cam–CO complex (Poulos and Raag, 1992; Raag and Poulos, 1989).

Nitric oxide (NO) is another diatomic gas which binds to cytochrome P450, but in contrast to O_2 and CO it also shows marked affinity for the oxidized form of the enzyme (Ebel et al., 1975; Hu and Kincaid, 1991). Like CO, it inhibits the enzyme, since both ligands occupy the position normally taken by O_2 (see Gray, 1983 for the analogous binding of these three XO gases). However, the mechanism of action of CO and NO are not identical since the P450(FeII)NO complex breaks down to a P420(FeII)NO complex with the Fe(II)-thiolate bond either severely distorted or completely broken (Duthu and Shertzer, 1979; O'Keeffe et al., 1978). The blue shift from 450 to 420 nm is due to the loss of electron transfer from the thiolate to the ferric ion (Section 3.2.1).

3.4.2 Substrate binding

Substrates bind to cytochrome P450 in a so-called hydrophobic pocket located near the catalytic site. Substrates are thus quite distinct from **ligands** whose binding primarily involves the iron atom (see previous and next sections). Substrate binding occurs primarily to the oxidized cytochrome P450, with rate constants in the range 10^4–10^5 M^{-1} s^{-1}, orders of magnitude faster than to the reduced enzyme (Blanck et al., 1977).

Upon substrate binding, the oxidized cytochrome P450 present in low-spin form changes to the high-spin form, detected in the absolute spectrum by a blue shift of the Soret peak (Fig. 3.7A). This change is best visualized in a difference spectrum (enzyme preparation in reference cuvette, enzyme preparation plus substrate in sample cuvette) where it appears as a trough at about 420 nm and a peak at 385–390 nm (Backes and Canady, 1981; Hall, 1986; Kumaki and Nebert, 1978; Kumaki et al., 1978; Schenkman et al., 1981). A difference spectrum of this type is

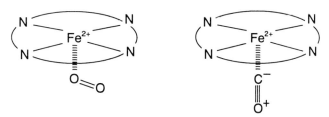

FIGURE 3.5 Simplified representation of molecular oxygen (A) and carbon monoxide (B) bound to a ferroporphyrin.

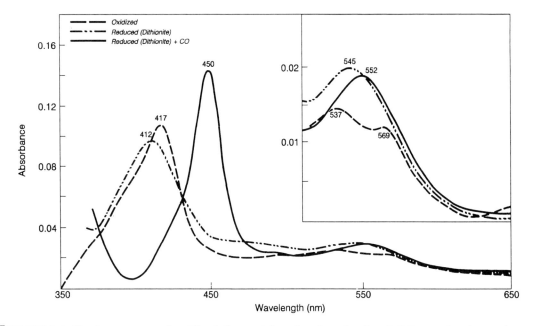

FIGURE 3.6 Absolute spectra of oxidized (low-spin), reduced, and reduced CO-complexed cytochrome P450 in microsomes from untreated male rats; the reference cuvette contained the same microsomal suspension in which cytochrome P450 (but not cytochrome b_5) had been destroyed by linoleic acid hydroperoxide. Reproduced from Nerland *et al.* (1981) with the permission of the copyright holder.

illustrated in Fig. 3.7B and is termed a **type I spectrum**. Because the proportion of enzyme molecules with bound substrate is proportional to the differential absorbance ($\Delta A = A_{390}-A_{420}$), the method provides a direct and non-destructive quantitation of the enzyme–substrate complex, and the dissociation constant of this complex (K_s) can thus be determined. The literature abounds in data of this type.

The **mechanism of substrate binding**, both *per se* and in contrast to ligand binding, is of great interest from a basic enzymological viewpoint and for a better understanding of structure–metabolism relationships. A limited number of examples show the binding of substrates to cytochrome P450 to be entropy-driven, in agreement with the hydrophobic nature of the interaction (Jänig *et al.*, 1977; Kühn-Velten, 1991). Indeed, the loss of the sixth ligand upon substrate binding should evoke an increase in entropy of the system, especially when that ligand is a water molecule or rather a cluster of water molecules. Thus, water displacement was observed conclusively upon binding of cholesterol to cytochrome P450scc (Jacobs *et al.*, 1987). The free energy of binding of hydrocarbons was found to be about −0.7 kcal mol^{-1} per methylene group,

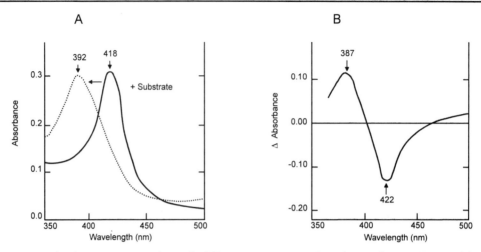

FIGURE 3.7 Absolute spectrum (A) and difference spectrum (B) of cytochrome P450 with bound substrate. Reproduced from Hall (1986) with the permission of the copyright holder.

a value similar to the free energy of partitioning of the same compounds between octanol and water, but larger than their free energy of microsomal partitioning (*ca* $-0.3 \text{ kcal mol}^{-1}$ per methylene unit) (Backes *et al.*, 1982). Clearly, octanol/water distribution is a good indicator of the binding of hydrocarbons to cytochrome P450, which involves a combination of Van der Waals interactions and hydration/dehydration processes.

Modern methods have yielded valuable insights into the **modes of binding** of substrates to cytochrome P450, an important factor which may contribute to both substrate selectivity and product regioselectivity of metabolic reactions. Indeed, the binding modes may be **productive** or **non-productive**, meaning that the target group(s) may or may not be properly positioned for catalysis (Tsubaki *et al.*, 1992). Distinct productive binding modes may also exist, each of which will direct catalytic attack to another target group. Thus, acetanilide, which is ring-hydroxylated by cytochrome P450LM4, was shown by NMR to bind with its phenyl ring in close proximity to the iron atom of this isozyme (Novak and Vatsis, 1982).

Site-directed mutagenesis studies are now contributing increasingly to an understanding of the role of specific amino acid residues in substrate binding, and more generally in enzymic mechanisms (e.g. Atkins and Sligar, 1988; Imai and Nakamura, 1988; Johnson, 1992; Johnson *et al.*, 1992; Koymans *et al.*, 1993). Here again, X-ray crystallographic studies have been most enlightening in unravelling the **3D-structure** of the cytochrome P450cam–camphor complex (Poulos, 1988; Poulos and Raag, 1989; Poulos *et al.*, 1985 and 1986). As shown in Fig. 3.8, camphor is bound distally to the thiolate ligand in the substrate and O_2 binding pocket, with its carbon-5 (5-*exo*-hydroxycamphor is the sole metabolite being formed) close to the catalytic site. Camphor binding involves a hydrogen bond with the phenolic group of Tyr-95, and Van der Waals interactions with the aliphatic and aromatic amino acids bordering the binding site, in particular Phe-87, Phe-98, Leu-244, Val-247, Thr-252, Val-295, as well as Ile-395 and Phe-193 which form a "cap" over the substrate molecule and thus do not appear in Fig. 3.8.

Using the known 3D-structure of CYP101, techniques of computational chemistry and molecular modelling are currently making a major impact on our understanding and visualization of substrate–enzyme recognition and structure–metabolism relationships. Thus, the binding and regioselectivity of reaction of (*R*)- and (*S*)-nicotine with CYP101 could be predicted and explained successfully (Jones *et al.*, 1993). Furthermore, the 3D-structure of CYP101 can be used as a starting template to model other cytochromes P450. This is exemplified by CYP17, whose

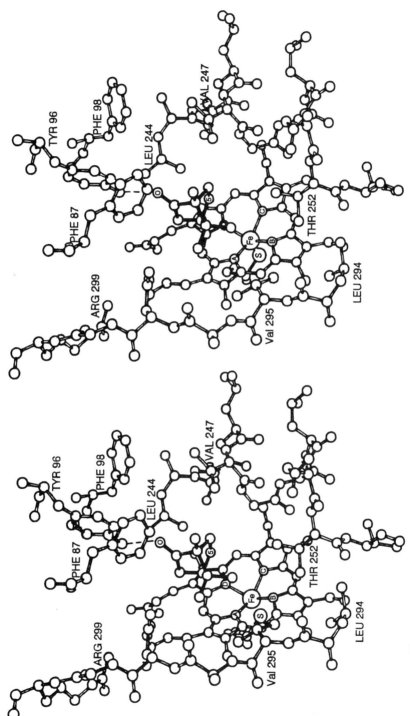

FIGURE 3.8 View of the substrate-binding site of cytochrome P450cam with bound camphor. To be visualized in 3D, this stereoscopic image must be altered in size by photocopying to reach a distance of about 6 cm between the same atoms. Reproduced from Poulos *et al.* (1985) with the permission of the copyright holder.

model thus constructed suggests the possibility of two modes of binding of steroid substrates at the active site (Laughton *et al.*, 1990). Studies of major therapeutic significance have unravelled the 3D topography and structure–metabolism relationships of CYP2D6, a human cytochrome P450 that metabolizes many basic drugs and is defective in so-called "poor metabolizers" (Koymans *et al.*, 1992).

3.4.3 Ligand binding

Cytochrome P450 ligands are compounds able to bind as a sixth ligand to the heme iron; this ability results from the presence of a functional group characterized by available electron lone-pair(s) (i.e. nucleophilic heteroatoms) or a (formal) negative charge (see Testa and Jenner, 1981, for an extensive review). The interaction of ligands with cytochrome P450 is thus primarily electrostatic in nature, and not unexpectedly appears mainly enthalpy-driven (Jänig *et al.*, 1977). Typical ligands include:

(a)   nitrogen-containing compounds such as primary amines and aromatic azaheterocyclic derivatives;
(b)   oxygen-containing compounds such as alcohols, phenols, ketones and ethers;
(c)   and certain anions such as cyanide.

Nitrogen-containing compounds are stronger ligands than oxygenated compounds; when they bind to oxidized cytochrome P450, they shift the high-spin form and the O-liganded low-spin form to an N-liganded low-spin form. This results in a marked red shift of the Soret band; the difference spectrum exhibits a peak around 425–430 nm and a trough at about 390 or 410 nm, and is called a **type II spectrum**. As a typical example, the binding spectrum of a pyridine derivative is shown in Fig. 3.9, which also demonstrates the concentration dependence of the phenomenon (Repond *et al.*, 1986).

Oxygenated compounds, being weaker ligands, will as a rule produce a detectable binding spectrum only when interacting with oxidized high-spin cytochrome P450 and thereby eliciting a shift to the low-spin form (Andersson and Dawson, 1984). Again a red shift of the Soret band is produced, the difference spectrum exhibiting a peak at about 420 nm and a trough at 385–390 nm. Such a difference spectrum being the mirror image of a type I spectrum is often called a **reverse type I (RI) spectrum**, or alternatively—and more adequately—a **modified type II (MII) spectrum**. The binding spectrum of cianidanol (a polyphenolic flavonoid) with native rat liver microsomes is shown in Fig. 3.10 as a representative example (Beyeler *et al.*, 1983).

The various binding spectra and the spin shifts discussed above are summarized in Fig. 3.11; abundant additional information can be found in a number of reviews (e.g. Griffin *et al.*, 1975; Kumaki and Nebert, 1978; Mannering, 1981; Ruckpaul and Rein, 1984; Schenkman *et al.*, 1981). It is clear however that the type of spectrum elicited depends as much on the interacting compound as on the enzyme preparation; when a ligand coordinates through an oxygen atom the spectrum of a low-spin cytochrome P450 will remain unchanged (White and Coon, 1982). Further confusion is due to the ability of many compounds to act both as substrates and ligands (productive versus non-productive binding modes), producing either a type I or a type II/MII spectrum depending on their concentration and on the particular enzyme preparation being used (Kumaki *et al.*, 1978). Thus, when hexobarbital interacts with rat liver microsomes it elicits a type I spectral change at low concentrations, and a modified type II spectral change at higher concentrations. Also, various nitrosamines produce either a type I or a modified type II spectral change with liver microsomes of mice pretreated with phenobarbital or 3-methylcholanthrene,

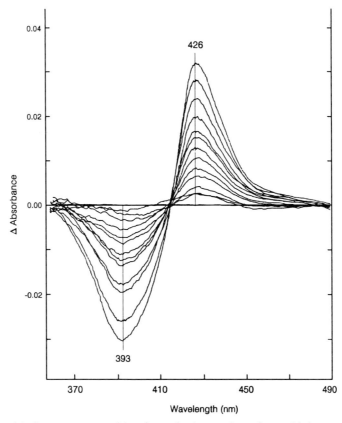

FIGURE 3.9 Type II binding spectra resulting from the interaction of 4-pyridylpentanamide (0.4–28 μM) with a microsomal suspension (initial cytochrome P450 concentration 3.1 μM) from phenobarbital-induced rats. Reproduced from Repond *et al.* (1986) with the permission of the copyright holder.

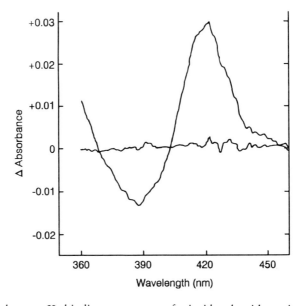

FIGURE 3.10 Modified type II binding spectrum of cianidanol with native rat liver microsomes. Reproduced from Beyeler *et al.* (1983) with the permission of the copyright holder.

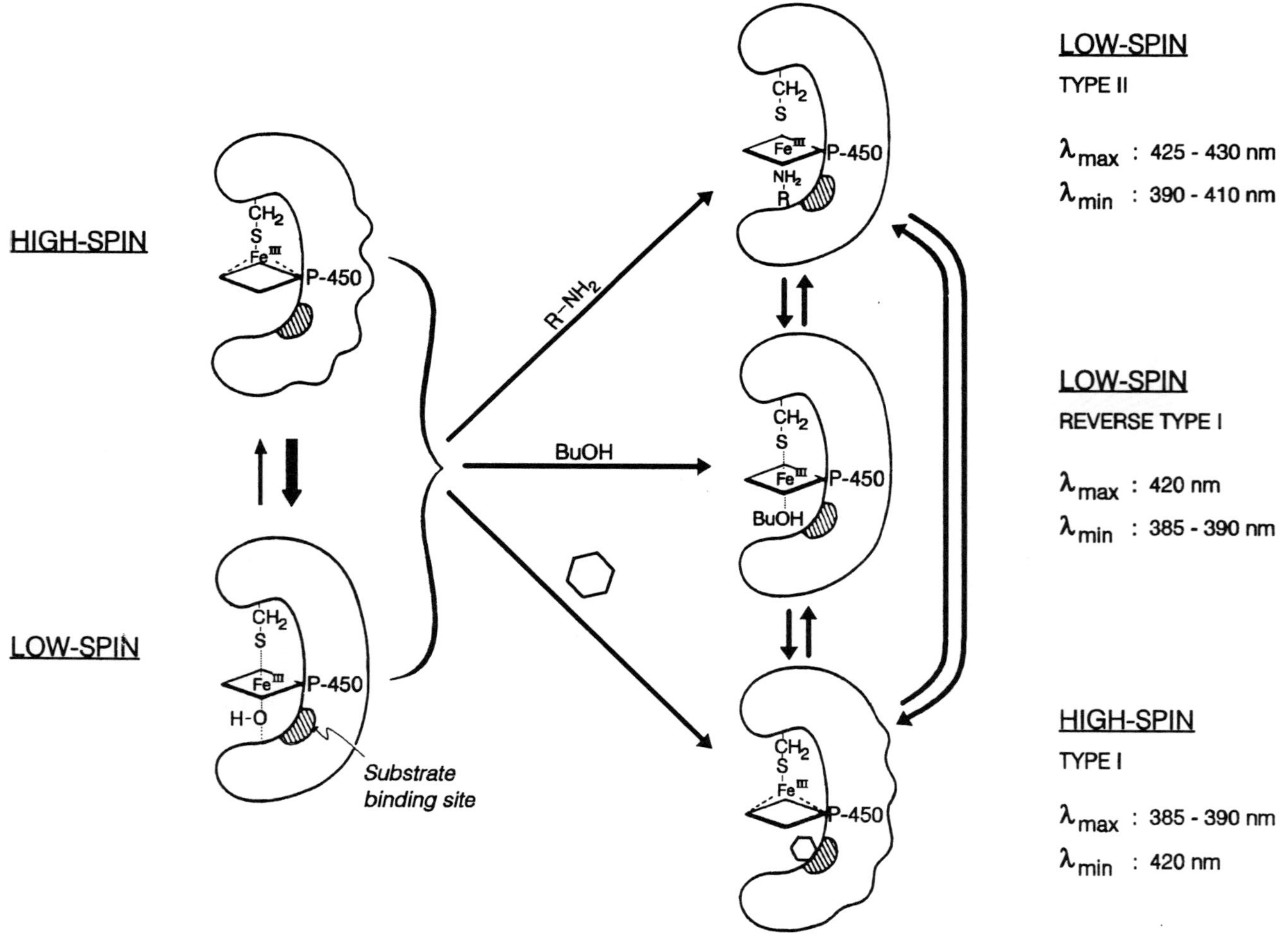

FIGURE 3.11 Schematic representation of the interaction of stronger ligands (e.g. primary amines), weaker ligands (e.g. butanol) and substrates (e.g. cyclohexane) with cytochrome P450, resulting in type II, modified type II (reverse type I), and type I difference spectra, respectively. Reproduced from Mannering (1981) with the permission of the copyright holder.

respectively (Appel et al., 1979). Similarly, there are two binding sites of pyridine in cytochrome P450cam, namely the iron atom and the camphor binding site (Ristau and Jung, 1991).

While oxygenated ligands bind only to oxidized cytochrome P450, some stronger ligands of the pyridine and imidazole type also interact with the reduced form of the enzyme, the resulting complexes being characterized by a Soret band around 445–450 nm. For example, the well-known cytochrome P450 inhibitor metyrapone (**3.I**) binds with comparable avidity to oxidized and reduced states of phenobarbital-inducible cytochromes P450 alike (reviewed in Testa and Jenner, 1981). Also, the rate constants of association of pyridine are about $10^4 \text{ M}^{-1} \text{ s}^{-1}$ to both the ferric and ferrous forms, while those of imidazole are about 100 and $10 \text{ M}^{-1} \text{ s}^{-1}$, respectively (Blanck et al., 1977). **Isocyanides (3.II)**, notably ethyl isocyanide, are able to bind to the oxidized (type II spectrum) and reduced (Soret band at 455 nm) forms of cytochrome P450; the electronic similarity of these compounds to carbon monoxide is obvious (see Fig. 3.5) (see Testa and Jenner, 1981).

3.I

3.II

Some **anions** are strong ligands of the heme iron, most notably the cyanide ion which elicits a modified type II spectrum with oxidized cytochrome P450; it has less affinity for the reduced enzyme (Sono and Dawson, 1982).

3.4.4 Direct acting inhibitors of cytochrome P450

Inhibition of cytochrome P450 activity involves a variety of mechanisms which can, rather schematically, be classified as follows:

- **Case A**: Action on the enzymatic macromolecule itself (inhibition in the proper sense), or **Case B**: elsewhere (effect on the membrane, on the electron transfer systems, or on the synthesis or degradation of the enzyme);
- The action at the enzyme (case A) can be mediated by the compound under consideration (direct inhibition, **Case A.1**) or by a metabolite generated *in situ* (mechanism-based inhibition, **Case A.2**).

Case B results from effects on the environment, interactions and regulation of the enzyme and falls outside the scope of this volume. As for case A.2, it is a consequence of cytochrome P450-mediated reactions and will be documented as necessary in the relevant chapters. The present section is thus devoted to case A.1, direct inhibition of cytochrome P450.

Any two substrates competing for the same active site will inhibit each other's metabolism to an extent which depends on their relative concentrations and affinities. This description fits straightforward cases of **competitive inhibition** as well as more complex situations encountered in enzyme systems; it will not be further discussed here. As far as **cytochrome P450 ligands** are concerned, their inhibitory action results from a mechanism which is both specific and, often, highly effective, leading to marked pharmacodynamic effects in a number of cases (Murray,

1987). Indeed, cytochrome P450 ligands will inhibit metabolism by displacement of the substrate and/or by keeping the enzyme in a low-spin form that cannot be reduced by cytochrome P450-reductase.

It is therefore tempting to venture the prediction that the stronger the ligand capacity, the more potent the inhibitory effect, provided steric hindrance does not interfere with access and binding to the iron atom. This is verified when comparing globally the two classes of oxygenated and nitrogenated ligands (see the many data compiled by Testa and Jenner, 1981). However, such a model fails to account for differences between homologous ligands, the inhibitory potency of which is often dependent upon **additional interactions** with the active site, particularly hydrophobic ones. For example, a large series of variously hydroxylated and O-alkylated **flavonoids** (both of natural and semisynthetic origin) were shown to be effective inhibitors of cytochrome P450-mediated reactions (Beyeler *et al.*, 1988). Spectral and kinetic data and structure–activity relationships were all consistent with the hypothesis that the compounds inhibit the enzyme by binding not only to the Fe(III) atom (via their more accessible and acidic 7-hydroxyl group), but simultaneously also to a lipophilic site in or near the substrate-binding pocket. These interactions are depicted in Fig. 3.12 using cianidanol and its O-alkylated derivatives as example.

Oxygenated ligands include phenols as well as some alcohols, ethers and ketones. For example, naphthoquinones of natural origin were shown to be ligands and inhibitors of cytochrome P450 (Muto *et al.*, 1987). Many xenobiotic metabolites being **phenols** (see Chapter 4), they must be viewed as potential inhibitors of the reaction leading to their formation. Such a mechanism creates the possibility of a **negative feedback** which might have greater significance in *in vitro* incubations than under physiological conditions. The inhibitory capacity of phenolic metabolites is illustrated by the twelve regioisomeric monophenols of benzo[*a*]pyrene (**3.III**), several of which are produced by microsomal oxidation. These compounds were shown to inhibit

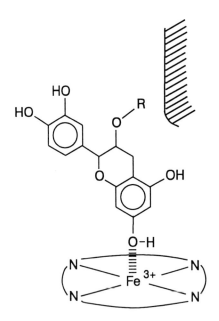

FIGURE 3.12 Proposed mode of binding of cianidanol and its derivatives to cytochrome P450, showing an electrostatic interaction (ligand binding) and a lipophilic interaction. Reproduced from Beyeler *et al.* (1988) with the permission of the copyright holder.

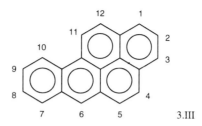

3.III

the cytochrome P450c-mediated oxidation of the parent compound with K_i values ranging from 0.02 to 1.5 μM (Turner *et al.*, 1985).

Some classes of **nitrogenated compounds**, besides being good ligands of cytochrome P450, also display potent inhibitory activity. Metyrapone (**3.I**), mentioned above, is remarkably active, notably towards CYP2B enzymes. Crystallographic studies of the cytochrome P450cam–metyrapone complex have revealed that the two nitrogen atoms of metyrapone both contribute to the binding, N(1) as an iron ligand and N(2) as an H-bond acceptor from Tyr-96 (Poulos and Howard, 1987). The latter interaction closely resembles that experienced by the camphor substrate. This example again demonstrates that the binding of directly acting cytochrome P450 inhibitors is frequently more complex than might be predicted by linear reasoning. Important drugs that are active nitrogenated inhibitors include imidazole antimycotic agents, quinoline antimalarial agents, quinolone antibiotics and H_2-receptor antagonists (Edwards *et al.*, 1988; Murray, 1987; Rekka *et al.*, 1988; Rodrigues *et al.*, 1987; Sheets *et al.*, 1986).

3.5 OXYGEN ACTIVATION BY CYTOCHROME P450

The **catalytic cycle of cytochrome P450** in its monooxygenase function involves a number of steps which can be summarized as follows (Björkhem, 1977; Blanck and Smettan, 1978; Castro, 1980; Estabrook *et al.*, 1982; Gander and Mannering, 1980; Guengerich, 1991; Hawkins and Dawson, 1992; Koymans *et al.*, 1993b; Lewis, 1986; Ortiz de Montellano, 1986; Schenkman and Gibson, 1981; Sligar *et al.*, 1984; White and Coon, 1980):

(a)   binding of the substrate to the ferric form of the enzyme, followed by a shift to the high-spin form (reaction **a** in Fig. 3.13);
(b)   first reduction step to the ferrous form (reaction **b** in Fig. 3.13);
(c)   binding of molecular oxygen (reaction **c** in Fig. 3.13);
(d)   second reduction step (reaction **e** in Fig. 3.13);
(e)   splitting of the dioxygen molecule, i.e. oxygen activation (reaction **g** in Fig. 3.13);
(f)   substrate oxidation and product release (reaction **i** in Fig. 3.13).

A detailed discussion of substrate oxidation will be found in Chapters 4–8 and 11, while other cytochrome P450-mediated reactions (peroxidatic reactions and reductions) are presented in Chapters 10 and 12, respectively. The present section examines the other steps, up to and including oxygen activation.

A simplified representation of the monooxygenase catalytic cycle is given in Fig. 3.13. The electron transport systems responsible for the two reduction steps as shown in this figure are discussed later in Section 3.6. To help the reader, some of the reduced forms of oxygen to be discussed in this and following chapters are presented in Fig. 3.14 (Estabrook, 1984).

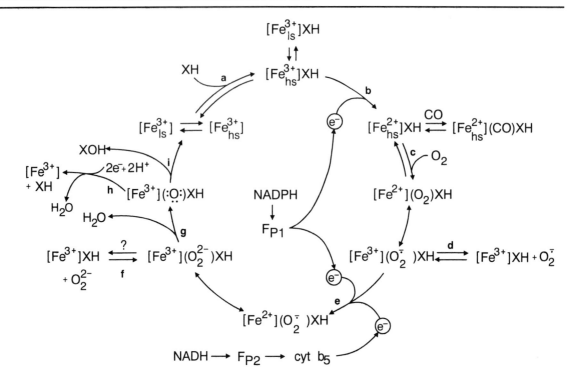

FIGURE 3.13 Catalytic cycle of cytochrome P450 associated with monooxygenation reactions. $[Fe^{3+}]$ = ferricytochrome P450; hs = high spin; ls = low spin; $[Fe^{2+}]$ = ferrocytochrome P450; F_{P1} = NADPH-cytochrome P450 reductase; F_{P2} = NADH-cytochrome b_5 reductase; cyt b_5 = cytochrome b_5; XH = substrate. Reproduced from Mesnil *et al.* (1984).

3.5.1 Substrate binding and the first reduction step

The details of substrate binding to oxidized cytochrome P450 have been discussed in Section 3.4.2, as well as the substrate-induced shift to the high-spin form (reaction **a** in Fig. 3.13). This shift is of critical importance for the enzymatic reaction to proceed, since it permits the first reduction step to occur (see below), and should in fact be viewed as a control mechanism on the function of the enzyme (Backes and Eyer, 1989).

The first reduction equivalent for microsomal and mitochondrial cytochrome P450 comes from NADPH (reaction **b** in Fig. 3.13), but from NADH for cytochrome P450cam. The microsomal enzyme is not reduced directly by NADPH; a flavoprotein known as NADPH-cytochrome P450 reductase (redox potential $-270\,mV$) is essential as an electron transfer system (Section 3.6).

Microsomal ferricytochrome P450 preparations where the low-spin form predominates have a midpoint potential ranging approximately from -360 to $-300\,mV$, while that of NADPH is $-320\,mV$, implying that enzyme reduction is not favoured (Guengerich, 1983; Schenkman and Gibson, 1981). Upon shift to the high-spin form, the midpoint potential becomes more positive, up to about $-175\,mV$ for a cytochrome P450 preparation containing only the high-spin form (Sligar *et al.*, 1979). High-spin ferricytochrome P450 is thus reduced very rapidly as compared to the low-spin form (Backes *et al.*, 1985; Rein *et al.*, 1979).

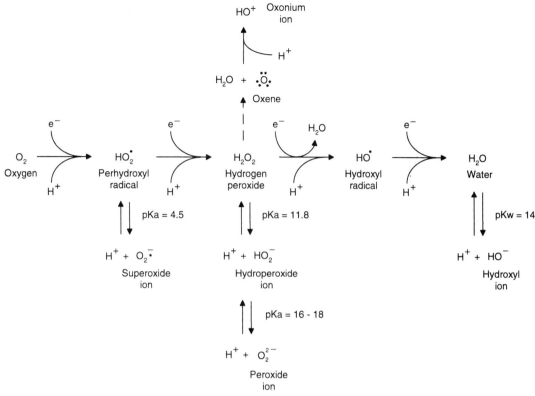

FIGURE 3.14 Steps in sequential reduction of oxygen. Reproduced from Estabrook (1984) with the permission of the copyright holder.

3.5.2 Binding of molecular oxygen and the second reduction step

As discussed in Section 3.4.1, molecular oxygen has a strong affinity for the reduced form of cytochrome P450 (reaction **c** in Fig. 3.13). Two possible resonance structures of this oxygenated complex are $Fe(II)O_2$ and $Fe(III)O_2^{\bullet-}$ (see Fig. 3.5). The latter form best accounts for the reactivity of the complex, in particular the second reduction step and the possible release of $O_2^{\bullet-}$, the superoxide anion-radical (see Section 3.5.3). The thiolate ligand plays a determining role in increasing the electron density on the two oxygen atoms, in particular the distal one, and in allowing O–O bond cleavage (Section 3.5.4) (Higuchi *et al.*, 1990; Rein *et al.*, 1984).

The **ferrous–dioxygen complex** represents a branching point in the catalytic cycle of cytochrome P450. For the monooxygenation reaction to occur, the second electron must be delivered rapidly, otherwise the complex dissociates with release of superoxide (reaction **d** in Fig. 3.13) (see also Section 3.5.3) (White and Coon, 1980). As far as microsomal cytochromes P450 are concerned, this second electron originates either from NADPH or from NADH (redox potential −320 mV) (reaction **e** in Fig. 3.13). In the former case, the electron transfer is again mediated by NADPH-cytochrome P450 reductase (Sections 3.5.1 and 3.6.1). When the reduction equivalent comes from NADH, it first serves to reduce another flavoprotein, NADH-cytochrome b_5 reductase (redox potential −290 mV), before being transferred to cytochrome b_5 (redox potential +30 mV), which in turn reduces the cytochrome P450 (Lewis, 1986). This second electron transfer system is also discussed in Section 3.6.

The origin of the second reduction equivalent, i.e. NADPH-cytochrome P450 reductase or cytochrome b_5, depends on the cytochrome P450 isozyme involved and thus, in microsomal preparations, on the substrate being investigated (Jansson and Schenkman, 1985; Jansson *et al.*, 1987; Kuwahara and Mannering, 1985; Peterson and Prough, 1986).

The doubly reduced cytochrome P450–oxygen–substrate complex can have several possible resonance structures, e.g. $Fe(IV)O_2^{3-}$, $Fe(III)O_2^{2-}$, $Fe(II)O_2^{\bullet-}$, and $Fe(I)O_2$ (Alexander and Goff, 1982). The reactivity of this complex is partly explained by the second resonance structure, i.e. that with bound peroxide anion.

3.5.3 Liberation of reduced dioxygen species

Following reduction, the oxycytochrome P450 complex can liberate reduced dioxygen, thereby escaping the monooxygenation cycle. A priori, two possibilities exist as shown in Fig. 3.13, namely release of **superoxide anion-radical** $O_2^{\bullet-}$ from the $Fe(III)O_2^{\bullet-}$ complex (reaction **d** in Fig. 3.13), or release of peroxide anion O_2^{2-} which protonates to **hydrogen peroxide** H_2O_2 (reaction **f** in Fig. 3.13). The former possibility appears to account for most or all of the activated dioxygen released from cytochrome P450 (Estabrook *et al.*, 1979; Kuthan and Ullrich, 1982; White and Coon, 1980).

Release of activated dioxygen species from cytochrome P450 is commonly observed in *in vitro* metabolic studies (Auclair *et al.*, 1978; Estabrook *et al.*, 1979) and is considered an autoxidative decomposition of the oxygenated enzyme (Oprian *et al.*, 1983). This is a **two-electron oxidase function** of cytochrome P450, and it is favoured by a number of factors, in particular the absence of substrate or the binding of poor substrates (e.g. some barbiturates) or pseudo-substrates such as perfluoroalkanes (Bast, 1986; De Matteis *et al.*, 1991; Kuthan and Ullrich, 1982). Such compounds bind with good affinity to the substrate binding site, but the ternary P450–substrate–dioxygen complex is destabilized to some extent, and substrate oxygenation becomes **uncoupled** from electron transfer. Other factors also play a role, e.g. lipid membrane environment and oxygen concentration. The nature of the isozyme is of great importance, as seen for example with the Thr252Ala mutant of cytochrome P450cam (Martinis *et al.*, 1989; Raag *et al.*, 1991). CYP2E1 is known to exhibit a higher rate of oxidase activity compared to other cytochromes P450, a phenomenon of potential toxicological significance in subjects with high levels of the enzyme (Koop and Kienle, 1993). While the oxidase activity of cytochrome P450 is commonly investigated *in vitro*, there is every reason to believe that it occurs *in vivo* also (Kuthan and Ullrich, 1982).

Much of the confusion about the nature of the activated dioxygen species which are released comes from the reactivity of the superoxide anion-radical. This is a topic of great biological significance which can only be fleetingly acknowledged here. Three reactions of particular significance must be mentioned: (a) the disproportionation of superoxide to hydrogen peroxide and molecular oxygen (Eq. 3.1); (b) the generation of the **hydroxyl radical** ($HO^{\bullet}$) from H_2O_2 and $O_2^{\bullet-}$ (Eq. 3.2); and (c) the production of **singlet oxygen** ($^1O_2$) from $O_2^{\bullet-}$ and $HO^{\bullet}$ (Eq. 3.3):

$$2O_2^{\bullet-} + 2H^+ \rightarrow H_2O_2 + O_2 \qquad (Eq. 3.1)$$

$$H_2O_2 + O_2^{\bullet-} \rightarrow O_2 + HO^- + HO^{\bullet} \qquad (Eq. 3.2)$$

$$O_2^{\bullet-} + HO^{\bullet} \rightarrow {}^1O_2 + HO^- \qquad (Eq. 3.3)$$

Other such reactions have been characterized and also account for the postenzymatic formation of reduced oxygen species (Bielski and Allen, 1977; Duchstein and Gurk, 1992; Gorman and Rodgers, 1981; Ingelman-Sundberg and Hagbjörk, 1982; Ingelman-Sundberg and Johansson, 1984a; Koppenol, 1976; Sawyer and Valentine, 1981; Trager, 1982; Wilshire and Sawyer, 1979).

Eq. 3.2 is the **Haber–Weiss reaction** which, although thermodynamically favourable, is kinetically slow. The role of transition metal ions (e.g. iron Fe^{3+}/Fe^{2+} and copper Cu^{2+}/Cu^{+}) is of noteworthy biological significance in catalyzing the Haber–Weiss reaction (metal-catalyzed Haber–Weiss reaction) (Aust *et al.*, 1985; Kadiiska *et al.*, 1992), e.g.:

$$O_2^{\bullet-} + Fe^{3+} \rightarrow O_2 + Fe^{2+} \tag{Eq. 3.4}$$

$$Fe^{2+} + H_2O_2 \rightarrow Fe^{3+} + HO^- + HO^\bullet \tag{Eq. 3.5}$$

Eq. 3.5 is the **Fenton reaction**, namely the transition metal-catalyzed breakdown of hydrogen peroxide. Note that the Fenton reaction can also break down hydroperoxides (ROOH), yielding HO^- and $RO^\bullet$. These activated oxygen species are responsible for the biological damage caused by molecular oxygen, e.g. **lipid peroxidation** (Section 10.5) and **oxidative degradation of proteins** (Bus and Gibson, 1979; Buettner, 1993; Dix and Aikens, 1993; Halliwell and Gutteridge, 1984; Iwasaki, 1990; Kappus, 1985; Naqui *et al.*, 1986; Packer, 1984; Singh, 1982; Stadtman, 1986, 1988 and 1990; Stadtman and Oliver, 1991). This renders all the more important those enzymes which deactivate hydroperoxides (various peroxidases, see Chapter 10), hydrogen peroxide (e.g. catalase and glutathione peroxidase, see Section 10.4), and superoxide [superoxide: superoxide oxidoreductase; superoxide dismutase; EC 1.15.1.1] (Calabrese and Canada, 1989; Canada and Calabrese, 1989; Deby and Goutier, 1990; McCord, 1979).

3.5.4 Formation and nature of the reactive atomic oxygen species

The monooxygenase reaction implies the transfer to the substrate of an activated **atom** of oxygen (reaction **i** in Fig. 3.13), a reaction that necessitates splitting of the reduced dioxygen (reaction **g** in Fig. 3.13). This reaction is perhaps the least understood step in the cycle, and our present view is still hypothetical in part. From a thermodynamic viewpoint, cleavage of the hydroperoxide anion is favoured over that of molecular oxygen, yet it remains largely endothermic (Jung and Ristau, 1978). As critically discussed by a number of authors, it is likely that the splitting of molecular oxygen is catalyzed by acylation of the iron-bound peroxide, the acyl moiety presumably being a free carboxyl group from a neighbouring amino acid (Sligar *et al.*, 1984; Trager, 1984; White and Coon, 1980). A distal charge relay mechanism may also be implicated (Gerber and Sligar, 1992). A simplified representation of a reasonable mechanism, the so-called **oxenoid pathway**, is shown in Fig. 3.15. Following acylation, irreversible heterolytic cleavage of the peroxide O–O bond occurs, the two electrons departing with the carboxylate anion. Note that this reaction of acylation is accompanied by formation of a water molecule, which together with the oxygenated substrate comprises the two products of the monooxygenase reaction.

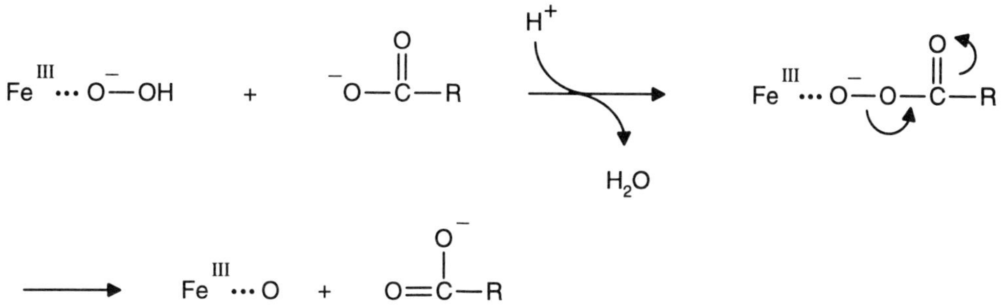

FIGURE 3.15 The "oxenoid pathway", a possible mechanism accounting for peroxide O–O cleavage to form the reactive oxygen atom in cytochrome P450-mediated monooxygenation reactions.

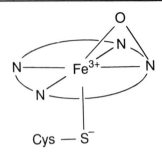

FIGURE 3.16 Minimal energy structure of the $[FeO]^{3+}$ oxo–heme complex as calculated by Jørgensen (1986).

The nature of the activated oxygen atom has been the object of numerous studies (Alexander and Goff, 1982; Dolphin, 1985; Groves, 1985; Rahimtula *et al.*, 1974; White and Coon, 1980). Formally, a number of **resonance structures** can be written for the P450–monooxygen complex generated by dioxygen cleavage, e.g. $PFe(V)O^{2-}$, $P^{+\bullet}Fe(IV)O^{2-}$, $PFe(IV)O^{-}$, $PFe(III)O$, where P is the porphyrin, and Fe(V) and Fe(IV) are the perferryl and ferryl oxidation states, respectively. In the PFe(III)O resonance structure, the oxygen atom is called **oxene**; it is neutral but has only six electrons in its outer layer. In the present book, this oxidation state of the P450–monooxygen complex will be symbolized as $[FeO]^{3+}$. Its one-electron reduced state(s) will be symbolized as $[FeO]^{2+}$ or $[FeOH]^{3+}$ in the following chapters.

The stereoelectronic structure of the $[FeO]^{3+}$ complex may well be more complex than implied by the resonance forms mentioned above. Indeed, quantum mechanical calculations, supported by X-ray structures of synthetic oxo-metal porphyrin compounds, show that the oxygen atom is bent to a significant degree towards one of the four nitrogen atoms (Fig. 3.16). An optimal structure has been calculated with bond lengths of about 1.9 Å (Fe–O) and 1.4 Å (N–O) (Jørgensen, 1986). The bent structure shown in Fig. 3.16 is attractively compatible with the known reactivity of cytochrome P450, in particular hydroxylation of unactivated C–H bonds and stereospecific olefin epoxidation (Chapter 4).

The mechanisms by which substrates are oxygenated, hydroxylated or oxidized by the activated oxygen atom, in particular the "**oxygen rebound mechanism**", will be discussed at length in the following chapters. Here, we wish to point out that, under some *in vitro* conditions, the $[FeO]^{3+}$ complex is found to undergo a further two-electron reduction, water being liberated as a result (reaction **h** in Fig. 3.13). This reaction corresponds to a **four-electron oxidase activity** of cytochrome P450. Evidence for this activity derives in part from experiments on stoichiometry showing that the production of metabolite(s) and H_2O_2 is not sufficient to account for the consumption of NADPH and O_2 (Gorsky *et al.*, 1984). It can even be rationalized from studies with deuterated norcamphor analogues that the more resistant the substrate to hydroxylation, the higher the four-electron oxidase activity (Atkins and Sligar, 1987).

Thus, the four-electron reductase activity of cytochrome P450 results from uncoupling in the enzyme–substrate–oxene ternary complex, due to the fact that the substrate is to some extent resistant to catalytic attack. This uncoupling must be distinguished from the comparable phenomenon occurring in the P450–substrate–dioxygen complex (see Section 3.5.3).

3.5.5 Other sources of oxygen. Outlook

Up to this point, the only source of oxygen we have considered in the catalytic function of cytochrome P450 is molecular oxygen. However, other sources do exist. The splitting of peroxides with transfer of one oxygen atom to a substrate constitutes the **peroxidase function** of cytochrome P450 to be discussed in Section 10.2. Both the monooxygenase and the peroxidatic functions imply peroxide cleavage, followed by transfer of the retained atom of oxygen to the substrate without exchange with an oxygen atom from H_2O, as has been repeatedly shown using oxygen isotopes.

However, there exists a further source of oxygen, namely compounds able to act as oxygen atom donors, e.g. iodosobenzene (**3.IV**) (Gustafsson *et al.*, 1982; Lichtenberger *et al.*, 1976). Here, the oxygen atom is transferred directly to the ferricytochrome P450–substrate complex, and substrate oxygenation occurs without NADPH and O_2. In this reaction, cytochrome P450 acts as an **oxene transferase**, a function of interest under *in vitro* conditions but which, to date, does not appear to have physiological significance.

3.IV

From a mechanistic viewpoint, it is significant to note that the $[FeO]^{3+}$ oxo–heme complex formed from cytochrome P450 and iodosobenzene exchanges its oxygen atom with H_2O, in contrast to the situation when the same complex is derived from molecular oxygen or peroxides (see above). Mechanistic or kinetic factors have been evoked to account for this difference (Heimbrook and Sligar, 1981; Macdonald *et al.*, 1982).

In summary, a number of functions of cytochrome P450 have been considered above (Persson *et al.*, 1990). Their global reactions and stoichiometry are:

monooxygenase function

$$XH + O_2 + 2e^- + 2H^+ \rightarrow XOH + H_2O \qquad \text{(Eq. 3.6)}$$

two-electron oxidase function

$$O_2 + 2e^- + 2H^+ \rightarrow H_2O_2 \qquad \text{(Eq. 3.7)}$$

four-electron oxidase function

$$O_2 + 4e^- + 4H^+ \rightarrow 2H_2O \qquad \text{(Eq. 3.8)}$$

oxene transferase function

$$XH + RO \rightarrow XOH + R \qquad \text{(Eq. 3.9)}$$

peroxidase function

$$XH + ROOH \rightarrow XOH + ROH \qquad \text{(Eq. 3.10)}$$

where XH is the substrate. The **reductase function** of cytochrome P450 is not listed here (Chapter 12).

3.6 ELECTRON TRANSFER SYSTEMS IN CYTOCHROME P450 MONOOXYGENASES

Previous sections in this chapter have alluded to the various electron transfer systems operating in cytochrome P450 monooxygenases, without giving details or explanations. Now that the biochemistry and biomechanisms of cytochrome P450 have been clarified, we examine the

TABLE 3.3 *Electron transport pathways in various cytochrome P450 systems* (modified from Lewis and Moereels, 1992; Nebert *et al.*, 1989b)

	2e⁻ donor	2e⁻ acceptor	1e⁻ transducer		1e⁻ acceptor
Bacterial	NADH	→ Putidaredoxin reductase	→ Putidaredoxin	→	P450
Fungal	NADPH	→ Cytochrome P450 reductase		→	P450
Microsomal	NADPH	→ Cytochrome P450 reductase		→	P450
	NADH	→ Cytochrome b_5 reductase	→ Cytochrome b_5	→	P450
Mitochondrial	NADPH	→ Adrenodoxin reductase	→ Adrenodoxin	→	P450

components of the electron transfer systems and their interactions with the terminal oxidase/oxygenase. Such systems differ among groups of P450 families, as summarized in Table 3.3 (Dreyer, 1984; Koymans *et al.*, 1993b; Lu and West, 1978; Nebert *et al.*, 1989b). The electron transport system in bacteria falls outside the scope of this book and will not be discussed here. Note however that it differs from all other systems.

3.6.1 NADPH-Cytochrome P450 reductase

NADPH-cytochrome P450 reductase [NADPH:ferrihemoprotein oxidoreductase; also known as NADPH-cytochrome *c* reductase; EC 1.6.2.4] is the major oxidoreductase transferring electrons to microsomal cytochrome P450. Various forms of this flavoprotein have been characterized with molecular weights in the range 68,000 to 78,000; some primary structures have been elucidated (Guengerich, 1978; Haniu *et al.*, 1989; Masters and Okita, 1980; Porter and Kasper, 1985; Strobel *et al.*, 1989; Yamano *et al.*, 1989). Site-directed mutagenesis and other techniques have begun to shed light on the critical role of some amino acid residues in catalysis, cofactor binding, and binding to P450 (Nadler and Strobel, 1991; Shen *et al.*, 1991; Strobel *et al.*, 1989).

NADPH-cytochrome P450 reductase is distinct from many other flavoproteins in that it contains one molecule each of **FAD** (flavin-adenine dinucleotide) and **FMN** (riboflavin 5′-phosphate) per polypeptide chain. The preferred source of reducing equivalents is NADPH (K_m in the micromolar range), but NADH can also act as an electron donor (K_m in the millimolar range) (Kurzban *et al.*, 1990; Noshiro and Omura, 1978; Sem and Kasper, 1992; Strobel *et al.*, 1980). Both are two-electron donors. The two physiological electron acceptors are cytochrome P450 and the soluble cytochrome *c*, a small metalloprotein that acts as an electron carrier in the respiratory chain of all aerobic organisms (Guenthner *et al.*, 1980; Peterson and Prough, 1986).

The **electron flow** within NADPH-cytochrome P450 reductase has intrigued scientists for many years due to the complexity of the possible electronic states. Indeed, the existence of semiquinones allows the enzyme to exist in five possible states of oxidation and nine possible electronic states (Oprian and Coon, 1982):

- oxidized [(FAD)(FMN)];
- one-electron reduced [(FAD)(FMNH•)] and [(FADH•)(FMN)];
- two-electron reduced [(FAD)(FMNH₂)], [(FADH•)(FMNH•)] and [(FADH₂)(FMN)];
- three-electron reduced [(FADH•)(FMNH₂)] and [(FADH₂)(FMNH•)];
- four-electron reduced [(FADH₂)(FMNH₂)].

FAD being the low-potential flavin acts as the acceptor of the two electrons from NADPH, whereas the high-potential flavin FMN serves as electron carrier to cytochrome P450. The rate of transfer of the first electron to cytochrome P450 appears controlled by the rate of complex formation between the two enzymes (Eyer and Backes, 1992). Apparently the two-, three- and four-electron reduced enzyme can transfer electrons to cytochrome P450, but there is evidence that ferricytochrome P450 is reduced during the catalytic cycle by the reductase in the $[(FADH^\bullet)(FMNH_2)]$ state. The latter, having reached the $[(FADH^\bullet)(FMNH^\bullet)]$ state, then equilibrates with the $[(FAD)(FMNH_2)]$ state and could donate another electron to the oxyferrous cytochrome P450 (Guengerich, 1983; Iyanagi et al., 1981).

Beside acting as an electron carrier, NADPH-cytochrome P450 reductase may also mediate **enzymatic reductions** (Chapter 12). Here, we note only that the enzyme may be a significant locus of **molecular oxygen reduction** to superoxide, which in turn leads to the hydroxyl radical as explained in Section 3.5.3 (Lai et al., 1979; Winston and Cederbaum, 1983).

3.6.2   NADH-cytochrome b_5 reductase and cytochrome b_5

NADH-cytochrome b_5 reductase [NADH:ferricytochrome-b_5 oxidoreductase; EC 1.6.2.2] is a flavoprotein containing one molecule of **FAD** as the prosthetic group. Its physiological role is to accept two electrons from NADH to reach a two-electron reduced state, and then to reduce two equivalents of cytochrome b_5 in successive one-electron steps (Iyanagi et al., 1984; Shirabe et al., 1991; Yubisui et al., 1991).

Many details of the structure and redox properties of **cytochrome b_5**, a 16 kDa hemoprotein, are known (Funk et al., 1990; Hagihara and Furuya, 1978; Lee et al., 1990; Ozols, 1989a; Peterson and Prough, 1986; Reid et al., 1982; Stayton et al., 1988; Strittmatter and Dailey, 1982; Yoo and Steggles, 1988; Zhang and Somerville, 1988). This enzyme is a one-electron reductase towards a number of acyl-coenzyme A desaturases, as well as other enzymes involved in the biosynthesis of fatty acids and cholesterol (Oshino, 1978; Strittmatter and Dailey, 1982; Wendoloski et al., 1987). As mentioned in Section 3.5.2, cytochrome b_5 can be the carrier of the second electron in cytochrome P450-mediated reactions and in some cases it may play an obligatory role; in many situations, however, both electrons reach the oxygenase through NADPH-cytochrome P450 reductase (Canova-Davis et al., 1985).

The above description treats the two electron-transport chains as independent from each other. In fact, there is evidence to indicate that the physiological situation may not always be so straightforward (Noshiro and Omura, 1978; Noshiro et al., 1980). In particular, circumstances have been found when cytochrome b_5 is reduced by NADPH-cytochrome P450 reductase (Ingelman-Sundberg and Johansson, 1984b). The functional interaction between NADPH-cytochrome P450 reductase and the two cytochromes (i.e. b_5 and P450) has also been characterized and involves different mechanisms and distinct binding domains on the reductase (Tamburini and Schenkman, 1986). A scheme summarizing the major reactions of electron transfer in the microsomal cytochrome P450 monooxygenase system is shown in Fig. 3.17; rate constants corresponding to such a scheme have been measured in a well-defined system (Taniguchi et al., 1984). Note that this figure, and the entire discussion above, presents the electron transport chains in an analytical and not systemic perspective. In other words, the monooxygenase system is "laid flat", and the complexity of the interactions and opportunities for feedback regulation are all but ignored. Examining the monooxygenase system in situ, i.e. in the membrane of the endoplasmic reticulum, somewhat enlarges the perspective (see Section 3.6.3).

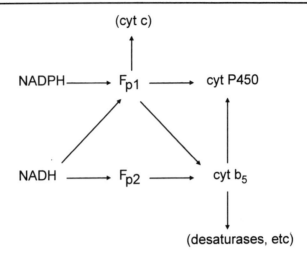

FIGURE 3.17 Main routes of electron flow in the microsomal cytochrome P450 monooxygenase system (cyt *c* = cytochrome *c*; other abbreviations see Figure 3.13).

3.6.3 Organization of cytochrome P450 monooxygenases in the endoplasmic reticulum

When reconstituting monooxygenase activities, it is not sufficient to mix a purified cytochrome P450 and a purified reductase to obtain a functional system. A third constituent is indispensable, namely **phospholipids** or analogous lipid-like compounds which provide a molecular medium that mimics the membrane. This is one indication among others that the membrane of the endoplasmic reticulum (which is "minced" to form microsomes upon tissue homogenization) plays a major role in cytochrome P450-mediated reactions. Many essential details on the endoplasmic reticulum membrane can be found in a comprehensive review by DePierre and Dallner (1975), while cytochrome P450 organization and membrane interactions have been aptly reviewed (Black, 1992; Edwards *et al.*, 1991; Ingelman-Sundberg, 1986; Ozols, 1989b).

The **membrane topology** of cytochrome P450 monooxygenases has been rationalized on the basis of their known primary structure, calculated secondary structure and modelled tertiary structure. Thus, cytochrome P450 has been envisaged as a thick triangle lying flat on the membrane surface, with the heme parallel to the membrane surface and the substrate binding site below the heme and facing the membrane. One or two NH$_2$-terminal transmembrane segments anchor the protein to the membrane bilayer, the remainder of the protein, from residue about 50 to the COOH terminus, being exposed on the cytosolic side of the membrane (Fig. 3.18) (Brown and Black, 1989; Chen and Zhou, 1992; Kunz *et al.*, 1991; Nelson and Strobel, 1988; Vergères *et al.*, 1989 and 1991). Similarly, NADPH-cytochrome P450 reductase contains a segment with high hydrophobicity, most likely to be transmembranal, and two flanking hydrophilic segments, one of which contains the FAD and FMN moieties and must be cytoplasmic (Black and Coon, 1982; Centero and Gutiérrez-Merino, 1992). Membranal and cytoplasmic segments have also been postulated for cytochrome b_5 (Strittmatter and Dailey, 1982). The cytochromes and reductases of the monooxygenase system thus appear to be anchored in the membrane and have their catalytic portion protruding into the cytosolic space.

Cytochrome P450 accounts for a significant proportion of liver microsomal proteins (up to 15%), and the number of molecules of this hemoprotein can be about 7 to 30 times greater than that of the reductase (McManus *et al.*, 1987; Yang, 1977). The enzymes of the cytochrome P450

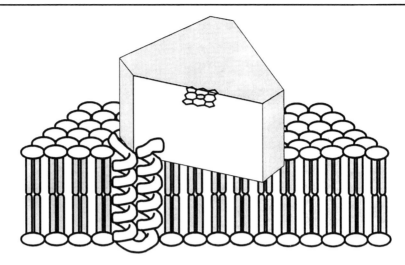

FIGURE 3.18 A model of microsomal cytochrome P450 structure and membrane topology. Reproduced from Nelson and Strobel (1988) with the permission of the copyright holder. For a more detailed picture, see Edwards *et al.* (1991).

monooxygenase system are viewed as being distributed, seemingly at random, in the membranal plane of the endoplasmic reticulum/microsome (an appropriate image may be that of floating icebergs); it is the lateral mobility of these enzymes that brings them into contact (Taniguchi *et al.*, 1984).

For a **functional interaction** (i.e. electron transfer) to take place, two constituents must form a binary complex via their respective specific binding domains. Such 1/1 complexes, which are transient and not stable, have been characterized for cytochrome P450/NADPH-cytochrome P450 reductase, cytochrome b_5/NADPH-cytochrome P450 reductase, and cytochrome P450/ cytochrome b_5 (e.g. Hlavica, 1984; Miwa and Lu, 1984; Tamburini *et al.*, 1986). In the case of cytochrome b_5, the functional complex appears to be ternary, involving also the reductase and cytochrome P450 (Ingelman-Sundberg, 1986). The fact that the formation of such functional complexes necessitates the presence of phospholipids is of major significance, implying that the membrane serves not merely as a medium but plays an active role in the process (Müller-Enoch *et al.*, 1984; Ruckpaul, 1978). The influence of the membrane on the spin state of cytochrome P450 may be one of the contributing factors. Also, the coupling of cytochrome P450 with the electron carriers is rendered functional by conformational changes which may be favoured by the membrane environment (Hlavica, 1984).

In addition to the complexes mentioned above, associations between cytochrome P450 enzymes have also been characterized (Alston *et al.*, 1991; Hildebrandt *et al.*, 1989). The **quaternary structure** of cytochrome P450 is still poorly understood, but it has implications for its catalytic efficiency, in particular by modulating substrate binding and facilitating metabolite flux for consecutive reactions.

In conclusion, it appears that electron flow in the cytochrome P450 monooxygenase system is controlled by a number of factors, including conformational state, degree of oxidation, spin state, bound substrate, and phospholipids. Such factors are, at least in part, interdependent, allowing for a self-regulating system possibly of a hypercyclic nature. Much current research work, being analytical and reductionistic, falls short of unravelling the functional and systemic dimensions of monooxygenases, but it would be unfair not to mention some quite informative kinetic and thermodynamic studies (e.g. Hlavica, 1984; Müller-Enoch *et al.*, 1984; Tamburini and Gibson, 1983; Taniguchi *et al.*, 1984).

3.6.4 Electron transfer in mitochondrial cytochrome P450 monooxygenases

Mitochondrial and bacterial cytochromes P450 are reduced by their own electron carrier systems, different from those coupled to microsomal cytochrome P450 (Table 3.3). An in-depth discussion of bacterial monooxygenases beyond the content of Table 3.2 falls outside the scope of this book (see the extensive review by Sligar and Murray, 1986). In contrast, **mitochondrial cytochrome P450 monooxygenases** are highly relevant and their presentation follows (Honeck, 1978; Jefcoate, 1986). The CYP11 family contains the major mitochondrial cytochromes P450, e.g. P450 11A1 and P450 11B1 (see Table 3.2). In comparison with microsomal cytochromes P450, mitochondrial cytochromes P450 generally exhibit a high degree of both substrate and product selectivity and hence may have a lower potential of metabolizing xenobiotics. Yet they are now receiving increasing attention as targets of mechanism-based enzyme inhibitors of therapeutic interest.

The electron carrier system reducing mitochondrial cytochromes P450 and cytochrome *c* comprises two enzymes, namely **adrenodoxin reductase** [ferredoxin:NADP$^+$ oxidoreductase; EC 1.18.1.2, formerly EC 1.6.7.1] and adrenal ferredoxin (**adrenodoxin**). Both are soluble, single-subunit proteins with molecular weights close to 52,000 and 12,000, respectively. Adrenodoxin reductase contains a single FAD as cofactor and exhibits a very high selectivity for NADPH from which it receives two electrons. Adrenodoxin is a non-haem iron protein which belongs to the group of iron–sulfur proteins; its active centre consists of two iron atoms, each coordinated by two cysteinyl sulfurs and bridged by two sulfur atoms, as shown in Fig. 3.19. While both iron atoms are in the ferric state in the oxidized enzyme, only a single electron can be introduced into a delocalized molecular orbital extending over the whole Fe$_2$S$_2$ cluster.

The **electron transfer** from NADPH to mitochondrial cytochrome P450 thus involves two single-electron steps:

- NADPH reduces the reductase to the FADH$_2$ state;
- adrenodoxin receives one electron from the reductase (which reaches the one-electron reduced FADH$^\bullet$ state);
- the reduced adrenodoxin supplies the first electron to cytochrome P450;
- adrenodoxin receives the second electron from the reductase in its FADH$^\bullet$ state and transfers it to the oxyferric cytochrome P450.

Many details of the adrenodoxin reductase–adrenodoxin complex and of the adrenodoxin–cytochrome P450 complex have been elucidated (e.g. Ichikawa and Hiwatashi, 1982; Lambeth and Kamin, 1979). One aspect of particular interest is the "**shuttle mechanism**" whereby the

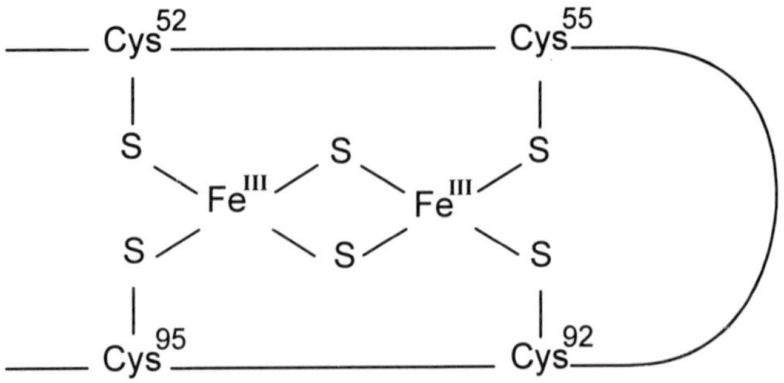

FIGURE 3.19 Active site of adrenodoxin showing the central Fe$_2$S$_2$ cluster coordinated to four cysteinyl sulfur atoms.

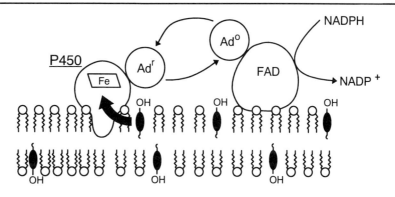

FIGURE 3.20 Electron transfer system in mitochondrial P450 11A1, showing also the transfer as discussed in the text.

reduced adrenodoxin dissociates from adrenodoxin reductase before forming a functional complex with cytochrome P450, thus effectively acting as an electron shuttle between the reductase and the oxygenase. This mechanism is illustrated in Fig. 3.20 and represents yet another difference between cytochrome b_5 and adrenodoxin.

3.7 FLAVIN-CONTAINING MONOOXYGENASES

The second monooxygenase system introduced in Section 3.1 and of significance in xenobiotic metabolism is the **microsomal flavin-containing monooxygenase** [N,N-dimethylaniline, NADPH:oxygen oxidoreductase (N-oxide-forming); EC 1.14.13.8], also known as FAD-containing monooxygenase and "Ziegler's enzyme", often abbreviated as FMO or MFMO, and previously called microsomal dimethylaniline monooxygenase or amine oxidase. These microsomal enzymes belong to the large class of flavoproteins and are very similar in properties to certain bacterial flavoprotein monooxygenases found in bacteria, e.g. *p*-hydroxybenzoate hydroxylase, salicylate hydroxylase, cyclohexanone oxygenase and luciferase (Bruice, 1980; Ghisla and Massey, 1989; Gunsalus *et al.*, 1975; Walsh, 1980a and 1980b).

The microsomal FAD-containing monooxygenases mediate a number of reactions of oxygenation (e.g. N- and S-oxygenation) which will be discussed further in Chapters 5 and 7.

FMOs are proteins whose apparent molecular weight is in the range 52,000 to 64,000 and which contain a single molecule of FAD as the prosthetic group (Ziegler, 1980 and 1988). A number of **isozymes** have been separated, their expression being markedly tissue- and species-dependent (Hodgson and Levi, 1988 and 1992; Lawton *et al.*, 1991; Lemoine *et al.*, 1990; Sausen *et al.*, 1993; Tynes and Hodgson, 1985; Tynes and Philpot, 1987; Williams *et al.*, 1985). Thus, a single form has apparently been detected in the liver and lung of the mouse and hamster; rat liver and lung also seem to contain a single isozyme which differs from the mouse and hamster form; the guinea-pig liver form may closely resemble the mouse and hamster isozyme, while three seemingly unique forms exist in the rabbit lung, and three other forms in the guinea-pig lung (Tynes and Philpot, 1987).

Molecular biology is now helping to clarify this picture. For example, a 535 amino acid FMO isolated from rabbit liver was found to have 87% homology with the FMO from pig liver, but only 56% homology with another 535 amino acid FMO from rabbit lung (Lawton *et al.*, 1990). An FMO present in low abundance in human liver appears orthologous to the pig and rabbit hepatic enzyme and has been named FMO1 (Dolphin *et al.*, 1991; Gasser *et al.*, 1990). The

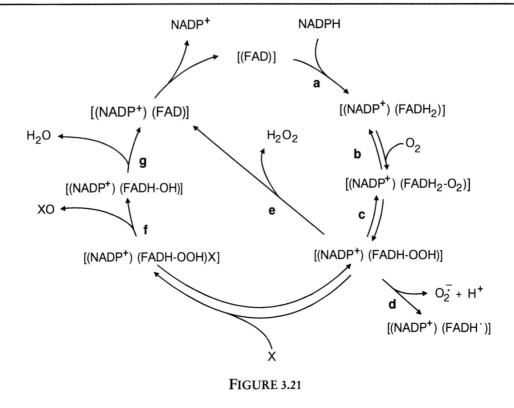

FIGURE 3.21

major human liver FMO is the FMO2 form which has about 50% homology with FMO1 (Lomri *et al.*, 1992, 1993a and 1993b). The per cent homology among the various forms of FMO has recently been found to define a single gene family consisting of at least five subfamilies, each containing a single gene (Philpot, 1992). Using a nomenclature similar to that characterizing cytochromes P450, it has been suggested that the FMO enzymes be designated **FMO 1A1, 1B1, 1C1, 1D1**, and **1E1**. The forms 1A1, 1D1 and 1E1 are found in humans. In addition to the five gene subfamilies *1A*, *1B*, *1C*, *1D* and *1F*, one and possibly two more genes remain to be characterized (Lawton and Philpot, 1993).

The **catalytic cycle of FMO** begins with the binding of NADPH and reduction of the flavin to $FADH_2$ (reaction **a** in Fig. 3.21) (Poulsen and Ziegler, 1979; Ziegler, 1993). Although NADH can replace NADPH with little effect on the V_{max} of oxygenation reactions, its affinity is markedly less (Beaty and Ballou, 1981a). $NADP^+$ is not released until the end of the cycle due to the low dissociation constant of the FMO–$NADP^+$ complex, a feature whose significance will be discussed below. Molecular oxygen then binds to the complex and is reduced to a hydroperoxide form (reactions **b** and **c** in Fig. 3.21), a probable mechanism being that shown in Eqs 3.10 to 3.12:

$$(FADH_2) \rightleftarrows (FADH^-) + H^+ \quad\quad\quad\quad \text{(Eq. 3.10)}$$

$$(FADH^-) + O_2 \rightarrow (FADH^\bullet O_2^\bullet) \quad\quad\quad\quad \text{(Eq. 3.11)}$$

$$(FADH^\bullet\text{--}O_2^{\bullet-}) + H^+ \rightarrow (FADH\text{--}OOH) \quad\quad\quad\quad \text{(Eq. 3.12)}$$

The FADH–OOH complex is the 4α-hydroperoxyflavin (**3.V** in Fig. 3.22), a stable intermediate in the absence of a substrate (Ballou, 1982; Hemmerich and Wessiak, 1976; Jones and Ballou,

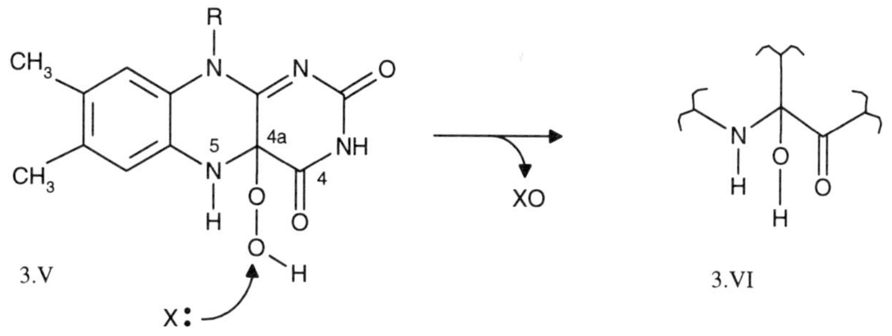

FIGURE 3.22

1986). The bound $NADP^+$ is required for the stability of the hydroperoxyflavin; the mechanism of this effect is not known but may involve stabilization of the N(5) proton (Ballou, 1982). However, this stability is only relative, since the release of superoxide and hydrogen peroxide is documented (reactions **d** and **e** in Fig. 3.21) (Hemmerich and Wessiak, 1976; Patton *et al.*, 1980), the probable mechanism being shown in Fig. 3.21.

In the presence of a nucleophilic substrate (X:), attack occurs on the distal oxygen atom to yield the oxygenated product (reaction **f** in Fig. 3.21; Fig. 3.22) with water molecules apparently playing a critical role in the transition state (Bach *et al.*, 1990; Ballou, 1982; Beaty and Ballou, 1981b; Jones and Ballou, 1986; Muranishi *et al.*, 1989). By analogy with organic peracids, the 4α-hydroperoxyflavin can also oxygenate electrophiles. After oxygenation of either nucleophiles or electrophiles, the flavin product is the 4α-hydroxyflavin (**3.VI** in Fig. 3.22). The latter compound, which is known to chemists as a pseudobase (i.e. formally resulting from addition of HO^- rather than loss of H^+), breaks down with release of water (reaction **g** in Fig. 3.21); this step may well be rate-limiting in the catalytic cycle of FMO (Jones and Ballou, 1986).

Many if not all reactions of FMO can also be catalyzed by cytochrome P450. *In vitro* and *in vivo*, the relative importance of the two contributions will be a function of a number of factors such as enzyme concentrations and substrate specificity. The FMO-catalyzed reactions will be discussed in Chapters 5 and 7.

3.8 REFERENCES

Alexander L.S. and Goff H.M. (1982). Chemicals, cancer, and cytochrome P-450. *J. Chem. Educ.* **59**, 179–182.

Alston K., Robinson R.C., Park S.S., Gelboin H.V. and Friedman F.K. (1991). Interactions among cytochromes P-450 in the endoplasmic reticulum. *J. Biol. Chem.* **266**, 735–739.

Andersson L.A. and Dawson J.H. (1984). The influence of oxygen donor ligation on the spectroscopic properties of ferric cytochrome P-450: ester, ether and ketone coordination to the haem iron. *Xenobiotica* **14**, 49–61.

Appel K.E., Ruf H.H., Mahr B., Schwarz M., Rickart R. and Kunz W. (1979). Binding of nitrosamines to cytochrome P-450 of liver microsomes. *Chem-Biol. Interact.* **28**, 17–33.

Armstrong R.N., Pinto-Coelho C., Ryan D.E., Thomas P.E. and Levin W. (1983). On the glycosylation state of five rat hepatic microsomal cytochrome P-450 isozymes. *J. Biol. Chem.* **258**, 2106–2108.

Aström A. and DePierre J.W. (1986). Rat-liver cytochrome P-450: purification, characterization, multiplicity and induction. *Biochim. Biophys. Acta* **853**, 1–27.

Atkins W.M. and Sligar S.G. (1987). Metabolic switching in cytochrome P-450$_{cam}$: deuterium isotope effects on regiospecificity and the monooxygenase/oxidase ratio. *J. Amer. Chem. Soc.* **109**, 3754–3760.

Atkins W.M. and Sligar S.G. (1988). The roles of active site hydrogen bonding in cytochrome P-450$_{cam}$ as revealed by site-directed mutagenesis. *J. Biol. Chem.* **263**, 18,842–18,849.

Auclair C., de Prost D. and Hakim J. (1978) Superoxide anion production by liver microsomes from phenobarbital treated rats. *Biochem. Pharmacol.* **27**, 355–358.

Aust S.D., Morehouse L.A. and Thomas C.E. (1985). Role of metals in oxygen radical reactions. *J. Free Radic. Biol. Med.* **1**, 3–25.

Bach R.D., McDouall J.J.W., Owensby A.L. and Schlegel H.B. (1990). Potential for water catalysis in flavin-mediated hydroxylation. A theoretical study. *J. Amer. Chem. Soc.* **112**, 7064–7065.

Backes W.L. and Canady W.J. (1981). Methods for the evaluation of hydrophobic substrate binding to cytochrome P-450. *Pharmacol. Ther.* **12**, 133–158.

Backes W.L. and Eyer C.S. (1989). Cytochrome P-450 LM2 reduction. Substrate effects on the rate of reductase-LM2 association. *J. Biol. Chem.* **264**, 6252–6259.

Backes W.L., Hogaboom M. and Canady W.J. (1982). The true hydrophobicity of microsomal cytochrome P-450 in the rat. Size dependence of the free energy of binding of a series of hydrocarbon substrates from the aqueous phase to the enzyme and to the membrane as derived from spectral binding data. *J. Biol. Chem.* **257**, 4063–4070.

Backes W.L., Tamburini P.P., Jansson I., Gibson G.G., Sligar S.G. and Schenkman J.B. (1985). Kinetics of cytochrome P-450 reduction: evidence for faster reduction of the high-spin ferric state. *Biochemistry* **24**, 5130–5136.

Ballou D.P. (1982). Flavoprotein monooxygenases. In *Flavins and Flavoproteins* (eds Massey V. and Williams C.H.). pp. 301–310. Elsevier, Amsterdam.

Bast A. (1986). Is formation of reactive oxygen by cytochrome P-450 perilous and predictable? *Trends Pharmacol. Sci.* **7**, 266–270.

Beaty N.B. and Ballou D.P. (1981a). The reductive half-reaction of liver microsomal FAD-containing mono-oxygenase. *J. Biol. Chem.* **256**, 4611–4618.

Beaty N.B. and Ballou D.P. (1981b). The oxidative half-reaction of liver microsomal FAD-containing mono-oxygenase. *J. Biol. Chem.* **256**, 4619–4625.

Beaune P.H., Kremers P.G., Kaminsky L.S., de Graeve J., Albert A. and Guengerich F.P. (1986). Comparison of monooxygenase activities and cytochrome P-450 isozyme concentrations in human liver microsomes. *Drug Metab. Disposit.* **14**, 437–442.

Beyeler S., Testa B. and Perrissoud D. (1983). The effect of cianidanol on rat hepatic monooxygenase activities. *Arzneim-Forsch (Drug Res.)* **33**, 564–567.

Beyeler S., Testa B. and Perrissoud D. (1988). Flavonoids as inhibitors of rat liver monooxygenase activities. *Biochem. Pharmacol.* **37**, 1971–1979.

Bielski B.H.J. and Allen A.O. (1977). Mechanism of the disproportionation of superoxide radicals. *J. Phys. Chem.* **81**, 1048–1050.

Björkhem I. (1977). Rate limiting step in microsomal cytochrome P-450 catalyzed hydroxylations. *Pharmacol. Ther. Part A* **1**, 327–348.

Black S.D. (1992). Membrane topology of the mammalian P450 cytochromes. *FASEB J.* **6**, 680–685.

Black S.D. and Coon M.J. (1982). Structural features of liver microsomal NADPH-cytochrome P-450 reductase.

Hydrophobic domain, hydrophilic domain, and connecting regions. *J. Biol. Chem.* **257**, 5929–5938.

Black S.D. and Coon M.J. (1985). Studies on the identity of the heme-binding cysteinyl residue in rabbit liver microsomal cytochrome P-450 isozyme 2. *Biochem. Biophys. Res. Commun.* **128**, 82–89.

Black S.D. and Coon M.J. (1986). Comparative structures of P-450 cytochromes. In *Cytochrome P-450. Structure, Mechanism, and Biochemistry* (ed. Ortiz de Montellano P.R.). pp. 161–216. Plenum Press, New York.

Blanck J. and Smettan G. (1978). The cytochrome P-450 reaction mechanism—kinetic aspects. *Pharmazie* **33**, 321–324.

Blanck J., Smettan G., Jänig G.R. and Ruckpaul K. (1977). Substrate binding kinetics and its role in the cytochrome P-450 hydroxylation sequence. *Croat. Chem. Acta* **49**, 271–277.

Boobis A.R. and Davies D.S. (1984). Human cytochromes P-450. *Xenobiotica* **14**, 151–185.

Brown C.A. and Black S.D. (1989). Membrane topology of mammalian cytochrome P-450 from liver endoplasmic reticulum. *J. Biol. Chem.* **264**, 4442–4449.

Bruice T.C. (1980). Mechanisms of flavin catalysis. *Acc. Chem. Res.* **13**, 256–262.

Bus J.S. and Gibson J.E. (1979). Lipid peroxidation and its role in toxicology. In *Reviews in Biochemical Toxicology*, Vol. 1 (eds Hodgson E., Bend J.R. and Philpot R.M.). pp. 125–149. Elsevier, Amsterdam.

Buettner G.R. (1993). The pecking order of free radicals and antioxidants. Lipid peroxidation, α-tocopherol and ascorbate. *Arch. Biochem. Biophys.* **300**, 535–543.

Calabrese E.J. and Canada A.T. (1989). Catalase: its role in xenobiotic detoxification. *Pharmacol. Ther.* **44**, 297–307.

Canada A.T. and Calabrese E.J. (1989). Superoxide dismutase: its role in xenobiotic detoxification. *Pharmacol. Ther.* **44**, 285–295.

Canova-Davis E., Chiang J.Y.L. and Waskell L. (1985). Obligatory role of cytochrome b_5 in the microsomal metabolism of methoxyflurane. *Biochem. Pharmacol.* **34**, 1907–1912.

Castro C.E. (1980). Mechanisms of reaction of hemeproteins with oxygen and hydrogen peroxide in the oxidation of organic substrates. *Pharmacol. Ther.* **10**, 171–189.

Caughey W.S. and Ibers J.A. (1977). Crystal and molecular structure of the free base porphyrin, protoporphyrin IX dimethyl ester. *J. Amer. Chem. Soc.* **99**, 6639–6645.

Centero F. and Gutiérrez-Merino C. (1992). Location of functional centres in the microsomal cytochrome P450 system. *Biochemistry* **31**, 8473–8481.

Chen S. and Zhou D. (1992). Functional domains of aromatase cytochrome P450 inferred from comparative analyses of amino acid sequences and substantiated by site-directed mutagenesis experiments. *J. Biol. Chem.* **267**, 22,587–22,594.

Cholerton S., Daly A.K. and Idle J.R. (1992). The role of individual human cytochromes P450 in drug metabolism and clinical response. *Trends Pharmacol. Sci.* **13**, 434–439.

Collman J.P., Sorrell T.N., Dawson J.H., Trudell J.R.,

Bunnenberg E. and Djerassi C. (1976a). Magnetic circular dichroism of ferrous carbonyl adducts of cytochromes P-450 and P-420 and their synthetic models: Further evidence for mercaptide as the fifth ligand to iron. *Proc. Natl. Acad. Sci. USA* **73**, 6–10.

Collman J.P., Brauman J.I., Halbert T.R. and Suslick K.S. (1976b). Nature of O_2 and CO binding to metalloporphyrins and heme proteins. *Proc. Natl. Acad. Sci. USA* **73**, 3333–3337.

Coon M.J. and Persson A.V. (1980). Microsomal cytochrome P-450: a central catalyst in detoxication reactions. In *Enzymatic Basis of Detoxication*, Vol. 1 (ed. Jakoby W.B.). pp. 117–134. Academic Press, New York.

Coon M.J. and Porter T.D. (1988). The cytochrome P-450 gene superfamily. In *Toxicological and Immunological Aspects of Drug Metabolism and Environmental Chemicals* (eds Estabrook R.W., Lindenlaub E., Oesch F. and de Weck A.L.). pp. 11–25. Schattauer, Stuttgart.

Coon M.J., Ding X., Pernecky S.J. and Vaz A.D.N. (1992). Cytochrome P450: progress and predictions. *FASEB J.* **6**, 669–673.

Cramer S.P., Dawson J.H., Hodgson K.O. and Hager L.P. (1978). Studies on the ferric forms of cytochrome P-450 and chloroperoxidase by extended X-ray absorption fine structure. Characterization of the Fe–N and Fe–S distances. *J. Amer. Chem. Soc.* **100**, 7282–7290.

Dawson J.H., Andersson L.A. and Sono M. (1982). Spectroscopic investigations of ferric cytochrome P-450-CAM ligand complexes. *J. Biol. Chem.* **257**, 3606–3617.

Deby C. and Goutier R. (1990). New perspectives on the biochemistry of superoxide anion and the efficiency of superoxide dismutase. *Biochem. Pharmacol.* **39**, 399–405.

De Matteis F., Dawson S.J., Boobis A.R. and Comoglio A. (1991). Inducible bilirubin-degrading system of rat liver microsomes: role of cytochrome P450IA1. *Molec. Pharmacol.* **40**, 686–691.

DePierre J.W. and Dallner G. (1975). Structural aspects of the membrane of the endoplasmic reticulum. *Biochim. Biophys. Acta* **415**, 411–472.

Dix T.A. and Aikens J. (1993). Mechanisms and biological relevance of lipid peroxidation initiation. *Chem. Res. Toxicol.* **6**, 2–18.

Dolphin D. (1985). Cytochrome P_{450}: substrate and prosthetic-group free radicals generated during the enzymatic cycle. *Phil. Trans. R Soc. Lond.* B **311**, 579–591.

Dolphin C., Shephard E.A., Povey S., Palmer C.N.A., Ziegler D.M., Ayesh R., Smith R.L. and Phillips I.R. (1991). Cloning, primary sequence, and chromosomal mapping of a human flavin-containing monooxygenase (FMO1). *J. Biol. Chem.* **266**, 12,379–12,385.

Dreyer J.L. (1984). Electron transfer in biological systems: an overview. *Experientia* **40**, 653–675.

Duchstein H.J. and Gurka H.J. (1992). Activated species of oxygen: a challenge to modern pharmaceutical chemistry. *Arch Pharm.* **325**, 129–146.

Duthu G.S. and Shertzer H.G. (1979). Effect of nitrite on rabbit liver mixed-function oxidase activity. *Drug Metab. Disposit.* **7**, 263–269.

Ebel R.E., O'Keeffe D.H. and Peterson J.A. (1975). Nitric oxide complexes of cytochrome P-450. *FEBS Lett* **55**, 198–201.

Edwards D.J., Bowles S.K., Svensson C.K. and Rybak M.J. (1988). Inhibition of drug metabolism by quinolone antibiotics. *Clin. Pharmacokin.* **15**, 194–204.

Edwards R.J., Murray B.P., Singleton A.M. and Boobis A.R. (1991). Orientation of cytochromes P450 in the endoplasmic reticulum. *Biochemistry* **30**, 71–76.

Estabrook R.W. (1984). Cytochrome P-450 and oxygenation reactions: a status report. In *Drug Metabolism and Drug Toxicity* (eds Mitchell J.R. and Horning M.G.). pp. 1–20. Raven Press, New York.

Estabrook R.W., Kawano S., Werringloer J., Kuthan H., Tsuji H., Graf H. and Ullrich V. (1979). Oxycytochrome P-450: its breakdown to superoxide for the formation of hydrogen peroxide. *Acta Biol. Med. Germ.* **38**, 423–434.

Estabrook R.W., Chacos N., Martin-Wixtrom C. and Capdevila J. (1982). Cytochrome P-450: a versatile vehicle of variable veracity. In *Oxygenases and Oxygen Metabolism* (eds Nozaki M., Yamamoto S., Ishimura Y., Coon M.J., Ernster L. and Estabrook R.W.). pp. 371–381. Academic Press, New York.

Eyer C.S. and Backes W.L. (1992). Relationship between the rate of reductase-cytochrome P450 complex formation and the rate of 1st electron transfer. *Arch Biochem. Biophys.* **293**, 231–240.

Fuji-Kuriyama Y., Kimura H., Higashi Y., Sogawa K., Shimizu T., Hatano M. and Gotoh O. (1989). Molecular similarity and diversity of cytochrome P-450 molecules. In *Xenobiotic Metabolism and Disposition* (eds Kato R., Estabrook R.W. and Cayen M.N.). pp. 11–19. Taylor & Francis, London.

Funk W.D., Lo T.P., Mauk M.R., Brayer G.D., MacGillivray R.T.A. and Mauk A.G. (1990). Mutagenic, electrochemical, and crystallographic investigation on the cytochrome b_5 oxidation–reduction equilibrium: involvement of asparagine-57, serine-64, and heme propionate-7. *Biochemistry* **29**, 5500–5508.

Gander J.E. and Mannering G.J. (1980). Kinetics of hepatic cytochrome P-450-dependent monooxygenase systems. *Pharmacol. Ther.* **10**, 191–221.

Gasser R., Negishi M. and Philpot R.M. (1988). Primary structure of multiple forms of cytochrome P-450 isozyme 2 derived from rabbit pulmonary and hepatic cDNAs. *Molec. Pharmacol.* **33**, 22–30.

Gasser R., Tynes R.E., Lawton M.P., Korsmeyer K.K., Ziegler D.M. and Philpot R.M. (1990). The flavin-containing monooxygenase expressed in pig liver: primary sequence, distribution, and evidence for a single gene. *Biochemistry* **29**, 119–124.

Gelboin H.V. and Friedman F.K. (1985). Monoclonal antibodies for studies on xenobiotic and endobiotic metabolism. Cytochromes P-450 as paradigm. *Biochem. Pharmacol.* **34**, 2225–2234.

Gerber N.C. and Sligar S.G. (1992). Catalytic mechanism of cytochrome P-450: evidence for a distal charge relay. *J. Amer. Chem. Soc.* **114**, 8742–8743.

Ghisla S. and Massey V. (1989). Mechanisms of

flavoprotein-catalyzed reactions. *Eur. J. Biochem.* **181**, 1–17.

Gonzalez F.J. (1989). The molecular biology of cytochrome P450s. *Pharmacol. Rev.* **40**, 243–288.

Gonzalez F.J. (1990). Molecular genetics of the P-450 superfamily. *Pharmacol. Ther.* **45**, 1–38.

Gonzalez F.J. (1992). Human cytochromes P450: problems and prospects. *Trends Pharmacol. Sci.* **13**, 346–352.

Gorman A.A. and Rodgers M.A.J. (1981). Singlet molecular oxygen. *Chem. Soc. Rev.* **10**, 205–231.

Gorsky L.D., Koop D.R. and Coon M.J. (1984). On the stoichiometry of the oxidase and monooxygenase reactions catalyzed by liver microsomal cytochrome P-450. Products of oxygen reduction. *J. Biol. Chem.* **259**, 6812–6817.

Gotoh O., Tagashira Y., Iizuka T. and Fujii-Kuriyama Y. (1983). Structural characteristics of cytochrome P-450. Possible location of the heme-binding cysteine in determined amino-acid sequences. *J. Biochem.* **93**, 807–817.

Gray R.D. (1982). Kinetics and mechanism of carbon monoxide binding to purified cytochrome P-450 isozymes. *J. Biol. Chem.* **257**, 1086–1094.

Gray R.D. (1983). Kinetics and mechanism of CO binding to cytochromes P-450$_{LM2}$ and P-450$_{LM4}$. Effect of phospholipid, non-ionic detergent, and substrate binding. *J. Biol. Chem.* **258**, 3764–3768.

Griffin B.W., Peterson J.A., Werringloer J. and Estabrook R.W. (1975). Chemistry of soluble and membrane-bound cytochrome P-450. *Ann. N.Y. Acad. Sci.* **244**, 107–131.

Groves J.T. (1985). Key elements of the chemistry of cytochrome P-450. The oxygen rebound mechanism. *J. Chem. Educat.* **62**, 928–931.

Guengerich F.P. (1978). Comparison of highly purified cytochromes P-450 and NADPH-cytochrome P-450 reductases by peptide mapping. *Biochem. Biophys. Res. Commun.* **82**, 820–827.

Guengerich F.P. (1979). Isolation and purification of cytochrome P-450 and the existence of multiple forms. *Pharmacol. Ther.* **6**, 99–121.

Guengerich F.P. (1983). Oxidation–reduction properties of rat liver cytochromes P-450 and NADPH-cytochrome P-450 reductase related to catalysis in reconstituted systems. *Biochemistry* **22**, 2811–2820.

Guengerich F.P. (1989). Polymorphism of cytochrome P-450 in humans. *Trends Pharmacol. Sci.* **10**, 107–109.

Guengerich F.P. (1990). Characterization of roles of human cytochrome P-450 enzymes in carcinogen metabolism. *Asia Pacific J. Pharmacol.* **5**, 327–345.

Guengerich F.P. (1991). Reactions and significance of cytochrome P-450 enzymes. *J. Biol. Chem.* **266**, 10,019–10,022.

Guengerich F.P. (1992a). Human cytochrome P-450 enzymes. *Life Sci.* **50**, 1471–1478.

Guengerich F.P. (1992b). Characterization of human cytochrome P450 enzymes. *FASEB J.* **6**, 745–748.

Guengerich F.P., Bork R.W., Ged C., Bellew T.M., Umbenhauer D.R., Muto T., Beaune P.H., Shinriki N., Srivastava P.K. and Lloyd R.S. (1989). Characterization

of human liver cytochrome P-450 proteins, mRNAs, and genes. In *Xenobiotic Metabolism and Disposition* (eds Kato R., Estabrook R.W. and Cayen M.N.). pp. 3–10. Taylor & Francis, London.

Guenthner T.M., Kahl G.F. and Nebert D.W. (1980). NADPH-cytochrome P-450 reductase: preferential inhibition by ellipticine and other type II compounds having little effect on NADPH-cytochrome c reductase. *Biochem. Pharmacol.* **29**, 89–95.

Gunsalus I.C., Pederson T.C. and Sligar S.G. (1975). Oxygenase-catalyzed biological hydroxylations. *Ann. Rev. Biochem.* **44**, 377–407.

Gustafsson J.Å., Rondahl L. and Bergman J. (1979). Iodosylbenzene derivatives as oxygen donors in cytochrome P-450 catalyzed steroid hydroxylations. *Biochemistry* **18**, 865–870.

Hagihara B. and Furuya E. (1978). Chemistry and physical properties of cytochrome b_5. *Pharmacol. Ther A* **2**, 537–550.

Hahn J.E., Hodgson K.O., Andersson L.A. and Dawson J.H. (1982). Endogenous cysteine ligation in ferric and ferrous cytochrome P-450. Direct evidence from X-ray absorption spectroscopy. *J. Biol. Chem.* **257**, 10,934–10,941.

Hall P.F. (1986). Cytochromes P-450 and the regulation of steroid synthesis. *Steroids* **48**, 131–196.

Halliwell B. and Gutteridge J.M.C. (1984). Oxygen toxicity, oxygen radicals, transition metals and disease. *Biochem. J.* **219**, 1–14.

Haniu M., Armes L.G., Tanaka M., Yasunobu K.T., Shastry B.S., Wagner G.C. and Gunsalus I.C. (1982). The primary structure of the monooxygenase cytochrome P450$_{cam}$. *Biochem. Biophys. Res. Commun.* **105**, 889–894.

Haniu M., Ryan D.E., Levin W. and Shively J.E. (1986). The primary structure of cytochrome P-450d purified from rat liver microsomes: prediction of helical regions and domain analysis. *Arch. Biochem. Biophys.* **244**, 323–337.

Haniu M., McManus M.E., Birkett D.J., Lee T.D. and Shively J.E. (1989). Structural and functional analysis of NADPH-cytochrome P-450 reductase from human liver: complete sequence of human enzyme and NADPH-binding sites. *Biochemistry* **28**, 8639–8645.

Hanson L.K., Sligar S.G. and Gunsalus I.C. (1977). Electronic structure of cytochrome P450. *Croat Chem. Acta* **49**, 237–250.

Hasegawa T. (1983). The recognition of a soluble cytochrome P450 in rat liver. *FEBS Lett.* **155**, 257–262.

Hawkins B.K. and Dawson J.H. (1992). Oxygen activation by heme-containing monooxygenases: cytochrome P-450 and secondary amine monooxygenase. Active site structures and mechanisms. *Front Biotransform* **7**, 216–278.

Heimbrook D.C. and Sligar S.G. (1981). Multiple mechanisms of cytochrome P-450-catalyzed substrate hydroxylations. *Biochem. Biophys. Res. Commun.* **99**, 530–535.

Heinemann F.S. and Ozols J. (1983). The complete amino acid sequence of rabbit phenobarbital-induced liver microsomal cytochrome P-450. *J. Biol. Chem.* **258**, 4195–4201.

Hemmerich P. and Wessiak A. (1976). The structural chemistry of flavin-dependent oxygen activation. In *Flavins and Flavoproteins* (ed. Singer T.P.). pp. 9–22. Elsevier, Amsterdam.

Higuchi T., Uzu S. and Hirobe M. (1990). Synthesis of a highly stable iron porphyrin coordinated by alkyl-thiolate anion as a model for cytochrome P-450 and its catalytic activity in O–O bond cleavage. *J. Amer. Chem. Soc.* **112**, 7051–7053.

Hildebrandt P., Garda H., Stier A., Bachmanova G.I., Kanaeva I.P. and Archakov A.I. (1989). Protein–protein interactions in microsomal cytochrome P-450 isozyme LM2 and their effect on substrate binding. *Eur. J. Biochem.* **186**, 383–388.

Hlavica P. (1984). On the function of cytochrome b_5 in the cytochrome P-450-dependent oxygenase system. *Arch. Biochem. Biophys.* **228**, 600–608.

Hodgson E. and Levi P.E. (1988). Species, organ and cellular variation in the flavin-containing monooxygenase. *Drug Metab. Drug Interact.* **6**, 219–233.

Hodgson E. and Levi P.E. (1992). The role of the flavin-containing monooxygenase (EC 1.14.13.8) in the metabolism and mode of action of agricultural chemicals. *Xenobiotica* **22**, 1175–1183.

Holton T.A., Brugliera F., Lester D.R., Tanaka Y., Hyland C.D., Menting J.G.T., Lu C.Y., Fracy E., Stevenson T.W. and Cornish E.C. (1993). Cloning and expression of cytochrome P450 genes controlling flower colour. *Nature* **366**, 276–279.

Honeck H. (1978). The mixed function monooxygenase systems of the adrenal cortex. *Pharmazie* **33**, 317–321.

Hu S. and Kincaid J.R. (1991). Resonance Raman spectra of the nitric oxide adducts of ferrous cytochrome P450cam in the presence of various substrates. *J. Amer. Chem. Soc.* **113**, 9760–9766.

Iba M.M. and Mannering G.J. (1987). NADPH- and linoleic acid hydroperoxide-induced lipid peroxidation and destruction of cytochrome P-450 in hepatic microsomes. *Biochem. Pharmacol.* **36**, 1447–1455.

Iba M.M., Gander J.E. and Mannering G.J. (1993). Lipid peroxidation–cytochrome P450 interactions. Use of linoleic acid hydroperoxide in the characterization of the spin-state of membrane-bound P450. *Xenobiotica* **23**, 227–239.

Ichikawa Y. and Hiwatashi A. (1982). The role of the sugar regions of components of the cytochrome P-450-linked mixed-function oxidase (monooxygenase) system of bovine adrenocortical mitochondria. *Biochim. Biophys. Acta* **705**, 82–91.

Imai Y. and Nakamura M. (1988). The importance of threonine-301 from cytochrome P-450 (laurate (ω-1)-hydroxylase and testosterone 16α-hydroxylase) in substrate binding as demonstrated by site-directed mutagenesis. *FEBS Lett.* **234**, 313–316.

Ingelman-Sundberg M. (1986). Cytochrome P450 organization and membrane interactions. In *Cytochrome P-450. Structure, Mechanism, and Biochemistry* (ed.

Ortiz de Montellano P.R.). pp. 119–160. Plenum Press, New York.

Ingelman-Sundberg M. and Hagbjörk A.L. (1982). On the significance of the cytochrome P-450-dependent hydroxyl radical-mediated oxygenation mechanism. *Xenobiotica* **12**, 673–686.

Ingelman-Sundberg M. and Johansson I. (1984a). Mechanisms of hydroxyl radical formation and ethanol oxidation by ethanol-inducible and other forms of rabbit liver microsomal cytochromes P-450. *J. Biol. Chem.* **259**, 6447–6458.

Ingelman-Sundberg M. and Johansson I. (1984b). Electron flow and complex formation during cytochrome P-450-catalyzed hydroxylation reactions in reconstituted membrane vesicles. *Acat. Chem. Scand.* **38**, 845–851.

International Union of Biochemistry and Molecular Biology (1992). *Enzyme Nomenclature 1992.* Academic Press, San Diego, USA.

Ioannides C. and Parke D.V. (1987). The cytochromes P-448—a unique family of enzymes involved in chemical toxicity and carcinogenesis. *Biochem. Pharmacol.* **36**, 4197–4207.

Iwasaki K. (1990). Reactive oxygen and glomerular dysfunction. *Xenobiotica* **20**, 909–914.

Iyanagi T., Makino R. and Anan F.K. (1981). Studies on the microsomal mixed-function oxidase system: mechanism of action of hepatic NADPH-cytochrome P-450 reductase. *Biochemistry* **20**, 1722–1730.

Iyanagi T., Watanabe S. and Anan K.F. (1984). One-electron oxidation–reduction properties of hepatic NADH-cytochrome b_5 reductase. *Biochemistry* **23**, 1418–1425.

Jacobs R.E., Singh J. and Vickery L.E. (1987). NMR studies of cytochrome P-450$_{scc}$. Effects of steroid binding on water proton access to the active site of the ferric enzyme. *Biochemistry* **26**, 4541–4545.

Jänig G.R., Misselwitz R., Zirwer D., Buder E., Rein H. and Ruckpaul K. (1977). Differentiation between type I and type II substrate binding to cytochrome P-450 by temperature studies. *Croat Chem. Acta* **49**, 263–270.

Jänig G.R., Makower A., Rabe H., Bernhardt R. and Ruckpaul K. (1984). Chemical modification of cytochrome P-450 LM2. Characterization of tyrosine as axial heme iron ligand *trans* to thiolate. *Biochim. Biophys. Acta* **787**, 8–18.

Jansson I. and Schenkman J.B. (1987). Influence of cytochrome b_5 on the stoichiometry of the different oxidative reactions catalyzed by liver microsomal cytochrome P-450. *Drug Metab. Disposit.* **15**, 344–348.

Jansson I., Tamburini P.P., Favreau L.V. and Schenkman J.B. (1985). The interaction of cytochrome b_5 with four cytochrome P-450 enzymes from the untreated rat. *Drug Metab. Disposit* **13**, 453–458.

Jefcoate C.R. (1986). Cytochrome P-450 enzymes in sterol biosynthesis and metabolism. In *Cytochrome P-450. Structure, Mechanism, and Biochemistry* (ed. Ortiz de Montellano P.R.). pp. 387–428. Plenum Press, New York.

Johnson E.F. (1992). Mapping determinants of the substrate selectivities of P450 enzymes by site-directed mutagenesis. *Trends Pharmacol. Sci.* **13**, 122–126.

Johnson E.F., Kronbach T. and Hsu M.H. (1992). Analysis of the catalytic specificity of cytochrome P450 enzymes through site-directed mutagenesis. *FASEB J.* **6**, 700–705.

Jones K.C. and Ballou D.P. (1986). Reactions of the 4α-hydroperoxide of liver microsomal flavin-containing monooxygenase with nucleophilic and electrophilic substrates. *J. Biol. Chem.* **261**, 2553–2559.

Jones J.P., Trager W.F. and Carlson T.J. (1993). The binding and regioselectivity of reaction of (*R*)- and (*S*)-nicotine with cytochrome P450cam: parallel experimental and theoretical studies. *J. Amer. Chem. Soc.* **115**, 381–387.

Jørgensen K.A. (1986). Does an unusual structure of oxo-iron porphyrins cause its stereoselective properties? *Acta Schem. Scand. B* **40**, 512–514.

Jung C. and Ristau O. (1978). Mechanism of the cytochrome P-450 catalyzed hydroxylation— Thermodynamical aspects and the nature of the active oxygen species. *Pharmazie* **33**, 329–331.

Jung C., Friedrich J. and Ristau O. (1979). Quantum chemical interpretation of the spectral properties of the CO and O_2 complexes of haemoglobin and cytochrome P-450. *Acta Biol. Med. Germ.* **38**, 363–377.

Kadiiska M.B., Hanna P.M., Hernandez L. and Mason R.P. (1992). *In vivo* evidence of hydroxyl radical formation after acute copper and ascorbic acid intake: electron spin resonance spin-trapping investigation. *Molec. Pharmacol.* **42**, 723–729.

Kapke G.F. and Baron J. (1980). Hepatic mitochondrial cholesterol hydroxylase activity—a cytochrome P-450-catalyzed monooxygenation refractory to cobaltous chloride. *Biochem. Pharmacol.* **29**, 845–847.

Kappus H. (1985). Lipid peroxidation: mechanisms, analysis, enzymology and biological relevance. In *Oxidative Stress* (ed. Sies H.). pp. 273–310. Academic Press, London.

Koch J.A. and Waxman D.J. (1991). P450 phosphorylation in isolated hepatocytes and *in vivo*. In *Cytochrome P450* (eds Waterman M.R. and Johnson E.F.). pp. 305–315. Academic Press, San Diego.

Koop D.R. and Kienle E. (1993). Stoichiometry of P450 2E1-dependent fatty acid metabolism. In *ISSX Proceedings*, Vol. 4. International Society for the Study of Xenobiotics. p. 128. Bethesda, MD, USA.

Koppenol W.H. (1976). Reactions involving singlet oxygen and the superoxide 1 anion. *Nature* **262**, 420–421.

Korzekwa K.R. and Jones J.P. (1993). Predicting the cytochrome-P450 mediated metabolism of xenobiotics. *Pharmacogenetics* **3**, 1–18.

Koymans L., Vermeulen N.P.E., van Acker S.A.B.E., te Koppele J.M., Heykants J.J.P., Lavrijsen K., Meuldermans W. and Donné-Op den Kelder G.M. (1992). A predictive model for substrates of cytochrome P450-debrisoquine (2D6). *Chem. Res. Toxicol.* **5**, 211–219.

Koymans L., Vermeulen N.P.E., Baarslag A. and Donné-Op den Kelder G.M. (1993a). A preliminary 3D model for cytochrome P450 2D6 constructed by homology model building. *J. Comput.-Aided Molec. Design* **7**, 281–289.

Koymans L., Donné-Op den Kelder G.M., te Koppele J.M. and Vermeulen N.P.E. (1993b). Cytochromes P450: Their active-site structure and mechanism of oxidation. *Drug Metab. Rev.* **25**, 325–387.

Kühn-Velten W.N. (1991). Thermodynamics and modulation of progesterone microcompartmentation and hydrophobic interaction with cytochrome P450XVII based on quantification of local ligand concentrations in a complex multi-component system. *Eur. J. Biochem.* **197**, 381–390.

Kumaki K. and Nebert D.W. (1978). Spectral evidence for weak ligand in sixth position of hepatic microsomal cytochrome P-450 low spin ferric iron *in vivo*. *Pharmacology* **17**, 262–279.

Kumaki K., Sato M., Kon H. and Nebert D.W. (1978). Correlation of type I, type II, and reverse type I difference spectra with absolute changes in spin state of hepatic microsomal cytochrome P-450 iron from five mammalian species. *J. Biol. Chem.* **253**, 1048–1058.

Kunz B.C., Vergères G., Winterhalter K.H. and Richter C. (1991). Chemical modification of rat liver microsomal cytochrome P-450: study of enzymic properties and membrane topology. *Biochim. Biophys. Acta* **1063**, 226–234.

Kurzban G.P., Howarth J., Palmer G. and Strobel H.W. (1990). NADPH-cytochrome P-450 reductase. Physical properties and redox behavior in the absence of the FAD moiety. *J. Biol. Chem.* **265**, 12,272–12,279.

Kuthan H. and Ullrich V. (1982). Oxidase and oxygenase function of the microsomal cytochrome P450 monooxygenase system. *Eur. J. Biochem.* **126**, 583–588.

Kuwahara S.I. and Mannering G.J. (1985). Evidence for a predominantly NADH-dependent O-dealkylating system in rat hepatic microsomes. *Biochem. Pharmacol.* **34**, 4215–4228.

LaBella F.S. (1991). Cytochrome P450 enzymes: ubiquitous "receptors" for drugs. *Can. J. Physiol. Pharmacol.* **69**, 1129–1132.

Lai C.S., Grover T.A. and Piette L.H. (1979). Hydroxyl radical production in a purified NADPH-cytochrome *c* (P-450) reductase system. *Arch. Biochem. Biophys.* **193**, 373–378.

Lambeth J.D. and Kamin H. (1979). Adrenodoxin reductase•adrenodoxin complex. *J. Biol. Chem.* **254**, 2766–2774.

Laughton C.A., Neidle S., Zvelebil M.J.J.M. and Sternberg M.J.E. (1990). A molecular model for the enzyme cytochrome P450$_{17\alpha}$, a major target for the chemotherapy of prostatic cancer. *Biochem. Biophys. Res. Commun.* **171**, 1160–1167.

Lawton M.P. and Philpot R.M. (1993). Molecular genetics of the flavin-dependent monooxygenases. *Pharmacogenetics* **3**, 40–44.

Lawton M.P., Gasser R., Tynes R.E., Hodgson E. and Philpot R.M. (1990). The flavin-containing monooxygenase enzymes expressed in rabbit liver and lung are products of related but distinctly different genes. *J. Biol.*

Chem. **265**, 5855–5861.

Lawton M.P., Kronbach T., Johnson E.F. and Philpot R.M. (1991). Properties of expressed and native flavin-containing monooxygenases: evidence of multiple forms in rabbit liver and lung. *Molec. Pharmacol.* **40**, 692–698.

Lee K.B., La Mar G.N., Kehres L.A., Fujinari E.M., Smith K.M., Pochapsky T.C. and Sligar S.G. (1990). ^{1}H NMR Study of the influence of hydrophobic contacts on protein-prosthetic group recognition in bovine and rat ferricytochrome b_5. *Biochemistry* **29**, 9623–9631.

Lemoine A., Johann M. and Cresteil T. (1990). Evidence for the presence of distinct flavin-containing monooxygenases in human tissues. *Arch. Biochem. Biophys.* **276**, 336–342.

Lewis D.F.V. (1986). Physical methods in the study of the active site geometry of cytochromes P-450. *Drug Metab. Rev.* **17**, 1–66.

Lewis D.F.V. and Moereels H. (1992). The sequence homologies of cytochromes P-450 and active-site geometries. *J. Comput.-Aided Molec. Design* **6**, 235–252.

Lichtenberger F., Nastainczyk W. and Ullrich V. (1976). Cytochrome P-450 as an oxene transferase. *Biochem. Biophys. Res. Commun.* **70**, 939–946.

Lomri N., Gu Q. and Cashman J.R. (1992). Molecular cloning of the flavin-containing monooxygenase (form II) cDNA from adult human liver. *Proc. Natl. Acad. Sci. USA* **89**, 1685–1689.

Lomri N., Yang Z. and Cashman J.R. (1993a). Expression in *Escherichia coli* of the flavin-containing monooxygenase D (form II) from adult human liver: Determination of a distinct tertiary amine substrate specificity. *Chem. Res. Toxicol.* **6**, 425–429.

Lomri N., Yang Z. and Cashman J.R. (1993b). Regio- and stereoselective oxygenation by adult human liver flavin-containing monooxygenase 3. Comparison with forms 1 and 2. *Chem. Res. Toxicol.* **6**, 800–807.

Lu A.Y.H. (1979). Multiplicity of liver drug metabolizing enzymes. *Drug Metab. Rev.* **10**, 187–208.

Lu A.Y.H. and West S.B. (1980). Reconstituted mammalian mixed-function oxidases: requirements, specificities and other properties. *Pharmacol. Ther. A* **2**, 337–358.

Macdonald T.L., Burka L.T., Wright S.T. and Guengerich F.P. (1982). Mechanisms of hydroxylation by cytochrome P-450: exchange of iron–oxygen intermediates with water. *Biochem. Biophys. Res. Commun.* **104**, 620–625.

Mannering G.J. (1981). Hepatic cytochrome P-450-linked drug-metabolizing systems. In *Concepts in Drug Metabolism*, Part B (eds Jenner P. and Testa B.). pp. 53–166. Dekker, New York.

Martinis S.A., Atkins W.M., Stayton P.S. and Sligar S.G. (1989). A conserved residue of cytochrome P-450 is involved in heme-oxygen stability and activation. *J. Amer. Chem. Soc.* **111**, 9252–9253.

Masters B.S.S. and Okita R.T. (1980). The history, properties, and function of NADPH-cytochrome P450 reductase. *Pharmacol. Ther.* **9**, 227–244.

McCord J.M. (1979). Superoxide, superoxide dismutase and oxygen toxicity. In *Reviews in Biochemical Toxicology*, Vol. 1 (eds Hodgson E., Bend J.R. and Philpot R.M.). pp. 109–124. Elsevier, Amsterdam.

McManus M.E., Hall P. de la M., Stupans I., Brennan J., Burgess W., Robson R. and Birkett D.J. (1987). Immunohistochemical localization and quantitation of NADPH-cytochrome P-450 reductase in human liver. *Molec. Pharmacol.* **32**, 189–194.

Mesnil M. and Testa B. (1984). Xenobiotic metabolism by brain monooxygenases and other enzymes. In *Advances in Drug Research*, Vol. 13 (ed. Testa B.). pp. 95–207. Academic Press, London.

Miners J., Birkett D.J., Drew R. and McManus M., eds (1988). *Microsomes and Drug Oxidations*. Taylor & Francis, London.

Miwa G.T. and Lu A.Y.H. (1984). The association of cytochrome P-450 and NADPH-cytochrome P-450 reductase in phospholipid membranes. *Arch. Biochem. Biophys.* **234**, 161–166.

Müller-Enoch D., Churchill P., Fleischer S. and Guengerich F.P. (1984). Interaction of liver microsomal cytochrome P-450 and NADPH-cytochrome P-450 reductase in the presence and absence of lipid. *J. Biol. Chem.* **259**, 8174–8182.

Muranishi S.I., Oda T. and Masui Y. (1989). Flavin-catalyzed oxidation of amines and sulfur compounds with hydrogen peroxide. *J. Amer. Chem. Soc.* **111**, 5002–5003.

Murray M. (1987). Mechanisms of the inhibition of cytochrome P-450-mediated drug oxidation by therapeutic agents. *Drug Metab. Rev.* **18**, 55–81.

Muto N., Inouye K., Inada A., Nakanishi T. and Tan L. (1987). Inhibition of cytochrome P-450-linked monooxygenase systems by naphthoquinones. *Biochem. Biophys. Res. Comm.* **146**, 487–494.

Nadler S.G. and Strobel H.W. (1991). Identification and characterization of an NADPH-cytochrome P450 reductase derived peptide involved in binding to cytochrome P450. *Arch. Biochem. Biophys.* **290**, 277–284.

Naqui A., Chance B. and Cadenas E. (1986). Reactive oxygen intermediates in biochemistry. *Annu. Rev. Biochem.* **55**, 137–166.

Nebert D.W. and Negishi M. (1982). Multiple forms of cytochrome P-450 and the importance of molecular biology and evolution. *Biochem. Pharmacol.* **31**, 2311–2317.

Nebert D.W. and Gonzalez F.J. (1985). Cytochrome P450 gene expression and regulation. *Trends Pharmacol. Sci.* **6**, 160–164.

Nebert D.W. and Gonzalez F.J. (1987). P450 genes: Structure, evolution, and regulation. *Annu. Rev. Biochem.* **56**, 945–993.

Nebert D.W., Adesnik M., Coon M.J., Estabrook R.W., Gonzalez F.J., Guengerich F.P., Gunsalus I.C., Johnson E.F., Kemper B., Levin W., Phillips I.R., Sato R. and Waterman M.R. (1987). The P450 gene superfamily: recommended nomenclature. *DNA* **6**, 1–11.

Nebert D.W., Nelson D.R., Adesnik M., Coon M.J., Estabrook R.W., Gonzalez F.J., Guengerich F.P., Gunsalus I.C., Johnson E.F., Kemper B., Levin W., Phillips

I.R., Sato R. and Waterman M.R. (1989a). The P450 superfamily: updated listing of all genes and recommended nomenclature for the chromosomal loci. *DNA* **8**, 1–13.

Nebert D.W., Nelson D.R. and Feyereisen R. (1989b). Evolution of the cytochrome P450 genes. *Xenobiotica* **19**, 1149–1160.

Nebert D.W., Nelson D.R., Coon M.J., Estabrook R.W., Feyereisen R., Fujii-Kuriyama Y., Gonzalez F.J., Guengerich F.P., Gunsalus I.C., Johnson E.F., Loper J.C., Sato R., Waterman M.R. and Waxman D.J. (1991). The P450 superfamily: update on new sequences, gene mapping, and recommended nomenclature. *DNA Cell Biol.* **10**, 1–14.

Nelson D.R. and Strobel H.W. (1988). On the membrane topology of vertebrate cytochrome P-450 proteins. *J. Biol. Chem.* **263**, 6038–6050.

Nelson D.R. and Strobel H.W. (1989). Secondary structure prediction of 52 membrane-bound cytochromes P450 shows a strong structural similarity to P450$_{cam}$. *Biochemistry* **28**, 656–660.

Nelson D.R., Kamataki T., Waxman D.J., Guengerich F.P., Estabrook R.W., Feyereisen R., Gonzalez F.J., Coon M.J., Gunsalus I.C., Gotoh O., Okuda K. and Nebert D.W. (1993). The P450 superfamily: Update on new sequences, gene mapping, accession numbers, early trivial names of enzymes, and nomenclature. *DNA Cell Biol.* **12**, 1–51.

Nerland D.E., Iba M.M. and Mannering G.J. (1981). Use of linoleic acid hydroperoxide in the determination of absolute spectra of membrane-bound cytochrome P-450. *Molec. Pharmacol.* **19**, 162–167.

Noshiro M. and Omura T. (1978). Immunological study on the electron pathway from NADH to cytochrome P-450 of liver microsomes. *J. Biochem.* **83**, 61–77.

Noshiro M., Harada N. and Omura T. (1980). Immunological study on the route of electron transfer from NADH and NADPH to cytochrome P-450 of liver microsomes. *J. Biochem.* **88**, 1521–1535.

Novak R.F. and Vatsis K.P. (1982). ^{1}H Fourier transform NMR relaxation rate studies on the interaction of acetanilide with purified isozymes of rabbit liver microsomal cytochrome P-450 and with cytochrome b_5. *Molec. Pharmacol.* **21**, 701–709.

O'Keeffe D.H., Ebel R.E. and Peterson J.A. (1978). Studies of the oxygen binding site of cytochrome P-450. Nitric oxide as a spin-label probe. *J. Biol. Chem.* **253**, 3509–3516.

Omura T. and Sato R. (1964). The carbon monoxide-binding pigment of liver microsomes. *J. Biol. Chem.* **239**, 2370–2385.

Omura T., Sadano H., Hasegawa T., Yoshida Y. and Kominami S. (1984). Hemoprotein H-450 identified as a form of cytochrome P-450 having an endogenous ligand at the 6th coordination position in the heme. *J. Biochem.* **96**, 1491–1500.

Oprian D.D. and Coon M.J. (1982). Oxidation–reduction states of FMN and FAD in NADPH-cytochrome P-450 reductase during reduction of NADPH. *J. Biol. Chem.* **257**, 8935–8944.

Oprian D.D., Gorsky L.D. and Coon M.J. (1983). Properties of the oxygenated form of liver microsomal cytochrome P-450. *J. Biol. Chem.* **258**, 8684–8691.

Ortiz de Montellano P.R., Editor (1986). *Cytochrome P-450. Structure, Mechanism, and Biochemistry*. Plenum Press, New York.

Ortiz de Montellano P.R., Kunze K.L. and Beilan H.S. (1983). Chiral orientation of prosthetic heme in the cytochrome P-450 active site. *J. Biol. Chem.* **258**, 45–48.

Oshino N. (1978). Cytochrome b_5 and its physiological significance. *Pharmacol. Ther. A* **2**, 477–515.

Ozols J. (1989a). Structure of cytochrome b_5 and its topology in the microsomal membrane. *Biochim. Biophys. Acta* **997**, 121–130.

Ozols J. (1989b). Orientation of microsomal membranes proteins. *Drug Metab. Rev.* **20**, 497–510.

Ozols J., Heinemann F.S. and Johnson E.F. (1985). The complete amino acid sequence of a constitutive form of liver microsomal cytochrome P-450. *J. Biol. Chem.* **260**, 5427–5434.

Packer L., ed. (1984). *Oxygen Radicals in Biological Systems*. Academic Press, Orlando, USA.

Patton S.E., Rosen G.M. and Rauckman E.J. (1980). Superoxide production by purified hamster hepatic nuclei. *Molec. Pharmacol.* **18**, 588–593.

Persson J.O., Terelius Y. and Ingelman-Sundberg M. (1990). Cytochrome P-450-dependent formation of reactive oxygen radicals: isozyme-specific inhibition of P-450-mediated reduction of oxygen and carbon tetrachloride. *Xenobiotica* **20**, 887–900.

Peterson J.A. and Prough R.A. (1986). Cytochrome P-450 reductase and cytochrome b_5 in cytochrome P-450 catalysis. In *Cytochrome P-450. Structure, Mechanism, and Biochemistry* (ed. Ortiz de Montellano P.R.). pp. 89–117. Plenum Press, New York.

Philpot R.M. (1992). The identities of the major cytochrome P450 and flavin-containing monooxygenases expressed in lung. In *Abstracts of the Fourth North American ISSX Meeting*, Bal Harbour, FL, November 2–6, 1992, Abstract 213.

Porter T.D. and Kasper C.B. (1985). Coding nucleotide sequence of rat NADPH-cytochrome P-450 oxidoreductase cDNA and identification of flavin-binding domains. *Proc. Natl. Acad. Sci. USA* **82**, 973–977.

Porter T.D. and Coon M.J. (1991). Cytochrome P-450—Multiplicity of isoforms, substrates, and catalytic and regulatory mechanisms. *J. Biol. Chem.* **266**, 13,469–13,472.

Poulos T.L. (1986). The crystal structure of cytochrome P-450$_{cam}$. In *Cytochrome P-450. Structure, Mechanism, and Biochemistry* (ed. Ortiz de Montellano P.R.). pp. 505–523. Plenum Press, New York.

Poulos T.L. (1988). Cytochrome P-450: molecular architecture, mechanism and prospects for rational inhibitor design. *Pharm. Res.* **5**, 67–75.

Poulos T.L. (1991). Modeling of mammalian P450s on the basis of P450cam X-ray structure. In *Cytochrome P450* (eds Waterman M.R. and Johnson E.F.). pp. 11–30. Academic Press, San Diego.

Poulos T.L. and Howard A.J. (1987). Crystal structure of

metyrapone- and phenylimidazole-inhibited complexes of cytochrome P-450$_{cam}$. *Biochemistry* **26**, 8165–8174.

Poulos T.L. and Raag R. (1992). Cytochrome P450$_{cam}$: crystallography, oxygen activation, and electron transfer. *FASEB J.* **6**, 674–679.

Poulos T.L., Finzel B.C., Gunsalus I.C., Wagner G.C. and Kraut J. (1985). The 2.6-Å crystal structure of *Pseudomonas putida* cytochrome P-450. *J. Biol. Chem.* **260**, 16,122–16,130.

Poulos T.L., Finzel B.C. and Howard A.J. (1986). Crystal structure of substrate-free *Pseudomonas putida* cytochrome P-450. *Biochemistry* **25**, 5314–5322.

Poulsen L.L. and Ziegler D.M. (1979). The liver microsomal FAD-containing monooxygenase. Spectral characterization and kinetic studies. *J. Biol. Chem.* **254**, 6449–6455.

Precious W.Y. and Barrett J. (1989). Xenobiotic metabolism in helminths. *Parasitol. Today* **5**, 156–160.

Puga A. and Nebert D.W. (1990). Evolution of the P450 gene superfamily and regulation of the murine *Cyp1a1* gene. *Biochem. Soc. Trans.* **18**, 7–10.

Raag R. and Poulos T.L. (1989). Crystal structure of the carbon monoxide–substrate–cytochrome P-450$_{cam}$ ternary complex. *Biochemistry* **28**, 7586–7592.

Raag R., Martinis S.A., Sligar S.G. and Poulos T.L. (1991). Crystal structure of the cytochrome P450$_{CAM}$ active site mutant Thr252Ala. *Biochemistry* **30**, 11,420–11,429.

Rahimtula A.D., O'Brien P.J., Hrycay E.G., Peterson J.A. and Estabrook R.W. (1974). Possible higher valence states of cytochrome P-450 during oxidative reactions. *Biochem. Biophys. Res. Commun.* **60**, 695–702.

Reid L.S., Taniguchi V.T., Gray H.B. and Mauk A.G. (1982). Oxidation–reduction equilibrium of cytochrome b_5. *J. Amer. Chem. Soc.* **104**, 7516–7519.

Rein H., Ristau O., Misselwitz R., Buder E. and Ruckpaul K. (1979). The importance of the spin equilibrium in cytochrome P-450 for the reduction rate of the heme iron. *Acta Biol. Med. Germ.* **38**, 187–200.

Rein H., Jung C., Ristau O. and Friedrich J. (1984). Biophysical properties of cytochrome P-450, analysis of the reaction mechanism—thermodynamic aspect. In *Cytochrome P-450* (eds Ruckpaul K. and Rein H.). pp. 163–249. Akademie Verlag, Berlin.

Rekka E., Sterk G.J., Timmerman H. and Bast A. (1988). Identification of structural characteristics of some potential H$_2$-receptor antagonists that determine the interaction with hepatic P-450. *Chem. Biol. Interact.* **67**, 117–127.

Repond C., Bulgheroni A., Meyer U.A., Mayer J.M. and Testa B. (1986). Dual binding of pyridylalkanamides top microsomal cytochrome P-450. *Biochem. Pharmacol.* **35**, 2233–2240.

Ristau O. and Jung C. (1991). Binding sites of pyridine in cytochrome P-450cam. *Biochim. Biophys. Acta* **1078**, 321–325.

Rodrigues A.D., Gibson G.G., Ioannides C. and Parke D.V. (1987). Interactions of imidazole antifungal agents with purified cytochrome P-450 proteins. *Biochem. Pharmacol.* **36**, 4277–4281.

Ruckpaul K. (1978). The molecular organization of the liver microsomal monooxygenatic system. *Pharmazie* **33**, 310–312.

Ruckpaul K. and Rein H., eds (1984). *Cytochrome P-450.* Akademie Verlag, Berlin.

Ruf H.H., Wende P. and Ullrich V. (1979). Models for ferric cytochrome P-450. Characterization of hemin mercaptide complexes by electronic and ESR spectra. *J. Inorg. Biochem.* **11**, 189–204.

Sausen P.S., Duescher R.J. and Elfarra A.A. (1993). Further characterization and purification of the flavin-dependent S-benzyl-L-cysteine S-oxidase activities of rat liver and kidney microsomes. *Molec. Pharmacol.* **43**, 388–396.

Sawyer D.T. and Valentine J.S. (1981). How super is superoxide? *Acc. Chem. Res.* **14**, 393–400.

Scheidt W.R. and Reed C.A. (1981). Spin-state/stereochemical relationships in iron porphyrins: implications for the hemoproteins. *Chem. Rev.* **81**, 543–555.

Schenkman J.B. and Gibson G.G. (1981). Status of the cytochrome P-450 cycle. *Trends Pharmacol. Sci.* **2**, 150–152.

Schenkman J.B., Sligar S.G. and Cinti D.L. (1981). Substrate interaction with cytochrome P-450. *Pharmacol. Ther.* **12**, 43–71.

Sem D.S. and Kasper C.B. (1992). Geometric relationship between the nicotinamide and isoalloxazine rings in NADPH-cytochrome P-450 oxidoreductase: implications for the classification of evolutionary and functionally related flavoproteins. *Biochemistry* **31**, 3391–3398.

Sheets J.J., Mason J.I., Wise C.A. and Estabrook R.W. (1986). Inhibition of rat liver microsomal cytochrome P-450 steroid hydroxylase reactions by imidazole antimycotic agents. *Biochem. Pharmacol.* **35**, 487–491.

Shen A.L., Christensen M.J. and Kasper C.B. (1991). NADPH-Cytochrome P450 oxidoreductase. The role of cysteine 566 in catalysis and cofactor binding. *J. Biol. Chem.* **266**, 19,976–19,980.

Shirabe K., Yubisui T., Nishino T. and Takeshita M. (1991). Role of cysteine residues in human NADH-cytochrome b_5 reductase studied by site-directed mutagenesis. *J. Biol. Chem.* **266**, 7531–7536.

Silver J. and Lukas B. (1984). Mössbauer studies on protoporphyrin IX iron(II) solutions containing sulphur ligands and their carbonyl adducts. Models for the active site of cytochrome P-450. *Inorg. Chim. Acta* **91**, 279–283.

Singh A. (1982). Chemical and biochemical aspects of superoxide radicals and related species of activated oxygen. *Can. J. Physiol. Pharmacol.* **60**, 1330–1345.

Sligar S.G. and Murray R.I. (1986). Cytochrome P-450$_{cam}$ and other bacterial P-450 enzymes. In *Cytochrome P-450. Structure, Mechanism, and Biochemistry* (ed. Ortiz de Montellano P.R.). pp. 429–503. Plenum Press, New York.

Sligar S.G., Cinti D.L., Gibson G.G. and Schenkman J.B. (1979). Spin state control of the hepatic cytochrome P-450 redox potential. *Biochem. Biophys. Res. Commun.* **90**, 925–932.

Sligar S.G., Gelb M.H. and Heimbrook D.C. (1984).

Bio-organic chemistry and cytochrome P-450-dependent catalysis. *Xenobiotica* 14, 63–86.

Smith D.A. and Jones B.C. (1992). Speculations on the substrate structure–activity relationships (SSAR) of cytochrome P450 enzymes. *Biochem. Pharmacol.* 44, 2089–2098.

Sono M. and Dawson J.H. (1982). Formation of low spin complexes of ferric cytochrome P-450-CAM with anionic ligands. *J. Biol. Chem.* 257, 5496–5502.

Soucek P. and Gut I. (1992). Cytochromes P-450 in rats: structures, functions, properties and relevant human forms. *Xenobiotica* 22, 83–103.

Stadtman E.R. (1986). Oxidation of proteins by mixed-function oxidation system: implication in protein turn-over, ageing, and neutrophil function. *Trends Biochem. Sci.* 11, 11–12.

Stadtman E.R. (1988). Protein modification in aging. *J. Gerontol.* 43, B112–B120.

Stadtman E.R. (1990). Metal ion-catalyzed oxidation of protein: biochemical mechanism and biological conse-quences. *Free Rad. Biol. Med.* 9, 315–325.

Stadtman E.R. and Oliver C.N. (1991). Metal-catalyzed oxidation of proteins. Physiological consequences. *J. Biol. Chem.* 266, 2005–2008.

Stayton P.S., Fisher M.T. and Sligar S.G. (1988). Deter-mination of cytochrome b_5 association reactions. *J. Biol. Chem.* 263. 13,544–13,548.

Strittmatter P. and Dailey H.A. (1982). Essential structural features and orientation of cytochrome b_5 in membranes. In *Membranes and Transport*, vol. 1 (ed. Martonosi A.N.). pp. 71–82. Plenum, New York.

Strobel H.W., Dignam J.D. and Gum J.R. (1980). NADPH-cytochrome P-450 reductase and its role in the mixed function oxidase reaction. *Pharmacol. Ther.* 8, 525–537.

Strobel H.W., Nadler S.G. and Nelson D.R. (1989). Cytochrome P450: cytochrome P-450 reductase interac-tions. *Drug Metab. Rev.* 20, 519–533.

Tamburini P.P. and Gibson G.G. (1983). Thermodynamic studies of the protein–protein interactions between cytochrome P-450 and cytochrome b_5. Evidence for a central role of the cytochrome P-450 spin state in the coupling of substrate and cytochrome b_5 binding to the terminal hemoprotein. *J. Biol. Chem.* 258, 13,444–13,452.

Tamburini P.P. and Schenkman J.B. (1986). Differences in the mechanism of functional interaction between NADPH-cytochrome P-450 reductase and its redox partners. *Molec. Pharmacol.* 30, 178–185.

Tamburini P.P., MacFarquhar S. and Schenkman J.B. (1986). Evidence for binary complex formations between cytochrome P-450, cytochrome b_5 and NADPH-cytochrome P-450 reductase of hepatic microsomes. *Biochem. Biophys. Res. Commun.* 134, 519–526.

Tang S.C., Koch S., Papaefthymiou G.C., Foner S., Frankel R.B., Ibers J.A. and Holm R.H. (1976). Axial ligation modes in iron(III) porphyrins. Models for the oxidized reaction states of cytochrome P-450 enzymes and the molecular structure of iron(III) protoporphyrin IX dimethyl ester *p*-nitrobenzenethiolate. *J. Amer.*

Chem. Soc. 98, 2414–2434.

Taniguchi H., Imai Y. and Sato R. (1984). Role of the electron transfer system in microsomal drug mono-oxygenase reaction catalyzed by cytochrome P-450. *Arch. Biochem. Biophys.* 232, 585–596.

Tarr G.E., Black S.D., Fujita V.S. and Coon M.J. (1983). Complete amino acid sequence and predicted membrane topology of phenobarbital-induced cytochrome P-450 (isozyme 2) from rabbit liver microsomes. *Proc. Natl. Acad. Sci. USA* 80, 6552–6556.

Testa B. and Jenner P. (1981). Inhibitors of cytochrome P-450s and their mechanism of action. *Drug Metab. Rev.* 12, 1–117.

Trager W.F. (1982). The postenzymatic chemistry of activated oxygen. *Drug Metab. Rev.* 13, 51–69.

Traylor T.G., White D.K., Campbell D.H. and Berzinis A.P. (1981). Electronic effects on the binding of diox-ygen and carbon monoxide to hemes. *J. Amer. Chem. Soc.* 103, 4932–4936.

Tsubaki M., Yoshikawa S., Ichikawa Y. and Yu N.T. (1992). Effects of cholesterol side-chain groups and adrenodoxin binding on the vibrational modes of carbon monoxide bound to cytochrome P450scc: implications of the productive and nonproductive substrate bindings. *Biochemistry* 31, 8991–8999.

Tuck S.F., Hiroya K., Shimizu T., Hatano M. and Ortiz de Montellano P. (1993). The cytochrome P450 1A2 active site: topology and perturbations caused by glutamic acid-318 and threonine-319 mutations. *Biochemistry* 32, 2548–2553.

Turner C.R., Marcus C.B. and Jefcoate C.R. (1985). Selectivity in the binding of hydroxylated ben-zo[*a*]pyrene derivatives to cytochrome P-450c. *Bio-chemistry* 24, 5124–5130.

Tynes R.E. and Hodgson E. (1985). Catalytic activity and substrate specificity of the flavin-containing monooxyge-nase in microsomal systems: characterization of the hepatic, pulmonary and renal enzymes of the mouse, rabbit and rat. *Arch. Biochem. Biophys.* 240, 77–93.

Tynes R.E. and Philpot R.M. (1987). Tissue- and species-dependent expression of multiple forms of mammalian microsomal flavin-containing monooxygenase. *Molec. Pharmacol.* 31, 569–574.

Ullrich V. and Kremers P. (1977). Multiple forms of cytochrome P-450 in the microsomal monooxygenase system. *Arch. Toxicol.* 39, 41–50.

Vergères G., Winterhalter K.H. and Richter C. (1989). Identification of the membrane anchor of microsomal rat liver cytochrome P-450. *Biochemistry* 28, 3650–3655.

Vergères G., Winterhalter K.H. and Richter C. (1991). Localization of the N-terminal methionine of rat liver cytochrome P-450 in the lumen of the endoplasmic reticulum. *Biochim. Biophys. Acta* 1063, 235–241.

Vijayakumar S. and Salerno J.C. (1992). Molecular modeling of the 3D structure of cytochrome P450$_{scc}$. *Biochim. Biophys. Acta* 1160, 281–286.

Walsh C. (1980a). Scope and mechanism of enzymatic monooxygenation reactions. *Ann. Rep. Med. Chem.* 15, 207–216.

Walsh C. (1980b). Flavin coenzymes: at the crossroads of

biological redox chemistry. *Acc. Chem. Res.* **13**, 148–155.

Wang P.P., Beaune P., Kaminsky L.S., Dannan G.A., Kadlubar F.F., Larrey D. and Guengerich F.P. (1983). Purification and characterization of six cytochrome P-450 isozymes from human liver microsomes. *Biochemistry* **22**, 5375–5383.

Waterman M.R. and Johnson E.F., eds (1991). *Cytochrome P450.* 716 pages. Academic Press, San Diego.

Wendoloski J.J., Matthew J.B., Weber P.C. and Salemme F.R. (1987). Molecular dynamics of a cytochrome *c*–cytochrome *b*$_5$ electron transfer complex. *Science* **238**, 794–797.

White R.E. and Coon M.J. (1980). Oxygen activation by cytochrome P-450. *Annu. Rev. Biochem.* **49**, 315–356.

White R.E. and Coon M.J. (1982). Heme ligand replacement reactions of cytochrome P-450. Characterization of the bonding atom of the axial ligand trans to thiolate as oxygen. *J. Biol. Chem.* **257**, 3073–3083.

Wickramasinghe R.H. and Villee C.A. (1975). Early role during chemical evolution for cytochrome P-450 in oxygen detoxification. *Nature* **256**, 509–511.

Williams D.E., Hale S.E., Muerhoff A.S. and Masters B.S.S. (1985). Rabbit lung flavin-containing monooxygenase. Purification, characterization, and induction during pregnancy. *Molec. Pharmacol.* **28**, 381–390.

Wilshire J. and Sawyer D.T. (1979). Redox chemistry of dioxygen species. *Acc. Chem. Res.* **12**, 105–110.

Winston G.W. and Cederbaum A.I. (1983). NADPH-dependent production of oxy radicals by purified components of the rat liver mixed function oxidase system. I. Oxidation of hydroxyl radical scavenging agents. *J. Biol. Chem.* **258**, 1508–1513.

Wrighton S.A., Campanile C., Thomas P.E., Maines S.L., Watkins P.B., Parker G., Mendez-Picon G., Haniu M., Shively J.E., Lewin W. and Guzelian P.S. (1986). Identification of a human liver cytochrome P-450 homologous to the major isosafrole-inducible cytochrome P-450

in the rat. *Molec. Pharmacol.* **29**, 405–410.

Wrighton S.A. and Stevens J.C. (1992). The human hepatic cytochromes P450 involved in drug metabolism. *Crit. Rev. Toxicol.* **22**, 1–21.

Yamano S., Aoyama T., McBride O.W., Hardwick J.P., Gelboin H.V. and Gonzalez F.J. (1989). Human NADPH-P450 oxidoreductase: complementary DNA cloning, sequence and vaccinia virus-mediated expression and localization of the CYPOR gene to chromosome 7. *Molec. Pharmacol.* **36**, 83–88.

Yang C.S. (1977). Organization and interaction of monooxygenase enzymes in microsomal membrane. *Life Sci.* **21**, 1047–1057.

Yoo M. and Steggles A.W. (1988). The complete nucleotide sequence of human liver cytochrome *b*$_5$ mRNA. *Biochem. Biophys. Res. Commun.* **156**, 576–581.

Yubisui T., Shirabe K., Takeshita M., Kobayashi Y., Fukumaki Y., Sakaki Y. and Takano T. (1991). Structural role of serine 127 in the NADH-binding site of human NADH-cytochrome *b*$_5$ reductase. *J. Biol. Chem.* **266**, 66–77.

Zhang H. and Somerville C. (1988). The primary structure of chicken liver cytochrome *b*$_5$ deduced from the DNA sequence of a cDNA clone. *Arch. Biochem. Biophys.* **264**, 343–347.

Ziegler D.M. (1980). Microsomal flavin-containing monooxygenase: Oxygenation of nucleophilic nitrogen and sulfur compounds. In *Enzymatic Basis of Detoxication*, Vol. 1 (ed. Jakoby W.B.). pp. 201–227. Academic Press, New York.

Ziegler D.M. (1988). Flavin-containing monooxygenases: catalytic mechanism and substrate specificities. *Drug Metab. Rev.* **19**, 1–32.

Ziegler D.M. (1993). Recent studies on the structure and function of multisubstrate flavin-containing monooxygenases. *Annu. Rev. Pharmacol. Toxicol.* **33**, 179–199.

chapter 4

CARBON OXIDATIONS CATALYZED BY CYTOCHROMES P450

Contents

4.1 INTRODUCTION

Having examined in the previous chapter the enzymatic and biochemical features of mono-oxygenases and particularly cytochrome P450, we shall now take a more chemical point of view and discuss the characteristics of substrates, reaction mechanisms, and products. This will be done in a series of chapters which will present many of the reactions catalyzed by cytochrome P450 and flavin-containing monooxygenase (FMO) (see section 3.7 Coon *et al.*, 1992; Guengerich, 1991; Guengerich and Macdonald, 1990; Koymans *et al.*, 1993; Ortiz de Montellano, 1984).

Oxidations of carbon atoms mediated by cytochrome P450 represent a convenient yet deceptively simple starting point. Carbon atoms in organic compounds differ greatly in their hybridization and molecular environment, and these characteristics are of utmost relevance as far as reactivity towards monooxygenases is concerned. This is duly acknowledged in the structure of Chapters 4–9. In the present chapter, we consider only carbon atoms connected to other carbons and/or to hydrogen atoms. From the viewpoint of monooxygenases, the reactivity of such carbons is often different from that of carbons linked to heteroatoms, as discussed in Chapters 6–9. However, it would be wrong to infer from the above that the present chapter is restricted to unactivated carbons; carbons adjacent to C–C double bonds (allylic position) or aromatic rings (benzylic position) are particularly interesting and in fact share some analogies with heteroatom-adjacent carbons.

4.2 OXIDATION OF sp³-HYBRIDIZED CARBON ATOMS

4.2.1 Reaction mechanism of C-sp³ hydroxylation

The overall cytochrome P450-mediated hydroxylation of sp³-hybridized carbons is described by Eq. 4.1:

$$RR'R''C-H + [O] \rightarrow RR'R''C-O-H \qquad \text{(Eq. 4.1)}$$

and represents the substitution of a hydrogen atom by a hydroxyl group. Targets of this reaction are methyl (CH_3), methylene (CH_2), and methine (CH) groups, yielding primary, secondary or tertiary alcoholic groups, respectively. The resulting metabolites may then undergo further metabolism as discussed in other chapters, e.g. dehydrogenation (Chapter 2); oxygenation (Chapter 7); or conjugation (see the volume in this series, *Biochemistry of Conjugation Reactions*). Note that a quaternary C-sp³ is inert in such a reaction, a point implicit in the discussions to follow.

The reaction of C-sp³ hydroxylation displays a number of noteworthy features; for example, its often marked regio- and stereoselectivity (see Section 6) must be contrasted with the apparently unlimited structural variety of its substrates. It is only natural therefore that biochemists rapidly became intrigued by the chemical mechanism of the reaction and have been hard at work to unravel its intricacies.

An important early contribution to our understanding of the reaction mechanism was the work of McMahon and colleagues with **ethylbenzene** (**4.I**). In rat liver preparations, this model compound was hydroxylated with high regioselectivity in the benzylic position and marked enantioselectivity to give predominantly (+)-(*R*)-1-phenylethanol (**4.II**) (*R/S* ratio 6/1). Incubating the labelled, chiral substrate (+)-(*S*)-[1-²H]ethylbenzene (**4.III**) afforded (+)-(*R*)-[1-²H]-1-

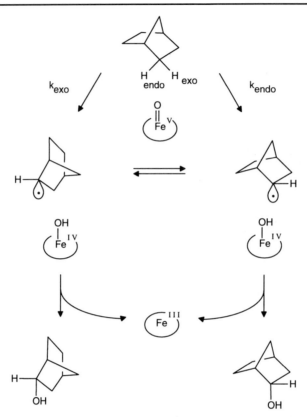

FIGURE 4.1 The oxygen rebound mechanism of cytochrome P450-mediated C-sp³ hydroxylation, as first deduced from the oxidation of norbornane to *exo-* and *endo-*2-norborneol (left and right route, respectively) (modified from Groves *et al.*, 1978).

phenylethanol (**4.IV**) as the major metabolite (*R/S* ratio 11/1; deuterium retention 86%) (McMahon *et al.*, 1969). Thus the reaction proceeded predominantly with retention of configuration, and this was taken as important evidence to indicate the mechanism to be one of front side displacement, in other words **insertion** of the oxene atom into the C–H bond (the formation and nature of oxene are discussed in Section 3.5).

Later studies on the hydroxylation of **norbornane** by a reconstituted cytochrome P450 system challenged this interpretation. The unlabelled substrate afforded *exo-* and *endo-*2-norborneol in a 3.4/1 ratio (Fig. 4.1), but the use of various deuterated isotopomers showed the reaction to display a very large isotope effect ($k_H/k_D = 11.5 \pm 1$) and to involve a significant amount of epimerization in the hydroxylation process (Groves *et al.*, 1978). These results imply a **homolytic hydrogen abstraction** as the rate-determining step, leading to an intermediate carbon radical that undergoes partial epimerization (Fig. 4.1). Similar conclusions were reached upon reinvestigation of the cytochrome P450LM2-mediated hydroxylation of ethylbenzene, (*S*)- and (*R*)-(1-²H)ethylbenzene, and (1-²H₂)ethylbenzene; here again the existence of a discrete tricoordinate carbon intermediate was inferred (White *et al.*, 1986).

The intrinsic primary isotope effect measured by Groves *et al.* (1978) affords primary evidence for the postulated mechanism of hydrogen abstraction. Thus, semiempirical quantum mechanical calculations have indicated the kinetic isotope effect to be about 1.6 for the reaction of singlet oxygen insertion, and 8–9 for the triplet oxygen reaction proceeding via a hydrogen radical abstraction–recombination mechanism (Shea *et al.*, 1983). The latter value corresponds well with the isotope effect reported above, and even better with the primary isotope effect of 7.3–7.9

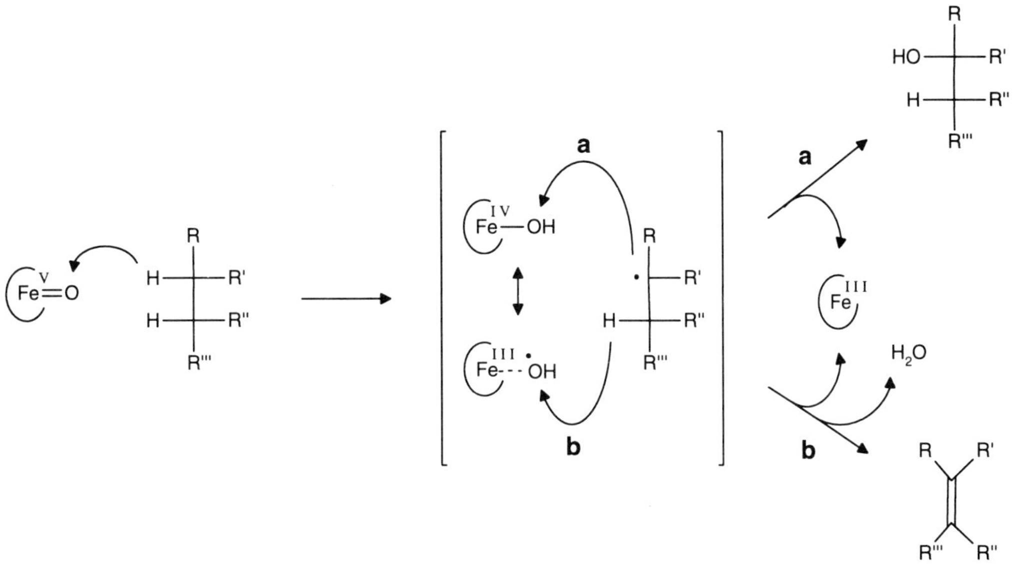

FIGURE 4.2 Cytochrome P450-catalyzed oxidation of sp³-carbon atoms resulting in hydroxylation or desaturation. Following hydrogen abstraction, there is competition between oxygen rebound (reaction **a**) leading to a hydroxylated metabolite, and abstraction of a second hydrogen (reaction **b**) leading to an olefin.

measured by a highly refined method for the CYP2B1-catalyzed ω-hydroxylation of n-octane (Jones and Trager, 1987).

The mechanism of hydrogen radical abstraction has come to be known as the **oxygen rebound mechanism** and has been extensively studied and discussed (reaction **a** in Fig. 4.2) (Champion, 1989; Dolphin, 1985; Groves, 1985; Guengerich and Macdonald, 1984 and 1990; Ortiz de Montellano, 1987; Ortiz de Montellano and Stearns, 1989; Sligar *et al.*, 1984). The perferryl-oxygen intermediate, or perhaps another form of the oxo-heme complex discussed in Section 3.5.4, is postulated to be responsible for homolytic cleavage of the C–H bond. This transforms the substrate into a carbon-centred free radical, while the enzyme becomes an iron-hydroxide intermediate in which the hydroxyl radical can be bound more or less tightly (Ingold, 1989). Collapse of this complex to form the hydroxylated product is presumably a cage reaction with a low-energy barrier. However, the **stereoselectivity** often observed in such hydroxylations appears contrary to the expected behaviour of a radical process (which would involve very extensive epimerization) and has for example been attributed to steric constraints within the active site (Guengerich and Macdonald, 1984; White *et al.*, 1986).

This stereochemical puzzle remained irritatingly unresolved until Ortiz de Montellano, in studies of particular elegance, demonstrated that the radical pair collapses with stereochemical specificity at a rate in excess of $10^9 \, s^{-1}$ (Ortiz de Montellano, 1987; Ortiz de Montellano and Stearns, 1987). In other words, and to quote Ortiz de Montellano (1987), "the enzymatic hydroxylation consequently masquerades as a concerted process because the carbon radical intermediate is trapped by the iron-coordinated hydroxyl radical before it can rearrange or break out of the solvent cage". The last part of this sentence is also of utmost significance as it explains why cytochrome P450-mediated C-sp³ hydroxylation is usually not a toxication reaction liberating carbon-centred free radicals. The experiment that allowed the rate of collapse to be estimated was the internal timing provided by the rearrangement of cytochrome P450-generated radicals of ring-strained hydrocarbon probes, e.g. **bicyclo[2.1.0]pentane** (Fig. 4.3). The bicyclo[2.1.0]pentyl radical undergoes two reactions, namely hydroxylation (reaction **a** in Fig.

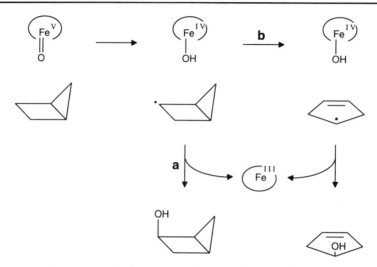

FIGURE 4.3 Competition between radical recombination (reaction **a**) and ring opening (reaction **b**) in the cytochrome P450-catalyzed hydroxylation of bicyclo[2.1.0]pentane to *endo*-bicyclo[2.1.0]pentan-2-ol and 3-cyclopentenol, respectively (modified from Ortiz de Montellano, 1987).

4.3) and rearrangement to the 3-cyclopropenyl radical (reaction **b** in Fig. 4.3). Rearrangement proceeds with a rate constant of $10^9\,s^{-1}$ or faster, yet the two metabolites *endo*-bicyclo[2.1.0]pentan-2-ol and 3-cyclopentanol (Fig. 4.3) were obtained in a 7/1 ratio indicating that little rearrangement had occurred (Ortiz de Montellano and Stearns, 1987). The rate constant for oxygen rebound has later been refined to $k_{OH} = 1.7 \times 10^{10}\,M^{-1}\,s^{-1}$ (Bowry *et al.*, 1989; Ingold, 1989)

No rearrangement of the carbon-centred radical exists in Fig. 4.2 whereas such a reaction is evidenced in Fig. 4.3 (reaction **b**). In our present state of knowledge, **rearrangement** of the carbon-centred radical intermediate is the exception rather than the rule, but a number of informative examples can be found in the literature which involve C–C bond cleavage and/or formation (Hakamatsuka *et al.*, 1991; Ortiz de Montellano, 1989):

- opening of strained alicycles (e.g. Fig. 4.3);
- ring closure;
- ring contraction;
- ring enlargement (e.g. Section 4.5);
- C-demethylation (Section 7.6);
- migration of an aryl group.

From the discussion above, it can be inferred that because of the efficiency of the rebound reaction, radical rearrangement must be extremely fast to occur at all. In particular, **radical delocalization** may be critical. Hence the chemical nature of the substrate will understandably condition the relative importance of hydroxylation and rearrangement. But enzymatic factors may also operate, and much remains to be done to understand them.

4.2.2 Reaction mechanism of C-sp³ desaturation

An additional reaction of the carbon-centred radical intermediate is desaturation to yield an olefin (reaction **b**, Fig. 4.2). An obvious prerequisite for the reaction is the presence in the substrate of two vicinal hydrogens, but other, poorly understood chemical properties may also be of importance.

An example of particular toxicological interest is **ethyl carbamate** (**4.V**), a carcinogen activated by oxidation to vinyl carbamate (**4.VI**) and then to an epoxide which reacts with nucleic acids. It has been demonstrated that CYP2E1 abstracts a hydrogen radical from the terminal carbon, yielding a C-centred radical as precursor of both 2-hydroxyethyl carbamate and vinyl carbamate (**4.VI**) (Guengerich and Kim, 1991). These metabolites were formed when ethyl carbamate was incubated with human liver microsomes.

4.V   4.VI

A few additional examples of desaturation will be discussed in subsequent sections.

4.2.3 Oxidation of non-activated C-sp³ atoms in alkyl groups

Hydroxylation of activated (i.e. adjacent to heteroatoms or conjugated systems) or non-activated sp³ carbons is one of the reactions most frequently encountered in xenobiotic metabolism. An impressive variety of alkyl and cycloalkyl groups are known to be targets of the reaction, a few of which will be presented here. For the sake of clarity, non-activated and activated carbons will be discussed separately, although the difference in reactivity between the two types is a quantitative rather than qualitative one.

The relative importance of C-hydroxylation at different positions in a molecule (i.e. the regioselectivity) depends on a number of factors such as the strength of the C–H bonds and their steric environment (which together are expressed in the reactivity of these bonds). Thus, the relative ability of a C–H bond to undergo cytochrome P450-catalyzed hydrogen abstraction can be estimated from the relative stability and ionization potential of the resulting radical (Korzekwa *et al.*, 1990a). Subtle topographical differences in the active site of cytochrome P450 isozymes can also contribute markedly to substrate and product selectivities.

Simple alkanes provide interesting illustrations of these principles. Thus, **n-hexane** yields three distinct primary metabolites, namely the three positional isomers of hexanol. With two purified phenobarbital-inducible cytochromes P450, 2-hexanol was formed preferentially, the turnover number decreasing in the series 2-hexanol > 3-hexanol > 1-hexanol; with a β-naphthflavone-inducible isozyme, 3-hexanol had the highest turnover number (Toftgård *et al.*, 1986). This is only part of the story, however, as n-hexane is further transformed into a variety of relevant metabolites, some of which have toxic potential. A partial metabolic scheme of n-hexane is shown in Fig. 4.4. Note in particular the further metabolism of 2-hexanol, which can be dehydrogenated reversibly to the ketone or be further hydroxylated to yield 2,5-hexanediol. A branching point is represented by 5-hydroxy-2-hexanone which leads to the neurotoxic 2,5-hexanedione (Perbellini *et al.*, 1982) (see also Section 4.2.6). Analogous metabolites were found in the urine of humans exposed to n-heptane (Perbellini *et al.*, 1986).

How enzymatic factors can override chemical reactivity is seen in the reaction mechanism of CYP4A1, the isozyme that hydroxylates **lauric acid** in the terminal position (ω-position). Indeed,

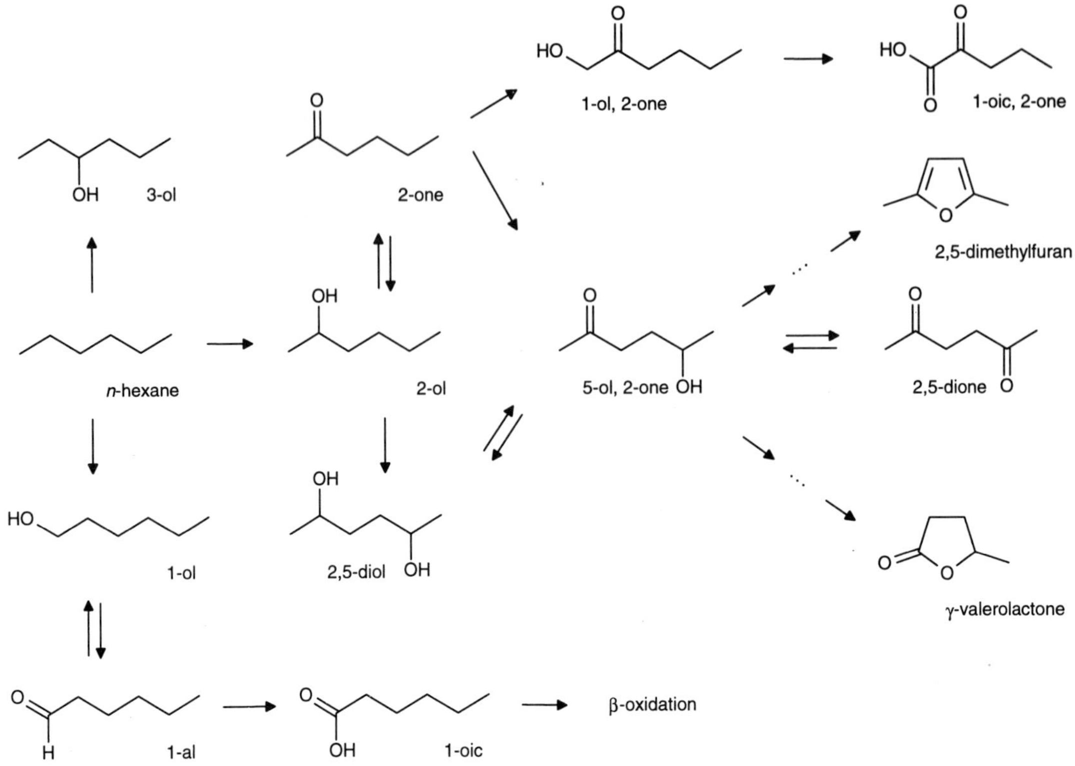

FIGURE 4.4 Partial metabolic scheme of *n*-hexane (modified from Perbellini *et al.*, 1982).

the active site of this isozyme is so efficiently structured that it suppresses $(\omega - 1)$-hydroxylation to deliver the oxygen atom to the apparently disfavoured ω-position (CaJacob *et al.*, 1988).

Valproic acid (4.VII, VA) is an important drug whose metabolism is of particular biochemical and toxicological interest (Baillie, 1992; Nau, 1990). Besides β-oxidation to be discussed in a future volume, cytochrome P450-mediated hydroxylation occurs at the ω-, $(\omega - 1)$- and $(\omega - 2)$-positions to yield the 5-, 4- and 3-hydroxylated metabolites and products of further metabolism (Abbott *et al.*, 1986; Collins *et al.*, 1991; Dickinson *et al.*, 1989; Prickett and Baillie,

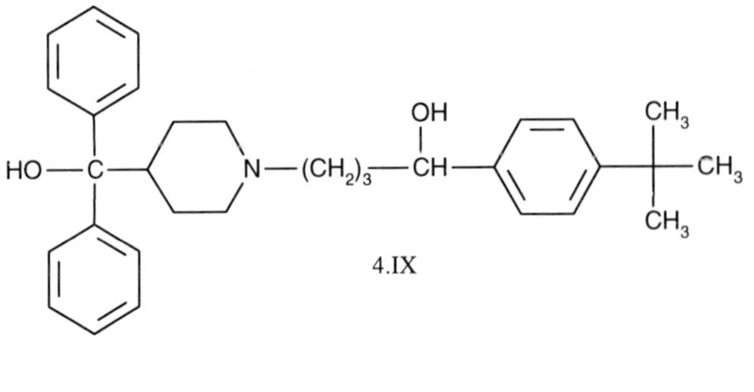

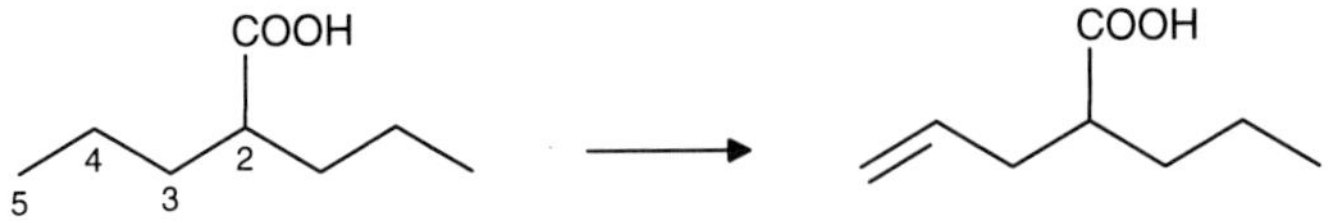

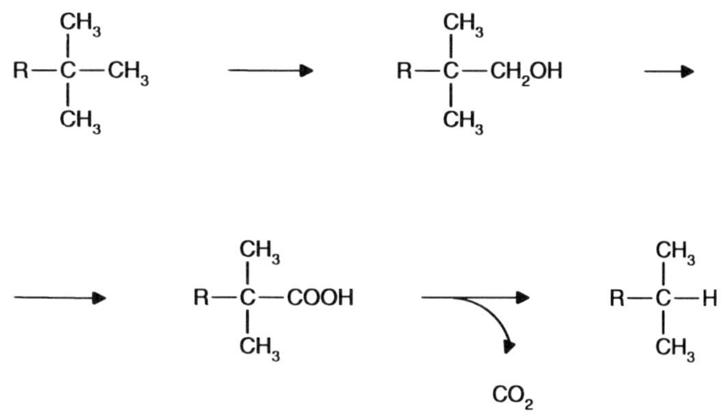

$$
\begin{array}{ccc}
\underset{\underset{CH_3}{|}}{\overset{\overset{CH_3}{|}}{R-C-CH_3}} & \longrightarrow & \underset{\underset{CH_3}{|}}{\overset{\overset{CH_3}{|}}{R-C-CH_2OH}} \longrightarrow \cdots\cdots
\end{array}
$$

$$
\longrightarrow \quad \underset{\underset{CH_3}{|}}{\overset{\overset{CH_3}{|}}{R-C-COOH}} \quad \longrightarrow \quad \underset{\underset{CH_3}{|}}{\overset{\overset{CH_3}{|}}{R-C-H}}
$$

$$
CO_2
$$

FIGURE 4.5 Sequential steps in the metabolic transformation of *tert*-butyl groups.

1984; Rettenmeier *et al.*, 1987 and 1989). Fatty acids and prostanoids undergo analogous cytochrome P450-mediated hydroxylations, the physiological significance of which is as yet incompletely understood. In addition to being hydroxylated, VA also undergoes cytochrome P450-mediated desaturation (Section 4.2.2) to 2-*n*-propyl-4-pentenoic acid (**4.VIII**, also known as Δ^4-VA) (Baillie, 1992; Kassahun and Baillie, 1993; Rettie *et al.*, 1987 and 1988). It was concluded that the C-5 and C-5 centred radicals of VA are precursors not only of the 5- and 4-hydroxylated metabolites, respectively, but also of Δ^4-VA. Further oxidation of Δ^4-VA is discussed in Section 4.4.2.

Methyl groups in a variety of positions (e.g. in branched alkyl groups and on alicycles) undergo cytochrome P450-catalyzed hydroxylation. Cases where the attachment is to a heteroatom (i.e. demethylation) or to an unsaturated system will be discussed later. Here, we first mention the **tert-butyl substituent**, since it can be hydroxylated at one of its CH_3 groups, as documented for mabuterol (Horiba *et al.*, 1984). Such a hydroxylated metabolite may be further oxidized to the acid (see Fig. 4.5), as documented for finasteride, terfenadine and other drugs (Carlin *et al.*, 1992; Garteiz *et al.*, 1982). In the case of the antihistaminic drug terfenadine (**4.IX**), the acid formed by oxidation of a methyl group is the major metabolite in human urine; CYP3A enzymes mediate the first oxidation step (Chan *et al.*, 1991; Yun *et al.*, 1993). The pathway *tert*-butyl oxidation may continue with a decarboxylation to yield an isopropyl group, as postulated for N-*tert*-butylnorchlorcyclizine (Kamm and Szuna, 1973) (Fig. 4.5).

Another interesting case, and one of particular biochemical and physiological significance, is offered by the 10-methyl group in androgens (i.e. C-19). Here, the methyl group is adjacent to a quaternary C-sp^3 and is oxidized to formic acid by the aromatase cytochrome P450 system (e.g. Kellis and Vickery, 1987). This is in fact a reaction of C-demethylation leading to ring A aromatization and estrogen formation, as discussed in more detail in Section 7.6.

Barbiturates bear **alkyl side-chains** that experience only limited activation since they are attached to a quaternary C-sp^3. With these compounds, side-chains of four carbons or more are usually hydroxylated preferentially at the ($\omega - 1$)-position (penultimate carbon), while hydroxylation of the terminal carbon is preferred for 3-carbon chains (reviewed in Testa and Jenner, 1976). Thus, about 40% of a dose of butobarbital (**4.X**) or pentobarbital (**4.XI**) were recovered in human urine as 3'-oxidized metabolites (3'-hydroxy and 3'-oxo), while the 4'-oxidized metabolites (4'-hydroxy and the ω-acid) represented *ca* 4% and 10% of a dose, respectively (Al Sharifi *et al.*, 1983). In contrast, secbutobarbital (**4.XII**) yields about 1/4 to 1/3 of a dose as the ω-acid, while only 2–3% is accounted for by the sum of the 2'-hydroxy and 2'-oxo metabolites (Gilbert *et al.*, 1975).

4.X   R = $-CH_2CH_2CH_2CH_3$ (3', 4')

4.XI   R = $-CHCH_2CH_2CH_3$
                  |
                  CH_3

4.XII   R = $-CHCH_2CH_3$ (2', 3')
                  |
                  CH_3

Hydroxylation reactions at carbons alpha to heteroatoms (N, O and S) will be examined in separate chapters (i.e. Chapters 6 and 7) since they lead to metabolic pathways differing markedly from those discussed here. Carbons alpha to heteroatoms are highly favoured positions of oxidative attack as will be seen, but it is interesting in this section to consider hydroxylation at other positions in **heteroatom-attached alkyl groups**. That hydroxylation at the β-position, the γ-position, or at further removed positions occurs is documented by a variety of studies. Thus, β-hydroxylation (i.e. ω-hydroxylation) of the ethyl group is a minor but genuine metabolic reaction of phenacetin (**4.XIII**), leading to the urinary excretion of the corresponding acid (4-acetamidophenoxyacetic acid, **4.XIV**); the relative importance of this reaction is strongly dependent on biological factors, being for example markedly increased by phenobarbital induction (Fischbach and Lenk, 1985). Also, the excretion of **4.XIV** is much smaller in humans than in the rat (Dittmann and Renner, 1977). Comparable observations were made with chlorpropamide (**4.XV**), which undergoes β-hydroxylation (i.e. $(\omega - 1)$-hydroxylation) of its *n*-propyl group as the major metabolic route in humans, α- and γ-hydroxylation being minor routes (Thomas and Judy, 1972). In contrast, α-hydroxylation (i.e. N-dealkylation, see Chapter 6) is a major pathway in rats.

4.XIII

4.XIV

4.XV

4.2.4 Oxidation of non-activated C-sp³ atoms in cycloalkyl groups

Cycloalkyl groups are of interest in the present context because they appear as substituents in a number of drugs and other xenobiotics, and because their relative rigidity is a useful feature when assessing structural factors that influence metabolic hydroxylation. In this area, studies of particular significance have been published. Thus, large differences in the pattern of hydroxylation of D-camphor (**4.XVI**), adamantanone (**4.XVII**) and adamantane (**4.XVIII**) were noted following incubation with cytochrome P450cam (CYP101) and cytochrome P450LM2 (CYP2B4) (White *et al.*, 1984). With CYP101 as the catalyst, each substrate yielded a single metabolite, namely 5-*exo*-hydroxycamphor, 5-hydroxyadamantanone, and 1-adamantanol; these metabolites result from attack at topographically congruent positions and imply a rather rigid enzyme-substrate complex (Raag and Poulos, 1991). In particular, the substrate is tightly bound to CYP101 by Tyr-96 (H-bonding), Val-247 and Val-295 (steric constraint), as revealed by artificial mutants of CYP101 (Atkins and Sligar, 1989). In contrast to wild-type CYP101, two or three products were formed from CYP2B4, namely 3-*endo*-, 5-*exo*-, and 5-*endo*-hydroxycamphor, 4-*anti*- and 5-hydroxyadamantanone, and 1- and 2-adamantanol. This distribution of products reflects the rank order of chemical reactivity of the various positions of hydroxylation, suggesting considerable freedom of movement of the substrate in the complex, and exposure of most of the hydrogens to enzymatic attack (see also Collins and Loew, 1988).

| 4.XVI | 4.XVII | 4.XVIII | 4.XIX |

Even more informative is the metabolism of **methylcyclohexane (4.XIX)**, a substrate containing primary, secondary and tertiary carbons, i.e. one CH_3, five CH_2 and one CH group. Hydroxylation by CYP2B4 gave a mixture of primary, secondary and tertiary methylcyclohexanols; after statistical correction of the percent distribution of the three types of hydrogens, the ratio of primary, secondary and tertiary alcohols was found to be 0.07/1/1.25 (White *et al.*, 1979). The ratio of primary to secondary alcohols is in accord with a selective hydrogen abstraction step. In contrast, the ratio of tertiary to secondary alcohols is lower than expected from a simple consideration of the C–H bond strength, indicating that a strong steric effect restricts access of the oxidant to the tertiary hydrogen. This postulate was supported by the fact that the ratio of 2-hydroxylation to the sum of 3- and 4-hydroxylation was only 0.026 when a statistical probability predicts a ratio of 0.67, indicating marked steric hindrance at the 2-position also (White *et al.*, 1979).

Two groups of cycloalkane derivatives, namely **steroid hormones** and **terpenes**, deserve special mention due to the physiological and toxicological significance of their regioselective and stereoselective hydroxylations catalyzed by cytochrome P450 (e.g. Santhanakrishnan, 1984; Swinney *et al.*, 1987; Waxman, 1988).

Various drugs contain cycloalkyl groups, their hydroxylation being documented in a number of cases. For example, the compound **MK-473 (4.XX)** was hydroxylated on the cyclopentyl group in humans and laboratory animals; oxidation occurred predominantly at the *trans*-3'- and *cis*-4'-position, but a small proportion of 1'-hydroxylation was also seen (Zacchei *et al.*, 1978). **Phencyclidine (4.XXI)** is also an interesting compound in the present context due to its cyclohexyl and piperidyl groups. Two monohydroxylated derivatives, 4-hydroxy- and 4'-hydroxyphencyclidine, were major urinary metabolites, the ratio of the two products being 2:1 and 4:1 in humans and dogs, respectively (Lin *et al.*, 1975).

A large variety of more complex saturated cyclic systems have also been investigated, two of which are presented here. Hydroxylation of a seven-membered ring is exemplified by **tolazamide (4.XXII)**, a hypoglycaemic agent. In humans, the 4'-hydroxylated derivative was a major urinary metabolite; no other ring-hydroxylated products were seen (Thomas *et al.*, 1978). Another hypoglycaemic drug, **gliclazide (4.XXIII)**, offers the example of a more complex cyclic system, yet hydroxylation at the most accessible positions was again characterized. Indeed, the 3-azabicyclo[3.3.0]oct-3-yl group was hydroxylated in humans at the 6β-, 7β- and 7α-position, the relative importance of the reactions decreasing in this order (Oida *et al.*, 1985).

Whether relatively simple or more complex, alicyclic groups always provide challenging opportunities for biochemists to unravel the regioselectivity, stereoselectivity, and other structural intricacies of hydroxylation reactions. But valuable information is also obtained from less ambitious studies, as is frequently the case. While the examples reported above leave many questions unanswered, they nevertheless indicate that a large variety of cycloalkyl groups can be hydroxylated, the most accessible positions being consistently preferred.

4.2.5 Oxidation of benzylic positions

A number of unsaturated functional groups direct hydroxylation to adjacent sp^3 carbons, the resulting regioselectivity being high or low, depending on a number of chemical and biological factors. The following unsaturated systems have been found to activate adjacent carbon atoms:

- aromatic rings (activation of benzylic positions);
- carbon–carbon double bonds (activation of allylic positions);
- carbonyl groups in ketones and amides;
- carbon–carbon triple bonds;
- cyano groups.

As compared to the beta- and gamma-positions, these alpha-positions have in common larger electron densities in the C–H bonds, and smaller electron densities in the C atoms (Testa and Mihailova, 1978; Testa *et al.*, 1979). These results from molecular orbital calculations appear as interesting electronic indices for predicting regioselective aliphatic hydroxylations. In addition, they are compatible with attack by the electrophilic oxene and with radical stabilization in the transition state.

The simplest model compound for **benzylic hydroxylation** is **toluene (4.XXIV)**, a xenobiotic undergoing cytochrome P450-mediated hydroxylation; this is followed by dehydrogenase-catalyzed dehydrogenation to benzaldehyde and benzoic acid which, as a conjugate, accounts for about 80% of a dose in humans (Parke, 1968). A number of cytochromes P450 can catalyze benzyl alcohol formation from toluene, namely CYP1A1, 1A2, 2B1, 2B2, 2C6, 2C11 and 2E1, their relative contributions depending on various biological factors (Nakajima *et*

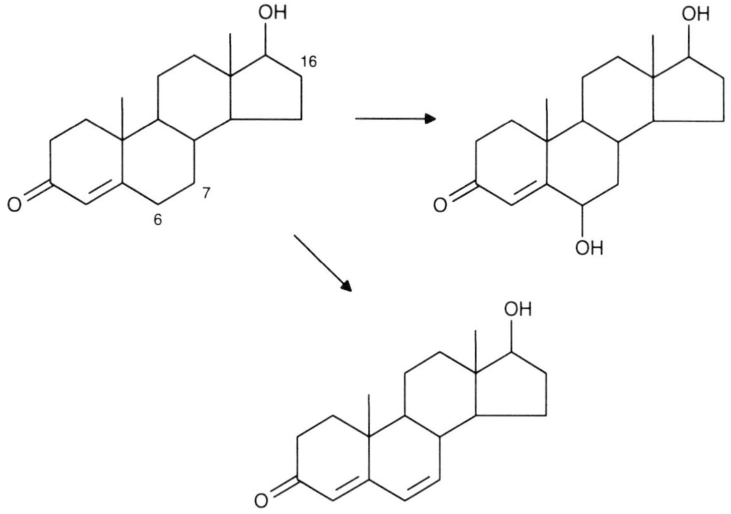

FIGURE 4.6 Cytochrome P450-catalyzed oxidation of testosterone to its 6β-hydroxylated and 6,7-desaturated metabolites.

al., 1991). Note that toluene is also ring-hydroxylated to isomeric cresols, the ratio of products depending on intrinsic reactivities (benzylic position > aromatic ring) and on the rate of dissociation of the enzyme–product complex (arene oxide > benzyl alcohol) (Hanzlik and Ling, 1990).

In the three isomeric **xylenes** (dimethylbenzenes), only one of the two methyl groups is oxidized to a methylbenzoic acid (toluic acid). Intermediate aldehydes may in some cases result in toxicity, as documented for *p*-methylbenzaldehyde which caused loss of pulmonary mono-oxygenases in rats administered *p*-xylene (Patel *et al.*, 1978). Drugs that undergo significant oxidation of a methyl group in a toluyl moiety include tolbutamide (CYP2C8, 2C9, 2C10), tolazamide (**4.XXII**), gliclazide (**4.XXIII**) and zolpidem (Ascalone *et al.*, 1992; Oida *et al.*, 1985; Srivastava *et al.*, 1991; Thomas *et al.*, 1978; Veronese *et al.*, 1990).

Methyl groups adjacent to some aromatic heterocycles appear to be oxidized just as readily as toluene and xylenes. This was seen for example with various monomethyl- and dimethylpyridines (**4.XXV**, X = CH) and pyrazines (**4.XXV**, X = N) which in the rat underwent methyl oxidation for almost all or a major fraction of a dose (Hawksworth and Scheline, 1975). An example of therapeutic relevance is that of **midazolam** (**4.XXVI**), the methyl group of which is hydroxylated to yield 1′-hydroxymidazolam. This compound is the major metabolite found in the plasma of humans dosed with the drug or formed *in vitro* by human hepatocytes or hepatic microsomes, CYP3A4 being predominantly involved (Fabre *et al.*, 1988; Kronbach *et al.*, 1989).

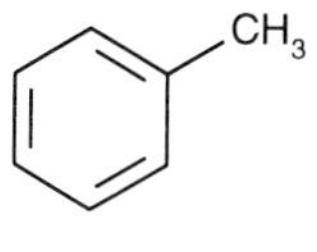

4.XXIV 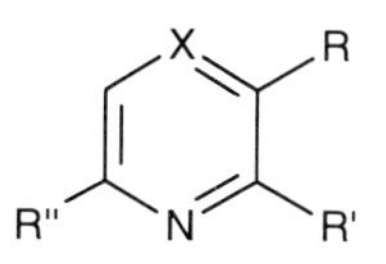   4.XXV 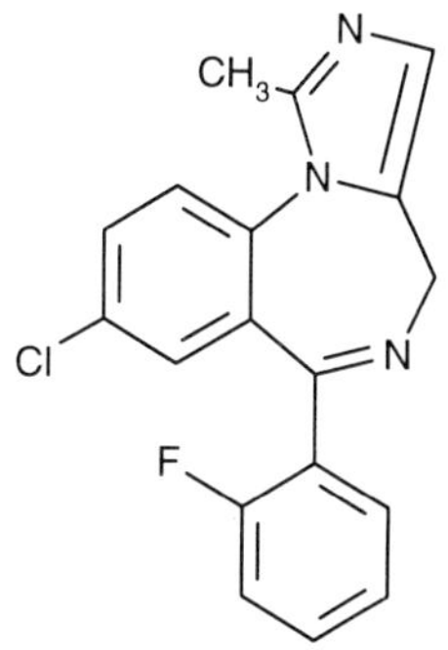   4.XXVI

For side-chains larger than a methyl group, regioselective benzylic hydroxylation also displays stereoselectivity as discussed in Section 4.2.1 for ethylbenzene (**4.I**). The influence of electronic factors on benzylic hydroxylation is nicely illustrated by monosubstituted 1,3-**diphenylpropanes (4.XXVII)** which are characterized by two benzylic positions. In rat liver microsomes, the ratio of the isomeric benzylic alcohols at positions 1 and 3 was found to be markedly influenced by the electronic character of the *para* substituent (Hjelmeland *et al.*, 1977). Specifically, this ratio was 50/50 for X = CH$_3$, 30/70 for X = F, and 5/95 for X = CF$_3$. In other words, hydroxylation is oriented away from electron-withdrawing groups and this effect increases with the strength of the substituent effect, as might be expected in view of the electrophilic nature of cytochrome P450-mediated hydroxylations.

4.XXVII

4.XXVIII

4.XXIX

4.XXX

Benzylic hydroxylation is also a significant reaction in the metabolism of a number of drugs, the position being in a chain or a ring. Thus, **metoprolol (4.XXVIII)** undergoes 1′-hydroxylation in rat liver microsomes, the diastereomeric benzylic metabolites having predominantly the 1′R configuration (Shetty and Nelson, 1988). An example of benzylic positions included in a ring is provided by **nortriptyline (4.XXIX)**. This drug undergoes marked benzylic hydroxylation in humans to yield the two diastereomeric (*E*)- and (*Z*)-10-hydroxynortriptyline, each of which is chiral (Mellström *et al.*, 1983; Nusser *et al.*, 1988). **Debrisoquine (4.XXX)** similarly undergoes marked 4-hydroxylation in humans and animals (Idle *et al.*, 1979); the two other methylene groups are also oxidized to yield ring-opened, acidic metabolites (Allen *et al.*, 1976). The benzylic hydroxylation of debrisoquine is under genetic control in humans (CYP2D6), very high to complete product enantioselectivity to (+)-(*S*)-4-hydroxydebrisoquine existing in extensive metabolizers (Eichelbaum, 1988; Eichelbaum *et al.*, 1988).

4.2.6 Oxidation of C-sp^3 atoms adjacent to other unsaturated systems

A number of examples in the literature document the hydroxylation of **allylic positions** in side-chains or cycloalkenyl groups. The first case is illustrated by 2-*n*-propyl-4-pentenoic acid (**4.VIII**), a metabolite of valproic acid (**4.VII**, see Section 4.2.3) which is further oxidized by 3-hydroxylation (Prickett and Baillie, 1986). The same reaction has been characterized for **estragole (4.XXXI)**; the complex biotransformation of this compound in rats and mice yields the

1'-hydroxylated derivative as an important metabolite (Anthony *et al.*, 1987). Interestingly, the 1'-methylene is simultaneously an allylic and a benzylic position, the increased reactivity of which underlies the role of the 1'-hydroxy metabolite in the genotoxicity and carcinogenicity of estragole and other allylbenzenes.

Eugenol (**4.XXXII**) is another allylbenzene of interest. In addition to the 1'-hydroxy metabolite and a number of other minor products of oxidation, humans dosed with this natural compound excreted *trans*-isoeugenol (**4.XXXIII**) as an important urinary metabolite; small amounts of *cis*-isoeugenol were also excreted (Fischer *et al.*, 1990). The mechanism of such a reaction of **double-bond migration** is poorly understood but we have noted that an increase in stability is achieved, isoeugenol being thermodynamically more stable than eugenol due to the conjugated double bond. A possible mechanism involves delocalization of the unpaired electron in an intermediate radical (Tsai *et al.*, 1994).

4.XXXI

4.XXXIV

4.XXXII

4.XXXIII

In **cyclohexene** also, a marked preference for the allylic position relative to the other methylene groups exists; indeed, a reconstituted CYP2B4 system yielded 2-cyclohexen-1-ol as the only product of C-sp^3 oxidation (White *et al.*, 1979). Note that allylic hydroxylation, both endo- and exocyclic, is an important metabolic reaction for a number of **terpenes** containing the cyclohexene ring (Santhanakrishnan, 1984), e.g. (+)-limonene (Kodama *et al.*, 1976). Similarly, the cyclohexene ring of **retinoic acid** is oxidized at its allylic position (Vanden Bossche and Willemsens, 1991). An example of medicinal relevance is **hexobarbital** (**4.XXXIV**), a major metabolic route of which involves 3'-hydroxylation followed by dehydrogenation to the 3'-keto metabolite. Since the drug is chiral and the 3'-carbon is prochiral, the hydroxylation reaction displays a complex pattern of substrate and product stereoselectivities which appears markedly influenced by biological factors (Van der Graaff *et al.*, 1988).

Testosterone is hydroxylated by cytochromes P450 in a number of positions, in particular 2β, 6β, 15β, 16α and 16β. Of relevance here is the allylic oxidation at the 6-position. When incubated with liver microsomes of dexamethasone-treated rats, the hormone yielded the 6β-hydroxylated and the 6,7-desaturated metabolites (Fig. 4.6) (Nagata *et al.*, 1986). Conclusive proof was provided that desaturation does not result from dehydration of 6β- or 7-hydroxytestosterone, but that these two metabolites are formed simultaneously by the same isozymes. Later studies using CYP2A1 confirmed a double hydrogen abstraction mechanism as discussed in Section 4.2.2, the first abstraction being that of the 6α-hydrogen (Korzekwa *et al.*,

1990b). The cases reported in Section 4.2 suggest that reactions of desaturation may not be as rare as believed and that additional examples await discovery.

Carbons adjacent to carbonyl groups are also known to be hydroxylated by cytochrome P450, although the number of documented examples is relatively limited. The simplest ketone is **acetone** (**4.XXXV**), which in rat liver microsomes is hydroxylated to acetol (**4.XXXVI**) with low affinity (K_m 0.8 mM) and slow velocity (V_{max} 0.25 nmol min^{-1} mg proteins^{-1}) (Johansson et al., 1986). Some properties of this acetone monooxygenase have been reported (Casazza et al., 1984). Turning our attention to a higher homologue, we find **2-hexanone** (see Section 4.2.3 and Fig. 4.4), an interesting chemical which produces peripheral neuropathy in laboratory animals, and its metabolite 2,5-hexanedione. In the rat, three major metabolic routes have been characterized for 2-hexanone, namely keto reduction, oxidation at C-1 (α-position), and oxidation at C-5 [($\omega - 1$)-position] (DiVincenzo et al., 1977). This last route is precisely the one leading to 2,5-hexanedione and other metabolites of known or potential toxicity. In contrast, α-hydroxylation leads to 2-ketohexanoic acid and then to the two parallel routes of decarboxylation and transamination. This pathway is viewed as the detoxication mechanism of 2-hexanone.

$$CH_3\text{---}CO\text{---}CH_3 \longrightarrow CH_3\text{---}CO\text{---}CH_2OH$$

4.XXXV   **4.XXXVI**

$$Cl\text{---}\langle\text{ring}\rangle\text{---}NHCO\text{---}(CH_2)_n\text{---}CH_3$$

4.XXXVII

Regioselective hydroxylation is also documented for carbon atoms adjacent to the carbonyl group of amides. In an elegant study, Lenk (1979) investigated the regioselective hydroxylation of acyl groups in **4-chloroanilides** (**4.XXXVII**, $n = 0$ to 3) using liver microsomes from rabbit pretreated with various inducers of cytochrome P450. While phenobarbital-inducible cytochromes P450 showed a preference for the (ω)- and ($\omega - 1$)-position, 3-methylcholanthrene induction predominantly increased α-hydroxylation in the acetyl, propionyl and butyryl residues.

An even higher selectivity for the α-position is evident in the metabolism of **glutethimide** (**4.XXXVIII**) in humans. The drug yields a number of hydroxylated products, 4-hydroxyglutethimide (in free and conjugated form) being the major plasmatic and urinary metabolite (Kennedy et al., 1978; Stillwell, 1975). This metabolite is a more active sedative-hypnotic agent than the parent drug, and is believed to account for much or most of the severe symptoms displayed by intoxicated patients.

Carbons adjacent to acetylenic groups also appear to be preferred targets of cytochrome P450, as suggested by a few examples such as **N-(5-pyrrolidinopent-3-ynyl)-succinimide** (**4.XXXIX**). Formation of the 2'-hydroxylated metabolite in rat liver preparations was demonstrated in addition to ring-oxidized products, in particular the 3-hydroxy derivative relevant to the previous paragraph (Lindeke et al., 1978).

The last case of regioselective hydroxylation to be discussed here is that of **C-sp^3 atoms adjacent to a cyano group**. **Acetonitrile** (**4.XL**, R = H), the simplest compound, is thus metabolized to cyanide in a reaction whose first step is mediated by CYP2E1 (Feierman and Cederbaum, 1989; Freeman and Hayes, 1988). The evidence points to a cyanohydrin derivative as the intermediate generated by cytochrome P450 and broken down to cyanide by catalase (catalase

4.XXXVIII   4.XXXIX

4.XL

is discussed in Section 10.4). Earlier studies had already concluded that the breakdown of the intermediate cyanohydrin is mainly an enzymatic process in which mitochondria appear to play a role (Floreani *et al.*, 1981).

Formation of cyanide is also documented from **higher nitriles** (**4.XL**, R = alkyl) as well as for other derivatives of similar structure (Silver *et al.*, 1982; Tanii and Hashimoto, 1984), confirming regioselective α-hydroxylation. As expected from the above, benzonitrile with no hydrogen on the α-carbon does not liberate cyanide (Tanii and Hashimoto, 1984).

4.3 OXIDATION OF sp²-HYBRIDIZED CARBON ATOMS IN AROMATIC RINGS

The cytochrome P450-mediated oxidation of C-sp^2 atoms is a highly complex metabolic route leading to a great variety of products that are either unstable intermediates or stable metabolites (e.g. phenols). Note that the chemical reactivity of the intermediates (e.g. epoxides) depends heavily on the chemical nature of the target group and molecular properties of the substrate, and that this reactivity in turn conditions the nature and ratio of the stable metabolites generated. Far from discussing innumerable details, the pages to follow aim at a reasonable balance between clarity and comprehensiveness.

4.3.1 Reaction mechanisms of aromatic ring oxidation

Phenols are the most stable and the most frequently excreted **products of aromatic ring oxidation** mediated by cytochrome P450. Other relatively stable metabolites include:

- Dihydrodiols, formed by epoxide hydrolase-mediated hydration of epoxides, see Volume 2;
- Catechols, formed either by dehydrogenation of dihydrodiols (see Section 2.5) or by hydroxylation of phenols as discussed in Section 4.3.2;
- Quinones, resulting from the oxidation of phenols (see Chapter 7).

The **mechanism of ring oxygenation** remained obscure for many years and it is only in the last few years that it has become reasonably well understood. The reaction involves loss of aromaticity due to the formation of tetrahedral transition states (Fig. 4.7), and it is only for end-products like phenols that aromaticity is recovered. Interesting data have been reported suggesting the first step in the reaction to be a one-electron oxidation by the activated

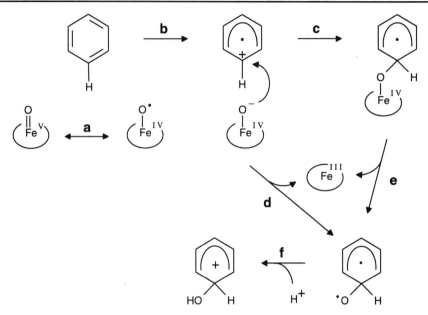

FIGURE 4.7 First steps in the cytochrome P450-catalyzed oxidation of aromatic rings. Three possible oxygenated intermediates are shown, formed by reactions **c**, **d** and/or **e**, and **f**. Assuming that Fe–O cleavage precedes any other rearrangement, only the biradical and cationic oxygenated intermediates at the bottom of this figure are examined in Fig. 4.8.

cytochrome P450–oxygen complex (reaction **b** in Fig. 4.7) (Ackland, 1993; Cavalieri and Rogan, 1992; Cavalieri *et al.*, 1988). Substituents containing an electron lone pair (e.g. a halogen) are known to accelerate ring oxidation, presumably because they facilitate this first step (Guengerich and Macdonald, 1984). The product of reaction **b** in Fig. 4.7 is a **cation-radical** that binds the activated oxygen atom by reaction **c** and/or **d**. Kinetic studies have indicated the involvement of a positively charged transition state in the rate-determining step, perhaps the product of reaction **b** or **c** in Fig. 4.7 (Burka *et al.*, 1983).

In discussing subsequent chemical events, we shall assume that Fe–O cleavage precedes further rearrangements (Korzekwa *et al.*, 1985) and restrict the discussion to the two oxygenated intermediates shown at the bottom of Fig. 4.7. Fig. 4.8 (for X = H) continues Fig. 4.7, but it is also meant to convey additional mechanistic information for X = ^{2}H or ^{3}H. As shown in Fig. 4.8 (and as supported by experimental and theoretical evidence), three products can be formed by rearrangement of the diradical or its protonated form, namely an **epoxide** (formed by reaction **g**), a **cyclohexadienone** (formed by reaction **h**), and a **phenol** (formed by reactions **k**, **l** or **m**) (Korzekwa *et al.*, 1985; Swinney *et al.*, 1984). An interesting feature is that some of these rearrangement reactions involve migration of the geminal hydrogen atom, as seen when X is a deuterium or tritium (Fig. 4.8). This displacement, which also affects the lower halogens, is known as the **NIH shift** and will be discussed in Section 4.3.2.

Careful theoretical studies have provided evidence for **two possible rearrangement pathways** (Korzekwa *et al.*, 1985). The biradical pathways show little or no substituent effects and the order of reaction rates is epoxide (reaction **g**) > ketone (reaction **h**) > phenol. The cationic pathways show marked substituent effects and the order of reaction rates is reversed with phenol (reaction **k**) > ketone (reaction **j**) > epoxide. Two important intermediates in Fig. 4.8 are the epoxide and the cyclohexadienone. The significance of epoxides of aromatic rings (**arene oxides**) was recognized in the late Sixties by workers at the NIH (National Institutes of Health in Bethesda, Maryland, USA) (Boyd and Jerina, 1985; Garner, 1976; Jerina *et al.*, 1969; and ref.

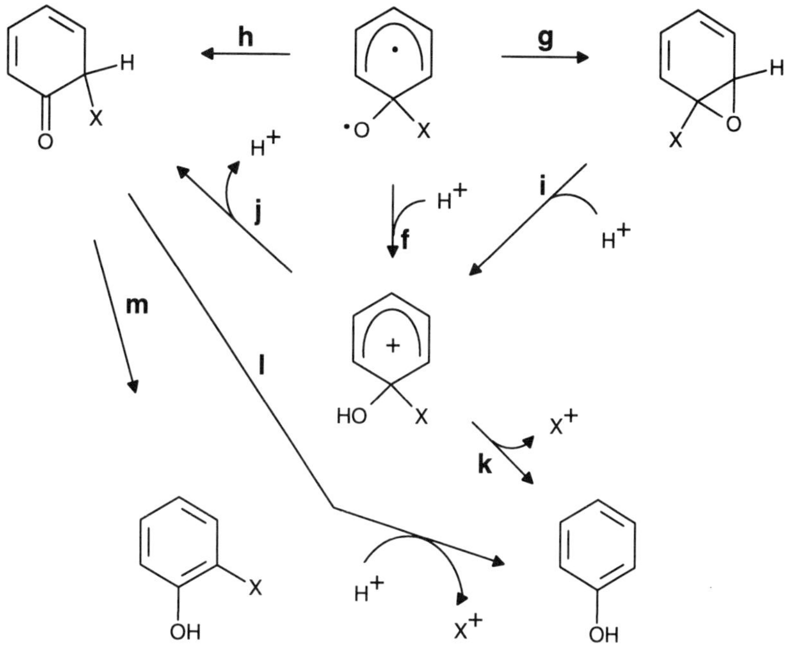

FIGURE 4.8 Biradical and cationic pathways leading to the formation of stable phenolic metabolites. A label (X = ^{2}H or ^{3}H) geminal to the oxygen atom may either be lost or displaced (NIH shift).

therein). The role of **cyclohexadienones** as intermediates was recognized more recently (Bush and Trager, 1982; Hinson *et al.*, 1985).

Arene oxides are usually highly unstable and undergo ring opening by a mechanism of general acid catalysis, ultimately leading to phenols (Bartok and Lang, 1985; Boyd and Jerina, 1985; Bruice and Bruice, 1976; Chao and Berchtold, 1981). Such a reaction may proceed according to two pathways, namely a direct (reactions **i** and **k** in Fig. 4.8) and an indirect aromatic hydroxylation (reactions **j**, **l** and **m** in Fig. 4.8) (Hanzlik *et al.*, 1984). The former pathway involves the complete loss of geminal label, while the latter involves the complete shift of the geminal label upon ketone formation (reaction **i** in Fig. 4.8), followed by its partial loss (reactions **l** vs. **m** in Fig. 4.8). As examples of arene oxide instability, the metabolite naphthalene-1,2-oxide has a half-life of less than 3 minutes in water at neutral pH, while the half-life of bromobenzene-3,4-oxide in blood at 37°C is about 13 seconds (Jerina *et al.*, 1969; Lau *et al.*, 1984). More stable epoxides are those of polycyclic aromatic hydrocarbons and olefins, as discussed later (Sections 4.3.3 and 4.3.5, respectively).

As documented by the above, a unitary mechanism of arene oxidation has now been uncovered and appears fairly well understood. The mechanism itself results from the reaction of oxygen activation characteristic of cytochrome P450 and should therefore be identical for all isozymes. With its numerous bifurcation points and intertwined paths, the mechanism is a highly intricate one, and the nature of the end-products generated will depend on both the properties of the substrate and the protein environment of the active site, inasmuch as they may favour one path over another. This view is a rather recent one, since a previous mechanistic model assumed that *ortho*- and *para*-phenols resulted from initial epoxidation, while *meta*-phenols were produced by direct hydroxylation. It was only in the early Eighties that elegant experimental studies challenged this view (Bush and Trager, 1982).

However, a **second mechanism of arene oxidation** operates, at least *in vitro*. Indeed, there is evidence that the cytochrome P450-catalyzed oxidation of simple aromatic compounds such as

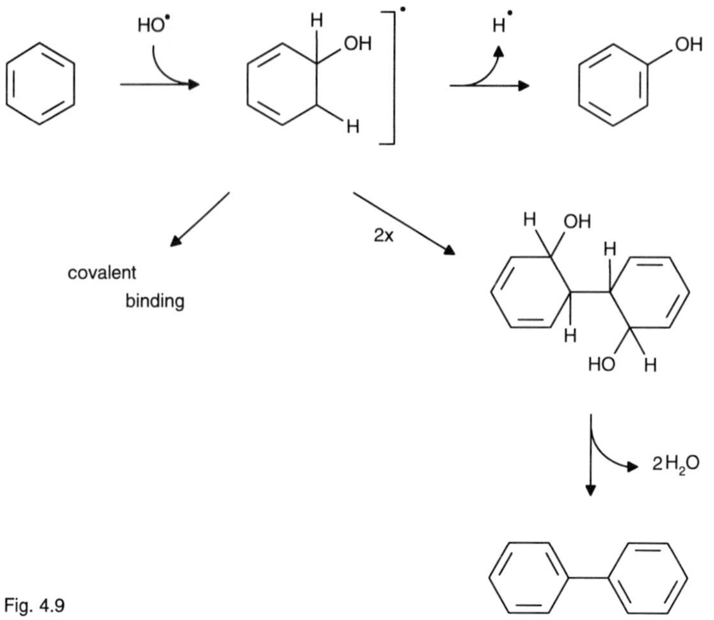

Fig. 4.9

FIGURE 4.9 Mechanism of hydroxyl radical-mediated oxidation of benzene to phenol, biphenyl, and adducts (Johansson and Ingelman-Sundberg, 1983).

benzene and aniline can in fact be mediated by hydroxyl radicals formed in a modified Haber–Weiss reaction between hydrogen peroxide and superoxide (Section 3.5.3) (Ingelman-Sundberg and Ekström, 1982; Johansson and Ingelman-Sundberg, 1983). These findings imply that the unitary mechanism discussed above may not be the only one or may be insufficiently understood. In the case of **benzene**, the hydroxyl-mediated oxidation leads to the hydroxycyclohexadienyl radical which, beside forming phenol and biphenyl, is a reactive intermediate responsible for covalent binding (Fig. 4.9).

4.3.2 NIH shift, regioselectivity and stereoselectivity in aryl oxidation of model compounds and drugs

The **NIH shift** mentioned in the previous section and explained in Fig. 4.8 is documented for a number of substrate molecules containing deuterium or tritium substituents on their aromatic ring(s). Its mechanism has been discussed in detail by Trager (1980), and quantum-mechanical calculations have revealed additional particulars (Tsuda et al., 1986). As is apparent from Fig. 4.8, hydroxylation at the labelled position will generate two phenols, one where the label has undergone migration, and one which has lost the label. In addition, oxidative attack and hydroxylation ortho to the label will also lead to both retention and loss of the label. These situations are exemplified in the metabolism of **[1,3,5-^{2}H$_3$]benzene** (Fig. 4.10). Four monophenolic metabolites were obtained following incubation with rat liver microsomes. The two trideuterated phenols each accounted for about 40% of the sum of monophenolic metabolites, while the two dideuterated phenols each accounted for 10% (Hinson et al., 1985). An NIH shift had occurred giving rise to [2,3,5-^{2}H$_3$]phenol, while ipso and ortho loss can be seen by the formation of [3,5-^{2}H$_2$]phenol and [2,4-^{2}H$_2$]phenol, respectively.

Beside deuterium and tritium, the NIH shift may also affect fluoro, chloro and bromo substituents. This fact is clearly significant as far as drugs are concerned, yet relevant examples are

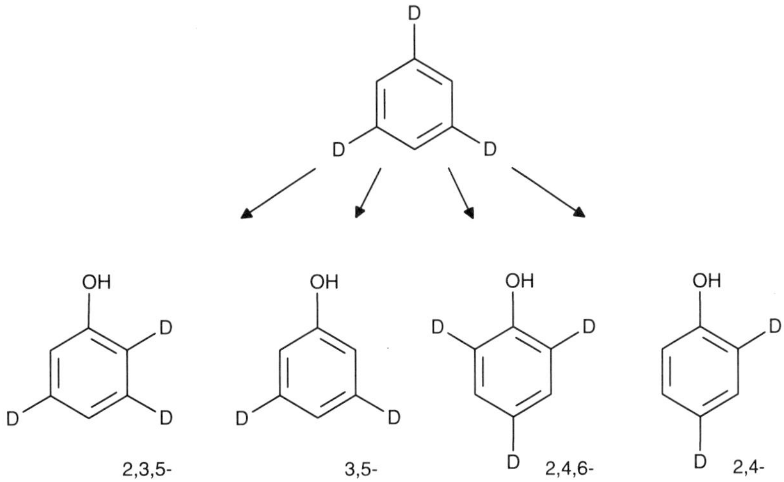

FIGURE 4.10 Rat liver microsomal metabolism of [1,3,5-^{2}H$_3$]benzene, showing displacement or loss of deuterium (Hinson *et al.*, 1985).

few. An informative case involving model compounds is that of **4,4′-dihalogenobiphenyls** (**4.XLI**, X = Cl, Br or I) (Safe *et al.*, 1976). The chloro and bromo analogues led to the following metabolites in decreasing order of importance: the 3-hydroxylated derivative (neither loss nor displacement of the 4-halogeno substituent), the 4-phenol (loss of the 4-halogeno substituent), and the 3-halogeno-4-hydroxy analogue (shift of the halogeno substituent). In contrast, the diiodo analogue gave the 3-hydroxylated derivative as the only metabolite, indicating absence of an NIH shift for this bulky substituent. Loss of an aromatic fluoro substituent is seen for example in the metabolism of **2-** and mainly **4-fluoroestradiol**, a significant portion of which is hydroxylated at the 2- and 4-position, respectively, without displacement of the halogen atom (Ashburn *et al.*, 1993; Li *et al.*, 1985).

Migration of nitro (see below) and methyl groups has also been reported (Walsh *et al.*, 1993).

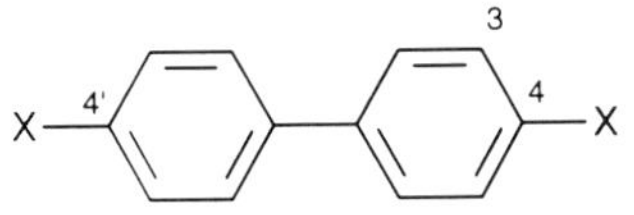

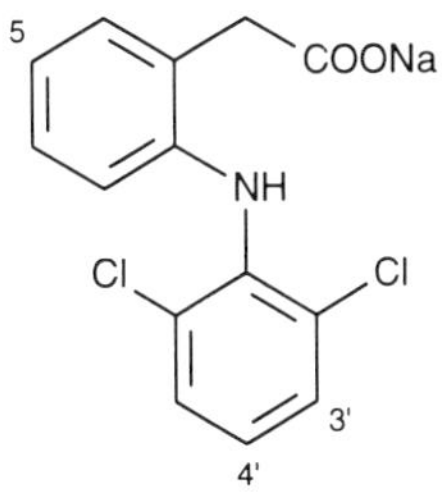

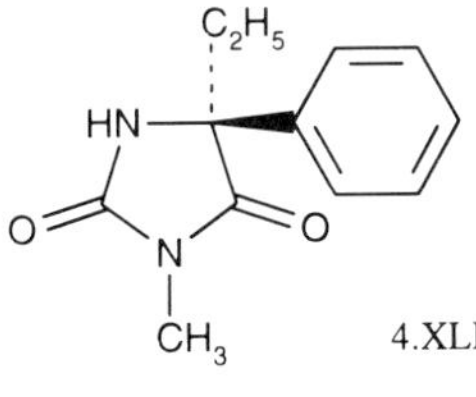

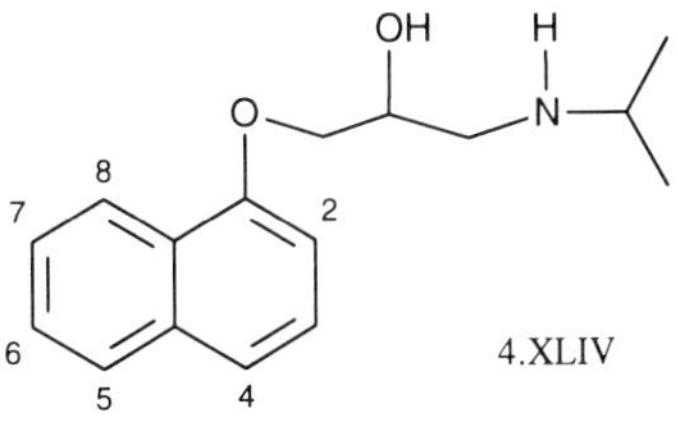

Product regioselectivity is an important feature of aromatic hydroxylation. Thus, the metabolism of *chlorobenzene* by hepatic microsomes and solubilized cytochrome P450 systems lead to the three isomeric chlorophenols, with the *para-* and *ortho*-isomers being largely predominant in most cases (Selander *et al.*, 1975). In agreement with knowledge available at that time, three distinct pathways were postulated, namely 2,3- and 3,4-epoxidation leading to 2- and 4-chlorophenol, respectively, and direct formation of 3-chlorophenol. The latter route is no longer compatible with our current understanding of the mechanism of *meta* hydroxylation (Swinney *et al.*, 1984). With **debrisoquine (4.XXX)**, while alicyclic hydroxylation predominates, aromatic oxidation also occurs with 5-hydroxy, 6-hydroxy, 7-hydroxy- and 8-hydroxy-debrisoquine all accounting for a minor fraction of the dose in humans (Idle *et al.*, 1979).

An interesting drug as far as regioselectivity is concerned is the anti-inflammatory agent **diclofenac (4.XLII)**. Only three of the seven possible positions are hydroxylated, their order of importance in the baboon being $3' > 4' = 5$ (Faigle *et al.*, 1988). Even more important in quantitative terms is 3'-hydroxy-4'-methoxydiclofenac, indicating that the dichloroanilino moiety is markedly more susceptible to aryl hydroxylation than the *ortho*-aminophenylacetate moiety. **Substrate enantioselectivity** in aromatic hydroxylation is seen with a number of drugs, **(S)-mephenytoin (4.XLIII)** being a case in point. One or more cytochromes P450 in the 2C subfamily catalyze the *para*-hydroxylation of mephenytoin with high efficacy and a marked preference for the (S)-enantiomer; the reaction attracts much interest because it displays polymorphism in humans (Srivastava *et al.*, 1991; Yasumori *et al.*, 1991).

A more complex situation is encountered in the metabolism of **propranolol (4.XLIV)** (see also Fig. 1.1 in Section 1.2). Here, as in a number of drugs such as other β-blockers and warfarin (see Rettie *et al.*, 1992), product regioselectivity is combined with substrate enantioselectivity. In rat urine, 4-hydroxy-, 7-hydroxy-, 5-hydroxy- and 2-hydroxypropranolol represented 66, 26, 7 and 1% of total monophenolic metabolites. While 4-hydroxylation showed no apparent substrate stereoselectivity, the 7- and 5-hydroxylations were selective for (+)-(R)-propranolol (20/1 ratio) and (-)-(S)-propranolol (3/1 ratio), respectively (Walle *et al.*, 1982). In humans, CYP2D6 is mainly responsible for 4-hydroxylation as a major route of propranolol metabolism, with a marked selectivity for the (R)-enantiomer (Ward *et al.*, 1989).

Product enantioselectivity in aryl oxidation is traditionally illustrated with **phenytoin (4.XLV)**, a prochiral drug displaying two enantiotopic phenyl rings. Phenyl hydroxylation in humans is mediated by a cytochrome P4502C enzyme and occurs almost exclusively in the *para*-position, the *S/R* ratio of the two enantiomeric metabolites being about 10/1 (Butler *et al.*, 1976; Poupaert *et al.*, 1975). In contrast, the *meta*-phenol is formed preferentially in dogs and is

4.XLV

4.XLVI

4.XLVII

the pure (R)-enantiomer (Butler *et al.*, 1976). There is evidence that the *meta-* and *para*-phenol are both formed from the 3,4-oxide (Moustafa *et al.*, 1983).

A complex case of **substrate–product stereoselectivity** was seen in the rat liver microsomal oxidation of **terodiline (4.XLVI)** (Lindeke *et al.*, 1987). The prochiral C-4 becomes chiral upon hydroxylation of an enantiotopic phenyl ring, but the product stereoselectivity of the process was found to vary markedly for (2R)- and (2S)-terolidine. While the former yielded the (2R;4S)- and (2R;4R)-metabolite in a 20/1 ratio, the (2S;4R)/(2S;4S) ratio was 3/2 for the (S)-substrate.

The **hydroxylation of phenols** deserves special mention. For example, phenol itself is metabolized by rat liver microsomes to hydroquinone and catechol in a 20/1 ratio, CYP2E1 playing an important role as a benzene and phenol hydroxylase (Koop *et al.*, 1989; Sawahata and Neal, 1983). For substituted phenols, the nature of the hydroxylated metabolite(s) will depend on chemical and other factors, as shown by the hydroxylation of *para*-nitrophenol to 4-nitrocatechol, a reaction catalyzed almost exclusively by CYP2E1 (Koop, 1986). As a rule, it appears that when the position *para* to the first hydroxyl group is free, it will generally be hydroxylated faster than the *ortho*-position, as indicated above by phenol. Similarly, about 50% of a dose of salicylamide (**4.XLVII**) administered to mice was recovered as 5-hydroxylated metabolites (i.e. gentisamide and its conjugates), but only about 20% of the dose underwent 3-hydroxylation (Howell *et al.*, 1988).

The **formation of catechol** metabolites is interesting in its own right as it can occur by two distinct pathways as represented in Fig. 4.11. The use of oxygen isotope can allow the two pathways to be distinguished, and it was found for example that the catechol metabolite of phenytoin (**4.XLV**) is formed mainly via two consecutive hydroxylations in mouse liver

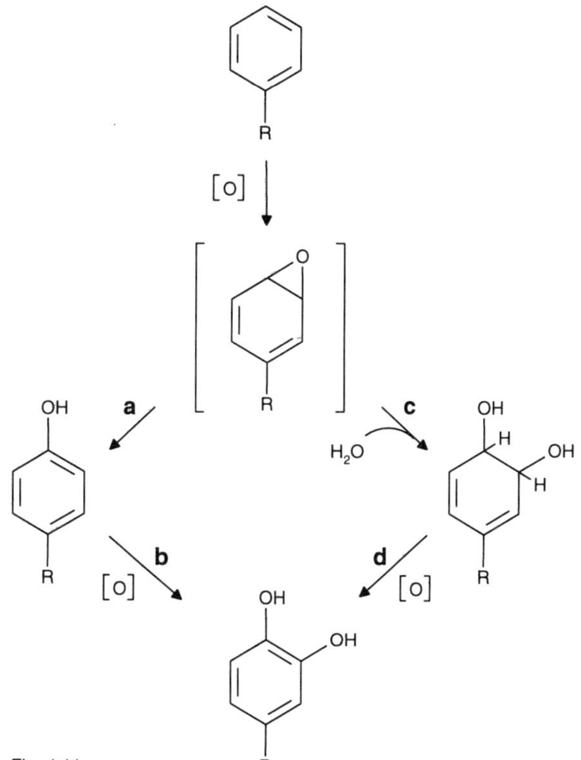

Fig. 4.11

FIGURE 4.11 Formation of catechol metabolites occurring either by two consecutive reactions of hydroxylation (reactions **a** and **b**), or via a dihydrodiol (reaction **c**, see the volume concerning the Biochemistry of Hydration Reactions) which is then dehydrogenated (reaction **d**, see Section 2.5).

microsomes (Billings and Fischer, 1985). In contrast, the oxidation of bromobenzene to 4-bromocatechol in isolated rat hepatocytes occurs mainly via the dihydrodiol (Dankovic et al., 1985).

The formation of polyphenols such as hydroquinones and catechols is of additional interest in that these compounds can be further oxidized to quinones. This is discussed in Section 7.6 in connection with the **oxidation of the oxygen atom** in phenols.

Propranolol (4.XLIV) offers another example of a drug undergoing aromatic dihydroxylation. In rat liver microsomes, the following dihydroxylated metabolites were formed from propranolol in decreasing order of importance: 4,6 > 3,4 > 3,7 > 5,6 > 4,8. The former two metabolites arose selectively from (S)-propranolol, while the latter three arose selectively from (R)-propranolol (Talaat and Nelson, 1988). Among the four monohydroxylated metabolites (see above), 4-hydroxy- and 5-hydroxypropranolol were poor substrates for a second hydroxylation, while 2-hydroxy and 7-hydroxypropranolol were the best. These last two compounds were precursors of 2,3-dihydroxy- and 3,7-dihydroxypropranolol, respectively. Three dihydroxylated metabolites were also found in the urine of humans dosed with propranolol, namely the 4,6-, 4,8- and 3,4-derivatives (Talaat and Nelson, 1988).

4.3.3 Oxidation of polyhalogenated benzenes, polycyclic aromatic hydrocarbons, and aromatic heterocycles

For a long time, **polyhalogenated aromatic compounds** have been considered to be poor substrates of cytochrome P450, steric hindrance preventing oxidative attack on the aromatic positions. This inertness is indeed verified, in particular *in vivo*, for a number of highly lipophilic compounds such as polyhalogenated biphenyls. However, recent studies have found significant oxidation of some **polyhalogenated benzenes** both *in vitro* and *in vivo*, pretreatment with dexamethasome (a strong inducer of CYP3A1) markedly increasing activity.

For example, **1,2,4-trichlorobenzene (4.XLVIII)** incubated with rat liver microsomes was oxidized to a variety of metabolites including 2,4,5- and 2,3,6-trichlorophenol as major products, and 2,4,6-, 2,3,5- and 2,3,4-trichlorophenol as minor products (den Besten et al., 1991). The formation of these metabolites implies oxidative attack at various ring positions (in particular the hindered 3-position to yield 2,3,6-trichlorophenol), followed in some cases by the shift of a chloro substituent (to yield 2,3,4- and 2,4,6-trichlorophenol). Similarly, **pentachlorobenzene (4.XLIX)** was metabolized to pentachlorophenol by oxidation of the hindered, unsubstituted ring position, and to tetrachlorophenols and tetrachlorohydroquinones by loss of a chloro substituent (for the mechanism, see Fig. 4.8). Note that halogen oxidation must have occurred if the lost chlorine atom is indeed cationic as suggested by Fig. 4.8. Halogen oxidation is discussed in Section 11.5.

4.XLVIII   4.XLIX

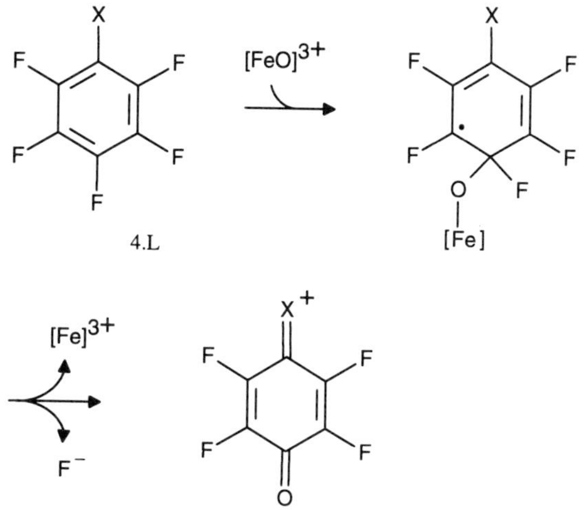

FIGURE 4.12 Mechanism of cytochrome P450-catalyzed oxidation of pentafluoroaniline (**4.L**, X = NH$_2$) and pentafluorochlorobenzene (**4.L**, X = Cl) to yield a reactive quinone-like primary metabolite (**4.LI**) (Rietjens and Vervoort, 1992; Rietjens *et al.*, 1990 and 1993).

Similar results (i.e. formation of phenols following dehalogenation) were also seen with **hexasubstituted benzenes** such as pentafluoroaniline (**4.L**, X = NH$_2$, in Fig. 4.12) and pentafluorochlorobenzene (**4.L**, X = Cl, in Fig. 4.12) (Rietjens and Vervoort, 1992; Rietjens *et al.*, 1990 and 1993). With these compounds, defluorination involved the substituent *para* to the chloro or amino group, respectively, the postulated mechanism implying loss of a fluorine anion and formation of a quinone-like product (**4.LI**) as the primary metabolite (Fig. 4.12). The fact that the fluorine is lost as an anion is compatible with a mechanism of dehalogenation different from that shown in Fig. 4.8. As for the quinone-like product, it can undergo reduction to the phenol, or react covalently with cellular nucleophiles such as glutathione or macromolecules. Note that other anilines containing a smaller number of fluoro substituents were also substrates of this reaction, and that a mechanism of initial N-oxidation also appears to lead to ring hydroxylated products (see Section 5.5).

Polycyclic aromatic hydrocarbons (PAHs) have been the objects of intense study due to their toxicological significance. A number of these compounds display high carcinogenic potencies following their toxication to reactive metabolites called ultimate carcinogens (Cavalieri and Rogan, 1992; Harvey, 1981; Levin *et al.*, 1982; Yang, 1988; Yang *et al.*, 1985). Three steric-electronic regions are commonly seen in PAHs, namely the sterically hindered **bay region** (B-region), the **K-region** which is the most electron-rich region in the molecule, and the **M-region** whose *trans*-dihydrodiol is the metabolic precursor of the bay-region dihydrodiol-epoxide (also called diol-epoxide). **Benzo[a]pyrene**, one of the most carcinogenic PAHs, aptly illustrates the regio- and stereoselectivity of the cytochrome P450-mediated oxidations undergone by these compounds. Three major epoxides have been characterized as shown in Fig. 4.13, namely the (4S;5R)-epoxide (a K-region epoxide), the (7R;8S)-epoxide (an M-region epoxide) and the (9S;10R)-epoxide (a bay-region epoxide) (Yang, 1988). These last two epoxides were formed with very high stereoselectivity.

The epoxides thus formed vary in their chemical stability, an approximate rule being that the higher the electron density in the double bond being oxygenated, the higher the stability of the resulting epoxide. Thus, the K-region epoxides tend to be more stable than non-K-region epoxides. However, all these epoxides undergo highly stereoselective hydration mediated by epoxide hydrolase (see the volume concerning the Biochemistry of Hydration Reactions),

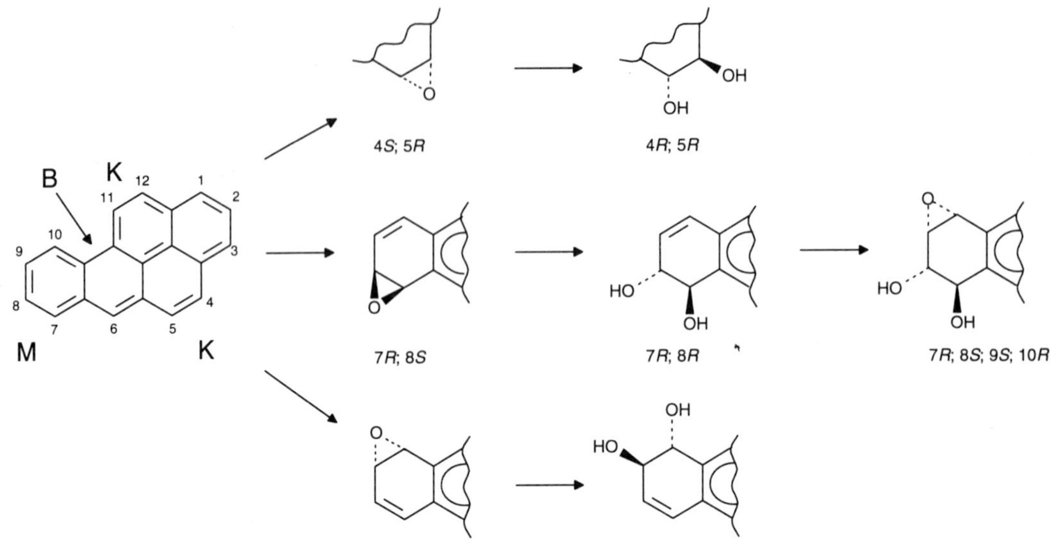

FIGURE 4.13 Chemical structure and relevant metabolic routes of benzo[*a*]pyrene. The figure shows the B-, K- and M-regions, the formation of the three major epoxide metabolites, their hydration by epoxide hydrolase to dihydrodiols (Volume 2), and the epoxidation of the M-region dihydrodiol to a dihydrodiol-epoxide considered to be the ultimate carcinogens.

yielding the dihydrodiols shown in Fig. 4.13. The M-region epoxide is of particular toxicological significance since its dihydrodiol is the metabolic precursor of the ultimate carcinogen (*7R;8S*)-dihydrodiol-(*9S;10R*)-epoxide. The reactivity of diol-epoxides is explained in terms of their rearrangement to a triol carbonium ion (**4.LII**) which will then react covalently with nucleophilic sites in, e.g., nucleic acids (Harvey, 1981; Lehr and Jerina, 1977; Lowe and Silverman, 1981; Sayer *et al.*, 1989).

It is even possible that epoxidation of PAHs is not limited to peripheral bonds since the carcinogen 15,16-dihydro-11-methyl-cyclopenta[*a*]phenanthren-17-one (**4.LIII**) has been shown

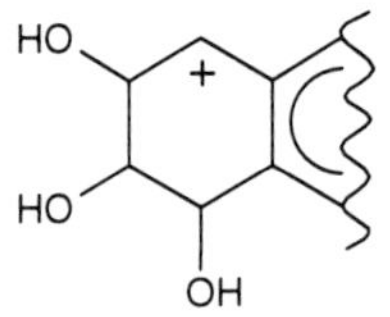

4.LII

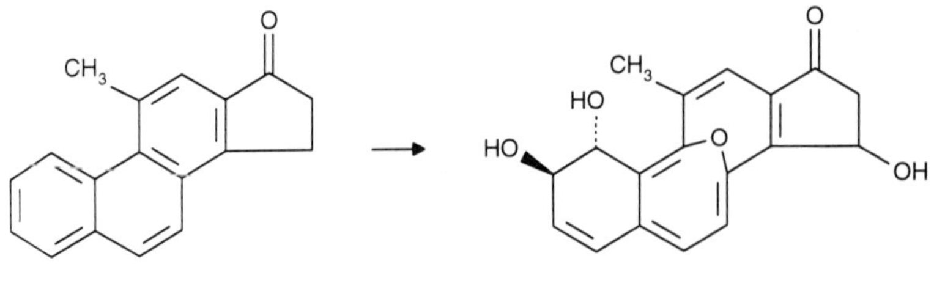

4.LIII

4.LIV

to yield the **bridgehead epoxide (4.LIV)** as the major rat urinary metabolite (Vore and Coombs, 1977). However, the question has not been answered whether compound **4.LIV** is an actual metabolite or a rearrangement product.

Metabolic oxidation is amply documented for a large variety of **aromatic heterocycles** (Damani, 1988). Involvement of cytochrome P450 is proven in some cases and assumed in others, but we shall see in Chapter 9 that xanthine oxidase and aldehyde oxidase may also be involved as they mediate the $C(\alpha)$-oxidation of some azaheterocycles.

Pyridine (4.LV) for example is hydroxylated in the 2- and 4-position in various human tissues (Wilke *et al.*, 1989); the involvement of different forms of cytochrome P450 was indicated. Note that these metabolites undergo tautomeric rearrangement and were characterized as 2- and 4-pyridone, respectively. Other **6-membered azaheterocycles** are similarly oxidized. Thus, pyrazinamide (**4.LVI**) is hydroxylated in the 5-position, a significant proportion of the dose being recovered as 5-hydroxypyrazinamide and 5-hydroxypyrazinoic acid in the urine of rats. The same reaction occurs in humans (Whitehouse *et al.*, 1987). Additionally, the sulfonamide derivative **4.LVII** is hydroxylated in the rat on both the benzene ring (*para*-position) and the pyrimidine ring (5'-position), the latter reaction largely predominating over the former one (Paulson and Feil, 1987).

Five-membered heterocycles can also be substrates of cytochrome P450, e.g. pyrazole (Section 2.2) which is oxidized to 4-hydroxypyrazole by CYP2E1 (Feierman and Cederbaum, 1987). An intriguing case is that of **tinidazole (4.LVIII)**, a nitroimidazole derivative metabolized in the dog by nitro-group migration and ring hydroxylation (Wood *et al.*, 1985). The resulting metabolite (**4.LIX**) was characterized by X-ray crystallography of its ammonium salt; it is tempting to speculate that an NIH shift accounts for its formation.

The **furan ring** can yield a number of metabolites following cytochrome P450-mediated oxidation. Two distinct routes appear likely, as shown in Fig. 4.14 (Kobayashi *et al.*, 1987). 4,5-Epoxidation leads to a 5-hydroxylated metabolite (reaction **a** in Fig. 4.14) which rearranges to a lactone; hydrolytic ring opening then leads to a γ-keto acid (Le Fur and Labaune, 1985). The

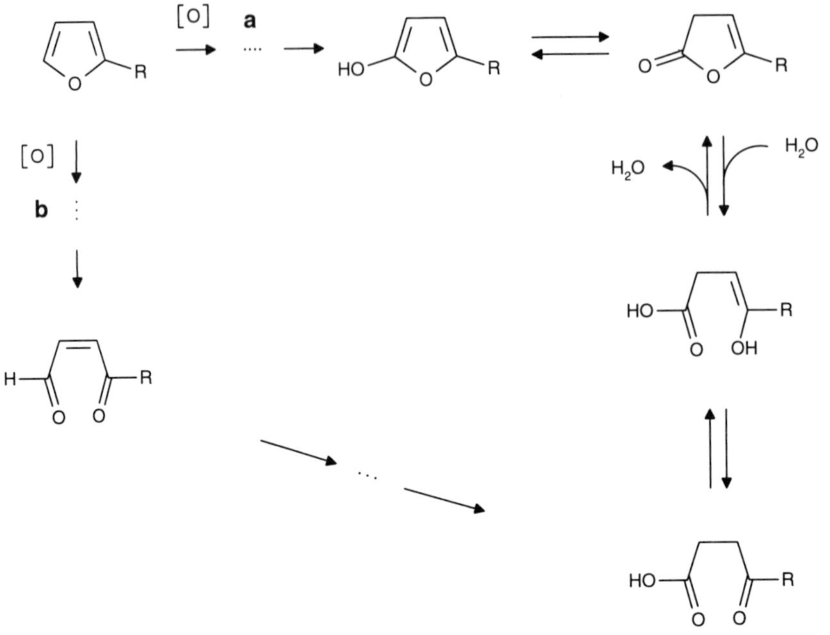

FIGURE 4.14 Cytochrome P450-mediated metabolism of the furan ring involving either 5-hydroxylation (reaction **a**) or oxidative ring opening (reaction **b**) to a reactive unsaturated keto-aldehyde (Kobayashi *et al.*, 1987).

second route is one of toxication; it involves an oxidative ring opening (reaction **b** in Fig. 4.14) to form an unsaturated keto-aldehyde. Metabolites of this type, which have been characterized for toxic methylfurans and for menthofuran, are reactive electrophiles binding covalently to tissue macromolecules (Ravindranath *et al.*, 1984; Thomassen *et al.*, 1992). Less detail is available on the metabolic fate of the **thiophene ring**. In a few drugs, 5-hydroxylation and even complete oxidative removal of a thienyl ring have been demonstrated (Mansuy *et al.*, 1984a; Mori *et al.*, 1985).

4.4 OXIDATION OF sp²-HYBRIDIZED CARBON ATOMS IN OLEFINIC BONDS

4.4.1 Mechanism of oxidation of olefinic bonds

Non-aromatic carbon–carbon double bonds, be they isolated or conjugated, undergo cytochrome P450-catalyzed oxidation to epoxides and a few other products. While the reaction is documented for a large variety of xenobiotics, it also involves endogenous substrates, e.g. the various epoxidations of arachidonic acid (Fitzpatrick and Murphy, 1989; Garner, 1976; Laniado-Schwartzman *et al.*, 1988).

The **mechanism of olefin oxidation**, which took years to be reasonably well understood, has much in common with arene oxidation (Fig. 4.15) (Collman *et al.*, 1990; Dolphin, 1985; Guengerich and Macdonald, 1984, 1990; Miller *et al.*, 1992; Ostovic and Bruice, 1989; Sharer *et al.*, 1992; White, 1990). Instead of being a straightforward oxene insertion into an olefinic bond as postulated earlier, the reaction involves two distinct formations of C–O bonds (reactions **a** and **b** in Fig. 4.15). Following the formation of the **first C–O bond** (reaction **a**), a number of

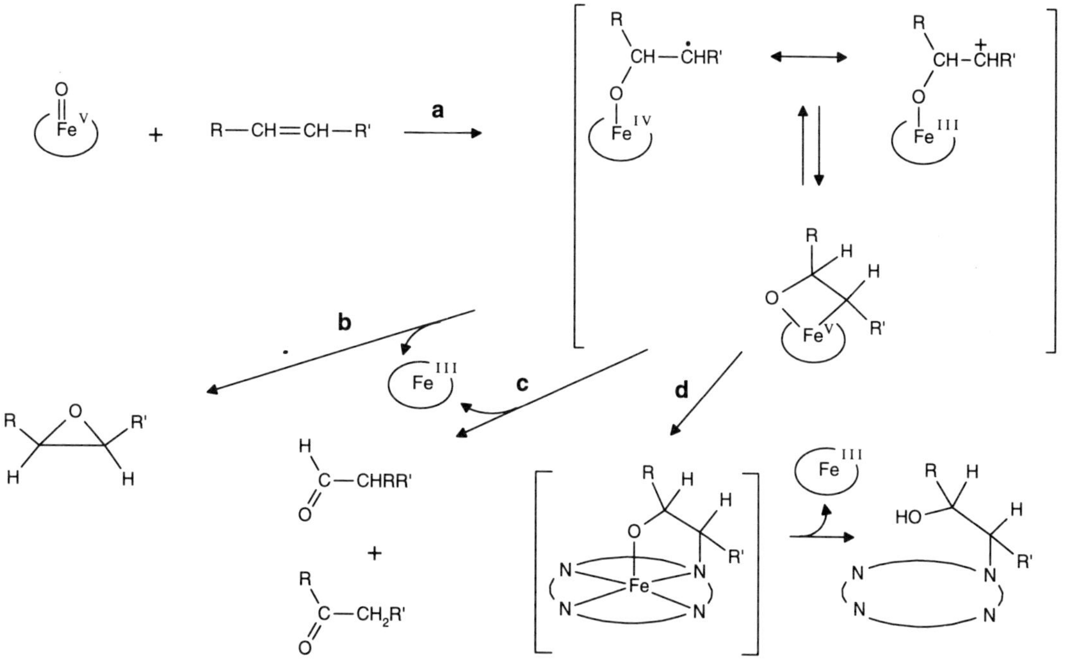

FIGURE 4.15 Currently accepted mechanism of cytochrome P450-catalyzed oxidation of olefinic bonds as exemplified by 1,2-disubstituted ethylene derivatives. Following formation of the first C–O bond (reaction **a**), three pathways lead to epoxides (pathway **b**), carbonyl derivatives (pathway **c**), and heme alkylation (pathway **d**).

intermediates have been postulated to arise, three of which are shown in Fig. 4.15. Rather than being mutually exclusive, it is likely that these three intermediates interconvert and have each a role to play, albeit to a variable extent depending on the groups attached to the olefinic bond (Mansuy *et al.*, 1984b). Studies have demonstrated the importance of the radical, the carbocation and/or the cyclic intermediate (i.e. a metallooxetane) shown in Fig. 4.15 (Castellino and Bruice, 1988; Collman *et al.*, 1985; Groves *et al.*, 1986; Ortiz de Montellano *et al.*, 1982). In addition, quantum mechanical calculations have suggested variants to these intermediates (Jørgensen, 1987).

Whatever the intermediate(s) involved, three reactions lead to generally stable products. Formation of the **second C–O bond** (pathway **b**, Fig. 4.15) generates the epoxide, which is often the predominant or sole product characterized. Such rearrangement occurs without group migration, and under physiological conditions of pH and temperature the chemical stability of epoxides of olefins is often quite marked (for a general review on the chemistry of oxiranes see Bartók and Láng, 1985). A second pathway (pathway **c**) leads to carbonyl derivatives, as documented by the formation of 1-phenyl-1-butanone and 1-phenyl-2-butanone from *trans*-1-phenyl-1-butene (Liebler and Guengerich, 1983). Pathway **c** may be accompanied by group migration (e.g. deuterium, chlorine), as illustrated in Section 4.4.2.

In addition to the formation of epoxides and carbonyl derivatives, compounds containing olefinic bonds may also react according to pathway **d** and bind covalently to heme, forming N-alkylporphyrins often characterized as abnormal ("green") pigments (Dolphin, 1984; Ortiz de Montellano, 1988 and 1991; Ortiz de Montellano and Correia, 1983; Ortiz de Montellano *et al.*, 1980). One type of such adducts is shown in Fig. 4.15 (Artaud *et al.*, 1987). This is one of the many mechanisms by which compounds (sometimes but not adequately called "suicide-substrates") can act as **irreversible mechanism-based inactivators** of enzymes (Testa, 1990).

The relative importance of pathway **d** depends extensively on steric and electronic factors of the substrate (Luke *et al.*, 1990; Ortiz de Montellano and Mico, 1980). Thus, the oxidation of styrene, cyclohexene and 3-hexene does not result in cytochrome P450 destruction, whereas 4-ethyl-1-hexene, 1-heptene, 3-methyl-1-octene, methyl 2-isopropyl-4-pentenoate, and 3-isopropyl-5-hexen-2-one caused cytochrome P450 loss and green pigments formation. A close analogue of the latter two compounds, **allylisopropylacetamide** (AIA, 2-isopropyl-4-pentenamide, **4.LX**), is also highly active and the molecular mechanism by which it alkylates porphyrins has been elucidated (Ortiz de Montellano *et al.*, 1984). Some 5-allylbarbiturates, e.g. secobarbital, behave similarly. From an enzymic point of view, it was shown that allyl substrates administered to rats can alkylate not only the heme but also the apoprotein of some cytochromes P450 (Bornheim *et al.*, 1987; Lunetta *et al.*, 1989).

4.LX

4.LXI

The role of heme N-alkylation may well be more complex than hitherto postulated. Indeed, there is now some evidence to suggest that the transient species formed by pathway **d** (shown in square brackets in Fig. 4.15) not only leads to cytochrome P450 destruction as discussed in the previous paragraphs, but may also act as a catalyst in a reaction of **hemin-catalyzed epoxidation**, as indicated for norbornene (Traylor *et al.*, 1987).

Some **allenic substrates**, e.g. 1,1-dimethylallene and 17α-propadienyl-19-nortestosterone (**4.LXI**), were also shown to destroy cytochrome P450 by forming heme adducts (Ortiz de Montellano and Kunze, 1980a).

4.4.2 Oxidation of olefinic bonds in drugs and other xenobiotics

Despite its apparent simplicity, the epoxidation of alkenes may display interesting and informative aspects of substrate and product regioselectivity and stereoselectivity. The epoxidation of even simple prochiral alkenes (e.g. propene, 1-butene, 1,3-butadiene, 2-methyl-1-butene, *cis*- and *trans*-2-pentene) and chiral alkenes (e.g. 3-methyl-1-pentene, *cis*- and *trans*-4-methyl-2-hexene) was found to proceed *in vitro* with species- and induction-dependent stereoselectivities, suggesting the involvement of several CYP enzymes (Wistuba *et al.*, 1989).

Olefinic epoxidation is of some importance in the metabolism of **terpinoids**. Thus, (+)-limonene (**4.LXII**) was oxidized by rat liver microsomes to the 1,2- and 8,9-epoxide in a 1/4 ratio, demonstrating the epoxidation of both alkenyl and cycloalkenyl groups (Watabe *et al.*, 1981). The **regioselectivity** in the oxidation of limonene is interesting in its own right and is believed to be caused by steric factors. Note that in such studies epoxides may not be detected in unchanged form due to rapid epoxide hydrolase-mediated hydration (see the volume concerning the Biochemistry of Hydration and Dehydration Reactions); their characterization then requires addition to the incubation medium of an inhibitor of epoxide hydrolase (e.g. 1,2-epoxy-3,3,3-trichloropropene).

The halogenated insecticide **aldrin** is also a substrate for epoxidation of its endocyclic

4.LXII   4.LXIII

4.LXIV

olefinic bond. Rat liver cytochromes P450 vary extensively in their capacity to mediate the reaction, with the highest activities being displayed by such enzymes as CYP2C11 (constitutive) and CYP2C6 (phenobarbital-inducible). In contrast, no or negligible activity was seen with CYP2C12 and CYP1A1 (Wolff and Guengerich, 1987).

A number of drugs or metabolites form olefinic epoxides which can be stable or rearrange intramolecularly. In humans, **carbamazepine** (**4.LXIII**) yields over 30 metabolites, among which the 10,11-epoxide is not only a predominant one, but is also pharmacologically active (Lertratanangkoon and Horning, 1982; Rambeck et al., 1987). In fact, epoxidation followed by enzymatic hydration is a major pathway in the human metabolism of tricyclic drugs of this type (Frigerio and Pantarotto, 1976). In contrast, the olefinic epoxide of the anti-inflammatory agent alclofenac (**4.LXIV**) is a very minor metabolite which accounts for 0.01% or less of a dose in humans (Slack and Ford-Hutchinson, 1980). It is interesting to note that this epoxide was found to break down in urine (pH 5, 37°C) with a half-life of 35 h.

Rearrangement reactions of epoxides include the formation of the lactone **4.LXV** from the epoxide of 2-n-propyl-4-pentenoic acid (**4.VIII**), the Δ^4-unsaturated metabolite of valproic acid (Section 4.2.3) (Porubek et al., 1988; Prickett and Baillie, 1986). A comparable intramolecular nucleophilic reaction has been reported for hexobarbital (**4.XXXIV**); following its epoxidation in the rat, the cyclized product **4.LXVI** was characterized. Note that the diol formed from this epoxide is also unstable and loses its 5-alkenyl substituent (Takenoshita et al., 1993; Vermeulen et al., 1981).

4.LXV   4.LXVI

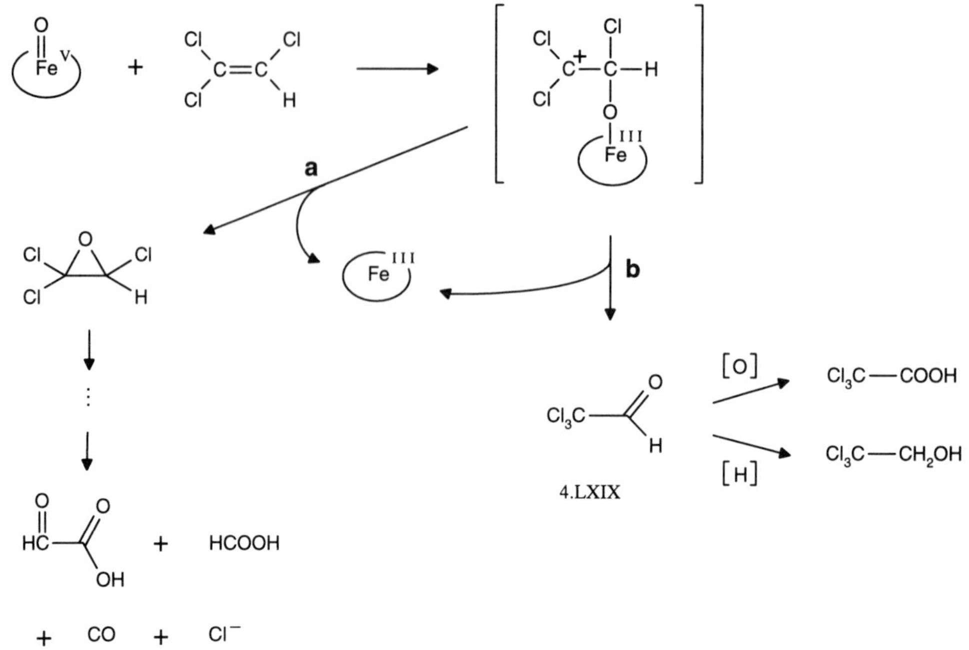

FIGURE 4.16 Postulated mechanism of cytochrome P450-catalyzed oxidation of trichloroethene. Reaction **a** leads to trichloroethene oxide and then to dechlorinated metabolites such as glyoxylic acid, formic acid and carbon monoxide. Reaction **b** involves halogen migration to chloral (**4.LXIX**) and its metabolites (modified from Miller and Guengerich, 1982).

4.4.3 Oxidation of halogenated alkenes

Olefinic groups bearing halogen atoms are also monooxygenated by cytochrome P450, but the particular reactivity of metabolic intermediates calls for a separate discussion. The many industrial uses of halogenated alkenes and the genotoxicity of some of these compounds (Jones and Mackrodt, 1983) render their metabolic toxication and detoxication of major significance. Thus, the hepatoxicity of 1,1-dichloro-2,2-difluoroethene (**4.LXVII**) in the rat was ascribed to an undetected reactive metabolite formed by oxidation; the stable product generated by this oxidative pathway was chlorodifluoroacetic acid (**4.LXVIII**), a metabolite demonstrating halogen migration (Commandeur *et al.*, 1987).

A number of authors have assumed the epoxide to be the reactive intermediate undergoing halogen migration (Anders, 1984; Henschler, 1985). However, conclusive evidence now exists that the mechanism is more complex and resembles that discussed in Section 4.4.1 (Fig. 4.15). Indeed, it could be demonstrated using **trichloroethene** as a substrate (Fig. 4.16) that a carbocation must be the intermediate which either collapses to the epoxide (reaction **a** in Fig. 4.16) or undergoes chlorine migration (reaction **b** in Fig. 4.16) to chloral (**4.LXIX** in Fig. 4.16), the major metabolite formed in microsomal preparations (Miller and Guengerich, 1982). *In vivo*, chloral undergoes hydrogenation to trichloroethanol and dehydrogenation to trichloroacetic acid; these reactions are discussed in Chapter 2. As for the epoxide, it is further transformed upon release of chloride anions to such metabolites as glyoxylic acid, formic acid, and carbon monoxide.

The interest of the mechanism outlined in Fig. 4.16 is that it can also explain the **loss of cytochrome P450** caused by a number of halogenated alkenes. In a series of chlorofluoroethenes, release of fluoride and covalent binding to cytochrome P450 were not correlated (Baker *et al.*,

1987). This fact is compatible with differential reactivity of the carbocation intermediate either to collapse to the epoxide (i.e. in analogy with reaction **a** in Fig. 4.16) and then to release fluoride, or to destroy heme (in analogy with reaction **d** in Fig. 4.15).

4.5 OXIDATION OF sp-HYBRIDIZED CARBON ATOMS IN ACETYLENIC BONDS

Triple carbon–carbon bonds as found in alkynes, rather than being metabolically inert as believed earlier, undergo cytochrome P450-mediated oxidation to a number of metabolites. In addition, a large variety of acetylenic derivatives, be they drugs or other xenobiotics, share with chemicals belonging to many other classes the property of being mechanism-based irreversible inactivators of cytochrome P450 (Ortiz de Montellano, 1984; Ortiz de Montellano and Correia, 1983; White, 1984).

The **mechanism of alkyne oxidation** has received less attention than that of alkene oxidation, and as a result our understanding of the former reaction is still more fragmentary than that of the latter. Nevertheless, a realistic if partial picture is now emerging, as shown in simplified form in Fig. 4.17. The lay-out of this figure is meant to emphasize analogies with olefin oxidation, although we recognize that some of these analogies might prove misleading.

A number of reactive intermediates have been postulated to be generated and/or to interconvert following bond formation between an acetylenic carbon atom and the oxygen atom (reaction **a** in Fig. 4.17). In addition to the radical, the carbocation and the metallooxetene shown in Fig. 4.17, a cation-radical and a carbene have also been postulated (Komives and Ortiz de Montellano, 1987; Ortiz de Montellano and Komives, 1985; Ortiz de Montellano and Kunze, 1980b and 1982; Ortiz de Montellano et al., 1982). Three pathways appear to account for the formation of metabolites or adducts of alkynes. Pathway **d** (Fig. 4.17) leads to heme alkylation,

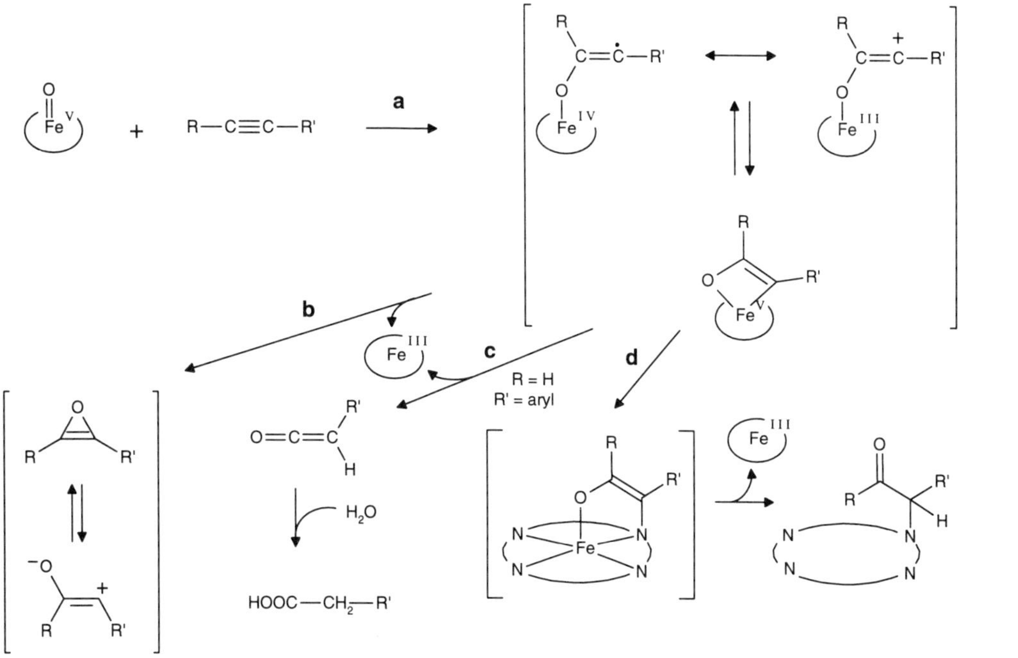

FIGURE 4.17 Postulated mechanism of cytochrome P450-mediated oxidation of acetylenic derivatives, leading to reactive intermediates (pathway **b**), ketenes (pathway **c**) which hydrolyze to arylacetic acids, and heme alkylation (pathway **d**).

destruction of cytochrome P450 and formation of abnormal "green" pigments (Ortiz de Montellano and Kunze, 1980b and 1981a). In this context, interesting structure–reactivity relationships have been reported. Among **1-alkynes**, 1-pentyne and 1-octadecyne were marginally active while 1-heptyne, 1-decyne and 1-tridecyne caused marked cytochrome P450 destruction (White, 1980). Among **positional isomers**, 2-decyne was as active as 1-decyne while 3-decyne was moderately active and 5-decyne was inactive, showing that a terminal ethynyl group is particularly reactive, while sterically hindered carbon–carbon triple bonds in non-terminal positions are inactive. In addition, polar derivatives appeared inactive (White, 1980). **Aryl-acetylenes** (see also below) may also be active mechanism-based inactivators of, e.g., CYP1A2, 2B1 and 2E1 depending on the size of the aromatic ring and the placement of the ethynyl group (Hammon *et al.*, 1989; Hopkins *et al.*, 1992; Roberts *et al.*, 1993).

Compounds possessing **geminal hydroxyl and ethynyl groups**, e.g. 1-ethynylcyclohexanol (**4.LXX**), 1-ethynylcyclopentanol and 3-methyl-1-pentyn-3-ol were also found to cause loss of cytochrome P450 (Ortiz de Montellano and Kunze, 1980b). Such compounds are of particular interest because they model the D-ring of a number of medicinal **17α-ethynyl steroids**, e.g. norethindrone (**4.LXXI**) and 17α-ethynylestradiol. There is indeed ample evidence that such steroids are potent mechanism-based irreversible inactivators of cytochrome P450 (Blakey and White, 1986; Guengerich, 1990a; Ortiz de Montellano *et al.*, 1979; Schmid *et al.*, 1983; White, 1978). In human liver microsomes, CYP3A4 was found to be the isozyme selectively destroyed by 17α-ethynylestradiol and analogues (Guengerich, 1988 and 1990b).

4.LXVII   4.LXVIII

The acetylenic oxidation of 17α-ethynyl steroids is not restricted to heme alkylation (pathway **d** in Fig. 4.17), but also results in D-homoannulation following **pathway b** (Fig. 4.17). Thus, the reactive intermediate(s) produced from pathway **b** rearrange(s) to D-homosteroids (steroids with a six-membered D-ring) according to the reaction shown in Fig. 4.18 (Ortiz de Montellano *et al.*, 1979; Schmid *et al.*, 1983).

4.LXX   4.LXXI

4.LXXII

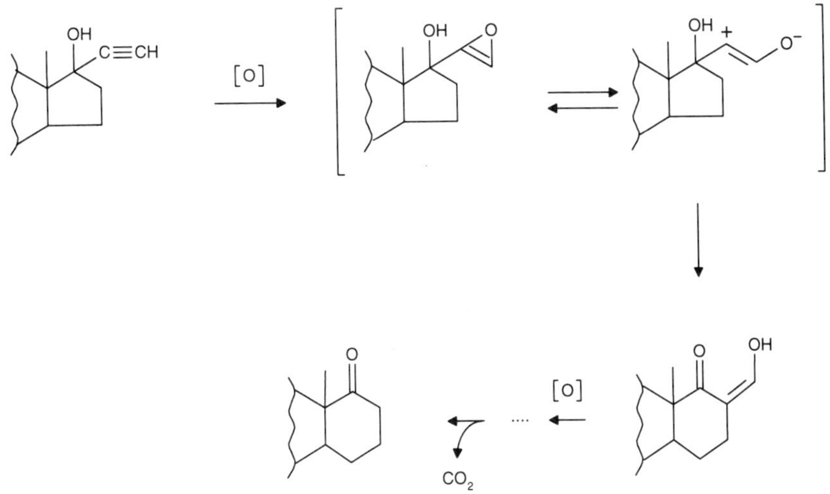

FIGURE 4.18 Postulated mechanism of D-homoannulation of 17α-ethynyl steroids, with reactive intermediate(s) formed by pathway **b** in Fig. 4.17 (modified from Ortiz de Montellano *et al.*, 1979; Schmid *et al.*, 1983).

Pathway c in Fig. 4.17 is exemplified by the oxidation of **arylacetylenes** (Fig. 4.17, R = H, R′ = aryl). Indeed, the cytochrome P450-mediated oxidation of such compounds leads both to heme alkylation (see above) and formation of an arylacetic acid metabolite (Fig. 4.17). For phenylacetylene incubated with hepatic microsomes from phenobarbital-treated rats, the partition ratio between metabolite formation and enzyme inactivation was found to be 26 (Ortiz de Montellano and Komives, 1985). The mechanism of arylacetic acid formation has particular toxicological significance; it is understood to involve formation of a **ketene** upon shift of the acetylenic hydrogen from C-2 to C-1, followed by non-enzymatic addition of water (Ortiz de Montellano and Kunze, 1980c and 1981b). Such ketenes are indeed reactive electrophiles, and they are suspected to account for at least part of the toxicity of arylacetylenes (Wade *et al.*, 1980).

Acetylenic oxidation is much more pronounced in ethynylbiphenyl derivatives than in ethynylbenzenes. In fact, the dose of 4-ethynylbiphenyl (**4.LXXII**) administered to rats and rabbits was completely accounted for as biphenyl-4-ylacetic acid and 4′-hydroxybiphenyl-4-ylacetic acid (Wade *et al.*, 1979). Extensive oxidation of the 2′-fluoro derivative was also reported (Sullivan *et al.*, 1979). It is interesting to note that a few ethynylbiphenyls were investigated as potential prodrugs of anti-inflammatory biphenylacetic acids until toxicity problems interrupted their development.

4.6 REFERENCES

Abbott F.S., Kassam J., Orr J.M. and Farrell K. (1986). The effect of aspirin on valproic acid metabolism. *Clin. Pharmacol. Ther.* **40**, 94–100.

Ackland M.J. (1993). Correlation between site specificity and electrophilic frontier values in the metabolic hydroxylation of biphenyl, di-aromatic and CYP2D6 substrates: a molecular modelling study. *Xenobiotica* **23**, 1135–1144.

Allen J.G., Brown A.N. and Marten T.R. (1976). Metabolism of debrisoquine sulphate in rat, dog and man. *Xenobiotica* **6**, 405–409.

Al Sharifi M.A., Gilbert J.N.T. and Powell J.W. (1983). 4′-Hydroxylated derivatives as urinary metabolites of two barbiturates. *Xenobiotica* **13**, 179–183.

Anders M.W. (1984). Biotransformation of halogenated hydrocarbons. In *Drug Metabolism and Drug Toxicity* (eds Mitchell J.R. and Horning M.G.). pp. 55–70. Raven Press, New York.

Anthony A., Caldwell J., Hutt A.J. and Smith R.L. (1987). Metabolism of estragole in rat and mouse and influence of dose size on excretion of the proximate carcinogen 1′-hydroxyestragole. *Fd. Chem. Toxicol.* **25**, 799–806.

Artaud I., Devocelle L., Battioni J.P., Girault J.P. and Mansuy D. (1987). Suicidal inactivation of iron porphyrins catalysts during alk-1-ene oxidation: isolation of a new type of N-alkylporphyrins. *J. Amer. Chem. Soc.* **109**, 3782–3783.

Ascalone V., Flaminio L., Guinebault P., Thenot J.P. and Morselli P.L. (1992). Determination of zolpidem, a new sleep-inducing agent, and its metabolites in biological fluids—Pharmacokinetics, drug metabolism and overdosing investigations in humans. *J. Chromatogr. Biomed. Appl.* **581**, 237–250.

Ashburn S.P., Han X. and Liehr J.G. (1993). Microsomal hydroxylation of 2- and 4-fluoroestradiol to catechol metabolites and their conversion to methyl esters: catechol estrogens as possible mediators of hormonal carcinogenesis. *Molec. Pharmacol.* **43**, 534–541.

Atkins W.M. and Sligar S.G. (1989). Molecular recognition in cytochrome P-450: Alteration of regioselective alkane hydroxylation via protein engineering. *J. Amer. Chem. Soc.* **111**, 2715–2717.

Baillie T.A. (1992). Metabolism of valproate to hepatotoxic intermediates. *Pharm. Weekbl. Sci. Ed.* **14**, 122–125.

Baker M.T., Bates J.N. and Leff S.V. (1987). Comparative defluorination and cytochrome P450 loss by the microsomal metabolism of fluoro- and fluorochloroethenes. *Drug Metab. Disposit.* **15**, 499–503.

Bartók M. and Láng K.L. (1985). Oxiranes. In *Small Ring Heterocycles*, Part 3 (ed. Hassner A.). pp. 1–196. Wiley, New York.

Billings R.E. and Fischer L.J. (1985). Oxygen-18 incorporation studies of the metabolism of phenytoin to the catechol. *Drug Metab. Disposit.* **13**, 312–317.

Blakey D.C. and White I.N.H. (1986). Destruction of cytochrome P-450 and formation of green pigments by contraceptive steroids in rat hepatocyte suspensions. *Biochem. Pharmacol.* **35**, 1561–1567.

Bornheim L.M., Underwood M.C., Caldera P., Rettie A.E., Trager W.F., Wrighton S.A. and Correia M.A. (1987). Inactivation of multiple hepatic cytochrome P-450 isozymes in rats by allylisopropylacetamide: mechanistic implications. *Molec. Pharmacol.* **32**, 299–308.

Bowry V.W., Lusztyk J. and Ingold K.U. (1989). Calibration of the bicyclo[2.1.0]pent-2-yl radical ring opening and an oxygen rebound constant for cytochrome P-450. *J. Amer. Chem. Soc.* **111**, 1927–1928.

Boyd D.R. and Jerina D.M. (1985). Arene oxides-oxepines. In *Small Ring Heterocycles*, Part 3 (ed. Hassner A). pp. 197–282. Wiley, New York.

Bruice P.Y. and Bruice T.C. (1976). Modes of acid catalysis in the aromatization of arene oxides. *J. Amer. Chem. Soc.* **98**, 2023–2025.

Burka L.T., Plucinski T.M. and Macdonald T.L. (1983). Mechanisms of hydroxylation by cytochrome P-450: Metabolism of monohalobenzenes by phenobarbital-induced microsomes. *Proc. Natl. Acad. Sci. USA* **80**, 6680–6684.

Bush E.D. and Trager W.F. (1982). Evidence against an abstraction or direct insertion mechanism for cytochrome P-450 catalysed *meta* hydroxylation. *Biochem. Biophys. Res. Commun.* **104**, 626–632.

Butler T.C., Dudley K.H., Johnson D. and Roberts S.B. (1976). Studies on the metabolism of 5,5-diphenylhydantoin relating principally to the stereoselectivity of the hydroxylation reactions in man and the dog. *J. Pharmacol. Exp. Ther.* **199**, 82–92.

CaJacob C.A., Chan W.K., Shephard E. and Ortiz de Montellano P.R. (1988). The catalytic site of rat hepatic lauric acid ω-hydroxylase. *J. Biol. Chem.* **263**, 18,640–18,649.

Carlin J.R., Höglund P., Eriksson L.O., Christofalo P., Gregoire S.L., Taylor A.M. and Andersson K.E. (1992). Disposition and pharmacokinetics of [^{14}C]finasteride after oral administration in humans. *Drug Metab. Disposit.* **20**, 148–155.

Casazza J.P., Felver M.E. and Veech R.L. (1984). The metabolism of acetone in rat. *J. Biol. Chem.* **259**, 231–236.

Castellino A.J. and Bruice T.C. (1988). Intermediates in the epoxidation of alkenes by cytochrome P-450 models. I. *cis*-Stilbene as a mechanistic probe. *J. Amer. Chem. Soc.* **110**, 158–162.

Cavalieri E.L. and Rogan E.G. (1992). The approach to understanding aromatic hydrocarbon carcinogenesis—The central role of radical cations in metabolic activation. *Pharmacol. Therap.* **55**, 183–199.

Champion P.M. (1989). Elementary electronic excitations and the mechanism of cytochrome P450. *J. Amer. Chem. Soc.* **111**, 3433–3434.

Chan K.Y., George R.C., Chen T.M. and Okerholm R.A. (1991). Direct enantiomeric separation of terfenadine and its major acid metabolite by HPLC and the lack of stereoselective terfenadine enantiomer biotransformation in man. *J. Chromatogr. Biomed. Appl.* **571**, 291–297.

Chao H.S.I. and Berchtold G.A. (1981). Aromatization of arene 1,2-oxides. Comparison of the aromatization pathways of 1-carboxy-, 1-carbomethoxy-, 1-formyl-, 1-(hydroxymethyl)-, and 1-(2-hydroxy-2- propyl)benzene oxide. *J. Amer. Chem. Soc.* **103**, 898–902.

Collins J.R. and Loew G.H. (1988). Theoretical study of the product specificity in the hydroxylation of camphor, norcamphor, 5,5-difluoro-camphor and pericyclocamphanone by cytochrome P-450$_{cam}$. *J. Biol. Chem.* **263**, 3164–3170.

Collins J.R., Camper D.L. and Loew G.H. (1991). Valproic acid metabolism by cytochrome P450: A theoretical study of stereoelectronic modulators of product distribution. *J. Amer. Chem. Soc.* **113**, 2736–2743.

Collman J.P., Kodadek T., Raybuck S.A., Brauman J.I. and Papazian L.M. (1985). Mechanism of oxygen atom transfer from high valent iron prophyrins to olefins: implications to the biological epoxidation of olefins by cytochrome P-450. *J. Amer. Chem. Soc.* **107**, 4343–4345.

Collman J.P., Hampton P.D. and Brauman J.I. (1990). Suicide inactivation of cytochrome P-450 model compounds by terminal olefins. *J. Amer. Chem. Soc.* **112**, 2977–2986 and 2986–2998.

Commandeur J.N.M., Oostendorp R.A.J., Schoofs P.R.,

Xu B. and Vermeulen N.P.E. (1987). Nephrotoxicity and hepatoxicity of 1,1-dichloro-2,2-difluoroethylene in the rat. *Biochem. Pharmacol.* **36**, 4229–4237.

Coon M.J., Ding X., Pernecky S.J. and Vaz A.D.N. (1992). Cytochrome P450: progress and predictions. *FASEB J.* **6**, 669–673.

Damani L.A. (1988). Chemical reactivity considerations in the metabolism of N-heteroaromatics. *Drug Metab. Drug Interact.* **6**, 149–158.

Dankovic D., Billings R.E., Seifert W. and Stillwell W.G. (1985). Bromobenzene metabolism in isolated rat hepatocytes. *Molec. Pharmacol.* **27**, 287–295.

den Besten C., Smink M.C.C, de Vries E.J. and van Bladeren P.J. (1991). Metabolic activation of 1,2,4-trichlorobenzene and pentachlorobenzene by rat liver microsomes—a major role for quinone metabolites. *Toxicol. Appl. Pharmacol.* **108**, 223–233.

Dickinson R.G., Hooper W.D., Dunstan P.R. and Eadie M.J. (1989). Urinary excretion of valproate and some metabolites in chronically treated patients. *Therap. Drug. Monit.* **11**, 127–133.

Dittmann B. and Renner G. (1977). 4-Acetaminophenoxyacetic acid, a new urinary metabolite of phenacetin. *N. S. Arch. Pharmacol.* **296**, 87–89.

DiVincenzo G.D., Hamilton M.L., Kaplan C.J. and Dedinas J. (1977). Metabolic fate and disposition of ^{14}C-labelled methyl *n*-butyl ketone in the rat. *Toxicol. Appl. Pharmacol.* **41**, 547–560.

Dolphin D. (1985). Cytochrome P450: substrate and prosthetic-group free radicals generated during the enzymatic cycle. *Phil. Trans. R. Soc. Lond. B* **311**, 579–591.

Eichelbaum M. (1988). Pharmacokinetic and pharmacodynamic consequences of stereoselective drug metabolism in man. *Biochem. Pharmacol.* **37**, 93–96.

Eichelbaum M., Bertilsson L., Küpfer A., Steiner E. and Meese C.O. (1988). Enantioselectivity of 4-hydroxylation in extensive and poor metabolizers of debrisoquine. *Brit. J. Clin. Pharmacol.* **25**, 505–508.

Fabre G., Rahmani R., Placidi M., Combalbert J., Covo J., Cano J.P., Coulange C., Ducros M. and Rampal M. (1988). Characterization of midazolam metabolism using human hepatic microsomal fractions and hepatocytes in suspension obtained by perfusing whole human livers. *Biochem. Pharmacol.* **37**, 4389–4397.

Faigle J.W., Böttcher I., Godbillon J., Kriemler H.P., Schlumpf E., Schneider W., Schweizer A., Stierlin H. and Winkler T. (1988). A new metabolite of diclofenac sodium in human plasma. *Xenobiotica* **18**, 1191–1197.

Feierman D.E. and Cederbaum A.I. (1987). Oxidation of the alcohol dehydrogenase inhibitor pyrazole to 4-hydroxypyrazole by microsomes. *Drug Metab. Disposit.* **15**, 634–639.

Feierman D.E. and Cederbaum A.I. (1989). Role of cytochrome P-450 IIE1 and catalase in the oxidation of acetonitrile to cyanide. *Chem. Res. Toxicol.* **2**, 359–366.

Fischbach T. and Lenk W. (1985). Additional routes in the metabolism of phenacetin. *Xenobiotica* **15**, 149–164.

Fischer I.U., von Unruh G.E. and Dengler H.J. (1990). The metabolism of eugenol in man. *Xenobiotica* **20**, 209–222.

Fitzpatrick F.A. and Murphy R.C. (1989). Cytochrome P-450 metabolism of arachidonic acid: Formation and biological actions of "epoxygenase"-derived eicosanoids. *Pharmacol. Rev.* **40**, 229–241.

Floreani M., Carpenedo F., Santi R. and Contessa A.R. (1981). Metabolism of succinonitrile in liver: studies on the systems involved in cyanide release. *Eur. J. Drug Metab. Pharmacokinet.* **6**, 135–140.

Freeman J.J. and Hayes E.P. (1988). Microsomal metabolism of acetonitrile to cyanide. *Biochem. Pharmacol.* **37**, 1153–1159.

Frigerio A. and Pantarotto C. (1976). Epoxide-diol pathway in the metabolism of tricyclic drugs. *J. Pharm. Pharmacol.* **28**, 665–666.

Garner R.C. (1976). The role of epoxides in bioactivation and carcinogenesis. In *Progress in Drug Metabolism*, Vol. 1 (eds Bridges J.W. and Chasseaud L.F.). pp. 77–128. Wiley, London.

Garteiz D.A., Hook R.H., Walker B.J. and Okerholm R.A. (1982). Pharmacokinetics and biotransformation studies of terfenadine in man. *Arzneim-Forsch (Drug Res.)* **32**, 1185–1190.

Gilbert J.N.T., Powell J.W. and Templeton J. (1975). A study of the human metabolism of secbutobarbitone. *J. Pharm. Pharmacol.* **27**, 923–927.

Groves J.T. (1985). Key elements of the chemistry of cytochrome P-450. The oxygen rebound mechanism. *J. Chem. Educ.* **62**, 928–931.

Groves J.T. and Watanabe Y. (1986). On the mechanism of olefin epoxidation by oxo-iron porphyrins. Direct observation of an intermediate. *J. Amer. Chem. Soc.* **108**, 507–508.

Groves J.T., McClusky G.A., White R.E. and Coon M.J. (1978). Aliphatic hydroxylation by a highly purified liver microsomal cytochrome P-450. Evidence for a carbon radical intermediate. *Biochem. Biophys. Res. Commun.* **81**, 154–160.

Guengerich F.P. (1988). Oxidation of 17α-ethynylestradiol by human liver cytochrome P-450. *Molec. Pharmacol.* **33**, 500–508.

Guengerich F.P. (1990a). Metabolism of 17α-ethynylestradiol in humans. *Life Sci.* **47**, 1981–1988.

Guengerich F.P. (1990b). Mechanism-based inactivation of human liver microsomal cytochrome P-450 IIIA4 by gestogene. *Chem. Res. Toxicol.* **3**, 363–371.

Guengerich F.P. (1991). Reactions and significance of cytochrome P-450 enzymes. *J. Biol. Chem.* **266**, 10,019–10,022.

Guengerich F.P. and Macdonald T.L. (1984). Chemical mechanisms of catalysis by cytochromes P-450: a unified view. *Acc. Chem. Res.* **17**, 9–16.

Guengerich F.P. and Macdonald T.L. (1990). Mechanism of cytochrome P-450 catalysis. *FASEB J.* **4**, 2453–2459.

Guengerich F.P. and Kim D.H. (1991). Enzymatic oxidation of ethyl carbamate to vinyl carbamate and its role as an intermediate in the formation of 1,N^6-ethenoadenosine. *Chem. Res. Toxicol.* **4**, 413–421.

Hakamatsuka T., Faisal Hashim M., Ebizuka Y. and Sankawa U. (1991). P-450-Dependent oxidative rearrangement in isoflavone biosynthesis: reconstitution of

P450 and NADPH:P-450 reductase. *Tetrahedron* **47**, 5969–5978.

Hammons G.J., Alworth W.L., Hopkins N.E., Guengerich F.P. and Kadlubar F.F. (1989). 2-Ethynylnaphthalene as a mechanism-based inactivator of the cytochrome P-450 catalyzed N-oxidation of 2-naphthylamine. *Chem. Res. Toxicol.* **2**, 367–374.

Hanzlik R.P. and Ling K.H.J. (1990). Active site dynamics of toluene hydroxylation by cytochrome P-450. *J. Org. Chem.* **55**, 3992–3997.

Hanzlik R.P., Hogberg K. and Judson C.M. (1984). Microsomal hydroxylation of specifically deuterated monosubstituted benzenes. Evidence for direct aromatic hydroxylation. *Biochemistry* **23**, 3048–3055.

Harvey R.G. (1981). Activated metabolites of carcinogenic hydrocarbons. *Acc. Chem. Res.* **14**, 218–226.

Hawksworth G. and Scheline R.R. (1975). Metabolism in the rat of some pyrazine derivatives having flavour importance in foods. *Xenobiotica* **5**, 389–399.

Henschler D. (1985). Halogenated alkenes and alkynes. In *Bioactivation of Foreign Compounds* (ed. Anders M.W.). pp. 317–347. Academic Press, Orlando.

Hinson J.A., Freeman J.P., Potter D.W., Mitchum R.K. and Evans F.E. (1985). Mechanism of microsomal metabolism of benzene to phenol. *Molec. Pharmacol.* **27**, 574–577.

Hjelmeland L.M., Aronow L. and Trudell J.R. (1977). Intramolecular determination of substituent effects in hydroxylations catalyzed by cytochrome P-450. *Molec. Pharmacol.* **13**, 634–639.

Hopkins N.E., Foroozesh M.K., Li L., Callaghan P. and Alworth W.L. (1992). The effects of the size of the ring system and placement of the ethynyl group on mechanism-based inhibition of P450 1A2 and 2E1 by ethynyl substituted polycyclic aromatic hydrocarbons. In *Abstracts of the Fourth North American ISSX Meeting*, Bal Harbour, FL, November 2–6, 1992, p. 47.

Horiba M., Murai T., Nomura K., Yuge T., Sanai K. and Osada E. (1984). Pharmacokinetic studies of mabuterol, a new selective β_2-stimulant. *Arzneim-Forsch. (Drug Res.)* **34**, 1668–1679.

Howell S.R., Kotkoskie L.A., Dills R.L. and Klaassen C.D. (1988). 3-Hydroxylation of salicylamide in mice. *J. Pharm. Sci.* **77**, 309–313.

Idle J.R., Mahgoub A., Angelo M.M., Dring L.G., Lancaster R. and Smith R.L. (1979). The metabolism of [^{14}C]-debrisoquine in man. *Brit. J. Clin. Pharmacol.* **7**, 257–266.

Ingelman-Sundberg M. and Ekström G. (1982). Aniline is hydroxylated by the cytochrome P-450-dependent hydroxyl radical-mediated oxygenation mechanism. *Biochem. Biophys. Res. Commun.* **106**, 625–631.

Ingold K.U. (1989). At the organic chemistry/bioscience interface: Rate processes in complex systems. *Aldrichimica Acta* **22**, 69–73.

Jerina D.M., Daly J.W., Witkop B., Zaltzman-Nirenberg P. and Udenfriend S. (1969). 1,2-Naphthalene oxide as an intermediate in the microsomal hydroxylation of naphthalene. *Biochemistry* **9**, 147–156.

Johansson I. and Ingelman-Sundberg M. (1983). Hydroxyl-mediated, cytochrome P-450-dependent metabolic activation of benzene in microsomes and reconstituted enzyme systems from rabbit liver. *J. Biol. Chem.* **258**, 7311–7316.

Johansson I., Eliasson E., Norsten C. and Ingelman-Sundberg M. (1986). Hydroxylation of acetone by ethanol- and acetone-inducible cytochrome P-450 in liver microsomes and reconstituted membranes. *FEBS Lett.* **196**, 59–64.

Jones J.P. and Trager W.F. (1987). The separation of the intramolecular isotope effect for the cytochrome P-450 catalyzed hydroxylation of n-octane into its primary and secondary components. *J. Amer. Chem. Soc.* **109**, 2171–2173.

Jones R.B. and Mackrodt W.C. (1983). Structure-genotoxicity relationship for aliphatic epoxides. *Biochem. Pharmacol.* **32**, 2359–2362.

Jørgensen K.A. (1987). On the mechanism of stereoselective epoxidation of alkenes by oxo-iron prophyrins. *J. Amer. Chem. Soc.* **109**, 698–705.

Kamm J.J. and Szuna A. (1973). Studies on an unusual N-dealkylation reaction. II. Characteristics of the enzyme system and proposed pathway for the reaction. *J. Pharmacol. Exp. Ther.* **184**, 729–738.

Kassahun K. and Baillie T.A. (1993). Cytochrome P450-mediated dehydrogenation of 2-n-propyl-2-(E)-pentenoic acid, a pharmacologically active metabolite of valproic acid, in rat liver microsomal preparations. *Drug Metab. Disposit.* **21**, 242–248.

Kellis J.T. and Vickery L.E. (1987). The active site of aromatase cytochrome P-450. *J. Biol. Chem.* **262**, 8840–8844.

Kennedy K.A., Ambre J.J. and Fischer L.J. (1978). A selected ion monitoring method for glutethimide and six metabolites: application to blood and urine from humans intoxicated with glutethimide. *Biomed. Mass Spectrom.* **5**, 679–685.

Kobayashi T., Sugihara J. and Harigaya S. (1987). Mechanism of metabolic cleavage of a furan ring. *Drug Metab. Disposit.* **15**, 877–881.

Kodama R., Yano T., Furukawa K., Noda K. and Ide H. (1976). Studies on the metabolism of d-limonene (p-mentha-1,8-diene). IV. Isolation and characterization of new metabolites and species differences in metabolism. *Xenobiotica* **6**, 377–389.

Komives E.A. and Ortiz de Montellano P.R. (1987). Mechanism of oxidation of π bonds by cytochrome P-450. Electronic requirements of the transition state in the turnover of phenylacetylene. *J. Biol. Chem.* **262**, 9793–9802.

Koop D.R. (1986). Hydroxylation of p-nitrophenol by rabbit ethanol-inducible cytochrome P-450 isozyme 3a. *Molec. Pharmacol.* **29**, 399–404.

Koop D.R., Laethem C.L. and Schnier G.G. (1989). Identification of ethanol-inducible P450 isozyme 3a (P450IIE1) as a benzene and phenol hydroxylase. *Toxicol. Appl. Pharmacol.* **98**, 278–288.

Korzekwa K., Trager W., Gouterman M., Spangler D. and

Loew G.H. (1985). Cytochrome P450 mediated aromatic oxidation: a theoretical study. *J. Amer. Chem. Soc.* **107**, 4273–4279.

Korzekwa K.R., Jones J.P. and Gillette J.R. (1990a). Theoretical studies on cytochrome P-450 mediated hydroxylation: A predictive model for hydrogen atom abstractions. *J. Amer. Chem. Soc.* **112**, 7042–7046.

Korzekwa K.R., Trager W.F., Nagata K., Parkinson A. and Gillette J.R. (1990b). Isotope effect studies on the mechanism of the cytochrome P-450IIA1-catalyzed formation of Δ6-testosterone from testosterone. *Drug Metab. Disposit.* **18**, 974–979.

Koymans L., Donné-Op den Kelder G.M., te Koppele J.M. and Vermeulen N.P.E. (1993). Cytochromes P450: Their active-site structure and mechanism of oxidation. *Drug Metab. Rev.* **25**, 325–387.

Kronbach T., Mathys D., Umeno M., Gonzalez F.J. and Meyer U.A. (1989). Oxidation of midazolam and triazolam by human liver cytochrome P450IIIA4. *Molec. Pharmacol.* **36**, 89–96.

Laniado-Schwartzman M., Davis K.L., McGiff J.C., Levere R.D. and Abraham N.G. (1988). Purification and characterization of cytochrome P-450-dependent arachidonic acid epoxygenase from human liver. *J. Biol. Chem.* **263**, 2536–2542.

Lau S.S., Monks T.J., Greene K.E. and Gillette J.R. (1984). Detection and half-life of bromobenzene-3,4-oxide in blood. *Xenobiotica* **14**, 539–543.

Le Fur J.M. and Labaune J.P. (1985). Metabolic pathway by cleavage of a furan ring. *Xenobiotica* **15**, 567–577.

Lehr R.E. and Jerina D.M. (1977). Metabolic activations of polycyclic hydrocarbons. Structure–activity relationships. *Arch. Toxicol.* **39**, 1–6.

Lenk W. (1979). Mixed function oxygenation of the lower fatty acyl residues—I. Hydroxylation of the acetic, propionic, butyric, and valeric residues by rabbit liver microsomes. *Biochem. Pharmacol.* **28**, 2149–2159.

Lertratanangkoon K. and Horning M.G. (1982). Metabolism of carbamazepine. *Drug Metab. Rev.* **10**, 1–10.

Levin W., Wood A., Chang R., Ryan D., Thomas P., Yagi H., Thakker D., Vyas K., Boyd C., Chu S.Y., Conney A. and Jerina D. (1982). Oxidative metabolism of polycyclic aromatic hydrocarbons to ultimate carcinogens. *Drug Metab. Rev.* **13**, 555–580.

Li J.J., Purdy R.H., Appelman E.H., Klicka J.K. and Li S.A. (1985). Catechol formation of fluoro- and bromo-substituted estradiols by hamster liver microsomes. Evidence for dehalogenation. *Molec. Pharmacol.* **27**, 559–565.

Liebler D.C. and Guengerich F.P. (1983). Olefin oxidation by cytochrome P-450: evidence for group migration in catalytic intermediates formed with vinylidene chloride and *trans*-1-phenyl-1-butene. *Biochemistry* **22**, 5482–5489.

Lin D.C.K., Fentiman Jr A.F., Foltz R.L., Forney Jr R.D. and Sunshine I. (1975). Quantification of phencyclidine in body fluids by GC/CI/MS and identification of two metabolites. *Biomed. Mass Spectrom.* **2**, 206–214.

Lindeke B., Hallström G. and Anderson E. (1978). Enzymic oxidation α to the acetylenic group in the metabolism of N-(5-pyrrolidinopent-3-ynyl)-succinimide (BL 14) *in vitro*. *Xenobiotica* **8**, 341–348.

Lowe J.P. and Silverman B.D. (1981). Simple molecular orbital explanation for "bay-region" carcinogenic reactivity. *J. Amer. Chem. Soc.* **103**, 2852–2855.

Luke B.T., Collins J.R., Loew G.H. and McLean A.D. (1990). Theoretical investigations of terminal alkenes as putative suicide substrates of cytochrome P-450. *J. Amer. Chem. Soc.* **112**, 8686–8691.

Lunetta J.M., Sugiyama K. and Correia M.A. (1989). Secobarbital-mediated inactivation of rat liver cytochrome P450$_b$: a mechanistic reappraisal. *Molec. Pharmacol.* **35**, 10–17.

Mansuy D., Dansette P.M., Foures C., Jaouen M., Moinet G. and Bayer N. (1984a). Metabolic hydroxylation of the thiophene ring: isolation of 5-hydroxy-tienilic acid as a major urinary metabolite of tienilic acid in man and rat. *Biochem. Pharmacol.* **33**, 1429–1435.

Mansuy D., Leclaire J., Fontecave M. and Momenteau M. (1984b). Oxidation of monosubstituted olefins by cytochromes P-450 and heme models: evidence for the formation of aldehydes in addition to epoxides and allylic alcohols. *Biochem. Biophys. Res. Commun.* **119**, 319–325.

McMahon R.E., Sullivan H.R., Craig J.C. and Pereira W.E. Jr (1969). The microsomal oxygenation of ethylbenzene: isotopic, stereochemical, and induction studies. *Arch. Biochem. Biophys.* **132**, 575–577.

Mellström B., Bertilsson L., Birgersson C., Göransson M. and Von Bahr C. (1983). E- and Z-10-Hydroxylation of nortriptyline by human liver microsomes—Methods and characterization. *Drug Metab. Disposit.* **11**, 115–119.

Miller R.E. and Guengerich F.P. (1982). Oxidation of trichloroethylene by liver microsomal cytochrome P-450: evidence for chlorine migration in a transition state not involving trichloroethylene oxide. *Biochemistry* **21**, 1090–1097.

Miller V.P., Fruetel J.A. and Ortiz de Montellano P.R. (1992). Cytochrome P450(cam)-catalyzed oxidation of a hypersensitive radical probe. *Arch. Biochem. Biophys.* **298**, 697–702.

Mori Y., Kuroda N., Sakai Y., Yokoya F., Toyoshi K. and Baba S. (1985). Species differences in the metabolism of suprofen in laboratory animals and man. *Drug Metab. Disposit.* **13**, 239–245.

Moustafa M.A.A., Claesen M., Adline J., Vandervorst D. and Poupaert J.H. (1983). Evidence for an arene-3,4-oxide as a metabolic intermediate in the *meta*- and *para*-hydroxylation of phenytoin in the dog. *Drug Metab. Disposit.* **11**, 574–580.

Nagata K., Liberato D.J., Gillette J.R. and Sasame H.A. (1986). An unusual metabolite of testosterone: 17β-Hydroxy-4,6-androstadien-3-one. *Drug Metab. Disposit.* **14**, 559–565.

Nakajima T., Wang R.S., Elovaara E., Park S.S., Gelboin H.V., Hietanen E. and Vainio H. (1991). Monoclonal antibody-directed characterization of cytochrome P450 isozymes responsible for toluene metabolism in rat liver.

Biochem. Pharmacol. **41**, 395–404.

Nau H. (1990). Pharmacokinetic aspects of drug tera-togenesis: species differences and structure–activity relationships of the anticonvulsant valproic acid. *Acta Pharm. Jugosl.* **40**, 291–300.

Nusser E., Nill K. and Breyer-Pfaff U. (1988). Enantio-selective formation and disposition of (*E*)- and (*Z*)-10-hydroxynortriptyline. *Drug Metab. Disposit.* **16**, 509–511.

Oida T., Yoshida K., Kagemoto A., Sekine Y. and Higashijima T. (1985). The metabolism of gliclazide in man. *Xenobiotica* **15**, 87–96.

Ortiz de Montellano P.R. (1984). The inactivation of cytochrome P-450. *Ann. Rep. Med. Chem.* **19**, 201–211.

Ortiz de Montellano P.R. (1987). Control of the catalytic activity of prosthetic heme by the structure of hemoproteins. *Acc. Chem. Res.* **20**, 289–294.

Ortiz de Montellano P.R. (1988). Suicide substrates for drug metabolizing enzymes: mechanisms and biological consequences. In *Progress in Drug Metabolism*, Vol. 11 (ed. Gibson G.G.). pp. 99–148. Taylor & Francis, London.

Ortiz de Montellano P.R. (1989). Cytochrome P-450 catalysis: radical intermediates and dehydrogenation reactions. *Trends Pharmacol. Sci.* **10**, 354–359.

Ortiz de Montellano P.R. (1991). Mechanism-based in-activation of cytochrome P450: isolation and character-ization of N-alkyl heme adducts. In *Cytochrome P450* (eds Waterman M.R. and Johnson E.F.). pp. 533–540. Academic Press, San Diego.

Ortiz de Montellano P.R. and Komives E.A. (1985). Branchpoint for heme alkylation and metabolite forma-tion in the oxidation of arylacetylenes by cytochrome P-450. *J. Biol. Chem.* **260**, 3330–3336.

Ortiz de Montellano P.R. and Kunze K.L. (1980a). In-activation of hepatic cytochrome P-450 by allenic sub-strates. *Biochem. Biophys. Res. Commun.* **94**, 443–449.

Ortiz de Montellano P.R. and Kunze K.L. (1980b). Self-catalyzed inactivation of hepatic cytochrome P-450 by ethynyl substrates. *J. Biol. Chem.* **255**, 5587–5585.

Ortiz de Montellano P.R. and Kunze K.L. (1980c). Occurrence of a 1,2 shift during enzymatic and chemical oxidation of a terminal acetylene. *J. Amer. Chem. Soc.* **102**, 7373–7375.

Ortiz de Montellano P.R. and Kunze K.L. (1981a). Cytochrome P-450 inactivation: structure of the pros-thetic heme adduct with propyne. *Biochemistry* **20**, 7266–7271.

Ortiz de Montellano P.R. and Kunze K.L. (1981b). Shift of the acetylenic hydrogen during chemical and enzymatic oxidation of the biphenylacetylene triple bond. *Arch. Biochem. Biophys.* **209**, 710–712.

Ortiz de Montellano P.R. and Mico B.A. (1980). Destruc-tion of cytochrome P-450 by ethylene and other olefins. *Molec. Pharmacol.* **18**, 128–135.

Ortiz de Montellano P.R. and Correia M.A. (1983). Suicidal destruction of cytochrome P-450 during oxida-tive drug metabolism. *Ann. Rev. Pharmacol. Toxicol.* **23**, 481–503.

Ortiz de Montellano P.R. and Stearns R.A. (1987). Timing of the radical recombination step in cytochrome P-450 catalysis with ring-strained probes. *J. Amer. Chem. Soc.* **109**, 3415–3420.

Ortiz de Montellano P.R. and Stearns R.A. (1989). Radical intermediates in the cytochrome P-450-catalyzed oxida-tion of aliphatic hydrocarbons. *Drug Metab. Rev.* **20**, 183–191.

Ortiz de Montellano P.R., Kunze K.L., Yost G.S. and Mico B.A. (1979). Self-catalyzed destruction of cytochrome P-450: Covalent binding of ethynyl sterols to prosthetic heme. *Proc. Natl. Acad. Sci. USA* **76**, 746–749.

Ortiz de Montellano P.R., Kunze K.L. and Mico B.A. (1980). Destruction of cytochrome P-450 by olefins: N-alkylation of prosthetic heme. *Molec. Pharmacol.* **18**, 602–605.

Ortiz de Montellano P.R., Kunze K.L., Beilan H.S. and Wheeler C. (1982). Destruction of cytochrome P-450 by vinyl fluoride, fluroxene, and acetylene. Evidence for a radical intermediate in olefin oxidation. *Biochemistry* **21**, 1331–1339.

Ortiz de Montellano P.R., Stearns R.A. and Langry K.C. (1984). The allyl-isopropylacetamide and novonal pros-thetic heme adducts. *Molec. Pharmacol.* **25**, 310–317.

Ostovic D. and Bruice T.C. (1989). Intermediates in the epoxidation of alkenes by cytochrome P-450 models. 5. Epoxidation of alkenes catalyzed by a sterically hindered (*meso*-tetrakis(2,6-dibromophenyl)porphinato)iron-(III) chloride. *J. Amer. Chem. Soc.* **111**, 6511–6517.

Parke D.V. (1968). *The Biochemistry of Foreign Com-pounds*, Pergamon, Oxford, p. 218.

Patel J.M., Harper C. and Drew R.T. (1978). The biotrans-formation of *p*-xylene to a toxic aldehyde. *Drug Metab. Disposit.* **6**, 368–374.

Paulson G.D. and Feil V.J. (1987). The disposition of N-(4,6-dimethyl-2-pyrimidinyl)benzene[U-^{14}C]sul-fonamide in the rat. *Drug Metab. Disposit.* **15**, 671–675.

Perbellini L., Amantini M.C., Brugnone F. and Frontali N. (1982). Urinary excretion of *n*-hexane metabolites. A comparative study in rat, rabbit and monkey. *Arch. Toxicol.* **50**, 203–215.

Perbellini L., Brugnone F., Cocheo V., De Rosa E. and Bartolucci G.B. (1986). Identification of the *n*-heptane metabolites in rat and human urine. *Arch. Toxicol.* **58**, 229–234.

Porubek D.J., Barnes H., Theodore L.J. and Baillie T.A. (1988). Enantio-selective synthesis and preliminary metabolic studies of the optical isomers of 2-*n*-propyl-4-pentoic acid, a hepatotoxic metabolite of valproic acid. *Chem. Res. Toxicol.* **1**, 343–348.

Poupaert J.H., Cavalier R., Claesen M.H. and Dumont P.A. (1975). Absolute configuration of the major metabolite of 5,5-diphenylhydantoin, 5-(4′-hydroxy-phenyl)-5-phenylhydantoin. *J. Med. Chem.* **18**, 1268–1271.

Prickett K.S. and Baillie T.A. (1984). Metabolism of valproic acid by hepatic microsomal cytochrome P450. *Biochem. Biophys. Res. Comm.* **122**, 1166–1173.

Prickett K.S. and Baillie T.A. (1986). Metabolism of unsaturated derivatives of valproic acid in rat liver microsomes and destruction of cytochrome P-450. *Drug Metab. Disposit.* **14**, 221–229.

Raag R. and Poulos T.L. (1991). Crystal structure of cytochrome P450$_{CAM}$ complexed with camphane, thiocamphor, and adamantane: Factors controlling P450 substrate hydroxylation. *Biochemistry* **30**, 2674–2684.

Rambeck B., May T. and Juergens U. (1987). Serum concentrations of carbamazepine and its epoxide and diol metabolites in epileptic patients: the influence of dose and comedication. *Therap. Drug Monit.* **9**, 298–303.

Ravindranath V., Burka L.T. and Boyd M.R. (1984). Reactive metabolites from the bioactivation of toxic methylfurans. *Science* **224**, 884–886.

Rettenmeier A.W., Gordon W.P., Barnes H. and Baillie T.A. (1987). Studies on the metabolic fate of valproic acid in the rat using stable isotope techniques. *Xenobiotica* **17**, 1147–1157.

Rettenmeier A.W., Howald W.N., Levy R.H., Witek D.J., Gordon W.P., Porubek D.J. and Baillie T.A. (1989). Quantitative metabolic profiling of valproic acid in humans using automated GC/MS techniques. *Biomed. Environm. Mass Spectrom.* **18**, 192–199.

Rettie A.E., Rettenmeier A.W., Howald W.N. and Baillie T.A. (1987). Cytochrome P-450-catalyzed formation of Δ^4-VPA, a toxic metabolite of valproic acid. *Science* **235**, 890–893.

Rettie A.E., Boberg M., Rettenmeier A.W. and Baillie T.A. (1988). Cytochrome P-450-catalyzed desaturation of valproic acid *in vitro*. *J. Biol. Chem.* **263**, 13,733–13,738.

Rettie A.E., Korzekwa K.R., Kunze K.L., Lawrence R.F., Eddy A.C., Aoyama T., Gelboin H.V., Gonzalez F.J. and Trager W.F. (1992). Hydroxylation of warfarin by human cDNA-expressed cytochrome P-450: a role for P-4502C9 in the etiology of (S)-warfarin interactions. *Chem. Res. Toxicol.* **5**, 54–59.

Rietjens I.M.C.M. and Vervoort J. (1992). A new hypothesis for the mechanism for cytochrome P-450 dependent aerobic conversion of hexahalogenated benzenes to pentahalogenated phenols. *Chem. Res. Toxicol.* **5**, 10–19.

Rietjens I.M.C.M., Tyrakowska B., Veeger C. and Vervoort J. (1990). Reaction pathways for biodehalogenation of fluorinated anilines. *Eur. J. Biochem.* **194**, 945–954.

Rietjens I.M.C.M., Soffers A.E.M.F., Veeger C. and Vervoort J. (1993). Regioselectivity of cytochrome P-450 catalyzed hydroxylation of fluorobenzenes predicted by calculated frontier orbital substrate characteristics. *Biochemistry* **32**, 4801–4812.

Roberts E.S., Hopkins N.E., Alworth W.L. and Hollenberg P.F. (1993). Mechanism-based inactivation of cytochrome P450 2B1 by 2-ethynylnaphthalene: Identification of an active-site peptide. *Chem. Res. Toxicol.* **6**, 470–479.

Safe S., Jones D. and Hutzinger O. (1976). Metabolism of 4,4′-dihalogeno-biphenyls. *J. Chem. Soc.* **PTI**, 357–359.

Santhanakrishnan T.S. (1984). Biohydroxylation of terpenes in mammals. *Tetrahedron* **40**, 3597–3609.

Sawahata T. and Neal R.A. (1983). Biotransformation of phenol to hydroquinone and catechol by rat liver microsomes. *Molec. Pharmacol.* **23**, 453–460.

Sayer J.M., Whalen D.L. and Jerina D.M. (1989). Chemical strategies for the inactivation of bay-region diol epoxides, ultimate carcinogens derived from polycyclic aromatic hydrocarbons. *Drug Metab. Rev.* **20**, 155–182.

Schmid S.E., Au W.Y.W., Hill D.E., Kadlubar F.F. and Slikker W. Jr (1983). Cytochrome P450-dependent oxidation of the 17α-ethynyl group of synthetic steroids. *Drug Metab. Disposit.* **11**, 531–536.

Selander H.G., Jerina D.M. and Daly J.W. (1975). Metabolism of chlorobenzene with hepatic microsomes and solubilized cytochrome P450 systems. *Arch. Biochem. Biophys.* **168**, 309–321.

Sharer J.E., Duescher R.J. and Elfarra A.A. (1992). Species and tissue differences in the microsomal oxidation of 1,3-butadiene and the glutathione conjugation of butadiene monoxide in mice and rats. *Drug Metab. Disposit.* **20**, 658–664.

Shea J.P., Nelson S.D. and Ford G.P. (1983). MNDO calculation of kinetic isotope effects in model cytochrome P-450 oxidations. *J. Amer. Chem. Soc.* **105**, 5451–5454.

Shetty H.U. and Nelson W.L. (1988). Chemical aspects of metoprolol metabolism. *J. Med. Chem.* **31**, 55–59.

Silver E.H., Kuttab S.H., Hasan T. and Hassan M. (1982). Structural considerations in the metabolism of nitriles to cyanide *in vivo*. *Drug Metab. Disposit.* **10**, 495–498.

Sligar S.G., Gelb M.H. and Heimbrook D.C. (1984). Bio-organic chemistry and cytochrome P450-dependent catalysis. *Xenobiotica* **14**, 63–86.

Srivastava P.K., Yun C.H., Beaune P.H., Ged C. and Guengerich F.P. (1991). Separation of human liver microsomal tolbutamide hydroxylase and (S)-mephenytoin 4′-hydroxylase cytochrome P-450 enzymes. *Molec. Pharmacol,* **40**, 69–79.

Stillwell W.G. (1975). Metabolism of glutethimide in the human. *Res. Commun. Chem. Pathol. Pharmacol.* **12**, 25–41.

Sullivan H.R., Roffey P. and McMahon R.E. (1979). Biotransformation of 4′-ethynyl-2-fluorobiphenyl in the rat. *Drug Metab. Disposit.* **7**, 76–80.

Swinney D.C., Howald W.N. and Trager W.F. (1984). Intramolecular isotope effects associated with *meta*-hydroxylation of biphenyl catalyzed by cytochrome P450. *Biochem. Biophys. Res. Commun.* **118**, 867–872.

Swinney D.C., Ryan D.E., Thomas P.E. and Levin W. (1987). Regioselective progesterone hydroxylation catalyzed by eleven rat hepatic cytochrome P-450 isozymes. *Biochemistry* **26**, 7073–7083.

Takenoshita R., Nakamura T. and Toki S. (1993). Hexobarbital metabolism: a new metabolic pathway to produce 1,5-dimethylbarbituric acid and cyclohexenone-glutathione adduct via 3′-oxohexobarbital. *Xenobiotica* **23**, 925–934.

Talaat R.E. and Nelson W.L. (1988). Regioisomeric aromatic dihydroxylation of propranolol. *Drug Metab. Disposit.* **16**, 207–216.

Tanii H. and Hashimoto K. (1984). Studies on the mechanism of acute toxicity of nitriles in mice. *Arch. Toxicol.* **55**, 47–54.

Testa B. (1990). Mechanisms of inhibition of xenobiotic-metabolizing enzymes. *Xenobiotica* **20**, 1129–1137.

Testa B. and Jenner P. (1976). The concept of regioselectivity in drug metabolism. *J. Pharm. Pharmacol.* **28**, 731–744.

Testa B. and Mihailova D. (1978). An *ab initio* study of electronic factors in metabolic hydroxylation of aliphatic carbon atoms. *J. Med. Chem.* **21**, 683–686.

Testa B., Mihailova D. and Natcheva R. (1979). Electronic indices of alkyl substituents undergoing regioselective metabolic hydroxylation. *Eur. J. Med. Chem.* **14**, 295–299.

Thomas R.C. and Judy R.W. (1972). Metabolic fate of chlorpropamide in man and in the rat. *J. Med. Chem.* **15**, 964–968.

Thomas R.C., Duchamp D.J., Judy R.W. and Ikeda G.J. (1978). Metabolic fate of tolazamide in man and in the rat. *J. Med. Chem.* **21**, 725–732.

Thomassen D., Knebel N., Slattery J.T., McClanahan R.H. and Nelson S.D. (1992). Reactive intermediates in the oxidation of menthofuran by cytochromes P450. *Chem. Res. Toxicol.* **5**, 123–130.

Toftgård R., Haaparanta T., Eng L. and Halpert J. (1986). Rat lung and liver microsomal cytochrome P-450 isozymes involved in the hydroxylation of *n*-hexane. *Biochem. Pharmacol.* **35**, 3733–3738.

Trager W.F. (1980). Oxidative functionalization reactions. In *Concepts in Drug Metabolism*, Part A (eds Jenner P. and Testa B.). pp. 177–209. Dekker, New York.

Traylor T.G., Nakano T., Miksztal A.R. and Dunlap B.E. (1987). Transient formation of N-alkylhemins during hemin-catalyzed epoxidation of norbornene. Evidence concerning the mechanism of epoxidation. *J. Amer. Chem. Soc.* **109**, 3625–3632.

Tsai R.S., Carrupt P.A., Testa B. and Caldwell J. (1994). Structure–genotoxicity relationships of allylbenzenes and propenylbenzenes: A quantum chemical study. *Chem. Res. Toxicol.* **7**, 73–76.

Tsuda M., Oikawa S., Okamura Y., Kimura K., Urabe T. and Nakajima M. (1986). Quantum-chemical elucidation of the mechanism of the NIH-shift during aryl hydroxylation catalyzed by cytochrome P-450. *Chem. Pharm. Bull.* **34**, 4457–4466.

Vanden Bossche H. and Willemsens G. (1991). Retinoic acid and cytochrome P-450. In *Retinoids: 10 Years On* (ed. Saurat J.H.). pp. 79–88. Karger, Basel.

Van der Graaff M., Vermeulen N.P.E. and Breimer D.D. (1988). Disposition of hexobarbital: 15 years of an intriguing model substrate. *Drug Metab. Rev.* **19**, 109–164.

Vermeulen N.P.E., Breimer D.D., Holthuis J., Mol C., Bakker B.H. and Van der Gen A. (1981). The metabolic fate of 1′,2′-epoxyhexobarbital in the rat. *Xenobiotica* **11**, 547–557.

Veronese M.E., McManus M.E., Laupattarakasem P., Miners J.O. and Birkett D.J. (1990). Tolbutamide hydroxylation by human, rabbit and rat liver microsomes and by purified forms of cytochrome P-450. *Drug Metab. Disposit.* **18**, 356–361.

Wade A., Symons A.M., Martin L. and Parke D.V. (1979). Metabolic oxidation of the ethynyl group in 4-ethynylbiphenyl. *Biochem. J.* **184**, 509–517.

Wade A., Symons A.M., Martin L. and Parke D.V. (1980). The metabolic oxidation of the ethynyl group in 4-ethynylbiphenyl *in vitro. Biochem. J.* **188**, 867–872.

Walle T., Oatis J.E. Jr, Walle U.K. and Knapp D.R. (1982). New ring-hydroxylated metabolites of propranolol. *Drug Metab. Disposit.* **10**, 122–127.

Walsh J.S., Patanella J.E., Facchine K.L., Halm K.A., Unger S.E., Sinhabatu A.K. and Levesque D. (1993). Biotransformation pathways of GR87442. Novel imidazole oxidation pathways involving 1,2-methyl shifts, and their replication with P450 model systems. In *ISSX Proceedings*, Vol. 4, p. 82. International Society for the Study of Xenobiotics, Bethesda, MD, USA.

Ward S.A., Walle T., Walle U.K., Wilkinson G.R. and Branch R.A. (1989). Propranolol's metabolism is determined by both mephenytoin and debrisoquin hydroxylase activities. *Clin. Pharmacol. Therap.* **45**, 72–79.

Watabe T., Hiratsuka A., Ozawa N. and Isobe M. (1981). A comparative study on the metabolism of d-limonene and 4-vinylcyclohex-1-ene by hepatic microsomes. *Xenobiotica* **11**, 333–344.

Waxman D.J. (1988). Interaction of hepatic cytochromes P-450 with steroid hormones. Regioselectivity and stereospecificity of steroid metabolism and hormonal regulation of rat P-450 enzyme expression. *Biochem. Pharmacol.* **37**, 71–84.

White I.N.H. (1978). Metabolic activation of acetylenic substituents to derivatives in the rat causing the loss of hepatic cytochrome. P-450 and haem. *Biochem. J.* **174**, 853–861.

White I.N.H. (1980). Structure–activity relationships in the destruction of cytochrome P-450 mediated by certain ethynyl-substituted compounds in rats. *Biochem. Pharmacol.* **29**, 3253–3255.

White I.N.H. (1984). Suicidal destruction of cytochrome P-450 by ethynyl substituted compounds. *Pharm. Res.* **1**, 141–148.

White P.W. (1990). Mechanistic studies and selective catalysis with cytochrome P-450 model systems. *BioOrg. Chem.* **18**, 440–456.

White R.E., Groves J.T. and McClusky G.A. (1979). Electronic and steric factors in regioselective hydroxylation catalyzed by purified cytochrome P-450. *Acta Biol. Med. Germ.* **38**, 475–482.

White R.E., McCarthy M.B., Egeberg K.D. and Sligar S.G. (1984). Regioselectivity in the cytochrome P-450: control by protein constraints and by chemical reactivity. *Arch. Biochem. Biophys.* **228**, 493–502.

White R.E., Miller J.P., Favreau L.V. and Bhattacharyya A. (1986). Stereochemical dynamics of aliphatic hydroxylation by cytochrome P-450. *J. Amer. Chem. Soc.* **108**, 6024–6031.

Whitehouse L.W., Lodge B.A., By A.W. and Thomas B.T. (1987). Metabolic disposition of pyrazinamide in the rat: identification of a novel *in vivo* metabolite common to both rat and human. *Biopharm. Drug Disposit.* **8**, 307–318.

Wilke T.J., Jondorf W.R. and Powis G. (1989). Oxidative metabolism of ^{14}C-pyridine by human and rat tissue subcellular fractions. *Xenobiotica* **19**, 1013–1022.

Wistuba D., Nowotny H.P., Träger O. and Schurig V. (1989). Cytochrome P-450-catalyzed asymmetric epoxidation of simple prochiral and chiral aliphatic alkenes: species dependence and effect of enzyme induction on enantioselective oxirane formation. *Chirality* **1**, 127–136.

Wolff T. and Guengerich F.P. (1987). Rat liver cytochrome P450 isozymes as catalysts of aldrin epoxidation in reconstituted monooxygenase systems and microsomes. *Biochem. Pharmacol.* **36**, 2581–2588.

Wood S.G., Scott P.W., Chasseaud L.F., Faulkner J.K., Matthews R.W. and Henrick K. (1985). A novel metabolite of tinidazole involving nitro-group migration. *Xenobiotica* **15**, 107–113.

Yang S.K. (1988). Stereoselectivity of cytochrome P-450 isozymes and epoxide hydrolase in the metabolism of polycyclic hydrocarbons. *Biochem. Pharmacol.* **37**, 61–70.

Yang S.K., Mushtaq M. and Chiu P.L. (1985). Stereoselective metabolism and activation of polycyclic aromatic hydrocarbons. In *Polycyclic Hydrocarbons and Carcinogenesis* (ed. Harvey R.G.). pp. 19–34. American Chemical Society, Washington DC.

Yasumori T., Yamazoe Y. and Kato R. (1991). Cytochrome P-450 human-2 (P-450IIC9) in mephenytoin hydroxylation polymorphism in human livers: Differences in substrate and stereoselectivities among microheterogeneous P-450IIC species expressed in yeast. *J. Biochem.* **109**, 711–717.

Yun C.H., Okerholm R.A. and Guengerich F.P. (1993). Oxidation of the antihistaminic drug terfenadine in human liver microsomes. Role of cytochrome P450 3A(4) in N-dealkylation and C-hydroxylation. *Drug Metab. Disposit.* **21**, 403–409.

Zacchei A.G., Wishousky T.I., Arison B.H. and Hitzenberger G. (1978). The metabolism of (2-cyclopentyl-6,7-dichloro-2-methyl-1-oxo-5-indanyloxy)acetic acid in chimpanzee and man. *Drug Metab. Disposit.* **6**, 303–312.

chapter 5

MONOOXYGENASE-CATALYZED NITROGEN OXIDATIONS

Contents

5.1 INTRODUCTION

There are a great many nitrogen-containing functionalities, and their chemistry is rich indeed. It is only reasonable, therefore, to expect a corresponding diversity in the biotransformation reactions which these functional groups undergo when belonging to a xenobiotic molecule, and this is confirmed by the abundance of data published in the last few decades. Nitrogenated groups, being substrates for reactions of oxidation, reduction, hydrolysis and conjugation, will be encountered throughout this volume and the ones following (Cho, 1988). Besides the diversity of these reactions, their pharmacological and toxicological significance also accounts for the attention they receive (Prough *et al.*, 1988; Quon, 1988).

     With some exceptions, such as 1,4-dihydropyridines (Section 5.4) and hydrazines (Section 5.7), the present chapter focuses on the reactions of **N-oxygenation**, a particular example of the reactions of N-oxidation (Bridges *et al.*, 1972; Cho and Lindeke, 1988; Gorrod, 1978a; Gorrod and Damani, 1985; Testa and Jenner, 1976). Indeed, most metabolites discussed in this chapter result from the addition of one or two oxygen atoms. Oxidations of the N–C unit, often but not always initiated by C-oxidation and resulting in N–C cleavage, constitute the topic of Chapter 6. As a gateway into the biochemistry of organic nitrogen molecules, some readers may find it useful to consider a classification of the functional groups encountered in the present and following chapters. Such **N-containing groups** are classified in Table 5.1 according to the formal oxidation state of the nitrogen atom, the zero oxidation state being that of elemental nitrogen (Lindeke, 1982). However, this is not the classification criterion adopted by some textbooks and reviews which, often implicitly and not always consistently, consider the overall oxidation states of the nitrogen and adjacent carbon(s), and the number of redox equivalents leading from one group to another. Such a classification was used by Testa and Jenner (1976) and is presented in an expanded form in Table 5.2.

A number of enzyme systems mediate N-oxidation, and cytochrome P450 and flavin-containing monooxygenase (FMO) are most prominent within our current knowledge of xenobiotic metabolism. The present chapter is restricted to these two monooxygenase systems, other systems such as monoamine oxidase and peroxidases being considered in Chapters 9 and 10, respectively.

When discussing a given route or metabolite, a recurrent question concerns the **nature of the monooxygenase system involved**. For N-oxidation, the answer to this question is not straightforward and often meets with marked experimental difficulties. General rules have been sought for more than two decades, a first approximation being based on the pK_a of the substrates (Gorrod, 1973). Briefly, it was proposed that:

- basic amines (pK_a 8–11) are N-oxidized by flavin-containing monooxygenase (FMO);
- non-basic nitrogenous groups (amides) are N-oxidized by cytochrome P450, subsequently shown to be mainly CYP1 enzymes;
- weak bases (pK_a 1–7) are substrates for both systems.

More recent evidence has indicated that the pK_a hypothesis alone cannot account for all observations and that structural factors also play a marked role (Clement, 1985; Gorrod 1978b and 1978c; Ziegler 1984 and 1988). A number of observations are summarized in Table 5.3, bearing in mind that generalizations of this type may be, in some cases, misleadingly simplistic. While exceptions do exist within chemical series, the role biological factors play is often underestimated. Hence, the pyrrolizidine alkaloid senecionine, a tertiary amine, is oxidized to the N-oxide by FMO in pig liver microsomes, but by CYP2C11 in rat liver microsomes (Williams *et al.*, 1989).

One major distinction between the cytochrome P450 and the flavin-containing monooxygenases is their **mechanisms of N-oxygenation** (Damani, 1988; Kurebayashi, 1989; Ziegler, 1984 and 1985) (Fig. 5.1). As discussed in Sections 3.5 and 4.2, cytochrome P450 initiates oxidation of C-sp^3 atoms by a homolytic hydrogen abstraction. This can be represented as pathway **A1** in Fig. 5.1; should an adjacent nitrogen atom be present as shown in Fig. 5.1, the outcome of the reaction will be N–C cleavage (Chapter 6). But the nitrogen atom may itself undergo direct oxidation by a single-electron abstraction step. This is the radical mechanism by which cytochrome P450 mediates N-oxidation. The nitrogen cation-radical thus formed may react with the activated oxygen atom in the active site of the enzyme (Section 3.5), forming an N-oxygenated product (pathway **A2** in Fig. 5.1), or it can rearrange to a C-centred radical. Clearly N-oxygenation will be a minor option if the molecular properties of the substrate are such that they favour rearrangement to the C-centred radical and N–C cleavage (see later). This implies that the lack of N-oxygenation of a given compound by cytochrome P450 does not necessarily mean lack of N-oxidation, an inference that few authors seem to have stated explicitly.

In contrast to cytochrome P450, FMO acts by direct addition of an activated, electrophilic

TABLE 5.1 *Formal oxidation states of the nitrogen atom in N-containing functional groups* (Electropositive atoms bonded to the nitrogen decrease its oxidation state, while more electronegative atoms cause an increase) (Modified and enlarged from Lindeke, 1982)

Oxidation state	Functional groups			
- 3	C—N—C (with C below)	C—NH-C	C—NH$_2$	amines and amides
	C=N—C	C=NH		imines
	C≡N			nitriles
-2	C—N—C (•+, with C below)	C—NH-C (•+)		radicals
	C—NH-NH-C	C—NH-NH$_2$		hydrazines and hydrazides
-1	C—N—OH (with C below)	C—NHOH		hydroxylamines and hydroxylamides
	C=N—OH			oximes
	C=N→O (with C below)			nitrones
	C—N→O (with C above and below)			N-oxides
	C—N=N—C			azo compounds
	C—N=NH			diazenes
0	C—N=N—C (with O above)			azoxy compounds
	C—N—N=O (with C below)	C—NH—N=O		nitrosamines
	C—N—O• (with C below)			nitroxides
+1	C—N=O			nitroso compounds
	C—N=N—C (with O above and O below)			nitroso dimers
+2	C—NO$_2^{\overline{\cdot}}$			nitro anion radicals
+3	C—NO$_2$			nitro compounds

TABLE 5.2 *Overall oxidation states of the C–N unit in N-containing functional groups* (In contrast to Table 5.1, C–N here means that the carbon atom is sp³-hybridized and linked to H or C atoms)

Redox steps	Functional groups			

	C—N—C
	    |
	    C
		C—NH-C	C—NH$_2$	amines

1e⁻/N	C—NH—NH—C	C—NH-NH$_2$		hydrazines
1e⁻/N				

	C—N—OH
	    |
	    C
		C—NHOH		hydroxylamines

	C
	    |
	C—N→O
	    |
	    C
				N-oxides

	C—N=N—C			azo compounds
	C—N=NH			diazenes
	C=N—C	C=NH		imines
	C—N—C | | OH C	C—NH-C | OH	C—NH$_2$ | OH	carbinolamines

	C=N—C
	   +|
	    C
				iminium species

1e⁻/N	O ↑ C—N=N—C			azoxy compounds

	C—N—N=O
	    |
	    C
		C—NH—N=O		nitrosamines

	C—N—O
	    |
	    C
				nitroxides

1e⁻/N	C—N=O			nitroso compounds (and nitroso dimers)
	C=N—OH			oximes

	C=N→O
	    |
	    C
				nitrones

	C—N—C || || O C	C—NH-C || O	C—NH$_2$ || O	amides
	C≡N			nitriles

TABLE 5.2 continued.

$1e^-/N$		
	$C—NO_2^{\bullet -}$	nitro anion-radicals
	C(=O)—NH—NH—C C(=O)—NH—NH_2	hydrazides
$1e^-/N$		
	$C—NO_2$	nitro compounds
	C(=O)—N(—C)—OH C(=O)—NHOH	hydroxylamides
	C(=O)—N^+—C	nitrenium species

oxygen atom (pathway **B** in Fig. 5.1), as discussed in Section 3.7 (Ball and Bruice, 1980). No intermediate radical is formed, and *a priori* no N–C cleavage is to be expected. But what is predictable, and indeed frequently confirmed (as discussed below), is a relationship between the nucleophilicity of nitrogen atoms and their oxygenation.

5.2 N-OXYGENATION OF TERTIARY AMINES

Three major groups of tertiary amines can be distinguished in metabolic N-oxygenation, namely the aromatic azaheterocycles (i.e. pyridine and analogues), and the tertiary amines *sensu stricto* which can be further subdivided into acyclic and cyclic ones. All three groups form **N-oxides** (also called amine oxides) which are characterized by a high polarity and a marked reduction in pK_a relative to the parent amine. Traditionally, the semipolar N–O bond in N-oxides is represented either by an arrow (N→O), or with formal charge separation (N^+–O^-).

Inasmuch as N-oxygenation by FAD-containing monooxygenase involves the direct addition of an electrophilic oxygen, one can expect that nucleophilicity (and thus basicity) of the amino group will be a facilitating factor. While this principle alone may fail in a number of cases when comparing rates of N-oxygenation of different tertiary amines, it could be of value in predicting regioselectivity, i.e. the relative reactivity of two or more target groups within a substrate molecule. Indeed, as illustrated below, N-oxygenation occurs at the more basic of two tertiary amino groups belonging to the same compound. Yet such a mechanistic interpretation neglects the fact that in most drugs of this type the two target sites are an aliphatic tertiary amino group and an aromatic heterocycle, which will in many cases be oxygenated by FAD-containing monooxygenase and cytochrome P450, respectively. In such cases, therefore, regioselectivity must be accounted for by the relative activity of the two monooxygenases rather than by differences in target site nucleophilicity and pK_a.

5.2.1 Tertiary heteroaromatic amines

Aromatic heterocyclic amines, which are usually of intermediate basicity (the pK_a of pyridine is close to 5.3), are N-oxygenated principally by cytochrome P450 (Table 5.3). However, there are

TABLE 5.3 *Simplified substrate specificities of P450 and FMO in catalyzing reactions of N-oxidation* (compiled from references cited in the text)

Functional groups	Monooxygenases[*]	
	P450	FMO
Amines		
Primary amines		
alkylamines	yes	no
arylamines	yes	no
arylalkylamines	yes	no
Secondary amines		
dialkylamines	no	yes
diarylamines	yes	no
arylalkylamines	yes	yes
alicyclic amines	no	yes
Tertiary amines		
trialkylamines	no	yes
aryldialkylamines	no	yes
alicyclic amines	no	yes
heteroaromatic amines	yes	no
1,4-Dihydropyridines	yes	no
Amides		
N-alkylamides	no	no
N-arylamides	yes	no
Hydrazines		
monosubstituted hydrazines	yes	yes
1,2-disubstituted hydrazines	yes	yes
1,1-disubstituted hydrazines	yes	yes
Benzamidines		
N-unsubstituted benzamidines	yes	no
N-alkylbenzamidines	no	no
Guanidines	yes	no

[*]"No" does not exclude weak activity and/or a few exceptions due e.g. to species differences.

also reports of some *in vitro* reactions being catalyzed by the FAD-containing monooxygenase (Miwa and Walsh, 1988).

Pyridine N-oxide (**5.I**) is thus an important metabolite of **pyridine** and accounts for 10% or more of a dose in a number of species (Damani, 1985). In rabbit liver, for example, two cytochromes P450 are mainly responsible for the N-oxygenation of pyridine, namely CYP2E1 as a high-affinity enzyme playing the major role at low substrate concentrations, and CYP4B as low-affinity enzymes playing the major role at high substrate concentrations (Kim *et al.*, 1991). Other early discovered substrates include nicotinamide (**5.II**), nikethamide (**5.III**), and quinoline

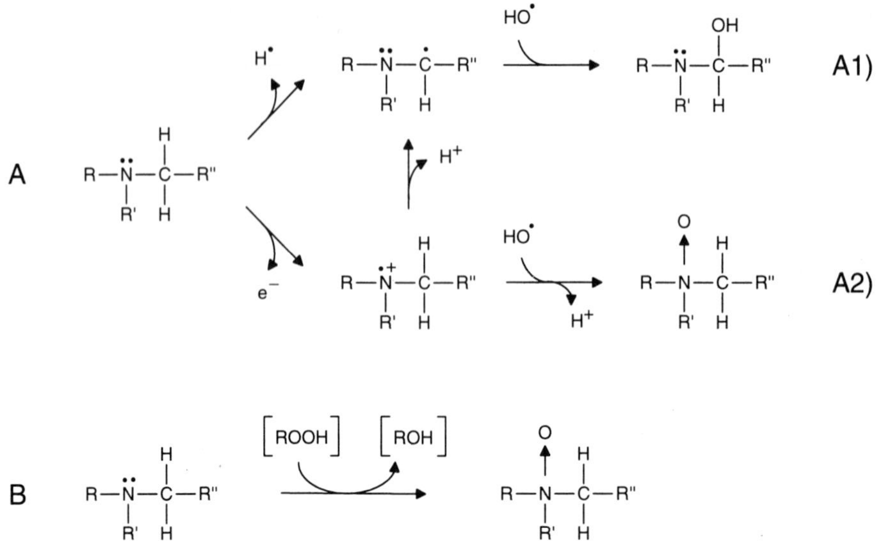

FIGURE 5.1 Mechanisms of N-oxidation and N-oxygenation mediated by cytochrome P450 (pathway **A2**) and flavin-containing monooxygenase (pathway **B**). Cytochrome P450 forms an N- and/or a C-centred radical, the products being either N- or C-oxygenated (pathways **A2** or **A1**, respectively).

(**5.IV**) (Damani, 1985). N-Oxygenation of a number of relatively lipophilic 3-substituted pyridines has been reported (e.g. 3-methyl-, 3-ethyl-, 3-chloro-, 3-bromo-, 3-acetyl- and 3-cyanopyridine), while no N-oxide formation was detected for some polar analogues such as 3-amino-, 3-acetamido-, 3-hydroxypyridine, nicotinic acid and 3-pyridylcarbinol (Cowan *et al.*, 1978).

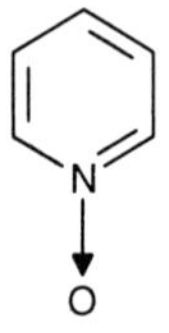

5.I

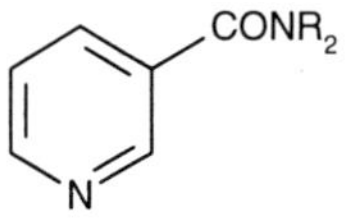

R = -H 5.II

R = $-CH_2CH_3$ 5.III

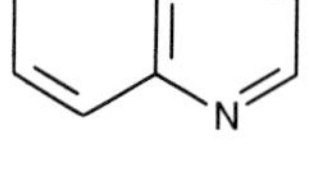

5.IV

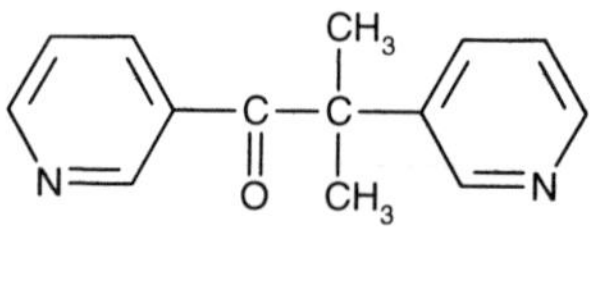

5.V

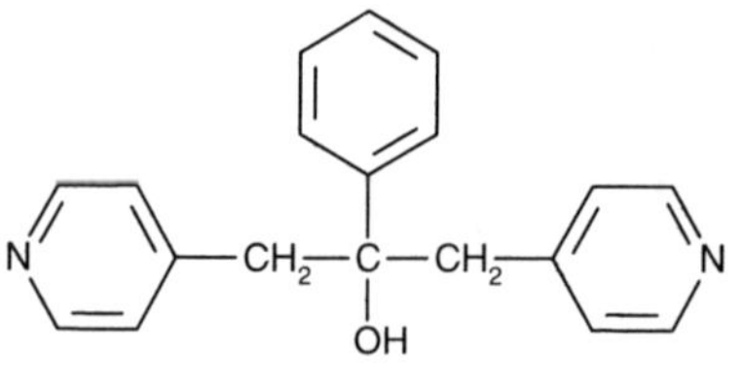

5.VI

A few interesting cases of regioselective and stereoselective N-oxygenation have been reported for compounds containing two pyridine rings. Thus, metyrapone (**5.V**) yielded two N-oxides, rats and their liver microsomes predominantly N-oxygenating the pyridine ring adjacent to the carbonyl group (De Graeve *et al.*, 1979; Usansky and Damani, 1992). The prochiral dipyridyl compound **5.VI** was N-oxidized as a major metabolic route in humans, dogs and rats; interestingly, the metabolite was levorotatory and enantiomerically pure, indicating very high or complete product enantioselectivity (Schwartz *et al.*, 1978).

5.2.2 Tertiary acyclic amines

A few **trialkylamines** (e.g. trimethylamine) and **aryldialkylamines** (e.g. N,N-dimethyl- and N,N-diethylaniline) are known to be N-oxygenated, in particular by microsomal preparations or purified FAD-containing monooxygenases from various tissues and animal species (Sabourin and Hodgson, 1984; Tynes and Hodgson, 1985; Ziegler, 1988). For example, the FAD-containing monooxygenase is the main system responsible for the N-oxygenation of N,N-dimethylaniline (**5.VII**) in human tissues (Lemoine *et al.*, 1990; McManus *et al.*, 1987a).

5.VII

$$Aryl-(CH_2)_n-N(CH_3)_2$$

5.VIII

An important number of drugs belong to the group of **N,N-dimethylarylalkylamines** (**5.VIII**) for which N-oxygenation is often a significant metabolic route. N-Oxygenation decreases by 3–4 units the pK_a of the parent drugs, which usually lie in the range 9–10. The N-oxides, while very seldom displaying pharmacological activities when examined *in vitro* (e.g. in receptor binding assays), may nevertheless be active *in vivo* as a consequence of reduction to the parent amine (Chapter 12).

Ziegler (1988) has published an extensive compilation of data on the N-oxygenation of amines, many of them of medicinal interest, by porcine liver FAD-containing monooxygenase. These studies were performed in the presence of a positive effector (e.g. *n*-octylamine or 2,4-dichloro-6-phenylphenoxyethylamine) which increases the velocity of the rate-limiting step. Under such conditions, V_{max} for all substrates is essentially the same, while the reported K_m values show 200-fold variations (Table 5.4). Comprehensive **structure–metabolism relationships** do not appear to be available, but some trends are apparent (Rose and Castagnoli, 1983; Ziegler, 1988). Thus, the best substrates are clearly lipophilic amines. N-Oxygenation is blocked by the presence of a second ionizable group (cationic or anionic) besides the basic amino function. An additional factor to consider is the fact that various FAD-containing monooxygenases may display different substrate specificities, as seen for example with a series of phenothiazines with dimethylaminoalkyl side-chains of different length (C_2 to C_7); while the porcine liver FMO metabolized all substrates with identical K_m and k_{cat} values, rabbit lung FMO oxidized only the two higher homologues (Nagata *et al.*, 1990).

Imipramine (5.IX) is a typical drug in the present context; while the N-oxide represents only a small percentage of the dose in human urine, it must nevertheless be considered as a

TABLE 5.4 *Substrate specificity of porcine liver FAD-containing monooxygenase for the N-oxygenation of various amines* (V_{max} values 730–750 nmol min^{-1} (mg protein)$^{-1}$) (Cashman and Ziegler, 1986; Ziegler, 1988)

	K_m (μM)		K_m (μM)
Tertiary amines			
Acyclic		*Secondary amines*	
Amitriptyline	98	*Acyclic*	
Benzphetamine	130	Desipramine	250
Brompheniramine	200	N-Methylaniline	30
Chlorpromazine	9	N-Methyloctylamine	400
Clorgyline	2	Nortryptyline	500
Deprenyl	49	*Alicyclic*	
Diphenhydramine	160	Desmethyltrifluoperazine	9
Imipramine (**5.IX**)	22	Perazine	8000
Pargyline (**5.XII**)	65		
Promazine	66	*Hydrazines*	
Trifluopromazine	20	*Monosubstituted*	
Alicyclic		Methylhydrazine	35,000
Fluphenazine	12	Butylhydrazine	6900
Guanethidine (**5.XXIV**)	170	Phenylhydrazine	3000
Prochlorperazine	3	Benzylhydrazine	7000
MPTP (**5.XX**)	32	*1,1-Disubstituted*	
Trifluoperazine	13	1,1-Dimethylhydrazine	430
		1-Methyl-1-phenylhydrazine	80
		N-Aminopyrrolidine	100
		N-Aminopiperidine	30
		N-Aminomorpholine	610
		1,2-Disubstituted	
		1,2-Dimethylhydrazine	12,100
		1-Methyl-2-benzylhydrazine	2000
		Procarbazine	5700

significant metabolite due to the large number of competitive pathways and to N-oxide reduction (Bickel, 1969). A comparable compound is **zimeldine**, which is extensively metabolized in humans and laboratory animals. Although both the aliphatic and the aromatic nitrogen are N-oxygenated, the aliphatic N-oxide was found to be excreted in considerable amounts in rat and dog urine (Lundström *et al.*, 1981). Zimeldine exists as the (*Z*) and (*E*) diastereomers, the former being displayed as **5.X**. In microsomal preparations, both diastereomers were metabolized with clear substrate stereoselectivity to the corresponding aliphatic N-oxide, the *Z/E* ratio in the rates of reaction being 1/2 in rat liver microsomes and 1/0.4 in hog liver microsomes (Cashman *et al.*, 1988). Interestingly, the *in vitro* metabolism of zimeldine was compared to that of its higher homologue homozimeldine, the (*E*) diastereomer of which is displayed as **5.XI**. The same *Z/E* ratios were found for homozimeldine, but the rates of reaction were two to three times faster than those of zimeldine; the greater basicity of the former was suggested to account for this difference (Cashman *et al.*, 1988).

As already mentioned above, the pK_a argument may be a misleading one when comparing and rationalizing the N-oxidation of amines. It is for example interesting that **pargyline (5.XII)**, which with a pK_a of 6.6 is a hundred- to a thousandfold less basic than many medicinal amines, is

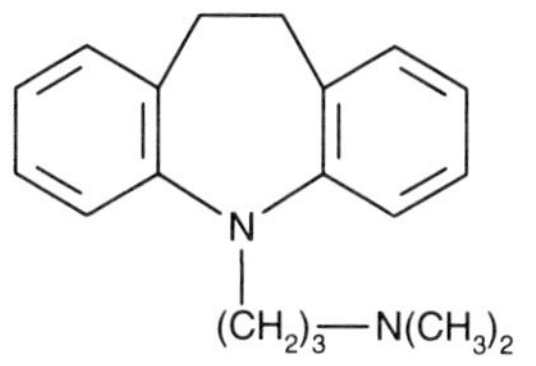

5.IX

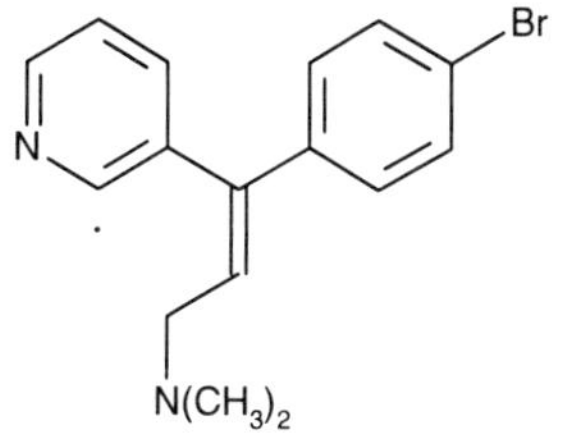

5.X

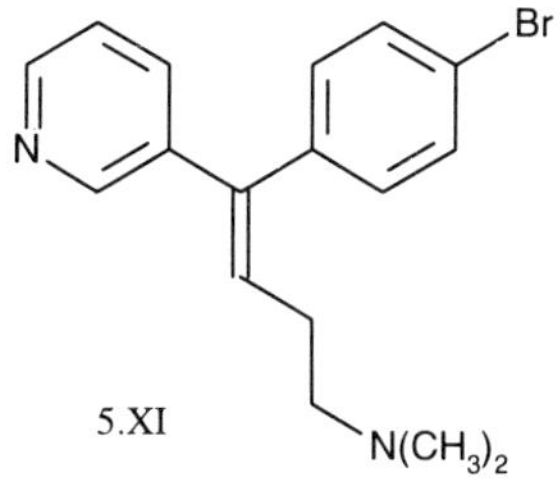

5.XI

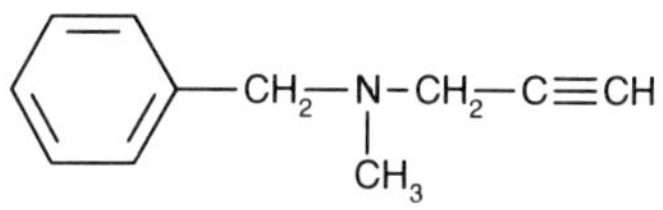

5.XII

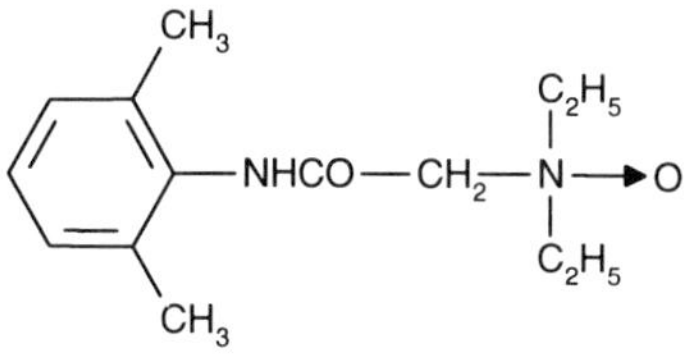

5.XIII

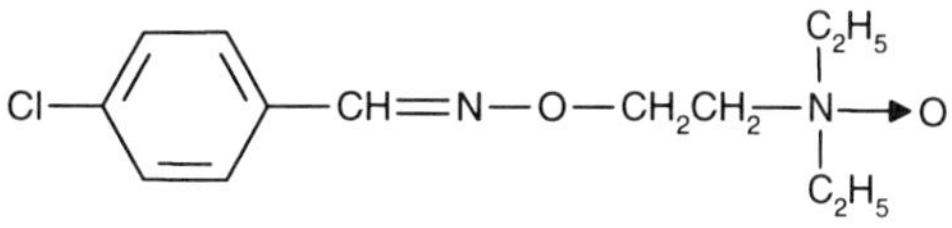

5.XIV

rapidly and predominantly N-oxygenated by FAD-containing monooxygenase in rat liver microsomes (Weli and Lindeke, 1985) (Table 5.4). A drug bearing some analogy with pargyline is verapamil, an N,N-di(arylalkyl)-N-methyl derivative which is effectively and stereoselectively N-oxygenated by the FAD-containing monooxygenase in rat and hog liver microsomes (Cashman, 1989).

Most of the compounds discussed so far are N,N-dimethylamino derivatives, but even the more hindered molecules like pargyline and verapamil contain an N-methyl group. For years, it was believed that more encumbered tertiary amino groups, particularly **N,N-diethylamino derivatives**, could not yield N-oxide metabolites due to steric hindrance (Testa and Jenner, 1976). As a rule, N,N-dimethylamino derivatives are far better substrates of N-oxygenation than their N,N-diethylamino homologues, although some xenobiotics belonging to the latter class are now known to produce small amounts of N-oxides. Examples include (E)-clomiphene N-oxide and

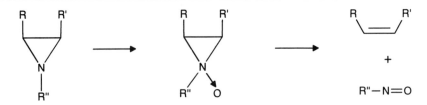

FIGURE 5.2 Fragmentation of aziridines to an olefin and a nitrosoalkane following their N-oxygenation (Hata *et al.*, 1976).

lidocaine N-oxide (**5.XIII**) formed in rat liver microsomes, and the N-oxide of O-(diethylaminoethyl)-4-chlorobenzaldoxime (**5.XIV**), which is the major urinary metabolite of this analgesic agent in dogs (Kirkpatrick *et al.*, 1977; Patterson *et al.*, 1986; Ruenitz *et al.*, 1983).

5.2.3 Tertiary alicyclic amines

N-Alkylated alicyclic amines represent another group of substrates that form N-oxides. A large variety of cyclic systems have been investigated, and some important ones are discussed here (Oelschläger and Al Shaik, 1985). Starting with the smallest ring system, **aziridines** form unstable N-oxides which break down to olefin and nitrosoalkane according to Fig. 5.2 (Hata *et al.*, 1976). The reaction has been characterized in rat liver microsomes for a number of N-alkyl-2-arylaziridines, and is in line with the known instability of azirine N-oxides. Interestingly, the fragmentation reactivity and the cytotoxic activity of N-methyl-2-phenylaziridines are related, the resulting nitrosomethane probably playing an important part in the *in vitro* toxicity of the compounds (Hata *et al.*, 1978).

  N-Oxygenation of four-membered alicyclic amines is illustrated by zetidoline (**5.XV**), an **azetidine** derivative of a type seldom encountered in medicinal chemistry. Its N-oxide was formed in moderate amounts following incubation with rat liver microsomes (Assandri *et al.*, 1986). An interesting and much studied **pyrrolidine** derivative is **nicotine**, whose natural and active enantiomer is the (−)-(S)-form. In liver microsomes from a number of species, (2'S)-nicotine is N-oxidized more to *cis*-(1'R;2'S)-nicotine-1'-N-oxide (**5.XVI**) than to *trans*-(1'S;2'S)-nicotine-1'-N-oxide (**5.XVII**) (Jenner *et al.*, 1973; Testa *et al.*, 1976). In contrast, no product enantioselectivity was seen with porcine liver FMO (Damani *et al.*, 1988). With (2'R)-nicotine, preferential formation of *trans*-(1'R;2'R)-nicotine-1'-N-oxide was observed in the presence of liver microsomes from various species or FAD-containing monooxygenase. In addition to these substrate and product stereoselectivities, nicotine metabolism also displays regioselectivity, since it is the pyrrolidinyl ring (pK_a 7.9), rather than the pyridinyl ring (pK_a 3.1) which is N-oxygenated. The basicity rule (see above) is further verified by the fact that in the case of cotinine, the basic pyridinyl ring rather than the non-basic lactam ring is N-oxygenated to yield cotinine-1-N-oxide (**5.XVIII**) (Dagne and Castagnoli, 1972).

  Six-membered alicyclic amines occur relatively frequently in pharmaco- and xenochemistry. **Piperidine** derivatives are exemplified by the analgesic pethidine (**5.XIX**), whose N-oxide is one of the minor metabolites found in the urine of humans dosed with the drug (Mitchard *et al.*, 1972). The case of **morphine**, also an N-methylpiperidine derivative forming an N-oxide, is of particular relevance. However, detection of the latter in rat urine was possible only after co-administration of tacrine, a compound inhibiting competitive metabolic routes of morphine and possibly also further metabolism of the N-oxide (Heimans *et al.*, 1971). This example indicates that further metabolism of N-oxides, particularly their reduction back to the parent

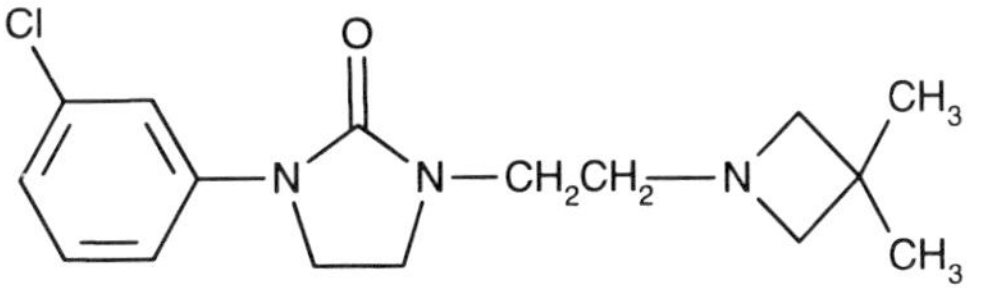

5.XV

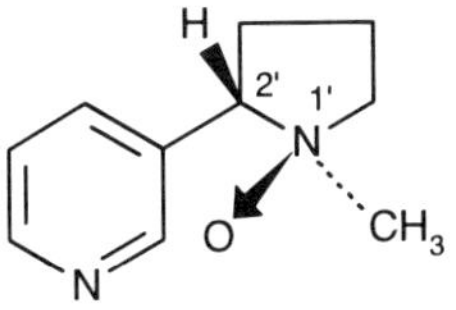

5.XVI

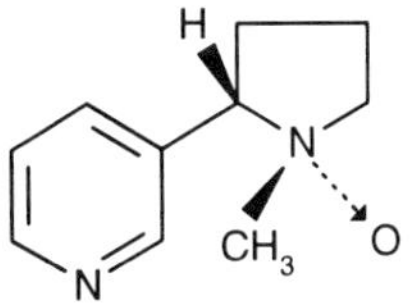

5.XVII

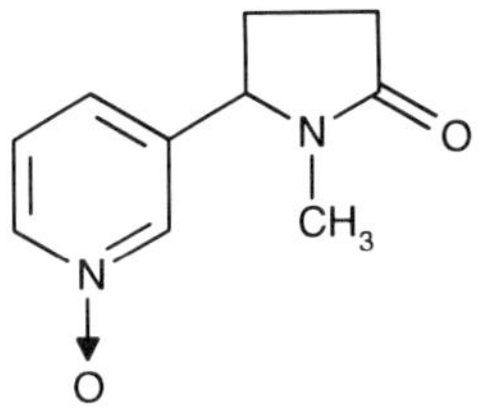

5.XVIII

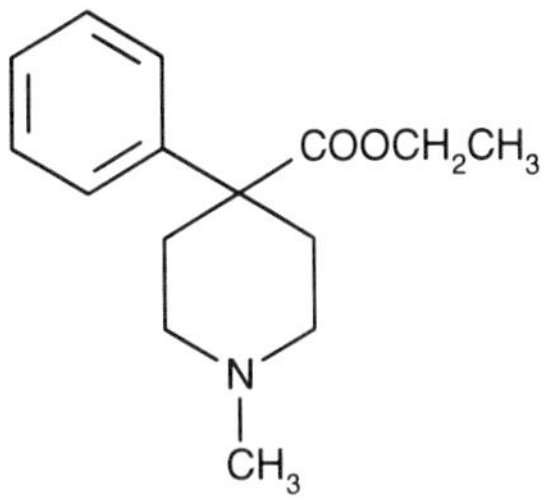

5.XIX

amine (Chapter 12), may be confused with a lack of formation. *In vitro*, morphine and a number of alkaloids and derivatives (codeine, ethylmorphine, thebaine, oxycodone, atropine, scopolamine, cocaine and strychnine) were found to be good substrates of guinea-pig liver FMO, while others were poor substrates (oxymorphone, nalorphine, naloxone and brucine) (Yuno *et al.*, 1990).

A xenobiotic that has attracted considerable attention in recent years is 1-methyl-4-phenyl-1,2,3,6-tetrahydropyridine (**MPTP, 5.XX**), a neurotoxin causing Parkinsonism in humans and primates (Maret *et al.*, 1990). Its metabolic toxication is mediated by monoamine oxidase (see Section 9.4), while detoxication occurs via monooxygenase-catalyzed reactions, namely N-demethylation and N-oxygenation. The FAD-containing monooxygenase in the purified form or in hepatic microsomes of rodent or human origin is highly active in forming MPTP-N-oxide (Cashman, 1988; Cashman and Ziegler, 1986; Chiba *et al.*, 1988).

Other six-membered alicycles of relevance in the present context are piperazine and morpholine. A number of drugs contain an **N-alkylpiperazino** moiety, and their N-oxygenation is documented in several but not all cases (Oelschläger and Al Shaik, 1985; Ziegler, 1988). An example where N-oxygenation is particularly marked is tiaramide (**5.XXI** without the N-oxide oxygen and with R = CH$_2$CH$_2$OH). This anti-inflammatory agent yields two N-oxides in humans and various animal species. In the urine of humans receiving the drug, one N-oxide (**5.XXI** with R = CH$_2$CH$_2$OH) is a minor metabolite, while the other (**5.XXI** with R = CH$_2$COOH) accounts for about 1/3 of a dose (Klunk *et al.*, 1982; Noguchi *et al.*, 1982). N-Oxygenation of a **morpholino** moiety is also known to occur in a few cases, e.g. with the local

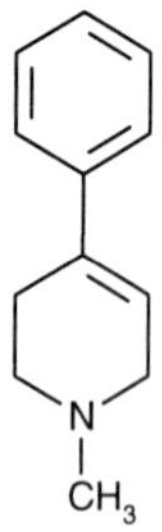

5.XX

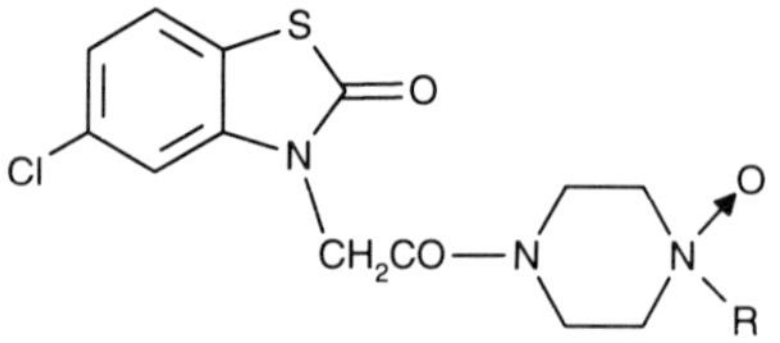

5.XXI

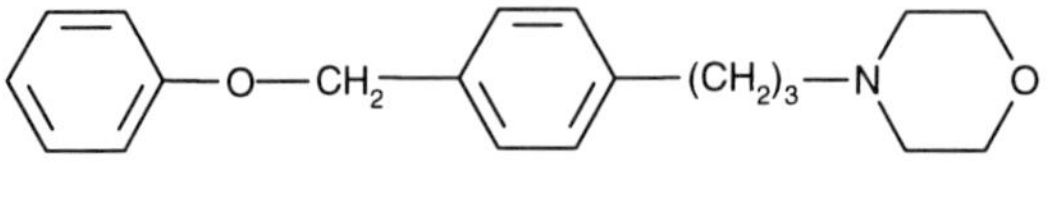

5.XXII

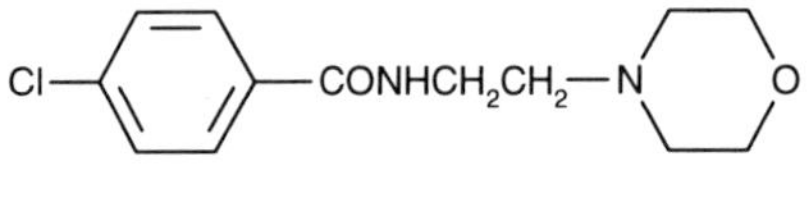

5.XXIII 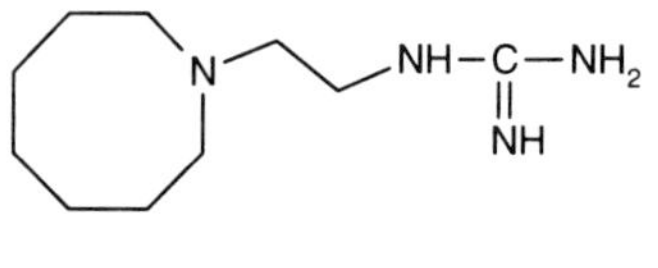   5.XXIV

anaesthetic fomocaine (**5.XXII**) and the MAO inhibitor moclobemide (**5.XXIII**) (Oelschläger *et al.*, 1975; Øie *et al.*, 1992).

Larger rings may also undergo N-oxygenation, although examples are scarce indeed! In this context, an interesting compound is the **octahydroazocine** derivative guanethidine (**5.XXIV**), an antihypertensive agent whose tertiary amino group undergoes N-oxidation in human liver microsomes, the reaction being catalyzed by FAD-containing monooxygenase (McManus *et al.*, 1987b). In contrast, the guanidino group in guanethidine appears inert towards N-oxidation (see Section 5.8).

5.3 N-OXYGENATION OF PRIMARY AND SECONDARY ALIPHATIC AND ALICYCLIC AMINES

5.3.1 Formation of hydroxylamines

Primary and secondary amines have in common the fact that the primary products of their N-oxygenation are hydroxylamines (Table 5.1). What distinguishes these two classes of amines, metabolically speaking, is the nature of the monooxygenase system primarily responsible for their N-oxygenation. As a rule, primary amines are substrates of cytochrome P450 rather than FAD-containing monooxygenase, in contrast to secondary amines which display the opposite enzyme selectivity (Table 5.3) (Sabourin and Hodgson, 1984; Tynes and Hodgson, 1985).

A large number of secondary amines, and a few primary amines, have been shown to yield hydroxylamines *in vitro* and/or *in vivo*, as documented by a large compilation of qualitative data

(Coutts and Beckett, 1977). As far as **primary amines** are concerned, a number of studies demonstrate the *in vitro* N-hydroxylation of amphetamine, but the best substrate appears to be the anorectic agent phentermine (**5.XXV**), whose N-oxidation yields the hydroxylamine **5.XXVI** as a major metabolite in rabbit urine as well as in rat liver microsomes (Beckett and Bélanger, 1978; Duncan and Cho, 1982; Sum and Cho, 1977). The reaction is definitively catalyzed by cytochrome P450, and this compound is particularly interesting in that the absence of any hydrogen on the alpha-carbon atom restricts the outcome of initial N-oxidation to pathway **A2** in Fig. 5.1. The magnitude of phentermine N-oxygenation is a proof of the efficiency of initial cytochrome P450-mediated N-oxidation, and it clearly suggests that it must be the predominance of pathway **A1** over **A2** (Fig. 5.1) which prevents many primary arylalkylamines from forming notable amounts of hydroxylamines.

In general, **secondary amines** are good substrates of FAD-containing monooxygenase, and known examples of compounds forming secondary hydroxylamines include arylalkylamines and alicyclic amines of some of the types discussed in Section 5.2.3 (Coutts and Beckett, 1977). To illustrate this point, a few kinetic data are presented in Table 5.4. A possible exception to this rule is norbenzphetamine (**5.XXIX**), the N-demethylated metabolite of benzphetamine, which yields the hydroxylamine **5.XXX** in rat liver microsomes in a reaction believed to be catalyzed by cytochrome P450 (Jeffrey and Mannering, 1983) (Section 5.3.2).

Secondary amines are reactive with 4α-hydroperoxyflavin, a model FAD-containing monooxygenase, and the second-order rate constant of hydroxylamine formation has been found to increase linearly with the pK_a of the substrates in agreement with the nucleophilicity rule discussed in the beginning of Section 5.2 (Ball and Bruice, 1980). Interestingly, linear relationships with identical slopes hold for tertiary amines and for secondary hydroxylamines. These linear free-energy relationships further indicate that, once pK_a has been accounted for, secondary hydroxylamines are about ten times more reactive towards the 4α-hydroperoxyflavin than tertiary amines, which themselves are about ten times more reactive than secondary amines.

5.3.2 Formation of other N-oxidized metabolites

Seen globally, the N-oxidation of primary and secondary amines is an intricate process generating a plethora of potential metabolites (Cho, 1988). What renders the problem even more complex is the possible occurrence of two phenomena, namely: (a) oxidation by reactive oxygen species formed by monooxygenases; and (b) autoxidation reactions (i.e. non-enzymatic oxidations)

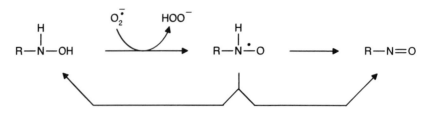

FIGURE 5.3 One-electron steps in the oxidation of primary hydroxylamines to a nitroso compound via the nitroxide.

during incubation (*in vitro* work) or analysis (*in vitro* and *in vivo* work) (Beckett *et al.*, 1977; Beckett *et al.*, 1979; Cho and Fukuto, 1988; Lindeke, 1982; Testa and Jenner, 1978).

To start with a **primary amine** of comparatively simple behaviour, **phentermine (5.XXV)** yielded the nitroso derivative **(5.XXVII)** in the rabbit beside the hydroxylamine **(5.XXVI)** mentioned above (Beckett and Bélanger, 1978). Under *in vitro* conditions (rat liver microsomes), N-hydroxyphentermine **(5.XXVI)** was further oxidized to the nitro derivative **(5.XXVIII)**, a reaction mediated by the cytochrome P450-generated superoxide radical (Maynard and Cho, 1981) (Section 3.5). Mechanistic studies suggested that superoxide abstracts a hydrogen radical from **5.XXVI** to produce a **nitroxide** and hydrogen peroxide. The nitroxide then disproportionates to **5.XXVI** and the **nitroso derivative 5.XXVII**, and the latter is then oxidized to the **nitro derivative 5.XXVIII** by molecular oxygen and/or by hydrogen peroxide (Fukuto *et al.*, 1985). This mechanism of hydroxylamine oxidation is depicted in Fig. 5.3, but it does not exclude the possibility of an enzymatic, non-dismutative one-electron oxidation of the nitroxide to the nitroso derivative.

The comparatively simple metabolic pattern of phentermine is due to the absence of an abstractable hydrogen atom adjacent to the alpha-carbon. When such a hydrogen atom is present (Fig. 5.4), oxidation of the hydroxylamine (reaction **c** in Fig. 5.4) yields two tautomers, namely a **nitroso compound** and an **oxime**, with the tautomeric equilibrium (reaction **e** in Fig. 5.4) largely or exclusively favouring the latter product (Lindeke, 1982). Thus, **N-hydroxyamphetamine** (**5.XXX** in Fig. 5.4, R = benzyl, R′ = methyl) was converted to phenylacetone oxime (**5.XXXII** in Fig. 5.4, R = benzyl, R′ = methyl) as the main metabolite in rat liver microsomes (Matsumoto and Cho, 1982), the reaction being partly due to autoxidation (Lindeke *et al.*, 1975).

Another relevant equilibrium is that between a **nitroso compound** and its **dimer** (see Table 5.1) (Lindeke, 1982). Yet another possibility is the coupling of a hydroxylamine and a nitroso monomer to form an **azoxy derivative** (see Table 5.1); such a reaction was characterized during the incubation of phenylethylamine with rabbit liver microsomes and appeared completely dependent on the presence of divalent manganese (Fiala *et al.*, 1981).

Whatever the biochemical interest of these various reactions, it must be stressed they were detected during *in vitro* studies. Thus, the *in vivo* relevance of such metabolites as nitroso dimers and azoxy compounds remains to be demonstrated.

Fig. 5.4 presents a few other reactions that have been characterized. Reactions **b** and **d,** which respectively form an **imine (5.XXXI)** and an **oxime (5.XXXII)**, were seen upon incubation of 1-(2-tolyl)-1-phenylmethylamine (**5.XXIX** in Fig. 5.4, R = 2-tolyl, R′ = phenyl) with liver microsomes of various animal species (Gorrod and Raman, 1989). Cytochrome P450 did not appear to be involved, suggesting that the mechanism of reaction **b** in Fig. 5.4 is not related to the formation of iminium ions from carbinolamines as discussed in Chapter 6. Confirmatory and mechanistic studies are needed to assess the significance of reaction **b**; as for reaction **d,** it has formal analogies with amidine N-oxygenation discussed in Section 5.8. A number of acetophenone imines (**5.XXXI** in Fig. 5.4, R = substituted phenyl; R′ = methyl) were thus found to yield

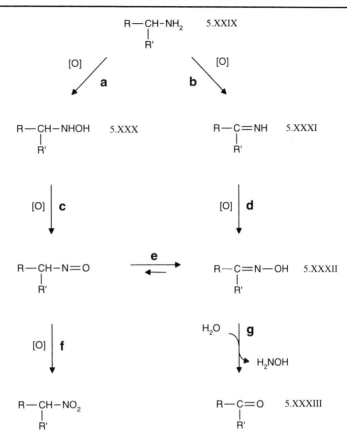

FIGURE 5.4 Frequently and occasionally characterized reactions during N-oxygenation and N-oxidation of primary arylalkylamines.

the diastereomeric (Z)-oxime and (E)-oxime in liver microsomes of rabbits and other species; oxime formation was strongly product stereoselective for the (E)-forms (Gorrod and Christou, 1986). Reactions **f** and **g** in Fig. 5.4 were seen in the *in vitro* metabolism of amphetamine-like compounds (Beckett and Jones, 1977; Coutts and Beckett, 1977; Coutts *et al.*, 1976); while reaction **f** is identical to the formation of the phentermine nitro derivative discussed above, reaction **g** represents a mechanism of deamination distinct from carbinolamine hydrolysis discussed in Chapter 6.

Recent studies now suggest that other reactions in addition to those shown in Fig. 5.4 could occur with some substrates. Indeed, *n*-butyraldoxime (**5.XXXII** in Fig. 5.4, R = *n*-C$_3$H$_7$, R' = H), in addition to yielding nitrobutane, also underwent a Beckmann-type dehydration catalyzed by cytochrome P450 to form **butyronitrile** (*n*-C$_3$H$_7$–CN) (DeMaster *et al.*, 1993). As for **nitroalkanes**, they may react with the hydroxyl radical and perhaps other reactive oxygen species (Bors *et al.*, 1993).

The oxidation of **secondary hydroxylamines** differs from that of primary hydroxylamines, **nitrones** being formed. The reaction is very effectively catalyzed by FAD-containing mono-oxygenase as discussed in Section 5.3 (Cashman *et al.*, 1990). Using 4α-hydroperoxyflavin to model this enzyme, Ball and Bruice (1980) established the reaction mechanism shown in Fig. 5.5, where a mixture of nitrones is formed via dehydration of a common intermediate. An example of medicinal relevance is that of **norbenzphetamine** (**5.XXXIV**), whose hydroxylamine **5.XXXV** is

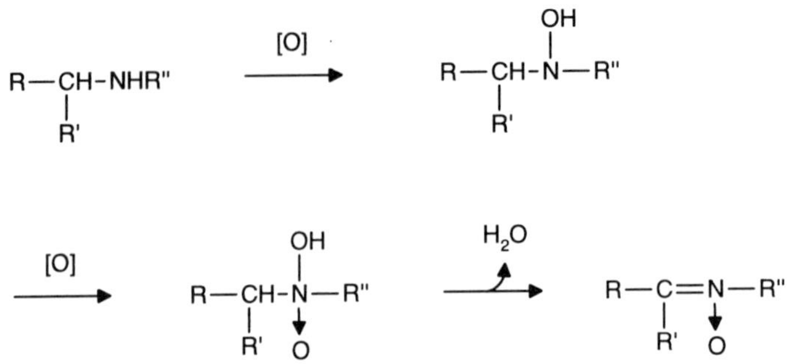

FIGURE 5.5 N-Oxidation of secondary amines to hydroxylamines, and then to nitrones via a hypothetical hydroxylamine oxide, as catalyzed by a 4α-hydroperoxyflavin (Ball and Bruice, 1980).

oxidized to the nitrone **5.XXXVI** by FMO (Jeffrey and Mannering, 1983). Interestingly, the nitrone is further oxidized to 2-nitroso-1-phenylpropane (**5.XXXVII**), a reaction catalyzed by cytochrome P450. Formally, such a reaction is an N-oxidation accompanied by N-dealkylation (Chapter 6). The formation and significance of a nitrone have also been documented in the *in vitro* metabolism of N-methylamphetamine; during extraction, the nitrone showed a marked tendency to break down to 1-phenyl-2-propanone oxime (Coutts and Kovach, 1977).

The picture emerging thus far is of **primary amines** undergoing cytochrome P450-mediated N-oxygenation to hydroxylamines, followed by two single-electron oxidation steps (the first of which is catalyzed by cytochrome P450-released superoxide) to the nitroso/oxime (Fig. 5.3); oxidation of the latter to the nitro derivative has seldom been reported. As far as **secondary amines** are concerned, their oxidation is catalyzed mainly by FAD-containing monooxygenase and involves two monooxygenation steps, first to a hydroxylamine and then to isomeric nitrones (Fig. 5.5). Nitrones in turn can be oxidized to the nitroso derivatives, but the reaction is catalyzed by cytochrome P450. In addition, there are a few reports showing that secondary hydroxylamines can be oxidized by monooxygenases (directly or by released superoxide) to form **nitroxides** (see above). Thus, a number of secondary hydroxylamines in the presence of the purified pig liver flavin-containing monooxygenase are transformed to their nitroxides which, when sufficiently stable, can be used as spin-labelled probes, e.g. TEMPO (**5.XXXVIII**) (Rauckman *et al.*, 1979). It is also interesting to note that **N-hydroxynorcocaine**, a secondary hydroxylamine formed by cytochrome P450 from cocaine, is further oxidized to norcocaine nitroxide and other reactive metabolites possibly accounting for the hepatotoxicity of this chemical (Boelsterli and Göldlin, 1991; Kloss *et al.*, 1984; Lloyd *et al.*, 1993).

5.XXXIV

5.XXXV

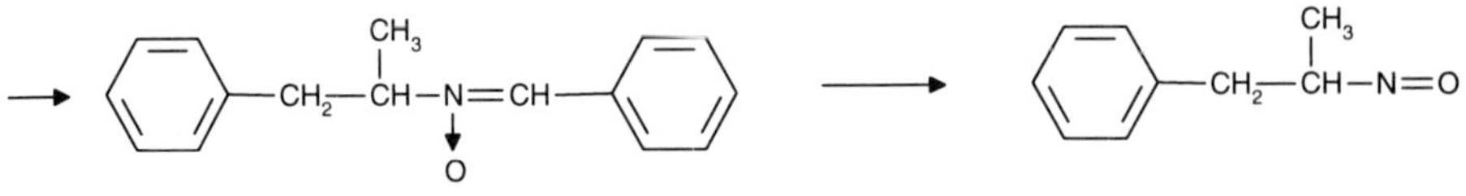

5.XXXVI

5.XXXVII

5.XXXVIII

$CH_3CH_2CH_2 \!-\! C \!-\! COOCH_2CH_2N(CH_2CH_3)_2$

5.XXXIX

$$\left[P450\!-\!Fe^{2+} \!\leftarrow\! \underset{\underset{O}{\parallel}}{N}\!-\!R \right]$$

5.XL

One biologically and pharmacologically significant consequence of N-oxygenation is the **formation of complexes** between some metabolic intermediates (MI) and cytochrome P450 enzymes, resulting in a mechanism-based, usually reversible inhibition of the latter (Franklin, 1977; Lindeke and Paulsen-Sörman, 1988; Testa and Jenner, 1981). A large variety of nitrogenous compounds of medicinal interest are N-oxidized to complex-forming MI, e.g. primary, secondary and tertiary amines in the amphetamine group, the well-known inhibitor **SKF-525A** (2-diethylaminoethyl 2,2-diphenylvalerate, **5.XXXIX**) and analogous lipophilic tertiary amines, aromatic azaheterocyclic compounds, as well as some aromatic amines, hydroxylamines, nitroso and nitro compounds, nitrones, N-oxides, and nitrosamines. In addition, some **macrolide antibiotics** bind as MI to CYP3A enzymes and inhibit them, e.g. erythromycin and troleandomycin (Babany *et al.*, 1988; Delaforge *et al.*, 1983; Pershing and Franklin, 1982; Roos *et al.*, 1993; Tinel *et al.*, 1989).

Such complex formation occurs with cytochrome P450 in the reduced state and can be detected by difference spectra with a maximum at 453–457 nm and 445–450 nm for MI formed from aliphatic and aromatic amines, respectively. The fact that amines and hydroxylamines must be oxidized to form complexes, while nitro compounds must be reduced indicates, together with other evidence, that nitroso derivatives are the metabolic intermediates responsible for complex formation (Lindeke and Paulsen-Sörman, 1988; Mansuy *et al.*, 1978a). The mode of binding of such MI to reduced cytochrome P450 involves the nitrogen atom interacting with the iron cation (**5.XL**). Note, however, that complex formation with other MI, e.g. nitroxides, cannot be excluded. For tertiary and some secondary amines, N-dealkylation is necessary for formation of the interacting metabolites. As discussed above, cytochrome P450 is involved in the oxidation of primary hydroxylamines and nitrones to the nitroso derivatives; this means that the ligand thus formed can bind directly (without being released) to the catalytic isoenzyme and inhibit it.

5.4 OXIDATION OF 1,4-DIHYDROPYRIDINES

4-Substituted-1,4-dihydropyridines (Fig. 5.6) are compounds of particular interest. 4-Aryl substitution affords drugs belonging to a major class of calcium channel blockers, while 4-alkyl

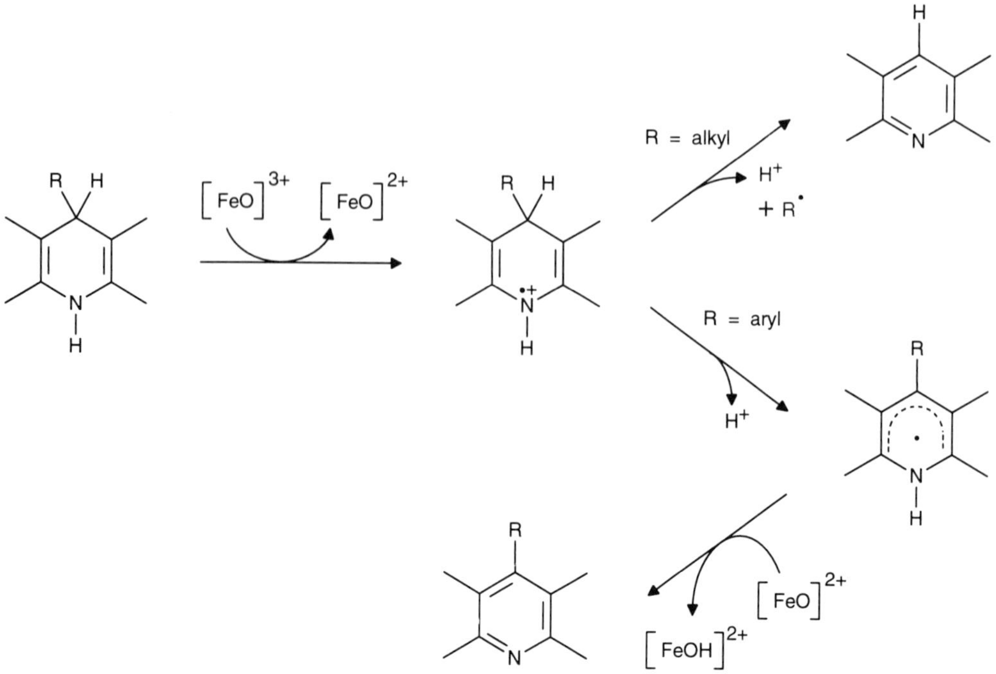

FIGURE 5.6 Postulated pathways in the aromatization of 4-alkyl- and 4-aryl-1,4-dihydropyridines (Augusto *et al.*, 1982; Böcker and Guengerich, 1986; Guengerich and Böcker, 1988).

substitution yields irreversible cytochrome P450 inhibitors (mechanism-based inactivators) of value as biochemical tools. These compounds, despite being secondary amines, are substrates of cytochrome P450 (Table 5.3) undergoing **aromatization** by a mechanism now fairly well understood (Augusto *et al.*, 1982; Böcker and Guengerich, 1986; Guengerich and Böcker, 1988; Ortiz de Montellano, 1989).

The **reaction mechanism** (Fig. 5.6) is initiated by a one-electron oxidation of the nitrogen atom, yielding an aminium radical whose fate depends on the nature of the 4-substituent. When the 4-substituent is an **alkyl group** (e.g. ethyl, propyl, isopropyl, butyl, isobutyl or benzyl), the radical cation aromatizes by ejecting the alkyl group as a radical. Biochemical effects of this alkyl radical are discussed below. When the 4-substituent is an **aryl group** (e.g. phenyl, substituted phenyl, 1- or 2-naphthyl), there is a very low probability of its existence as a radical. Thus, loss of the 4-proton occurs, the resulting hydropyridine radical being stabilized by delocalization as shown. A second one-electron oxidation now takes place, also catalyzed by cytochrome P450, and produces the 4-arylpyridine metabolite. This mechanism of aromatization is supported by very low kinetic isotope effects when the 4-position is labelled with a deuterium or tritium atom (Guengerich, 1990). This aromatization reaction also exhibits low substrate enantioselectivity (Guengerich and Böcker, 1988).

Most of the **4-alkylated analogues** investigated as mechanism-based inactivators of cytochrome P450 have been 4-alkyl-3,5-dicarbethoxy-2,6-dimethyl-1,4-dihydropyridines (**5.XLI**), with R often being methyl or ethyl (Kennedy and Mason, 1990; Lee *et al.*, 1988). Selective inactivation of CYP1A1, CYP2C11, CYP3A and CYP4A has been reported, an inactivation caused by different, isozyme-specific reactions of heme alkylation as well as loss or alteration of apoprotein in some cases. Such inactivation results in the inhibition of a number of

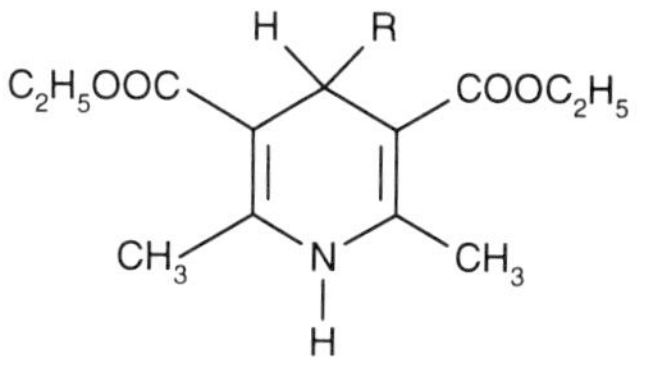

5.XLI

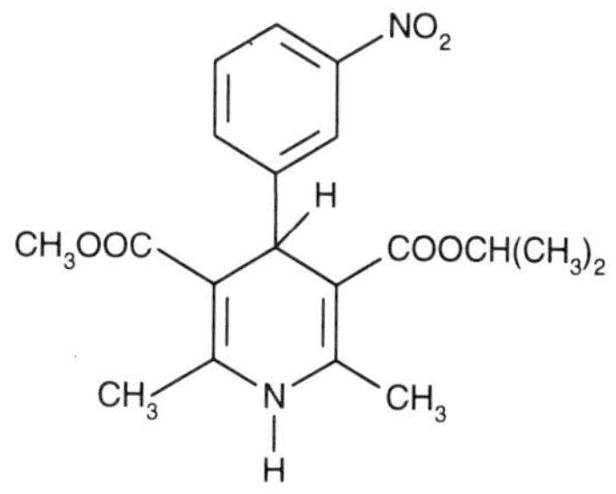

5.XLII

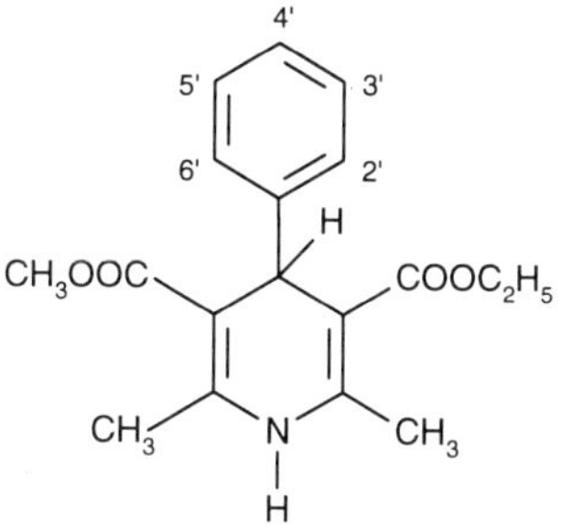

5.XLIII

isozyme-specific activities (Böcker and Guengerich, 1986; Correia *et al.*, 1987; Riddick *et al.*, 1990a and 1990b; Sugiyama *et al.*, 1989).

For the **1,4-dihydropyridine calcium channel blockers**, numerous studies document their aromatization to the pyridine metabolite under a variety of *in vitro* and *in vivo* conditions, the reaction in humans being catalyzed mainly by CYP3A4 sometimes called nifedipine oxidase (Ferenczy and Norris, 1989; Guengerich *et al.*, 1991). Thus, only traces of **nivaldipine (5.XLII)** are excreted in rats dosed with the drug, by far most of a dose being excreted as metabolites containing the pyridine moiety (Terashita *et al.*, 1989). This is compatible with studies in rat and dog liver microsomes showing that the reaction of aromatization is the first step in the biotransformation of the drug (Niwa *et al.*, 1989). Similar results have been reported for **felodipine** (2′,3′-dichloro-**5.XLIII**) (Bäärnhielm *et al.*, 1984). Among a large series of felodipine analogues (**5.XLIII**), the fastest rate of aromatization was seen with 2′,6′-disubstituted derivatives, and the slowest rates with, e.g. 2′,3′-, 2′,4′-, 3′,4′- and 3′,5′-disubstituted derivatives. These variations were correlated with electronic properties of the substrates (Bäärnhielm and Westerlund, 1986).

5.5 N-OXYGENATION OF PRIMARY AND SECONDARY AROMATIC AMINES

Tertiary aromatic amines have been discussed in Section 5.2 together with aliphatic amines, so this section will consider only primary and secondary aromatic amines. Their major N-oxygenated metabolites are the hydroxylamine derivatives, the formation of which has been known for many years (Testa and Jenner, 1976 and 1978).

5.5.1 Secondary aromatic amines

By analogy with their aliphatic analogues, secondary aromatic amines are N-oxidized to the corresponding **hydroxylamines** and **nitrones**, but the production of these metabolites can be expected to be strongly dependent on biological conditions and substrate properties. Thus, the microsomal metabolism of N-benzylaniline (**5.XLIV**, X = H) and N-benzyl-4-toluidine (**5.XLIV**, X = CH$_3$) under a variety of biological conditions led exclusively to the nitrone metabolite (**5.XLVI**); only with N-benzyl-4-chloroaniline (**5.XLIV**, X = Cl) was the intermediate hydroxylamine (**5.XLV**) detected (Gooderham and Gorrod, 1985). The N-oxygenation of secondary aromatic amines is usually mediated by the FAD-containing monooxygenase, witness N-methylaniline (Table 5.4), but the enzymatic situation may be more complex. For example, the N-oxygenation of N-benzyl-4-chloroaniline (**5.XLIV**, X = Cl) and 4-fluoro-N-methylaniline involves both FMO and cytochrome P450, suggesting that the contribution of both enzymes is determined by their relative amounts in the biological system, and by substrate properties (Boersma *et al.*, 1993; Gooderham and Gorrod, 1985).

5.XLIV

5.XLV   5.XLVI

For a secondary aromatic amine such as 4-fluoro-N-methylaniline, there are some indications that the hydroxylamino metabolite may lose its fluoro atom and rearrange to *para*-N-methylaminophenol (Boersma *et al.*, 1993). This is certainly an interesting reaction whose substrate selectivity and mechanism should be better known.

5.5.2 Primary arylamines

In contrast to the scarcity of data pertaining to the N-oxygenation of secondary aromatic amines, the metabolism of primary arylamines has received considerable attention due to the toxicological significance of these xenobiotics (Dipple *et al.*, 1985; Frederick *et al.*, 1985; Kadlubar *et al.*, 1992; Prough *et al.*, 1988; Quon, 1988). Here, the *a priori* products of N-oxygenation are **hydroxylamines** and **nitroso** compounds, in analogy with metabolites of primary aliphatic amines lacking a hydrogen atom on the alpha-carbon. However, the nitroso metabolites may not be formed or escape detection for a number of reasons. For example, the N-oxygenation of a large variety of 4-substituted anilines by hepatic microsomes from various animal species led exclusively to the corresponding hydroxylamines, no nitrosoarenes being detected (Smith and Gorrod, 1978).

An interesting drug in this context is **procainamide (5.XLVII)**, which is metabolized to the hydroxylamine in rat and human liver microsomes. Failure to detect this metabolite *in vivo* may well be due to its reactivity (Budinski *et al.*, 1987). Indeed, this hydroxylamine undergoes non-enzymatic oxidation to the nitroso compound, the latter reacting covalently with glutathione and thiol groups in proteins to form **sulfinamide adducts** (see Lindeke, 1982, and the volume in this series, *Biochemistry of Conjugation Reactions*). It has been postulated that this reaction may be responsible for procainamide-induced lupus (Uetrecht, 1985). Another possibility for nitroso metabolites escaping detection is their coupling with a hydroxylamine to form an **azoxy derivative** (see Section 5.3.2 and Table 5.1), or with the parent primary amine to form an **azo compound** (Tyrakowska *et al.*, 1993).

$$H_2N-\langle\bigcirc\rangle-CONHCH_2CH_2N(CH_2CH_3)_2 \qquad 5.XLVII$$

5.XLVIII

As a rule, the N-oxygenation of primary arylamines to the hydroxylamino and nitroso metabolites is mediated by cytochrome P450, particularly by enzymes of the P4501A subfamily. Other cytochromes P450 are involved in the oxidation of some primary arylamines, for example CYP3A4 which catalyzes the N-hydroxylation of dapsone in human liver (Fleming *et al.*, 1992). In analogy with the primary arylalkylamines discussed in Section 5.3, the nitroso metabolites of primary arylamines will form **complexes with reduced cytochrome P450** (Mansuy *et al.*, 1978b). Interestingly, nitrosoarenes such as nitrosobenzene react with cytochrome P450 in the iron(III) state, in the absence of any exogenous reducing agent, to produce the iron(II)–nitrosobenzene complex; this ligand apparently is capable of inducing autoreduction of the iron atom, possibly by oxidation of the axial bound thiolate group (Fukuto *et al.*, 1986). The fact that the nitrosoarene–iron porphyrin complexes are markedly less stable than the nitrosoalkane–iron porphyrin complexes is also noteworthy.

The N-oxygenation by the FAD-containing monooxygenase requires high nucleophilicity of the amino group (Section 5.2), so that primary arylamines are excluded. This renders all the more interesting the fact that 2-naphthylamine (**5.XLVIII**), besides being a substrate of CYP1A, was found to be N-hydroxylated by the flavin-containing monooxygenase in pig liver microsomes (Poulsen *et al.*, 1976). This reactivity has been explained in terms of the imino tautomer being a reactive form of 2-naphthylamine and having a degree of nucleophilicity comparable to that of other known substrates of this enzyme.

Arylhydroxylamines can also be oxidized by hemoglobin, as discussed in Section 9.2.

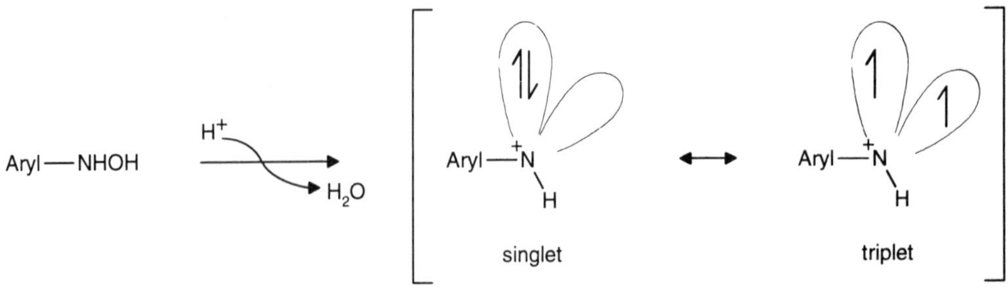

FIGURE 5.7 One of the postulated breakdown reactions of arylhydroxylamines leading to the formation of nitrenium ions, and the singlet and triplet states of the latter (Hartman and Schlegel, 1981).

The toxicological significance of primary arylamines, in particular the carcinogenic and mutagenic potential of polycyclic arylamines, rests on complex sequences of toxication and detoxication pathways (especially N-acetylation) which will be considered in the volume, *Biochemistry of Conjugation Reactions*. Of particular significance here is the involvement of highly reactive **nitrenium ions** (aryl-N$^+$-H) (Ford and Herman, 1992; Wild, 1993). For example, there is evidence that a nitrenium ion is responsible for the covalent binding of nitrofurazone to DNA (Streeter and Hoener, 1988); it is postulated that this nitrenium ion is formed from the hydroxylamino metabolite according to the reaction shown in Fig. 5.7, although we will see in Section 5.6 and in another volume that such nitrenium ions are formed more readily from hydroxylamides and particularly from their O-sulfates and O-glucuronides.

The statement that nitrenium ions are highly reactive needs to be qualified, following a theoretical study which suggests a differential role for the singlet and triplet states (Fig. 5.7) (Hartman and Schlegel, 1981). An empirical correlation was established for a number of primary arylamines between, on the one side, the energy separation of the singlet and triplet states of the nitrenium ion, and on the other side the carcinogenic or mutagenic potential of the parent amine. Briefly, the nitrenium ions of non-toxic amines were found to exist preferentially in the **triplet state**. In contrast, the nitrenium ions of mutagenic/carcinogenic amines were characterized by **singlet states** of similar or greater stability than the triplet states. It was therefore suggested that nitrenium ions must exist and react in the singlet state for the initiation of the mutagenic/carcinogenic process. Nitrenium ion reactivity will be discussed further in Section 5.6.

5.5.3 Amino azaheterocycles

Amino azaheterocycles are compounds that pose a particular problem in connection with their N-oxygenation and potential toxicity. The tertiary nitrogen atom and the primary amino group are targets for N-oxide and hydroxylamine formation, respectively (Fig. 5.8).

While N-oxide formation (reaction **a** in Fig. 5.8) is associated with detoxication, hydroxylamine formation (reaction **b** in Fig. 5.8) is considered as a route of toxication. Factors controlling this regioselectivity are complex and poorly understood, but the role of an **amine–imine tautomerism** (Fig. 5.8) as one of the chemical determinants of the reaction has been repeatedly underlined (Gorrod, 1985a, 1985b and 1987). Thus, the antibacterial drug **trimethoprim (5.XLIX)**, a 2,4-diamino-6-substituted pyrimidine, is not N-hydroxylated but forms the two isomeric N-oxides in the 1- and 3-position (Gorrod, 1985b). The 6-substituent was also found to play a marked role in influencing N-oxide formation from compounds of this type (El-Ghomari and Gorrod, 1987). Compounds known to be N-hydroxylated rather than forming N-oxides include

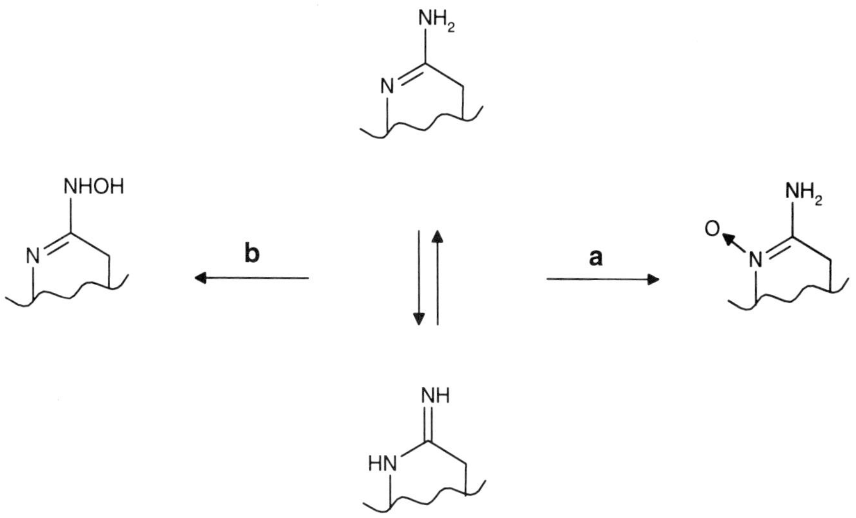

FIGURE 5.8 Amine–imine tautomeric equilibrium of azaheterocyclic amines and their N-oxygenation to N-oxides (reaction **a**, associated with detoxication) and hydroxylamines (reaction **b**, associated with toxication) (Gorrod, 1985a, 1985b and 1987).

carcinogens occurring as **amino acid pyrolysates** in cooked or charred foods, for example the mutagenic and carcinogenic compound IQ (**5.L**, 2-amino-3-methylimidazo[4,5-*f*]quinoline) (Aeschbacher and Turesky, 1991; Felton and Knize, 1991; Kerdar *et al.*, 1993; Sugimura, 1988; Turesky, 1990). Another example involves the recently discovered N-hydroxylation of the purine base **adenine** (**5.LI**), by 3-methylcholanthrene-induced rat liver microsomes, to 6-N-hydroxylaminopurine, a compound known to be genotoxic and carcinogenic (Clement and Kunze, 1990). For such heterocyclic hydroxylamines, nitrenium ion formation is again considered as the step leading to the ultimate mutagen and carcinogen (Ford and Griffin, 1992).

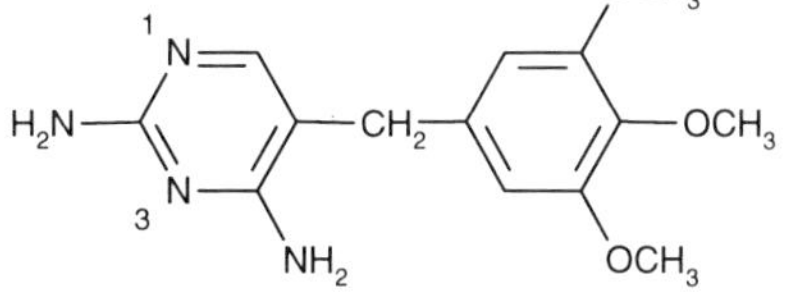

5.XLIX

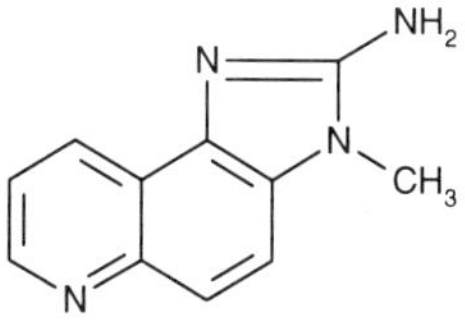

5.L

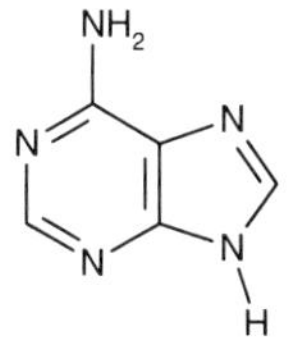

5.LI

5.6 N-OXYGENATION OF AROMATIC AMIDES

As a rule, **aliphatic amides** are not N-hydroxylated (Table 5.3.). Earlier studies reported the N-hydroxylation of some carbamates such as urethane (**5.LII**, R = ethyl), but this has not been confirmed in later investigations (Damani, 1982; Marsden and Gorrod, 1985).

While **tertiary aromatic amides** are not N-oxidized, **secondary aromatic amides** (N-arylamides) constitute an important group of cytochrome P450 substrates whose N-oxidation leads to **N-hydroxylamines** (**5.LIII**), also known as **hydroxamic acids**. The **catalytic mechanism** of their formation has been shown to involve **H• abstraction** from NH to form an N-centred radical, followed by radical combination with HO• (oxygen rebound) (Koymans *et al.*, 1993a). Because the N-centred radical is resonance-stabilized, the lone electron may delocalize to the *ortho* and *para* position, leading to phenols and quinone imines in analogy with the reactions discussed in Section 4.3 (see Fig. 4.8) (Koymans *et al.*, 1993b).

The formation of N-hydroxylamines is documented for a number of compounds, in particular some drugs and carcinogenic N-arylamides (Dipple *et al.*, 1985). For example, when **phenacetin** (**5.LIV**, R = ethyl) and two homologues (R = methyl and *n*-butyl) were incubated with mice liver microsomes, they were N-hydroxylated at a rate approximately proportional to the lipophilicity of the substrate (Kapetanovic *et al.*, 1979). The reaction was clearly mediated by CYP1A enzymes, a finding repeatedly reported for toxic N-arylamides, for example the carcinogenic 2-acetylaminofluorene (**5.LV**) (Thorgeirsson *et al.*, 1984). Phenacetin N-hydroxylation is also of great toxicological significance since it leads to reactive intermediates as shown in Fig. 5.9 (see below).

The **structure–metabolism relationships** for N-hydroxylation were investigated for a series of 4′-substituted *trans*-4-acetamidostilbenes (**5.LVI**) using hamster liver microsomes (Hanna *et al.*, 1980). Electronegative substituents such as halogens, CN and CF$_3$ caused a reduction in the

5.LII

5.LIII

5.LIV

5.LV

5.LVI

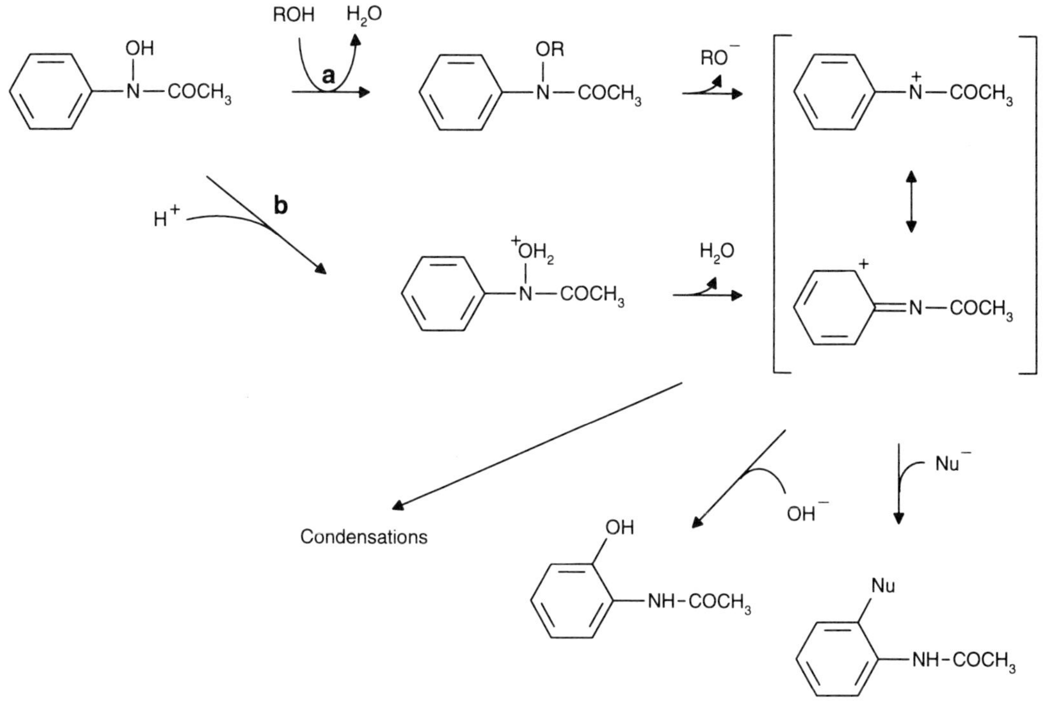

FIGURE 5.9 Mechanisms of formation of nitrenium ions from arylhydroxamic acids (via O-conjugation, reaction **a**, or via dehydroxylation, reaction **b**), and their reactivity as electrophiles to form condensation products, phenols, or adducts with biological nucleophiles.

rate of N-hydroxylation (consistent with the mechanism of H• abstraction discussed above), but there was also a favourable influence of lipophilicity. A compound whose N-hydroxylation has attracted considerable attention is **acetaminophen** (**5.LIV**, R = H, paracetamol). By analogy with the toxication of phenacetin (see above), the hepatoxicity of this analgesic drug was postulated to be initiated by N-hydroxylation. This hypothesis has not been verified, and it is now known that acetaminophen is not N-hydroxylated, the ultimate toxic metabolite, N-acetyl-p-benzoquinone imine, being formed by a reaction of oxygen oxidation (see Section 7.6) (Calder *et al.*, 1981). The same absence of N-hydroxylation is documented for *meta*-hydroxyacetanilide, a positional isomer of acetaminophen (Rashed *et al.*, 1989).

Hydroxamic acids are acidic in nature and considerably more stable than N-arylhydroxylamines (Damani, 1982; Lindeke, 1982; Ziegler, 1984). For example, while the autoxidation of N-hydroxy-4-chloroaniline was comparatively fast and led to such products as 4-chlorophenyl nitroxide, 4-chloronitrosobenzene, 4,4'-azoxy*bis*chlorobenzene and 4-chloronitrobenzene, the autoxidation of N-hydroxy-4-chloroacetanilide was very slow (Lenk and Riedl, 1989). But reactions other than oxidation occur, in particular proton-catalyzed dehydroxylation/dehydration to form **nitrenium ions** (pathway **b** in Fig. 5.9) (Nelson, 1985). Under biological conditions, however, a more efficient route to nitrenium ions is via O-conjugation (formation of O-sulfates or O-glucuronides, see volume on conjugations) (pathway **a** in Fig. 5.9). These electrophilic nitrenium ions and the transition state by which they are formed are resonance-stabilized. Nitrenium ions will react in the *ortho* or *para* position with hydroxyl ions to form phenols, or with endogenous nucleophiles such as macromolecules to form adducts; they may also yield condensation products (Fig. 5.9) (Campbell *et al.*, 1991; Koymans *et* *al.*, 1990; Lindeke, 1982; Sternson and Gammans, 1975; Testa and Jenner, 1978; Thorgeirsson *et al.*, 1984).

5.7 N-OXIDATION OF HYDRAZINES AND N-OXYGENATION OF AZO DERIVATIVES

A limited number of hydrazines (alkyl, aryl and acyl hydrazines) have medicinal value, but a large number of others are markedly toxic, being for example recognized as carcinogens or hepatotoxins (Dipple *et al.*, 1985; Moloney and Prough, 1983; Prough and Moloney, 1985; Prough *et al.*, 1988; Tweedie *et al.*, 1987). The more data are accumulated, the clearer it becomes that the biotransformation of hydrazines is complex indeed. Yet despite many published studies and a few authoritative reviews, one cannot escape the feeling that our knowledge of the toxication and detoxication routes followed by these compounds is still too fragmentary to allow a global picture of the underlying mechanisms and structural factors influencing them. A complicating biological factor is certainly the fact that most classes of hydrazines can be metabolized by both the cytochrome P450 and the FAD-containing monooxygenase systems (Table 5.3); in the former case, N-dealkylation (Chapter 6) by oxidation of carbon atoms adjacent to the nitrogen functionality (alpha-carbons) are competing reactions.

From a metabolic viewpoint, it is useful to distinguish between unsymmetrical hydrazines (1-substituted and 1,1-disubstituted) and 1,2-disubstituted hydrazines.

5.7.1   1-Substituted hydrazines

1-Substituted hydrazines (**5.LVII** in Fig. 5.10, R = alkyl, aryl or acyl) yield unstable monoazo compounds (**diazenes, 5.LVIII** in Fig. 5.10); the underlying mechanism most likely involves two single-electron N-oxidation steps rather than N-oxygenation (Lindeke, 1982). The diazene can then decompose to the radical R•, or more likely undergoes a further one-electron oxidation step (reaction **a** in Fig. 5.10) before breaking down to N_2 and R• (Battioni *et al.*, 1983a). For example, the ethyl radical was observed by electron spin resonance following incubation of ethylhydrazine (**5.LVII** in Fig. 5.10, R = ethyl) with rat liver microsomes; in the case of acetylhydrazine (**5.LVII** in Fig. 5.10, R = acetyl), a radical was also observed but its chemical nature was not established (Augusto *et al.*, 1981). In addition to these N-oxidation steps, it is also possible for diazenes to rearrange to **hydrazones** when an alpha-hydrogen is present (reaction **b** in Fig. 5.10); hydrazones can then undergo hydrolysis to hydrazine and a carbonyl derivative, a reaction of N-dealkylation (see Chapter 6) (Ziegler, 1984).

Similarly, the monoamine oxidase inhibitor **phenelzine** (**5.LVII** in Fig. 5.10, R = 2-phenylethyl) was found to be metabolized by rat liver microsomes to the phenylethyl radical; the latter formed ethylbenzene and reacted with molecular oxygen to yield numerous other metabolites such as 2-phenylethanol, 2-phenylacetaldehyde, benzaldehyde, benzylalcohol, and toluene (Ortiz de Montellano and Watanabe, 1987). In addition, the phenylethyl radical also reacted covalently with the prosthetic heme of cytochrome P450, forming the **adduct** N-(2-phenylethyl)protoporphyrin IX and inactivating the enzyme (Ortiz de Montellano *et al.*, 1983). In fact, a number of alkyl-, aryl- and acylhydrazines behave as **mechanism-based inactivators** of some cytochromes P450 (e.g. Tuck and Ortiz de Montellano, 1992). Another derivative of medicinal interest, the antihypertensive drug **hydralazine** (**5.LIX**), is also metabolized by radical pathways, losing the hydrazino moiety to yield phthalazine as a major metabolite in rat liver microsomes (LaCagnin *et al.*, 1986).

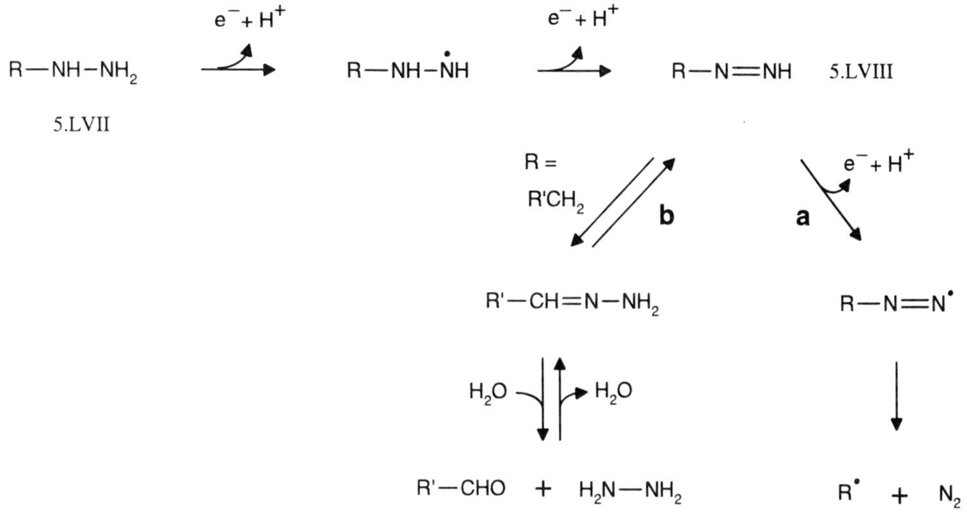

FIGURE 5.10 Postulated reaction mechanisms in the N-oxidation of 1-substituted hydrazines.

Under carefully controlled *in vitro* conditions, in particular the absence or minimal amounts of O_2, **alkyl-** and **aryldiazenes** form two types of spectrally detectable **complexes with cytochrome P450**. Whether generated as metabolites of hydrazines or added directly to cytochrome P450 preparations, alkyl- and aryldiazenes give complexes with ferrocytochrome P450 characterized by a Soret peak in the 446–448 nm region; the structure of such complexes

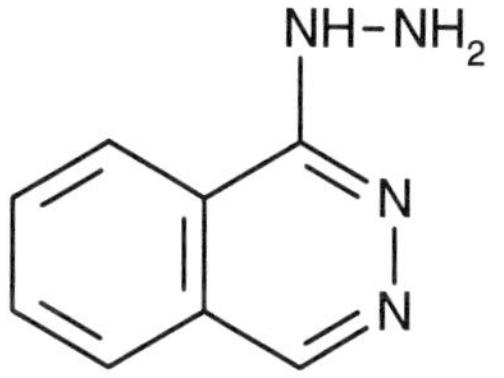

5.LIX

[P450–Fe(II)(NH=NR)] is shown in Fig. 5.11 and can be understood by the fact that diazenes are isoelectronic with nitroso compounds, dioxygen, carbon monoxide, etc. Note that the complexes formed from aryldiazenes are markedly less stable than those formed from alkyldiazenes. Careful one-electron oxidation of these diazene–iron(II) complexes led to complexes with a Soret peak in the 480 nm region and having a σ-alkyl or σ-aryl P450–Fe(III)–R structure (Fig. 5.11) (Battioni *et al.*, 1983a and 1983b; Moloney *et al.*, 1984). Their rearrangement may then produce the alkylated porphyrins mentioned above (e.g. Tuck and Ortiz de Montellano, 1992).

5.7.2 1,1-Disubstituted hydrazines

The **mechanism of N-oxidation** of 1,1-disubstituted hydrazines is also quite complex and far from being well understood (Fig. 5.12). Two-electron oxidation, or N-hydroxylation followed by dehydration, yields a diazene intermediate which may also be drawn as a nitrene resonance form. When one or more alpha-hydrogens are present, the diazene seems to exist in tautomeric

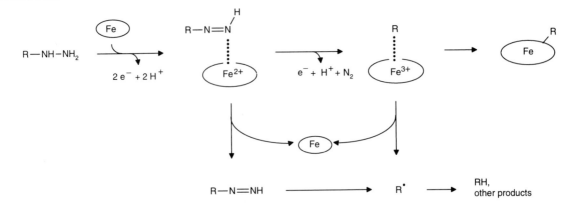

FIGURE 5.11 Complexes formed from the interactions of hydrazines and diazenes with cytochrome P450. First, a diazene–iron(II) complex is formed, followed by a σ-alkyl- or σ-aryliron(III) complex. The latter rearranges to an alkylated porphyrin (modified from Battioni *et al.*, 1983a; Moloney *et al.*, 1984).

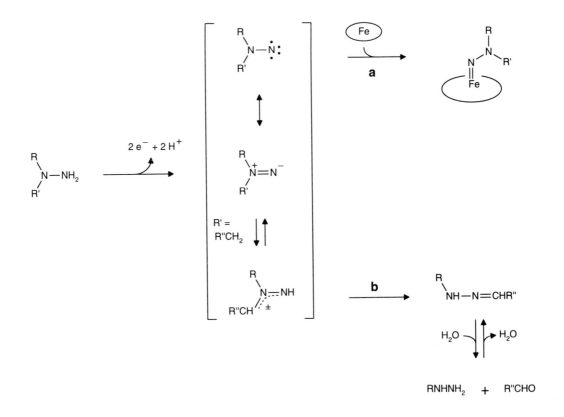

FIGURE 5.12 Postulated pathways in the oxidation of 1,1-disubstituted hydrazines. The intermediate resulting from N-oxidation may be drawn as a diazene (centre) or nitrene (top) resonance form; it may also exist in tautomeric equilibrium with an azomethinimine (bottom). The nitrene intermediate may form an iron–nitrene complex with cytochrome P450 (reaction **a**), while the azomethinimine can rearrange to a hydrazone (reaction **b**) that hydrolyzes as shown.

equilibrium with an azomethinimine which rearranges to a hydrazone (reaction **b** in Fig. 5.12), as documented for 1,1-dimethylhydrazine (Prough *et al.*, 1981). The formaldehyde methylhydrazone was then found to undergo hydrolysis to release methylhydrazine and formaldehyde, again a reaction of N-dealkylation. In addition, a number of 1,1-disubstituted hydrazines, but not 1-substituted or 1,2-disubstituted hydrazines, are able to form an iron–nitrene complex (reaction **a** in Fig. 5.12); presumably the reaction is favoured for substrates that cannot form a hydrazone, namely when the two substituents are part of a ring (e.g. 1-aminopiperidine) or when an alpha-hydrogen is lacking (Hines and Prough, 1980; Mansuy *et al.*, 1982).

5.LX   5.LXI

It is likely that the metabolism of 1,1-disubstituted hydrazines has some surprises in store considering the formation of **N-nitrosodiphenylamine** (**5.LXI**) from 1,1-diphenylhydrazine (**5.LX**) by rat liver microsomes (Tatsumi *et al.*, 1984). The reaction was catalyzed by a superoxide radical released from NADPH-cytochrome P450 reductase, and it is noteworthy that this substrate has no alpha-hydrogen, preventing hydrazone formation.

Interestingly, NADPH-cytochrome P450 reductase was also found to catalyze the one-electron oxidation of hydrazine to the hydrazine radical (**5.LXII**), the first step towards the ultimate metabolite N_2 (Noda *et al.*, 1988).

5.7.3 1,2-Disubstituted hydrazines and azo derivatives

The metabolism of **1,2-disubstituted hydrazines** again differs from that of other hydrazines. Here, products of N-oxidation are comparatively stable azo derivatives (**5.LXIII** in Fig. 5.13) whose further biotransformation as metabolites or xenobiotics is discussed below.

Azo compounds containing a hydrogen on one alpha-carbon may undergo tautomeric equilibrium to **hydrazones** followed by hydrolysis (pathway **a** in Fig. 5.13) (Ziegler, 1984). 1,2-Dimethylhydrazine for example is N-oxidized to azomethane (Erikson and Prough, 1986). Azo formation and subsequent N–C cleavage reactions are documented for the antitumour agent **procarbazine** (**5.LXIV**) (Weinkaum and Shiba, 1978), although the mechanism of N-dealkylation may involve alpha-carbon hydroxylation (see Chapter 6) rather than hydrazone hydrolysis.

5.LXIV

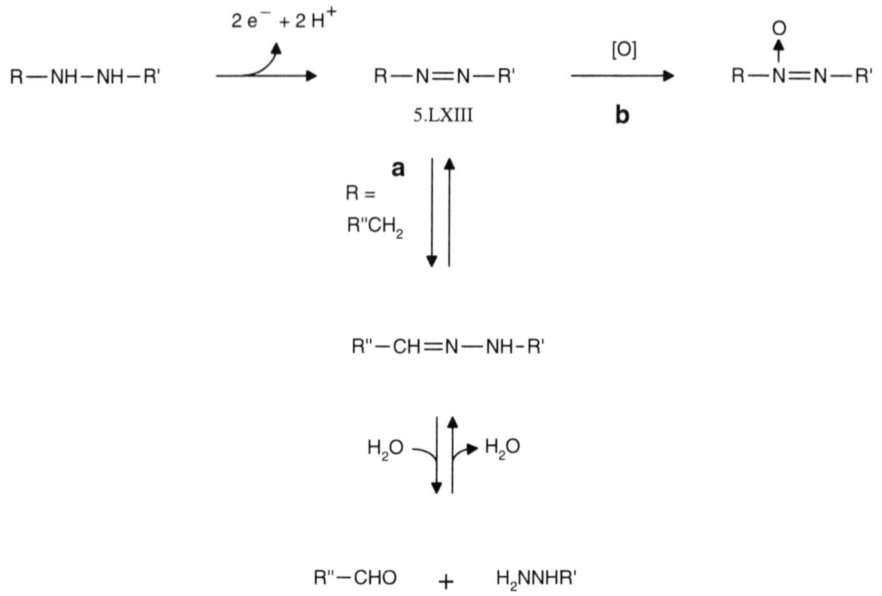

$$R{-}NH{-}NH{-}R' \xrightarrow{\;2\,e^- + 2\,H^+\;} \underset{\text{5.LXIII}}{R{-}N{=}N{-}R'} \xrightarrow[\;\textbf{b}\;]{[O]} R{-}\overset{\overset{\displaystyle O}{\uparrow}}{N}{=}N{-}R'$$

$$\textbf{a} \;\Big\updownarrow\quad \begin{array}{l} R = \\ R''CH_2 \end{array}$$

$$R''{-}CH{=}N{-}NH{-}R'$$

$$H_2O \;\Big\downarrow\Big\downarrow\; H_2O$$

$$R''{-}CHO \;+\; H_2NNHR'$$

FIGURE 5.13 Oxidative metabolism of 1,2-disubstituted hydrazines to azo derivatives (**5.LXIII**). The latter may in some cases rearrange to hydrolyzable hydrazones (reaction **a**), or can be further N-oxygenated to azoxy derivatives (reaction **b**).

Azo compounds can also be N-oxygenated to the corresponding **azoxy derivatives**, as exemplified by azoxymethane (reaction **b** in Fig. 5.13, R = R′ = methyl) (Dipple *et al.*, 1985). Similarly, procarbazine yielded the two isomeric azoxy metabolites in rat liver preparations (Weinkaum and Shiba, 1978). A number of alkyl azo and azoxy derivatives, despite their chemical stability, are potent carcinogens; this toxicity results from further activation by alpha-carbon hydroxylation (Chapter 6) (Dipple *et al.*, 1985). In contrast, a number of aromatic azo compounds with a *para*-amino group (aminoazobenzenes) are carcinogenic due to the activation of the amino group, while the azo group undergoes reduction (Section 12.4) (Dipple *et al.*, 1985; Quon, 1988).

5.8 N-OXYGENATION OF AMIDINES AND GUANIDINES

A number of **benzamidines**, a group of strong bases with pK_a values in the range 11–12, were investigated as potential monooxygenase substrates to assess better the structural factors influencing N-oxygenation. Careful studies show that benzamidines (**5.LXV** in Fig. 5.14) are N-oxygenated to **benzamidoximes** of Z-configuration (**5.LXVI** in Fig. 5.14) when R = H or phenyl (Clement, 1983, 1984, 1985 and 1989; Clement and Zimmermann, 1987a; Clement *et al.*, 1989, 1993a and 1993b). The reaction is mediated by cytochrome P450 (Table 5.3), in particular CYP2C3, and is believed to result from initial N-oxidation of the primary NH₂ group, followed by tautomeric rearrangement to the oxime (pathway **A** in Fig. 5.14). A typical compound in this respect is the trypanocidal agent **diminazene** (**5.LXVIII**), a diamidine that was N-oxygenated by rabbit liver homogenates to the mono- and di-amidoxime (Clement *et al.*, 1992).

When R = phenyl in **5.LXV** (Fig. 5.14), N-oxygenation is thought to be made possible by a tautomeric rearrangement of the imine to the primary amine (Fig. 5.14). In contrast, when R =

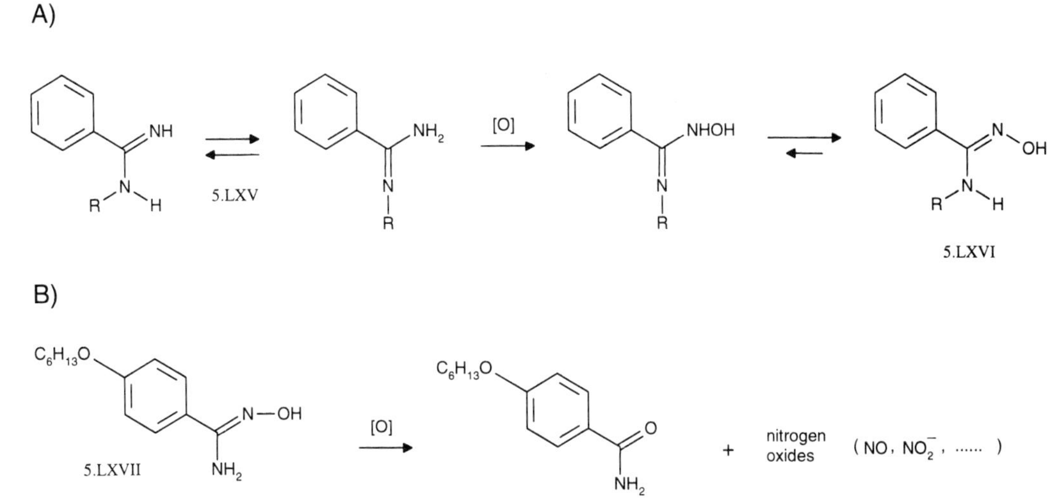

A)

B)

FIGURE 5.14 Pathway **A**: Cytochrome P450-catalyzed N-oxygenation of benzamidines (**5.LXV**) to benzamidoximes (**5.LXVI**), and the tautomeric equilibria involving the substrate and the product. Pathway **B**: Cytochrome P450-catalyzed oxidation of an arylamidoxime (**5.LXVIII**) to the amide and nitrogen oxides, in particular nitric oxide (NO) (Andronik-Lion *et al.*, 1992).

methyl or other alkyls in **5.LXV** (Fig. 5.14), the imine-to-amine tautomeric equilibrium very strongly favours the imine, perhaps explaining why N-alkylated benzamidines are not N-oxygenated but rather N-dealkylated (Clement and Zimmermann, 1987b).

Regarding the **benzamidoximes** of structure **5.LXVI** (Fig. 5.14), there was until recently no evidence of their further N-oxidation or hydrolysis to amides, although metabolic reduction back to the benzamidines has been detected (Clement, 1989). However, recent findings have demonstrated the ability of cytochrome P450, and particularly CYP3A, to oxidize an aromatic amidoxime such as **5.LXVII** (pathway **B** in Fig. 5.14) (Andronik-Lion *et al.*, 1992). The resulting metabolites are the benzamide and nitrogen oxides, most notably **nitric oxide** (NO; see below). Nitric oxide is an essential mammalian mediator, and it has been suggested that compounds containing amidine or amidoxime functions could act as precursors of NO *in vivo* after *in situ* oxidation by cytochrome P450 (Andronik-Lion *et al.*, 1992) (Section 12.4).

For many years, and in contrast to benzamidines, **guanidines** (**5.LXIX**) were believed to be resistant to N-oxygenation whatever the nature of the substituents. **Debrisoquine** (**4.XXX** in Chapter 4) was taken as an example of such a complete absence of reactivity (Clement, 1985 and 1986). It is only very recently that the CYP2C3-dependent N-hydroxylation of debrisoquine has been demonstrated for the first time in the presence of competitive inhibitors of the microsomal NADH-dependent reductase that very effectively retroreduces N-hydroxydebrisoquine (Clement *et al.*, 1993c). This metabolite has been shown to decouple monooxygenases, thus liberating $O_2^{\bullet-}$ which further transforms it into the corresponding urea derivative (i.e. a reaction comparable to pathway **B** in Fig. 5.14).

Such an N-oxidation of a xenobiotic guanidino derivative is comparable to the activation of the guanidino group in L-arginine (**5.LXX**). Indeed, L-arginine is the physiological precursor of nitric oxide to which it is oxidized by **nitric oxide synthase** [L-arginine, NADPH:oxygen oxidoreductase (nitric-oxide-forming); EC 1.14.13.39]. This enzyme is a complex hemoprotein displaying similarities with cytochrome P450 and particularly CYP102 (see Table 3.2 in Chapter 3). L-Arginine oxidation by nitric oxide synthase occurs in two steps, forming first N$^\omega$-hydroxy-L-arginine and then citrulline and nitric oxide in a sequence of reactions similar to that shown in pathways **A** and **B** (Fig. 5.14) (Feldman *et al.*, 1993; White and Marletta, 1992).

5.LXVIII

5.LXIX

5.LXX

5.9 REFERENCES

Aeschbacher H.U. and Turesky R.J. (1991). Mammalian cell mutagenicity and metabolism of heterocyclic aromatic amines. *Mutat. Res.* **259**, 235–250.

Andronik-Lion V., Boucher J.L., Delaforge M., Henry Y. and Mansuy D. (1992). Formation of nitric oxide by cytochrome P450-catalyzed oxidation of aromatic amidoximes. *Biochem. Biophys. Res. Commun.* **185**, 452–458.

Assandri A., Galliani G., Zerilli L., Tuan G., Tarzia G. and Barone D. (1986). Zetidoline metabolism by rat liver microsomes. Formation of metabolites with potential neuroleptic activity. *Biochem. Pharmacol.* **35**, 1459–1467.

Augusto O., Ortiz de Montellano P.R. and Quintanilha A. (1981). Spin-trapping of free radicals formed during microsomal metabolism of ethylhydrazine and acetylhydrazine. *Biochem. Biophys. Res. Commun.* **101**, 1324–1330.

Augusto O., Beilan H.S. and Ortiz de Montellano P.R. (1982). The catalytic mechanism of cytochrome P-450. Spin-trapping evidence for one-electron substrate oxidation. *J. Biol. Chem.* **257**, 11,288–11,295.

Bäärnhielm C., Skanberg I. and Borg K.O. (1984). Cytochrome P-450-dependent oxidation of felodipine—a 1,4-dihydropyridine—to the corresponding pyridine. *Xenobiotica* **14**, 719–726.

Bäärnhielm C. and Westerlund C. (1986). Quantitative relationships between structure and microsomal oxidation rate of 1,4-dihydropyridines. *Chem.-Biol. Interact.* **58**, 277–288.

Babany G., Larrey D. and Pessayre D. (1988). Macrolide antibiotics as inducers and inhibitors of cytochrome

P-450 in experimental animals and man. In *Progress in Drug Metabolism*, Vol. 11 (ed. Gibson G.G.). pp. 61–98. Taylor & Francis, London.

Ball S. and Bruice T.C. (1980). Oxidation of amines by 4α-hydroxyperoxy-flavin. *J. Amer. Chem. Soc.* **102**, 6498–6503.

Battioni P., Mahy J.P., Delaforge M. and Mansuy D. (1983a). Reaction of monosubstituted hydrazines and diazenes with rat-liver cytochrome P450. *Eur. J. Biochem.* **134**, 241–248.

Battioni P., Mahy J.P., Gillet G. and Mansuy D. (1983b). Iron porphyrin dependent oxidation of methyl- and phenylhydrazine: isolation of iron(II)–diazene and σ-alkyliron(III) (or aryliron(III)) complexes. *J. Amer. Chem. Soc.* **105**, 1399–1401.

Beckett A.H. and Jones G.R. (1977). Metabolic oxidation of aralkyl oximes to nitro compounds by fortified 9000g liver supernatants from various species. *J. Pharm. Pharmacol.* **29**, 416–421.

Beckett A.H. and Bélanger P.M. (1978). The disposition of phentermine and its N-oxidized metabolic products in the rabbit. *Xenobiotica* **8**, 555–560.

Beckett A.H., Purkaystha A.R. and Morgan P.H. (1977). Oxidation of aliphatic hydroxylamines in aqueous solutions. *J. Pharm. Pharmacol.* **29**, 15–21.

Beckett A.H., Navas G.E., Hutt A.J. and Farag M. (1979). Disappearing N-hydroxy compounds. *J. Pharm. Pharmacol.* **31**, 476–477.

Bickel M.H. (1969). The pharmacology and biochemistry of N-oxides. *Pharmacol. Rev.* **21**, 325–355.

Bock K.W. (1992). Metabolic polymorphism affecting

activation of toxic and mutagenic arylamines. *Trends Pharmacol. Sci.* **13**, 223–226.

Böcker R.H. and Guengerich F.P. (1986). Oxidation of 4-aryl- and 4-alkyl-substituted 2,6-dimethyl-3,5-*bis*(alkoxycarbonyl)-1,4-dihydropyridines by human liver microsomes and immunochemical evidence for the involvement of a form of cytochrome P-450. *J. Med. Chem.* **29**, 1596–1603.

Boelsterli U.A. and Göldlin C. (1991). Biomechanisms of cocaine-induced hepatocyte injury mediated by the formation of reactive metabolites. *Arch. Toxicol.* **65**, 351–360.

Boersma M.G., Cnubben N.H.P., Van Berkel W.J.H., Blom M., Vervoort J. and Rietjens I.M.C.M. (1993). Role of cytochromes P-450 and flavin-containing monooxygenase in the biotransformation of 4-fluoro-N-methylaniline. *Drug Metab. Disposit.* **21**, 218–230.

Bors W., Michel C., Dalke C., Stettmaier K., Saran M. and Andrae U. (1993). Radical intermediates during the oxidation of nitropropanes. The formation of NO_2 from 2-nitropropane, its reactivity with nucleosides, and implications for the genotoxicity of 2-nitropropane. *Chem. Res. Toxicol.* **6**, 302–309.

Bridges J.W., Gorrod J.W. and Parke D.V., eds (1972). *Biological Oxidation of Nitrogen in Organic Molecules.* Taylor & Francis, London.

Budinski R.A., Roberts S.M., Coats E.A., Adams L. and Hess E.V. (1987). The formation of procainamide hydroxylamine by rat and human liver microsomes. *Drug Metab. Disposit.* **15**, 37–43.

Calder I.C., Hart S.J., Healey K. and Ham K.N. (1981). N-Hydroxyacetaminophen: a postulated toxic metabolite of acetaminophen. *J. Med. Chem.* **24**, 988–993.

Campbell J.J., Glover S.A., Hammond G.P. and Rowbottom C.A. (1991). Evidence for the formation of nitrenium ions in the acid-catalysed solvolysis of mutagenic N-acetoxy-N-alkoxybenzamides. *J. Chem. Soc. Perkin. Trans. 2*, 2067–2079.

Cashman J.R. (1988). Facile N-oxygenation of 1-methyl-4-phenyl-1,2,3,6-tetrahydropyridine by the flavin-containing monooxygenase. *J. Med. Chem.* **31**, 1258–1261.

Cashman J.R. (1989). Enantioselective N-oxygenation of verapamil by the hepatic flavin-containing monooxygenase. *Molec. Pharmacol.* **36**, 497–503.

Cashman J.R. and Ziegler D.M. (1986). Contribution of N-oxygenation to the metabolism of MPTP (1-methyl-4-phenyl-1,2,3,6-tetrahydropyridine) by various liver preparations. *Molec. Pharmacol.* **29**, 163–167.

Cashman J.R., Proudfoot J., Pate D.W. and Högberg T. (1988). Stereoselective N-oxygenation of zimeldine and homozimeldine by the flavin-containing monooxygenase. *Drug Metab. Disposit.* **16**, 616–622.

Cashman J.R., Yang Z.C. and Högberg T. (1990). Oxidation of N-hydroxynorzimeldine to a stable nitrone by hepatic monooxygenases. *Chem. Res. Toxicol.* **3**, 428–432.

Chiba K., Kubota E., Miyakawa T., Kato Y. and Ishizaki T. (1988). Characterization of hepatic microsomal metabolism as an *in vivo* detoxication pathway of 1-methyl-4-phenyl-1,2,3,6-tetrahydropyridine in mice. *J. Pharmacol. Exp. Ther.* **246**, 1108–1115.

Cho A.K. (1988). Metabolic disposition of nitrogen functionalities. In *Biotransformation of Organic Nitrogen Compounds* (eds Cho A.K. and Lindeke B.). pp. 184–212. Karger, Basel.

Cho A.K. and Fukuto J.M. (1988). Chemistry of organic nitrogen compounds. In *Biotransformation of Organic Nitrogen Compounds* (eds Cho A.K. and Lindeke B.). pp. 6–26. Karger, Basel.

Cho A.K. and Lindeke B., eds (1988). *Biotransformation of Organic Nitrogen Compounds.* Karger, Basel.

Clement B. (1983). The N-oxidation of benzamidines *in vitro*. *Xenobiotica* **13**, 467–473.

Clement B. (1984) *In vitro* Untersuchungen zur mikrosomalen N-Oxidation N-substituierter Benzamidine. *Arch. Pharm.* **317**, 925–933.

Clement B. (1985). The biological N-oxidation of amidines and guanidines. In *Biological Oxidation of Nitrogen in Organic Molecules. Chemistry, Toxicology and Pharmacology* (eds Gorrod J.W. and Damani L.A.). pp. 253–266. Horwood, Chichester.

Clement B. (1986). *In vitro* Untersuchungen zur mikrosomalen N-Oxidation einiger Guanidine. *Arch. Pharm.* **319**, 961–968.

Clement B. (1989). Structural requirements of microsomal N-oxygenations derived from studies on amidines. *Drug Metab. Drug. Interact.* **7**, 87–108.

Clement B. and Kunze T. (1990). Hepatic microsomal N-hydroxylation of adenine to 6-hydroxyaminopurine. *Biochem. Pharmacol.* **39**, 925–933.

Clement B. and Zimmermann M. (1987a). Characteristics of the microsomal N-hydroxylation of benzamidine to benzamidoxime. *Xenobiotica* **17**, 659–667.

Clement B. and Zimmermann M. (1987b). Hepatic microsomal N-demethylation of N-methylbenzamidine. N-Dealkylation vs N-oxygenation of amidines. *Biochem. Pharmacol.* **36**, 3127–3133.

Clement B., Zimmermann M. and Schmitt S. (1989). Biotransformation des Benzamidins und des Benzamidoxims durch mikrosomale Enzyme vom Kaninchen. *Arch. Pharm.* **322**, 431–435.

Clement B., Immel M. and Raether W. (1992). Metabolic N-hydroxylation of diminazene *in vitro*. *Arzneim-Forsch. (Drug Res.)* **42**, 1497–1504.

Clement B., Immel M., Schmitt S. and Steinmann U. (1993a). Biotransformations of benzamidine and benzamidoxime *in vivo*. *Arch Pharm.* **326**, 807–812.

Clement B., Jung F. and Pfunder H. (1993b). N-Hydroxylation of benzamidine to benzamidoxime by a reconstituted cytochrome P-450 oxidase system from rabbit liver: involvement of cytochrome P-450 IIC3. *Molec. Pharmacol.* **43**, 335–342.

Clement B., Schultze-Mosgau M.H. and Wohlers H. (1993c). Cytochrome P450 dependent N-hydroxylation of a guanidine (debrisoquine), microsomal catalysed reduction and further oxidation of the N-hydroxyguanidine metabolite to the urea derivative. *Biochem. Pharmacol.* **46**, 2249–2267.

Correia M.A., Decker C., Sugiyama K., Caldera P.,

Bornheim L., Wrighton S.A., Rettie A.E. and Trager W.F. (1987). Degradation of rat hepatic cytochrome P-450 heme by 3,5-dicarbethoxy-2,6-dimethyl-4-ethyl-1,4-dihydropyridine to irreversibly bound protein adducts. *Arch. Biochem. Biophys.* **258**, 436–451.

Coutts R.T. and Beckett A.H. (1977). Metabolic N-oxidation of primary and secondary aliphatic medicinal amines. *Drug Metab. Rev.* **6**, 51–104.

Coutts R.T. and Kovach S.H. (1977). Metabolism *in vitro* of N-methylamphetamine with rat liver homogenates. *Biochem. Pharmacol.* **26**, 1043–1049.

Coutts R.T., Dawe R., Dawson G.W. and Kovach S.H. (1976). *In vitro* metabolism of 1-phenyl-2-propanone oxime in rat liver homogenates. *Drug Metab. Disposit.* **4**, 35–39.

Cowan D.A., Damani L.A. and Gorrod J.W. (1978). Metabolic N-oxidation of 3-substituted pyridines. Identification of products by mass spectrometry. *Biomed. Mass Spectrom.* **5**, 551–556.

Dagne E. and Castagnoli N. Jr (1972). Cotinine N-oxide, a new metabolite of nicotine. *J. Med. Chem.* **15**, 840–841.

Damani L.A. (1982). Oxidation at nitrogen centers. In *Metabolic Basis of Detoxication* (eds Jakoby W.B., Bend J.R. and Caldwell J.). pp. 127–149. Academic Press, New York.

Damani L.A. (1985). Oxidation of tertiary heteroaromatic amines. In *Biological Oxidation of Nitrogen in Organic Molecules. Chemistry, Toxicology and Pharmacology* (eds Gorrod J.W. and Damani L.A.). pp. 205–218. Horwood, Chichester.

Damani L.A. (1988). The flavin-containing mono-oxygenase as an amine oxidase. In *Metabolism of Xenobiotics* (eds Gorrod J.W., Oelschläger H. and Caldwell J.). pp. 59–70. Taylor & Francis, London.

Damani L.A., Pool W.F., Crooks P.A., Kaderlik R.K. and Ziegler D.M. (1988). Stereoselectivity in the N′-oxidation of nicotine isomers by flavin-containing monooxygenase. *Molec. Pharmacol.* **33**, 702–705.

De Graeve J., Gielen J.E., Kahl G.F., Tüttenberg K.H., Kahl R. and Maume B. (1979). Formation of two metyrapone N-oxides by rat liver microsomes. *Drug Metab. Disposit.* **7**, 166–170.

Delaforge M., Jaouen M. and Mansuy D. (1983). Dual effects of macrolide antibiotics on rat liver cytochrome P-450. Induction and formation of metabolite-complexes: a structure–activity relationship. *Biochem. Pharmacol.* **32**, 2309–2318.

DeMaster E.G., Shirota F.N. and Nagasawa H.T. (1992). A Beckmann-type dehydration of *n*-butyraldoxime catalyzed by cytochrome P-450. *J. Org. Chem.* **57**, 5074–5075.

Dipple A., Michejda C.J. and Weisburger E.K. (1985). Metabolism of chemical carcinogens. *Pharmacol. Ther.* **27**, 265–296.

Duncan J.D. and Cho A.K. (1982). N-Oxidation of phentermine to N-hydroxy-phentermine by a reconstituted cytochrome P-450 oxidase system from rabbit liver. *Molec. Pharmacol.* **22**, 235–238.

El-Ghomari K. and Gorrod J.W. (1987). Metabolic N-

oxygenation of 2,4-diamino-6-substituted pyrimidines. *Eur. J. Drug Metab. Pharmacokin.* **12**, 253–258.

Erikson J.M. and Prough R.A. (1986). Oxidative metabolism of some hydrazine derivatives by rat liver and lung tissue fractions. *J. Biochem. Toxicol.* **1**, 41–52.

Feldman P.L., Griffith O.W. and Stuehr D.J. (1993). The surprising life of nitric oxide. *Chem. Engineer News* **71**(51), 26–38.

Felton J.S. and Knize M.G. (1991). Occurrence, identification, and bacterial mutagenicity of heterocyclic amines in cooked foods. *Mutat. Res.* **259**, 205–217.

Ferenczy G.G. and Norris G.M. (1989). The active site of cytochrome P-450 nifedipine oxidase: a model-building study. *J. Molec. Graphics* **7**, 206–211.

Fiala E.S., Kohl N.E., Hecht S.S., Yang J.J. and Shimada T. (1981). The formation of azoxy-2-phenylethane during the biological oxidation of phenylethylamine by rabbit liver microsomes. *Carcinogenesis* **2**, 165–173.

Fleming C.M., Branch R.A., Wilkinson G.R. and Guengerich F.P. (1992). Human liver microsomal N-hydroxylation of dapsone by cytochrome P-4503A4. *Molec. Pharmacol.* **41**, 975–980.

Ford G.P. and Herman P.S. (1992). Relative stabilities of nitrenium ions derived from polycyclic aromatic amines. Relationships to mutagenicity. *Chem.-Biol. Interact.* **81**, 1–18.

Ford G.P. and Griffin G.R. (1992). Relative stabilities of nitrenium ions derived from heterocyclic amine food carcinogens. Relationships to mutagenicity. *Chem.-Biol. Interact.* **81**, 19–33.

Franklin M.R. (1977). Inhibition of mixed-function oxidations by substrates forming reduced cytochrome P-450 metabolic-intermediate complexes. *Pharmacol. Ther. A* **2**, 227–245.

Frederick C.B., Hammons G.J., Beland F.A., Yamazoe Y., Guengerich F.P., Zenser T.V., Ziegler D.M. and Kadlubar F.F. (1985). N-Oxidation of primary aromatic amines in relation to chemical carcinogenesis. In *Biological Oxidation of Nitrogen in Organic Molecules. Chemistry, Toxicology and Pharmacology* (eds Gorrod J.W. and Damani L.A.). pp. 131–148. Horwood, Chichester.

Fukuto J.M., Di Stefano E.W., Burstyn J.N., Valentine J.S. and Cho A.K. (1985). Mechanism of oxidation of N-hydroxyphentermine by superoxide. *Biochemistry* **24**, 4161–4167.

Fukuto J.M., Brady J.F., Burstyn J.N., VanAtta R.B., Valentine J.S. and Cho A.K. (1986). Direct formation of complexes between cytochrome P-450 and nitroso-arenes. *Biochemistry* **25**, 2714–2719.

Gooderham N.J. and Gorrod J.W. (1985). Microsomal N-oxidation of secondary aromatic amines. In *Biological Oxidation of Nitrogen in Organic Molecules. Chemistry, Toxicology and Pharmacology* (eds Gorrod J.W. and Damani L.A.). pp. 81–95. Horwood, Chichester.

Gorrod J.W. (1973). Differentiation of various types of biological oxidation of nitrogen in organic compounds. *Chem.-Biol. Interact.* **7**, 289–303.

Gorrod J.W., ed. (1978a). *Biological Oxidation of Nit-*

rogen. Elsevier/North Holland, Amsterdam.

Gorrod J.W. (1978b). Biological oxidation of nitrogen centres. *Hoppe-Seyler's Z Physiol. Chem.* **359**, 1088.

Gorrod J.W. (1978c). The current status of the pK_a concept in the differentiation of enzymic N-oxidation. In *Biological Oxidation of Nitrogen* (ed. Gorrod J.W.). pp. 201–210. Elsevier/North Holland, Amsterdam.

Gorrod J.W. (1985a). Chemical determinants of the enzymology of organic nitrogen oxidation. *Drug Metab. Disposit.* **13**, 283–286.

Gorrod J.W. (1985b). Amine–imine tautomerism as a determinant of the site of biological N-oxidation. In *Biological Oxidation of Nitrogen in Organic Molecules. Chemistry, Toxicology and Pharmacology* (eds Gorrod J.W. and Damani L.A.). pp. 219–230. Horwood, Chichester.

Gorrod J.W. (1987). The *in vitro* metabolism of amino azaheterocycles. In *Drug Metabolism—from Molecules to Man* (eds Benford D.J., Bridges J.W. and Gibson G.G.). pp. 456–461. Taylor & Francis, London.

Gorrod J.W. and Damani L.A., eds (1985). *Biological Oxidation of Nitrogen in Organic Molecules. Chemistry, Toxicology and Pharmacology.* Horwood, Chichester.

Gorrod J.W. and Christou M. (1986). Metabolic N-hydroxylation of substituted acetophenone imines. I. Evidence for formation of isomeric oximes. *Xenobiotica* **16**, 575–585.

Gorrod J.W. and Raman A. (1989). Imines as intermediates in oxidative aralkylamine metabolism. *Drug Metab. Rev.* **20**, 307–339.

Guengerich F.P. (1990). Low kinetic hydrogen isotope effects in the dehydrogenation of 1,4 - dihydro - 2,6 - dimethyl - 4 - (2 - nitrophenyl) - 3,5 - pyridinedicarboxylic acid dimethyl ester (nifedipine) by cytochrome P-450 enzymes are consistent with an electron/proton/electron transfer mechanism. *Chem. Res. Toxicol.* **3**, 21–26.

Guengerich F.P. and Böcker R.H. (1988). Cytochrome P-450-catalyzed dehydrogenation of 1,4-dihydropyridines. *J. Biol. Chem.* **263**, 8168–8175.

Guengerich F.P., Brian W.R., Iwasaki M., Sari M.A., Bäärnhielm C. and Berntsson P. (1991). Oxidation of dihydropyridine calcium channel blockers and analogues by human liver cytochrome P-450 IIIA4. *J. Med. Chem.* **34**, 1838–1844.

Hanna P.E., Gammans R.E., Sehon R.D. and Lee M.K. (1980). Metabolic N-hydroxylation. Use of substituent variation to modulate the *in vitro* biactivation of 4-acetamidostilbenes. *J. Med. Chem.* **23**, 1038–1044.

Hartman G.D. and Schlegel H.B. (1981). The relationship of the carcinogenic/mutagenic potential of arylamines to their singlet-triplet nitrenium ion energies. *Chem.-Biol. Interact.* **36**, 319–330.

Hata Y., Watanabe M., Matsubara T. and Touchi A. (1976). Fragmentation reaction of ylide. 5. A new metabolic reaction of aziridine derivatives. *J. Amer. Chem. Soc.* **98**, 6033–6036.

Hata Y., Watanabe M., Shiratori O. and Takase S. (1978). Cytotoxic activity and fragmentation of aziridines in microsomes. *Biochem. Biophys. Res. Commun.* **80**, 911–916.

Heimans R.L.H., Fennessy M.R. and Gaff G.A. (1971). Some aspects of the metabolism of morphine N-oxide. *J. Pharm. Pharmacol.* **23**, 831–836.

Hines R.N. and Prough R.A. (1980). The characterization of an inhibitory complex formed with cytochrome P-450 and a metabolite of 1,1-disubstituted hydrazines. *J. Pharmacol. Exp. Ther.* **214**, 80–86.

Jeffrey E.H. and Mannering G.J. (1983). Interaction of constitutive and phenobarbital-induced cytochrome P-450 isozymes during the sequential oxidation of benzphetamine. *Molec. Pharmacol.* **23**, 748–757.

Jenner P., Gorrod J.W. and Beckett A.H. (1973). Species variation in the metabolism of (R)-(+)- and (S)-(−)-nicotine by α-C- and N-oxidation *in vitro*. *Xenobiotica* **3**, 573–580.

Kadlubar F.F., Butler M.A., Kaderlik K.R., Chou H.C. and Lang N.P. (1992). Polymorphisms for aromatic amine metabolism in humans: relevance for human carcinogenesis. *Environm. Health Perspect.* **98**, 69–74.

Kapetanovic I.M., Strong J.M. and Mieyal J.J. (1979). Metabolic structure–activity relationships for a homologous series of phenacetin analogs. *J. Pharmacol. Exp. Ther.* **209**, 20–24.

Kennedy C.H. and Mason R.P. (1990). A reexamination of the cytochrome P-450-catalyzed free radical production from a dihydropyridine. *J. Biol. Chem.* **265**, 11,425–11,428.

Kerdar R.S., Dehner D. and Wild D. (1993). Reactivity and genotoxicity of arylnitrenium ions in bacterial and mammalian cells. *Toxicol. Lett.* **67**, 73–85.

Kim S.G., Philpot R.M. and Novak R.F. (1991). Pyridine effects on P450IIE1, IIB and IVB expression in rabbit liver: characterization of high- and low-affinity pyridine N-oxygenases. *J. Pharmacol. Exp. Therap.* **259**, 470–477.

Kirkpatrick D., Weston K.T., Hawkins D.R., Chasseaud L.F. and Elsom L.F. (1977). Identification of an N-oxide as the major metabolite of the analgesic O-(diethylaminoethyl)-4-chlorobenzaldoxime hydrochloride in dogs. *Xenobiotica* **7**, 747–755.

Kloss M.W., Rosen G.M. and Rauckman E.J. (1984). Biotransformation of norcocaine to norcocaine nitroxide by rat brain microsomes. *Psychopharmacology* **84**, 221–224.

Klunk L.J., Riska P.S. and Maynard D.E. (1982). The disposition and metabolism of ^{14}C-tiaramide•HCl in man. *Drug Metab. Disposit.* **10**, 241–245.

Koymans L., Van Lenthe J.H., Donné-Op den Kelder G.M. and Vermeulen N.P.E. (1990). Mechanisms of oxidation of phenacetin to reactive metabolites by cytochrome P450: A theoretical study involving radical intermediates. *Molec. Pharmacol.* **37**, 452–460.

Koymans L., Donné-Op den Kelder G.M., te Koppele J.M. and Vermeulen N.P.E. (1993a). Generalized cytochrome P450-mediated oxidation and oxygenation reactions in aromatic substrates with activated N–H, O–H, C–H, or S–H substituents. *Xenobiotica* **23**, 633–648.

Koymans L., Menge W.M.P.B., Van Lenthe J.H., Donné-Op den Kelder G.M., te Koppele J.M. and Vermeulen N.P.E. (1993b). A theoretical study on the oxidative metabolism of 4-chloroacetanilide by cytochrome P450: alternative mechanisms for migration of 4-substituents during enzymatic oxidation. *Recl. Trav. Chim. Pays-Bas* **112**, 186–190.

Kurebayashi H. (1989). Kinetic deuterium effects on deamination and N-hydroxylation of cyclohexylamine by rabbit liver microsomes. *Arch. Biochem. Biophys.* **270**, 320–329.

LaCagnin L.B., Colby H.D. and O'Donnell J.P. (1986). The oxidative metabolism of hydralazine by rat liver microsomes. *Drug Metab. Disposit.* **14**, 549–554.

Lee J.S., Jacobsen N.E. and Ortiz de Montellano P.R. (1988). 4-Alkyl radical extrusion in the cytochrome P-450-catalyzed oxidation of 4-alkyl-1,4-dihydropyridines. *Biochemistry* **27**, 7703–7710.

Lemoine A., Johann M. and Cresteil T. (1990). Evidence for the presence of distinct flavin-containing monooxygenases in human tissues. *Arch. Biochem. Biophys.* **276**, 336–342.

Lenk W. and Riedl M. (1989). N-Hydroxy-N-arylacetamides. V. Differences in the mechanism of haemoglobin oxidation *in vitro* by N-hydroxy-4-chloroacetanilide and N-hydroxy-4-chloroaniline. *Xenobiotica* **19**, 453–475.

Lindeke B. (1982). The non- and postenzymatic chemistry of N-oxygenated molecules. *Drug Metab. Rev.* **13**, 71–121.

Lindeke B. and Paulsen-Sörman U. (1988). Nitrogenous compounds as ligands to hemoproteins—the concept of metabolic-intermediary complexes. In *Biotransformation of Organic Nitrogen Compounds* (eds Cho A.K. and Lindeke B.). pp. 63–102. Karger, Basel.

Lindeke B., Anderson E., Lundkvist G., Jonsson U. and Eriksson S.O. (1975). Autoxidation of N-hydroxyamphetamine and N-hydroxyphentermine. *Acta Pharm. Suec.* **12**, 183–198.

Lloyd R.V., Shuster L. and Mason R.P. (1993). Reexamination of the microsomal transformation of N-hydroxynorcocaine to norcocaine nitroxide. *Molec. Pharmacol.* **43**, 645–648.

Lundström J., Högberg T., Gosztonyi T. and de Paulis T. (1981). Metabolism of zimeldine in rat, dog and man. *Arzneim-Forsch. (Drug Res.)* **31**, 486–494.

Mansuy D., Rouer E., Bacot C., Gans P., Chottard J.C. and Leroux J.P. (1978a). Interaction of aliphatic N-hydroxylamines with microsomal cytochrome P450: nature of the different derived complexes and inhibitory effects on monoxygenase activities. *Biochem. Pharmacol.* **27**, 1229–1237.

Mansuy D., Beaune P., Cresteil T., Bacot C., Chottard J.C. and Gans P. (1978b). Formation of complexes between microsomal cytochrome P-450-Fe(II) and nitrosoarenes obtained by oxidation of arylhydroxylamines or reduction of nitroarenes *in situ. Eur. J. Biochem.* **86**, 573–579.

Mansuy D., Battioni P. and Mahy J.P. (1982). Isolation of an iron-nitrene complex from the dioxygen and iron porphyrin dependent oxidation of a hydrazine. *J. Amer. Chem. Soc.* **104**, 4487–4489.

Maret G., Testa B., Jenner P., El Tayar N. and Carrupt P.A. (1990). The MPTP story: MAO activates tetrahydropyridine derivatives to toxins causing parkinsonism. *Drug Metab. Rev.* **22**, 291–332.

Marsden J.T. and Gorrod J.W. (1985). The failure to detect N-hydroxylation as a metabolic pathway for a series of carbamates. In *Biological Oxidation of Nitrogen in Organic Molecules. Chemistry, Toxicology and Pharmacology* (eds Gorrod J.W. and Damani L.A.). pp. 192–196. Horwood, Chichester.

Matsumoto R.M. and Cho A.K. (1982). Conversion of N-hydroxyamphetamine to phenylacetone oxime by rat liver microsomes. *Biochem. Pharmacol.* **31**, 105–108.

Maynard M.S. and Cho A.K. (1981). Oxidation of N-hydroxyphentermine to 2-methyl-2-nitro-1-phenyl-propane by liver microsomes. *Biochem. Pharmacol.* **30**, 111–1119.

McManus M.E., Stupans I., Burgess W., Koening J.A., de la M Hall P. and Birkett D.J. (1987a). Flavin-containing monooxygenase activity in human liver microsomes. *Drug Metab. Disposit.* **15**, 256–261.

McManus M.E., Davies D.S., Boobis A.R., Grantham P.H. and Wirth P.J. (1987b). Guanethidine N-oxidation in human liver microsomes. *J. Pharm. Pharmacol.* **39**, 1052–1055.

Mitchard M., Kendall M.J. and Chan K. (1971). Pethidine N-oxide: a metabolite in human urine. *J. Pharm. Pharmacol.* **24**, 915.

Miwa G.T. and Walsh J.S. (1988). Cytochrome P450 in nitrogen metabolism. In *Biotransformation of Organic Nitrogen Compounds* (eds Cho A.K. and Lindeke B.). pp. 27–62. Karger, Basel.

Moloney S.J. and Prough R.A. (1983). Biochemical toxicology of hydrazines. In *Reviews in Biochemical Toxicology*, Vol. 5 (eds Hodgson E., Bend J.R. and Philpot R.M.). pp. 313–348. Elsevier Biomedical, New York.

Moloney S.J., Snider B.J. and Prough R.A. (1984). The interactions of hydrazine derivatives with rat-hepatic cytochrome P-450. *Xenobiotica* **14**, 803–814.

Nelson S.D. (1985). Arylamines and arylamides: Oxidation mechanisms. In *Bioactivation of Foreign Compounds* (ed. Anders M.W.). pp. 349–374. Academic Press, Orlando.

Niwa T., Tokuma Y., Nakagawa K. and Noguchi H. (1989). Stereoselective oxidation of nivaldipine, a new dihydropyridine calcium antagonist, in rat and dog liver. *Drug Metab. Disposit.* **17**, 64–68.

Noda A., Noda H., Misaka A., Sumimoto H. and Tatsumi K. (1988). Hydrazine radical formation catalyzed by rat microsomal NADPH-cytochrome P450 reductase. *Biochem. Biophys. Res. Commun.* **153**, 256–260.

Noguchi H., Tada K. and Iwasaki K. (1982). Urinary metabolite profile of tiaramide in man and some animal species. *Xenobiotica* **12**, 211–220.

Oelschläger H. and Al Shaik M. (1985). Metabolic N-oxidation of alicyclic amines. In *Biological Oxidation of Nitrogen in Organic Molecules. Chemistry, Toxicology and Pharmacology* (eds Gorrod J.W. and Damani L.A.). pp. 60–75. Horwood, Chichester.

Oelschläger H.A.H., Temple D.J. and Temple C.F. (1975).

The metabolism of the local anaesthetic fomocaine in the rat and dog after oral application. *Xenobiotica* **5**, 309–323.

Øie S., Guentert T.W., Tolentino L. and Hermodsson G. (1992). Pharmacokinetics of moclobemide in male, virgin female, pregnant and nursing rats. *J. Pharm. Pharmacol.* **44**, 413–418.

Ortiz de Montellano P.R. (1989). Cytochrome P-450 catalysis: radical intermediates and dehydrogenation reactions. *Trends Pharmacol. Sci.* **10**, 354–359.

Ortiz de Montellano P.R. and Watanabe M.D. (1987). Free radical pathways in the *in vitro* hepatic metabolism of phenelzine. *Molec. Pharmacol.* **31**, 213–219.

Ortiz de Montellano P.R., Augusto O., Viola F. and Kunze K.L. (1983). Carbon radicals in the metabolism of alkyl hydrazines. *J. Biol. Chem.* **258**, 8623–8629.

Patterson L.H., Hall G., Nijar B.S., Khatra P.K. and Cowan D.A. (1986). *In vitro* metabolism of lignocaine to its N-oxide. *J. Pharm. Pharmacol.* **38**, 326.

Pershing L.K. and Franklin M.R. (1982). Cytochrome P-450 metabolic-intermediate complex formation and induction by macrolide antibiotics; a new class of agents. *Xenobiotica* **12**, 687–699.

Poulsen L.L., Masters B.S.S. and Ziegler D.M. (1976). Mechanism of 2-naphthylamine oxidation catalysed by pig liver microsomes. *Xenobiotica* **6**, 481–498.

Prough R.A. and Moloney S.J. (1985). Hydrazines. In *Bioactivation of Foreign Compounds* (ed. Anders M.W.). pp. 433–449. Academic Press, Orlando.

Prough R.A., Freeman P.C. and Hines R.N. (1981). The oxidation of hydrazine derivatives catalyzed by the purified liver microsomal FAD-containing monooxygenase. *J. Biol. Chem.* **256**, 4178–4184.

Prough R.A., Erikson J.M. and Wiebkin P. (1988). Nitrogen oxidation in toxicity. In *Biotransformation of Organic Nitrogen Compounds* (eds Cho A.K. and Lindeke B.). pp. 161–183. Karger, Basel.

Quon C.Y. (1988). Nitrogen oxidation in carcinogenesis. In *Biotransformation of Organic Nitrogen Compounds* (eds Cho A.K. and Lindeke B.). pp. 132–160. Karger, Basel.

Rashed M.S., Streeter A.J. and Nelson S.D. (1989). Investigations of the N-hydroxylation of 3'-hydroxyacetanilide, a non-hepatotoxic positional isomer of acetaminophen. *Drug Metab. Disposit.* **17**, 355–359.

Rauckman E.J., Rosen G.M. and Kitchell B.B. (1979). Superoxide radical as an intermediate in the oxidation of hydroxylamines by mixed function amine oxidase. *Molec. Pharmacol.* **15**, 131–137.

Riddick D.S., Park S.S., Gelboin H.V. and Marks G.S. (1990a). Effects of 4-alkyl analogues of 3,5-diethoxycarbonyl-1,4-dihydro-2,4,6-trimethylpyridine on hepatic cytochrome P-450 heme, apoproteins and catalytic activities following *in vivo* administration to rats. *Molec. Pharmacol.* **37**, 130–136.

Riddick D.S., McGilvray I. and Marks G.S. (1990b). Inactivation of rat liver microsomal steroid hydroxylations by 4-alkyl analogues of 3,5-diethoxycarbonyl-1,4-dihydro-2,4,6-trimethylpyridine. Evidence for selectivity

among steroid-inducible cytochrome-P450IIIA forms. *Can J. Physiol. Pharmacol.* **68**, 1533–1541.

Roos P.H., Golub-Ciosk B., Kallweit P., Kauczinski D. and Hanstein W.G. (1993). Formation of ligand and metabolite complexes as a means for selective quantitation of cytochrome P450 isozymes. *Biochem. Pharmacol.* **45**, 2239–2250.

Rose J. and Castagnoli N. Jr (1983). The metabolism of tertiary amines. *Med. Res. Rev.* **3**, 73–88.

Ruenitz P.C., Bagley J.R. and Mokler C.M. (1983). Metabolism of clomiphene in the rat. Estrogen receptor affinity and antiestrogen activity of clomiphene metabolites. *Biochem. Pharmacol.* **32**, 2941–2947.

Sabourin P.J. and Hodgson E. (1984). Characterization of the purified microsomal FAD-containing monooxygenase from mouse and pig liver. *Chem.-Biol. Interact.* **51**, 125–139.

Schwartz M.A., Williams T.H., Kolis S.J., Postma E. and Sasso G.J. (1978). Biotransformation of prochiral 2-phenyl-1,3-di(4-pyridyl)-2-propanol to a chiral N-oxide metabolite. *Drug Metab. Disposit.* **6**, 647–653.

Smith M.R. and Gorrod J.W. (1978). The microsomal N-oxidation of some primary aromatic amines. In *Biological Oxidation of Nitrogen* (ed. Gorrod J.W.). pp. 65–70. Elsevier/North Holland, Amsterdam.

Sternson L.A. and Gammans R.E. (1975). A mechanistic study of aromatic hydroxylamine rearrangement in the rat. *Bioorg. Chem.* **4**, 58–63.

Streeter A.J. and Hoener B.A. (1988). Evidence for the involvement of a nitrenium ion in the covalent binding of nitrofurazone to DNA. *Pharm. Res.* **5**, 434–436.

Sugimura T. (1988). New environmental carcinogens in daily life. *Trends Pharmacol. Sci.* **9**, 205–209.

Sugiyama K., Yao K., Rettie A.E. and Correia M.A. (1989). Inactivation of rat hepatic cytochrome P-450 isozymes by 3,5-dicarbethoxy-2,6-dimethyl-4-ethyl-1,4-dihydropyridine. *Chem. Res. Toxicol.* **2**, 400–410.

Sum C.Y. and Cho A.K. (1977). The N-hydroxylation of phentermine by rat liver microsomes. *Drug Metab. Disposit.* **5**, 464–468.

Tatsumi K., Kitamura S. and Sumida M. (1984). Formation of N-nitrosodiphenylamine from 1,1-diphenylhydrazine by rat liver microsomal preparations. *Biochem. Biophys. Res. Commun.* **118**, 958–963.

Terashita S., Tokuma Y., Sekiguchi M. and Noguchi H. (1989). Sex differences in the metabolism and excretion of nivaldipine, a new dihydropyridine calcium antagonist, in rats. *Xenobiotica* **19**, 1221–1229.

Testa B. and Jenner P. (1976). *Drug Metabolism. Chemical and Biochemical Aspects*. pp. 61–73. Dekker, New York.

Testa B. and Jenner P. (1978). Novel drug metabolites produced by functionalization reactions. Chemistry and toxicology. *Drug Metab. Rev.* **7**, 325–369.

Testa B. and Jenner P. (1981). Inhibitors of cytochrome P-450s and their mechanisms of action. *Drug Metab. Rev.* **12**, 1–117.

Testa B., Jenner P., Beckett A.H. and Gorrod J.W. (1976). A reappraisal of the stereoselective metabolism of nicotine to nicotine-1'-N-oxide. *Xenobiotica* **6**, 553–556.

Thorgeirsson S.S., McManus M.E. and Glowinski I.B. (1984). Metabolic processing of aromatic amides. In *Drug Metabolism and Drug Toxicity* (eds Mitchell J.R. and Horning M.G.). pp. 183–197. Raven, New York.

Tinel M., Descatoire V., Larrey D., Loeper J., Labbe G., Letteron P. and Pessayre D. (1989). Effects of clarithromycin on cytochrome P-450. Comparison with other macrolides. *J. Pharmacol. Exp. Ther.* **250**, 746–751.

Tuck S.F. and Ortiz de Montellano P.R. (1992). Topological mapping of the active sites of cytochrome-P4502B1 and cytochrome-P4502B2 by *in situ* rearrangement of aryl-iron complexes. *Biochemistry* **31**, 6911–6916.

Turesky R.J. (1990). Metabolism and biodisposition of heterocyclic amines. *Prog. Clin. Biol. Res.* **347**, 39–53.

Tweedie D.J., Erikson J.M. and Prough R.A. (1987). Metabolism of hydrazine anti-cancer agents. *Pharmacol. Therap.* **34**, 111–127.

Tynes R.E. and Hodgson E. (1985). Catalytic activity and substrate specificity of the flavin-containing monooxygenase in microsomal systems: characterization of the hepatic, pulmonary and renal enzymes of the mouse, rabbit and rat. *Arch. Biochem. Biophys.* **240**, 77–93.

Tyrakowska B., Boeren S., Guertsen B. and Rietjens I.M.C.M. (1993). Qualitative and quantitative influences of *ortho* chlorine substituents on the microsomal metabolism of 4-toluidines. *Drug Metab. Disposit.* **21**, 508–519.

Uetrecht J.P. (1985). Reactivity and possible significance of hydroxylamine and nitroso metabolites of procainamide. *J. Pharmacol. Exp. Ther.* **232**, 420–425.

Usansky J.I. and Damani L.A. (1992). The urinary metabolic profile of metyrapone in the rat. Identification of two novel isomeric metyrapol N-oxide metabolites. *Drug Metab. Disposit.* **20**, 64–69.

Weinkaum R.J. and Shiba D.A. (1978). Metabolic activation of procarbazine. *Life Sci.* **22**, 937–946.

Weli A.M. and Lindeke B. (1985). The metabolic fate of pargyline in rat liver microsomes. *Biochem. Pharmacol.* **34**, 1993–1998.

White K.A. and Marletta M.A. (1992). Nitric oxide synthase is a cytochrome P-450 type hemoprotein. *Biochemistry* **31**, 6627–6631.

Wild D. (1993). Arylnitrenium ions and the genotoxic potency of aromatic amines and nitro compounds. *Adv. Mutagen. Res.* **4**, 16–30.

Williams D.E., Reed R.L., Kedzierski B., Ziegler D.M. and Buhler D.R. (1989). The role of flavin-containing monooxygenase in the N-oxidation of the pyrrolizidine alkaloid senecionine. *Drug Metab. Disposit.* **17**, 380–392.

Yuno K., Yamada H., Oguri K. and Yoshimura H. (1990). Substrate specificity of guinea pig liver flavin-containing monooxygenase for morphine, tropane and strychnos alkaloids. *Biochem. Pharmacol.* **40**, 2380–2382.

Ziegler D.M. (1984). Metabolic oxygenation of organic nitrogen and sulfur compounds. In *Drug Metabolism and Drug Toxicity* (eds Mitchell J.R. and Horning M.G.). pp. 33–53. Raven, New York.

Ziegler D.M. (1985). Molecular basis of N-oxygenation of *sec-* and *tert*-amines. In *Biological Oxidation of Nitrogen in Organic Molecules. Chemistry, Toxicology and Pharmacology* (eds Gorrod J.W. and Damani L.A.). pp. 43–52. Horwood, Chichester.

Ziegler D.M. (1988). Flavin-containing monooxygenases: catalytic mechanism and substrate specificities. *Drug Metab. Rev.* **19**, 1–32.

chapter 6

MONOOXYGENASE-CATALYZED N–C CLEAVAGE

Contents

6.1 INTRODUCTION

Having in previous chapters examined separately the oxidation of carbon and nitrogen atoms, we can now turn our attention to the fate of the N–C moiety as a target of the monooxygenases. Here, the nitrogen atom is present in an amino or amido function, while the carbon atom is in the sp^3-hybridized state; one exception to this last condition is presented in Section 6.4. Note that cleavage of the N–C moiety will also be encountered in later chapters, being mediated for example by monoamine oxidase (Chapter 9), or hydrolytic enzymes in the case of amido groups (see Volume 2). Hydrolytic cleavage of some N=C moieties has been discussed in Sections 5.3 (oximes) and 5.7 (hydrazones).

The monooxygenase-mediated oxidation of the N–C moiety almost always involves **cytochrome P450**, and more often than not results in the cleavage of the N–C bond (Lindeke and Cho, 1982). Typical reactions are: (a) **N-dealkylations** (when the carbon atom is part of an alkyl group); (b) **deaminations** (when the amino group is detached from the remainder of the molecule); and (c) **opening of saturated azaheterocycles**. But, as we shall see, the distinction between N-dealkylation and deamination is not always straightforward and may even be quite arbitrary. Mechanistic differences between the three reaction types are more formal than genuine.

What may markedly differ, in contrast, are the **pharmacological and pharmacokinetic consequences** of N-dealkylation vs. deamination and ring opening. When N-dealkylation involves the loss of a small group such as methyl (N-demethylation) or ethyl (N-deethylation), it is usually found that the pharmacological activity of the nitrogen-retaining metabolite is comparable to that of the parent drug. In contrast, loss of the amino group or ring opening normally destroys the pharmacophore with qualitative changes in the pharmacodynamic profile.

6.2 N-DEMETHYLATION AND THE MECHANISMS OF OXIDATIVE N–C CLEAVAGE

The simplest case of oxidative N–C cleavage is N-demethylation. This is also a very well-documented reaction, both from a mechanistic viewpoint and from the great variety of substrates. For this reason, the mechanisms of oxidative N–C cleavage are discussed here using data obtained with the N-methyl moiety. Mechanistic peculiarities of N-dealkylation, deamination and ring opening, when they exist, will be mentioned in the relevant sections.

6.2.1 Mechanisms of oxidative N–C cleavage

A mechanistic scheme of N-demethylation is given in Fig. 6.1. The **"direct" path** involves **initial hydrogen abstraction** and subsequent alpha-carbon hydroxylation (reactions **a** and **b** in Fig. 6.1) by the classical oxygen rebound mechanism of cytochrome P450-mediated C-sp^3 hydroxylation

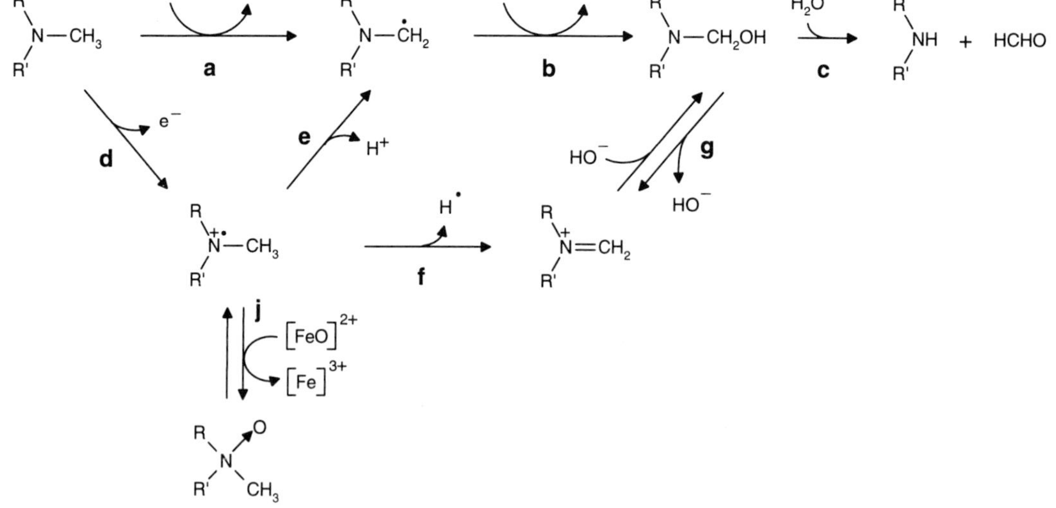

FIGURE 6.1 General mechanistic scheme of cytochrome P450-catalyzed N-demethylation and related reactions. Reactions **a**, **b** and **c** define the "direct" path (initial hydrogen abstraction).

(Section 4.2) (Burka *et al.*, 1985; Heimbrook *et al.*, 1984). The **carbinolamine** thus formed is quite unstable as a rule and hydrolyzes rapidly (reaction **c** in Fig. 6.1) to the demethylated amine and formaldehyde. The latter will be oxidized by dehydrogenases (Section 2.3) to formic acid and then to CO_2.

The **lack of stability of some carbinolamines**, however, is not so great as to prevent them from completely escaping detection. Thus, N-hydroxymethylcarbazole (**6.II**) was found as a metabolite of N-methylcarbazole (**6.I**) following incubation with liver microsomes of various animal species; this metabolite was also found as a conjugate (probably the O-glucuronide) in the urine of some species (Gorrod and Temple, 1976). Compound **6.II** decomposed spontaneously to carbazole and formaldehyde at pH 7.4 and 37°C, but the reaction was markedly accelerated in the presence of liver microsomes from various animal species. In a systematic study of N,N-dimethyl derivatives of arylamines (**6.III**), aryltriazenes (**6.IV**), arylformamidines (**6.V**) and arylureas (**6.VI**), their incubation with mouse liver microsomes resulted in formaldehyde production. Only in the case of arylureas (**6.VI**) were the formaldehyde progenitors (the carbinolamines) stable enough to be detectable by the colorimetric method used (Ross *et al.*, 1982). Interestingly, 1-(2,4,6-trichlorophenyl)-3,3-dimethyltriazene, a ring-substituted analogue of triazenes **6.IV**, yielded the O-glucuronide of its carbinolamine as a urinary metabolite in rats (Kolar and Carubelli, 1979). **Carbinolamines of aromatic amides** appear particularly stable, witness N-hydroxymethylbenzamide (**6.VII**) which has a half-live of about 10^4 min in buffer at pH 7.4 and 37°C (Ross *et al.*, 1983).

The above results suggest that electronic factors may account for an increase in the chemical stability of carbinolamines. Another factor may be operative, namely stabilization by intra-molecular hydrogen bonding. This is documented for **xanthine N-carbinols** as metabolic intermediates of methylxanthines (see Section 6.2.2) (Lander *et al.*, 1988). Thus, 1-hydroxy-methyltheobromine (**6.IX**, R = CH_2OH, R′ = R″ = CH_3), 3-hydroxymethylparaxanthine (**6.IX**,

R	= −CH₃	6.I
R	= −CH₂OH	6.II

6.III

6.IV

6.V

6.VI

R	= −CH₂OH	6.VII
R	= −CHO	6.VIII

6.IX

6.X

6.XI

6.XII

R′ = CH₂OH, R = R″ = CH₃) and 7-hydroxymethyltheophylline (**6.IX**, R″ = CH₂OH, R = R′ = CH₃) are stable enough to allow characterization (Lander *et al.*, 1988). The structure of the latter compound is displayed again as **6.X** to exemplify the internal hydrogen-bond.

Beside the N-demethylation pathway depicted as reactions **a**, **b** and **c** in Fig. 6.1, other reactions have been characterized in some cases and disproven in others. The formation of the C-centred radical via the aminium cation radical (reactions **d** and **e** in Fig. 6.1) has been discussed in Chapter 5 (Fig. 5.1). An intermediate playing a distinct role in some reactions of N-demethylation, and more generally N–C cleavage, is the **iminium ion** generated from the carbinolamine by reaction **g** (Fig. 6.1) (Burka *et al.*, 1985). This reaction does not occur with N-hydroxymethylcarbazole (**6.II**), the reason being the very low basicity of the parent amine (pK_a about −8) (Kedderis *et al.*, 1983; Overton *et al.*, 1985). In contrast, a number of rather basic amines were conclusively shown to yield the intermediate iminium ion, whose formation can be characterized indirectly by oxygen exchange with water, and directly by trapping with nucleophiles such as the cyanide anion (Overton *et al.*, 1985). Two representative examples are intermediates **6.XI** and **6.XII**, the iminium ions of nicotine and methapyrilene, respectively (Overton *et al.*, 1985; Ziegler *et al.*, 1981). These iminium ions being markedly electrophilic can react with nucleophiles and are thus potentially toxic intermediates (Overton *et al.*, 1985).

As indicated in Fig. 6.1, the possibility also exists for the iminium ion to be generated from the aminium cation radical (reaction **f**) itself formed by N-oxidation (reaction **d**) (Shannon and Bruice, 1981). In fact, it is now believed that the N-dealkylation of a number of basic amines involves **initial electron abstraction** (reactions **d** in Fig. 6.1), while the N-demethylation of amides has conclusively been shown to occur by initial hydrogen abstraction (reactions **a** and **b** in Fig. 6.1) (Constantino *et al.*, 1992; Hall and Hanzlik, 1990).

A role for **N-oxides** as intermediates in the N-dealkylation of tertiary amines has repeatedly been postulated (Bickel, 1969). While the rearrangement mechanisms implied by such processes are realistic, no convincing proof seems to exist that they are indeed involved in metabolic N-demethylation, and more generally N-dealkylation (Lindeke, 1982). What may occur, however, and has been documented by isotope effects, is a mechanism by which an N-oxide such as N,N-dimethylaniline N-oxide is **reduced** by cytochrome P450 (Section 12.4), thereby acting as an oxygen donor to the enzyme (Heimbrook *et al.*, 1984; Seto and Guengerich, 1993). The N-demethylation step follows immediately without the tertiary amine having had time to leave the active site. This reaction, however, had a very slow turnover number, and may well be restricted to a limited number of substrates and cytochromes P450 (Burka *et al.*, 1985). What can also be added to Fig. 6.1 is the fact that the aminium cation radical generated in reaction **d** is the intermediate by which cytochrome P450 forms N-oxides (Chapter 5, Figure 5.1, pathway A2); the reversibility of the reaction **j** (Fig. 6.1) follows from the above arguments (Burka *et al.*, 1985; Heimbrook *et al.*, 1984). **Cocaine (6.XIII)** serves as a good example for such a route. Besides undergoing direct cytochrome P450-catalyzed N-demethylation, cocaine was also found to be N-demethylated by a more complex route involving N-oxygenation by FAD-containing monooxygenase followed by cytochrome P450-mediated demethylation of the N-oxide via the iminium cation, as depicted in Fig. 6.1 (Kloss *et al.*, 1983).

6.XIII

6.XIV

Carbinolamines of relatively good stability may be substrates for dehydrogenases to yield **N-formyl derivatives** (formamides) (reaction **h** in Fig. 6.1), the latter then hydrolyzing to the demethylated amine and formic acid (reaction **i** in Fig. 6.1). Thus, N-hydroxymethylbenzamide (**6.VII**), whose stability is discussed above, did indeed yield N-formylbenzamide (**6.VIII**) in a reaction catalyzed by liver alcohol dehydrogenase (Ross *et al.*, 1983). In contrast to the carbinolamine, N-formylbenzamide at pH 7.4 and 37°C degraded rapidly to benzamide with a half-life of about 8 min. The same reaction has been characterized in the *in vivo* and *in vitro* N-demethylation of aminopyrine (Noda *et al.*, 1976). When investigated in its own right, the metabolism of aliphatic N-methylformamides (i.e. $-N(CH_3)CHO$) can be quite complex and lead to a variety of products several of which in fact retain the formyl moiety (Slatter *et al.*, 1989).

To end this section, let us briefly indicate that N-dealkylation reactions are not mediated exclusively by cytochrome P450. Indeed, **FAD-containing monooxygenases** may be involved in the N-demethylation (and more generally N-dealkylation) of secondary amines, as exemplified by methylamphetamine (Baba *et al.*, 1987). This compound is oxidized by the flavin-containing monooxygenase to the hydroxylamine and then to the nitrone (**6.XIV**) (see Fig. 5.5, Section 5.3), the latter undergoing non-enzymatic hydrolysis to yield formaldehyde and N-hydroxyamphetamine. This pathway affords another example of **N-dealkylation via hydrolysis** of an N=C moiety (see Section 6.1).

6.2.2 Substrate selectivity in N-demethylation reactions

Metabolic reactions of N-demethylation are displayed by a large variety of N-methylated amines, and seemingly by every type of $N-CH_3$ group that has been investigated. This is true for tertiary as well as secondary amines, but it is consistently found that tertiary amines are demethylated faster than secondary ones. In other words, in the sequence below, the first step is generally found to be faster than the second:

$$-N(CH_3)_2 \rightarrow -NH-CH_3 \rightarrow -NH_2$$

The first type of substrates to be considered here is that of aromatic amines, e.g. **N-methylated anilines**. For example, the demethylation of N,N-dimethylaniline was examined using four purified liver microsomal cytochromes P450, showing that rabbit CYP2B4 and rat CYP2B1 (i.e. phenobarbital-inducible forms) were markedly more active than rabbit CYP1A2 and rat CYP1A1 (Pandey *et al.*, 1989). In a different perspective, the N-demethylation of twelve *para*-substituted N,N-dimethylanilines (**6.XV**) was investigated in liver microsomes from phenobarbital-pretreated rats (Galliani *et al.*, 1984). Quantitative structure–metabolism relationships showed that the affinity (as expressed by K_m, the Michaelis constant) increased together with the lipophilicity of the substrate, while the maximal velocity of the reaction (V_{max}) increased with increasing lipophilicity of the substrate and decreasing electron-withdrawing power of the substituent X. The same electronic influence was seen on the k_{cat} of N-demethylation of N,N-dimethylanilines (Macdonald *et al.*, 1989). These findings are of interest in indicating that electron-withdrawing substituents deactivate substrates presumably by rendering the $-N(CH_3)_2$ group less susceptible to electrophilic attack.

Many important drugs are **N-methylated arylalkylamines** whose N-demethylation leads to metabolites with diminished lipophilicity but comparable basicity. In a series of N-methyl-2-phenylethylamines (**6.XVI**, R = methyl, ethyl, isopropyl, isobutyl and benzyl), N-demethylation by rat liver microsomes proceeded at comparable V_{max} values, while affinity (as assessed by K_m) increased with increasing lipophilicity (Duncan *et al.*, 1983). This relation may explain, at least in part, why secondary amines are N-demethylated more slowly than tertiary amines.

An interesting compound is **diltiazem (6.XVII)**, a calcium channel antagonist which undergoes a variety of metabolic reactions in humans and animals. The secondary amine was

6.XV

6.XVI

6.XVII

shown to be a major urinary metabolite in humans, whereas the primary amine was a minor metabolite (Sugawara *et al.*, 1988). In humans and rabbits, CYP3A are the major enzymes involved in the N-demethylation of diltiazem (Pichard *et al.*, 1990). This reaction is just as effective for arylalkylamines with complex ring systems, for example tricyclic neuroleptic and antidepressants, as repeatedly reported in the literature (e.g. Lemoine *et al.*, 1993; Ohmori *et al.*, 1993).

Beside amines, a number of **other nitrogen functionalities** are substrates for N-demethylation, as seen with amides, azo compounds, N-methylated aryltriazenes (**6.IV**), arylformamidines (**6.V**) and arylureas (**6.VI**) (Section 6.2.1). For example, the N-demethylation of 1-aryl-3,3-dimethyltriazenes (**6.IV**) by mouse liver microsomes was restricted to the loss of one methyl group only and was not markedly influenced by the nature of the *para*-substituent (Godin *et al.*, 1981). In such compounds, N-demethylation appears to follow the sequence of reactions **a**, **b** and **c** in Fig. 6.1 (Iley and Ruecroft, 1990).

A number of **saturated azaheterocycles** bearing an N-methyl group undergo extensive demethylation. This is true for smaller or larger heterocycles, whether or not part of a complex molecule. **Morphine** (**6.XVIII**, R = H) affords a good example of a piperidine ring enclosed in a complex molecule; its N-demethylation is amply documented in humans and animals. The same reaction was examined in rat liver microsomes for a homologous series of eleven 3-O-alkylmorphine analogues (**6.XVIII**, R = methyl (i.e. codeine) to decyl and dodecyl) (Duquette *et al.*, 1983). The K_m for the reaction declined with increasing chain length from 1 to 9 carbons, while the V_{max} increased to a maximum for the butyl analogue and then declined for longer chains; the decyl and dodecyl analogues were not N-demethylated, nor did they show any detectable binding spectrum. For the other analogues, a good correlation was seen between the type I binding dissociation constant and lipophilicity.

A drug such as the central analgesic **meptazinol** (**6.XIX**) undergoes a number of reactions of oxidation on its ethyl side-chain and azepine ring; the N-demethylated metabolite, although minor, nevertheless accounted for about 5% of a dose in humans (Murray *et al.*, 1989). Other examples of seven-membered azaheterocycles are provided by benzodiazepines, **diazepam** (**6.XX**)

6.XVIII

6.XIX

6.XX   R = —CH$_3$

6.XXIV   R = —CH$_2$—C≡CH

6.XXV   R = —CH$_2$—△

being a representative substrate. Its N-demethylation to the long-acting desmethyldiazepam is a major route in humans, together with C(3)-hydroxylation (Inaba *et al.*, 1988).

The N-demethylation of **caffeine** (**6.IX**, R = R′ = R″ = CH$_3$, see also Section 6.2.1) is of significance for a number of reasons such as the regioselectivity of the reaction and the pharmacological importance of the xenobiotic itself. Studies using human liver microsomes showed N(3)-demethylation (yielding paraxanthine) to markedly predominate over N(1)- and N(7)-demethylation (yielding theobromine and theophylline, respectively) whose rates were comparable (Grant *et al.*, 1987). CYP1A2 is the enzyme primarily responsible for the N(3)-demethylation of caffeine in human liver, while the formation of other demethylated metabolites is mediated, at least in part, by other P450 enzymes (Berthou *et al.*, 1991 and 1992; Butler *et al.*, 1989; Fuhr *et al.*, 1992; Kalow and Campbell, 1988). Following administration of caffeine to humans, the plasma concentrations and AUCs (areas-under-the-curve) of the parent compound and paraxanthine were comparable, whereas those of theophylline and theobromine tended to be one order of magnitude smaller (Kalow, 1985). There is thus a good concordance between *in vivo* and *in vitro* regioselectivity of caffeine N-demethylation.

6.3 N-DEALKYLATION AND DEAMINATION

6.3.1 N-Dealkylation of saturated alkyl groups

Several N-alkyl groups are known to be cleaved from a variety of exogenous substrates by N-dealkylation. The reaction has many similarities to N-demethylation (Section 6.2) and requires the presence of at least one hydrogen atom on the alpha-carbon. The alkyl group itself is oxidized and released as a carbonyl derivative (Fig. 6.2, pathway **A**).

Whether N-dealkylation proceeds faster or more slowly than N-demethylation depends on a number of biological factors as well as on the chemical nature of the N-substituent; as a rule, the N-dealkylation of simple alkyl groups bearing no functional group is slower than N-demethylation due to steric factors. When the metabolism of N-ethyl-N-methylaniline was investigated in rabbit liver microsomes, it was found that the first metabolic step of

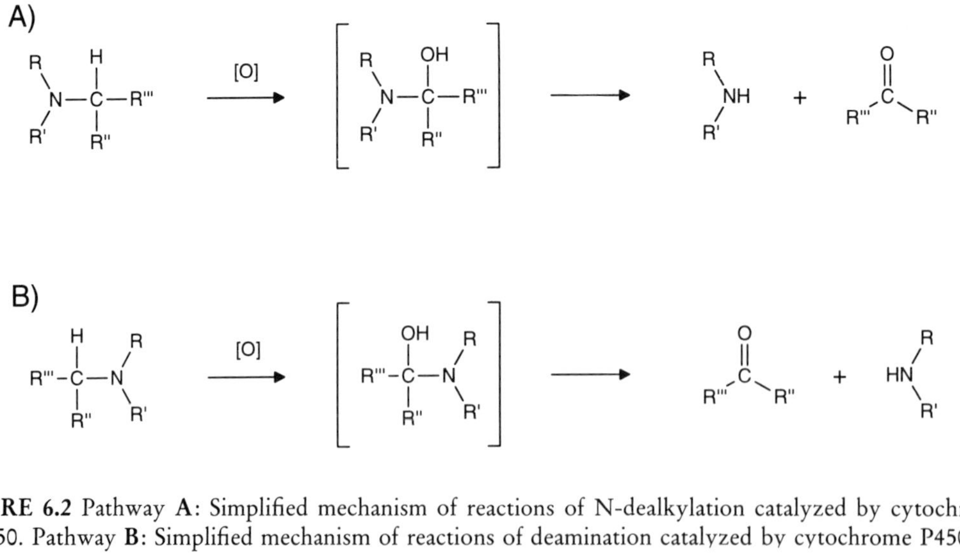

FIGURE 6.2 Pathway **A**: Simplified mechanism of reactions of N-dealkylation catalyzed by cytochrome P450. Pathway **B**: Simplified mechanism of reactions of deamination catalyzed by cytochrome P450.

6.XXI   6.XXII

N-demethylation was severalfold faster than N-deethylation; the second step to yield the primary amine was in turn much slower than the first (Gorrod *et al.*, 1975). Comparable results were reported for tertiary amides (Hall and Hanzlik, 1991).

N-Deethylation is a common reaction since a number of drugs bear an N-ethyl or N,N-diethyl group. Thus, the N-deethylation of **lidocaine (6.XXI)** was one of the first to be investigated from a mechanistic viewpoint and led to significant insights (Nelson *et al.*, 1975). For a substrate like N-propylamphetamine (**6.XXII**, R = H, R' = *n*-propyl), N-dealkylation was the major route in rat liver homogenates, but it is interesting to note that hydroxylation of the beta-carbon on the propyl substituent was also detected (Coutts *et al.*, 1976). Upon incubation of N-alkyl-N-methylanilines with rabbit liver microsomes, the rates of N-dealkylation followed the sequence **methyl > ethyl > *n*-propyl = *n*-butyl > isopropyl = isobutyl**; no N-dealkylation of *sec*-butyl and *tert*-butyl groups was seen (Gorrod *et al.*, 1979). The failure to remove the *sec*-butyl group is probably ascribable to steric hindrance preventing C(α)-hydroxylation, whereas the *tert*-butyl group, having no hydrogen on the alpha-carbon, cannot undergo hydroxylation at this position. Note however that a very few cases of slow N-dealkylation of a *tert*-butyl group have been detected; the reaction is believed to occur via loss of a methyl group by oxidative decarboxylation, in effect transforming the *tert*-butyl group into an isopropyl group (Section 4.2) (Kamm and Szuna, 1973).

6.3.2 N-Dealkylation of unsaturated and functionalized alkyl groups

Unsaturated substituents (e.g. arylalkyl, alkenyl and alkynyl groups) are also targets of N-dealkylation. The **N-benzyl** group is of relatively frequent occurrence in medicinal chemistry and is particularly sensitive to N-dealkylation (Hall and Hanzlik, 1991). Thus, the biotransformation of benzphetamine (**6.XXII**, R = methyl, R' = benzyl) was investigated under a variety of *in vitro* and *in vivo* conditions, allowing an interesting comparison between the two pathways of N-demethylation and N-debenzylation (Inoue *et al.*, 1983). The comparative effectiveness of N-debenzylation as compared to cleavage of alkyl substituents may be ascribed to the methylene group being activated by the phenyl ring (benzylic position, see Section 4.2.5). A similar activation accounts for reactions of N-dealkylation involving **allyl** (–CH$_2$–CH=CH$_2$) and particularly **propargyl** (–CH$_2$–C≡CH) groups. An interesting drug in this context is **pargyline** (**6.XXIII**), the metabolism of which was investigated in rat liver microsomes (Weli *et al.*, 1985). While N-oxygenation was the most effective route, the relative rates of the three reactions of N-dealkylation was **N-depropargylation > N-demethylation > N-debenzylation**. The importance of steric factors has been demonstrated by the fact that N-depropargylation and

6.XXIII

N-debenzylation were markedly decreased in homologues with a methyl group attached to the alpha-carbon of the propargyl or benzyl substituent, respectively.

The above example is one of **intramolecular** competition between metabolic routes, i.e. regioselective metabolism. **Intermolecular** comparison (i.e. substrate selectivity) may also lead to valuable conclusions provided the substrates are structurally very close, for example **diazepam (6.XX)** and **pinazepam (6.XXIV)**. N-Dealkylation of these two drugs to produce N-demethyldiazepam occurs at markedly different rates in rat liver microsomes, N-depropargylation of pinazepam being eightfold faster than N-demethylation of diazepam (Marcucci *et al.*, 1981). This result is in line with the metabolism of pargyline discussed above. The **cyclopropylmethyl** group, which is known to chemists to be partially unsaturated in character, is cleaved quite effectively from **prazepam (6.XXV)** in rats, but more slowly in humans and dogs (Viau *et al.*, 1973).

The N-cyclopropylmethyl substituent of pinazepam and a number of other drugs should not be confused with the **N-cyclopropyl** moiety, which is also oxidized by cytochrome P450, leading to its irreversible inhibition. This mechanism-based inhibition has been characterized for N-cyclopropylbenzylamines **(6.XXVI, R = H)** and N-cyclobutylbenzylamines, and was first thought to result from alpha-carbon hydroxylation. Later studies using N-(1-methylcyclopropyl)benzylamine **(6.XXVI, R = methyl)** and 1-phenylcyclobutylamine indicated one-electron oxidation of the nitrogen atom as a more likely mechanism, the N-centred radical rearranging by ring opening to form C-centred radicals themselves leading to enzyme adducts or oxygenated metabolites (Bondon *et al.*, 1989; Guengerich *et al.*, 1984; Hall and Hanzlik, 1991; Hanzlik and Tullman, 1982).

6.XXVI   6.XXVII

Functionalized substituents also undergo N-dealkylation, e.g. the **2-hydroxyethyl** (–CH$_2$CH$_2$OH) and **2-cyanoethyl** (–CH$_2$CH$_2$CN) groups. Another example is provided by the antimalarial drug **primaquine (6.XXVII)**, the side-chain of which is cleaved in humans by N-dealkylation to give 8-amino-6-methoxyquinoline (Baty *et al.*, 1975). More complex cases will be discussed in Section 6.3.4.

6.3.3 Oxidative deamination

Deamination is the reaction by which aliphatic amines lose their amino group. The mechanism of this metabolic route is presented in simplified form in Fig. 6.2, pathway **B**, showing its almost complete similarity with N-dealkylation. Examples of deamination reactions abound in the literature, beginning with the epoch-making paper of Axelrod (1955) on the *in vitro* metabolism of amphetamine **(6.XXII, R = R' = H)**. Its derivative ethylamphetamine **(6.XXII, R = H, R' = ethyl)** undergoes both N-deethylation and deamination; the latter reaction, which leads to the formation of phenylacetone (Fig. 6.2, pathway **B**, R = benzyl, R' = methyl), was found to

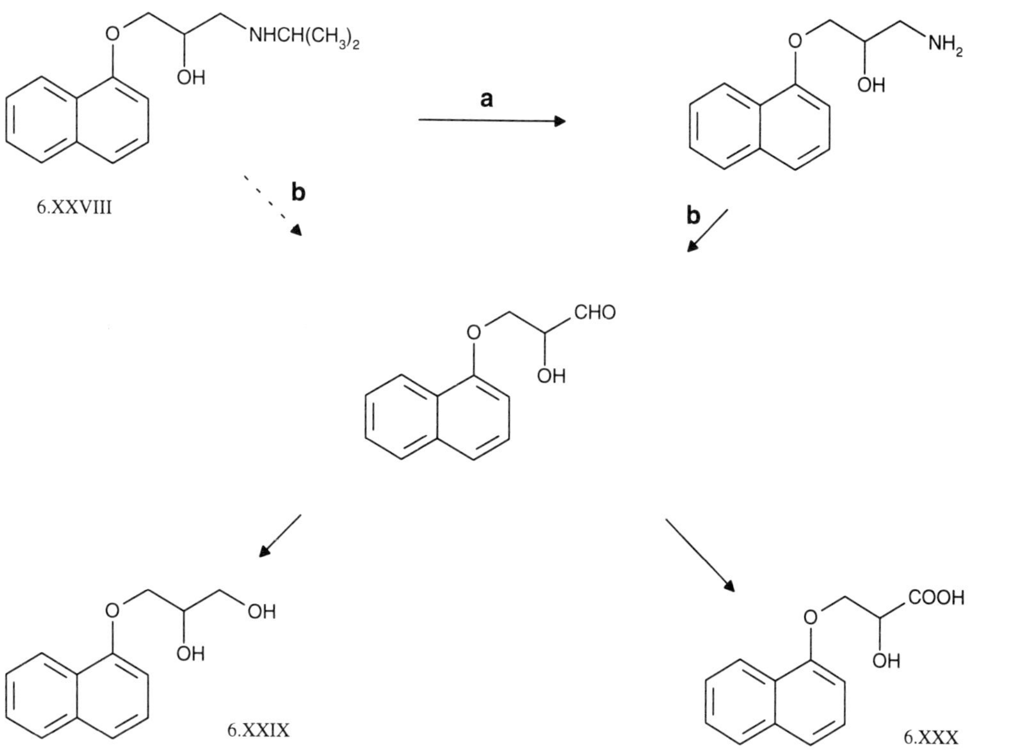

FIGURE 6.3 Reactions of N-dealkylation (reaction **a**) and deamination (reactions **b**) in the metabolism of propranolol (**6.XXVIII**), leading to the formation of a diol (**6.XXIX**) and an acid (**6.XXX**) metabolite.

proceed with higher affinity (lower K_m) but lower velocity than the former reaction in rabbit liver microsomes (Beckett and Haya, 1978).

Numerous other drugs with a basic side-chain undergo deamination, e.g. β-blockers, antihistamines and antipsychotics. These drugs are usually arylalkylamines with a **secondary or tertiary amino group**, deamination involving the parent drug and/or its N-dealkylated metabolite(s). When the alpha position is a methylene group, the resulting aldehyde is rapidly reduced to the primary alcohol and oxidized to the carboxylic acid (Chapter 2). Taking **propranolol (6.XXVIII** in Fig. 6.3) as an example, its major metabolic routes are N-dealkylation and deamination. Most of the dose being deaminated is first dealkylated, indicating that deamination of the parent drug is minor compared to that of deisopropylpropranolol. The aldehyde produced by deamination is rapidly reduced to 3-(1-naphthoxy)-1,2-propanediol (**6.XXIX** in Fig. 6.3) or oxidized to naphthoxylactic acid (**6.XXX** in Fig. 6.3). This oxidative degradation of the side-chain of propranolol is an important process in humans, accounting for 14–30% of a dose on chronic administration of the drug (Nelson and Bartels, 1984).

In the case of **diltiazem (6.XVII)**, deamination is also an important route in humans and rats, leading to the formation and excretion of **6.XXXI** and other metabolites with an acetic acid side-chain (Sugawara *et al.*, 1988).

Cycloalkylamines afford another example of the deamination of **primary amines**, witness the formation of cyclohexanone (**6.XXXIII**) from cyclohexylamine (**6.XXXII**). Among homologues and analogues, the rates of deamination in rabbit liver microsomes decreased in the

6.XXXI

6.XXXII   6.XXXIII

6.XXXIV   6.XXXV

following order: cyclopentylamine > cycloheptylamine = 1-aminotetralin (**6.XXXV**) > cyclohexylamine = 1-aminoindane (**6.XXXIV**) = 2-aminotetralin (**6.XXXV**) > 2-aminoindane (**6.XXXIV**) (Kurebayashi *et al.*, 1988). It is difficult to rationalize such data in terms of structure–metabolism relationships, except that the oxidation of the benzylic position could account for the faster deamination of the 1-amino derivatives of indane and tetralin relative to the 2-isomers.

As mentioned above and discussed in Section 5.3, deamination may also occur as a consequence of N-oxygenation, as seen with the **hydrolytic cleavage** of oximes to form carbonyl derivatives.

6.3.4 N-Dealkylation/deamination

When comparing pathways **A** and **B** in Fig. 6.2 (N-dealkylation and deamination, respectively), the only difference one can see is the point of view taken to describe the reaction, i.e. the viewpoint of the molecule versus that of the leaving group. When the reaction splits the substrate into two molecules of comparable size, the distinction between N-dealkylation and deamination becomes arbitrary and even meaningless. Such cases are not rare and are generally labelled as N-dealkylations for reasons of convenience.

A few representative examples are shown in Fig. 6.4. Thus, **terfenadine (6.XXXVI)**, a piperidine derivative, yielded the secondary amine shown in Fig. 6.4 as a major urinary metabolite in humans in a reaction catalyzed mainly by CYP3A enzymes (Garteiz *et al.*, 1982; Yun *et al.*, 1993). The same reaction gave rise to an N-monosubstituted piperazine from

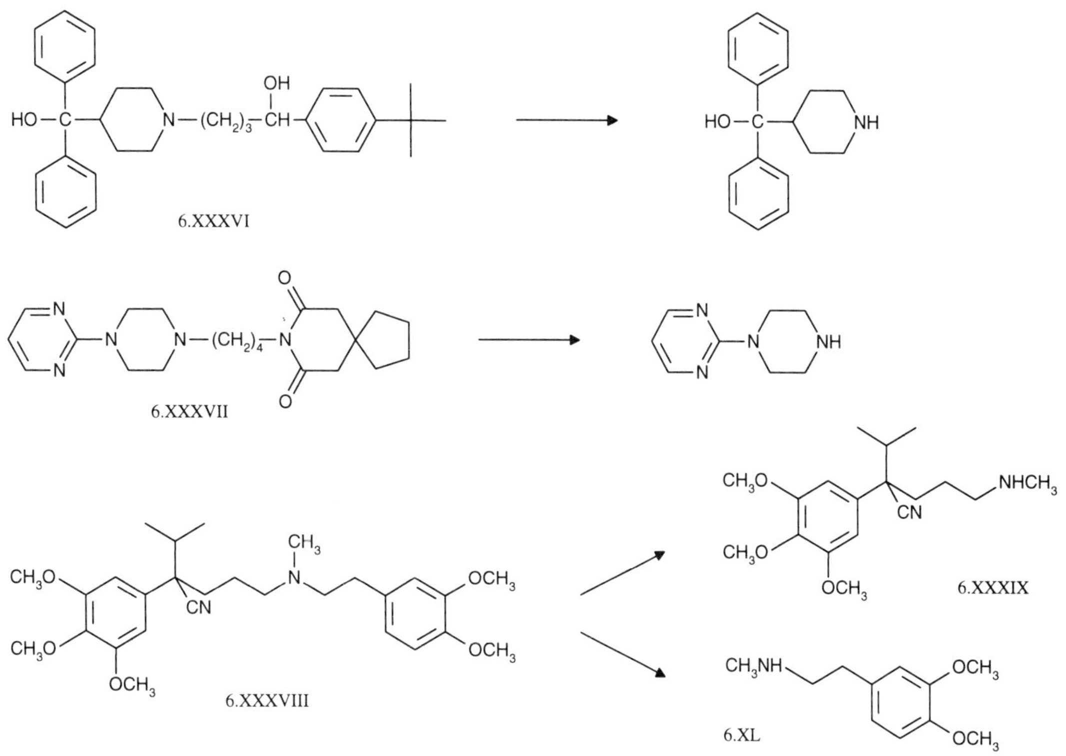

FIGURE 6.4 Some representative examples of reactions of N-dealkylation/deamination and the resulting amine metabolites. The substrates are terfenadine (**6.XXXVI**), buspirone (**6.XXXVII**) and gallopamil (**6.XXXVIII**). For further details see text.

buspirone (**6.XXXVII** in Fig. 6.4). This metabolite appeared in significant amounts in body fluids and tissues of rats dosed with the drug; it was also a major plasma and urine metabolite in humans (Caccia *et al.*, 1986). The third drug in Fig. 6.4 is **gallopamil** (**6.XXXVIII**), an analogue of verapamil. Three reactions of N-dealkylation are possible for this substrate and were quantitated in human and rat liver microsomes. While N-demethylation predominated, the formation of **6.XXXIX** (Fig. 6.4) by removal of the phenylethyl moiety was second in importance; the formation of the phenylethylamine derivative **6.XL** (Fig. 6.4) was very minor in rat liver microsomes and undetectable in human liver microsomes (Mutlib and Nelson, 1990). Note that the corresponding alcohol and carboxyl metabolites resulting from the two reactions of N-dealkylation (i.e. the deaminated products) were also detected and measured.

6.4 ALPHA-CARBON OXIDATION IN SATURATED AZAHETEROCYCLES

In saturated (and partly saturated) azaheterocycles, oxidative ring opening is analogous to N-dealkylation/deamination. This type of reaction has indeed been detected in numerous cases, but careful studies have always revealed a variety of metabolites and shown the complexity of underlying mechanisms. The general metabolic scheme of Fig. 6.1 is also valid for cytochrome P450-catalyzed alpha-carbon oxidation of azaheterocyclic compounds, but the cyclic nature of the substrate gives rise to additional metabolites. This is the case of two types of stable and often major metabolites, namely lactams and their corresponding ring-opened carboxylic acids. The formation of lactams occurs via the sequence of reactions **a**, **b** and **h** in Fig. 6.1, with reaction **g** also being involved. The formation of carboxylic acids occurs via reaction **c** rather than reaction **h** in Fig. 6.1.

6.4.1 Heterocycles containing one nitrogen atom

Formation of **lactams** is a common metabolic route of saturated azaheterocycles. For example, meptazinol (**6.XIX**) yielded the 7-oxo, but not the isomeric 2-oxo metabolite in humans (Murray *et al.*, 1989). For the well-known neurotoxin **MPTP** (**6.XLI**, 1-methyl-4-phenyl-1,2,3,6-tetrahydropyridine), oxidation to lactams is a reaction of detoxication. Three such metabolites (**6.XLII** mainly, but also the saturated piperidinone analogue and the 5,6-dihydropyridinone

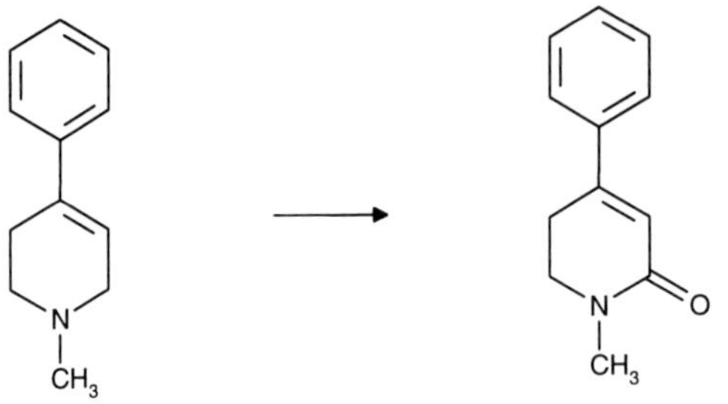

6.XLI

6.XLII

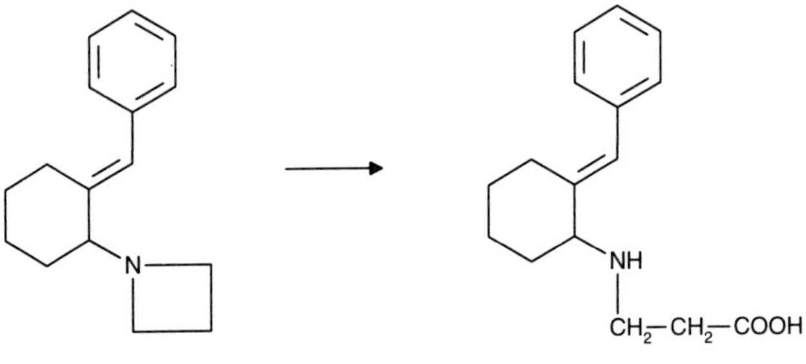

6.XLIII

6.XLIV

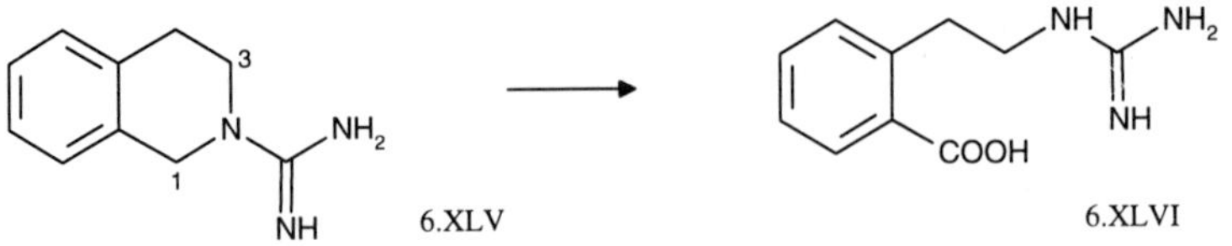

6.XLV

6.XLVI

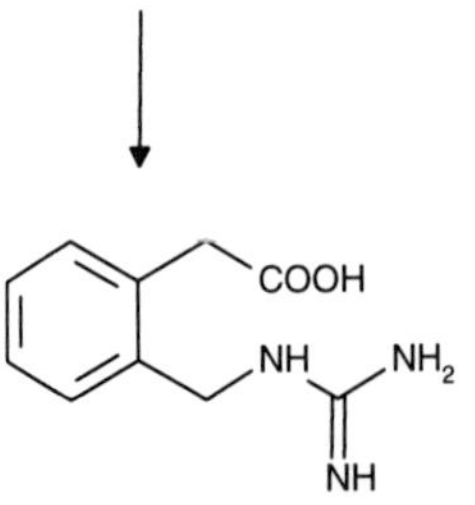

6.XLVII

derivative) were characterized in large amounts in the liver of rats dosed with the compound (Arora *et al.*, 1988).

An example of **ring opening** with formation of an amino acid can be found in the biotransformation of tazadolene (**6.XLIII**), the azetidine ring of which is opened to a β-alanine moiety, affording **6.XLIV** as a major *in vivo* metabolite in various animal species (Darlington *et al.*, 1987). Debrisoquine (**6.XLV**) is also of interest in the present context since C(1)–N and C(3)–N cleavage lead to benzoic acid and phenylacetic acid derivatives (**6.XLVI** and **6.XLVII**), respectively; these two acidic metabolites were characterized in the urine of humans and animals dosed with the drug (Allen *et al.*, 1976).

The acidic metabolites discussed above retain the total number of carbon atoms of the parent compound. However, it must be realized that they may not necessarily be metabolic end-points and that **oxidative chain shortening** may yield products markedly reduced in size. Thus, the antimalarial drug mefloquine (**6.XLVIII**) is transformed into the quinolinic acid **6.XLIX**, a major urinary metabolite in rats (Jauch *et al.*, 1980). Here, the entire piperidine ring is lost by unknown routes.

6.XLVIII   6.XLVIII

The above examples were chosen to illustrate the fact that saturated and partly unsaturated azaheterocycles of various sizes undergo alpha-carbon oxidation, but they say nothing about **mechanism(s) and metabolic intermediates** (Overton *et al.*, 1985). For this purpose, we now turn our attention to a few well-studied xenobiotics, beginning with nicotine (Fig. 6.5).

A major metabolic route of (**S**)-nicotine is C(5')-hydroxylation (reaction **a** in Fig. 6.5) leading to ring opening by C(5')-N cleavage. *A priori*, reaction **a** can be initiated by one-electron N-oxidation or C(5')-hydroxylation, but decisive proof in favour of one or the other mechanism may be difficult to obtain as the $\Delta^{1'(5')}$-**iminium ion** and the **5'-carbinolamine** exist in a pH-dependent equilibrium (reaction **b** in Fig. 6.5). The two forms co-exist in the neutral and weakly alkaline pH range, while only the carbinolamine exists in strongly alkaline media (Brandänge and Lindblom, 1979). Proof of the formation of nicotine $\Delta^{1'(5')}$-iminium species came from its trapping with cyanide to give 5'-cyanonicotine (Nguyen *et al.*, 1979; Peterson *et al.*, 1987). But whatever the mechanism of initial oxidative attack, formation of the iminium ion occurs with loss of the 5'-*pro-E* proton, indicating that the transition state at the active site of cytochrome P450 must be a highly ordered one (Peterson *et al.*, 1987).

The 5'-carbinolamine of nicotine exists in a **ring–chain tautomeric equilibrium** with an aldehyde (reaction **c** in Fig. 6.5) (Brandänge and Lindblom, 1979; Obach and Van Vunakis, 1988). Neither tautomer is stable metabolically, but they are both substrates for oxidases and/or dehydrogenases to yield a **lactam** (reaction **d** in Fig. 6.5) and an **amino acid** (reaction **e** in Fig. 6.5), respectively. Reaction **d** (Fig. 6.5) in particular is catalyzed by aldehyde oxidase (Section 9.5) (Hibberd and Gorrod, 1983; Obach and Van Vunakis, 1988); the lactam thus produced is

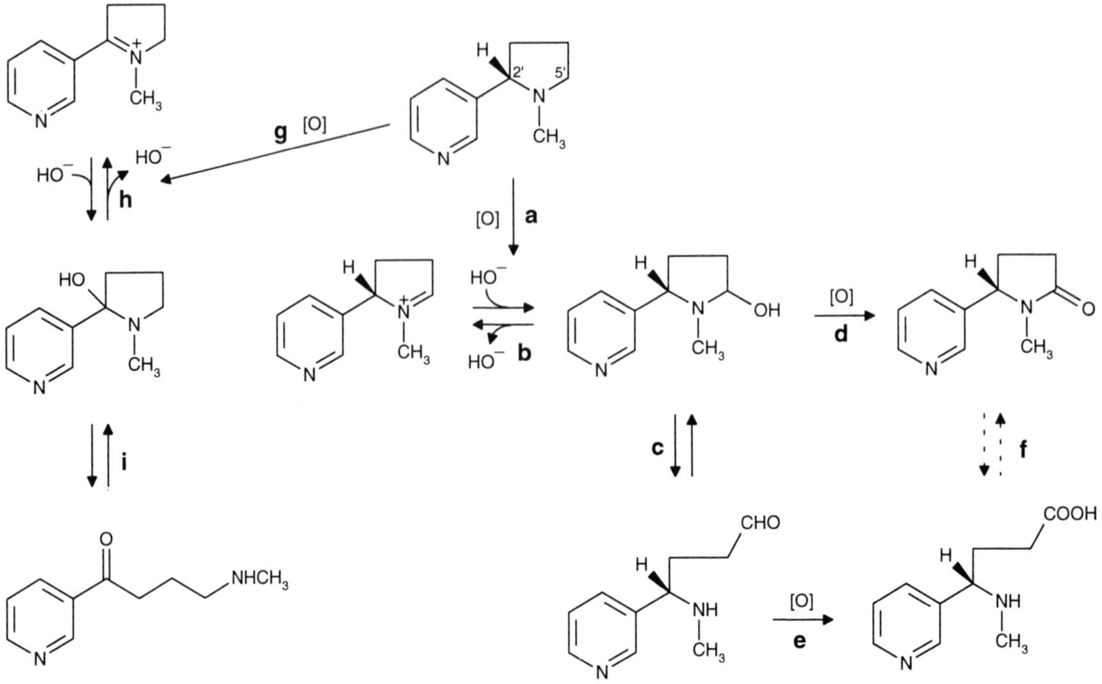

FIGURE 6.5 Mechanisms of monooxygenase-catalyzed oxidative opening of the pyrrolidine ring of (S)-nicotine. Reactions **a** and **g** lead to C(5')-N and C(2')-N cleavage, respectively.

cotinine, the major metabolite of nicotine under a variety of conditions. Note that cotinine and the corresponding amino acid could interconvert by hydration/dehydration (reaction **f** in Fig. 6.5), but reactions of this type appear negligible under physiological conditions, when detected at all.

A second nicotine iminium ion exists, namely the $\Delta^{1'(2')}$-**iminium** species formed by reaction **g** (Fig. 6.5). This is indeed a metabolic reaction of nicotine, and its products are also in two equilibria, namely an iminium–carbinolamine equilibrium (reaction **h** in Fig. 6.5), and a ring–chain equilibrium with a ketone, and not, as above, a secondary alcohol in equilibrium with lactam and the amino acid cannot be formed since the carbinolamine is a tertiary alcohol in ring-chain equilibrium with a ketone, and not, as above, a secondary alcohol in equilibrium with an aldehyde. Reaction **g** in Fig. 6.5 is also known to occur with cotinine, again producing a carbinolamine in equilibrium with a ketone (Nguyen et al., 1981).

Fig. 6.5 gives some indication that the nature of the metabolites produced by ring oxidation depends markedly on the chemical structure of the heterocycle. This can be verified by comparing the metabolism of nicotine (a 2-substituted pyrrolidine) with that of a 3-substituted pyrrolidine such as **3-(p-chlorophenyl)pyrrolidine**, a potential prodrug of baclofen (Fig. 6.6). In rat liver and brain preparations, hydroxylation of the 5-position of the pyrrolidine ring (reaction **a** in Fig. 6.6) ultimately led to the active drug baclofen (4-amino-3-(p-chlorophenyl)butyric acid), while hydroxylation of the 2-position (reaction **b** in Fig. 6.6) led to a positional isomer of baclofen (Wall and Baker, 1989). In rat brain homogenates, the 2- and 5-lactams were produced in amounts equivalent to those of the ring-openend amino acids, while in rat liver preparations the lactam pathways were largely predominant. Interestingly, route **a** in Fig. 6.6 was favoured over route **b**, presumably for reasons of steric accessibility.

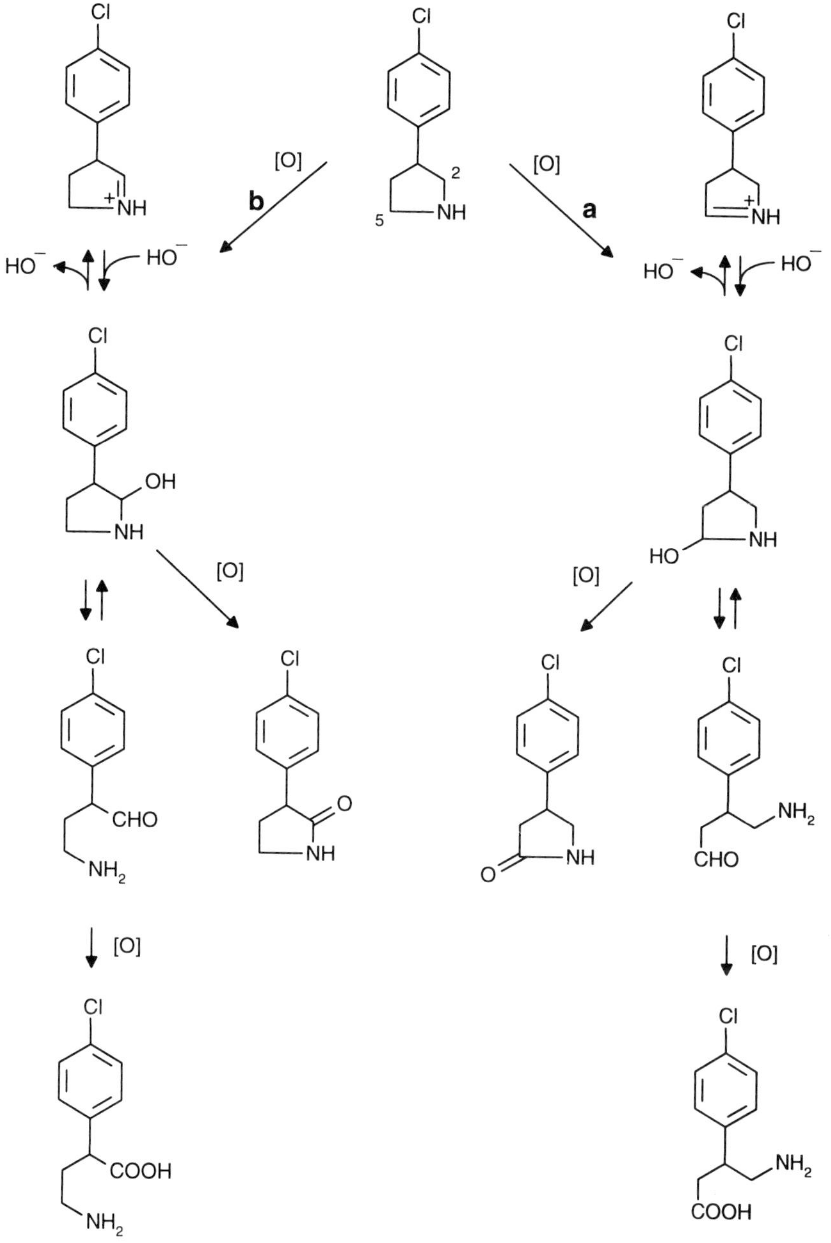

FIGURE 6.6 Postulated mechanisms of ring oxidation of 3-(*p*-chlorophenyl)pyrrolidine leading to the formation of isomeric lactams and ring-opened amino acids (Wall and Baker, 1989).

Nicotine (Fig. 6.5) and 3-(*p*-chlorophenyl)pyrrolidine (Fig. 6.6) are secondary cyclic amines substituted in position alpha (2-yl) or beta (3-yl) to the nitrogen atom. Overall, their oxidation is not different from that of tertiary cyclic amines with a substituent on the nitrogen atom (1-yl type), as exemplified by **phencyclidine**. The oxidative metabolism of the piperidine ring in phencyclidine is summarized in Fig. 6.7, a number of metabolites and intermediates shown having

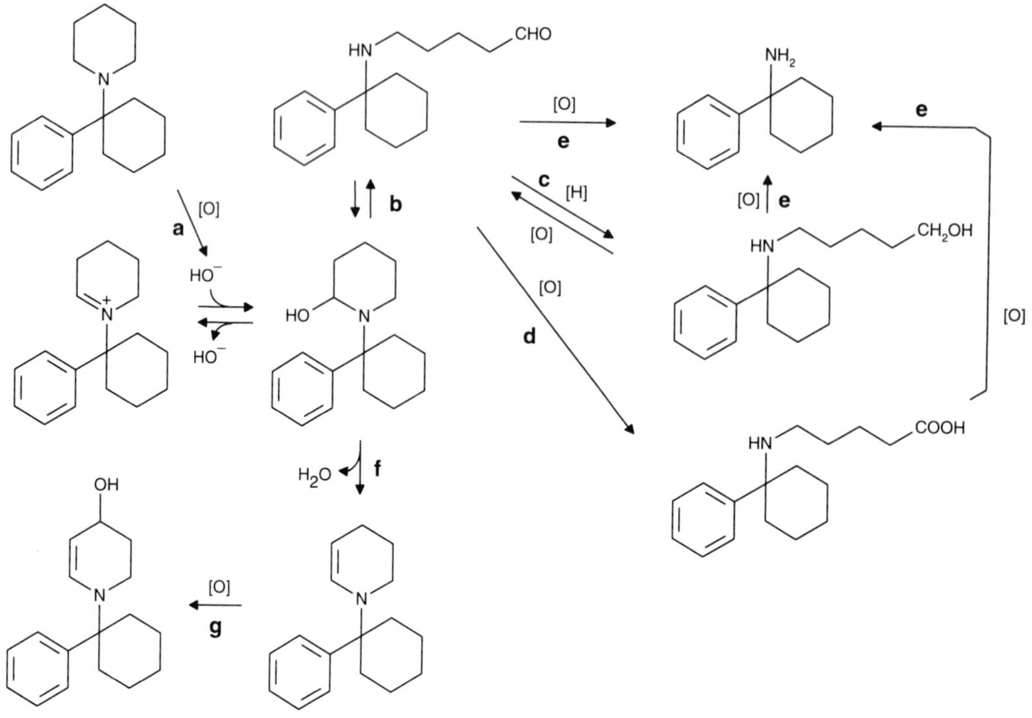

FIGURE 6.7 Metabolic scheme describing the various reactions of oxidation of the piperidine ring of phencyclidine.

toxicological significance (Hoag *et al.*, 1988; Ward *et al.*, 1982). This agent of abuse, beside a number of other metabolic routes, is oxidized in the 2-position (reaction **a** in Fig. 6.7) to form the iminium ion and the carbinolamine (Ward *et al.*, 1982). The ring–chain tautomerism of the carbinolamine (reaction **b** in Fig. 6.7) leads to the open-chain alcohol and carboxylic acid (reaction **c** and **d** in Fig. 6.7); these metabolites were formed under a number of conditions (Baker and Little, 1985; Baker *et al.*, 1981; Hallström *et al.*, 1983; Ward *et al.*, 1982). Interestingly, the corresponding lactam was not formed in mouse liver microsomes, nor does it appear to be a metabolite of phencyclidine under other biological conditions (Baker and Little, 1985). However, and in contrast to other nitrogen heterocycles, the formation of an **enamine** has also been documented, the postulated route being dehydration of the carbinolamine (reaction **f** in Fig. 6.7) (Hallström *et al.*, 1983). This enamine can be further oxidized to an allyl alcohol (reaction **g** in Fig. 6.7), and then to an enamine ketone and a 2,3-dihydropyridinium species (Hoag *et al.*, 1988). The metabolic formation of enamines from tertiary cyclic amines is an interesting phenomenon that deserves further investigation, in particular the possibility and mechanism of an enamine–iminium equilibrium (Sayre *et al.*, 1991).

Fig. 6.7 also displays another oxidative reaction involving the piperidine ring, namely **complete N-dealkylation** to form the primary amine 1-phenylcyclohexylamine (reactions **e** in Fig. 6.7). The reactions of N–C cleavage leading to this metabolite were investigated in rat liver microsomes and the rates compared with those of analogues. Thus, the rate of formation of 1-phenylcyclohexylamine decreases in the order phenylcyclohexyldiethylamine = phenylcyclo-hexylpyrrolidine > phenylcyclohexylpiperidine (phencyclidine) > phenylcyclohexylhexa-methyleneimine (Stefek *et al.*, 1990). In other words, ring opening and N-dealkylation decrease with increasing size of the heterocycle.

6.4.2 Azaheterocycles containing two or more heteroatoms

A variety of saturated (and partly saturated) azaheterocycles containing one or two additional heteroatoms are known to undergo cytochrome P450-mediated N–C cleavage and/or accompanying reactions. The cases presented below were chosen for their interest and representativeness.

The **imidazoline ring** is of rather common occurrence among diazaheterocyclic drugs, and its metabolic oxidation at an alpha-carbon has been repeatedly documented, the hypoglycaemic agent **midaglizole** (**6.L**) offering a particularly well-studied example. Following administration to rats, a number of metabolites (**6.LI–6.LV**) were excreted resulting from oxidation of the imidazoline ring (Fujimaki *et al.*, 1989). The imidazole derivative (**6.LI**) and the dilactam derivative (**6.LII**) were comparatively simple products of alpha-carbon oxidation, while ring opening led to a glycine derivative (**6.LIII**), an amidine (**6.LIV**) and an amide (**6.LV**).

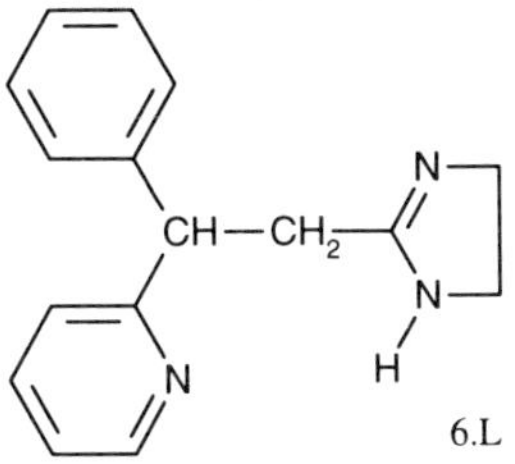

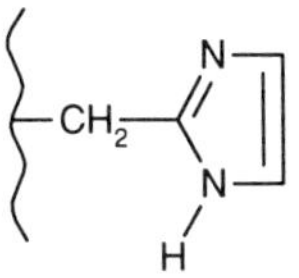

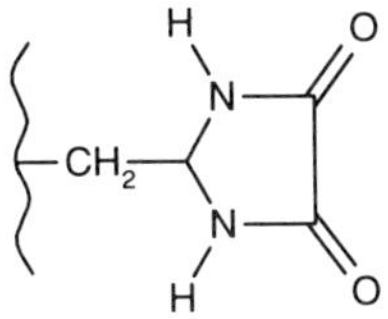

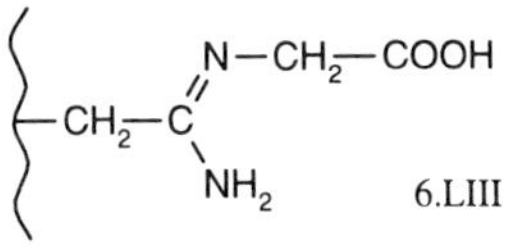

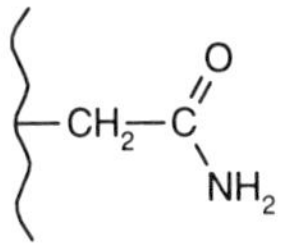

Piperazine-containing drugs offer another example of particular interest. A number of neuropharmacological agents, in particular tricyclic neuroleptics, are 1,4-disubstituted piperazines of structure **6.LVI** and **6.LVII** (see Fig. 6.8) that undergo metabolism to N-substituted and N,N'-disubstituted ethylenediamines. Chronic administration to rats and dogs of trifluoperazine, fluphenazine, prochlorperazine or perphenazine led to accumulation and long persistence in various tissues of metabolites containing the ethylenediamine moiety (Gaertner *et al.*, 1975). As stated by the authors of these studies, the possible toxicological significance of such findings should not be neglected.

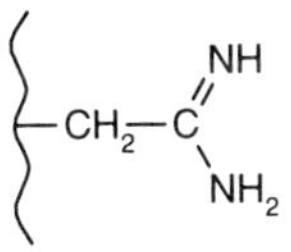

Primidone (Fig. 6.9), an antiepileptic prodrug, is well known for its biotransformation to two active metabolites, phenylethylmalonamide (**6.LVIII** in Fig. 6.9) and phenobarbital (**6.LIX** in Fig. 6.9). Converging evidence indicates that a common, C-hydroxylated precursor is either hydrolyzed to phenylethylmalonamide or dehydrogenated to phenobarbital. The two metabolites each account for about 40% of a dose of primidone in rabbits (Hunt and Miller, 1978).

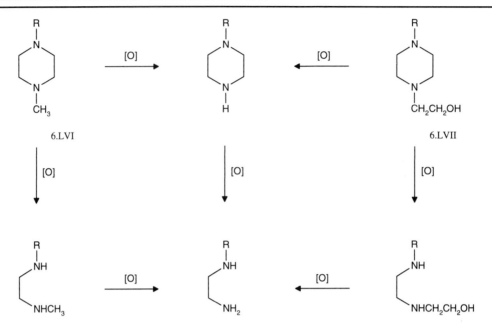

FIGURE 6.8 Partial metabolic scheme of piperazine-containing drugs of general structure **6.LVI** or **6.LVII** showing the formation of N-substituted and N,N'-disubstituted ethylenediamine derivatives.

Heterocycles containing both a nitrogen atom and another heteroatom are also of relevance in the present context, for example morpholine and **morpholine**-containing xenobiotics. Oxygenation of the morpholino moiety of emorfazone (**6.LX**) is a major reaction in guinea-pigs and other animal species. N–C Cleavage led to such metabolites as **6.LXI** and **6.LXII**, while O–C cleavage (Section 7.2) led to **6.LXIII** (Hayashi *et al.*, 1983). Similarly, the morpholino moiety in minaprine undergoes alpha-carbon oxidation and N–C cleavage in human and animal hepatocytes

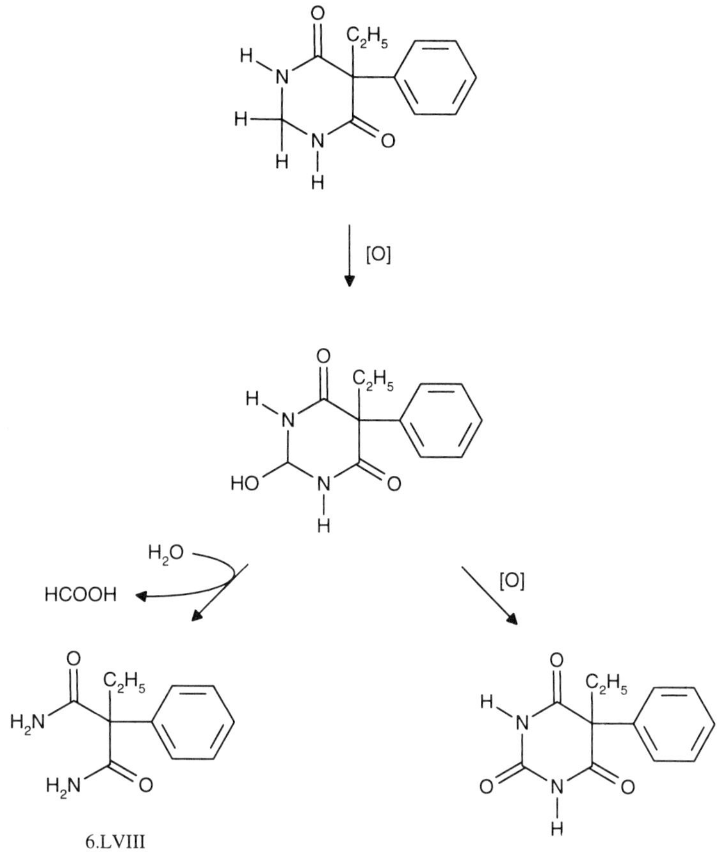

FIGURE 6.9 Metabolism of primidone to phenylethylmalonamide (**6.LVIII**) and phenobarbital (**6.LIX**) via a common precursor.

and liver microsomes (Lacarelle *et al.*, 1991). Another example is that of viloxazine, the morpholino ring of which was shown in humans and animals to be completely broken down to one- and two-carbon fragments which were utilized by endogenous metabolic pathways (Case, 1975).

More complex heterocyclic derivatives include the diuretic drug **hydrochlorothiazide** (**6.LXIV**), the carbon-3 of which is lost in humans with opening of the ring and production of a benzenedisulphonamide metabolite (Okuda *et al.*, 1987). Another compound of particular significance is the widely used anticancer drug **cyclophosphamide** (Fig. 6.10), since N–C oxidative ring cleavage underlies its activation and toxication mainly in hypoxic tumour cells, and its deactivation mainly in healthy cells. The initial metabolic reaction is oxidation to 4-hydroxycyclophosphamide (**6.LXV** in Fig. 6.10), a carbinolamine in equilibrium with its open-ring tautomer aldophosphamide (**6.LXVI** in Fig. 6.10) (Borch *et al.*, 1984; Zon *et al.*, 1984). Dehydrogenation of 4-hydroxycyclophosphamide and aldophosphamide, especially in healthy oxygen-rich cells, deactivates the drug to the urinary metabolites 4-oxocyclophosphamide (**6.LXVII** in Fig. 6.10) and carboxyphosphamide (**6.LXVIII** in Fig. 6.10), while aldophosphamide is also in a redox equilibrium with alcophosphamide (**6.LXIX** in Fig. 6.10), another urinary metabolite (Hong and Chang, 1987). In relatively anaerobic tumour cells, the biologically active metabolite phosphoramide mustard (**6.LXX** in Fig. 6.10) and the toxic metabolite acrolein

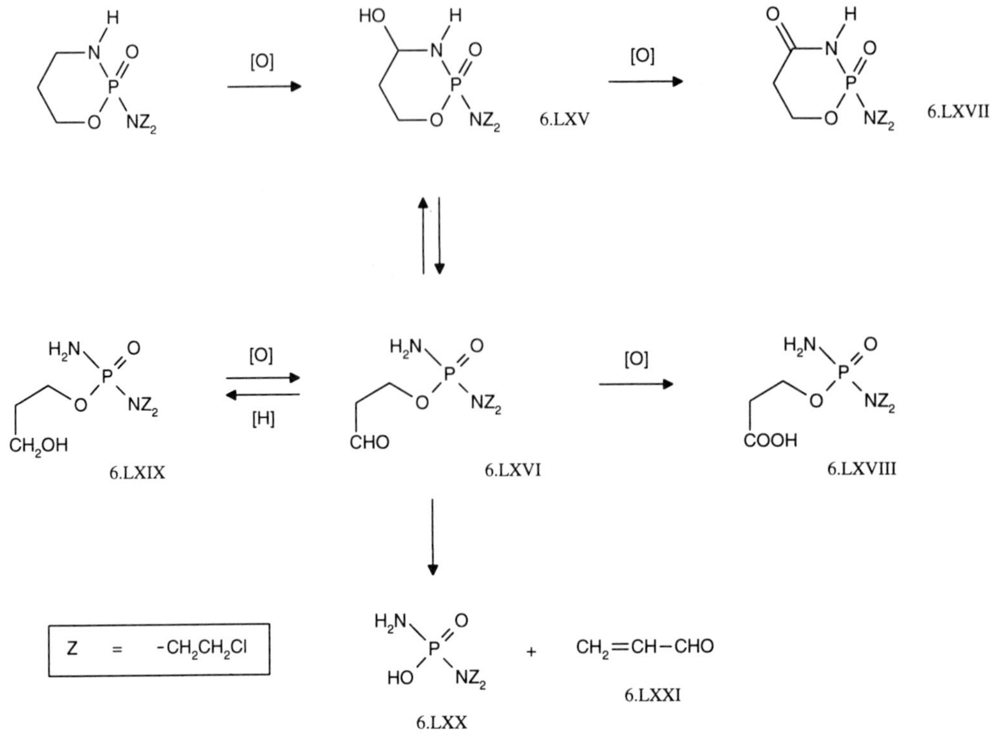

FIGURE 6.10 Partial metabolic scheme of the antitumour drug cyclophosphamide to the intermediates 4-hydroxycyclophosphamide (**6.LXV**) and aldophosphamide (**6.LXVI**), the urinary metabolites 4-oxocyclophosphamide (**6.LXVII**), carboxyphosphamide (**6.LXVIII**) and alcophosphamide (**6.LXIX**), the active metabolite phosphoramide mustard (**6.LXX**), and the toxic product acrolein (**6.LXXI**).

(**6.LXXI** in Fig. 6.10) are produced from aldophosphamide in a rate-limiting reaction of β-elimination (Struck *et al.*, 1975). It should be noted that 4-hydroxycyclophosphamide is also in a dehydration/hydration equilibrium with the corresponding imino form (Borch and Millard, 1987; Boyd *et al.*, 1987).

6.5 N–C CLEAVAGE IN NITROSAMINES AND NITROALKANES

Nitrosamines (N-nitroso derivatives) form a special group of xenobiotics whose biotransformation can lead to highly reactive intermediates often responsible for hepatotoxicity and carcinogenicity. Nitroalkanes, while also substrates for oxidative N–C cleavage, follow different reaction paths and as a class are less toxic than nitrosamines.

6.5.1 Nitrosamines

The occurrence of nitrosamines, as well as the chemistry of their formation and destruction and the factors influencing them, have been comprehensively reviewed and fall outside the scope of this work (e.g. Digenis and Issidorides, 1979; Douglass *et al.*, 1978). The toxication of dialkyl-

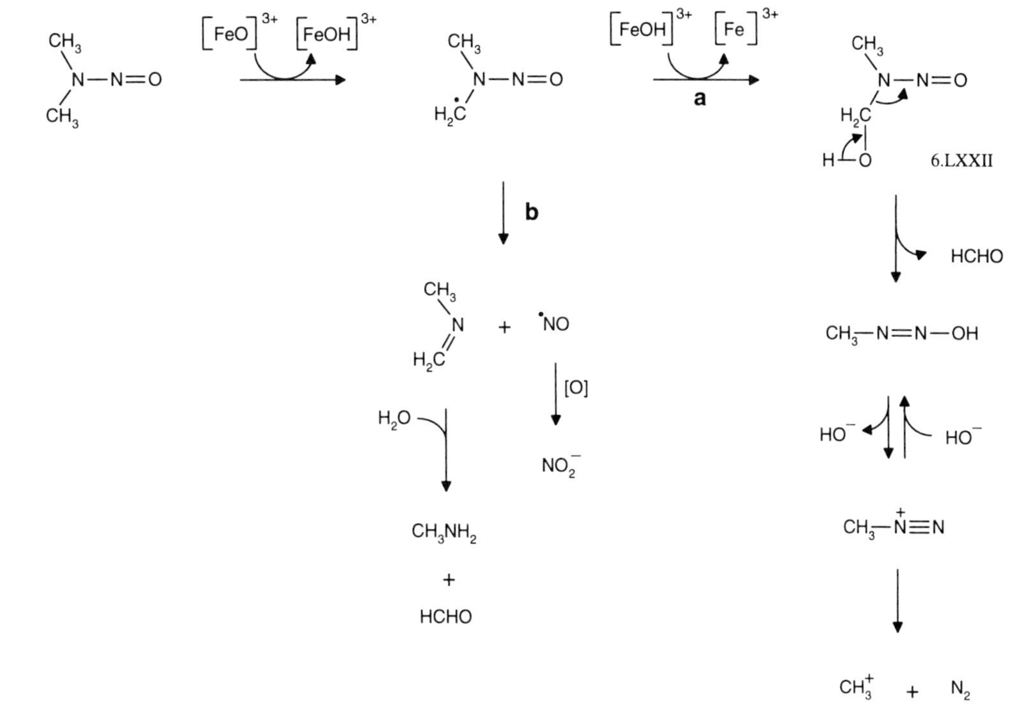

FIGURE 6.11 Toxication of dimethylnitrosamine to the methyl cation via a dealkylation pathway (reaction **a** and subsequent reactions). Also shown is the denitrosation pathway (reaction **b**).

and alkylarylnitrosamines is discussed here using as an example **dimethylnitrosamine**, a much studied and potent mutagen and carcinogen (Fig. 6.11). The compound is a substrate of CYP2E1, the ethanol-inducible form of cytochrome P450, and of other cytochromes P450 (Kawanishi *et al.*, 1992; Lauriault *et al.*, 1992; Yang *et al.*, 1990). Toxication begins with a traditional N-dealkylation via formation of a C-centred radical and an α-nitrosamino alcohol (reaction **a** and compound **6.LXXII** in Fig. 6.11) (oxygen-rebound mechanism, see Section 4.2). The latter intermediate decomposes rapidly, probably by a concerted mechanism, to yield formaldehyde and **diazomethane** as the actual N-dealkylated species. Further decomposition of the diazo compound under elimination of N_2 produces a carbonium ion, in this example the methyl cation (Lindeke, 1982).

Proof of the involvement of an intermediary radical comes among others from the occurrence of denitrosation (reaction **b** in Fig. 6.11) as a minor pathway in the microsomal metabolism of dimethylnitrosamine. Here, the C-centred radical escapes oxygen rebound and breaks down spontaneously to N-methylformamidine and nitric oxide; while the former hydrolyzes to methylamine and formaldehyde, the latter is oxidized to nitrite (Fig. 6.11). Confirmation of the mechanism of denitrosation shown in Fig. 6.11 was obtained by non-enzymatic models of cytochrome P450, for example the Fenton reaction where denitrosation is the exclusive outcome of dimethylnitrosamine oxidation (Heur *et al.*, 1989).

The **carbocation** produced by the decomposition of a diazoalkane (Fig. 6.11) may react as a strong electrophile on nucleophilic sites of biomolecules such as DNA, a molecular injury that initiates the sequence of events possibly leading to hepatotoxicity, carcinogenicity, or other toxic effects. In addition, alkyl cations can also be deactivated by loss of a proton to form alkenes, or by reaction with water to form alcohols, not to mention detoxication reactions with thiols (see

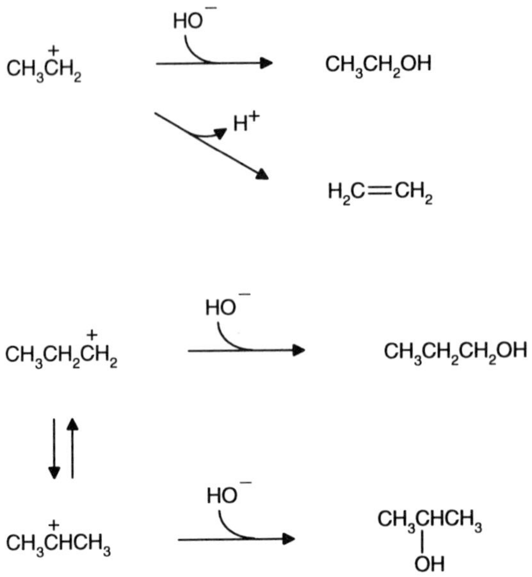
HO⁻
$CH_3\overset{+}{C}H_2$
CH_3CH_2OH
H+
$H_2C{=}CH_2$
HO⁻
$CH_3CH_2\overset{+}{C}H_2$
$CH_3CH_2CH_2OH$
HO⁻
$CH_3\overset{+}{C}HCH_3$
CH_3CHCH_3
OH

FIGURE 6.12 Formation of alkanols and alkenes from the ethyl and *n*-propyl cations produced in the microsomal metabolism of N-nitrosoethylamines and N-nitroso-*n*-propylamines (Ding and Coon, 1988; Park *et al.*, 1977).

the volume in this series, *Biochemistry of Conjugation Reactions*). Thus, various N-nitrosoethylamines were oxidized by some cytochromes P450 to the ethyl cation, which besides ethylating biomacromolecules could be detected as ethanol and ethylene (Fig. 6.12) (Ding and Coon, 1988). Similarly, the *n*-propyl cation produced from N-nitroso-N,N-di-*n*-propylamine reacted with water to give 1-propanol and 2-propanol in a 5:1 ratio (Fig. 6.12), while N-nitroso-N-*n*-propylurea (**6.LXXIII**) yielded 1-propanol and 2-propanol in a 6:4 ratio. The formation of the rearranged alcohol 2-propanol gave an additional and elegant proof for the involvement of carbocations in the toxication of nitrosamines (Park *et al.*, 1977).

Heterocyclic nitrosamines react comparably to N-nitrosodialkylamines, being hydroxylated at an alpha-carbon prior to yielding a diazohydroxide which decomposes to a carbonium ion. In the microsomal metabolism of the carcinogen **N-nitrosopyrrolidine** (Fig. 6.13), the carbonium ion was trapped with water (reaction **a** in Fig. 6.13) to produce 4-hydroxybutyraldehyde (**6.LXXIV** in Fig. 6.13) which is in equilibrium with 2-hydroxytetrahydrofuran, its cyclic hemiacetal. Rearrangement of the carbonium ion (reaction **b** in Fig. 6.13) additionally led to two stable metabolites, namely crotonaldehyde (**6.LXXV** in Fig. 6.13) and 3-hydroxybutyraldehyde. Note however that the latter was a minor product compared to **6.LXXIV** and **6.LXXV** (Wang *et al.*, 1988). N-Nitrosopiperidine, the higher homologue of N-nitrosopyrrolidine, similarly led to the formation of 5-hydroxypentanal (Leung *et al.*, 1978).

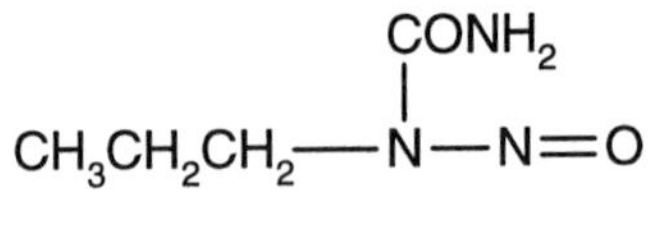
$CONH_2$
$CH_3CH_2CH_2{-}N{-}N{=}O$

6.LXXIII

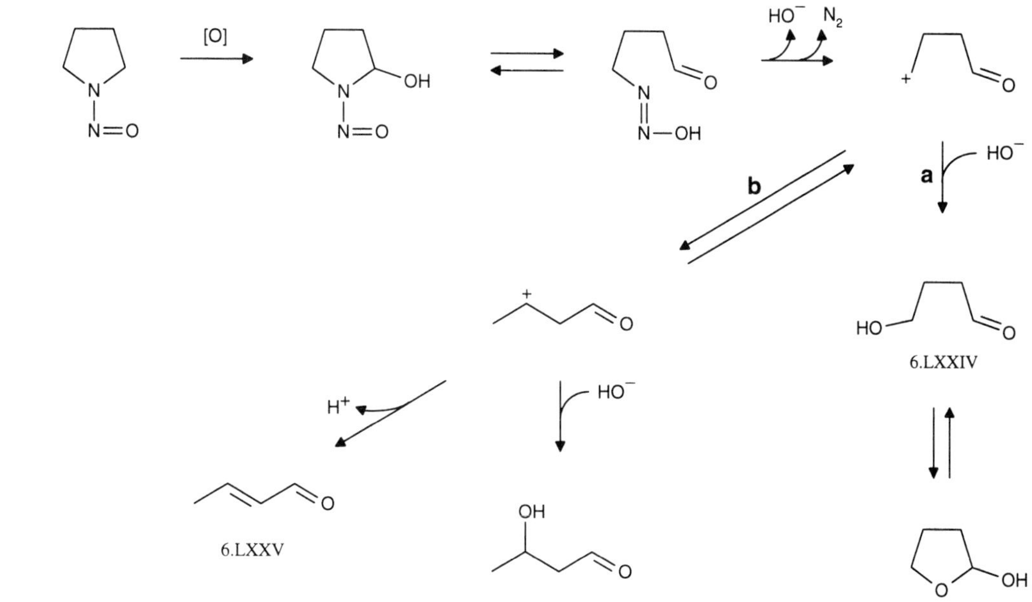

FIGURE 6.13 Cytochrome P450-catalyzed metabolism of N-nitrosopyrrolidine leading to carbonium ions which can react with water to produce 4-hydroxybutyraldehyde (**6.LXXIV**) and 3-hydroxybutyraldehyde, respectively. Crotonaldehyde (**6.LXXV**) was also produced by loss of a proton (Wang *et al.*, 1988).

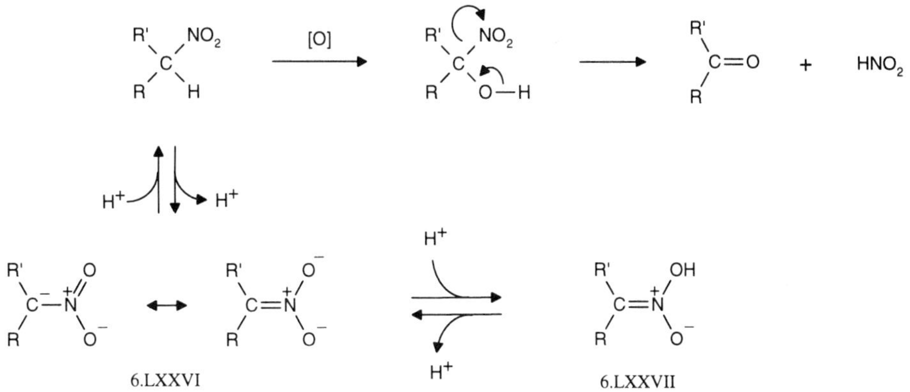

FIGURE 6.14 Hypothetical mechanism of cytochrome P450-mediated oxidative denitrification of nitroalkanes to carbonyl compounds and nitrite (Ullrich *et al.*, 1978). Also shown is the acid–base behaviour of nitroalkanes, which exist in equilibrium with nitronic acids (**6.LXXVII**) via nitronate ions (**6.LXXVI**) (Alston *et al.*, 1985).

6.5.2 Nitroalkanes

A limited number of nitroalkanes have been found in nature, while others are synthetic chemicals. Few, if any, of these xenobiotics are biologically inert, yet little is known about biotransformation reactions specific to the nitroalkyl moiety (Alston *et al.*, 1985). A simple and likely mechanism has been postulated following the cytochrome P450-mediated metabolism of 2-nitropropane (Fig. 6.14, R = R' = CH$_3$) to acetone and nitrite, involving the formation of an

α-hydroxynitroalkane which breaks down to nitrite and a carbonyl compound (Ullrich *et al.*, 1978).

The mechanism shown in Fig. 6.14 is perhaps too simple or not always relevant, considering that the nitroalkyl group displays a complex behaviour (Alston *et al.*, 1985). First, nitroalkanes are relatively strong acids (pK_a values in the range 7–10); deprotonation yields nitronate ions (**6.LXXVI** in Fig. 6.14) which may react as nucleophiles (or reductants) towards enzymes. The protonation of nitronate ions not only leads back to nitroalkanes, but can also afford nitronic acids (**6.LXXVII** in Fig. 6.14) which may react as electrophiles (or oxidants). As summarized by Lindeke (1982), cytochrome P450(FeIII) could also react with nitronic acids by catalyzing oxygen migration from N to C(α).

While the number of nitroalkanes investigated metabolically is very small, it is interesting to note that 2-nitro-1-phenylpropane (Fig. 6.14, R = benzyl, R′ = methyl), an *in vitro* metabolite of amphetamine, was transformed to phenylacetone by rabbit liver microsomes (Jonsson *et al.*, 1977).

6.6 N-DEARYLATION

Following administration of **N-phenyl-2-naphthylamine (6.LXXVIII)** to rats, 2-naphthylamine (**6.LXXIX**) was isolated as a slowly excreted metabolite, confirming earlier observations in humans and dogs (Laham and Potvin, 1983). This reaction of N–C cleavage is clearly an unusual one since in contrast to all other cases discussed above the carbon atom is sp^2- rather than sp^3-hybridized. The reaction is usually referred to as one of N-dephenylation, but the more general term of N-dearylation is also used here. To date, little is known on the mechanism of N-dearylation. A marked formal analogy exists with O-dearylation to be presented in Section 7.4, and the fragmental evidence available for both reactions may well be complementary.

Interestingly, the hepatic microsomal metabolism of N-phenyl-2-naphthylamine produced the 4′-hydroxylated metabolite, but no N-dephenylation was observed. However, subsequent oxidation of 4′-hydroxy-**6.LXXVIII** with hydrogen peroxide did result in the formation of 2-naphthylamine and 1,4-benzoquinone, suggesting the quinone imine **6.LXXX** to be the intermediate whose hydrolytic N=C cleavage leads to *in vivo* N-dephenylation (Anderson *et al.*, 1982).

A few examples of *in vivo* **N-dearylation of drugs** have appeared in the literature. Thus, a small part (about 15%) of a dose of the neuroleptic agent **zetidoline (6.LXXXI)** was found to undergo this reaction in humans (Assandri *et al.*, 1985). Here, formation of a quinone imine appears somewhat less likely since it would transform the tertiary nitrogen into a quaternary one. Because 4′-hydroxylation is the major metabolic route and subsequent 2′-hydroxylation was seen in rats, the authors have suggested the 2′,4′-dihydroxylated metabolite as the intermediate leading to N-dearylation. Another possible candidate is the 1′,2′-epoxy-4′-hydroxy precursor of the 2′,4′-dihydroxylated metabolite (see below and Section 7.4).

More than a quarter of a dose of the antiemetic agent mociprazine (6.LXXXII) is similarly N-dephenylated in dogs (Pognat *et al.*, 1986). N-Dearylation of aromatic azaheterocycles is also documented, e.g. N-depyridination of azaperone (6.LXXXIII), tripelennamine (6.LXXXIV, R = H) and pyrilamine (6.LXXXIV, R = OCH₃) (Heykants *et al.*, 1971; Yeh, 1990). Such examples show that we are far from understanding the substrate selectivity and mechanism of N-dearylation reactions, and can even postulate the involvement of more than one mechanism. In this context, the fate of the antileprosy drug **clofazimine (6.LXXXV)**, if correctly interpreted, could shed some mechanistic light. Two metabolites were isolated from the urine of leprosy patients, namely the 4′-hydroxylated analogue **6.LXXXVI** and the dearylated metabolite **6.LXXXVII** (as a glucuronide) (Feng *et al.*, 1981). Metabolite **6.LXXXVII** is particularly interesting because N–C cleavage occurred between N and the tricyclic system rather than the phenyl ring. This excludes an intermediate quinone imine formed from **6.LXXXVI**, while a mechanism of hydrolytic deamination appears unsupported. Perhaps a 3,4-epoxide could account for the N-dearylation/deamination of clofazimine, a mechanism postulated to explain the N-depyridination of tripelennamine (Yeh, 1990).

In summary, **two mechanisms** can be hypothesized to explain N-dearylation, as shown in Fig. 6.15. The first possibility is formation of an intermediate quinone imine followed by its hydrolytic cleavage (reaction **a** in Fig. 6.15), a pathway perhaps favoured for primary and secondary amines. The second possibility, perhaps favouring tertiary amines, is formation of an *ipso,ortho*-epoxide followed by its hydrolytic opening and rearrangement of the diol (reaction **b** in Fig. 6.15). Clearly more experimental work is needed to confirm or refute the mechanisms proposed in Fig. 6.15 (see also Section 7.4).

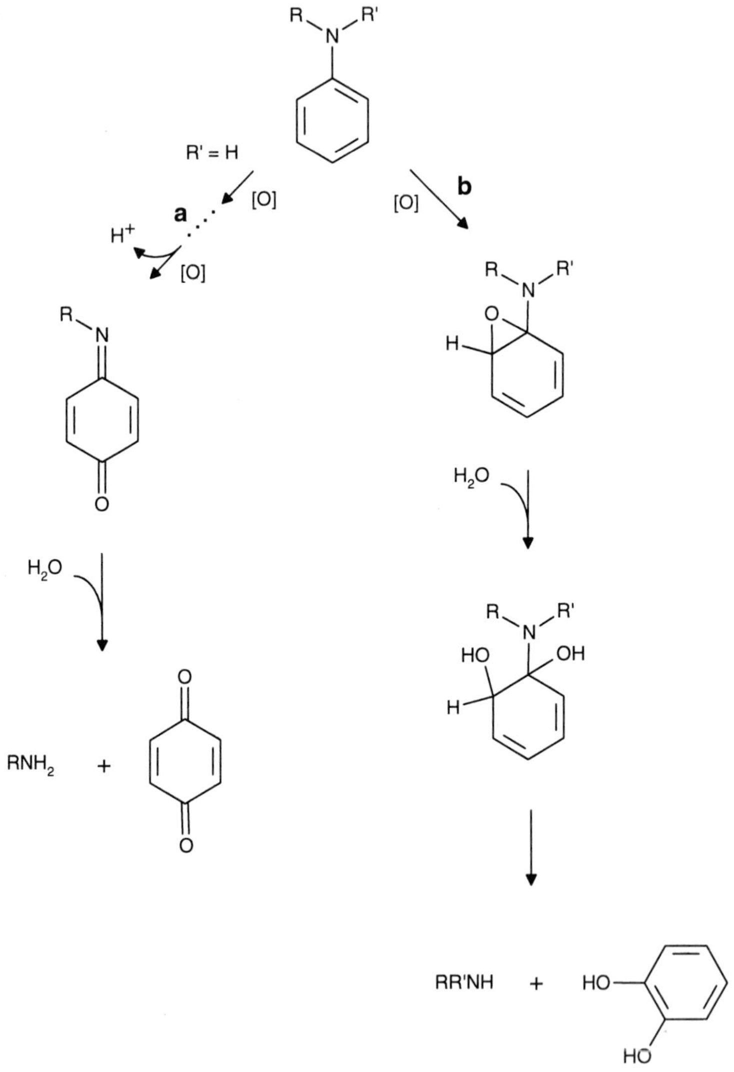

FIGURE 6.15 Hypothetical mechanisms proposed to explain oxidative N-dearylation. See text for further details.

6.7 REFERENCES

Allen J.G., Brown A.N. and Marten T.R. (1976). Metabolism of debrisoquine sulphate in rat, dog and man. *Xenobiotica* **6**, 405–409.

Alston T.A., Porter D.J.T. and Bright H.J. (1985). The bioorganic chemistry of the nitroalkyl group. *BioOrg. Chem.* **13**, 375–403.

Anderson M.M., Mitchum R.K. and Beland F.A. (1982). Hepatic microsomal metabolism and macromolecular binding of the antioxidant, N-phenyl-2-naphthylamine. *Xenobiotica* **12**, 31–43.

Arora P.K., Riachi N.J., Harik S.I. and Sayre L.M. (1988). Chemical oxidation of 1-methyl-4-phenyl-1,2,3,6-tetrahydropyridine (MPTP) and its *in vivo* metabolism in rat brain and liver. *Biochem. Biophys. Res. Commun.* **152**, 1339–1347.

Assandri A., Perazzi A., Ferrari P., Martinelli E., Ripamonti A., Tarzia G. and Tuan G. (1985). Metabolic fate of zetidoline, a new neuroleptic agent, in man. *Naunyn-Schmiedeberg's Arch. Pharmacol.* **328**, 341–347.

Axelrod J. (1955). The enzymatic deamination of amphetamine. *J. Biol. Chem.* **214**, 753–763.

Baba T., Yamada H., Oguri K. and Yoshimura H. (1987). Studies on N-demethylation of methamphetamine by means of purified guinea-pig liver flavin-containing monooxygenase. *Biochem. Pharmacol.* **36**, 4171–4173.

Baker J.K. and Little T.L. (1985). Metabolism of phencyclidine. The role of the carbinolamine intermediate in the formation of lactam and amino acid metabolites of nitrogen heterocycles. *J. Med. Chem.* **28**, 46–50.

Baker J.K., Wohlford J.G., Bradbury B.J. and Wirth P.W. (1981). Mammalian metabolism of phencyclidine. *J. Med. Chem.* **24**, 666–669.

Baty J.D., Price-Evans D.A. and Robinson P.A. (1975). The identification of 6-methoxy-8-aminoquinoline as a metabolite of primaquine in man. *Biomed. Mass Spectrum* **2**, 304–306.

Beckett A.H. and Haya K. (1978). The stereoselective metabolism of ethylamphetamine with fortified rabbit liver homogenates. *Xenobiotica* **8**, 85–96.

Berthou F., Flinois J.P., Ratanasavanh D., Beaune P., Riche C. and Guillouzo A. (1991). Evidence for the involvement of several cytochromes P-450 in the first steps of caffeine metabolism by human liver microsomes. *Drug Metab. Disposit.* **19**, 561–567.

Berthou F., Guillois B., Riche C., Dreano Y., Jacqz-Aigrain E. and Beaune P.H. (1992). Interspecies variatons in caffeine metabolism related to cytochrome P4501A enzymes. *Xenobiotica* **22**, 671–680.

Bickel M.H. (1969). The pharmacology and biochemistry of N-oxides. *Pharmacol. Rev.* **21**, 325–355.

Bondon A., Macdonald T.L., Harris T.M. and Guengerich F.P. (1989). Oxidation of cycloalkylamines by cytochrome P-450. Mechanism-based inactivation, adduct formation, ring expansion, and nitrone formation. *J. Biol. Chem.* **264**, 1988–1997.

Borch R.F. and Millard J.A. (1987). The mechanism of activation of 4-hydroxy-cyclophosphamide. *J. Med. Chem.* **30**, 427–431.

Borch R.F., Hoye T.R. and Swanson T.A. (1984). *In situ* preparation and fate of cis-4-hydroxycyclophosphamide and aldophosphamide. *J. Med. Chem.* **27**, 490–494.

Boyd V.L., Summers M.F., Ludeman S.M., Egan W., Zon G. and Regan J.B. (1987). NMR spectroscopic studies of intermediary metabolites of cyclophosphamide. 2. Direct observation, characterization, and reactivity studies of iminocyclophosphamide and related species. *J. Med. Chem.* **30**, 366–374.

Brandänge S. and Lindblom L. (1979). Synthesis, structure and stability of nicotine $\Delta^{1'(5')}$ iminium ion, an intermediary metabolite of nicotine. *Acta Chem. Scand. B* **33**, 187–191.

Brandänge S., Lindblom L., Pilotti Å. and Rodriguez B. (1983). Ring-chain tautomerism of pseudooxynicotine and some other iminium compounds. *Acta Chem. Scand.* **37**, 617–622.

Burka L.T., Guengerich F.P., Willard R.J. and Macdonald T.L. (1985). Mechanism of cytochrome P-450 catalysis. Mechanisms of N-dealkylation and amine oxide deoxygenation. *J. Amer. Chem. Soc.* **107**, 2549–2551.

Butler M.A., Iwasaki M., Guengerich F.P. and Kadlubar F.F. (1989). Human cytochrome P-450$_{PA}$ (P-450IA2), the phenacetin O-deethylase, is primarily responsible for the hepatic 3-demethylation of caffeine and N-oxidation of carcinogenic arylamines. *Proc. Natl Acad. Sci. USA* **86**, 7696–7700.

Caccia S., Conti I., Vigano G. and Garattini S. (1986). 1-(2-Pyrimidinyl)-piperazine as active metabolite of buspirone in man and rat. *Pharmacology* **33**, 46–51.

Case D.E. (1975). Incorporation into endogenous metabolic pathways of small fragments from viloxazine. *Xenobiotica* **5**, 133–143.

Constantino L., Rosa E. and Iley J. (1992). The microsomal demethylation of N,N-dimethylbenzamides. Substituent and kinetic deuterium effects. *Biochem. Pharmacol.* **44**, 651–658.

Coutts R.T., Dawson G.W. and Beckett A.H. (1976). *In vitro* metabolism of N-propylamphetamine by rat liver homogenates. *J. Pharm. Pharmacol.* **28**, 815–821.

Darlington W.H., Constable D.A., Baczynskyj L., Mizsak S.A., Scahill T.A., Dring L.G., McCall J.M. and Szmuszkovicz J. (1987). Isolation, identification and synthesis of a metabolite of tazadolene succinate. *Drug Design Delivery* **1**, 225–230.

Digenis G.A. and Issidorides C.H. (1979). Some biochemical aspects of N-nitroso compounds. *BioOrg. Chem.* **8**, 97–137.

Ding X. and Coon M.J. (1988). Cytochrome P-450-dependent formation of ethylene from N-nitrosoethylamines. *Drug Metab. Disposit.* **16**, 265–269.

Douglass M.L., Kabacoff B.L., Anderson G.A. and Cheng M.C. (1978). The chemistry of nitrosamine formation, inhibition and destruction. *J. Soc. Cosmet. Chem.* **29**, 581–605.

Duncan J.D., Hallström G., Paulsen-Sörman U., Lindeke

B. and Cho A.K. (1983). Effects of α-carbon substituents on the N-demethylation of N-methyl-2-phenylethylamines by rat liver microsomes. *Drug Metab. Disposit.* **11**, 15–20.

Duquette P.H., Erickson R.R. and Holtzman J.L. (1983). Role of substrate lipophilicity on the N-demethylation and type I binding of 3-O-alkylmorphine analogues. *J. Med. Chem.* **26**, 1343–1348.

Feng P.C.C., Fenselau C.C. and Jacobson R.R. (1981). Metabolism of clofazimine in leprosy patients. *Drug Metab. Disposit.* **9**, 521–524.

Fuhr U., Doehmer J., Battula N., Wölfel C., Kudla C., Keita Y. and Staib A.H. (1992). Biotransformation of caffeine and theophylline in mammalian cell lines genetically engineered for expression of single cytochrome P450 isoforms. *Biochem. Pharmacol.* **43**, 22–235.

Fujimaki M., Ishigaki N. and Hakusui H. (1989). Metabolic fate of the oral hypoglycaemic agent, midaglizole, in rats. *Xenobiotica* **19**, 609–625.

Gaertner H.J., Liomin G., Villumsen D., Bertele R. and Breyer U. (1975). Tissue metabolites of trifluoperazine, fluphenazine, prochlorperazine, and perphenazine. Kinetics in chronic treatment. *Drug Metab. Disposit.* **3**, 437–444.

Galliani G., Rindone B., Dagnino G. and Salmona M. (1984). Structure–activity relationships in the microsomal oxidation of tertiary amines. *Eur. J. Drug Metab. Pharmacokin.* **9**, 289–293.

Garteiz D.A., Hook R.H., Walker B.J. and Okerholm R.A. (1982). Pharmacokinetics and biotransformation studies of terfenadine in man. *Arzneim-Forsch. (Drug Res.)* **32**, 1185–1190.

Godin J.R.P., Vaughan K. and Renton K.W. (1981). Triazene metabolism. I. The effect of substituents in the aryl group on the kinetics of enzyme-catalysed N-demethylation of 1-aryl-3,3-dimethyltriazenes. *Can. J. Physiol. Pharmacol.* **59**, 1234–1238.

Gorrod J.W. and Temple D.J. (1976). The formation of an N-hydroxymethyl intermediate in the N-demethylation of N-methylcarbazole *in vitro* and *in vivo*. *Xenobiotica* **6**, 265–274.

Gorrod J.W., Temple D.J. and Beckett A.H. (1975). The metabolism of N-ethyl-N-methylaniline by rabbit liver microsomes. *Xenobiotica* **5**, 453–463.

Gorrod J.W., Temple D.J. and Beckett A.H. (1979). The N- and α-C-oxidation of N,N-dialkylanilines by rabbit liver microsomes *in vitro*. *Xenobiotica* **9**, 17–25.

Grant D.M., Campbell M.E., Tang B.K. and Kalow W. (1987). Biotransformation of caffeine by microsomes from human liver. *Biochem. Pharmacol.* **36**, 1251–1260.

Guengerich F.P., Willard R.J., Shea J.P., Richards L.E. and Macdonald T.L. (1984). Mechanism-based inactivation of cytochrome P-450 by heteroatom-substituted cyclopropylamines and formation of ring-opened products. *J. Amer. Chem. Soc.* **106**, 6446–6447.

Hall L.R. and Hanzlik R.P. (1990). Kinetic deuterium effects on the N-demethylation of tertiary amides by cytochrome P-450. *J. Biol. Chem.* **265**, 12,349–12,355.

Hall L.R. and Hanzlik R.P. (1991). N-Dealkylation of tertiary amides by cytochrome P-450. *Xenobiotica* **21**, 1127–1138.

Hallström G., Kammerer R.C., Nguyen C.H., Schmitz D.A., Di Stefano E.W. and Cho A.K. (1983). Phencyclidine metabolism *in vitro*. The formation of a carbinolamine and its metabolites by rabbit liver preparations. *Drug Metab. Disposit.* **11**, 47–53.

Hanzlik R.P. and Tullman R.H. (1982). Suicidal inactivation of cytochrome P-450 by cyclopropylamines. Evidence for cation-radical intermediates. *J. Amer. Chem. Soc.* **104**, 2048–2050.

Hayashi T., Amino M. and Ikoma Y. (1983). Changes of metabolism and substrate-binding spectrum of emorfazone between immature and mature guinea-pigs. *Xenobiotica* **13**, 461–466.

Heimbrook D.C., Murray R.I., Egeberg K.D., Sligar S.G., Nee M.W. and Bruice T.C. (1984). Demethylation of N,N-dimethylaniline and *p*-cyano-N,N-dimethylaniline and their N-oxides by cytochrome P450$_{LM2}$ and cytochrome P450$_{CAM}$. *J. Amer. Chem. Soc.* **106**, 1514–1515.

Heur Y.H., Streeter A.J., Nims R.W. and Keefer L.K. (1989). The Fenton degradation as a nonenzymatic model for microsomal denitrosation of N-nitrosodimethylamine. *Chem. Res. Toxicol.* **2**, 247–253.

Heykants J., Pardoel L. and Janssen P.A.J. (1971). On the distribution and metabolism of azaperone in the rat and pig. *Arzneim-Forsch. (Drug Res.)* **21**, 982–984.

Hibberd A.R. and Gorrod J.W. (1983). Enzymology of the metabolic pathway from nicotine to cotinine, *in vitro*. *Eur. J. Drug Metab. Pharmacokin.* **8**, 151–162.

Hoag M.K.P., Schmidt-Peets M., Lampen L., Trevor A. and Castagnoli N. Jr (1988). Metabolic studies on phencyclidine: characterization of a phencyclidine iminium ion metabolite. *Chem. Res. Toxicol.* **1**, 128–131.

Hong P.S. and Chan K.K. (1987). Identification and quantitation of alcophosphamide, a metabolite of cyclophosphamide, in the rat using CI/MS. *Biomed. Environm. Mass Spectrom.* **14**, 167–172.

Hunt R.J. and Miller K.W. (1978). Disposition of primidone, phenylethyl-malonamide, and phenobarbital in the rabbit. *Drug Metab. Disposit.* **6**, 75–81.

Iley J. and Ruecroft G. (1990). Mechanism of the microsomal demethylation of 1-aryl-3,3-dimethyltriazenes. *Biochem. Pharmacol.* **40**, 2123–2128.

Inaba T., Tait A., Nakano M., Mahon W.A. and Kalow W. (1988). Metabolism of diazepam *in vitro* by human liver. Independent variability of N-demethylation and C3-hydroxylation. *Drug Metab. Disposit.* **16**, 605–608.

Inoue T., Suzuki S. and Niwaguchi T. (1983). The metabolism of 1-phenyl-2-(N-methyl-N-benzylamino)propane (benzphetamine) *in vitro* in rats. *Xenobiotica* **13**, 241–249.

Jauch R., Griesser E. and Oesterhelt G. (1980). Metabolismus von Ro 21-5998 (Mefloquin) bei der Ratte. *Arzneim-Forsch. (Drug Res.)* **30**, 60–67.

Jonsson J., Kammerer R.C. and Cho A.K. (1977). Metabolism of 2-nitro-1-phenylpropane to phenylacetone by rabbit liver microsomes. *Res. Commun. Chem. Pathol.*

MONOOXYGENASE-CATALYZED N–C CLEAVAGE 233

Pharmacol. **18**, 75–82.

Kalow W. (1985). Variability of caffeine metabolism in humans. *Arzneim-Forsch. (Drug Res.)* **35**, 319–324.

Kalow W. and Campbell M. (1988). Biotransformation of caffeine by microsomes. *ISI Atlas Sci: Pharmacol.* **2**, 381–386.

Kamm J.J. and Szuna A. (1973). Studies on an unusual N-dealkylation reaction. II. *J. Pharmacol. Exp. Therap.* **184**, 729–738.

Kawanishi T., Ohno Y., Takanaka A., Kawano S., Yamazoe Y., Kato R. and Omori Y. (1992). N-Nitrosodialkylamine dealkylation in reconstituted systems containing cytochrome P-450 purified from phenobarbital and β-naphthoflavone-treated rats. *Arch. Toxicol.* **66**, 137–142.

Kedderis G.L., Dwyer L.A., Rickert D.E. and Hollenberg P.F. (1983). Source of the oxygen atom in the product of cytochrome P-450-catalyzed N-demethylation reactions. *Molec. Pharmacol.* **23**, 758–760.

Kloss M.W., Rosen G.M. and Rauckman E.J. (1983). N-Demethylation of cocaine to norcocaine. Evidence for participation by cytochrome P-450 and FAD-containing monooxygenase. *Molec. Pharmacol.* **23**, 482–485.

Kolar G.F. and Carubelli R. (1979). Urinary metabolite of 1-(2,4,6-trichlorophenyl)-3,3-dimethyltriazene with an intact diazoamino structure. *Cancer Lett.* **7**, 209–214.

Kurebayashi H., Tanaka A., Yamaha T. and Tatahashi A. (1988). Oxidative deamination of alicyclic primary amines by liver microsomes from rats and rabbits. *Xenobiotica* **18**, 1039–1048.

Lacarelle B., Marre F., Durand A., Davi H. and Rahmani R. (1991). Metabolism of minaprine in human and animal hepatocytes and liver microsomes—prediction of metabolism *in vivo*. *Xenobiotica* **21**, 317–329.

Laham S. and Potvin M. (1983). Biological conversion of N-phenyl-2-naphthylamine to 2-naphthylamine in the Sprague-Dawley rat. *Drug Chem. Toxicol.* **6**, 295–309.

Lander N., Soloway A.H., Minton J.P., Rawal B.D. and Gairola C.C. (1988). Potential metabolic mutagens of caffeine and various methylxanthines. *J. Pharm. Sci.* **77**, 955–958.

Lauriault V.V., Khan S. and O'Brien P.J. (1992). Hepatocyte cytotoxicity induced by various hepatotoxins mediated by cytochrome P-450IIE1: Protection with diethyldithiocarbamate administration. *Chem.-Biol. Interact.* **81**, 271–289.

Lemoine A., Gautier J.C., Azoulay D., Kiffel L., Belloc C., Guengerich F.P., Maurel P., Beaune P. and Leroux J.P. (1993). Major pathways of imipramine metabolism is catalyzed by cytochromes P-450 1A2 and P-450 3A4 in human liver. *Molec. Pharmacol.* **43**, 827–832.

Leung K.H., Park K.K. and Archer M.C. (1978). Alpha-hydroxylation in the metabolism of N-nitrosopiperidine by rat liver microsomes. Formation of 5-hydroxypentanal. *Res. Commun. Chem. Pathol. Pharmacol.* **19**, 201–211.

Lindeke B. (1982). The non- and postenzymatic chemistry of N-oxygenated molecules. *Drug Metab. Rev.* **13**, 71–121.

Lindeke B. and Cho A.K. (1982). N-Dealkylation and deamination. In *Metabolic Basis of Detoxication* (eds Jakoby W.B., Bend J.R. and Caldwell J.). pp. 105–126. Academic Press, New York.

Macdonald T.L., Gutheim W.G., Martin R.B. and Guengerich F.P. (1989). Oxidation of substituted N,N-dimethylanilines by cytochrome P-450: Estimation of the effective oxidation–reduction potential of cytochrome P-450. *Biochemistry* **28**, 2071–2077.

Marcucci F., Airoldi L., Zavattini G. and Mussini E. (1981). Metabolism of pinazepam by rat liver microsomes. *Eur. J. Drug Metab. Pharmacokin.* **6**, 109–114.

Murray G.R., Whiffin G.M., Franklin R.A. and Henry J.A. (1989). Quantitative aspects of the urinary excretion of meptazinol and its metabolites in human volunteers. *Xenobiotica* **19**, 669–675.

Mutlib A.E. and Nelson W.L. (1990). Pathways of gallopamil metabolism. Regiochemistry and enantioselectivity of the N-dealkylation processes. *Drug Metab. Disposit.* **18**, 331–337.

Nelson S.D., Pohl L.R. and Trager W.F. (1975). Primary and β-secondary deuterium isotope effects in N-deethylation reactions. *J. Med. Chem.* **18**, 1062–1065.

Nelson W.L. and Bartels M.J. (1984). N-Dealkylation of propranolol in rat, dog and man. Chemical and stereochemical aspects. *Drug Metab. Disposit.* **12**, 345–352.

Nguyen T.L., Gruenke L.D. and Castagnoli N. Jr (1979). Metabolic oxidation of nicotine to chemically reactive intermediates. *J. Med. Chem.* **22**, 259–263.

Nguyen T.L., Dagne E., Gruenke L., Bhargava H. and Castagnoli N. Jr (1981). The tautomeric structures of 5-hydroxycotinine, a secondary mammalian metabolite of nicotine. *J. Org. Chem.* **46**, 758–760.

Noda A., Goromaru T., Tsubone N., Matsuyama K. and Iguchi S. (1976). *In vivo* formation of 4-formylaminoantipyrine as a new metabolite of aminopyrine. *Chem. Pharm. Bull.* **24**, 1502–1505.

Obach R.S. and Van Vunakis H. (1988). Non-metabolic covalent binding of nicotine $\Delta^{1'(5')}$-iminium ion to liver microsomes and sulphhydryl-containing polyamino acids. *Biochem. Pharmacol.* **37**, 4601–4604.

Ohmori S., Takeda S., Rikihisa T., Kiuchi M., Kanakubo Y. and Kitada M. (1993). Studies on cytochrome P450 responsible for oxidative metabolism of imipramine in human liver microsomes. *Biol. Pharm. Bull.* **16**, 571–575.

Okuda T., Itoh S., Yamazaki M., Nakahama H., Fukuhara Y. and Orita Y. (1987). Biopharmaceutical studies of thiazide diuretics. III. *In vivo* formation of 2-amino-4-chloro-*m*-benzenedisulfonamide as a metabolite of hydrochlorothiazide in a patient. *Chem. Pharm. Bull.* **35**, 3516–3518.

Overton M., Hickman J.A., Threadgill M.D., Vaughan K. and Gescher A. (1985). The generation of potentially toxic, reactive iminium ions from the oxidative metabolism of xenobiotic N-alkyl compounds. *Biochem. Pharmacol.* **34**, 2055–2061.

Pandey R.N., Armstrong A.P. and Hollenberg P.F. (1989). Oxidative N-demethylation of N,N-dimethylaniline by purified isozymes of cytochrome P-450. *Biochem. Pharmacol.* **38**, 2181–2185.

Park K.K., Wishnok J.S. and Archer M.C. (1977). Mechanism of alkylation by N-nitroso compounds: detection of rearranged alcohol in the microsomal metabolism of N-nitrosodi-*n*-propylamine and base-catalyzed decomposition of N-*n*-propyl-N-nitrosourea. *Chem. Biol. Interact.* **18**, 349–354.

Peterson L.A., Trevor A. and Castagnoli N. Jr (1987). Stereochemical studies on the cytochrome P-450 catalyzed oxidation of (*S*)-nicotine to the (*S*)-nicotine $\Delta^{1'(5')}$-iminium species. *J. Med. Chem.* **30**, 249–254.

Pichard L., Gillet G., Fabre I., Dalet-Beluche I., Bonfils C., Thenot J.P. and Maurel P. (1990). Identification of the rabbit and human cytochromes P-450IIIA as the major enzymes involved in the N-demethylation of diltiazem. *Drug Metab. Disposit.* **18**, 711–719.

Pognat J.F., Enreille A., Chabard J.L., Busch N. and Berger J.A. (1986). N-Dephenylation of CERM 3517 (mociprazine) in Beagle dogs. *Drug Metab. Disposit.* **14**, 147–154.

Ross D., Farmer P.B., Gescher A., Hickman J.A. and Threadgill M.D. (1982). The formation and metabolism of N-hydroxymethyl compounds - I. The oxidative N-demethylation of N-dimethyl derivatives of arylamines, aryltriazenes, arylformamidines and arylureas including the herbicide monuron. *Biochem. Pharmacol.* **31**, 3621–3627.

Ross D., Farmer P.B., Gescher A., Hickman J.A. and Threadgill M.D. (1983). The metabolism of a stable N-hydromethyl derivative of a N-methylamide. *Life Sci.* **32**, 597–604.

Sayre L.M., Engelhart D.A., Venkataraman B., Babu M.K.M. and McCoy G.D. (1991). Generation and fate of enamines in the microsomal metabolism of cyclic tertiary amines. *Biochem. Biophys. Res. Commun.* **179**, 1368–1376.

Seto Y. and Guengerich F.P. (1993). Partitioning between N-dealkylation and N-oxygenation in the oxidation of N,N-dialkylarylamines catalyzed by cytochrome P450 2B1. *J. Biol. Chem.* **268**, 9986–9997.

Shannon P. and Bruice T.C. (1981). A novel P-450 model system for the N-dealkylation reaction. *J. Amer. Chem. Soc.* **103**, 4580–4582.

Slatter J.G., Mutlib A.E. and Abbott F.S. (1989). Biotransformation of aliphatic formamides: metabolites of (±)-N-methyl-N-(1-methyl-3,3-diphenylpropyl)formamides in rats. *Biomed. Environm. Mass Spectrom.* **18**, 690–701.

Stefek M., Ransom R.W., DiStefano E.W. and Cho A.K. (1990). The alpha carbon oxidation of some phencyclidine analogues by rat tissue and pharmacological implications. *Xenobiotica* **20**, 591–600.

Struck R.F., Kirk M.C., Witt M.H. and Laster W.R. Jr (1975). Isolation and mass spectral identification of blood metabolites of cyclophosphamide: evidence for phosphoramide mustard as the biologically active metabolite. *Biomed. Mass Spectrom.* **2**, 46–52.

Sugawara Y., Nakamura S., Usuki S., Ito Y., Suzuki T., Ohashi M. and Harigaya S. (1988). Metabolism of diltiazem. II. Metabolic profile in rat, dog and man. *J. Pharmacobio.-Dyn.* **11**, 224–233.

Ullrich V., Hermann G. and Weber P. (1978). Nitrite formation from 2-nitropropane by microsomal monooxygenases. *Biochem. Pharmacol.* **27**, 2301–2304.

Viau J.P., Epps J.E. and Di Carlo F.J. (1973). Prazepam metabolism in the rat. *J. Pharm. Sci.* **62**, 641–645.

Wall G.M. and Baker J.K. (1989). Metabolism of 3-(*p*-chlorophenyl)pyrrolidine. Structural effects in conversion of a prototype γ-aminobutyric acid prodrug to lactam and γ-aminobutyric acid type metabolites. *J. Med. Chem.* **32**, 1340–1348.

Wang M., Chung F.L. and Hecht S.S. (1988). Identification of crotonaldehyde as a hepatic microsomal metabolite formed by α-hydroxylation of the carcinogen N-nitrosopyrrolidine. *Chem. Res. Toxicol.* **1**, 28–31.

Ward D.P., Trevor A.J., Kalir A., Adams J.D., Baillie T.A. and Castagnoli N. Jr (1982). Metabolism of phencyclidine. The role of iminium ion formation in covalent binding to rabbit microsomal protein. *Drug Metab. Disposit.* **10**, 690–695.

Weli A.M., Backlund Höök B. and Lindeke B. (1985). N-Dealkylation and N-oxidation of two α-methyl-substituted pargyline analogues in rat liver microsomes. *Acta Pharm. Suec.* **22**, 249–264.

Yang C.S., Yoo J.S.H., Ishizaki H. and Hong J. (1990). Cytochrome P450IIE1: Roles in nitrosamine metabolism and mechanisms of regulation. *Drug Metab. Rev.* **22**, 147–159.

Yeh S.Y. (1990). N-Depyridination and N-dedimethylaminoethylation of tripelennamine and pyrilamine in the rat. *Drug Metab. Disposit.* **18**, 453–461.

Yun C.H., Okerholm R.A. and Guengerich F.P. (1993). Oxidation of the antihistaminic drug terfenadine in human liver microsomes. Role of cytochrome P-450 3A(4) in N-dealkylation and C-hydroxylation. *Drug Metab. Disposit.* **21**, 403–409.

Ziegler R., Ho B. and Castagnoli Jr N. (1981). Trapping of metabolically generated electrophilic species with cyanide ion: metabolism of methapyrilene. *J. Med. Chem.* **24**, 1133–1138.

Zon G., Ludeman S.M., Brandt J.A., Boyd V.L., Ozkan G., Egan W. and Shao K.L. (1984). NMR spectroscopic studies of intermediary metabolites of cyclophosphamide. *J. Med. Chem.* **27**, 466–485.

chapter 7

MONOOXYGENASE-CATALYZED OXIDATION OF OXYGEN- AND SULFUR-CONTAINING COMPOUNDS

Contents

7.1 INTRODUCTION

A vast number of xenobiotics possess oxygen- and/or sulfur-containing functional groups, which are subject to a variety of metabolic reactions. The dehydrogenation of alcohols and aldehydes, and the reduction of carbonyl compounds, have been treated in Chapter 2, while later chapters in this and subsequent volumes will examine the reduction, hydrolysis and conjugation of O- and S-containing xenobiotics. The present chapter is concerned with monooxygenase-mediated reactions including the oxidation of ethers, esters, alcohols, aldehydes and phenols, and the oxidation or oxygenation of thiols, thioethers, thiocarbonyls, and other sulfur derivatives.

While a few of the reactions discussed in this chapter are more or less specific (e.g. oxidation of thiols to disulfides, oxidative desulfuration), most of them (e.g. O- and S-dealkylation, O-dearylation, S-oxygenation) are comparable with those of nitrogenated compounds. As a consequence, the present chapter will refer extensively to previous ones, notably Chapters 4–6, thereby avoiding the need to dwell on mechanisms that the reader may easily piece together.

The cytochrome P450 and FAD-containing monooxygenase systems are both involved in the oxidation and oxygenation not only of nitrogenated moieties (Chapters 5 and 6), but also of sulfur-containing groups. In contrast, the mammalian monooxygenation of oxygen-containing groups appears to involve exclusively cytochrome P450, and we are aware of no evidence indicating the involvement of the FAD-containing monooxygenase.

7.2 O-DEALKYLATION

Most published examples of O-dealkylation involve medicinal aryl alkyl ethers, but xenobiotic dialkyl ethers and cyclic ethers are also of interest in this context. Diaryl ethers are altogether different, and the relevant reaction of O-dearylation will be considered separately in Section 7.4.

7.2.1 Mechanism of O-dealkylation and substrate selectivity of O-demethylation reactions

The reaction mechanism of cytochrome P450-catalyzed O-dealkylation has attracted far less interest than that of N-dealkylation (e.g. Al-Gailany *et al.*, 1975; Garland *et al.*, 1976; Lindsay Smith and Sleath, 1983; Lu *et al.*, 1984). The picture emerging at present is a classical one: that of alpha-carbon oxidation by hydrogen radical abstraction (reaction **a** in Fig. 7.1) followed by hydroxylation (reaction **b** in Fig. 7.1), in other words the well-known **oxygen rebound mechanism**. The resulting hydroxylated intermediate is a hemiacetal of low stability that rapidly hydrolyzes to the corresponding phenol (or alcohol) and a carbonyl compound such as formaldehyde. Fig. 7.1 is considerably simpler than the corresponding routes A1 and A2 (Fig. 6.1, Chapter 6) for N-dealkylation. Indeed, the possibility of an initial abstraction of one electron from the oxygen atom to yield the radical cation is not shown in Fig. 7.1, such a mechanism having been excluded in the O-demethylation of anisole (**7.I**), a model compound of particular interest (Lindsay Smith and Sleath, 1983). Nevertheless, the possibility exists that an electron abstraction can take place in some cases, as discussed in Section 7.6.1 (Guengerich *et al.*, 1984).

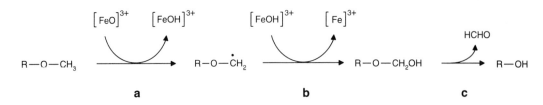

FIGURE 7.1 Mechanistic scheme for cytochrome P450-catalyzed O-demethylation (and more generally O-dealkylation).

Besides anisole, many **aromatic methyl ethers** are known to undergo O-demethylation, a number of which are of medicinal interest. For example, the antiarrhythmic drug encainide (**7.II**) undergoes several metabolic reactions in humans, O-demethylation in this compound greatly predominating over other routes such as N-demethylation, lactam formation and aromatic oxidation (Jajoo *et al.*, 1990). Another drug of particular importance is codeine (Chapter 6, **6.XVIII** with R = CH$_3$), which is O-demethylated to the active metabolite morphine. In humans, the reaction is mediated by the CYP2D6 also involved in dextromethorphan O-demethylation (Dayer *et al.*, 1988; Vree and Verwey-Van Wissen, 1992).

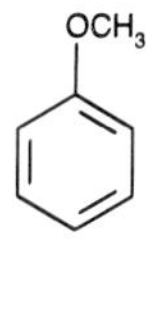

7.I 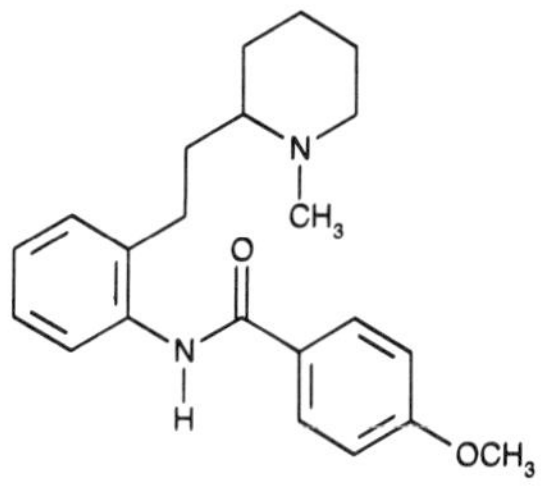   7.II

Informative cases of **substrate regioselectivity** and **enantioselectivity** have been uncovered in the metabolism of verapamil (**7.III**, R = H) and gallopamil (**7.III**, R = OCH$_3$) (see also Section 6.3). For example, the regioselectivity of O-demethylation of verapamil in rat and human liver microsomes was 4′ > 4 > 3, no reaction being detected at the 3′-position (Nelson *et al.*, 1988). With gallopamil, mono-O-demethylation can yield four monophenols, as the 3- and 5-positions are equivalent. O-Demethylation at these sites was less than at the 4-position. But in contrast to verapamil, gallopamil showed a predominance of 4-O-demethylation over 4′-O-demethylation (Mutlib and Nelson, 1990).

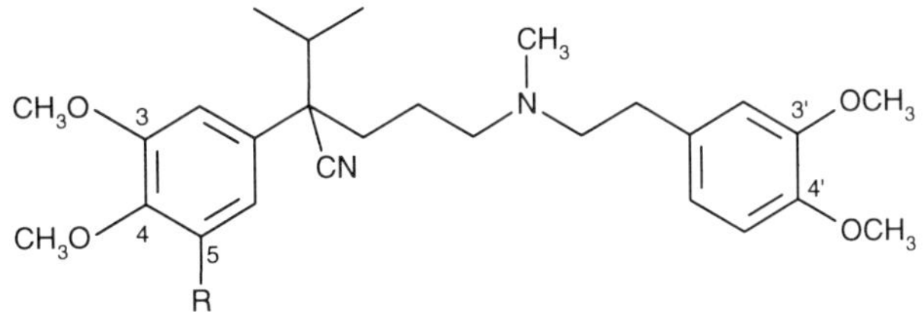

7.III

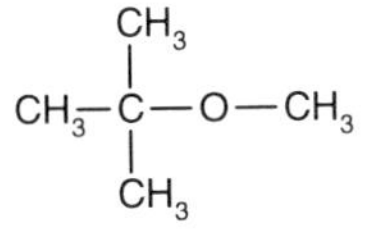

7.IV 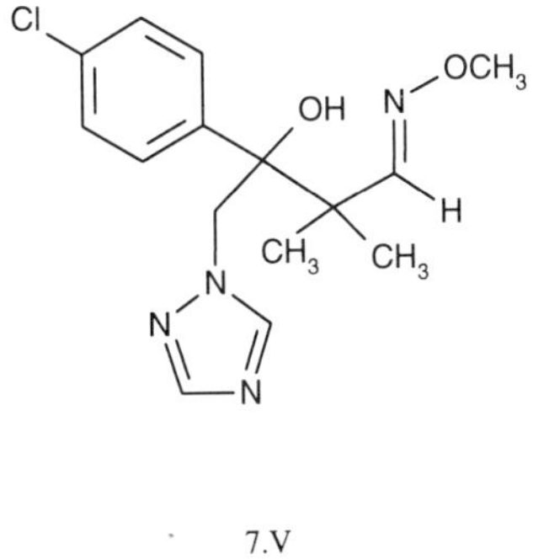   7.V

The biotransformation of a few **alkyl methyl ethers** has been investigated, a noteworthy example being methyl *tert*-butyl ether (**7.IV**). This octane booster used in gasoline has been shown to be O-demethylated in rat liver microsomes to *tert*-butanol and formaldehyde, the reaction being mediated in part by CYP2E1, the ethanol-inducible cytochrome P450 (Brady *et al.*, 1990). **Oxime O-methyl ethers**, despite their rare occurrence, are worth mentioning. Thus, the antifungal agent BAYr3783 (**7.V**) undergoes O-demethylation to the oxime as the major route in rats and dogs (Boberg *et al.*, 1990). Another similar example is that of 1-methoxyindole-3-carboxylic acid, where the nitrogen atom occupies an endocyclic position (Nwankwo, 1991).

7.2.2 Substrate selectivity in O-dealkylation reactions

Besides the methyl ethers discussed above, a variety of other **alkyl ethers** have been shown to undergo O-dealkylation. Thus, diethyl ether is a substrate of cytochrome P450, and particularly CYP2E1, yielding acetaldehyde as a metabolite (Brady *et al.*, 1988). The kinetic parameters of the reaction in rat liver microsomes indicate a relatively high efficiency. A drug also containing an **ethoxy group** is **phenacetin** (**7.VI**), the O-deethylation of which yields the well-known drug acetaminophen (see Section 7.6). The reaction is mediated by CYP1A2 (known as phenacetin O-deethylase) and CYP1A1 (aryl hydrocarbon hydroxylase), two enzymes inducible by polycyclic aromatic hydrocarbons (Sesardic *et al.*, 1990). A detailed investigation of the reaction in human liver microsomes has been reported (Gillam and Reilly, 1988). CYP1A1 is also involved in the O-deethylation of 7-ethoxyresorufin (**7.VII**, R = ethyl), a convenient substrate frequently used to monitor the induction of this enzyme (e.g. Ayrton *et al.*, 1990).

7.VI   7.VII   7.VIII

The rate of O-dealkylation of four model *para*-nitrophenyl alkyl ethers (alkyl = methyl, ethyl, isopropyl and *n*-butyl) was investigated in rat liver microsomes (Al-Gailany *et al.*, 1975). For the three linear homologues, affinity (spectral [K_s] and kinetic [K_m]) increased with chain length and lipophilicity, and so did maximal velocity (V_{max}). However, the isopropyl ether displayed the highest affinity and velocity, indicating it to be a better substrate than expected from simple lipophilicity arguments. Interestingly, another series of model compounds, namely 1-(4-acetylnaphthyl) alkyl ethers (**7.VIII**), did not yield comparable results under similar conditions (Hunter and Wilson, 1981). Here, maximal velocity decreased with increasing chain length and lipophilicity in the sequence *methyl* > *ethyl* > *propyl* = *isopropyl* > *butyl*; as for the differences in affinity, they appear unrelated to chain length. Thus, a comparison between these two series of aryl alkyl ethers shows how misleading it can be to generalize structure–metabolism relationships obtained from limited series of substrates. The major reason for this situation can be found in the different **substrate specificities** exhibited by the various cytochromes P450 that catalyze reactions of O-dealkylation. Both the alkoxy group and the aromatic nucleus of alkyl aryl ethers direct such substrates towards specific cytochromes P450 and influence the apparent affinity and catalytic rate of the reaction, as seen for example when comparing the O-dealkylation

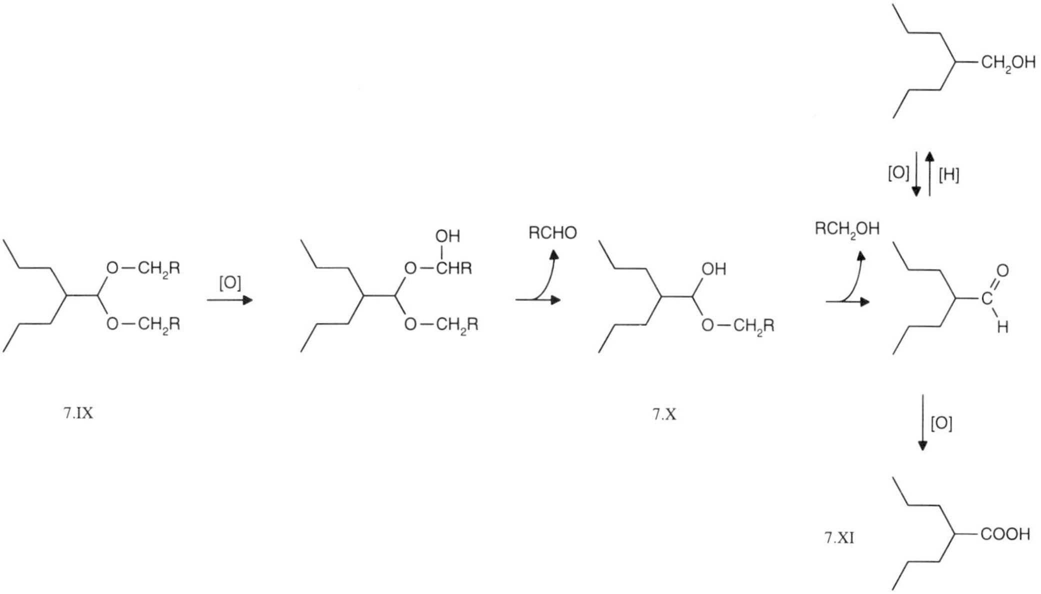

FIGURE 7.2 Activation by O-dealkylation of acetals as prodrugs of carboxylic acids, illustrated here with the conversion of 2-propylpentanal acetals (**7.IX**) to valproic acid (**7.XI**) via a hemiacetal (**7.X**) (Vicchio and Callery, 1989).

of **7-alkoxyresorufins** (**7.VII**), **7-alkoxycoumarins**, and **7-alkoxyquinolines** (Buters *et al.*, 1993; Mayer *et al.*, 1990; Nerurkar *et al.*, 1993). As a result of such substrate specificities, 7-alkoxyresorufins and analogous compounds are often used as probes of specific cytochromes P450.

Other moieties being cleaved by O-dealkylation include the **pentoxy, benzyloxy** and substituted benzyloxy groups (e.g. Rabovsky and Judy, 1987). More complex groups are also cleaved by O-dealkylation, a well-known example being that of the propanolamino side-chain of β-blockers such as propranolol (Chapter 6, Fig. 6.3). This drug yields 1-naphthol as a metabolite, although *in vitro* experiments suggested that O-dealkylation occurs less with the parent drug than with its deaminated metabolites, notably naphthoxylactic acid (**6.XXX** in Fig. 6.3) (Nelson and Bartels, 1984).

A particularly elegant exploitation of O-dealkylation has recently been proposed for the bioactivation of **prodrugs of medicinal acids**, as illustrated in Fig. 7.2 for valproic acid **7.XI** (Vicchio and Callery, 1989). O-Dealkylation of **acetals** (here 2-propylpentanal acetals, **7.IX**, R = methyl, ethyl or isopropyl in Fig. 7.2) yields a hemiacetal (**7.X** in Fig. 7.2) which hydrolyzes to the aldehyde, the latter then being dehydrogenated to the acid.

Cleavable O-alkyl groups are not the only ones of interest to drug designers. Indeed, **groups resistant to O-dealkylation** may also be desirable in some cases, although little research has been done in this direction. For example, the 2,2,2-trifluoroethoxy group (CF_3CH_2O-) was not cleaved when aromatic substrates containing this moiety were incubated with rat liver microsomes (Irurre *et al.*, 1993).

Cyclic ethers also can undergo alpha-carbon oxidation leading to ring opening and possibly lactone formation, in analogy with saturated azaheterocycles (Section 6.4). For example, **1,4-dioxane** (**7.XII**), an organic solvent, is metabolized in rats to β-hydroxyethoxyacetic acid (**7.XIII**) as the major urinary metabolite; this product is proof of C(α)-hydroxylation followed by ring opening and dehydrogenation (Braun and Young, 1977). In addition, there was evidence to

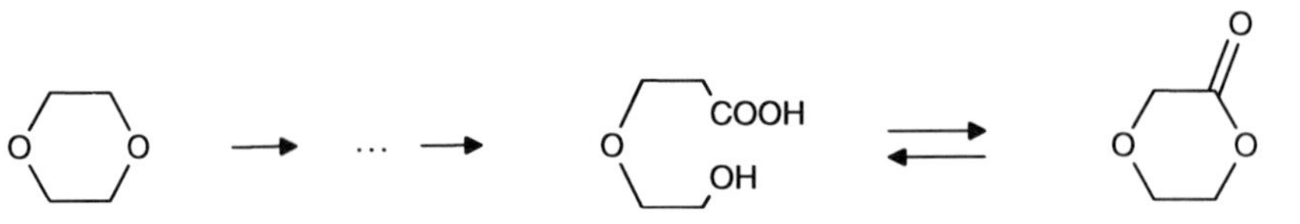

7.XII   7.XIII   7.XIV

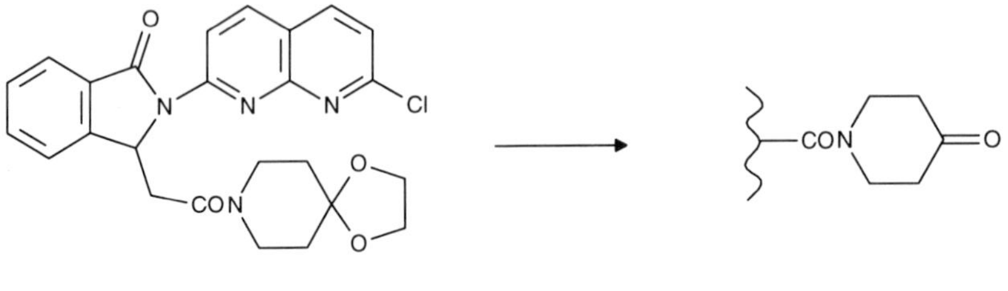

7.XV

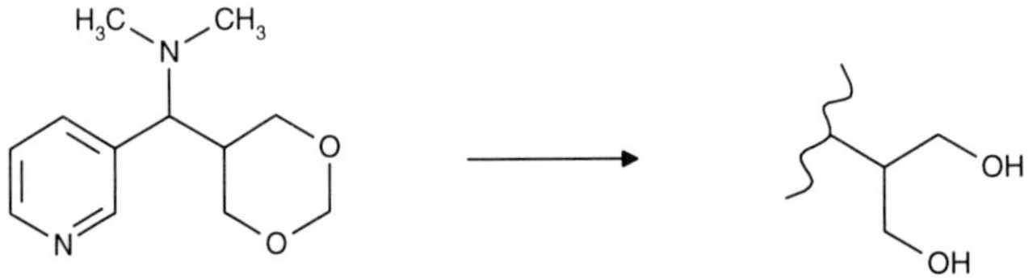

7.XVI

indicate a pH-dependent equilibrium between the hydroxyacid **7.XIII** and 1,4-dioxanone, the corresponding lactone (**7.XIV**). Opening of a **morpholine ring** by C(α)-hydroxylation has been discussed in Section 6.4 taking the morpholine ring of emorfazone (**6.LX**) as an example. As compared to N–C cleavage, O–C cleavage leading to the hydroxyacid **6.LXIII** occurred with higher affinity but lower velocity in guinea-pig liver microsomes (Hayashi *et al.*, 1983).

Cyclic acetals, i.e. 1,3-dioxo saturated heterocycles, may be metabolized like the acyclic acetals discussed above (Fig. 7.2). Oxidative ring opening unmasks a diol function or a carbonyl group depending which part of the substrate molecule is considered. Thus, the anxiolytic agent pazinaclone (**7.XV**) is transformed into the 4-oxopiperidino derivative (Hussein *et al.*, 1993). As for 3-[(dimethylamino)-(*m*-dioxan-5-yl)methyl]pyridine (**7.XVI**), it contains a 1,3-dioxane ring that undergoes opening to the diol by oxidative O-demethylenation; the reaction was characterized in humans, although it involved only a very small percent of the dose (Rubin *et al.*, 1979). This last example also serves as a transition with the next section.

7.3 O-DEMETHYLENATION OF 1,3-BENZODIOXOLES

1,3-Benzodioxoles, also called **methylenedioxybenzenes**, are a class of cyclic ethers whose O-dealkylation is of particular interest. The reaction is known as an O-demethylenation since it is the methylene group attached to the two oxygen atoms that is removed, thereby unmasking a catechol function. For example, the demethylenation of **methylenedioxymethamphetamine**

(**7.XVII**, MDMA) in rat liver and brain microsomes was shown to be catalyzed by cytochrome P450, yielding 3,4-dihydroxymethamphetamine (**7.XVIII**) (Hiramatsu *et al.*, 1990; Lin *et al.*, 1992). The rabbit enzyme CYP2B4 is particularly effective in catalyzing the O-demethylenation of methylenedioxybenzene (Fukuto *et al.*, 1991; Kumagai *et al.*, 1991 and 1992a). Another compound of interest is the antiepileptic agent **stiripentol** (**7.XIX**), whose biotransformation in humans yields a wealth of demethylenated metabolites accounting for almost half of a dose (Moreland *et al.*, 1986).

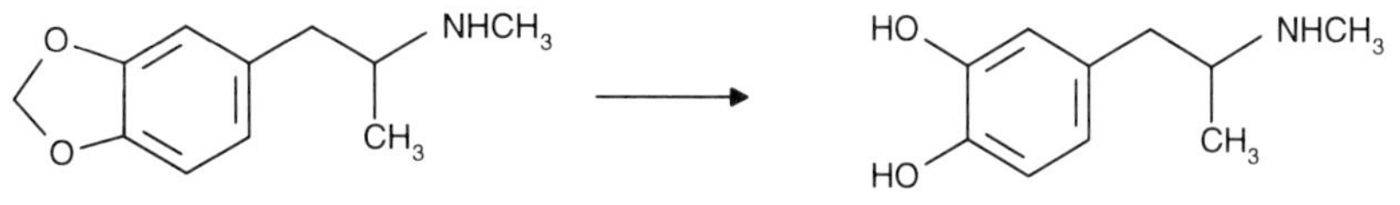

7.XVII   7.XVIII

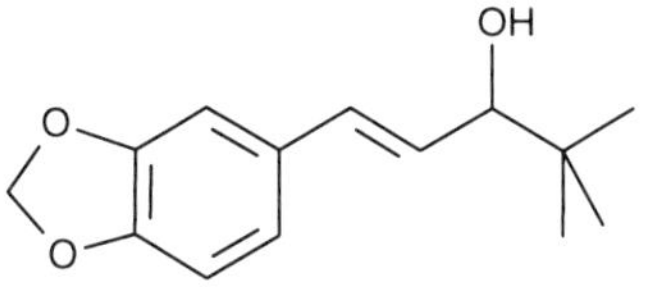

7.XIX

O-Demethylenation is thus a major reaction of stiripentol, a quite lipophilic compound. In contrast, such **hydrophilic xenobiotics** as piperonyl alcohol (**7.XX**) and piperonal (**7.XXI**) are poor substrates for the reaction (less than 1% of a dose in rats) (Klungsøyr and Scheline, 1984). Even more telling is the fact that highly polar acids containing the 3,4-methylenedioxyphenyl moiety (e.g. the benzoic acid analogue **7.XXII**) did not show the slightest evidence of catechol formation in rats. Clearly, a relationship exists between substrate lipophilicity and the extent of demethylenation (Klungsøyr and Scheline, 1981).

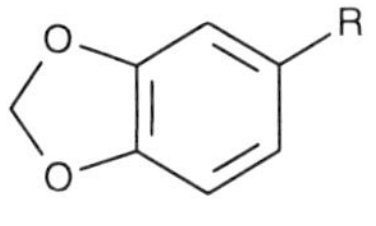

7.XX   R   = $-CH_2OH$

7.XXI   R   = $-CHO$

7.XXII R   = $-COOH$

7.XXIII R   = $-CH_2CH=CH_2$

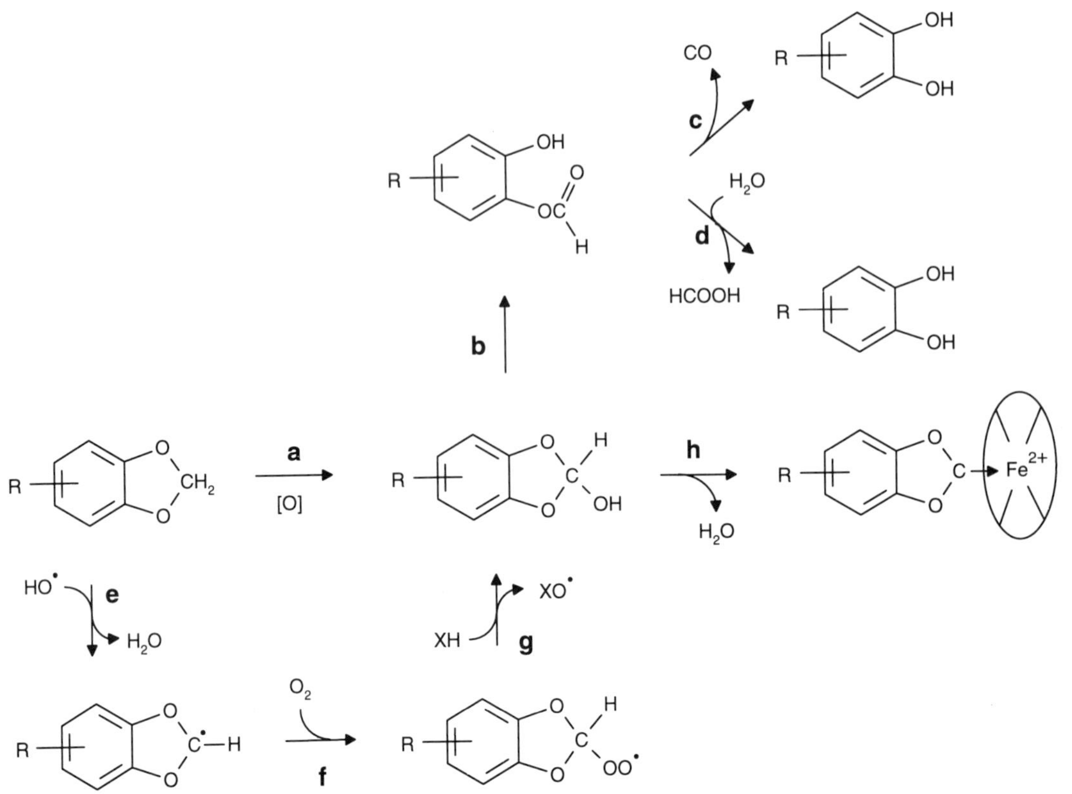

FIGURE 7.3 Reaction mechanisms of oxidative O-demethylenation of 1,3-benzodioxoles. The direct route leads to a catechol and carbon monoxide or formate (reactions **a–d**), while the hydroxyl radical produced by uncoupling mediates an indirect mechanism (reactions **e–g**). Also shown is the dehydration of the intermediate 2-hydroxy-1,3-benzodioxole producing a carbene which binds as a strong ligand to ferrocytochrome P450 (reaction **h**) (modified from Anders *et al.*, 1984; Lin *et al.*, 1992).

The methylene moiety cleaved from 1,3-benzodioxoles is recovered as carbon dioxide during *in vivo* studies, and as formic acid or carbon monoxide from *in vitro* incubations. These observations have led Anders and coworkers to propose the **direct reaction mechanism** shown in Fig. 7.3 (Anders *et al.*, 1984). Cytochrome P450-catalyzed oxidation yields a 2-hydroxy-1,3-benzodioxole intermediate (reaction **a** in Fig. 7.3) which undergoes ring scission (reaction **b** in Fig. 7.3) to a formate ester; decarbonylation of the latter (reaction **c** in Fig. 7.3) leads to carbon monoxide and catechol, while its hydrolysis (reaction **d** in Fig. 7.3) leads to formic acid and catechol. The fact that electron-withdrawing substituents in the 5- or 6-position of the ring favour carbon monoxide production is also of interest and could be explained in terms of increased monooxygenation of the methylene unit and/or to a chemoselectivity for reaction **c** over reaction **d** in Fig. 7.3 (Anders *et al.*, 1984).

In addition to the direct mechanism (reactions **a–d**) shown in Fig. 7.3, there is evidence to indicate that in some cases the cytochrome P450-catalyzed O-demethylenation of benzodioxoles may proceed indirectly. In such an **indirect reaction mechanism**, the hydroxyl radical (HO$^\bullet$) resulting from uncoupling (Section 3.5) pulls away a hydrogen radical from the methylene group to form a C-centred radical (reaction **e** in Fig. 7.3). Addition of molecular oxygen to the latter leads to a peroxyl radical (reaction **f** in Fig. 7.3) that can decompose to a 2-hydroxy-1,3-benzodioxole intermediate (reaction **g** in Fig. 7.3) by mechanisms discussed in Chapter 10

(Fukuto *et al.*, 1991; Lin *et al.*, 1992). A good substrate such as methylenedioxybenzene appears to be O-demethylenated by the direct mechanism, while poorer substrates such as MDMA (**7.XVII**) and methylenedioxyamphetamine (MDA) produce some uncoupling and thus react by both the direct and indirect routes.

Many 1,3-benzodioxoles display a marked **inhibitory activity** towards some cytochrome P450 isozymes, with which they form metabolic intermediate (MI) complexes (Franklin, 1977; Marcus *et al.*, 1985; Testa and Jenner, 1981). Formation of such MI complexes is characterized by an absorption maximum at about 437 nm with ferricytochrome P450, but with the reduced form of the enzyme two absorption maxima at about 427 and 455 nm are seen (Delaforge *et al.*, 1985; Murray *et al.*, 1985). The complexes are relatively stable, particularly those with ferrocytochrome P450. Converging evidence indicates that the metabolic intermediate acting as a strong ligand of the iron cation is a **carbene** (>C:) whose formation is explained by dehydration of the 2-hydroxy-1,3-benzodioxole intermediate (reaction **h** in Fig. 7.3). Methylenedioxybenzenes are thus classified as mechanism-based (indirect), reversible inhibitors of cytochrome P450 (Testa and Jenner, 1981).

Formation of an MI complex explains much of the cytochrome P450 inhibitory activity of methylenedioxybenzenes such as safrole (**7.XXIII**), a natural compound, and piperonyl butoxide, a synthetic potentiator of insecticides. The marked inhibition by stiripentol (**7.XIX**) of cytochrome P450-catalyzed reactions *in vitro* and *in vivo* is also accounted for by its activation to a complex-forming metabolic intermediate (Mesnil *et al.*, 1988).

7.4 O-Dearylation

The reaction of N-dearylation discussed in Section 6.6 finds its counterpart in oxidative O–C cleavage. Indeed, a few diaryl ethers are known to undergo O-dearylation, for example **3-phenoxybenzoic acid** (**7.XXIV**). This compound occurs as a mammalian metabolite of fluvalinate and some other pyrethroid insecticides, and it was shown to be further transformed in chickens to 3-hydroxybenzoic acid (**7.XXV**) as a major metabolite (Quistad *et al.*, 1988). However, the metabolic reaction leading from **7.XXIV** to **7.XXV** is not a direct one and involves first *para*-hydroxylation of the phenoxy moiety (Akhtar and Mahadevan, 1992).

7.XXIV

7.XXV

7.XXVI

An example of greater medicinal relevance is afforded by (−)-**3-phenoxy-N-methylmorphinan** (**7.XXVI**, PMM), a potent *in vivo* analgesic. When administered to dogs, this compound was oxidized in the phenyl ring to *para*-hydroxy-PMM and *meta*-methoxy-*para*-hydroxy-PMM. In addition, O-dephenylation occurred in rats as well as in dogs, where it accounted for approximately one half of the recovered dose, making this reaction a major one in dogs (Kamm *et al.*, 1979; Leinweber *et al.*, 1981). Because O-dephenylation yields the active opiate levorphanol, the possibility was mentioned that PMM may be a prodrug of the latter.

The fact that the phenyl ring in PMM is easily oxidized and that no ether cleavage occurred in an analogue having a pentafluorinated phenyl ring strongly suggested that O-dephenylation cannot occur without phenyl oxidation. Two **reaction mechanisms** have been mentioned in Section 6.6 in connection with N-dearylation, namely formation and hydrolysis of a quinone imine, or formation of an *ipso,ortho*-epoxide followed by rearrangement (Fig. 6.15). The same two mechanisms may conceivably operate in O-dearylation. Thus, *para*-hydroxylation followed by oxidation could yield a quinone-like intermediate that breaks down to benzoquinone and a phenol (reaction **a** in Fig. 7.4). Epoxidation appears as a plausible alternative and was first proposed by Kamm *et al.* (1979), who also suggested a subsequent conjugation with glutathione to explain the cleavage step. In fact, glutathione is not the only nucleophile which could lead to cleavage, the hydroxyl anion being another candidate. A proposed mechanism of O-dearylation by epoxidation is presented in simplified form as reaction **b** in Fig. 7.4, showing initial *ipso,ortho*-epoxidation followed by a nucleophilic attack at the *ipso*-carbon, a particularly electron-poor position. The subsequent step of rearrangement/cleavage may occur by more than one mechanism. Note that pathways **a** and **b** in Fig. 7.4 are not mutually exclusive since *para*-hydroxylation might favour *ipso,ortho*-epoxidation. Obviously Fig. 7.4 must remain hypothetical until detailed *in vitro* studies clarify the actual mechanism of the reaction and the structure of the metabolite(s) arising from the aromatic moiety being removed.

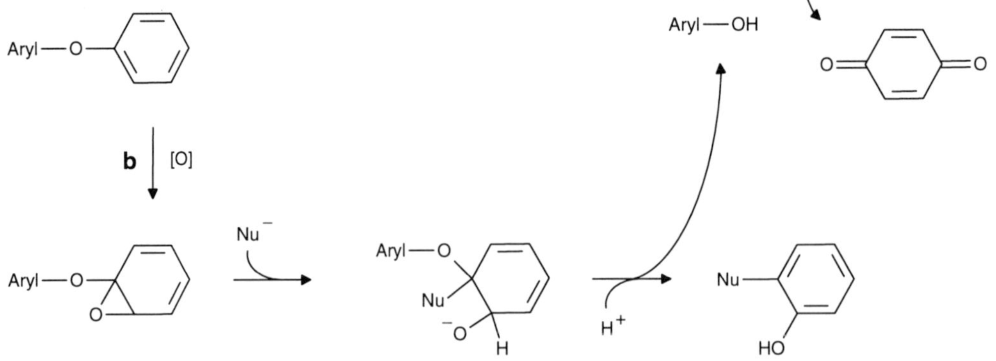

FIGURE 7.4 Hypothetical reaction mechanisms of cytochrome P450-catalyzed O-dearylation, shown in simplified form; Nu⁻ is a nucleophile such as HO⁻ or the glutathionyl anion (GS⁻) attacking the *ipso*-position of the postulated *ipso,ortho*-epoxide. As discussed in the text, pathways **a** and **b** are not mutually exclusive.

7.5 OXIDATIVE ESTER CLEAVAGE

Hydrolytic ester cleavage is a metabolic reaction of great significance which will be discussed and illustrated at length in the following volume. An alternative pathway is presented here, namely cytochrome P450-catalyzed oxidative ester cleavage. A few isolated observations of such a reaction were published several years ago, for example the oxidative deesterification of the herbicide flampropisopropyl (**7.XXVII**) to the acid **7.XXVIII** (Bedford *et al.*, 1978). In this study, the use of cofactors and inhibitors strongly suggested the existence of a cytochrome P450-mediated deesterification besides enzymatic hydrolysis. The proposed **mechanism** involves formation of the hydroxylated intermediate **7.XXIX** followed by its postenzymatic breakdown to the acid and acetone.

7.XXVII R = $-CH(CH_3)_2$

7.XXVIII R = $-H$

7.XXIX R = $-\overset{\overset{\displaystyle CH_3}{|}}{\underset{\underset{\displaystyle CH_3}{|}}{C}}-OH$

7.XXX

In recent years, these earlier findings have been confirmed by careful metabolic studies of 2,6-dimethyl-4-phenyl-3,5-pyridinedicarboxylic acid dialkyl esters (**7.XXX**). These compounds are metabolites formed by oxidation of **1,4-dihydropyridines** (see Section 5.4). Upon incubation of **7.XXX** with NADPH-fortified rat or human liver microsomes, the corresponding monoester was readily obtained, the diethyl and diisopropyl esters being better substrates than the dimethyl ester (Guengerich, 1987). When the alkyl group was perdeuterated, a large deuterium isotope effect was seen in the reaction. This, together with other evidence, has indicated that the reaction mechanism indeed involves **hydroxylation of the alpha-carbon** in the alkyl group.

Another mechanism of oxidative ester cleavage exists in compounds of this type, namely **intramolecular transesterification** to form a lactone. Specifically, 2,6-dimethyl-4-phenyl-3,5-pyridinedicarboxylic acid diethyl ester is oxidized to two metabolites, namely the monoester as discussed above (reaction **a** in Fig. 7.5), and the 2-hydroxymethyl analogue (reaction **b** in Fig. 7.5) which then undergoes deethylation by lactone formation (reaction **c** in Fig. 7.3) (Guengerich *et al.*, 1988). CYP1A1 and CYP2B1 were the most active among the various cytochromes P450 examined in catalyzing reactions **a** and **b** (Fig. 7.5), respectively. The *in vivo* significance of these reactions was demonstrated in rats dosed with the pyridine metabolite of nifedipine, and in rats and humans dosed with oxodipine (Flinois *et al.*, 1992; Funaki *et al.*, 1989).

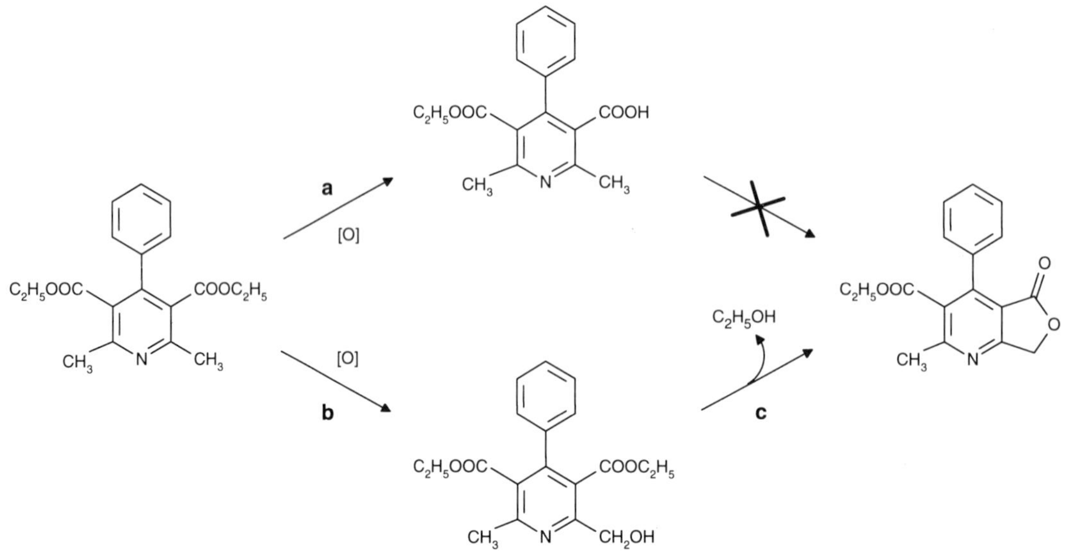

FIGURE 7.5 Oxidative deesterification of pyridinedicarboxylic acid diesters by hydroxylation of an alkyl group (reaction **a**), or formation of a 2-hydroxymethyl analogue followed by intramolecular transesterification to a lactone (reactions **b** and **c**) (Guengerich *et al.*, 1988).

Oxidative deesterification thus appears as an intriguing metabolic pathway, whose contribution may well remain unrecognized in a number of cases. As workers become aware of this route, they will begin assessing its relative importance in various reactions of ester cleavage. Note that Section 7.7 presents yet another oxidative mechanism of ester cleavage, namely one involving some thioesters.

7.6 CYTOCHROME P450-CATALYZED OXIDATION OF ALCOHOLS, ALDEHYDES, FORMAMIDES AND PHENOLS

A number of oxygenated compounds undergo monooxygenase-mediated oxidation in addition to other reactions discussed in previous chapters. Thus, the oxidation of some alcohols to carbonyl compounds can be mediated by cytochromes P450 in addition to or instead of alcohol dehydrogenases (Section 2.2). Similarly, some aldehydes can undergo cytochrome P450-catalyzed oxidation to carboxylic acids and then to decarboxylated products. Finally, the oxidation of some phenols to quinones or quinonoid compounds is a significant metabolic route that has little in common with the oxygenation of aromatic rings (Section 4.3).

7.6.1 Oxidation of alcohols

Two principal mechanisms are now recognized in the cytochrome P450-catalyzed oxidation of alcohols to carbonyl compounds, one mechanism depending on the hydroxyl radical, the second more closely resembling the usual functioning of this enzyme.

In microsomal preparations or reconstituted systems (cytochrome P450 plus NADPH-cytochrome P450 reductase plus phospholipids), ethanol and other primary **alcohols of low molecular weight** such as methanol, 1-propanol and 1-butanol are oxidized to the corresponding

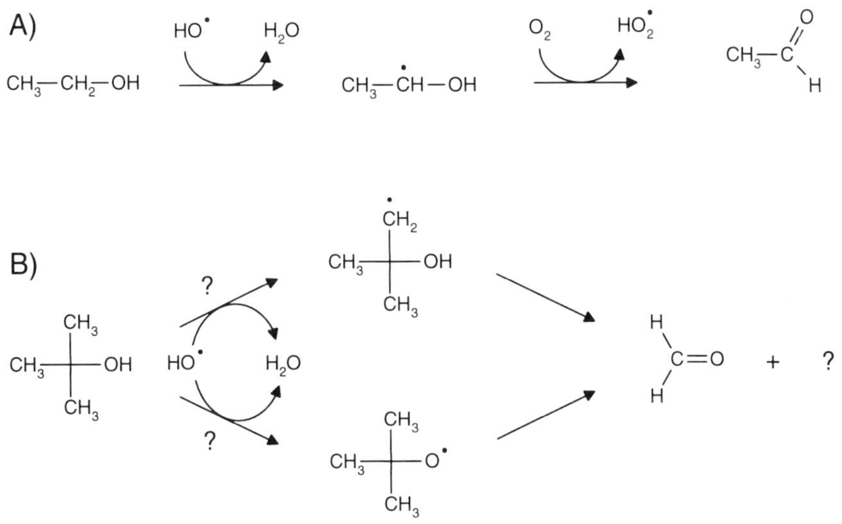

FIGURE 7.6 Postulated mechanisms of the cytochrome P450-catalyzed oxidation of ethanol to acetalde-hyde (pathway **A**) and of *tert*-butanol to formaldehyde and other products (pathway **B**) (Cederbaum and Cohen, 1980; Ingelman-Sundberg and Johansson, 1984).

aldehyde. The reaction is an indirect one in that it is mediated by the **hydroxyl radical** (HO•), as evidenced by the fact that hydroxyl radical scavengers (e.g. benzoate, dimethylsulphoxide, mannitol, thiourea) have a strong inhibitory effect (Cohen and Cederbaum, 1979 and 1980; Morgan *et al.*, 1982; Ohnishi and Lieber, 1978). In contrast, superoxide dismutase has no such inhibitory effect, ruling out a direct role for superoxide ($O_2^{\bullet-}$). The accelerating influence of added hydrogen peroxide provides evidence that the hydroxyl radical must be formed from reduced oxygen species released by the enzyme. Two mechanisms are often mentioned, namely the iron-catalyzed Haber–Weiss reaction and the Fenton reaction (see Section 3.5). The partial inhibitory effect of desferroxamine, an iron chelator, on the oxidation of alcohols suggests a role for either reaction (Ingelman-Sundberg and Johansson, 1984; Krikun and Cederbaum, 1984).

The oxidation of ethanol and homologues is mediated by a number of cytochromes P450 among which CYP2E1 is particularly active due to its capacity to reduce oxygen (Albano *et al.*, 1991; Morgan *et al.*, 1982). Kinetic isotope effects have indicated that cleavage of the C(1)–H bond appears to be a rate-determining step in the catalysis by CYP2E1, suggesting the **reaction mechanism** shown in pathway **A** (Fig. 7.6) (Ekström *et al.*, 1987; Ingelman-Sundberg and Johansson, 1984). More insight can be gained from the cytochrome P450-mediated oxidation of *tert*-butanol, itself a scavenger of hydroxyl radicals whose oxidation is inhibited by other hydroxyl radical scavengers. The fact that *tert*-butanol is also a substrate indicates that the reaction is not restricted to primary alcohols, as might wrongly be inferred from the above. Since *tert*-butanol does not have an alpha-hydrogen, hydrogen abstraction can produce a C-centred radical and/or an O-centred radical (pathway **B** in Fig. 7.6) which fragment to formaldehyde and other products (possibly acetone) (Cederbaum and Cohen, 1980). In such a reaction, *tert*-butanol undergoes **oxidative C-demethylation**.

Another interesting feature of the hydroxyl radical-mediated reaction was seen upon oxidation of **2-butanol**, a chiral compound. Microsomes from untreated rats did not discriminate between (+)- and (−)-2-butanol, but microsomes from ethanol-treated rats catalyzed the oxidation of (+)-2-butanol at rates twice those of (−)-2-butanol (Krikun and Cederbaum, 1984). The latter finding is not compatible with a reaction occurring outside the catalytic site, but suggests the involvement of a "**bound hydroxyl radical**".

In sum, the reaction discussed above involves the oxidation of **chiefly primary alcohols of low molecular weight**; the reagent seems to be a loosely bound hydroxyl radical produced from H_2O_2 generated by cytochrome P450 and mainly by CYP2E1. But in addition to this hydroxyl radical-mediated route, cytochrome P450 has also been shown conclusively to oxidize a number of usually secondary alcohols of relatively high molecular weight. These reactions, however, are inhibited neither by hydroxyl radical scavengers nor by desferroxamine, indicating a different mechanism.

Indeed, the oxidation of **large, secondary alcohols** partly resembles the **regular C-sp³ hydroxylation**, being initiated by a hydrogen abstraction on the oxygen-bearing carbon atom to form a carbon-centred radical. The best evidence for such a reaction comes from careful studies on the CYP2B1-mediated oxidation of **testosterone** (**7.XXXI** in Fig. 7.7) and epitestosterone (the 17α-hydroxy epimer) to androstenedione (**7.XXXII** in Fig. 7.7) (Wood *et al.*, 1988). With both substrates, abstraction of the 17-hydrogen was the rate-limiting step, which was followed either by the formation of a *gem*-diol by the regular oxygen rebound mechanism (reaction **a** in Fig. 7.7) or by loss of the hydroxyl hydrogen (reaction **b** in Fig. 7.7). Both reactions **a** and **b** in Fig. 7.7 appear open to the two substrates, with *gem*-diol formation seemingly predominating for epitestosterone. The same pathway(s) appear(s) to be involved in the cytochrome P450-mediated oxidation of the 7α- and 7β-hydroxylated metabolites of Δ⁸-tetrahydrocannabinol (Δ⁸-THC, **7.XXXIII**) to 7-oxo-Δ⁸-tetrahydrocannabinol (Narimatsu *et al.*, 1988). Note that the carbon-centred radical might also under adequate conditions add molecular oxygen to form a hydroperoxyl intermediate ultimately leading to a ketone, as seen in the hydroxyl radical-mediated conversion of morphine to morphinone (Kumagai *et al.*, 1992b).

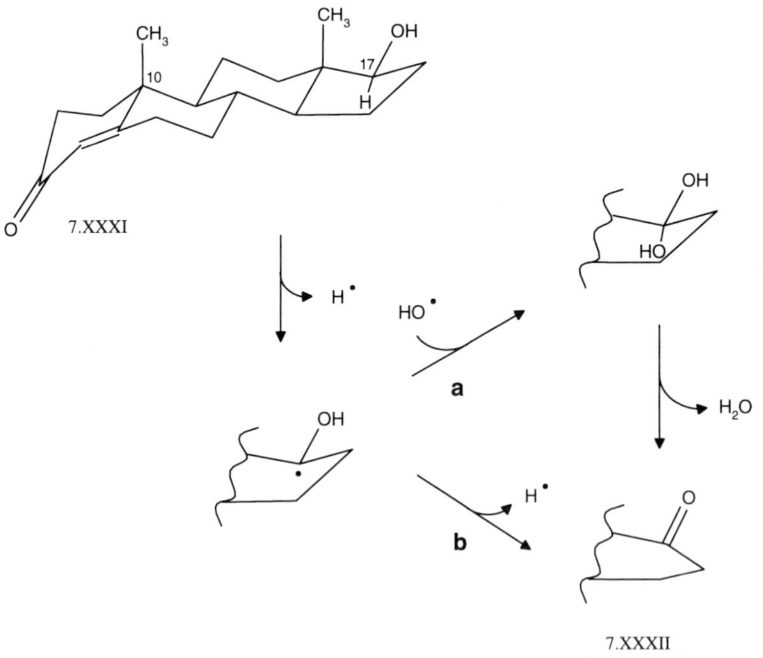

FIGURE 7.7 Postulated mechanism for the cytochrome P450-mediated oxidation of testosterone (**7.XXXI**) to androstenedione (**7.XXXII**) via oxygen rebound (reaction **a**) or dual hydrogen abstraction (reaction **b**) (Wood *et al.*, 1988).

Similar mechanisms might be involved in the oxidative breakdown of **cardiac glycosides**. Thus, digitoxin (i.e. digitoxigenin trisdigitoxoside) loses one and then a second digitoxose unit to yield the bis- and monodigitoxoside, respectively. The reactions are catalyzed by cytochrome P450, CYP3A in particular, and occur by initial oxidation of the axial hydroxyl group of the terminal sugar (Eberhart *et al.*, 1992; Thomas, 1990).

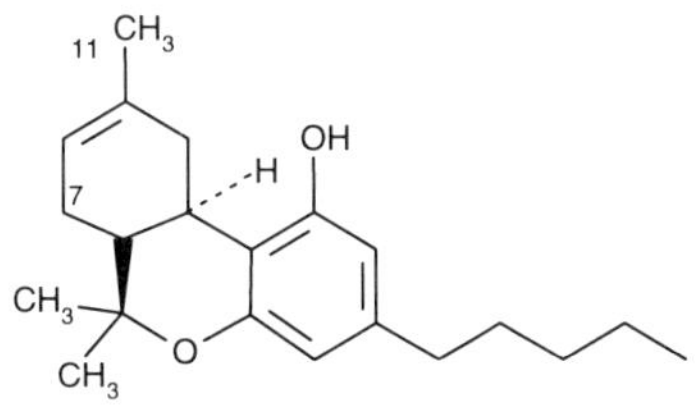

7.XXXIII

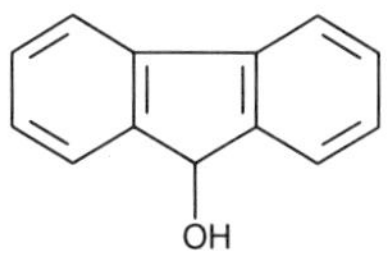

7.XXXIV

Cytochrome P450 was shown to be involved in the formation of fluoren-9-one from the model compound fluoren-9-ol (**7.XXXIV**) (Chen *et al.*, 1984). Alcohol oxidation was also seen in the *in vivo* metabolism of stiripentol (**7.XIX**) to the corresponding ketone, the reaction being catalyzed in part by cytochrome P450 (Zhang *et al.*, 1990). Similarly, CYP2D6 oxidizes the secondary alcohol metabolite of haloperidol back to the parent ketone (Tyndale *et al.*, 1991). All these substrates are secondary alcohols, but the possibility of primary alcohols also undergoing alpha-carbon hydroxylation should not be dismissed, e.g. the primary alcoholic group of chloramphenicol (Morris *et al.*, 1982).

There are now reasons to believe that direct (rather than hydroxyl radical mediated) oxidation of alcohols can also occur via **hydroxyl hydrogen abstraction** (homolytic O–H cleavage) rather than C–H cleavage. This is the case of the CYP2E1-catalyzed formation of formaldehyde from glycerol and a variety of other alcohol substrates, a **reaction of C–C cleavage** whose hypothetical mechanism is shown in Fig. 7.8 (Clejan and Cederbaum, 1991 and 1992; Winters and Cederbaum, 1990). Such a mechanism is the one postulated in the biotransformation of 20,22-dihydroxycholesterol to pregnenolone, a glycol cleavage reaction mediated by CYP11A1 (the enzyme catalyzing cholesterol side-chain cleavage) (Sligar *et al.*, 1984). The mechanistic details of this abstraction are not well understood; they may or may not begin with the **abstraction of an electron from the oxygen atom**, a reaction seen in the cytochrome P450-mediated oxidation of cyclopropyl benzyl ether (**7.XXXV**) and 1-methylcyclopropyl benzyl ether (**7.XXXVI**) (Guengerich *et al.*, 1984).

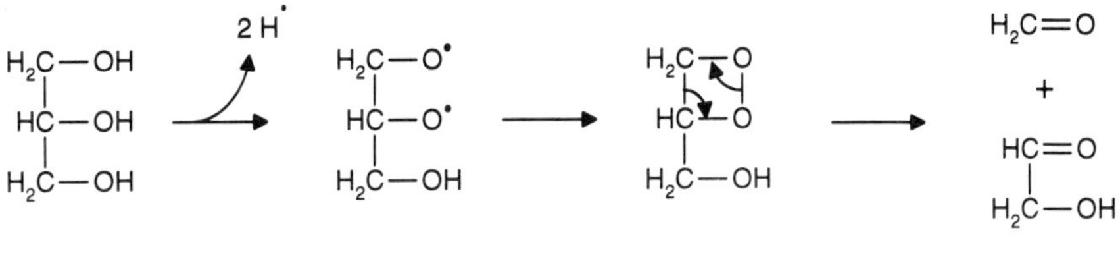

FIGURE 7.8 Hypothetical mechanism of the cytochrome P450-mediated oxidation of glycerol to formaldehyde and other metabolites (Sligar *et al.*, 1984; Winters and Cederbaum, 1990).

7.XXXV	R	=	—H
7.XXXVI	R	=	—CH$_3$

In conclusion, a broad survey of the literature indicates that there are three basic mechanisms in the cytochrome P450-catalyzed oxidation of alcohols, namely:

- alpha-hydrogen abstraction by a loosely bound hydroxyl radical;
- alpha-hydrogen abstraction by the iron-bound oxene;
- hydroxyl hydrogen abstraction.

Much remains to be done, however, to establish the mechanistic similarities and differences between these reactions, and in analogy with nitrogen oxidation, to understand the factors, enzymatic and molecular, which determine abstraction of an alpha-hydrogen, a hydroxyl hydrogen, or an electron of the oxygen atom.

7.6.2 Oxidation of aldehydes

The cytochrome P450-catalyzed oxidation of aldehydic groups may follow either of two pathways, namely oxygenation to a carboxylic acid or deformylation with olefin formation. As discussed below, the latter route is an important physiological reaction when catalyzed by aromatase (CYP19), the enzyme that converts androgens to estrogens (Graham-Lorence et al., 1991).

The microsomal, NADPH-dependent oxidation of aldehydes to the corresponding **carboxylic acid** is documented for a variety of substrates, e.g. 3-phenylpropionaldehyde, 4-isopropylbenzaldehyde (cuminaldehyde), 3,4-dimethoxybenzaldehyde, myrtenal and 9-anthraldehyde, as well as retinal (Roberts et al., 1992; Watanabe et al., 1990). Similarly, the 11-methyl group in Δ^8-THC (**7.XXXIII**), after being hydroxylated by cytochrome P450 to form 11-hydroxy-Δ^8-THC, can be oxidized to the aldehyde (11-oxo-Δ^8-THC) and then to the carboxylic acid (Δ^8-THC-11-oic acid), not only by dehydrogenases, but also by cytochrome P450 (Watanabe et al., 1991a and 1993; Yamamoto et al., 1988). In these examples, the oxygen atom being incorporated has been shown to originate from O_2 and not from H_2O. It was also found that the conversion of 11-oxo-Δ^8-THC to the acid is catalyzed by a number of cytochromes P450, i.e. 2C11 > 2C6 > 2A1 > 2A2 = 2C13 = 1A1 = 1A2 > 2B1, while the activity of 2B2 and 2E1 was not detectable (Watanabe et al., 1991b). A recent and therapeutically relevant example is that of losartan, an angiotensin II receptor antagonist whose –CH$_2$OH function is oxidized to a carboxylic group by both CYP3A4 and 2C (Stearns et al., 1993).

The second pathway, namely **deformylation with olefin formation**, has been observed with a number of branched aldehydes, e.g. trimethylacetaldehyde (**7.XXXVII**), 2-methylbutyraldehyde (**7.XXXIX**) and cyclohexanecarboxaldehyde (**7.XLI**) to form isobutylene (**7.XXXVIII**), 1-butene (**7.XL**) and cyclohexene (**7.XLII**), respectively (Roberts et al., 1991; Vaz et al., 1991). The most active cytochromes P450 were 2B4, 2C3, 2E1 and 3A6. Interestingly, unbranched aldehydes were not substrates.

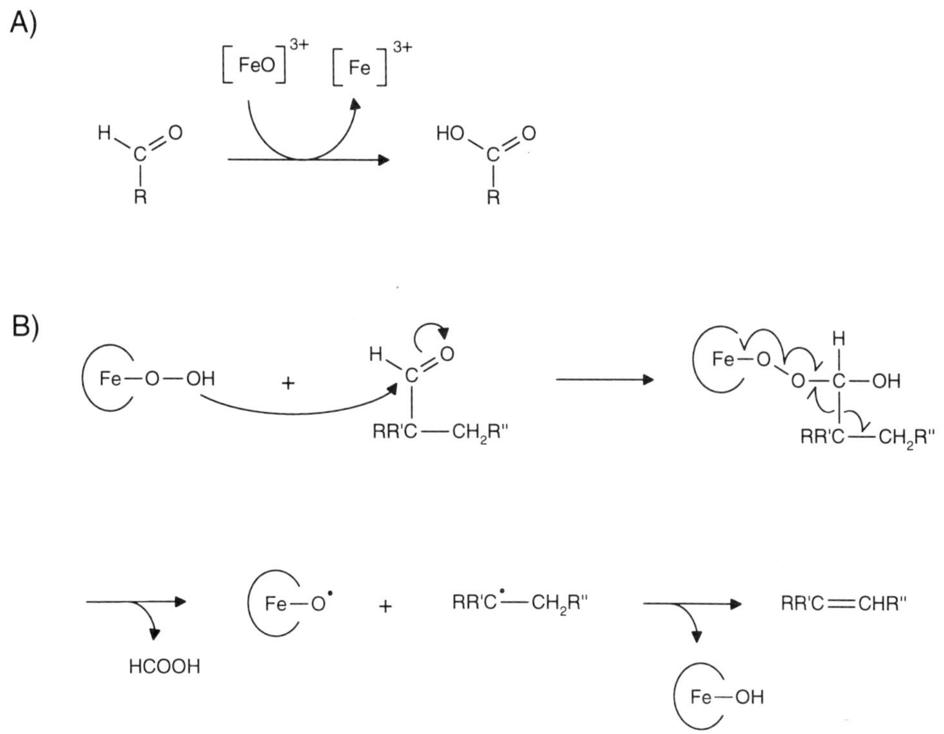

A)

B)

FIGURE 7.9 Postulated mechanisms in the oxidation of aldehydes catalyzed by cytochrome P450. Pathway **A**: Oxygenation to carboxylic acids. Pathway **B**: Stepwise mechanism leading to deformylation with olefin formation (Roberts *et al.*, 1991; Watanabe and Ishimura, 1989).

The **mechanisms of aldehyde oxidation** by cytochrome P450 have been explored by experimental and theoretical means (Korzekwa *et al.*, 1991; Roberts *et al.*, 1991; Vaz *et al.*, 1991; Watanabe and Ishimura, 1989). It thus appears likely that the $[FeO]^{3+}$ state of cytochrome P450 is responsible for aldehyde oxygenation to a carboxylic acid, a reaction which can thus be viewed formally as a hydroxylation (pathway **A** in Fig. 7.9). In contrast, the $[Fe^{3+}(O_2)^{2-}]$ state of

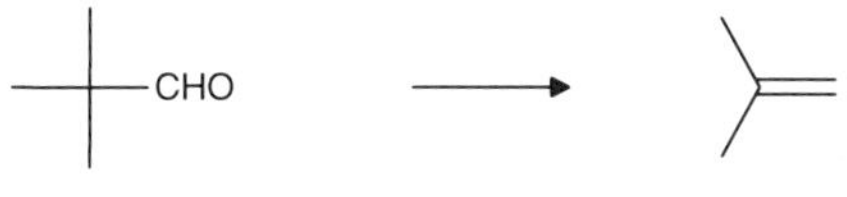

7.XXXVII   7.XXXVIII

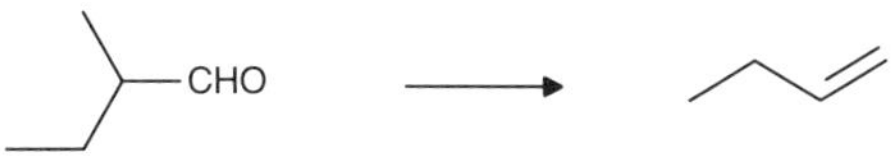

7.XXXIX   7.XL

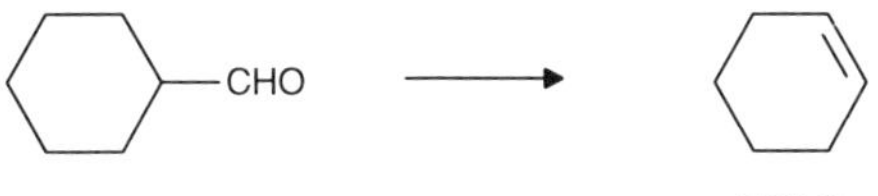

7.XLI   7.XLII

cytochrome P450 is believed to mediate deformylation. Here, two reaction mechanisms have been proposed, concerted and stepwise; the latter mechanism is shown as pathway **B** in Fig. 7.9 and involves homolytic cleavage of the O–O bond, loss of formic acid, and formation of a C-centred radical. The C–C double bond is then formed in analogy with the reaction of desaturation discussed in Section 4.2 (Fig. 4.2). Note that heterolytic cleavage of the O–O bond in the $[Fe^{3+}(O_2)^{2-}]$ state of cytochrome P450 (see Section 3.5) would form carboxylic acids rather than deformylated olefins, a hypothesis worth investigating.

Deformylation with olefin formation is an essential step in the **C-demethylation and aromatization of androgens** (e.g. testosterone) to estrogens (e.g. estradiol) catalyzed by aromatase (CYP19). Here, the methyl group on C(10) is sequentially oxidized by the same enzyme to a hydroxymethyl group and then a dihydroxymethyl group (a *gem*-diol) which dehydrates to a formyl group; oxidation of the latter results in deformylation and olefin formation (Akhtar *et al.*, 1993; Cole and Robinson, 1990). A similar pathway exists in the C(14α)-demethylation of lanosterol (Sono *et al.*, 1991).

7.6.3 Oxidation of formamides

Recent evidence indicates that **N-substituted formamides** are substrates of cytochrome P450 in a reaction that produces a highly toxic isocyanate metabolite. Thus, **N-methylformamide** yields the infamous methyl isocyanate as shown in Eq. 7.1:

$$CH_3-NH-COH \quad \rightarrow \quad CH_3-N=C=O \qquad \text{(Eq. 7.1)}$$

This reaction is catalyzed by CYP2E1, although its exact mechanism is not completely understood. Two pathways have been postulated, namely: (a) oxidation of the formyl group by hydrogen radical abstraction followed by NH oxidation again by hydrogen radical abstraction; and/or (b) N-hydroxylation followed by dehydration (Gescher, 1993; Hyland *et al.*, 1992; Mráz *et al.*, 1993). Formamide activation thus involves possibly C=O oxidation in analogy with aldehyde oxidation, and certainly also N-oxidation.

This reaction of oxidation does much to explain the toxicity of N,N-dimethylformamide, whose toxication begins with N-demethylation to N-methylformamide. Of medicinal relevance is the fact that larger molecules are also substrates of this reaction, witness the formamide **N-formylamphetamine** which was oxidized to 1-methyl-2-phenylethyl isocyanate by mitochondrial cytochrome P450 (Borel *et al.*, 1993).

7.6.4 Quinone and quinone imine formation

The oxidation of benzene derivatives to diphenolic metabolites (catechols and hydroquinones, see Section 4.3) does not stop there but may continues via **semiquinones to quinones**. Greenlee *et al.* (1981) were among the first to provide evidence that the chronic toxicity of **benzene** may be ascribed to the oxidation (presumably by **autoxidation**, i.e. one-electron oxidation steps mediated by molecular oxygen) of at least two of its metabolites, namely hydroquinone and 1,2,4-trihydroxybenzene, to the corresponding semiquinones and quinones (Fig. 7.10). These compounds, being reactive electrophiles, tend to bind covalently to a number of endogenous nucleophiles and may therefore be of toxicological significance. Two major routes of detoxication are conjugation with glutathione (see a subsequent volume) and reduction to the polyphenols (see Section 12.2) (Koster, 1991). However, it should be noted that covalent binding to macro-

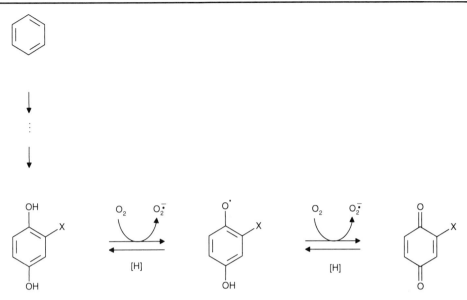

FIGURE 7.10 Formation by autoxidation of semiquinones and quinones from polyphenolic metabolites of benzene (X = H or OH) (Greenlee *et al.*, 1981).

molecules is not systematically associated with toxicity (Monks *et al.*, 1984). In addition, toxication to semiquinones and quinones may also be involved in the mechanism of action of antineoplastic phenols such as teniposide and etoposide (Relling *et al.*, 1992).

Besides benzene, a number of analogues are also known to yield quinones, but the **mechanism** of the oxidative steps leading from diphenol to semiquinone to quinone has not always been clarified. In the case of benzo[*a*]pyrene and possibly also bromobenzene, autoxidation appears to be involved (Buben *et al.*, 1988; Cavalieri *et al.*, 1988; Lesko *et al.*, 1975). In other cases, the oxidizing agent was shown to be the **superoxide anion radical**, which in the process undergoes a one-electron reduction to hydrogen peroxide. For example, the oxidation of 3,4-dihydroxymethamphetamine (**7.XVIII**) to the corresponding *ortho*-quinone in rat liver microsomes was mediated by superoxide resulting from uncoupling of cytochrome P450 (Hiramatsu *et al.*, 1990). The same reaction occurs for tetrachloro-1,4-hydroquinone (Fig. 7.11), and in the first step of the oxidation of *ortho*-dihydroxylated polycyclic aromatic hydrocarbons (Flowers-Geary *et al.*, 1993; van Ommen *et al.*, 1988).

In fact, the enzymology of quinone formation is quite complex as a variety of systems have the capacity to catalyze the reaction. Thus, **cytochrome P450** itself may play a direct role in some cases, as seen in the oxidation of 1-naphthol (**7.XLIII**) to 1,4-naphthoquinone (**7.XLIV**) and 1,2-naphthoquinone by a reconstituted system (D'Arcy Doherty *et al.*, 1985). The fact that the

7.XLIII   7.XLIV

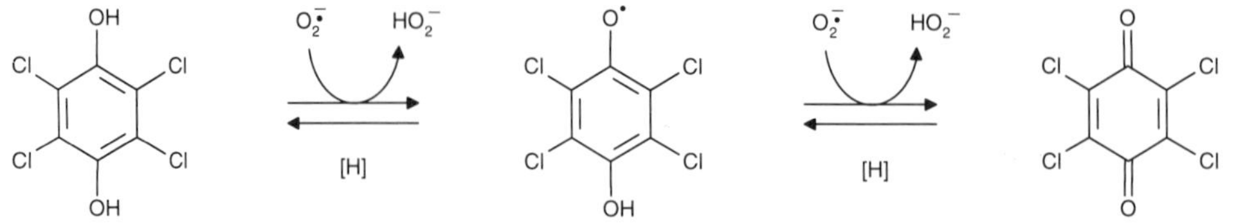

FIGURE 7.11 Mechanism of the superoxide-mediated oxidation of tetrachloro-1,4-hydroquinone to the corresponding quinone (van Ommen *et al.*, 1988).

reaction also occurred when the oxygen source was cumene hydroperoxide (a **peroxidase activity** of cytochrome P450 discussed in Section 10.2) argues against the involvement of superoxide. Similarly, CYP1A1 and to a lesser extent CYP1A2 in the presence of cumene hydroperoxide were effective in forming quinones from diethylstilbestrol or catecholestrogens (Roy *et al.*, 1992).

Quinone formation by the peroxidase activity of cytochrome P450 may not be fortuitous since a number of diphenols undergo one-electron oxidation steps mediated by various **peroxidases**, e.g. lactoperoxidase, prostaglandin synthetase and myeloperoxidase, as discussed in Chapter 10 (Chignell, 1985). For example, the oxidation of catechol in rat and human bone marrow cells is mediated by myeloperoxidase, resulting in covalent binding to proteins (Bhat *et al.*, 1988). This latter study suggests that it may be myeloperoxidase rather than autoxidation (see above, Greenlee *et al.*, 1981) that is responsible in bone marrow cells for the toxication of benzene metabolites to semiquinones and quinones.

Our understanding of the formation and reactivity of quinone metabolites has gained significantly from studying the metabolic fate of **acetaminophen** (paracetamol, **7.XLV** in Fig. 7.12), a well-known analgesic agent that causes life-threatening hepatotoxicity beyond threshold doses. The toxic metabolite of paracetamol is a **quinone imine**, namely N-acetyl-*p*-benzoquinone imine (NAPQI, **7.XLVI** in Fig. 7.12), the very high reactivity of which was first established directly by Dahlin and Nelson (1982).

The **mechanism** of acetaminophen oxidation has been the object of numerous investigations (Vermeulen *et al.*, 1992). The two main products are the catechol analogue (i.e. the 3-hydroxylated metabolite) and NAPQI (which is usually characterized as the glutathionyl conjugate). Acetaminophen oxidation displays a marked isozyme selectivity (with CYP1A1, 1A2,

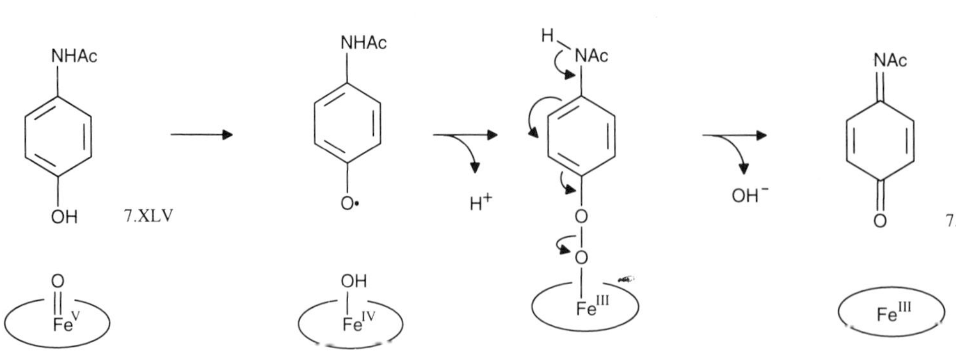

FIGURE 7.12 Postulated mechanism of the cytochrome P450-mediated oxidation of acetaminophen (**7.XLV**) to N-acetyl-*p*-quinone imine (NAPQI, **7.XLVI**). The semiquinone imine radical may be oxidized to NAPQI as shown, or may react via resonance forms to yield *p*-benzoquinone (from the radical centred on the *ipso*-carbon) or 3-hydroxyacetaminophen (from the radical centred on the *meta*-carbon) (Hoffmann *et al.*, 1990; Koymans *et al.*, 1989).

2E1 and 3A4 being particularly active), and it is particularly relevant that CYP1A1 binds acetaminophen so that its phenolic group comes in close proximity to the central iron ion (Harvison *et al.*, 1988; Patten *et al.*, 1993; van de Straat *et al.*, 1987). Quantum mechanical calculations have indicated that hydrogen abstraction proceeds from the hydroxyl group rather than from the amide group, the resulting radical being predominantly oxygen-centred (Koymans *et al.*, 1989). This would support the intermediacy of the semiquinone imine radical, but autoxidation of the latter was not detected (Bisby and Tabassum, 1988). In fact, it is now established that the cytochrome P450-catalyzed oxidation of acetaminophen to NAPQI occurs by two sequential single-electron steps and not by disproportionation of the semiquinone imine radical (Potter and Hinson, 1987; van de Straat *et al.*, 1988). The mechanism considered most likely to account for these results is shown in Fig. 7.12 (Hoffmann *et al.*, 1990; Koymans *et al.*, 1993). Note that the O-centred radical can rearrange to a C(3)- and a C(1)-centred radical; oxygenation of the former leads to the 3-hydroxylated metabolite, while oxygenation at C(1) of the latter radical leads to *p*-benzoquinone via N–C cleavage (N-dearylation, see Section 6.6).

Beside acetaminophen, the antimalarial **amodiaquine** (**7.XLVII**) has also been reported to form a quinone imine metabolite. The latter, which is responsible for the immunotoxicity of amodiaquine, appears to be generated by autoxidation and/or by peroxidases (Christie *et al.*, 1989).

Of further biological and toxicological interest is the oxidation of some 4-alkylphenols to **quinone methides**. These metabolites are strong alkylating agents which undergo Michael additions at the exocyclic methylene carbon, thereby binding covalently to soluble and macromolecular nucleophiles (Bolton *et al.*, 1993; Thompson *et al.*, 1992). This reaction of oxidation is exemplified by the antioxidant **butylated hydroxytoluene** (BHT, **7.XLVIII**) whose quinone methide (**7.XLIX**) presumably arises from the BHT phenoxy radical (Thompson *et al.*, 1987). The formation of this quinone methide was seen in hepatic and pulmonary microsomes from rats and mice, but the enzymatic and mechanistic aspects of the reaction deserve further investigations. In a series of congeners of BHT, namely 2-alkylated and 2,6-dialkylated 4-methylphenols, the enzymatic formation of quinone methides and their reactivity with nucleophiles were shown to correlate with hepatotoxicity (Bolton *et al.*, 1992).

7.XLVII

7.XLVIII   7.XLIX

It would be wrong to conclude from the above that the cytochrome P450-catalyzed oxidation of phenols is solely a reaction of toxication. Among the physiological roles of this reaction, we note that radicals formed by phenol oxidation may couple intramolecularly with high regio- and stereoselectivity, resulting in the endogenous synthesis of complex molecules. Many such examples are known in plant biochemistry. In contrast, only few examples of **intramolecular phenol oxidative coupling** have been reported for mammals, but their interest is such that they should stimulate many investigators. One very telling example is the recently discovered capacity of mammalian hepatic cytochrome P450 to form the morphine skeleton by cyclizing (R)-reticuline to salutaridine (Amann and Zenk, 1991) (see also Section 13.5).

7.7 OXIDATION OF THIOLS AND THIOETHERS

Sulfur chemistry is very rich and complex, and sulfur-containing compounds occupy a unique position in medicinal chemistry. Whether endogenous or exogenous, they undergo a variety of metabolic reactions, namely oxidations, reductions (Chapter 12), hydrolysis and conjugations (see the volumes in this series, *Biochemistry of Hydration and Dehydration Reactions* and *Biochemistry of Conjugation Reactions*) (James, 1988).

Metabolic oxidation of sulfur involves not only the organic derivatives and functional groups examined below, but also **inorganic sulfur** (Bartholomew et al., 1980; Gunnison et al., 1977; Sun et al., 1989; Togawa et al., 1990). The major metabolic reactions of inorganic sulfur oxygenation are presented in Eqs. 7.2–7.4 in simplified form and without consideration of stoichiometry. Thus, inorganic sulfide is oxidized to thiosulfate by mitochondrial enzymes, possibly via the highly unstable sulfoxylate which disproportionates to form thiosulfate:

$$S^{2-} \to [SO^{2-}] \to \tfrac{1}{2}S_2O_3^{2-} \qquad \text{(Eq. 7.2)}$$

Thiosulfate is then reductively cleaved by glutathione, an endogenous thiol, to some form of sulfide (which is recycled) and sulfite:

$$S_2O_3^{2-} \to S^{2-} + SO_3^{2-} \qquad \text{(Eq. 7.3)}$$

The latter is then oxidized to sulfate, the end-product in this sequence:

$$SO_3^{2-} \to SO_4^{2-} \qquad \text{(Eq. 7.4)}$$

To help the reader with the various **organic sulfur-containing groups** to be discussed below, a number of relevant moieties are presented in Table 7.1 in analogy with a comparable table of nitrogen-containing groups (Table 5.1) given in Chapter 5.

7.7.1 Oxidation of thiols and thioacids

Thiols (mercaptans) are good substrates for monooxygenases, and particularly for the FAD-containing monooxygenase (Damani, 1987; Poulsen, 1981; Ziegler, 1980, 1984, 1988a, 1988b and 1993). However, systematic and comprehensive comparisons between cytochrome P450 and the flavin-containing monooxygenase are not available, a further complication arising from the fact that thiols can also be oxidized by superoxide (Crank and Makin, 1984). A limited generalization suggests that the less marked the nucleophilic character of the sulfur atom, the greater the probability of its oxidation by cytochrome P450 (see Section 7.7.3) (Damani and Houdi, 1988).

TABLE 7.1 *Conventional oxidation states of the sulfur atom in S-containing functional groups* (electropositive atoms bonded to the sulfur atom decrease its oxidation state, while more electronegative atoms cause an increase) (Extended and modified from Damani, 1987)

Oxidation state	Functional groups	
- 2	C—S—C	thioethers (sulfides)
	C—SH	thiols (mercaptans)
	C—C—C C—C—N (‖S)	thiones and thioamides
	N—C—NH N—C=N (‖S, SH)	thioureas (thiocarbamides)
	C—SH (‖S)	dithioacids
	N—C—SH (‖S)	dithiocarbamic acids
	C—O—P—O—C C—P—O—C (O—C, ‖S)	phosphorothionates and phosphonothionates
- 1	C—S•	thiyl radicals
	C—S—S—C	disulfides
0	C—S—C (‖O)	sulfoxides
	C—S—OH	sulfenic acids
	C—C—C C—C—N (S=O)	sulfines
	C—C—C C—C—N (O, S)	oxathiiranes
	P (O, S)	oxathiaphosphiranes
	C—S—S—C (‖O)	thiosulfinates

(Table 7.1 cont'd)

+ 1	$C-\overset{\overset{O}{\|\|}}{S}-\overset{\overset{O}{\|\|}}{S}-C$	α-disulfoxides
	$C-\overset{\overset{O}{\|\|}}{\underset{\underset{O}{\|\|}}{S}}-S-C$	thiosulfonates
+ 2	$C-\overset{\overset{O}{\|\|}}{\underset{\underset{O}{\|\|}}{S}}-C$	sulfones
	$C-SO_2H$	sulfinic acids
	$C-C-C \atop O=S=O$ $C-C-N \atop O=S=O$	sulfenes
+ 4	$C-SO_3H$	sulfonic acids

The **chemical mechanism** of monooxygenase-mediated oxidation of thiols proceeds as shown in Fig. 7.13 to yield sulfenic acids (R–SOH). When FAD-containing monooxygenase is involved, the reaction is one of **direct oxygenation** (reaction **a** in Fig. 7.13), whereas cytochrome P450 is believed to mediate a **one-electron sulfur oxidation** yielding the **thiyl radical**, followed by oxygen transfer (reactions **b** and **c** in Fig. 7.13), in analogy with nitrogen oxidation (see Chapter 5; Fig. 5.1). To the best of our knowledge, the detailed mechanism of cytochrome P450-catalyzed thiol oxidation has been established in a few cases only (see later, spironolactone), a situation also characteristic of S-dealkylation (Section 7.7.2) and thioether oxygenation (Section 7.7.3). Nevertheless, a global consideration of thiol oxidation, S-dealkylation and thioether oxygenation gives strong support to the mechanisms shown in Figs. 7.13 and 7.14 (the latter being shown in Section 7.7.2).

Sulfenic acids are reactive electrophiles whose sulfur atom can be a centre of nucleophilic substitution by a thiol group to yield H_2O and a disulfide (reaction **d** in Fig. 7.13), the further fate of which will be discussed later. The competing reaction involves oxidation of the sulfenic acid to a sulfinic acid and then a sulfonic acid (reactions **e** and **f** in Fig. 7.13, respectively) (see later).

A variety of thiols have been studied as *in vitro* substrates of the FAD-containing monooxygenase, the product of the reaction being the symmetrical disulfide (Fig. 7.13, R = R′) since under these conditions the sulfenic acid will tend to react with excess substrate. Table 7.2 lists the K_m values of a few mercaptans metabolized under conditions where V_{max} values are comparable. Compounds such as thiophenol and 1,4-butanedithiol are even better substrates than the thiols listed in Table 7.2 (Ziegler, 1988a). While cysteamine (**7.L**) is a good substrate, other aminothiols such as piperazinylethanethiol have low affinities (Ziegler, 1988a). Interesting **structure–metabolism relationships** show that excellent substrates are characterized by a negative charge on a sulfur atom, e.g. dithioacids (Table 7.2) (Taylor and Ziegler, 1987). Although the metabolites were not isolated, it was found that they were dioxygenated products. In contrast to dithioacids, mercaptans having a carboxylate group near the target site were either substrates of lower affinity (e.g. thiosalicylic acid) or were not substrates at all (e.g. thioglycolic acid).

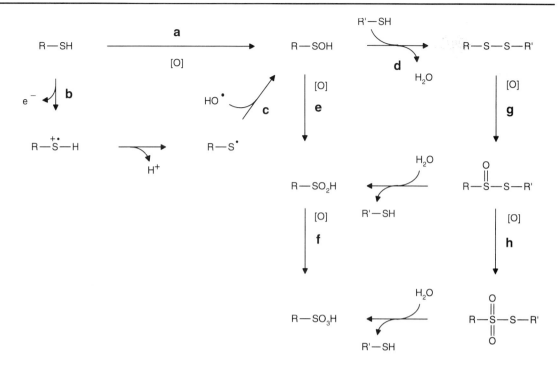

FIGURE 7.13 Metabolic scheme of the monooxygenase-catalyzed oxidation of thiols to disulfides, sulfinic acids and sulfonic acids. Sulfinic and sulfonic acids can also result from the hydrolysis of oxygenated disulfides, namely thiolsulfinates and thiolsulfonates, respectively.

TABLE 7.2 *Substrate selectivity of porcine liver FAD-containing monooxygenase for the oxidation of various sulfur-containing compounds* (V_{max} values usually in the range 0.3–0.4 μmol/min/mg protein) (Sabourin and Hodgson, 1984; Taylor and Ziegler, 1987)

	K_m (μM)		K_m (μM)
Thiols		*Disulfides*	
Butanethiol	78	Benzyl disulfide	5
Benzyl mercaptan	108	*trans*-1,2-Dithiane-4,5-diol	254
Dithiothreitol	296		
Cysteamine (**7.L**)	59	*Thioamides*	
		Thioacetamide (**7.LXXX**)	10
		Thiobenzamide (**7.LXXXI**)	3
Dithiobenzoic acids			
Dithiobenzoate	3	*Thioureas (thiocarbamides)*	
Dithiosalicylate	3	Thiourea	20
		Thiocarbanilide	13
Thioethers		Methimazole (**7.XCII**)	13
Dimethyl sulfide	11	2-Mercaptobenzimidazole	16
Thioanisole (**7.LXVII**, X = H)	2		
Benzyl methyl sulfide	2		
Diphenyl sulfide	24		

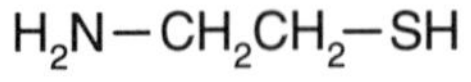

7.L

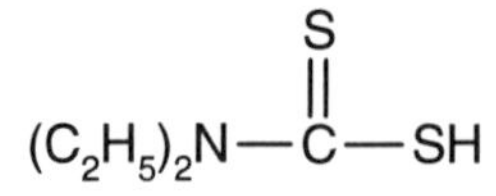

7.LI

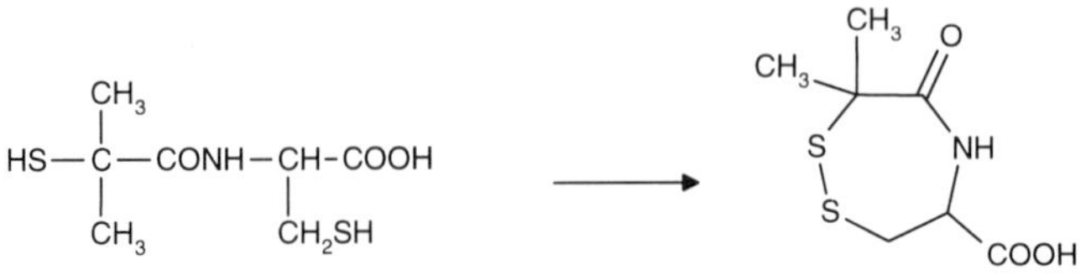

7.LII

7.LIII

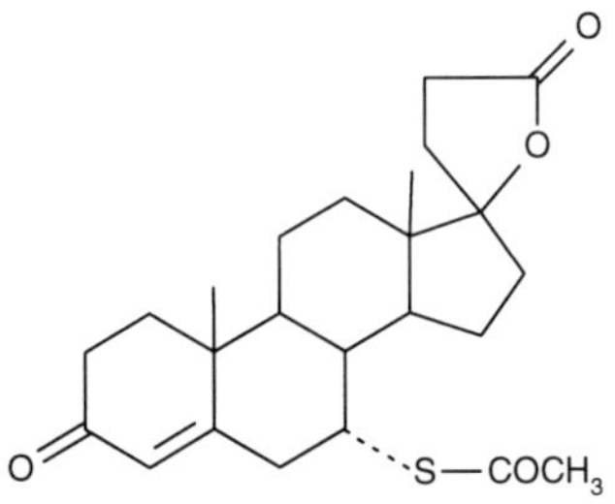

7.LIV

A compound of particular interest is **diethyldithiocarbamate** (**7.LI**), an *in vivo* metabolite resulting from the reductive S–S cleavage of disulfiram (see Section 12.5), a well-known inhibitor of liver acetaldehyde dehydrogenase. Interestingly, diethyldithiocarbamate can undergo S-oxidation back to disulfiram, the *in vitro* reaction being catalyzed largely by cytochrome P450 and partly by hydrogen peroxide generated during NADPH oxidation (Masuda and Nakamura, 1989). Diethyldithiocarbamate oxidation was accompanied by loss of cytochrome P450, suggested to be due to covalent binding of active sulfur to the hemoprotein.

Intramolecular formation of a disulfide from a dithiol, when sterically allowed, should proceed rapidly if only for reasons of entropy. Thus, the potential antirheumatic compound **7.LII** was found to be oxidized to the cyclic disulfide **7.LIII**, a significant *in vivo* metabolite in rats and dogs (Horiuchi *et al.*, 1985).

Spironolactone (**7.LIV**) is another sulfur-containing drug whose metabolism has been particularly informative. Indeed, the major metabolic route of this aldosterone antagonist is deacetylation to yield the 7α-thiol, this product being then S-oxidized by cytochrome P450 in liver microsomes from dexamethasone-induced rats (Decker *et al.*, 1989). The sulfinic and sulfonic acid metabolites were characterized, which points to the initial formation of a thiyl radical followed by oxygen rebound to yield the sulfenic acid (i.e. reactions **b** and **c** in Fig. 7.13). This metabolic pathway was accompanied by destruction of cytochrome P450, the key intermediate(s) possibly being the thiyl radical and/or the sulfenic acid and/or some activated form of oxygen. Direct S-oxygenation by FAD-containing monooxygenase is also a reaction of the 7α-thiol metabolite of spironolactone (Decker *et al.*, 1991).

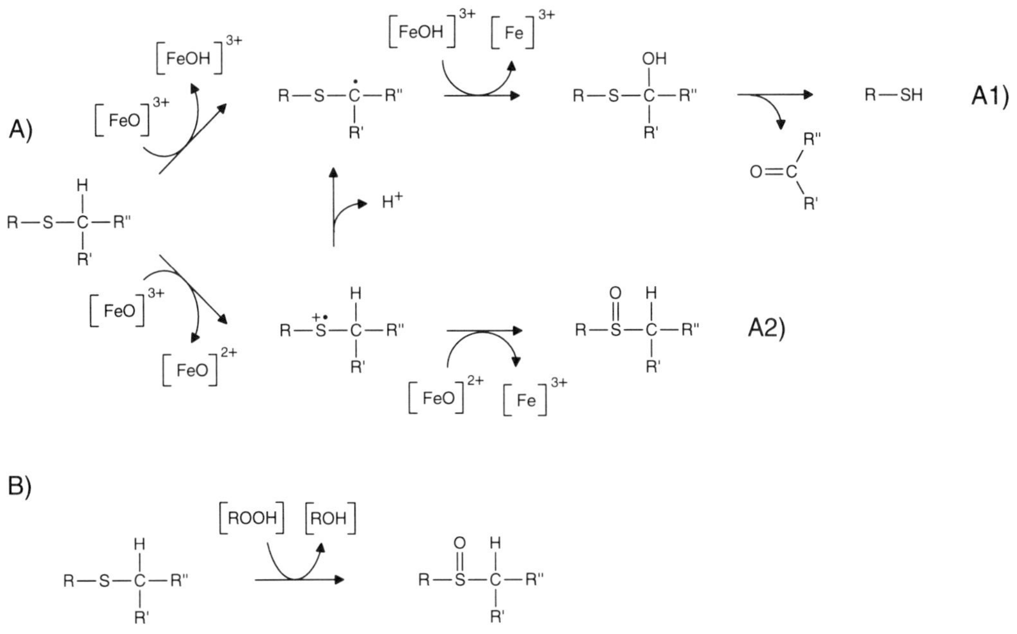

A)

A1)

A2)

B)

FIGURE 7.14 Postulated mechanisms of S-dealkylation (pathway **A1**) and S-oxygenation (pathways **A2** and **B**) catalyzed by cytochrome P450 (pathway **A**) and the FAD-containing monooxygenase (pathway **B**).

The above examples illustrate the variety of routes undergone by thiol-containing compounds, but do not allow a rationalization of the factors (molecular and enzymatic) that direct S-oxidation towards formation of disulfides or sulfinic and sulfonic acids. Additional thiol substrates, namely the tautomers of thioureas, will be considered in Section 7.8. Note that mixed disulfides formed from a xenobiotic and an endogenous molecule will be examined in a subsequent volume *Biochemistry of Conjugation Reactions*.

7.7.2 S-Dealkylation

Reactions of S-dealkylation occupy far fewer pages in the literature than reactions of N- and O-dealkylation. This is not due to these reactions being very slow and energetically unfavourable, but because the number of substrates tested is comparatively limited.

S-Dealkylations are cytochrome P450-catalyzed reactions the **mechanism(s)** of which can be schematized by pathway **A** in Fig. 7.14 (Oae *et al.*, 1985). As for N- and O-dealkylation, the intermediate undergoing S–C cleavage is a C(α)-hydroxylated metabolite (a hemimercaptal) which hydrolyzes to a thiol and a carbonyl compound. Hydroxylation of the alpha-carbon by oxygen rebound (pathway **A1**) is a possible route, but the C(α)-centred radical can also be formed by initial oxidation of the sulfur atom followed by expulsion of a proton. Analogies with the mechanism of N-dealkylation (Figs. 5.1 and 6.1) are compelling, although more intricacies have been discovered for N-dealkylation (Fig. 6.1) than for S-dealkylation.

A number of **interesting examples** of S-dealkylation have been published. Thus, 4-(*p*-chlorophenylthio)butanol (**7.LV**), a compound with antiallergic properties, yielded *p*-chlorothiophenol (**7.LVI**) as the major urinary metabolite in rats and dogs (Kucharczyk *et al.*, 1979). As for the hepatotrophic agent malotilate (**7.LVIII**), opening of its 1,3-dithiol ring led to the dithiol **7.LIX**. While this product was found only in small amounts in rat urine, its S-glucuronide was a major biliary metabolite, indicating the quantitative importance of S-dealkylation (Nakaoka *et al.*, 1989). Interestingly, a unique mechanism of S-dealkylation is conceivable here which would be initiated by epoxidation of the double bond followed by epoxide hydration to an unstable dihydrodiol.

Benzyl S-haloalkenyl sulfides of structure **7.LX** (see Fig. 7.15) are also substrates of cytochrome P450-catalyzed S-dealkylation, yielding unstable thiols of structure **7.LXII** (Vamvakas *et al.*, 1989). These latter rearrange to mutagenic thioacylating intermediates, either thioketenes (**7.LXIII**) and/or thioacyl chlorides (**7.LXIV**). In fact, the sulfides **7.LX** were prepared and investigated as models of S-haloalkenyl-L-cysteine conjugates (**7.LXI**), which are activated to the same unstable thiols **7.LXII** by the action of **cysteine-conjugate β-lyase** [L-cysteine-S-conjugate thiol-lyase (deaminating); EC 4.4.1.13] (Dekant *et al.*, 1988a and 1991). The latter is not a monooxygenase, but a pyridoxal phosphate-dependent enzyme found mainly in the kidney and which cleaves L-cysteine conjugates to thiols, NH_3 and pyruvic acid (Blagbrough *et al.*, 1990 and 1992; Dekant *et al.*, 1988b; Lertratanangkoon and Denney, 1993). The high renal activity of β-lyase accounts for the nephrotoxicity of a number of S-haloalkyl- and S-haloalkenyl-L-cysteine conjugates formed from glutathione in the liver (see the volume in this series, *Biochemistry of Conjugation Reactions*) but activated to thiols in the kidney.

β-Lyase is of interest not only from a toxicological viewpoint, but also in the perspective of **kidney-selective delivery** of thiol-containing drugs. Indeed, prodrugs have been designed and successfully tested that are substrates of the enzyme and are thus activated by S–C cleavage. The renal activation of S-(6-purinyl)-L-cysteine (**7.LXV**) to 6-mercaptopurine affords such an example (Elfarra and Hwang, 1993; Hwang and Elfarra, 1989 and 1991).

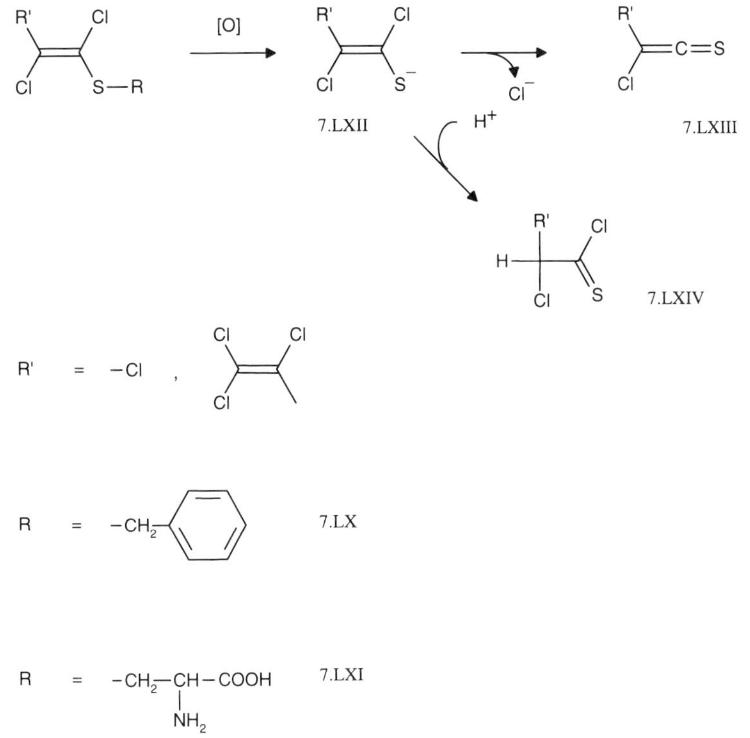

FIGURE 7.15 Cytochrome P450-catalyzed S-dealkylation of benzyl S-haloalkenyl sulfides (**7.LX**), and cysteine-conjugate β-lyase catalyzed S-dealkylation of S-haloalkenyl-L-cysteines (**7.LXI**), to unstable thiols (**7.LXII**) rearranging to mutagenic intermediates (Dekant *et al.*, 1988; Vamvakas *et al.*, 1989).

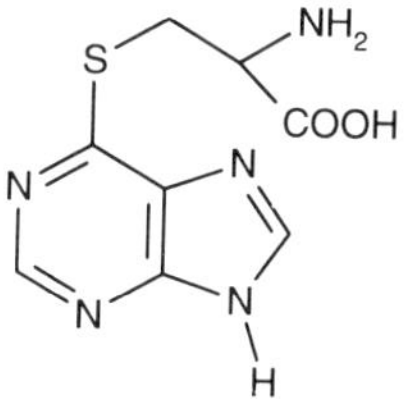

7.LXV

7.7.3 Oxygenation of thioethers to sulfoxides and sulfones

The metabolic formation of sulfoxides and sulfones involves many xenobiotics investigated over a number of decades (Mitchell and Waring, 1985). Besides the two microsomal monooxygenase systems to be discussed below, other enzyme systems can also mediate the sulfoxidation of some sulfides, e.g. some **peroxidases** (Chapter 10) and **cytosolic** (i.e. soluble) **cysteine oxidases**. The latter have for example been implicated in the sulfoxidation of the mucolytic agent S-carboxymethyl-L-cysteine (**7.LXVI**) whose structural analogy with the natural substrate is obvious (Waring *et al.*, 1986).

In Table 7.1, sulfoxides and sulfones are drawn with sulfur-oxygen double bonds. This representation, while not incorrect, does not fully explain the **polarized nature of this bond**, which is best understood as a resonance intermediate between a double bond and semipolar bond, both representations being acceptable:

$$S=O \quad \longleftrightarrow \quad S^{+}\text{–}O^{-}$$

The polarized character of the S=O bond explains the high polarity and hydrophilicity of sulfoxides. Interestingly, it is not always realized that sulfones are markedly less hydrophilic and more lipophilic than sulfoxydes due to partial cancellation of the two S=O vectors of dipolarity. The relative **hydrophilicity** of sulfoxides and **lipophilicity** of sulfones account for the differential pharmacokinetic behaviour of these two classes of metabolites.

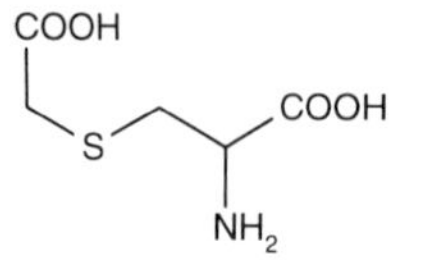

7.LXVI 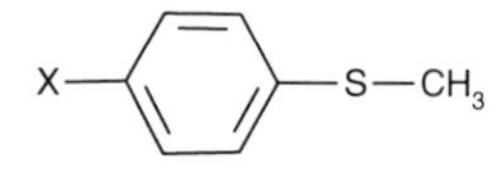   7.LXVII

The **mechanisms of sulfoxidation** are shown in Fig. 7.14. The reaction catalyzed by **cytochrome P450** (pathway **A2**) is initiated by a one-electron oxidation of the sulfur atom followed by transfer of the activated oxygen atom (oxygen rebound). Such a mechanism implies that the more readily a substrate can lose an electron, the more effective its cytochrome P450-catalyzed sulfoxidation. Indeed, a fair correlation was found for *para*-substituted thioanisoles (**7.LXVII**, X = H, CH$_3$, OCH$_3$, Cl, NO$_2$) between their V_{max} values (measured in a reconstituted cytochrome P450 system) and their one-electron oxidation potential (Watanabe *et al.*, 1982a). Note that chemically produced hydroxyl radicals are also very active in forming sulfoxides (Watanabe *et al.*, 1981), suggesting that hydroxyl radicals produced by monooxygenases may be involved in some cases.

A mechanism comparable to pathway **A2** in Fig. 7.14 operates in the cytochrome P450-catalyzed **oxygenation of sulfoxides to sulfones,** as presented in Fig. 7.16 (Watanabe *et al.*, 1982b). Here again, a correlation was found between V_{max} values of *para*-substituted phenyl methyl sulfoxides (**7.LXVIII**, X = H, CH$_3$, OCH$_3$, Cl) and their one-electron oxidation potential, in agreement with the proposed mechanism (Watanabe *et al.*, 1982b).

Besides being oxygenated to sulfones, sulfoxides can also be oxidized by **hydroxyl radicals** released by the cytochrome P450 monooxygenase system (see Section 7.6.1) (Cohen and Cederbaum, 1979 and 1980). Dimethyl sulfoxide (CH$_3$–SO–CH$_3$), a potent scavenger of hydroxyl radicals, is broken down by such a reaction to the sulfinic acid (CH$_3$SOOH) and the methyl radical ($^{\bullet}$CH$_3$); the latter may then abstract a hydrogen to form methane, dimerize to ethane, or react with molecular oxygen to yield ultimately formaldehyde (Klein *et al.*, 1981; Veltwisch *et al.*, 1980).

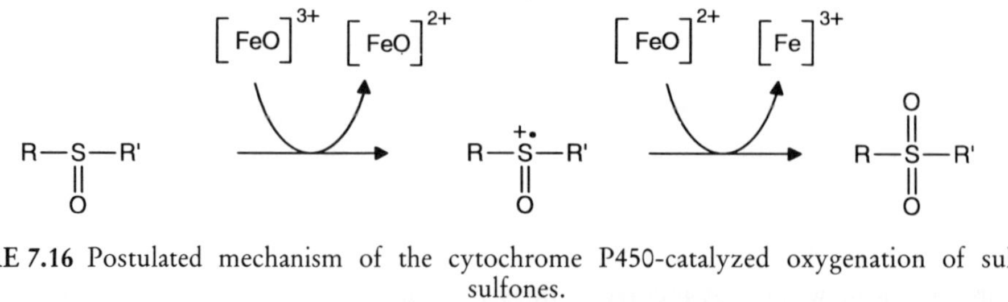

FIGURE 7.16 Postulated mechanism of the cytochrome P450-catalyzed oxygenation of sulfoxides to sulfones.

7.LXVIII   7.LXIX

In contrast to cytochrome P450, the **FAD-containing monooxygenase** forms sulfoxides and sulfones by a direct, electrophilic attack and transfer of the activated oxygen atom (pathway **B** in Fig. 7.14) (see Section 3.7). As a consequence, the **nucleophilicity** of the sulfur atom should be one of the factors controlling the rate of sulfoxidation. Thus, *para*-substituted 2-phenyl-1,3-oxathiolanes (**7.LXIX**, X = H, CH_3, OCH_3, Cl, NO_2) were oxygenated by purified pig and rat FAD-containing monooxygenases at rates negatively correlated with the electron-withdrawing power of the *para*-substituent (Cashman *et al.*, 1989). Other molecular properties, in particular steric factors, also markedly influence the rate of reaction, as demonstrated with a large series of thioether-containing pesticides (Hajjar and Hodgson, 1982). The oxygen atom being strongly electron-withdrawing, it makes sense that the oxygenation of sulfoxides to sulfones is generally much slower than the first oxygenation step (e.g. Cashman *et al.*, 1989; Light *et al.*, 1982).

From the above considerations, it can be concluded that a variety of molecular factors will determine the **relative substrate activity** of a given sulfide towards cytochrome P450 and FAD-containing monooxygenase. As a result, the conclusion that the flavin-containing monooxygenase prefers non-aromatic, more nucleophilic sulfides has limited validity (Damani and Hoodi, 1988; Hoodi and Damani, 1984). Even the few thioethers listed in Table 7.2 do not verify this generalization.

Since sulfoxides are configurationally stable, the sulfoxidation of sulfides with two different substituents creates a centre of chirality. A large number of studies document the **product enantioselectivity of S-oxygenation** catalyzed by cytochrome P450 or FAD-containing monooxygenase (e.g. Benoit *et al.*, 1992; Cashman *et al.*, 1989 and 1990; Park *et al.*, 1992; Takata *et al.*, 1983). Thus, 4-tolyl ethyl sulfide can yield the (+)-(*R*)- and (−)-(*S*)-sulfoxides (**7.LXX**, R = ethyl); the *R/S* ratio was 20/1 for purified hog liver FAD-containing monooxygenase and about 1/4 for purified cytochromes P450 (Light *et al.*, 1982; Waxman *et al.*, 1982). With purified

(*R*)   (*S*)

7.LXX

7.LXXI

FAD-containing monooxygenases, the *R/S* ratio decreased in 4-tolyl alkyl sulfoxides (**7.LXX**, R = methyl, ethyl, propyl and isopropyl) with increasing bulk of the alkyl group (Rettie *et al.*, 1990). With the 2-phenyl-1,3-oxathiolanes (**7.LXIX**) discussed above, it was found that FAD-containing monooxygenase specifically mediated the attack of the *pro-S* electron lone pair on the sulfur atom, while CYP2B1 showed a selectivity for the *pro-R* lone pair over the *pro-S* (Cashman *et al.*, 1990).

A number of **sulfur-containing drugs** are known to form sulfoxides and also sulfones in some cases (Damani, 1987; Ziegler, 1982 and 1988). This is for example the case with the anthelmintic drug albendazole (**7.LXXI**), which is sulfoxidized in pig liver microsomes by cytochrome P450 and, more slowly, by FAD-containing monooxygenase (Souhaili El Amri *et al.*, 1987). A different enantioselectivity was noted in various animal species, humans, dogs and sheep producing more (+)- than (−)-sulfoxide, while the reverse was seen in rats (Delatour *et al.*, 1990 and 1991).

Sulfoxidation is a major metabolic route of cimetidine (**7.LXXII**) in the rat, dog and human, with a marked product enantioselectivity for (−)-cimetidine S-oxide seen in human liver

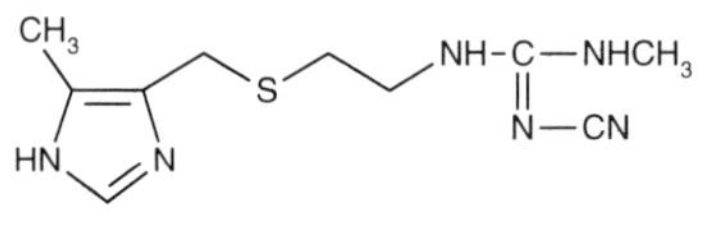

7.LXXII

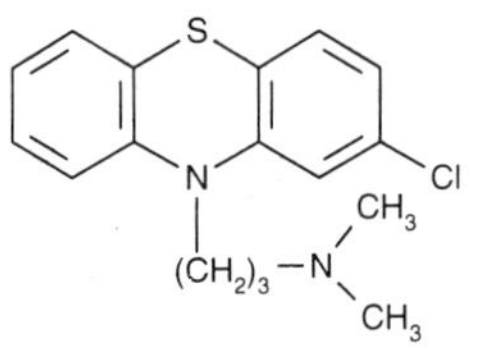

7.LXXIII

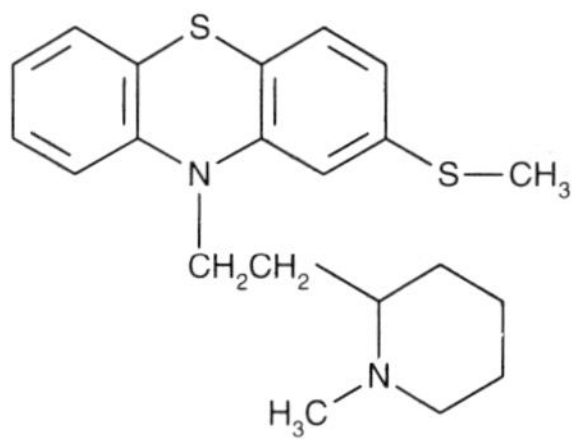

7.LXXIV

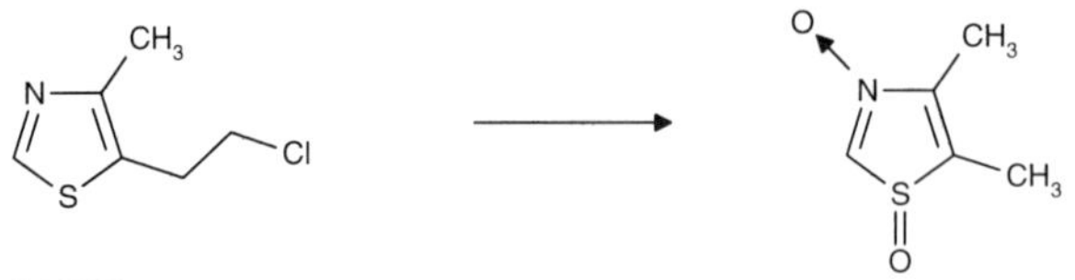

7.LXXV

7.LXXVI

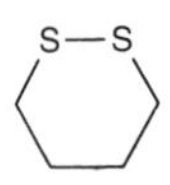

7.LXXVII

microsomes (Cashman *et al.*, 1993; Taylor *et al.*, 1978). Neuroleptic drugs such as chlorpromazine (**7.LXXIII**) and perazine form sulfoxide and sulfone metabolites in humans, while thioridazine (**7.LXXIV**) was reported to form ring sulfoxides as well as side-chain sulfoxides and sulfones in humans (Breyer-Pfaff *et al.*, 1978; Papadopoulos and Crammer, 1986). Another quite intriguing metabolite is the dioxide **7.LXXVI** (4,5-dimethyl-N-oxide-S-oxide) formed from the sedative chlormethiazole (**7.LXXV**) (Offen *et al.*, 1985). The compound 4-(*p*-chlorophenylthio)butanol (**7.LV**) discussed earlier also yielded small amounts of sulfones (**7.LVII**, *n* = 3 and 4) in rats and dogs (Kucharczyk *et al.*, 1979).

In analogy with sulfides, **disulfides** are also oxidized by monooxygenases. Stepwise oxygenation (see Table 7.1) leads to the corresponding **thiolsulfinate** and then to the **thiolsulfonate** probably via the α-disulfoxide (Fukushima *et al.*, 1978). Such compounds may be relatively unstable and decompose to various products. Thus, an unstable thiolsulfinate may disproportionate to the corresponding disulfide and thiolsulfonate. Thiolsulfinates, α-disulfoxides and thiolsulfonates may be hydrolytically cleaved to the corresponding thiol and sulfinic acid, sulfenic and sulfinic acids, and thiol and sulfonic acid, respectively (see Fig. 7.13) (Ziegler, 1980 and 1984). However, stable oxygenated disulfides do exist, e.g. cyclic disulfides such as 1,2-dithiane (**7.LXXVII**) which was oxygenated by rabbit liver microsomes and a purified cytochrome P450 preparation to the corresponding thiolsulfinate, while the latter under the same conditions yielded the thiolsulfonate at a comparatively slower rate (Fukushima *et al.*, 1978). The oxidation of disulfides by FAD-containing monooxygenase is exemplified in Table 7.2.

An interesting consequence of S-oxygenation has recently been discovered in the metabolism of dithiopyr, a herbicidal agent containing two methylthioester groups (R–CO–S–CH₃). Either group was cleaved *in vivo* and *in vitro* to yield a carboxylic acid, the involvement of monooxygenases rather than esterases being demonstrated (Feng and Solsten, 1991). The proposed mechanism of such an **oxidative thioester cleavage** involves formation of an unstable sulfoxide intermediate which hydrolyzes to the acid and (presumably) a sulfenic acid (Fig. 7.17) (compare with oxidative ester cleavage in Section 7.5).

7.8 SULFOXIDATION OF THIONES, THIOAMIDES AND THIOUREAS

Thiocarbonyl derivatives (i.e. compounds containing a carbon–sulfur double bond) can undergo quite complex reactions of S-oxygenation leading to a variety of products, some of which have marked toxicological significance (Neal, 1980; Ziegler, 1982 and 1984). Because of differences in reactivity and even products, a distinction is made here between the sulfur analogues of ketones (thiones in a narrow sense), amides (thioamides), and ureas (thioureas = thiocarbamides) (Table 7.1). Compounds containing a phosphorus–sulfur double bond are considered in Section 7.9.

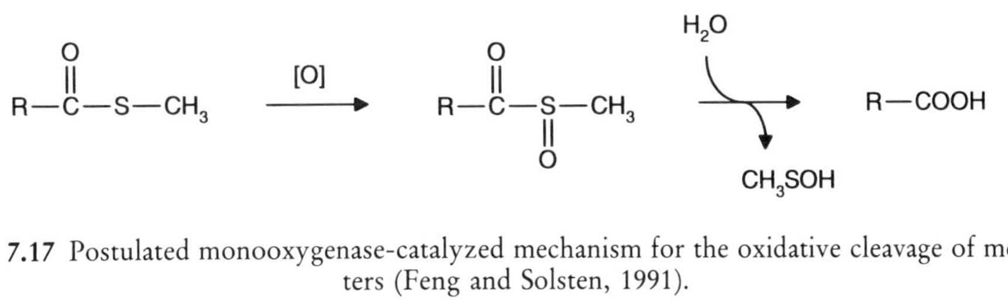

FIGURE 7.17 Postulated monooxygenase-catalyzed mechanism for the oxidative cleavage of methylthioesters (Feng and Solsten, 1991).

7.8.1 Thiones

The simplest xenobiotic thione is **carbon disulfide** (CS_2), a compound whose hepatotoxicity results in part from monooxygenase-mediated toxication (Dalvi, 1988). A number of studies document the cytochrome P450-catalyzed oxidation of carbon disulfide to carbonyl sulfide (COS, **7.LXXVIII** in Fig. 7.18) and carbon dioxide (e.g. Chengelis and Neal, 1979 and 1987; Dalvi and Neal, 1978). In untreated rats, for example, COS is the predominant metabolite excreted in the expired air, while phenobarbital-induced rats excreted mainly CO_2 (Dalvi and Neal, 1978). Recent *in vitro* studies have given evidence that the product of microsomal oxidation of CS_2 is not COS *per se*, but its hydrated form, monothiocarbonic acid (**7.LXXIX** in Fig. 7.18), suggesting the **mechanism** shown in Fig. 7.18 and discussed below (Chengelis and Neal, 1987).

First, cytochrome P450 generates an S-oxide (reaction **a** in Fig. 7.18) which can be represented in several canonical forms, an oxathiirane intermediate being also conceivable based on evidence obtained with thiophosphates (Section 7.9). Hydrolysis of this S-oxide (reaction **b** in Fig. 7.18) results in the formation of monothiocarbonic acid (**7.LXXIX** in Fig. 7.18) upon expulsion of a sulfur atom. The atomic species of sulfur expelled is not known (it may be an electrophilic intermediate analogous to oxene, see also below), but it must be fairly reactive since it has the capacity to react with thiol groups in proteins to produce hydrodisulfides (reaction **c** in Fig. 7.18). Carbon disulfide, and a wealth of other thiocarbonyl derivatives (thioamides as well as thioureas) and phosphorothionates, are known to be **mechanism-based, irreversible inhibitors** of cytochrome P450 (Hunter and Neal, 1975; Järvisalo *et al.*, 1977; Testa and Jenner, 1981). It is likely that the covalent binding of the sulfur atom to the apoenzyme accounts for most of the activity of these inhibitors.

Monothiocarbonic acid is in equilibrium with carbonyl sulfide (reaction **d** in Fig. 7.18), the reaction being catalyzed by **carbonic anhydrase**. In fact, acetazolamide, an inhibitor of carbonic

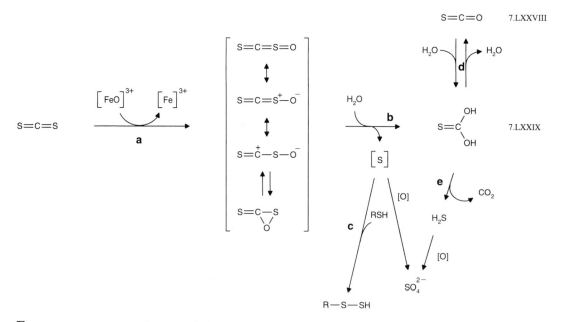

FIGURE 7.18 Main mechanism of the oxidative desulfuration of carbon disulfide to carbonyl sulfide (**7.LXXVIII**) and carbon dioxide. Also shown is the postulated mechanism by which the expelled sulfur atom binds to proteins (reaction **c**), making CS_2 a mechanism-based, irreversible inhibitor of cytochrome P450 (Modified from Chengelis and Neal, 1987; Testa and Jenner, 1981).

anhydrase, inhibited much of the metabolism of COS in rat hepatocytes (Chengelis and Neal, 1979). Because monothiocarbonic acid breaks down spontaneously to CO_2 and H_2S (reaction e in Fig. 7.18), the sequence of reactions d and e in Fig. 7.18 offers a mechanism for the formation of CO_2 from COS (Chengelis and Neal, 1987). However, cytochrome P450 also appears to catalyze the transformation of COS to CO_2 (Dalvi, 1988; Dalvi and Neal, 1978).

In overall terms, the transformation of CS_2 to COS and then to CO_2 involves the sequential replacement of the two sulfur atoms by oxygen. Such reactions, when occurring via oxidative mechanisms, are known as **oxidative desulfuration**. Beside CS_2, they have been investigated mainly for thioamides and thioureas, as discussed below. In addition, some **isothiocyanates** (R–N=C=S) have also been shown to be substrates of oxidative desulfuration to yield toxic isocyanates (R–N=C=O) (Lee, 1992).

7.8.2 Thioamides

The sulfoxidation of thioamides is of marked interest due to the potential toxicity of some metabolites, in particular their hepatotoxicity and carcinogenicity. A number of studies have examined the biotransformation of thioacetamide (**7.LXXX**) and thiobenzamide (**7.LXXXI**); as shown in Table 7.2, the two compounds are very good substrates of the FAD-containing monooxygenase (Sabourin and Hodgson, 1984). One reason for thioamides being such good substrates of this enzyme is that resonance (**7.LXXXII**) increases the nucleophilic character of the sulfur atom (Doerge and Corbett, 1984). However, thioamides are also S-oxygenated by cytochrome P450, and the same compound is often found to be oxidized by either or both monooxygenases depending on the biological preparation being used.

Available evidence indicates that the S-oxygenation of thioamides leads to a **sulfine** (i.e. the S-monooxide **7.LXXXIII**, reaction a in Fig. 7.19) and then to a **sulfene** (i.e. the S-dioxide **7.LXXXIV**, reaction c in Fig. 7.19). Unknown aspects remain in the mechanism underlying the chemical reactivity of these metabolites, and particularly of the highly reactive sulfenes (Damani, 1987; Snyder, 1973; Ziegler, 1982 and 1984). Thus, thioacetamide (**7.LXXX**) was metabolized by rat liver microsomes to the sulfine and then to the sulfene, the end-products being acetamide (i.e. the metabolite resulting from oxidative desulfuration), other polar compounds, and microsomal-bound material (adducts) (Porter and Neal, 1978). The formation of all these products required a double oxygenation, thus seemingly ruling out desulfuration of the S-monooxide **7.LXXXIII** (reaction b in Fig. 7.19). Two oxygenation steps were also necessary for thioacetamide to bind

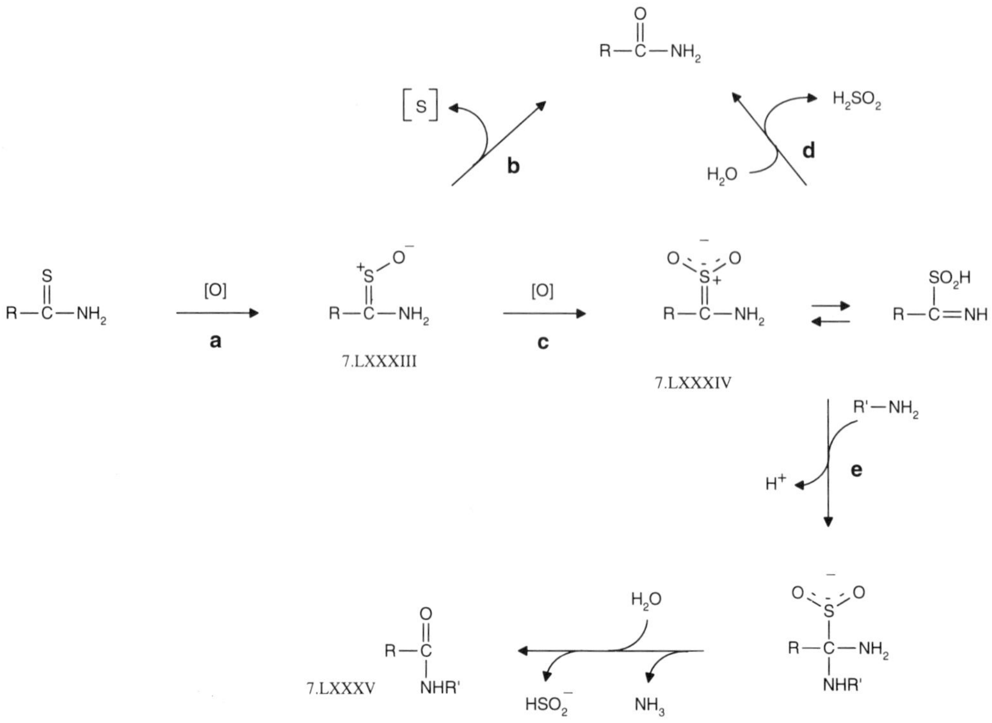

FIGURE 7.19 Metabolic scheme of the monooxygenase-mediated oxygenation of thioamides to sulfines (**7.LXXXIII**), sulfenes (**7.LXXXIV**) and amides. Also shown is the mechanism of protein acylation (reaction **e**) uncovered by Dyroff and Neal (1983).

covalently to DNA and other polynucleotides (Vadi and Neal, 1981). Studies of great importance have uncovered the mechanism by which thioacetamide S-dioxide reacts with some nucleophilic groups in macromolecules, specifically with the amino group of lysine in albumin (Dyroff and Neal, 1983). As shown in simplified form in Fig. 7.19 (reaction **e**), a double nucleophilic substitution (by the macromolecule and H_2O) results in the loss of ammonia and a sulfoxylate anion and in the acetylation of lysine (**7.LXXXV** in Fig. 7.19, R = CH_3, R' = albumin). Both cytochrome P450 and the FAD-containing monooxygenase mediate the two oxygenation steps (Vadi and Neal, 1981).

Thiobenzamide (**7.LXXXI**) can also be activated by both the FAD-containing monooxygenase and cytochrome P450, in particular CYP2E1 (Chieli *et al.*, 1990; Levi *et al.*, 1982). Here again, oxidative desulfuration to yield benzamide was shown to occur via reaction **d** in Fig. 7.19 but not reaction **b** (Hanzlik and Cashman, 1983). Unfortunately, the molecular factors influencing S-oxygenation, covalent binding and desulfuration are poorly understood. In this context, it is interesting to note that ring substituents in thiobenzamide (**7.LXXXI**) markedly affect toxicity. The influence of *para-* and *meta-*substituents is of electronic origin, toxicity increasing markedly with increasing electron donation; in contrast, *ortho-*substituted derivatives show little toxicity presumably due to steric shielding against the second oxygenation (Cashman *et al.*, 1983; Hanzlik *et al.*, 1980). These results are in agreement with oxygenation resulting in bioactivation. In addition, electronic and steric factors possibly also affect the relative importance of covalent binding (reaction **e** in Fig. 7.19) vs. desulfuration (reaction **d** and/or **b** in Fig. 7.19), but this remains to be investigated. It certainly is of interest that thioacetanilide (**7.LXXXVI**) is rapidly desulfurated in the rat to acetanilide, no sulfine being seen (Trennery and Waring, 1983). This suggests a direct desulfuration via reaction **b** (Fig. 7.19).

Some thioamides are known to **react like thiols** (Section 7.7.1) rather than thiones for the simple reason that they exist predominantly as the **thiol tautomer**. This is the case with 6-mercaptopurine (**7.LXXXVII**), which is metabolized by cytochrome P450 to the reactive sulfenic acid (reaction **a** in Fig. 7.13) and then to the sulfinic acid (reaction **e** in Fig. 7.13) (Abraham *et al.*, 1983; Hyslop and Jardine, 1981). The former metabolite binds avidly to thiol groups in proteins (reaction **d** in Fig. 7.13); binding to and recycling by glutathione (GSH) also occur (see a subsequent volume).

7.LXXXVI

7.LXXXVII

7.8.3 Thioureas

Little *a priori* reason is apparent to distinguish between thioamides and thioureas as far as their biotransformation is concerned. Both classes of compounds are substrates of cytochrome P450 and FAD-containing monooxygenases (see Table 7.2 for reactivities towards the latter system), and both can undergo double oxygenation of the sulfur atom. But while few thioamides react metabolically as thiol tautomers (e.g. 6-mercaptopurine discussed above), various reports indicate that the **thiol–thione tautomerism** must be taken into account for a number of thioureas (reaction **f** in Fig. 7.20). This difference may not be without consequence as far as postenzymatic reactions (i.e. the chemical reactivity of metabolites) are concerned.

Let us first consider **reactions typical of thiones**. The **oxidative desulfuration** of thioureas to the corresponding urea derivative tells us little about the underlying mechanism since the transformation can occur by two routes: rearrangement of a sulfine with loss of atomic sulfur (reaction **b** in Fig. 7.19), or hydrolysis of a sulfene/sulfinic acid (reaction **d** in Fig. 7.19 and reaction **k** in Fig. 7.20). A decisive element in this context is the chemical nature of the expelled sulfur, namely atomic sulfur (presumably the sulfur analogue of oxene) or sulfoxylic acid (H_2SO_2). Thus, the rodenticide α-naphthylthiourea (**7.LXXXVIII**) was metabolized by rat liver and lung microsomes to α-naphthylurea and atomic sulfur (Lee *et al.*, 1980). Liberation of the latter was proven by the reaction with cysteinyl residues in microsomal proteins to form hydrodisulfides (see reaction **c** in Fig. 7.18). Such a result brings evidence, but of course not proof, for the desulfuration of a sulfine intermediate (reaction **b** in Fig. 7.19). Metiamide (**7.LXXXIX**), the toxic predecessor of the H_2-histamine receptor antagonist cimetidine (**7.LXXII**), was also desulfurated, giving the urea analogue as a minor metabolite in rats and

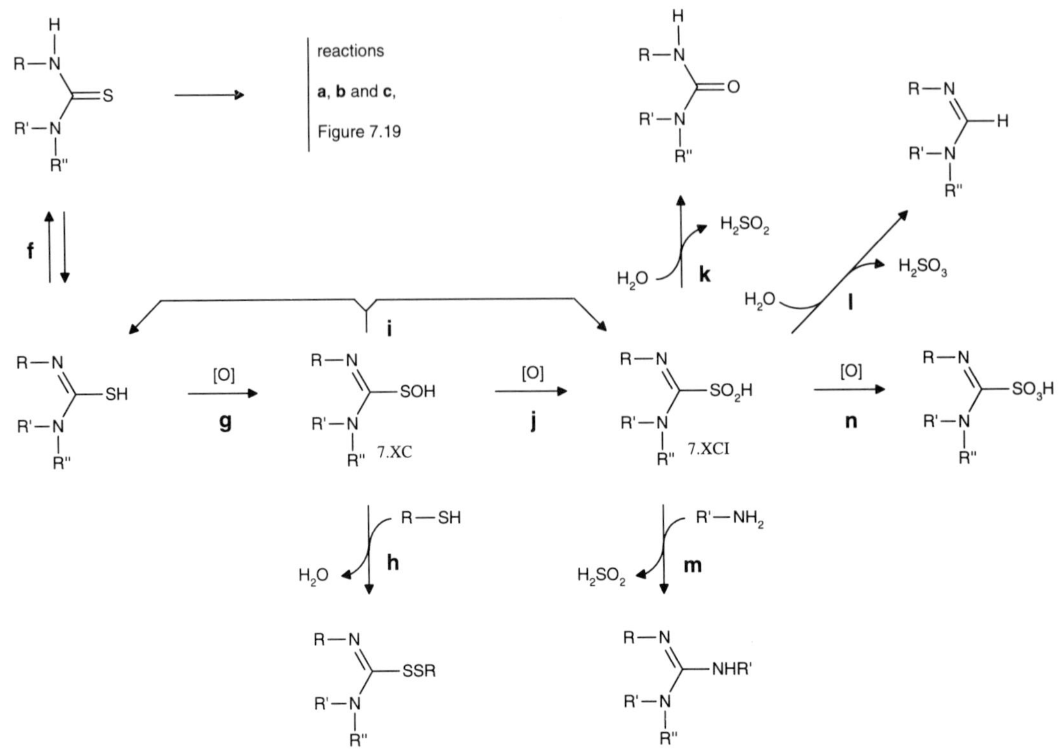

FIGURE 7.20 Metabolic scheme of the monooxygenase-catalyzed oxygenation of thiourea derivatives to formamidine sulfenic acids (**7.XC**), sulfinic acids (**7.XCI**), and sulfonic acids. Also shown are some postenzymatic reactions, namely: (a) for formamidine sulfenic acids, disproportionation (reaction **i**) and formation of disulfides (reaction **h**); (b) for formamidine sulfinic acids, hydrolyses (reactions **k** and **l**) and adduct formation with amino groups in proteins (reaction **m**).

humans, but in this case the pathway was not established (Taylor *et al.*, 1979). Interestingly, the major metabolite in rats, dogs and humans was the sulfoxide, indicating a regioselectivity for the thioether vs. the thiourea group.

In the light of available evidence, the capacity of thioureas to react as the **thiol tautomers** to form **formamidine sulfenic acids** (**7.XC**, reaction **g** in Fig. 7.20) and then **formamidine sulfinic**

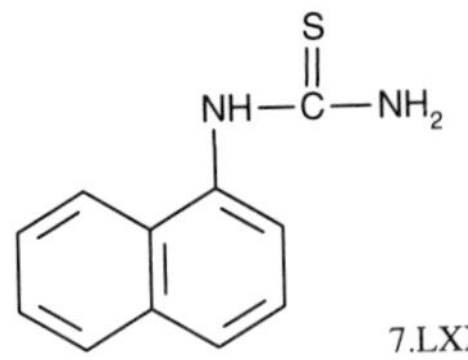

7.LXXXVIII

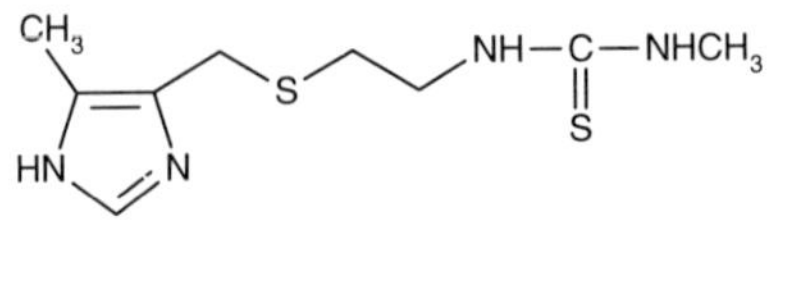

7.LXXXIX

acids (**7.XCI**, reaction **j** in Fig. 7.20) is noteworthy (Ziegler, 1980, 1982, 1984 and 1988). The reactivity of the formamidine sulfenic acids **7.XC** is analogous to that of other sulfenic acids as discussed in Section 7.7.1, resulting in the formation of **disulfides** (reaction **h** in Fig. 7.20) upon reaction with endogenous thiols such as glutathione and cysteinyl residues in proteins. The possibility of dimerization to formamidine disulfides should also be considered, especially since these potential metabolites have been shown to be some 50 to 100 times more toxic to isolated rat hepatocytes than the parent compounds (Jatoe *et al.*, 1988).

Another reaction of the formamidine sulfenates **7.XC** in Fig. 7.20 is their disproportionation to a thiol and a sulfinate (reaction **i** in Fig. 7.20), perhaps via a thiolsulfinate (see Fig. 7.13) (Poulsen *et al.*, 1979).

Very slow formation of **formamidine sulfonic acids** (reaction **n** in Fig. 7.20) was seen from phenylformamidine and ethyleneformamidine sulfinic acids (Poulsen *et al.*, 1979). Such sulfinic acids **7.XCI** in Fig. 7.20 can also undergo nucleophilic substitution with water to yield the corresponding urea derivative and sulfoxylic acid (reaction **k** in Fig. 7.20) or with nucleophilic groups in macromolecules resulting in covalent binding (reaction **m** in Fig. 7.20) (Ziegler, 1982 and 1988).

For such substrates as thiourea, methylthiourea, phenylthiourea, ethylenethiourea and thiocarbanilide, S-oxygenation was mediated exclusively by the FAD-containing monooxygenase in hog and hamster liver microsomes and perfused rat liver (Krieter *et al.*, 1984; Poulsen *et al.*, 1979). Furthermore, the molecular size of thiocarbamides has a marked influence on their affinity towards isoforms of the FAD-containing monooxygenase (Guo *et al.*, 1992). **2-Mercaptoimidazoles** (e.g. **7.XCII**) are cyclized thioureas existing mainly as the thiol tautomer by virtue of their aromaticity (note the analogy with 6-mercaptopurine **7.LXXXVII**). Their S-oxygenation is comparable to that of other thioureas, but the reactivity of the resulting imidazole sulfinates differs from that of formamidine sulfinates, in particular in their hydrolysis to an imidazole and sulfurous acid (H_2SO_3) (reaction **l** in Fig. 7.20) (Decker and Doerge, 1992; Ziegler, 1988). One compound of medicinal relevance is the antithyroid drug **methimazole** (**7.XCII**); formation of N-methylimidazole (**7.XCIII**) with release of sulfite/sulfurous acid was mediated mainly by the FAD-containing monooxygenase (Poulsen *et al.*, 1974). Cytochrome P450 also formed N-methylimidazole in addition to N-methylimidazolidinedione (**7.XCIV**); atomic sulfur was released during this reaction, suggesting both the thione and thiol tautomeric forms of methimazole to be S-oxygenated (Lee and Neal, 1978). Further insights into these reactions have been gained by the study of 1,3-dimethylbenzimidazoline-2-thione, an analogue unable to exist in thiol tautomeric form (Decker *et al.*, 1992).

7.XCII

7.XCIII

7.XCIV

7.9 OXIDATIVE DESULFURATION OF PHOSPHOROTHIONATES, PHOSPHONOTHIONATES AND ANALOGUES

Oxidative desulfuration is also documented for a number of xenobiotics containing a thiono-sulfur bonded to a phosphorus atom (Neal, 1980). These compounds are insecticides and inhibitors of acetylcholinesterase; they include (see also Table 7.1):

- phosphorothionates $(RO)(R'\dot{O})P{=}S(OR'')$;
- phosphorodithioates $(RO)(R'O)P{=}S(SR'')$;
- phosphonothionates $(RO)(R')P{=}S(OR'')$; and
- phosphonodithioates $(RO)(R')P{=}S(SR'')$.

Oxidative desulfuration transforms these thiophosphates and thiophosphonates into their oxon analogue, a reaction generally accompanied by a marked increase in activity and hence toxicity.

A derivative that has received particular attention is **parathion** (**7.XCV** in Fig. 7.21). Oxidation by cytochrome P450 (reaction **a** in Fig. 7.21) leads to an unstable monooxygenated species postulated to be an S-oxide existing in equilibrium with an **oxathiaphosphirane**, i.e. a trimembered ring structure analogous to an epoxide (reaction **b** in Fig. 7.21) (Kamataki *et al.*, 1976; Kexel *et al.*, 1977). Rearrangement of the latter intermediate can explain the formation of paraoxon (**7.XCVI** in Fig. 7.21) with concurrent loss of atomic sulfur. Good evidence indeed exists that sulfur is released in an atomic, activated form that binds covalently to apocytochrome P450 and inhibits the enzyme. Specifically, and as discussed in Section 7.8, the activated sulfur binds to the thiol group of cysteinyl residues, forming hydrodisulfides (RSSH) (Davis and Mende, 1977). In addition, covalent binding to proteins also involves tyrosine and amino acids with branched side-chains (isoleucine, leucine, and valine). This would suggest the atomic sulfur to be released in a singlet rather than triplet state (Halpert *et al.*, 1980).

Beside forming paraoxon, the monooxygenation of parathion can also be followed by hydrolysis (reaction **c** in Fig. 7.21) and leads to the formation of diethyl phosphate (**7.XCVII** in Fig. 7.21) and diethyl thiophosphate (**7.XCVIII** in Fig. 7.21) (Kamataki *et al.*, 1976; Kexel *et al.*, 1977). Indeed, the intermediate S-oxide is activated towards nucleophilic attack by H_2O or the hydroxyl anion.

Comparable reactions are documented for **fonofos** (O-ethyl S-phenyl ethyldithiophosphon-ate) (Menn *et al.*, 1976). Interestingly, this compound is a substrate of both cytochrome P450 and the FAD-containing monooxygenase, and it appears that a carbon–phosphorus bond is necessary for the latter enzyme to effect the desulfuration of organophosphorus derivatives (Kinsler *et al.*, 1988). Attack on the phosphorus rather than sulfur atom has been postulated.

A variety of organophosphorus insecticides contain a **side-chain with a thioether group**; the latter often but not always becomes a privileged target group for the FAD-containing monooxygenase, resulting in the formation of a stable sulfoxide of low toxicity (Hajjar and Hodgson, 1982). As a result of the predominance of this pathway, desulfuration (and toxication) of phosphorothionates and phosphorodithioates by cytochrome P450 becomes a minor route, as documented for **phorate** (**7.XCIX**) (Kinsler *et al.*, 1988). Schematically, insecticides such as

$$(C_2H_5O)_2\ \overset{\displaystyle S}{\overset{\|}{P}}{-}S{-}CH_2{-}S{-}C_2H_5$$

7.XCIX

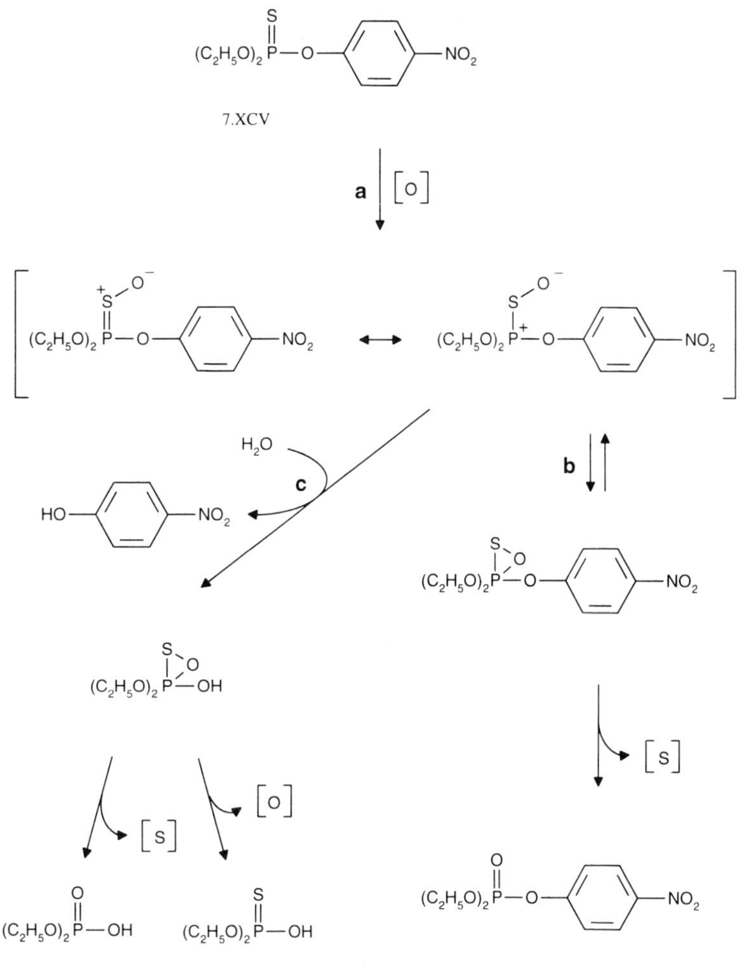

FIGURE 7.21 Postulated mechanisms of the oxidative desulfuration and hydrolysis of parathion (**7.XCV**) to paraoxon (**7.XCVI**), diethyl phosphate (**7.XCVII**) and diethyl thiophosphate (**7.XCVIII**) (modified from Testa and Jenner, 1978).

phorate are substrates for two competitive metabolic reactions, one of detoxication and the other of toxication, implying that toxicity may be markedly affected by biological factors influencing the relative importance of the two routes.

7.10 REFERENCES

Abraham R.T., Benson L.M. and Jardine I. (1983). Synthesis and pH-dependent stability of purine-6-sulfenic acid, a putative reactive metabolite of 6-thiopurine. *J. Med. Chem.* **26**, 1523–1526.

Akhtar M.H. and Mahadevan S. (1992). Diphenyl ether cleavage of 3-phenoxybenzoic acid by chicken kidney microsomal preparations. *Drug Metab. Disposit.* **20**, 356–359.

Akhtar M., Njar V.C.O. and Wright J.N. (1993). Mechanistic studies on aromatase and related C–C bond cleaving P-450 enzymes. *J. Ster. Biochem. Molec. Biol.* **44**, 375–387.

Albano E., Tomasi A., Persson J.O., Terelius Y., Goria-Gatti L., Ingelman-Sundberg M. and Dianzani M.U. (1991). Role of ethanol-inducible cytochrome P450 (P450IIE1) in catalysing the free radical activation of aliphatic alcohols. *Biochem. Pharmacol.* **41**, 1895–1902.

Al-Gailany K.A.S., Bridges J.W. and Netter K.J. (1975). The dealkylation of some *p*-nitrophenylalkyl ethers and their α-deuterated analogues by rat liver microsomes. *Biochem. Pharmacol.* **24**, 867–870.

Amann T. and Zenk M.H. (1991). Formation of the morphine precursor salutaridine is catalyzed by a cytochrome P-450 enzyme in mammalian liver. *Tetrahedron Lett.* **32**, 3675–3678.

Anders M.W., Sunram J.M. and Wilkinson W.F. (1984). Mechanism of the metabolism of 1,3-benzodioxoles to carbon monoxide. *Biochem. Pharmacol.* **33**, 577–580.

Ayrton A.D., McFarlane M., Walker R., Neville S. and Ioannides C. (1990). The induction of P 450 I proteins by aromatic amines may be related to their carcinogenic potential. *Carcinogenesis* **11**, 803–809.

Bartholomew T.C., Powell G.M., Dodgson K.S. and Curtis C.G. (1980). Oxidation of sodium sulphide by rat liver, lungs and kidney. *Biochem. Pharmacol.* **29**, 2431–2437.

Bedford C.T., Crayford J.V., Hutson D.H. and Wiggins D.E. (1978). An example of the oxidative de-esterification of an isopropyl ester. Its role in the metabolism of the herbicide flampropisopropyl. *Xenobiotica* **8**, 383–395.

Benoit E., Cresteil T., Rivière J.L. and Delatour P. (1992). Specific and enantioselective sulfoxidation of an aryl-trifluoromethyl sulfide by rat liver cytochromes P-450. *Drug Metab. Disposit.* **20**, 877–881.

Bhat R.V., Subrahmanyam V.V., Sadler A. and Ross D. (1988). Bioactivation of catechol in rat and human bone marrow cells. *Toxicol. Appl. Pharmacol.* **94**, 297–304.

Bisby R.H. and Tabassum N. (1988). Properties of the radicals formed by one-electron oxidation of acetaminophen—a pulse radiolysis study. *Biochem. Pharmacol.* **37**, 2731–2738.

Blagbrough I.S., Buckberry L.D., Bycroft B.W. and Shaw P.N. (1990). Human renal C–S lyase: structure–activity relationships of cytosolic and mitochondrial enzymes. *Toxicol. Lett.* **53**, 257–259.

Blagbrough I.S., Buckberry L.D., Bycroft B.W. and Shaw P.N. (1992). Structure–activity relationship studies of bovine C–S lyase enzymes. *Pharm. Pharmacol. Lett.* **1**, 93–96.

Boberg M., Karl W., Siefert H.M. and Wünsche C. (1990). Biotransformation of BAY r 3783 in rats and dogs. *XIIth European Workshop on Drug Metabolism*, Basel, September 16–21, Abstracts, p. 133.

Bolton J.L., Le Blanc J.C.Y. and Siu K.W.M. (1993). Reactions of quinone methides with proteins: analysis of myoglobin adduct formation by electrospray mass spectrometry. *Biol. Mass Spectrom.* **22**, 666–668.

Borel A.G., Tang W., Panesar S.K. and Abbott F.S. (1993). Delineating the involvement of hepatic mitochondrial cytochrome P-450 in the bioactivation of formamides. In *ISSX Proceedings*, Vol. 4. International Society for the Study of Xenobiotics, Bethesda, MD, USA, p. 41.

Boulton J.L., Valerio L.G. Jr and Thompson J.A. (1992). The enzymatic formation and chemical reactivity of

quinone methides correlate with alkylphenol-induced toxicity in rat hepatocytes. *Chem. Res. Toxicol.* **5**, 816–822.

Brady J.F., Lee M.J., Li M., Ishizaki H. and Yang C.S. (1988). Diethyl ether as a substrate for acetone/ethanol-inducible cytochrome P-450 and as an inducer for cytochrome(s) P-450. *Molec. Pharmacol.* **33**, 148–154.

Brady J.F., Xiao F., Ning S.M. and Yang C.S. (1990). Metabolism of methyl *tertiary*-butyl ether by rat hepatic microsomes. *Arch. Toxicol.* **64**, 157–160.

Braun W.H. and Young J.D. (1977). Identification of β-hydroxyethoxyacetic acid as the major urinary metabolite of 1,4-dioxane in the rat. *Toxicol. Appl. Pharmacol.* **39**, 33–38.

Breyer-Pfaff U., Kreft H., Rassner H. and Prox A. (1978). Formation of sulfone metabolites from chlorpromazine and perazine in man. *Drug Metab. Disposit.* **6**, 114–119.

Buben J.A., Narasimhan N. and Hanzlik R.P. (1988). Effects of chemical and enzymic probes on microsomal covalent binding of bromobenzene and derivatives. Evidence for quinones as reactive metabolites. *Xenobiotica* **18**, 501–510.

Buters J.T.M., Schiller C.D. and Chou R.C. (1993). A highly sensitive tool for the assay of cytochrome P450 enzyme activity in rat, dog and man. *Biochem. Pharmacol.* **46**, 1577–1584.

Cashman J.R., Parikh K.K., Traiger G.J. and Hanzlik R.P. (1983). Relative hepatotoxicity of *ortho* and *meta* mono-substituted thiobenzamides in the rat. *Chem.-Biol. Interact.* **45**, 341–347.

Cashman J.R., Proudfoot J, Ho Y.K., Chin M.S. and Olsen L.D. (1989). Chemical and enzymatic oxidation of 2-aryl-1,3-oxathiolanes: mechanism of the hepatic flavin-containing monooxygenase. *J. Amer. Chem. Soc.* **111**, 4844–4852.

Cashman J.R., Olsen L.D. and Bornhaim L.M. (1990). Enantioselective S-oxygenation by flavin-containing and cytochrome P-450 monooxygenases. *Chem. Res. Toxicol.* **3**, 344–349.

Cashman J.R., Park S.B., Yang Z.C., Washington C.B., Gomez D.Y., Giacomini K.M. and Brett C.M. (1993). Chemical, enzymic, and human enantioselective S-oxygenation of cimetidine. *Drug Metab. Disposit.* **21**, 587–597.

Cavalieri E.L., Rogan E.G., Cremonesi P. and Devanesan P.D. (1988). Radical cations as precursors in the metabolic formation of quinones from benzo[*a*]pyrene and 6-fluorobenzo[*a*]pyrene. *Biochem. Pharmacol.* **37**, 2173–2182.

Cederbaum A.I. and Cohen G. (1980). Oxidative de-methylation of *t*-butyl alcohol by rat liver microsomes. *Biochem. Biophys. Res. Commun.* **97**, 730–736.

Chen C., Lefers R.C., Brough E.L. and Gurka D.P. (1984). Metabolism of alcohol and ketone by cytochrome P-450 oxygenase: fluoren-9-ol & fluoren-9-one. *Drug Metab. Disposit.* **12**, 421–426.

Chengelis C.P. and Neal R.A. (1979). Hepatic carbonyl sulfide metabolism. *Biochem. Biophys. Res. Commun.* **90**, 993–999.

Chengelis C.P. and Neal R.A. (1987). Oxidative metabolism of carbon disulfide by isolated rat hepatocytes and microsomes. *Biochem. Pharmacol.* **36**, 363–368.

Chieli E., Saviozzi M., Puccini P., Longo V. and Gervasi P.G. (1990). Possible role of the acetone-inducible cytochrome P-450IIE1 in the metabolism and hepatotoxicity of thiobenzamide. *Arch. Toxicol.* **64**, 122–127.

Chignell C.F. (1985). Structure–activity relationships in the free-radical metabolism of xenobiotics. *Environm. Health Perspect.* **61**, 133–137.

Christie G., Breckenridge A.M. and Park B.K. (1989). Drug–protein conjugates—XVIII. Detection of antibodies towards the antimalarial amodiaquine and its quinone imine metabolite in man and the rat. *Biochem. Pharmacol.* **38**, 1451–14,458.

Clejan L.A. and Cederbaum A.I. (1991) Role of iron, hydrogen peroxide and reactive oxygen species in microsomal oxidation of glycerol to formaldehyde. *Arch. Biochem. Biophys.* **285**, 83–89.

Clejan L.A. and Cederbaum A.I. (1992). Structural determinants for alcohol substrates to be oxidized to formaldehyde by rat liver microsomes. *Arch. Biochem. Biophys.* **298**, 105–113.

Cohen G. and Cederbaum A.I. (1979). Chemical evidence for production of hydroxyl radicals during microsomal electron transfer. *Science* **204**, 66–68.

Cohen G. and Cederbaum A.I. (1980). Microsomal metabolism of hydroxyl radical scavenging agents: relationship to the microsomal oxidation of alcohols. *Arch. Biochem. Biophys.* **199**, 438–447.

Cole P.A. and Robinson C.H. (1990). Mechanism and inhibition of cytochrome P-450 aromatase. *J. Med. Chem.* **33**, 2933–2942.

Crank G. and Makin M.I.H. (1984). Oxidation of thiols by superoxide ion. *Austral. J. Chem.* **37**, 2331–2337.

Dahlin D.C. and Nelson S.D. (1982). Synthesis, decomposition kinetics, and preliminary toxicological studies of pure N-acetyl-*p*-benzoquinone imine, a proposed toxic metabolite of acetaminophen. *J. Med. Chem.* **25**, 885–886.

Dalvi R.R. (1988). Mechanism of the neurotoxic and hepatotoxic effects of carbon disulfide. *Drug Metab. Drug Interact.* **6**, 275–284.

Dalvi R.R. and Neal R.A. (1978). Metabolism *in vivo* of carbon disulfide to carbonyl sulfide and carbon dioxide in the rat. *Biochem. Pharmacol.* **27**, 1608–1609.

Damani L.A. (1987). Metabolism of sulphur-containing drugs. In *Drug Metabolism—From Microbes to Man* (eds Benford D.J., Bridges J.W. and Gibson G.G.). pp. 581–603. Taylor and Francis, London.

Damani L.A. and Hoodi A.A. (1988). Cytochrome P-450 and FAD-monooxygenase mediated S- and N-oxygenations. *Drug Metab. Drug Interact.* **6**, 235–244.

D'Arcy Doherty M., Makowski R., Gibson G.G. and Cohen G.M. (1985). Cytochrome P-450 dependent metabolic activation of 1-naphthol to naphthoquinones and covalent binding species. *Biochem. Pharmacol.* **34**, 2261–2267.

Davis J.E. and Mende T.J. (1977). A study of the binding

of sulfur to rat liver microsomes which occurs concurrently with the metabolism of parathion and paraoxon. *J. Pharmacol. Exp. Therap.* **201**, 490–497.

Dayer P., Desmeules J., Leemann T. and Striberni R. (1988). Bioactivation of the narcotic drug codeine in human liver is mediated by the polymorphic monooxygenase catalyzing debrisoquine 4-hydroxylation (cytochrome P-450 db1/bufI). *Biochem. Biophys. Res. Commun.* **152**, 411–416.

Decker C.J. and Doerge D.R. (1992). Covalent binding of ^{14}C- and ^{35}S-labelled thiocarbamides in rat hepatic microsomes. *Biochem. Pharmacol.* **43**, 881–888.

Decker C.J., Rashed M.S., Baillie T.A., Maltby D. and Correia M.A. (1989). Oxidative metabolism of spironolactone: evidence for the involvement of electrophilic thiosteroid species in drug-mediated destruction of rat hepatic cytochrome P450. *Biochemistry* **28**, 5128–5136.

Decker C.J., Cashman J.R., Sujiyama K., Maltby D. and Correia M.A. (1991). Formation of glutathionyl-spironolactone disulfide by rat liver cytochromes P450 or hog liver flavin-containing monooxygenases: a functional probe of two-electron oxidations of the thiosteroid? *Chem. Res. Toxicol.* **4**, 669–677.

Decker C.J., Doerge D.R. and Cashman J.R. (1992). Metabolism of benzimidazoline-2-thiones by rat hepatic microsomes and hog liver flavin-containing monooxygenase. *Chem. Res. Toxicol.* **5**, 726–733.

Dekant W., Berthold K., Vamvakas S. and Henschler D. (1988a). Thioacylating agents as ultimate intermediates in the β-lyase catalysed metabolism of S-(pentachlorobutadienyl)-L-cysteine. *Chem.-Biol. Interact.* **67**, 139–148.

Dekant W., Lash L.H. and Anders M.W. (1988b). Fate of glutathione conjugates and bioactivation of cysteine S-conjugates by cysteine conjugate β-lyase. In *Glutathione Conjugation. Mechanisms and Biological Significance* (eds Sies H. and Ketterer B.). pp. 415–447. Academic Press, London.

Dekant W., Urban G., Görsmann C. and Anders M.W. (1991). Thioketene formation from α-haloalkenyl 2-nitrophenyldisulfides: models for biological reactive intermediates of cytotoxic S-conjugates. *J. Amer. Chem. Soc.* **113**, 5120–5122.

Delaforge M., Ioannides C. and Parke D.V. (1985). Ligand-complex formation between cytochromes P-450 and P-448 and methylenedioxyphenyl compounds. *Xenobiotica* **15**, 333–342.

Delatour P., Benoit E., Caude M. and Tambute A. (1990). Species differences in the generation of the chiral sulfoxide metabolite of albendazole in sheep and rats. *Chirality* **2**, 156–160.

Delatour P., Benoit E., Besse S. and Boukraa A. (1991). Comparative enantioselectivity in the sulfoxidation of albendazole in man, dogs and rats. *Xenobiotica* **21**, 217–221.

Doerge D.R. and Corbett M.D. (1984). Hydroperoxy-flavin-mediated oxidations of organosulfur compounds. Model studies for the flavin monooxygenase. *Molec. Pharmacol.* **26**, 348–352.

Dyroff M.C. and Neal R.A. (1983). Studies of the mechanism of metabolism of thioacetamide S-oxide by rat liver microsomes. *Molec. Pharmacol.* 23, 219–227.

Eberhart D., Titzgerld K. and Parkinson A. (1992). Evidence for the involvement of a distinct form of cytochrome P450 3A in the oxidation of digitoxin by rat liver microsomes. *J. Biochem. Toxicol.* 7, 53–64.

Ekström G., Norsten C., Cronholm T. and Ingelman-Sundberg M. (1987). Cytochrome P-450 dependent ethanol oxidation. Kinetic isotope effects and absence of stereoselectivity. *Biochemistry* 26, 7348–7354.

Elfarra A.A. and Hwang I.Y. (1993). Targeting of 6-mercaptopurine to the kidneys. Metabolism and kidney-selectivity of S-(6-purinyl)-L-cysteine analogs in rats. *Drug Metab. Disposit.* 21, 841–845.

Feng P.C.C. and Solsten R.T. (1991). *In vitro* transformation of dithiopyr by rat liver enzymes: conversion of methylthioesters to acids by oxygenases. *Xenobiotica* 21, 1265–1271.

Flinois J.P., Chabin M., Egros F., Dufour A., de Waziers I., Mas-Chamberlin C. and Beaune P.H. (1992). Metabolism rate of oxodipine in rats and humans: comparison of *in vivo* and *in vitro* data. *J. Pharmacol. Exp. Therap.* 261, 381–386.

Flowers-Geary L., Harvey R.G. and Penning T.M. (1993). Cytotoxicity of polycyclic aromatic hydrocarbon *o*-quinone in rat and human hepatoma cells. *Chem. Res. Toxicol.* 6, 252–260.

Franklin M.R. (1977). Inhibition of mixed-function oxidations by substrates forming reduced cytochrome P-450 metabolic-intermediate complexes. *Pharmacol. Ther. A* 2, 227–241.

Fukushima D., Kim Y.H., Iyanagi T. and Oae S. (1978). Enzymatic oxidation of disulfides and thiolsulfinates by both rabbit liver microsomes and a reconstituted system with purified cytochrome P-450. *J. Biochem. (Tokyo)* 83, 1019–1027.

Fukuto J.M., Kumagai Y. and Cho A.K. (1991). Determination of the mechanism of demethylenation of (methylenedioxy)phenyl compounds by cytochrome P450 using deuterium isotope effects. *J. Med. Chem.* 34, 2871–2876.

Funaki T., Soons P.A., Guengerich F.P. and Breimer D.D. (1989). *In vivo* oxidative cleavage of a pyridine-carboxylic acid ester metabolite of nifedipine. *Biochem. Pharmacol.* 38, 4213–4216.

Garland W.A., Nelson S.D. and Sasame H.A. (1976). Primary and β-secondary deuterium isotope effects in the O-deethylation of phenacetin. *Biochem. Biophys. Res. Commun.* 72, 539–545.

Gescher A. (1993). Metabolism of N,N-dimethylformamide: key to the understanding of its toxicity. *Chem. Res. Toxicol.* 6, 245–251.

Gillam E.M.J. and Reilly P.E.B. (1988). Phenacetin O-deethylation by human liver microsomes: kinetics and propranolol inhibition. *Xenobiotica* 18, 95–104.

Graham-Lorence S., Khalil M.W., Lorence M.C., Mendelson C.R. and Simpson E.R. (1991). Structure–function relationships of human aromatase cytochrome P-450 using molecular modeling and site-directed mutagenesis. *J. Biol. Chem.* 266, 11,939–11,946.

Greenlee W.F., Sun J.D. and Bus J.S. (1981). A proposed mechanism of benzene toxicity: formation of reactive intermediates from polyphenol metabolites. *Toxicol. Appl. Pharmacol.* 59, 187–195.

Guengerich F.P. (1987). Oxidative cleavage of carboxylic esters by cytochrome P-450. *J. Biol. Chem.* 262, 8459–8462.

Guengerich F.P., Willard R.J., Shea J.P., Richards L.E. and Macdonald T.L. (1984). Mechanism-based inactivation of cytochrome P-450 by heteroatom-substituted cyclopropanes and formation of ring-opened products. *J. Amer. Chem. Soc.* 106, 6446–6447.

Guengerich F.P., Peterson L.A. and Böcker R.H. (1988). Cytochrome P-450-catalyzed hydroxylation and carboxylic acid ester cleavage of Hantzsch pyridine esters. *J. Biol. Chem.* 263, 8176–8183.

Gunnison A.F., Bresnahan C.A. and Palmes E.D. (1977). Comparative sulfite metabolism in the rat, rabbit, and rhesus monkey. *Toxicol. Appl. Pharmacol.* 42, 99–109.

Guo W.X.A., Poulsen L.L. and Ziegler D.M. (1992). Use of thiocarbamides as selective substrate probes for isoforms of flavin-containing monooxygenases. *Biochem. Pharmacol.* 44, 2029–2037.

Hajjar N.P. and Hodgson E. (1982). Sulfoxidation of thioether-containing pesticides by the flavin-adenine dinucleotide-dependent monooxygenase of pig liver microsomes. *Biochem. Pharmacol.* 31, 745–752.

Halpert J., Hammond D. and Neal R.A. (1980). Inactivation of purified rat liver cytochrome P-450 during the metabolism of parathion (diethyl *p*-nitrophenyl phosphorothionate). *J. Biol. Chem.* 255, 1080–1089.

Hanzlik R.P. and Cashman J.R. (1983). Microsomal metabolism of thiobenzamide and thiobenzamide S-oxide. *Drug Metab. Disposit.* 11, 201–205.

Hanzlik R.P., Cashman J.R. and Traiger G.J. (1980). Relative hepatotoxicity of substituted thiobenzamides and thiobenzamide-S-oxides in the rat. *Toxicol. Appl. Pharmacol.* 55, 260–272.

Harvison P.J., Guengerich F.P., Rashed M.S. and Nelson S.D. (1988). Cytochrome P-450 isozyme selectivity in the oxidation of acetaminophen. *Chem. Res. Toxicol.* 1, 47–52.

Hayashi T., Amino M. and Ikoma Y. (1983). Changes of metabolism and substrate-binding spectrum of emorfazone between immature and mature guinea-pigs. *Xenobiotica* 13, 461–466.

Hiramatsu M., Kumagai Y., Unger S.E. and Cho A.K. (1990). Metabolism of methylenedioxymethamphetamine: formation of dihydroxymethamphetamine and a quinone identified as its glutathione adduct. *J. Pharmacol. Exp. Therap.* 254, 521–527.

Hoffmann K.J., Axworthy D.B. and Baillie T.A. (1990). Mechanistic studies on the metabolic activation of acetaminophen *in vivo*. *Chem. Res. Toxicol.* 3, 204–211.

Hoodi A.A. and Damani L.A. (1984). Cytochrome P-450 and non P-450 sulphoxidations. *J. Pharm. Pharmacol.* 36, 62P.

Horiuchi M., Takashina H., Iwatani T. and Iso T. (1985). Study on metabolism of dithiol compound I. Isolation and identification of metabolites of N-(2-mercapto-2-methylpropanoyl)-L-cysteine (SA 96) in blood and urine of rat. *Yakugaku Zasshi* **105**, 665–670.

Hunter A.L. and Neal R.A. (1975). Inhibition of hepatic mixed-function oxidase activity *in vitro* and *in vivo* by various thiono-sulfur-containing compounds. *Biochem. Pharmacol.* **24**, 2199–2205.

Hunter W.H. and Wilson P. (1981). The hydroxylation and dealkylation of some naphthyl alkyl ethers by rat liver microsomes. *Xenobiotica* **11**, 179–188.

Hussein Z., Mulford D.J., Bopp B.A. and Granneman G.R. (1993). Differences in the stereoselective pharmaco-kinetics of pazinaclone (DN-2327), a new anxiolytic, and its active metabolite after intravenous and oral single doses to dogs. *Drug Metab. Disposit.* **21**, 805–810.

Hwang I.Y. and Elfarra A.A. (1989). Cysteine S-conjugates may act as kidney-selective prodrugs: formation of 6-mercaptopurine by the renal metabolism of S-(6-purinyl)-L-cysteine. *J. Pharmacol. Exp. Therap.* **251**, 448–454.

Hwang I.Y. and Elfarra A.A. (1991). Kidney-selective prodrugs of 6-mercaptopurine: biochemical basis of the kidney selectivity of S-(6-purinyl)-L-cysteine and met-abolism of new analogs in rats. *J. Pharmacol. Exp. Therap.* **258**, 171–177.

Hyland R., Gescher A., Thummel K., Schiller C., Jheeta P., Mynett K., Smith A.W and Mráz J. (1992). Metabolic oxidation and toxification of N-methylformamide catalyzed by the cytochrome P450 isoenzyme CYP2E1. *Molec. Pharmacol.* **41**, 259–266.

Hyslop R.M. and Jardine I. (1981). Metabolism of 6-thiopurines. I & II. *J. Pharmacol. Exp. Therap.* **218**, 621–628, 629–635.

Ingelman-Sundberg M. and Johansson I. (1984). Mechan-isms of hydroxyl radical formation and ethanol oxida-tion by ethanol-inducible and other forms of rabbit liver microsomal cytochrome P-450. *J. Biol. Chem.* **259**, 6447–6458.

Irurre Jr J., Casas J. and Messeguer A. (1993). Resistance of the 2,2,2-trifluoroethoxy aryl moiety to the cytochrome P-450 metabolism in rat liver microsomes. *Bioorg. Med. Chem. Lett.* **3**, 179–182.

Jajoo H.K., Majol R.F., LaBudde J.A. and Blair I.A. (1990). Structural characterization of urinary metabolites of the antiarrhythmic drug encainide in human subjects. *Drug Metab. Disposit.* **18**, 28–35.

James S.P. (1988). The biochemistry of endogenous orga-nosulphur compounds. *Drug Metab. Drug Interact.* **6**, 167–182.

Järvisalo J., Savolainen H., Elovaara E. and Vainio H. (1977). The *in vivo* toxicity of CS_2 to liver microsomes: Binding of labelled CS_2 and changes of the microsomal enzyme activities. *Acta Pharmacol. Toxicol.* **40**, 329–336.

Jatoe S.D., Lauriault V., McGirr L.G. and O'Brien P.J. (1988). The toxicity of disulfides to isolated hepatocytes and mitochondria. *Drug Metab. Drug Interact.* **6**, 395–412.

Kamataki T., Lee Lin M.C.M., Belcher D.H. and Neal R.A. (1976). Studies of the metabolism of parathion with an apparently fomogeneous preparation of rabbit liver cytochrome P-450. *Drug Metab. Disposit.* **4**, 180–189.

Kamm J.J., Szuna A. and Mohacsi E. (1979). Metabolism of 3-phenoxy-N-methylmorphinan (PMM): an unusual diaryl ether cleavage reaction. *Pharmacologist* **21**, 173.

Kexel H., Schmelz E. and Schmidt H.L. (1977). Oxygen transfer in microsomal oxidative desulfuration. In *Micro-somes and Drug Oxidations* (eds Ullrich V., Hildebrandt A., Roots J., Estabrook R. and Conney A.). pp. 269–274. Pergamon Press, New York.

Kinsler S., Levi P.E. and Hodgson E. (1988). Hepatic and extrahepatic microsomal oxidation of phorate by the cytochrome P-450 and FAD-containing monooxygenase systems in the mouse. *Pestic. Biochem. Physiol.* **31**, 54–60.

Klein S.M., Cohen G. and Cederbaum A.I. (1981). Pro-duction of formaldehyde during metabolism of dimethyl sulfoxide by hydroxyl radical generating systems. *Biochemistry* **20**, 6006–6012.

Klungsøyr J. and Scheline R.R. (1981). Metabolism in rats of several carboxylic acid derivatives containing the 3,4-methylenedioxyphenyl group. *Acta Pharmacol. Tox-icol.* **49**, 305–312.

Klungsøyr J. and Scheline R.R. (1984). Metabolism of piperonal and piperonyl alcohol in the rat with special reference to the scission of the 3,4-methylenedioxy group. *Acta Pharm. Suec.* **21**, 67–72.

Korzekwa K.R., Trager W.F., Smith S.J., Osawa Y. and Gillette J.R. (1991). Theoretical studies on the mechan-ism of conversion of androgens to estrogens by aroma-tase. *Biochemistry* **30**, 6155–6162.

Koster A.S. (1991). Bioreductive activation of quinones: a mixed blessing. *Pharm. Weekbl. Sci. Ed.* **13**, 123–126.

Koymans L., van Lenthe J.H., van de Straat R., Donné-Op den Kelder GM and Vermeulen NPE (1989). A theo-retical study on the metabolic activation of paracetamol by cytochrome P-450: indications for a uniform oxida-tion mechanism. *Chem. Res. Toxicol.* **2**, 60–66.

Koymans L., Donné-Op den Kelder G.M., te Koppele J.M. and Vermeulen N.P.E. (1993). Generalized cytochrome P450-mediated oxidation and oxygenation reactions in aromatic substrates with activated N–H, O–H, C–H, or S–H substituents. *Xenobiotica* **23**, 633–648.

Krieter P.A., Ziegler D.M., Hill K.E. and Burk R.F. (1984). Increased biliary GSSG efflux from rat livers perfused with thiocarbamide substrates for the flavin-containing monooxygenase. *Molec. Pharmacol.* **26**, 122–127.

Krikun G. and Cederbaum A.I. (1984). Stereochemical studies on the cytochrome P-450 and hydroxyl radical dependent pathways of 2-butanol oxidation by micro-somes from chow-fed, phenobarbital-treated, and ethanol-treated rats. *Biochemistry* **23**, 5489–5494.

Kucharczyk N., Edelson J., Sofia R.D., Ludwig B.J., Shahinian S., Schuster E., Ballard F.H., Yang J. and Myers G. (1979). Metabolism and pharmacokinetics of

4-(p-chlorophenylthio)butanol in the rat and dog. *Arzneim-Forsch. (Drug Res.)* **29**, 1550–1556.

Kumagai Y., Wickham K.A., Schmitz D.A. and Cho A.K. (1991). Metabolism of methylenedioxyphenyl compounds by rabbit liver preparations. Participation of different cytochrome P450 isozymes in the demethylenation reaction. *Biochem. Pharmacol.* **42**, 1061–1067.

Kumagai Y., Lin L.Y., Philpot R.M., Yamada H., Oguri K., Yoshimura H. and Cho A.K. (1992a). Regiochemical differences in cytochrome P450 isozymes responsible for the oxidation of methylenedioxyphenyl groups by rabbit liver. *Molec. Pharmacol.* **42**, 695–702.

Kumagai Y., Ikeda Y. and Toki S. (1992b). Hydroxyl radical-mediated conversion of morphine to morphinone. *Xenobiotica* **22**, 507–513.

Lee M.S. (1992). Oxidative conversion by rat liver microsomes of 2-naphthyl isothiocyanate to 2-naphthyl isocyanate, a genotoxicant. *Chem. Res. Toxicol.* **5**, 791–796.

Lee P.W. and Neal R.A. (1978). Metabolism of methimazole by rat liver cytochrome P-450-containing monooxygenases. *Drug Metab. Disposit.* **6**, 591–600.

Lee P.W., Arnau T. and Neal R.A. (1980). Metabolism of α-naphthylthiourea by rat liver and rat lung microsomes. *Toxicol. Appl. Pharmacol.* **53**, 164–173.

Leinweber F.J., Szuna A.J., Williams T.H., Sasso G.J. and DeBarbieri B.A. (1981). The metabolism of (−)-3-phenoxy-N-methylmorphinane in dogs. *Drug Metab. Disposit.* **9**, 284–291.

Lertratanangkoon K. and Denney D. (1993). Formation of phenol and thiocatechol metabolites from bromobenzene premercapturic acids through pyridoxal phosphate-dependent C–S lyase activity. *Biochem. Pharmacol.* **45**, 2513–2525.

Lesko S., Caspary W., Lorentzen R. and Ts'o P.O.P. (1975). Enzymic formation of 6-oxobenzo[a]pyrene radical in rat liver homogenates from carcinogenic benzo[a]pyrene. *Biochemistry* **14**, 3978–3984.

Levi P.E., Tynes R.E., Sabourin P.J. and Hodgson E. (1982). Is thiobenzamide a specific substrate for the microsomal FAD-containing monooxygenase? *Biochem. Biophys. Res. Commun.* **107**, 1314–1318.

Light D.R., Waxman D.J. and Walsh C. (1982). Studies on the chirality of sulfoxidation catalyzed by bacterial flavoenzyme cyclohexanone monooxygenase and hog liver flavin adenine dinucleotide containing monooxygenase. *Biochemistry* **21**, 2490–2498.

Lin L.Y., Kumagai Y. and Cho A.K. (1992). Enzymatic and chemical demethylenation of (methylenedioxy)amphetamine and (methylenedioxy)methamphetamine by rat brain microsomes. *Chem. Res. Toxicol.* **5**, 401–406.

Lindsay Smith J.R. and Sleath P.R. (1983). Model systems for cytochrome P450-dependent monooxygenases. Part 2. Kinetic isotope effects for the oxidative demethylation of anisole and [*Me*-²H₃]anisole by cytochrome P450 dependent monooxygenases and model systems. *J. Chem. Soc. Perkin Trans.* II, 621–628.

Lu A.Y.H., Harada N. and Miwa G.T. (1984). Rate-limiting steps in cytochrome P-450-catalysed reactions: studies on isotope effects in the O-de-ethylation of 7-ethoxycoumarin. *Xenobiotica* **14**, 19–26.

Marcus C.B., Murray M. and Wilkinson C.F. (1985). Spectral and inhibitory interactions of methylenedioxyphenyl and related compounds with purified isozymes of cytochrome P-450. *Xenobiotica* **15**, 351–362.

Masuda Y. and Nakamura Y. (1989). Oxidation of diethyldithiocarbamate to disulfiram by liver microsomal cytochrome P-450-containing monooxygenase system. *Res. Commun. Chem. Pathol. Pharmacol.* **66**, 57–67.

Mayer R.T., Netter K.J., Heubel F., Hahnemann B., Buchheister A., Mayer G.K. and Burke M.D. (1990). 7-Alkoxyquinolines: new fluorescent substrates for cytochrome P450 monooxygenases. *Biochem. Pharmacol.* **40**, 1645–1655.

Menn J.J., DeBaun J.R. and McBain J.B. (1976). Recent advances in the metabolism of organophosphorus insecticides. *Fed. Proc.* **35**, 2598–2602.

Mesnil M., Testa B. and Jenner P. (1988). *Ex vivo* inhibition of rat brain cytochrome P-450 activity by stiripentol. *Biochem. Pharmacol.* **37**, 3619–3622.

Mitchell S.C. and Waring R.H. (1985). The early history of xenobiotic sulfoxidation. *Drug Metab. Rev.* **16**, 255–284.

Monks T.J., Lau S.S. and Highet R.J. (1984). Formation of nontoxic reactive. metabolites of p-bromophenol. *Drug Metab. Disposit.* **12**, 432–437.

Moreland T.A., Astoin J., Lepage F., Tombret F., Lévy R.H. and Baillie T.A. (1986). The metabolic fate of stiripentol in man. *Drug Metab. Disposit.* **14**, 654–662.

Morgan A.T., Koop D.R. and Coon M.J. (1982). Catalytic activity of cytochrome P-450 isozyme 3a isolated from liver microsomes of ethanol-treated rabbits. *J. Biol. Chem.* **257**, 13,951–13,957.

Morris P.L., Burke T.R. Jr, George J.W. and Pohl L.R. (1982). A new pathway for the oxidative metabolism of chloramphenicol by rat liver microsomes. *Drug Metab. Disposit.* **10**, 439–445.

Mráz J., Jheeta P., Gescher A., Hyland R., Thummel K. and Threadgill M.D. (1993). Investigation of the mechanistic basis of N,N-dimethylformamide toxicity. Metabolism of N,N-dimethylformamide and its deuterated isotopomers by cytochrome P450 2E1. *Chem. Res. Toxicol.* **6**, 197–207.

Murray M., Wilkinson C.F. and Dube C.E. (1985). Induction of rat hepatic microsomal cytochrome P-450 and aryl hydrocarbon hydroxylase by 1,3-benzodioxole derivatives. *Xenobiotica* **15**, 361–368.

Mutlib A.E. and Nelson W.L. (1990). Pathways of gallopamil metabolism. Regiochemistry and enantioselectivity of the O-demethylation processes. *Drug Metab. Disposit.* **18**, 309–314.

Nakaoka M., Hakusui H. and Takegoshi T. (1989). Isolation and characterization of a new thio-glucuronide, a biliary metabolite of malotilate in rats. *Xenobiotica* **19**, 209–216.

Narimatsu S., Matsubara K., Shimonishi T., Watanabe K., Yamamoto I. and Yoshimura H. (1988). Enzymatic oxidation of 7-hydroxylated Δ⁸-tetrahydrocannabinol to 7-oxo-Δ⁸-tetrahydrocannabinol by hepatic microsomes of the guinea pig. *Drug Metab. Disposit.* **16**, 156–161.

Neal R.A. (1980). Microsomal metabolism of thiono-sulfur compounds: Mechanisms and toxicological significance.

In *Reviews in Biochemical Toxicology*, Volume 2 (eds Hodgson E., Bend J.R. and Philpot R.M.). pp. 131–171. Elsevier, New York.

Nelson W.L. and Bartels M.J. (1984). N-Dealkylation of propranolol in rat, dog, and man. Chemical and stereochemical aspects. *Drug Metab. Disposit.* 12, 345–352.

Nelson W.L., Olsen L.D., Beitner D.B. and Pallow R.J., Jr (1988). Regiochemistry and substrate stereoselectivity of O-demethylation of verapamil in the presence of the microsomal fraction from rat and human liver. *Drug Metab. Disposit.* 16, 184–188.

Nerurkar P.V., Park S.S., Thomas P.E., Nims R.W. and Lubet R.A. (1993). Methoxyresorufin and benzyloxyresorufin: Substrates preferentially metabolized by cytochromes P4501A2 and 2B, respectively, in the rat and mouse. *Biochem. Pharmacol.* 46, 933–943.

Nwankwo J.O. (1991). *In vitro* O-demethylation from a heterocyclic nitrogen: a novel metabolic reaction? *Xenobiotica* 21, 569–574.

Oae S., Mikami A., Matsuura T., Ogawa-Asada K., Watanabe Y., Fujimori K. and Iyanagi T. (1985). Comparison of sulfide oxygenation mechanism for liver microsomal FAD-containing monooxygenase with that for cytochrome P-450. *Biochem. Biophys. Res. Commun.* 131, 567–573.

Offen C.P., Frearson M.J., Wilson K. and Burnett D. (1985). 4,5-Dimethylthiazole-N-oxide-S-oxide: a metabolite of chlormethiazole in man. *Xenobiotica* 15, 503–511.

Ohnishi K. and Lieber C.S. (1978). Respective role of superoxide and hydroxyl radical in the activity of the reconstituted microsomal ethanol-oxidizing system. *Arch. Biochem. Biophys.* 191, 798–803.

Papadopoulos A.S. and Crammer J.L (1986). Sulphoxide metabolites of thioridazine in man. *Xenobiotica* 16, 1097–1107.

Park S.B., Osterloh J.D., Vamvakas S., Hashmi M., Anders M.W. and Cashman J.R. (1992). Flavin-containing monooxygenase-dependent stereoselective S-oxygenation and cytotoxicity of cysteine S-conjugates and mercapturates. *Chem. Res. Toxicol.* 5, 193–201.

Patten C.J., Thomas P.E., Guy R.L., Lee M,. Gonzalez F.J., Guengerich F.P. and Yang C.S. (1993). Cytochrome P450 enzymes involved in acetaminophen activation by rat and human liver microsomes and their kinetics. *Chem. Res. Toxicol.* 6, 511–518.

Porter W.R. and Neal R.A. (1978). Metabolism of thioacetamide and thioacetamide S-oxide by rat liver microsomes. *Drug Metab. Disposit.* 6, 379–388.

Potter D.W. and Hinson J.A. (1987). Mechanisms of acetaminophen oxidation to N-acetyl-*p*-benzoquinone imine by horseradish peroxidase and cytochrome P-450. *J. Biol. Chem.* 262, 966–973.

Poulsen L.L. (1981). Organic sulfur substrates for the microsomal flavin-containing monooxygenase. In *Reviews in Biochemical Toxicology*, Vol. 3 (eds Hodgson E., Bend J.R. and Philpot R.M.). pp. 33–49. Elsevier, New York.

Poulsen L.L., Hyslop R.M. and Ziegler D.M. (1974).

S-Oxidation of thioureylenes catalyzed by a microsomal flavoprotein mixed-function oxidase. *Biochem. Pharmacol.* 23, 3431–3440.

Poulsen L.L., Hyslop R.M. and Ziegler D.M. (1979). S-Oxygenation of N-substituted thioureas catalyzed by the pig liver microsomal FAD-containing monooxygenase. *Arch. Biochem. Biophys.* 198, 78–88.

Quistad G.B., Saunders A.L., Skinner W.S., Collier K.D., Sakai D.H. and Reuter C.C. (1988). O-Dephenylation and conjugation with benzoylornithine. New metabolic pathways for 3-phenoxybenzoic acid in chickens. *Drug Metab. Disposit.* 16, 818–822.

Rabovsky J. and Judy D.J. (1987). Cytochrome P-450-dependent alkoxyphenoxazone dealkylase activities in lung microsomes from untreated and β-naphthoflavone-treated rats. Effects of *in vitro* inhibitors. *Res. Commun. Chem. Pathol. Pharmacol.* 57, 375–387.

Relling M.V., Evans R., Dass C., Desiderio D.M. and Nemec J. (1992). Human cytochrome P450 metabolism of teniposide and etoposide. *J. Pharmacol. Exp. Therap.* 261, 491–496.

Rettie A.E., Bogucki B.D., Lim I. and Meier G.P. (1990). Stereoselective sulfoxidation of a series of alkyl *p*-tolyl sulfides by microsomal and purified flavin-containing monooxygenases. *Molec. Pharmacol.* 37, 643–651.

Roberts E.S., Vaz A.D.N. and Coon M.J. (1991). Catalysis by cytochrome P-450 of an oxidative reaction in xenobiotic aldehyde metabolism: deformylation with olefin formation. *Proc. Natl Acad. Sci. USA* 88, 8963–8966.

Roberts E.S., Vaz A.D.N. and Coon M.J. (1992). Role of isozymes of rabbit microsomal cytochrome P-450 in the metabolism of retinoic acid, retinol and retinal. *Molec. Pharmacol.* 41, 427–433.

Roy D., Bernhardt A., Strobel H.W. and Liehr J.G. (1992). Catalysis of the oxidation of steroid and stilbene estrogens to estrogen quinone metabolites by the β-naphthoflavone-inducible cytochrome P450 IA family. *Arch. Biochem. Biophys.* 296, 450–456.

Rubin A., Dhahir P.H., Crabtree R.E. and Henry D.P. (1979). The disposition of l-3-[(dimethylamino)-(*m*-dioxan-5-yl)methyl]pyridine in man. *Drug Metab. Disposit.* 7, 149–154.

Sabourin P.J. and Hodgson E. (1984). Characterization of the purified microsomal FAD-containing monooxygenase from mouse and pig liver. *Chem.-Biol. Interact.* 51, 125–139.

Sesardic D., Cole K.J., Edwards R.J., Davies D.S., Thomas P.E., Levin W. and Boobis A.R. (1990). The inducibility and catalytic activity of cytochromes P450c (P450IA1) and P450d (P450IA2) in rat tissues. *Biochem. Pharmacol.* 39, 499–506.

Sligar S.G., Gelb M.H. and Heimbrook D.C. (1984). Bio-organic chemistry and cytochrome P-450-dependent catalysis. *Xenobiotica* 14, 63–86.

Sono H., Sonoda Y. and Sato Y. (1991). Purification and characterization of cytochrome P-450$_{14DM}$ (lanosterol 14α-demethylase) from pig liver microsomes. *Biochim. Biophys. Acta* 1078, 388–394.

Souhaili El Amri H., Fargetton X., Delatour P. and Batt A.M. (1987). Sulphoxidation of albendazole by the

FAD-containing and cytochrome P-450 dependent mono-oxygenases from pig liver microsomes. *Xenobiotica* **17**, 1159–1168.

Snyder J.P. (1973). Sulfine and sulfene reactivity. *J. Org. Chem.* **38**, 3965–3967.

Stearns R.A., Chakravarty P.K., Chen R. and Lee Chiu S.H. (1993). Investigations into the mechanism of oxidation of losartan, an alcohol, to its active metabolite, a carboxylic acid derivative. In *ISSX Proceedings*, Vol. 4. International Society for the Study of Xenobiotics, Bethesda, MD, USA, p. 238.

Sun Y., Cotgreave I., Lindeke B. and Moldéus P. (1989). The metabolism of sulfite in liver. Stimulation of sulfate conjugation and effects on paracetamol and allyl alcohol toxicity. *Biochem. Pharmacol.* **38**, 4299–4305.

Takata T., Yamazaki M., Fujimori K., Kim Y.H., Iyanagi T. and Oae S. (1983). Enzymatic oxygenation of sulfides with cytochrome P-450 from rabbit liver. Stereochemistry of sulfoxide formation. *Bull. Chem. Soc. Japan* **56**, 2300–2310.

Taylor K.L. and Ziegler D.M. (1987). Studies on substrate specificity of the hog liver flavin-containing monooxygenase. Anionic organic sulfur compounds. *Biochem. Pharmacol.* **36**, 141–146.

Taylor D.C., Cresswell P.R. and Bartlett D.C. (1978). The metabolism and elimination of cimetidine, a histamine H_2-receptor antagonist, in the rat, dog, and man. *Drug Metab. Disposit.* **6**, 21–30.

Taylor D.C., Cresswell P.R. and Pepper E.S. (1979). The excretion and metabolism of metiamide in the rat, dog and man. *Drug Metab. Disposit.* **7**, 393–398.

Testa B. and Jenner P. (1978). Novel drug metabolites produced by functionalization reactions: Chemistry and toxicology. *Drug Metab. Rev.* **7**, 325–369.

Testa B. and Jenner P. (1981). Inhibitors of cytochrome P-450s and their mechanism of action. *Drug Metab. Rev.* **12**, 1–117.

Thomas R., Gray P. and Andrews J. (1990). Digitalis: Its mode of action, receptor, and structure-activity relationships. In *Advances in Drug Research*, Vol. 19 (ed. Testa B.). pp. 313–562. Academic Press, London.

Thompson D.C., Thompson J.A., Sugumaran M. and Moldéus P. (1992). Biological and toxicological consequences of quinone methide formation. *Chem.-Biol. Interact.* **86**, 129–162.

Thompson J.A., Malkinson A.M., Wand M.D., Mastovich S.L., Mead E.W., Schullek K.M. and Laudenschlager W.G (1987). Oxidative metabolism of butylated hydroxytoluene by hepatic and pulmonary microsomes from rats and mice. *Drug Metab. Disposit.* **15**, 833–840.

Togawa T., Tanabe S., Kato M., Koshiishi I., Toida T. and Imanari T. (1990). Metabolic pathways of sodium bisulfite injected intravenously in rabbits. *J. Pharmacobio.-Dynam.* **13**, 83–89.

Trennery P.N. and Waring R.H (1983). The metabolism of thioacetanilide in the rat. *Xenobiotica* **13**, 475–482.

Tyndale R.F., Kalow W. and Inaba T. (1991). Oxidation of reduced haloperidol to haloperidol—involvement of human P450IID6. *Brit. J. Clin. Pharmacol.* **31**, 655–660.

Vadi H.V. and Neal R.A. (1981). Microsomal activation of thioacetamide-S-oxide to a metabolite(s) that covalently binds to calf thymus DNA and other polynucleotides. *Chem.-Biol. Interact.* **35**, 25–38.

Vamvakas S., Dekant W. and Anders M.W. (1989). Mutagenicity of benzyl S-haloalkyl and S-haloalkenyl sulfides in the Ames-test. *Biochem. Pharmacol.* **38**, 935–939.

van de Straat R., de Vries J., de Boer H.J.R., Vromans R.M. and Vermeulen N.P.E. (1987). Relationships between paracetamol binding to and its oxidation by two cytochromes P-450 isozymes—a proton nuclear magnetic resonance and spectrophotometric study. *Xenobiotica* **17**, 1–9.

van de Straat R., Vromans R.M., Bosman P., de Vries J. and Vermeulen N.P.E. (1988). Cytochrome P-450-mediated oxidation of substrates by electron-transfer: role of oxygen radicals and of 1- and 2-electron oxidation of paracetamol. *Chem.-Biol. Interact.* **64**, 267–280.

van Ommen B., Voncken J.W., Müller F. and van Bladeren P.J. (1988). The oxidation of tetrachloro-1,4-hydroquinone by microsomes and purified cytochrome P450b. Implications for covalent binding to protein and involvement of reactive oxygen species. *Chem.-Biol. Interact.* **65**, 247–259.

Vaz A.D.N., Roberts E.S. and Coon M.J. (1991). Olefin formation in the oxidative deformylation of aldehydes by cytochrome P-450. Mechanistic implications for catalysis by oxygen-derived peroxide. *J. Amer. Chem. Soc.* **113**, 5886–5887.

Veltwisch D., Janata E. and Asmus K.D. (1980). Primary processes in the reaction of OH-radicals with sulphoxides. *J. Chem. Soc. Perkin Trans.* **II**, 146–153.

Vermeulen N.P.E., Bessems J.G.M. and van de Straat R. (1992). Molecular aspects of paracetamol-induced hepatotoxicity and its mechanism-based prevention. *Drug Metab. Rev.* **24**, 367–407.

Vicchio D. and Callery P.S. (1989). Metabolic conversion of 2-propylpentanal acetals to valproic acid *in vitro*. Model prodrugs of carboxylic acid agents. *Drug Metab. Disposit.* **17**, 513–517.

Vree T.B. and Verwey-Van Wissen C.P.W.G.M. (1992). Pharmacokinetics and metabolism of codeine in humans. *Biopharm. Drug Disposit.* **13**, 445–460.

Waring R.H., Mitchell S.C., O'Gorman J. and Fraser M. (1986). Cytosolic sulphoxidation of S-carboxymethyl-L-cysteine in mammals. *Biochem. Pharmacol.* **35**, 2999–3002.

Watanabe Y. and Ishimura Y. (1989). A model study on aromatase cytochrome P-450 reaction: transformation of androstene-3,17,19-trione to 10β-hydroxyestr-4-ene-3,17-dione. *J. Amer. Chem. Soc.* **111**, 8047–8049.

Watanabe Y., Numata T., Iyanagi T. and Oae S. (1981). Enzymatic oxidation of alkyl sulfides by cytochrome P-450 and hydroxyl radical. *Bull. Chem. Soc. Japan* **54**, 1163–1170.

Watanabe Y., Oae S. and Iyanagi T. (1982a). Mechanisms of enzymatic S-oxygenation of thioanisole derivatives and O-demethylation of anisole derivatives promoted by both microsomes and a reconstituted system with purified cytochrome P-450. *Bull. Chem. Soc. Japan* **55**, 188–195.

Watanabe Y., Iyanagi T. and Oae S. (1982b). One electron transfer mechanism in the enzymatic oxygenation of sulfoxide to sulfone promoted by a reconstituted system with purified cytochrome P-450. *Tetrahedron Lett.* **23**, 533–536.

Watanabe K., Narimatsu S., Yamamoto I. and Yoshimura H. (1990). Hepatic microsomal oxygenation of aldehydes to carboxylic acids. *Biochem. Biophys. Res. Commun.* **166**, 1308–1312.

Watanabe K., Narimatsu S., Yamamoto I. and Yoshimura H. (1991a). Oxygenation mechanism in conversion of aldehyde to carboxylic acid catalyzed by a cytochrome P-450 isozyme. *J. Biol. Chem.* **266**, 2709–2711.

Watanabe K., Matsunaga T., Narimatsu S., Yamamoto I., Imaoka S., Funae Y. and Yoshimura H. (1991b). Catalytic activity of cytochrome P450 isozymes purified from rat liver in converting 11-oxo-Δ^8-tetrahydrocannabinol to Δ^8-tetrahydrocannabinol-11-oic acid. *Biochem. Pharmacol.* **42**, 1255–1259.

Watanabe K., Narimatsu S., Matsunaga T., Yamamoto I. and Yoshimura H. (1993). A cytochrome P450 isozyme having aldehyde oxygenase activity plays a major role in metabolizing cannabinoids by mouse hepatic microsomes. *Biochem. Pharmacol.* **46**, 405–411.

Waxman D.J., Light D.R. and Walsh C. (1982). Chiral sulfoxidations catalyzed by rat liver cytochromes P-450. *Biochemistry* **21**, 2499–2507.

Winters D.K. and Cederbaum A.I. (1990). Oxidation of glycerol to formaldehyde by rat liver microsomes. Effects of cytochrome P-450 inducing agents. *Biochem. Pharmacol.* **39**, 697–705.

Wood A.W., Swinney D.C., Thomas P.E., Ryan D.E., Hall P.F., Levin W. and Garland W.A. (1988). Mechanism of androstenedione formation from testosterone and epitestosterone catalyzed by purified cytochrome P-450b. *J. Biol. Chem.* **263**, 17,322–17,332.

Yamamoto I., Watanabe K., Narimatsu S. and Yoshimura H. (1988). Oxygenation mechanism in the oxidation of xenobiotic aldehyde to carboxylic acid by mouse hepatic microsomes. *Biochem. Biophys. Res. Commun.* **153**, 779–782.

Zhang K., Lepage F., Cuvier G., Astoin J., Rashed M.S. and Baillie T.A. (1990). The metabolic fate of stiripentol in the rat. Studies on cytochrome P-450-mediated methylenedioxy ring cleavage and side chain isomerism. *Drug Metab. Disposit.* **18**, 794–803.

Ziegler D.M. (1980). Microsomal flavin-containing monooxygenase: oxygenation of nucleophilic nitrogen and sulfur compounds. In *Enzymatic Basis of Detoxication*, Volume 1 (ed. Jakoby W.B.). pp. 201–227. Academic Press, New York.

Ziegler D.M. (1982). Functional groups bearing sulfur. In *Metabolic Basis of Detoxication* (eds Jakobi W.B., Bend J.R. and Caldwell J.). pp. 171–184. Academic Press, New York.

Ziegler D.M. (1984). Metabolic oxygenation of organic nitrogen and sulfur compounds. In *Drug Metabolism and Drug Toxicity* (eds Mitchell J.R. and Horning M.G.). pp. 33–53. Raven Press, New York.

Ziegler D.M. (1988a). Functional groups activated by flavin-containing monooxygenases. In *Microsomes and Drug Oxidations* (eds Miners J., Birkett D.J., Drew R. and McManus M.). pp. 297–304. Taylor and Francis, London.

Ziegler D.M. (1988b). Flavin-containing monooxygenases: catalytic mechanism and substrate specificities. *Drug Metab. Rev.* **19**, 1–32.

Ziegler D.M. (1993). Recent studies on the structure and function of multisubstrate flavin-containing monooxygenases. *Annu. Rev. Pharmacol. Toxicol.* **33**, 179–199.

chapter 8

OXIDATIVE DEHALOGENATION AND DEALKYLATION OF ORGANOMETALLICS

Contents

8.1 INTRODUCTION

Previous chapters have examined monooxygenase-catalyzed reactions of heteroatom–carbon cleavage, in particular N–C cleavage (Chapter 6), and O- and S-dealkylation (Chapter 7). The present chapter is dedicated to two further reactions of this type, namely oxidative dehalogenation (halogen–C cleavage where C is sp^3-hybridized), and dealkylation of organometallic compounds. Clearly the two types of reactions are quite distinct, yet their grouping in the same chapter is not without justification. Note too that further cases of heteroatom–carbon cleavage will be encountered in future chapters.

8.2 OXIDATIVE DEHALOGENATION

This section is not the first one in which the reader encounters halogenated compounds. Indeed, the cytochrome P450-catalyzed oxidations of halogenated arenes and alkenes have been discussed in Sections 4.3 and 4.4, respectively. Here, we consider the oxidation of **sp^3-hybridized carbon atoms carrying one, two or three halogens and at least one hydrogen atom**. The reaction results in halogen–carbon cleavage, hence its designation as oxidative dehalogenation. In Chapter 11 is discussed another reaction of oxidative dehalogenation, namely that of halogenated

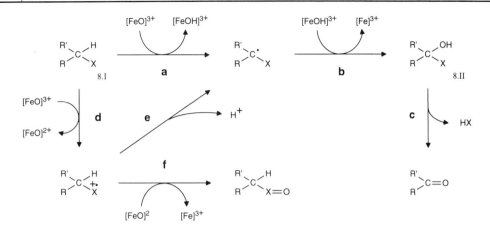

FIGURE 8.1 Generally accepted (reactions **a** to **c**) and hypothetical, additional (reactions **d** to **f**) mechanisms of oxidative dehalogenation catalyzed by cytochrome P450.

sp^3-carbons carrying no hydrogen, e.g. CCl_4. The same compounds may also undergo reductive dehalogenation, another important functionalization reaction of haloalkanes to be presented in Chapter 12.

Halogenated alkanes are of importance as general anaesthetics, while a number of other medicinal compounds contain haloalkyl groups (see Section 8.2.2). But much of the current interest in halogenated alkanes is centred on ozone-depleting **chlorofluorocarbons** (CFCs) and on the search for non-ozone-depleting substitutes such as **hydrochlorofluorocarbons** (HCFCs) and **hydrofluorocarbons** (HFCs).

8.2.1 Reaction mechanisms and oxidative dehalogenation of haloalkanes

The generally accepted mechanism of oxidative dehalogenation is shown in the upper part of Fig. 8.1. The reaction, which is catalyzed by cytochrome P450, is one of **alpha-carbon hydroxylation** proceeding by oxygen rebound, i.e. reactions **a** and **b** in Fig. 8.1 (Anders, 1984; Van Dyke and Gandolfi, 1975). The resulting metabolite is a *gem*-halohydrin (**8.II** in Fig. 8.1; with R = alkyl or aryl), an unstable intermediate that spontaneously loses HX to yield a carbonyl derivative (reaction **c** in Fig. 8.1). The latter will be either an **aldehyde** (R′ = H), a **ketone** (R′ = alkyl or aryl), or an **acyl halide** (R′ = halogen) (Anders, 1982a, 1982b and 1984; Anders and Pohl, 1985; Hales *et al.*, 1987).

In other words, the **end-product(s)** of oxidative dehalogenation of halogenated alkanes, and to a large extent their toxic potential, will depend on the chemical nature of the substrate. **Primary monohalogenated positions** (**8.I** in Fig. 8.1; R = alkyl or aryl, R′ = H) will be dehalogenated to an aldehyde group which can be further reduced to an alcohol function and oxidized to a carboxylic group by dehydrogenases (Chapter 2), while **secondary monohalogenated positions** (**8.I** in Fig. 8.1; R and R′ = alkyl or aryl) will yield a ketone group which can be further hydrogenated to a secondary alcohol function (Chapter 2). With **dihalomethyl groups** (**8.III** in Fig. 8.2; R = alkyl or aryl), the resulting carbonyl compounds are highly reactive acyl halides (**8.IV**) which will undergo non-enzymatic hydrolysis to the corresponding carboxylic acid (Fig. 8.2), or may acylate endogenous constituents (see later). Dihalomethanes (**8.III** in Fig. 8.2; R = H) and trihalomethanes (haloforms) (**8.III**, R = halogen) represent special cases and will be discussed separately.

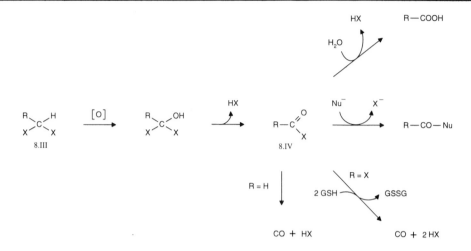

FIGURE 8.2 Formation of a carboxylic acid from a dihalomethyl group (**8.III**; R = alkyl or aryl) via oxidative dehalogenation followed by postenzymatic loss of hydrogen halide to an acyl halide and hydrolysis. The highly reactive intermediate acyl halide may also react with nucleophilic groups in macromolecules and form adducts. Also shown are the special cases of dihalomethanes (R = H) and haloforms (R = X), which both form carbon monoxide but through different mechanisms.

Conclusive evidence for alpha-carbon hydroxylation was obtained from the study of kinetic deuterium isotope effects, as in the oxidative dehalogenation of 1,1,2,2-tetrachloroethane (**8.V**) to dichloroacetic acid (**8.VI**) by rat liver microsomes (Hales *et al.*, 1987). Under the same conditions, the analogue 1,1,2-trichloroethane (**8.VIII**) was metabolized to chloroacetic acid (**8.IX**), indicating a regioselectivity favouring oxidation of the $-CHCl_2$ over the $-CH_2Cl$ group (Hales *et al.*, 1987). *In vivo* also, it had been found earlier that the metabolism of 1,1,2-trichloroethane proceeds mainly via chloroacetic acid, with a limited production of 2,2-dichloroethanol (indicating attack on the $-CH_2Cl$ group) and other metabolites resulting from other pathways (Yllner, 1971a).

Kinetic studies of the oxidative dehalogenation of various chloroethanes in rat liver microsomes have confirmed the **regioselectivity** of the $-CHCl_2$ over the $-CH_2Cl$ group noted above. Thus, as judged by V_{max} values and V_{max}/K_m ratios, 1,1-dichloroethane and 1,1,2,2-

$$CHCl_2\!-\!CHCl_2 \longrightarrow CHCl_2\!-\!COOH$$

  8.V   8.VI

$$CCl_2\!=\!CHCl$$

  8.VII

$$CH_2Cl\!-\!CHCl_2 \longrightarrow CH_2Cl\!-\!COOH$$

  8.VIII   8.IX

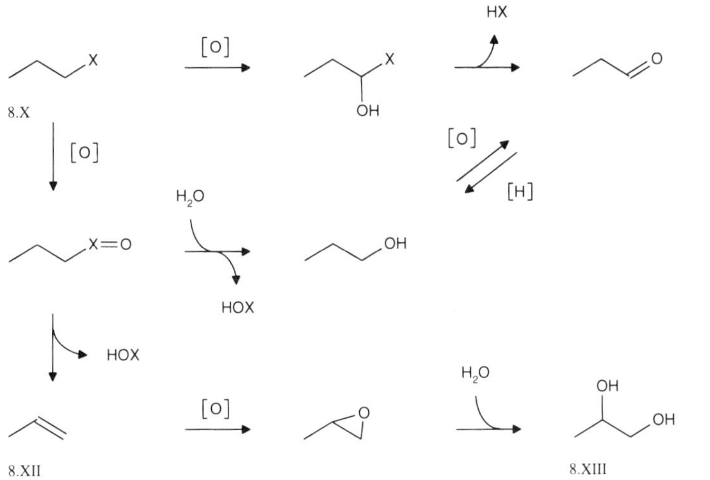

FIGURE 8.3 Partial scheme of the postulated metabolic reactions of 1-halopropanes (**8.X**; X = Cl, Br or I) in rat liver microsomes. Not shown are glutathione conjugations and adduct formation (Modified from Tachizawa *et al.*, 1982).

tetrachloroethane were far better substrates than 1,2-dichloroethane and 1,1,1-trifluoro-2-chloroethane. Electronic factors presumably account for this selectivity since for a larger series of chlorinated ethanes and propanes, maximal dechlorination was related to a narrowly defined optimal electron deficiency on the carbon atom being oxidized (Salmon *et al.*, 1981).

Reactions **a** to **c** in Fig. 8.1 are certainly the major routes of oxidative dehalogenation, but there may be others as far as monohalogenated positions are concerned. Indeed, careful studies have indicated that CYP2B1 may perhaps mediate direct, **one-electron oxidation of the halogen atom** in compounds such as cyclopropyl and 1-methylcyclopropyl chloride, bromide and iodide, leading to C-centred radicals that bind covalently to the enzyme (Guengerich *et al.*, 1984). If electron abstraction from the halogen atom (reaction **d** in Fig. 8.1) indeed occurs for some haloalkanes, then in analogy with N–C and S–C cleavage (Chapters 6 and 7) proton expulsion (reaction **e** in Fig. 8.1) would lead to a C-centred radical. Oxygen rebound to the heteroatomic centre (reaction **f** in Fig. 8.1) is also likely for sufficiently stable heteroatom-centred radicals, and its relative importance is expected to increase from chloride to bromide to iodide (Guengerich *et al.*, 1984). Halogen oxidation is discussed in more detail in Section 11.6.

In this context, a particularly relevant study is that of Tachizawa and colleagues (1982), who rationalized the rat liver microsomal metabolism of **1-halopropanes** (**8.X** in Fig. 8.3, X = Cl, Br or I) in terms of two pathways, namely oxidative dehalogenation and halogen oxygenation (Fig. 8.3). The former pathway led to propionic acid (**8.XI** in Fig. 8.3), the rate of formation of which increased in the order I < Cl < Br. The formation of a number of other metabolites (propene **8.XII**, 1,2-propanediol **8.XIII**, and glutathione conjugates) was explained by halogen oxygenation to a transient organohalide oxide which could undergo nucleophilic substitutions (e.g. by water to 1-propanol or by glutathione to conjugates) and β-elimination to propene; summing the rates of formation of these other metabolites suggests that halogen oxygenation indeed increased in the order Cl < Br < I.

The case of **dihalomethyl groups** (–CHX₂) deserves special mention because of the formation of highly reactive acyl halides. Such metabolites may bind to nucleophilic groups in macromolecules (Fig. 8.2), in particular the –NH₂ group of lysine, and elicit immunologically mediated liver damage (see also Section 8.2.2). Thus, 2,2-dichloro-1,1,1-trifluoroethane, a candidate substitute for CFCs, formed a trifluoroacetylated protein adduct in the liver of rats dosed with the compound (Harris *et al.*, 1991). These adducts were immunologically identical with trifluoroacetylated liver proteins associated with idiosyncratic hepatitis caused by halothane (see Section 8.2.2). In pentahaloethanes, the *in vivo* trifluoroacetylation of hepatic proteins and urinary excretion of trifluoroacetic acid decreased in the order $CF_3CHClBr = CF_3CHCl_2 \gg CF_3CHFCl > CF_3CHF_2$; these biological indices of metabolic toxication were shown to correlate with enthalpies of activation for alpha-hydroxylation (Harris *et al.*, 1992).

Dihalomethanes (**8.III** in Fig. 8.2, R = H) behave as expected in that they undergo alpha-carbon hydroxylation to a *gem*-halohydrin followed by dehydrohalogenation to an acyl halide, in this case a formyl halide (**8.IV** in Fig. 8.2, R = H). Formyl halides are known to decompose spontaneously to carbon monoxide and HX in a second step of dehydrohalogenation (Fig. 8.2) (Kubic and Anders, 1978). In rat liver microsomes, the oxidative metabolism of dihalomethanes to CO increased about eight-fold throughout the sequence $CH_2Cl_2 < CH_2BrCl < CH_2Br_2 < CH_2I_2$ (Kubic and Anders, 1975).

Haloforms (**8.III** in Fig. 8.2, R = X) are also oxidized by cytochrome P450 to carbon monoxide, the rates of reaction in rat liver microsomes increasing along the sequence $CHCl_3 = CHBrCl_2 < CHBr_2Cl < CHBr_3 < CHI_3$ (Ahmed *et al.*, 1977). Here, the acyl halide being formed is a dihalocarbonyl (**8.IV** in Fig. 8.2, R = X), for example phosgene ($Cl_2C=O$) in the case of chloroform (Pohl, 1979). Phosgene is a highly reactive and toxic compound, and its formation from $CHCl_3$ has been demonstrated in rats both *in vitro* and *in vivo* (Pohl *et al.*, 1979). The hepatoxicity of bromoform is also explained by the same mechanism, namely the formation of dibromocarbonyl which, like phosgene, binds covalently to macromolecules (Stevens and Anders, 1979). What differentiates dihalo- and trihalo-methanes is the mechanism of the reaction leading from the acyl halide to CO. For trihalomethanes, the reaction proceeds mainly with the involvement of glutathione (GSH, Fig. 8.2) (see the volume in this series, *Biochemistry of Conjugation Reactions*) (Stevens and Anders, 1979). In the context of the toxicity of chloroform, it is relevant to note that, at least in rats, its oxidative metabolism is mediated mainly by CYP2E1, the ethanol-inducible isozyme responsible for the metabolism and bioactivation of a large number of halogenated alkanes (Brady *et al.*, 1989; Koop, 1992; Raucy *et al.*, 1993).

In view of the toxicity of dihalomethyl groups (see above), it is easy to understand why much of the research on HCFCs and HFCs as CFC substitutes currently concentrates on compounds which do not contain a toxophoric $-CHX_2$ group, e.g. **1,1,1-trihaloethanes** and **1,1,1,2-tetrahaloethanes**. Relevant examples of the latter group include 1,1,1,2-tetrafluoroethane (**8.XIV**) and 1,2-dichloro-1,1-difluoroethane (**8.XVII**), whose initial hydroxylation (on the $-CH_2X$ group) is catalyzed mainly by CYP2E1. The major metabolites thus formed are the corresponding alcohols (**8.XV** and **8.XVIII**) and acids (**8.XVI** and **8.XIX**) (Harris and Anders,

$$CF_3-CH_2F\,\cdot \longrightarrow CF_3-CH_2OH \ + \ CF_3-COOH$$

8.XIV $\qquad\qquad\qquad\qquad$ 8.XV $\qquad\qquad$ 8.XVI

$$CF_2Cl-CH_2Cl \longrightarrow CF_2Cl-CH_2OH \ + \ CF_2Cl-COOH$$

8.XVII $\qquad\qquad\qquad\qquad$ 8.XVIII $\qquad\qquad$ 8.XIX

$$CCl_3-CHCl_2 \longrightarrow CCl_2=CCl_2$$

8.XX $\qquad\qquad\qquad\qquad$ 8.XXI

1991; Olson *et al.*, 1990 and 1991; Surbrook and Olson, 1992). A representative 1,1,1-trihaloethane is 1,1-dichloro-1-fluoroethane which as expected is oxidized by CYP2E1 to 1,1-dichloro-1-fluoroethanol (Loizou and Anders, 1993).

In Section 4.4, we have examined the oxidative **metabolism of haloalkenes**. It is important to realize that metabolism to haloalkenes is documented for a number of haloalkanes, leading to secondary metabolites by mechanisms (e.g. halogen migration) discussed in Section 4.4. Thus, mice dosed with 1,1,2,2-tetrachloroethane (**8.V**) excreted trichloroethanol and trichloroacetic acid as urinary metabolites whose formation implies trichloroethene (**8.VII**) as an intermediate. The latter metabolite was indeed characterized in the expired air of the same animals, its formation resulting from **non-enzymatic dehydrochlorination** (Yllner, 1971b). Pentachloroethane (**8.XX**) administered to mice similarly yielded tetrachloroethene (**8.XXI**) by a non-enzymatic reaction of dehydrochlorination. In addition, trichloroethene (**8.VII**) was also formed from pentachloroethane (**8.XX**) by loss of two chlorine atoms (**dechlorination**) (Yllner, 1971c), but the mechanism of the reaction does not appear to be known.

8.2.2 Compounds of medicinal interest

A number of compounds of medicinal interest feature one or more halogen atoms adjacent to sp^3-carbon atoms and are thus potential substrates for oxidative dehalogenation. This is the case of several **inhalation anaesthetics**, three of which will be discussed here.

Halothane (CF_3–CHClBr) undergoes cytochrome P450-catalyzed dehalogenation by both oxidative and reductive routes, the latter being discussed in Chapter 12. The compound can induce postanaesthetic jaundice or hepatitis, its reductive metabolism partly and perhaps mainly accounting for such unwanted effects (Sipes *et al.*, 1980). As for its oxidative metabolism, it occurs at the –CHClBr group as discussed above and leads to trifluoroacetic acid by the pathway shown in Fig. 8.2. Besides being hydrolyzed, the intermediate trifluoroacetyl halide may also react with endogenous molecules and macromolecules. Trifluoroacetylated liver proteins serve as antigens and are associated with (sometimes fatal) idiosyncratic hepatitis (Christen *et al.*, 1991a and 1991b; Gut *et al.*, 1993; Harris *et al.*, 1991). However, formation of protein adducts is not restricted to the liver, recent evidence indicating that the kidney is also able to activate halothane and 2,2-dichloro-1,1,1-trifluoroethane to a trifluoroacetylating reagent (Huwyler *et al.*, 1992). Furthermore, acylation of phospholipids led to the formation of N-trifluoroacetyl phosphatidyl ethanolamine in the liver microsomes of rabbits exposed to halothane, and to the excretion of N-trifluoroacetyl-2-aminoethanol in human urine (Cohen *et al.*, 1975; Müller and Stier, 1982).

Enflurane (**8.XXII**) displays two potential target sites for oxidative dehalogenation, namely the –CHF_2 and –CHClF groups. In agreement with the reaction sequence reported in the previous section, the latter group is the preferred (and in fact practically unique) site of dehalogenation to form the acid **8.XXIII** as a rat liver microsomal and human urinary metabolite (Burke *et al.*, 1980). As with halothane but to a smaller extent, the oxidation of enflurane leads to liver protein adducts. In this case, acylation is by the difluoromethoxydifluoroacetyl moiety (CHF_2–O–CF_2–CO–), yet the adducts are recognized by antibodies from patients with halothane hepatitis (Christ *et al.*, 1988a and 1988b). Furthermore, oxidative dehalogenation releases inorganic fluoride which is believed to be responsible, at least in part, for the nephrotoxicity of enflurane and analogues. It is therefore of potential significance that replacing the –CHFCl group of enflurane with a –$CFCl_2$ group produces an analogue that releases only minute amounts of

$$CHF_2\!-\!O\!-\!CF_2\!-\!CHFCl \longrightarrow CHF_2\!-\!O\!-\!CF_2\!-\!COOH$$

8.XXII   8.XXIII

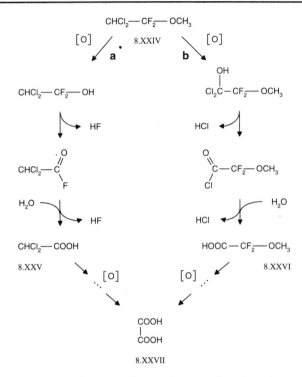

FIGURE 8.4 Major pathways in the metabolism of methoxyflurane (**8.XXIV**).

inorganic fluoride, in agreement with the very slow oxidation of the only remaining target site (the –CHF$_2$ group) (Burke *et al.*, 1981).

As for **methoxyflurane (8.XXIV** in Fig. 8.4), it presents two target sites for alpha-carbon oxidation, namely the methyl group whose hydroxylation results in O-demethylation (reaction **a** in Fig. 8.4) followed by a postenzymatic cascade to dichloroacetic acid (**8.XXV** in Fig. 8.4), and the dichloromethyl group whose dechlorination (reaction **b** in Fig. 8.4) leads to methoxy-difluoroacetic acid (**8.XXVI** in Fig. 8.4). Each of the two metabolites can then be further oxidized to oxalic acid (**8.XXVII** in Fig. 8.4) and other products. A metabolic study in rats indicated that at early times after methoxyflurane administration the major pathway was oxalic acid formation via initial O-demethylation (reaction **a** in Fig. 8.4). At later stages, the major pathway was reaction **b** to methoxydifluoroacetic acid (**8.XXVI**) which was mostly excreted unchanged (Selinsky *et al.*, 1988).

Administration of methoxyflurane to humans and animals can result in hepatitis and acute polyuric renal lesions. Both reactions **a** and **b** in Fig. 8.4 form an acyl halide that can acylate liver proteins and transform them into immunogens (Christ *et al.*, 1988a). As for nephrotoxicity, it is caused by inorganic fluoride (Cousins *et al.*, 1974). Inorganic fluoride can be released following O-demethylation of methoxyflurane and methoxydifluoroacetate (Fig. 8.4, **8.XXIV** and **8.XXVI**, respectively), but in view of the metabolic stability of the latter compound (see above), reaction **a** appears as the predominant source of fluoride from methoxyflurane.

As the above examples suggest, metabolic studies of model compounds, CFC substitutes and inhalation anaesthetics have led to a broad view of structure–toxicity relationships in haloalkanes and can help in the rational design of improved agents.

Drugs of other classes also present interesting examples of oxidative dehalogenation, in particular **fluorosteroids**. Thus, the synthetic corticosteroid flunisolide (**8.XXVIII**) displays a fluoro-substituent in the 6α-position. The compound was defluorinated in mouse liver microsomes to the 6-keto metabolite, the latter being further metabolized by hydrogenation to the 6β-hydroxy analogue. An additional metabolite was Δ^6-flunisolide, the formation of which was postulated to result from the dehydration of the unstable fluorohydrin (the 6-fluoro-6-hydroxy intermediate) generated by cytochrome P450 (Teitelbaum *et al.*, 1981). In humans given [^{14}C]flunisolide, the 6β-hydroxy metabolite accounts for 60–75% of urinary radioactivity, indicating the importance of the defluorination pathway (Tökes *et al.*, 1981).

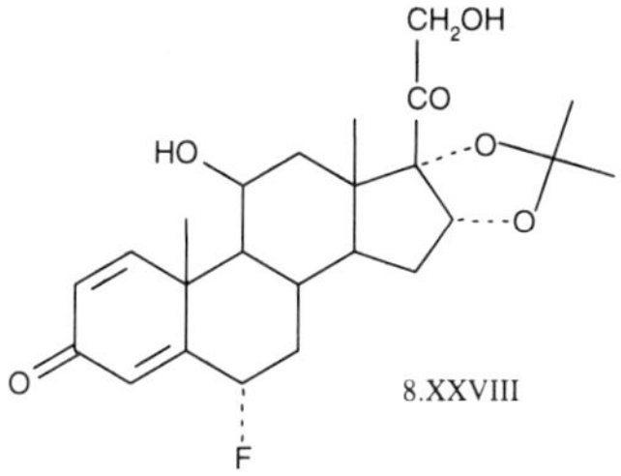

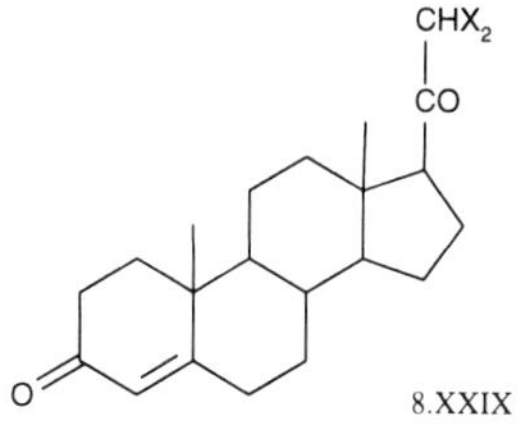

Another example of fluorosteroids is given by 21,21-dichloro- and 21,21-difluoroprogesterone (**8.XXIX**, X = Cl and F, respectively), two mechanism-based inactivators of adrenocortical cytochromes P450 (Stevens *et al.*, 1991). While the dichloro analogue inactivates both CYP17 and CYP21A1, the difluoro analogue appears more selective for CYP21A1. It has been postulated that inactivation is due to irreversible binding of the acyl halide (R–CO–CO–X) to the enzyme.

The last drug to be discussed here is the antibiotic **chloramphenicol** (**8.XXX** in Fig. 8.5),

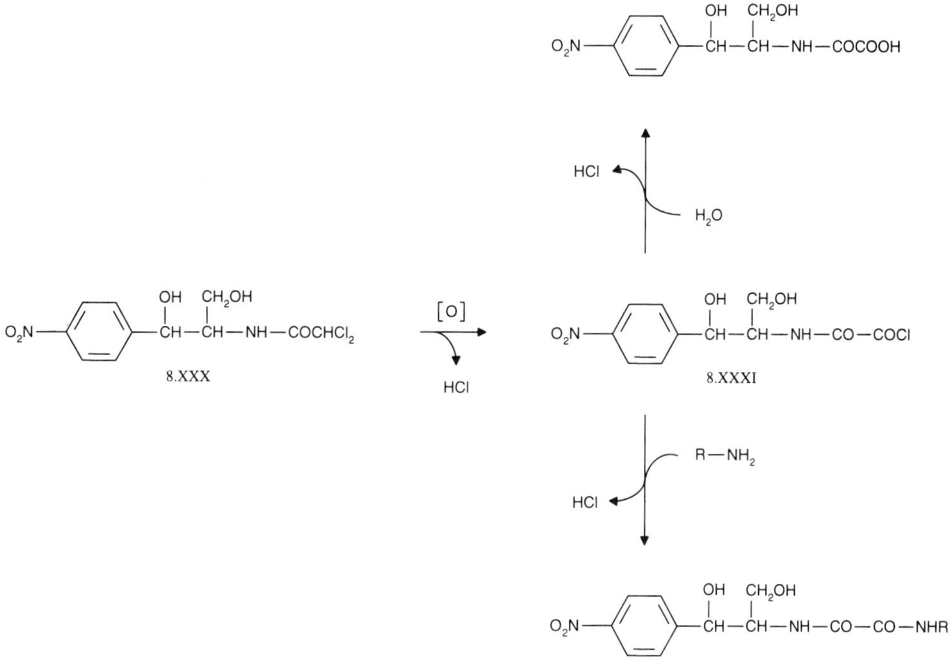

FIGURE 8.5 Partial metabolic scheme of chloramphenicol (**8.XXX**) showing its oxidative dechlorination to an intermediate oxamyl chloride (**8.XXXI**) which can be hydrolyzed to the corresponding oxamic acid derivative, or bind covalently to proteins and particularly to the terminal amino group of lysyl residues.

whose N-dichloroacetyl moiety is subject to cytochrome P450-mediated dechlorination. In conformity with the mechanism shown in Fig. 8.2, the reaction leads to an acyl chloride, in this case an oxamyl chloride (**8.XXXI** in Fig. 8.5), which can both hydrolyze to the oxamic acid derivative and acylate proteins. Phenobarbital pretreatment was necessary for these reactions to be characterized in rat liver microsomes (Pohl *et al.*, 1978). Protein acylation mainly involves cytochrome P450, implying that chloramphenicol is an irreversible inactivator of the enzyme. It has also been demonstrated that acylation of apocytochrome P450 occurs to the terminal amino group of lysyl residues (Halpert, 1981).

8.3   OXIDATIVE DEALKYLATION OF ORGANOMETALLIC COMPOUNDS

Many physicochemical properties of organometallic compounds depend on the ionic versus covalent character of their carbon–metal bond. Compounds whose carbon–metal bond has a marked ionic character (e.g. organosodium compounds) are highly unstable under biomimetic conditions and may even react explosively with water. Such organometallic compounds do not concern us here. In contrast, carbon–metal bonds of a predominantly covalent character (e.g. organomercurials) are of low polarity and comparably high stability. Much of the discussion to follow will focus on organometallic derivatives of some Group IV elements, namely silicon (Si), germanium (Ge), tin (Sn) and lead (Pb). Organomercury derivatives will also be briefly considered.

8.3.1   Oxidative dealkylation of organosilicon, organogermanium, organotin and organolead compounds

Silicon displays many similarities with carbon, and organosilicon compounds have various applications as chemicals and drugs. Little is known of the metabolic fate of such compounds except reactions of silicon oxidation (Chapter 11), and Si–C cleavage to be briefly examined here. Administration to rats of a silicon-containing carbamate (**8.XXXII**; R = CH$_3$) resulted in Si-depropylation and in the urinary excretion of a metabolite postulated to be a silanol derivative (**8.XXXIII**; R = CH$_3$); this metabolite was not characterized as such, but as the artefactual disiloxane **8.XXXIV** (R = CH$_3$) formed by condensation during the isolation procedure (Fessenden and Ahlfors, 1967). The same reaction was observed with the dicarbamate (**8.XXXII**; R = CH$_2$OCONH$_2$), but not with the analogue having the *n*-propyl group replaced by a methyl group. Furthermore, only methyl hydroxylation (to form **8.XXXVI**) but no Si–C cleavage were observed when phenyltrimethylsilane (**8.XXXV**) was given to rats (Fessenden and Hartman, 1970).

In compatibility with the possible absence of Si-demethylation, there were some indications that the mechanism of Si–C cleavage might result from an oxidation of the beta-carbon, followed by proton-catalyzed Si–C cleavage to produce propene and the silanol metabolite. Further details on such a reaction will be given when considering organotin compounds (see later Fig. 8.6).

The higher elements in Group IV are **germanium**, **tin** and **lead**, and metal–carbon cleavage is documented for each of these elements. Thus, rat liver microsomes were found to mediate the deethylation of a number of tri- and tetraethylmetallic compounds, the rate of the reaction decreasing in the order tetraethyllead > triethylgermanium chloride > tetraethyltin > triethyllead acetate > triethyltin bromide > tetraethylgermanium (Prough *et al.*, 1981). The reaction, conclusively a cytochrome P450-catalyzed one, was monitored by the formation of ethylene, but the mechanism of the reaction was not elucidated (see below for a possible explanation). Other

$$CH_3CH_2CH_2-\overset{\overset{\displaystyle CH_3}{|}}{\underset{\underset{\displaystyle R}{|}}{Si}}-CH_2OCONH_2 \quad \longrightarrow \quad HO-\overset{\overset{\displaystyle CH_3}{|}}{\underset{\underset{\displaystyle R}{|}}{Si}}-CH_2OCONH_2$$

8.XXXII   8.XXXIII

$$H_2NCOOCH_2-\overset{\overset{\displaystyle CH_3}{|}}{\underset{\underset{\displaystyle R}{|}}{Si}}-O-\overset{\overset{\displaystyle CH_3}{|}}{\underset{\underset{\displaystyle R}{|}}{Si}}-CH_2OCONH_2$$

8.XXXIV

$$Ph-\overset{\overset{\displaystyle CH_3}{|}}{\underset{\underset{\displaystyle CH_3}{|}}{Si}}-CH_3 \quad \longrightarrow \quad Ph-\overset{\overset{\displaystyle CH_3}{|}}{\underset{\underset{\displaystyle CH_3}{|}}{Si}}-CH_2OH$$

8.XXXV   8.XXXVI

organotin and organolead compounds were found to be dealkylated by liver microsomes (Casida *et al.*, 1971; Hathway, 1979a). Thus, the dealkylation of Et_3Sn^+, Pr_3Sn^+, Bu_3Sn^+, Pen_3Sn^+, Hex_3Sn^+ and $(cyclohexyl)_3Sn^+$ decreased with increasing size of the alkyl substituents but did not appear to be influenced by the counterion, i.e. acetate, chloride or hydroxide. In addition:

- Et_4Sn gave Et_3Sn^+ and Et_2Sn2^+,
- Bu_2Sn2^+ gave $BuSn^{3+}$,
- $(cyclohexyl)_2Sn^{+2}$ gave $(cyclohexyl)Sn^{+3}$, cyclohexanone and cyclohexanol,
- Et_4Pb gave Et_3Pb^+,
- Bu_3Pb^+ gave Bu_2Pb^{2+} and 1-butene,
- Ph_3Pb^+ was not metabolized.

Tetraethyllead has been particularly investigated in view of its technical importance as a gasoline additive; its *in vivo* metabolites in humans, rats and rabbits are triethyllead and inorganic lead. The compound binds as a substrate (Type I binding) to cytochrome P450; kinetic studies revealed the high activity of liver microsomes from 3-methylcholanthrene-treated rats in forming triethyllead (Ferreira da Silva *et al.*, 1983).

8.3.2 Mechanisms of oxidative Sn–C and Pb–C cleavage

Insights into the mechanism(s) of oxidative Sn–C cleavage can be found in a metabolic study of **tributyltin acetate** (**8.XXXVII** in Fig. 8.6) in rat liver microsomes (Fish *et al.*, 1976; Hathway, 1979a). It was found that all four carbon atoms in the butyl chain were hydroxylated, the $\alpha/\beta/\gamma/\delta$ ratio being approximatively 3/6/2/1. Such a regioselectivity reflects a marked influence of the tin atom (see below). More interesting in the present context is the reactivity of the β-hydroxylated and α-hydroxylated metabolites. The β-hydroxylated metabolite (formed by reaction **a** in Fig. 8.6) decomposed under acidic conditions to yield butene and a dibutyltin compound. The α-hydroxylated metabolite (formed by reaction **b** in Fig. 8.6) was even less stable and under physiological conditions of temperature and pH broke down to butanol and a dibutyltin compound. In sum, both the β- and α-hydroxylated metabolite can lead to Sn–C cleavage, but

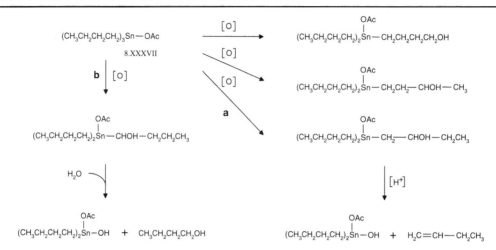

FIGURE 8.6 Metabolism of tributyltin acetate (**8.XXXVII**) in rat liver microsomes, showing the breakdown of the β-hydroxylated and α-hydroxylated metabolites under acidic and physiological conditions, respectively (modified from Fish *et al.*, 1976).

only the decomposition of the α-hydroxylated metabolite can be considered as a physiologically relevant post-enzymatic reaction. As for the breakdown products of the β-hydroxylated metabolite, they must be viewed as artifacts.

The study of Fish and coworkers (1976) thus proposes **two mechanisms** explaining the generation of alkenes and alkanols upon oxidative cleavage of organotin compounds. But whether these mechanisms are relevant to the metabolism of all organotin compounds and more generally of other organometallic compounds is not fully clarified. In any case, a connection is established between metal–carbon cleavage and the regioselectivity of carbon hydroxylation. The evidence available indicates that in organometallic compounds as in other organic compounds (see Section 4.2), carbon hydroxylation is influenced by electronic and steric factors.

The influence of **electronic factors** is seen for example in the fact that tetramethyllead was dealkylated 20 times faster than tetraethyllead, suggesting that the carbon adjacent to the lead atom possesses the highest reactivity (Ferreira de Silva and Diehl, 1985). Also, the decreasing dealkylation in the sequence $Et_4Pb > Et_4Sn > Et_4Ge$ is particularly interesting since it indicates that the rate of reaction decreases with increasing covalent character of the metal–carbon bond (Prough *et al.*, 1981, see Section 8.3.1). The influence of **steric factors** is for example evidenced by the metabolism of cyclohexyltriphenyltin (**8.XXXVIII**) (Fish *et al.*, 1977). In rat liver microsomes, this compound was hydroxylated mainly in the 4-position of the cyclohexyl ring (almost 90% of the fraction metabolized), with the 3-position accounting for about 10% and the 2-position for less than 2%. No 1-hydroxylation was seen, and this pattern of hydroxylation clearly reflects the marked steric hindrance caused by the triphenyltin group.

8.XXXVIII

8.3.3 Dealkylation of organomercurials

Alkylmercury compounds undergo *in vivo* cleavage of the Hg–C bond with release of inorganic mercury (Hg^{2+}) (Hathway, 1972, 1975 and 1979b). Examples include methylmercury and ethylmercury salts ($CH_3Hg^+X^-$ and $CH_3CH_2Hg^+X^-$, respectively), although the extent of dealkylation appears low in experimental animals (e.g. Magos and Butler, 1976). In contrast, a compound such as 2-methoxyethylmercury chloride ($CH_3OCH_2CH_2Hg^+Cl^-$) is rapidly and extensively dealkylated *in vivo* (Hathway, 1972 and 1979b).

Animals treated with methylmercury exhibit decreased hepatic monooxygenase activity due to degradation of cytochrome P450. However, the **enzymes** mediating organomercurial dealkylation and their mechanisms are not well understood. The dealkylation of ethylmercury and methylmercury was observed *in vitro* upon incubation with rat liver microsomes, and converging evidence indicated the involvement of the hydroxyl radical ($HO^\bullet$) possibly generated by NADPH-cytochrome P450 reductase (Suda and Hirayama, 1992). Phagocytic cells (see Chapter 10) also catalyze MeHg and EtHg dealkylation. In contrast, an organomercurial of another class, **phenylmercury**, was broken down by rat liver cytosol but not microsomes to inorganic mercury and benzene (Daniel *et al.*, 1972).

The dealkylation of organomercurials has significance in connection with the toxicity, and particularly neurotoxicity, elicited by these compounds. While both organic and inorganic mercury are toxic in their own right, there are indications that the metabolism of methylmercury may have a role in mediating brain damage (Gallagher and Lee, 1980; Vandewater *et al.*, 1983). The oxidation of inorganic mercury is discussed in Section 11.2.

8.4 REFERENCES

Ahmed A.E., Kubic V.L. and Anders M.W. (1977). Metabolism of haloforms to carbon monoxide. I. *In vitro* studies. *Drug Metab. Disposit.* **5**, 198–204.

Anders M.W. (1982a). Mechanisms of haloalkane and haloalkene biotransformation. *Trends Pharmacol. Sci.* **3**, 356–357.

Anders M.W. (1982b). Aliphatic halogenated hydrocarbons. In *Metabolic Basis of Detoxication* (eds Jakoby W.B., Bend J.R. and Caldwell J.). pp. 29–49. Academic Press, New York.

Anders M.W. (1984). Biotransformation of halogenated hydrocarbons. In *Drug Metabolism and Drug Toxicity* (eds Mitchell J.R. and Horning M.G.). pp. 55–70. Raven Press, New York.

Anders M.W. and Pohl L.R. (1985). Halogenated alkanes. In *Bioactivation of Foreign Compounds* (ed. Anders M.W.). pp. 283–315. Academic Press, Orlando.

Brady J.F., Li D., Ishizaki H., Lee M., Ning S.M., Xiao F. and Yang C.S. (1989). Induction of cytochromes P450IIE1 and P450IIB1 by secondary ketones and the role of P450IIE1 in chloroform metabolism. *Toxicol. Appl. Pharmacol.* **100**, 342–349.

Burke T.R. Jr, Martin J.L., George J.W. and Pohl L.R. (1980). Investigation of the metabolism of defluorination of enflurane in rat liver microsomes with specifically deuterated derivatives. *Biochem. Pharmacol.* **29**, 1623–1626.

Burke T.R. Jr, Branchflower R.V., Lees D.E. and Pohl L.R. (1981). Mechanism of defluorination of enflurane. Identification of an organic metabolite in rat and man. *Drug Metab. Disposit.* **9**, 19–24.

Casida J.E., Kimmel E.C., Holm B. and Widmark G.

(1971). Oxidative dealkylation of tetra-, tri-, and dialkyltins and tetra- and trialkylleads by liver microsomes. *Acta Chem. Scand.* **25**, 1497–1499.

Christ D.D., Kenna J.G., Kammerer W., Satoh H. and Pohl L.R. (1988a). Enflurane metabolism produces covalently bound liver adducts recognized by antibodies from patients with halothane hepatitis. *Anesthesiology* **69**, 833–838.

Christ D.D., Satoh H., Kenna J.G. and Pohl L.R. (1988b). Potential metabolic basis for enflurane hepatitis and the apparent cross-sensitization between enflurane and halothane. *Drug Metab. Disposit.* **16**, 135–140.

Christen U., Bürgin M. and Gut J. (1991a). Halothane metabolism: Kupffer cells carry and partially process trifluoroacetylated protein adducts. *Biochem. Biophys. Res. Commun.* **175**, 256–262.

Christen U., Bürgin M. and Gut J. (1991b). Halothane metabolism: immunological evidence for molecular mimicry of trifluoroacetylated liver protein adducts by constitutive polypeptides. *Molec. Pharmacol.* **40**, 390–400.

Cohen E.N., Trudell J.R., Edmunds H.N. and Watson E. (1975). Urinary metabolites of halothane in man. *Anesthesiology* **43**, 392–401.

Cousins M.J., Mazze R.I., Kosek J.C., Hitt B.A. and Love F.V. (1974). The etiology of methoxyflurane nephrotoxicity. *J. Pharmacol. Exp. Therap.* **190**, 530–541.

Daniel J.W., Gage J.C. and Lefevre P.A. (1972). The metabolism of phenylmercury by the rat. *Biochem. J.* **129**, 961–967.

Ferreira da Silva D. and Diehl H. (1985). Metabolism of tetraorganolead compounds by rat-liver microsomal monooxygenase. III. Enzymic dealkylation of tetramethyl lead compared with tetraethyl lead. *Xenobiotica* **15**, 789–797.

Ferreira da Silva D., Schröder U. and Diehl H. (1983). Metabolism of tetraorganolead compounds by rat-liver microsomal monooxygenase. II. Enzymic dealkylation of tetraethyl lead. *Xenobiotica* **13**, 583–590.

Fessenden R.J. and Ahlfors C. (1967). The metabolic fate of some silicon-containing carbamates. *J. Med. Chem.* **10**, 810–812.

Fessenden R.J. and Hartman R.A. (1970). Metabolic fate of phenyltrimethylsilane and phenyldimethylsilane. *J. Med. Chem.* **13**, 52–54.

Fish R.H., Kimmel E.C. and Casida J.E. (1976). Bioorganotin chemistry: reactions of tributyltin derivatives with a cytochrome P-450 dependent monooxygenase enzyme system. *J. Organometal. Chem.* **118**, 41–54.

Fish R.H., Casida J.E. and Kimmel E.C. (1977). Bioorganotin chemistry: situs and stereoselectivity in the reaction of cyclohexyltriphenyltin with a cytochrome P-450 dependent monooxygenase enzyme system. *Tetrahedron. Lett.* 3515–3518.

Gallagher P.J. and Lee R.L. (1980). The role of biotransformation in organic mercury neurotoxicity. *Toxicology* **15**, 129–134.

Guengerich F.P., Willard R.J., Shea J.P., Richards L.E. and Macdonald T.L. (1984). Mechanism-based inactivation of cytochrome P-450 by heteroatom-substituted cyclopropanes and formation of ring-opened products. *J. Amer. Chem. Soc.* **106**, 6446–6447.

Gut J., Christen U. and Huwyler J. (1993). Mechanisms of halothane toxicity: novel insights. *Pharmacol. Therap.* **58**, 133–155.

Hales D.B., Ho B. and Thompson J.A. (1987). Inter- and intramolecular deuterium isotope effects on the cytochrome P-450-catalyzed oxidative dehalogenation of 1,1,2,2-tetrachloroethane. *Biochem. Biophys. Res. Commun.* **149**, 319–325.

Halpert J. (1981). Covalent modification of lysine during the suicide inactivation of rat liver cytochrome P-450 by chloramphenicol. *Biochem. Pharmacol.* **30**, 875–881.

Harris J.W. and Anders M.W. (1991). Metabolism of the hydrochlorofluorocarbon 1,2-dichloro-1,1-difluoroethane. *Chem. Res. Toxicol.* **4**, 180–186.

Harris J.W., Pohl L.R., Martin J.L. and Anders M.W. (1991). Tissue acylation by the chlorofluorocarbon substitute 2,2-dichloro-1,1,1-trifluoroethane. *Proc. Natl Acad. Sci. USA* **88**, 1407–1410.

Harris J.W., Jones J.P., Martin J.L., LaRosa A.C., Olson M.J., Pohl L.R. and Anders M.W. (1992). Pentahaloethane-based chlorofluorocarbon substitutes and halothane: Correlation of *in vivo* hepatic protein trifluoroacetylation and urinary trifluoroacetic acid excretion with calculated enthalpies of activation. *Chem. Res. Toxicol.* **5**, 720–725.

Hathway D.E. (1972). *Foreign Compound Metabolism in Mammals*, Volume 2. pp. 155–157, 313. The Chemical Society, London.

Hathway D.E. (1975). *Foreign Compound Metabolism in*

Mammals, Volume 3. pp. 427, 496. The Chemical Society, London.

Hathway D.E. (1979a). *Foreign Compound Metabolism in Mammals*, Volume 5. pp. 522–523. The Chemical Society, London.

Hathway D.E. (1979b). *Foreign Compound Metabolism in Mammals*, Volume 5. pp. 488–489. The Chemical Society, London.

Huwyler J., Aeschlimann D., Christen U. and Gut J. (1992). The kidney as a novel target tissue for protein adduct formation associated with metabolism of halothane and the candidate chlorofluorocarbon replacement 2,2-dichloro-1,1,1-trifluoroethane. *Eur. J. Biochem.* **207**, 229–238.

Koop D.R. (1992). Oxidative and reductive metabolism of cytochrome P450 2E1. *FASEB J.* **6**, 724–730.

Kubic V.L. and Anders M.W. (1975). Metabolism of dihalomethanes to carbon monoxide. II. *In vitro* studies. *Drug Metab. Disposit.* **3**, 104–112.

Kubic V.L. and Anders M.W. (1978). Metabolism of dihalomethanes to carbon monoxide. II. Studies on the mechanism of the reaction. *Biochem. Pharmacol.* **27**, 2349–2355.

Loizou G.D. and Anders M.W. (1993). Gas-uptake pharmacokinetics and biotransformation of 1,1-dichloro-1-fluoroethane (HCFC-141b). *Drug Metab. Disposit.* **21**, 634–639.

Magos L. and Butler W.H. (1976). The kinetics of methylmercury administered repeatedly to rats. *Arch. Toxicol.* **35**, 25–39.

Müller R. and Stier A. (1982). Modification of liver microsomal lipids by halothane metabolites: a multi nuclear NMR spectroscopy study. *Naun-Schmied Arch. Pharmacol.* **321**, 234–237.

Olson M.J., Reidy C.A., Johnson J.T. and Pederson T.C. (1990). Oxidative defluorination of 1,1,1,2-tetrafluoroethane by rat liver microsomes. *Drug Metab. Disposit.* **18**, 992–998.

Olson M.J., Kim S.G., Reidy C.A., Johnson J.T. and Novak R.F. (1991). Oxidation of 1,1,1,2-tetrafluoroethane by rat liver microsomes is catalyzed primarily by cytochrome P-450IIE1. *Drug Metab. Disposit.* **19**, 298–303.

Pohl L.R. (1979). Biochemical toxicology of chloroform. In *Reviews in Biochemical Toxicology*, Vol. 1 (eds Hodgson E., Bend J.R. and Philpot R.M.). pp. 79–107. Elsevier/North Holland, New York.

Pohl L.R., Nelson S.D. and Krishna G. (1978). Investigation of the mechanism of the metabolic activation of chloramphenicol by rat liver microsomes. Identification of a new metabolite. *Biochem. Pharmacol.* **27**, 491–496.

Pohl L.R., George J.W., Martin J.L. and Krishna G. (1979). Deuterium isotope effect in *in vivo* bioactivation of chloroform to phosgene. *Biochem. Pharmacol.* **28**, 561–563.

Prough R.A., Stalmach M.A., Wiebkin P. and Bridges J.W. (1981). The microsomal metabolism of the organometallic derivatives of the Group-IV elements, germanium, tin and lead. *Biochem. J.* **196**, 763–770.

Raucy J.L., Kraner J.C. and Lasker J.M. (1993). Bioactivation of halogenated hydrocarbons by cytochrome P4502E1. *Crit. Rev. Toxicol.* **23**, 1–20.

Salmon A.G., Jones R.B. and Mackrodt W.C. (1981). Microsomal dechlorination of chloroethanes: structure–activity relationships. *Xenobiotica* **11**, 723–734.

Selinski B.S., Perlman M.E. and London R.E. (1988). *In vivo* nuclear magnetic resonance studies of hepatic methoxyflurane metabolism. II. A reevaluation of hepatic metabolic pathways. *Molec. Pharmacol.* **33**, 567–573.

Sipes I.G., Gandolfi A.J., Pohl L.R., Krishna G. and Brown B.R. Jr (1980). Comparison of the biotransformation and hepatotoxicity of halothane and deuterated halothane. *J. Pharmacol. Exp. Therap.* **214**, 716–720.

Stevens J.L. and Anders M.W. (1979). Metabolism of haloforms to carbon monoxide. III. Studies on the mechanism of the reaction. *Biochem. Pharmacol.* **28**, 3189–3194.

Stevens J.C., Jaw J.Y., Peng C.T. and Halpert J. (1991). Mechanism-based inactivation of bovine adrenal cytochromes P450 C-21 and P450 17α by 17β-substituted steroids. *Biochemistry* **30**, 3649–3658.

Suda I. and Hirayama K. (1992). Degradation of methyl and ethyl mercury into inorganic mercury by hydroxyl radical produced from rat liver microsomes. *Arch. Toxicol.* **66**, 398–402.

Surbrook S.E. Jr and Olson M.J. (1992). Dominant role of cytochrome P-450 2E1 in human hepatic microsomal oxidation of the CFC-substitute 1,1,1,2-tetrafluoroethane. *Drug Metab. Disposit.* **20**, 518–524.

Tachizawa H., Macdonald T.L. and Neal R.A. (1982). Rat liver microsomal metabolism of propyl halides. *Molec. Pharmacol.* **22**, 745–751.

Teitelbaum P.J., Chu N.I., Cho D., Tökés L., Patterson J.W., Wagner P.J. and Chaplin M.D. (1981). Mechanism for the oxidative defluorination of flunisolide. *J. Pharmacol. Exp. Therap.* **218**, 16–22.

Tökes L., Cho D., Maddox M.L., Chaplin M.D. and Chu N.I. (1981). Isolation and identification of an oxidatively defluorinated metabolite of flunisolide in man. *Drug Metab. Disposit.* **9**, 485–486.

Vandewater L.J.S., Racz W.J., Norris A.R. and Buncel E. (1983). Methylmercury distribution, metabolism, and neurotoxicity in the mouse brain. *Can. J. Physiol. Pharmacol.* **61**, 1487–1493.

Van Dyke R.A. and Gandolfi A.J. (1975). Characterization of a microsomal dechlorination system. *Molec. Pharmacol.* **11**, 809–817.

Yllner S. (1971a). Metabolism of 1,1,2-trichloroethane-1,2-^{14}C in the mouse. *Acta Pharmacol. Toxicol.* **30**, 248–256.

Yllner S. (1971b). Metabolism of 1,1,2,2-tetrachloroethane-^{14}C in the mouse. *Acta Pharmacol. Toxicol.* **29**, 499–512.

Yllner S. (1971c). Metabolism of pentachloroethane in the mouse. *Acta Pharmacol. Toxicol.* **29**, 481–489.

chapter 9

OXIDATIONS CATALYZED BY VARIOUS OXIDASES AND MONO-OXYGENASES

Contents

9.1 INTRODUCTION

Having considered in Chapters 3 to 8 a number of reactions catalyzed by cytochrome P450 and the FAD-containing monooxygenase, we now proceed to discuss some other enzyme systems of perhaps lesser quantitative importance in xenobiotic metabolism. These enzymes share the characteristic that for many years, their involvement in xenobiotic metabolism was considered to be marginal, a view superseded by many recent findings of particular toxicological and therapeutic significance. To allow a better transition from previous chapters, we begin with hemoglobin, a hemoprotein having some resemblance with cytochrome P450, before continuing with dopamine monooxygenase and then various oxidases.

9.2 REACTIONS CATALYZED BY HEMOGLOBIN

Hemoglobin is the well-known oxygen carrier macromolecule in the blood. In addition to this essential physiological function, hemoglobin has also been found to display enzyme-like activities in mediating a number of biotransformation reactions, some of which have toxicological significance. These reactions include carbon hydroxylation (Section 9.2.2) and nitrogen oxidation (Section 9.2.3). Two good reviews are available on the biochemistry and enzyme-like activities of hemoglobin (Cossum, 1988; Mieyal, 1985).

9.2.1 The biochemistry of hemoglobin

Hemoglobin is found in high concentrations in the cytosol of erythrocytes. It is a tetramer, each subunit (MW about 16,000) being a hemoprotein whose prosthetic group (like that of cytochrome P450) is iron-protoporphyrin IX. Multiple forms (e.g. HbA, HbA_2, HbS) and variants have been described, some of which have pathological consequences. Like cytochrome P450 (and all hemoproteins), hemoglobin in its reduced (i.e. Fe^{2+}), physiological state has a strong affinity for diatomic gases, but in contrast to cytochrome P450 its fifth axial heme ligand is a histidine nitrogen rather than a cysteine thiolate. This influences the redox potential of the iron atom and increases the stability of the ferrohemoprotein–O_2 complex by markedly decreasing the rate of autoxidation. The Fe^{3+}/Fe^{2+} equilibrium, which is functional in cytochrome P450, has toxicological implications for hemoglobin since it results in the formation of the ferric, inactive state (known as methemoglobin).

   Two **electron transport systems** exist in erythrocytes to maintain hemoglobin in the reduced state. In the primary pathway, electrons originate with NADH and are transferred to an FAD-containing reductase, then to cytochrome b_5, and ultimately to methemoglobin. A secondary, NADPH-dependent system exists involving two sequential reductases which can be replaced *in vitro* by NADPH-cytochrome P450 reductase. It is in such reconstituted conditions (hemoglobin or erythrocytes plus NADPH plus NADPH-cytochrome P450 reductase) that the highest monooxygenase activities of hemoglobin have been found *in vitro* (Mieyal, 1985; Mieyal et al., 1976; Starke et al., 1984).

   Myoglobin, the monomeric oxygen-carrier hemoprotein of muscles and heart, displays enzymic activities resembling those of hemoglobin (Mieyal, 1985).

9.2.2 Reactions of carbon oxidation

Among the various reactions of biotransformation catalyzed by hemoglobin, that most investigated is the hydroxylation of **aniline** (**9.I**; R = H) to *p*-aminophenol (**9.I**; R = OH), as seen for example in human red cells and whole blood (Blisard and Mieyal, 1979; Tomoda et al., 1977). The monooxygenasic activity of intact tetrameric hemoglobin is predominantly due to the β-subunits (Ferraiolo and Mieyal, 1982).

   Mechanistically, analogies with and differences from cytochrome P450-catalyzed monooxygenation have been found. A first difference is that the reaction of hydroxylation is exclusive for the *para*-position. In the absence of an electron donor, the incubation of aniline with oxyferrohemoglobin did not lead to substrate hydroxylation but markedly accelerated hemoglobin autoxidation. When an electron donor was added (e.g. NADPH plus NADPH-cytochrome P450 reductase), aniline hydroxylation (but not *p*-nitroanisole O-demethylation) proceeded readily after a lag time (Mieyal, 1985). This led to the suggestion that aniline binds before O_2 to hemoglobin, and that subsequent one-electron reduction and protonation generate a ternary complex of structure [XH–Hb^{3+}–OOH$^-$], where XH is the substrate and –OOH$^-$ is bound peroxide anion (Mieyal, 1985; Mieyal et al., 1976). A comparable type of complex is formed in the catalytic cycle of cytochrome P450 (i.e. [XH–Fe^{3+}–OOH$^-$], see Section 3.5), but whether the mechanism of O–O cleavage is identical for the two complexes is not fully elucidated. Another open question is the nature of the active oxygen species generated in the catalytic cycle of hemoglobin; an oxenoid species has been postulated but proof still appears to be lacking.

9.I   9.II   9.III

para-Hydroxylation also occurs with aniline derivatives and analogues such as o-toluidine, m-toluidine, N-methylaniline (Table 9.1, Starke et al., 1984), and with phenol (Mieyal, 1985). Another reaction involving **C-sp^2 atoms** is the epoxidation of styrene to styrene oxide (**9.II**) which occurs in human blood red cells where it is catalyzed by oxyhemoglobin (Belvedere and Tursi, 1981). In contrast to other known examples of hemoglobin-mediated monooxygenation, the epoxidation of styrene was reported to be only marginally stimulated by NADPH and NADH.

Aliphatic hydroxylation reactions, e.g. the oxidation of cyclohexane to cyclohexanol, are also catalyzed by oxyhemoglobin. The K_m for the reaction (1 mM) was similar to that for the reaction catalyzed by CYP2B4, but the turnover number (0.052 min^{-1}) was less than 1/500 that

TABLE 9.1 *Carbon hydroxylation reactions catalyzed by isolated hemoglobin; a few values for cytochrome P450 isozymes are reported for comparison purposes* (Starke et al., 1984)

Substrate	Reaction	K_m (mM)	Turnover number (min^{-1})	
			Hemoglobin	CYP
Aniline	p-hydroxylation	5.7	0.064	1.0 (2B4) 0.4 (1A2)
o-Toluidine	p-hydroxylation	65.4	0.068	
m-Toluidine	p-hydroxylation	87.0	0.004	
N-Methylaniline	p-hydroxylation	3.6	0.025	
	N-demethylation	0.52	0.16	
Benzphetamine	N-demethylation	0.42	0.11	56.8 (2B4) 4.9 (1A2)
Anisole	O-demethylation	0.89	0.44	
p-Anisidine	O-demethylation	36.4	0.66	
p-Nitroanisole	O-demethylation	0.094	0.21	5.7 (2B4) 3.4 (1A2)

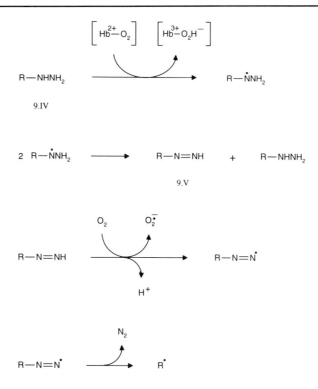

FIGURE 9.1 Enzymatic and postenzymatic mechanisms of the oxidation of phenylhydrazine (**9.IV**; R = phenyl) and phenelzine (**9.IV**; R = phenylethyl) by hemoglobin. (Modified from Maples *et al.*, 1988a and 1988b).

for the cytochrome P450 reaction (30 min^{-1}) (Starke and Mieyal, 1989). Other hydroxylation reactions of hemoglobin include demethylations, the K_m values and turnover numbers of which are given in Table 9.1. Thus, the N-demethylation of N-methylaniline displayed typical Michaelis–Menten kinetics and was almost 50 times more efficient than its *p*-hydroxylation (Starke *et al.*, 1984; Stecca *et al.*, 1992). As far as O-demethylation is concerned, anisole (**9.III**; R = H) and *p*-nitroanisole (**9.III**; R = NO$_2$) had a higher affinity than *p*-anisidine (**9.III**, R = NH$_2$). Comparison of turnover numbers with those of CYP2B4 and 1A2 show 6- to 500-fold smaller values.

9.2.3 Reactions of nitrogen oxidation

The oxidations of hydrazines and hydroxylamines are two reactions catalyzed by hemoglobin that have received particular attention since they induce the oxidative denaturation of hemoglobin.

The reaction of phenylhydrazine (**9.IV**; R = phenyl in Fig. 9.1) with erythrocytes has been an object of study for over a century. By denaturing hemoglobin, some **hydrazine derivatives** induce hemolytic anaemia, but the underlying molecular mechanisms have only recently been understood. Thus, there is convincing evidence to indicate that phenylhydrazine and phenelzine (**9.IV**, R = phenylethyl in Fig. 9.1) are oxidized by hemoglobin (Itano and Matteson, 1982; Maples *et al.*, 1988a and 1988b). One-electron oxidation by oxyhemoglobin and deprotonation lead to an N-centred hydrazinyl radical which disproportionates to the parent hydrazine and a **diazene** (**9.V** in Fig. 9.1). This diazene is rapidly oxidized by molecular oxygen to an unstable diazenyl radical which decomposes to N_2 and a phenyl or phenylethyl radical, respectively. This aryl or arylalkyl radical is the molecular species which denaturates hemoglobin by reacting with a cysteinyl thiol group and generating a hemoglobin-thiyl free radical (Hb–S$^\bullet$) (Mason and Maples, 1990). Other denaturation reactions occur; in particular, the superoxide anion generated during diazene oxidation can oxidize hemoglobin to methemoglobin.

Iproniazid (**9.VI**) is another hydrazine-based drug similarly oxidized by hemoglobin; in contrast, no radical formation was detected with isoniazid and hydralazine (Maples *et al.*, 1988b).

CONHNH—

9.VI

A number of **aromatic amines** are also substrates of hemoglobin. Thus, 2-aminofluorene was oxygenated by human red blood cell cytosol to the hydroxylamine (Duverger-van Bogaert *et al.*, 1992). The reaction may continue, because as shown in Fig. 9.2 **arylhydroxylamines** and **arylhydroxylamides** (**9.VII** in Fig. 9.2) can be substrates for oxyhemoglobin-catalyzed one-electron oxidation (reaction **a** in Fig. 9.2) to the corresponding nitroxide radical (**9.VIII** in Fig. 9.2). In the process, hemoglobin is oxidized to methemoglobin with bound hydrogen peroxide anion, this complex liberating methemoglobin and hydrogen peroxide (reaction **b** in Fig. 9.2). As for the nitroxide, its further fate depends largely on whether the parent compound is an arylhydroxylamine or an N-hydroxy-N-arylacetamide. In the latter case, fast reduction back to the parent compound is catalyzed by oxyhemoglobin, which is oxidized in the process to methemoglobin (reaction **c** in Fig. 9.2). In such a reaction, the arylhydroxylamide acts as a genuine catalyst which oxidizes two molecules of hemoglobin to methemoglobin in each cycle (Heilmair *et al.*, 1987; Lenk and Riedl, 1989). Among a series of arylhydroxylamides, N-hydroxy-4-chloroacetamide proved the most active, and N-hydroxyacetanilide the least, in oxidizing hemoglobin.

For **arylhydroxylamines** (reaction **d** in Fig. 9.2), the reaction of the nitroxide with oxyhemoglobin results in oxidation of the latter to an arylnitroso derivative (**9.IX** in Fig. 9.2), oxygen being reduced to superoxide (Harrison and Jollow, 1987; Lenk and Riedl, 1989). **Nitroso metabolites** can also be formed by postenzymatic oxidation of the arylhydroxylamines, the mediator being hydrogen peroxide liberated in reaction **b** (Fig. 9.2). Postenzymatic reactions of the arylnitroso metabolites have also been characterized, in particular formation of nitro derivatives and ferroheme–nitrosoarene complexes, and covalent binding to thiol groups in hemoglobin (Heilmair *et al.*, 1991; Lenk and Riedl, 1989; Sabbioni, 1992).

9.3 REACTIONS CATALYZED BY DOPAMINE β-MONOOXYGENASE

Dopamine β-monooxygenase (DBM), also called dopamine β-hydroxylase, is an apparently highly specialized enzyme the physiological role of which is to catalyze the hydroxylation of dopamine (**9.X**) to (−)-(*R*)-noradrenaline (**9.XI**). However, it has been recognized for at least three decades that DBM is also able to β-hydroxylate a large variety of exogenous and endogenous phenylethylamines (van der Schoot and Creveling, 1965). In addition, the enzyme is attracting considerable interest as a target for inhibitors which would lower noradrenaline levels

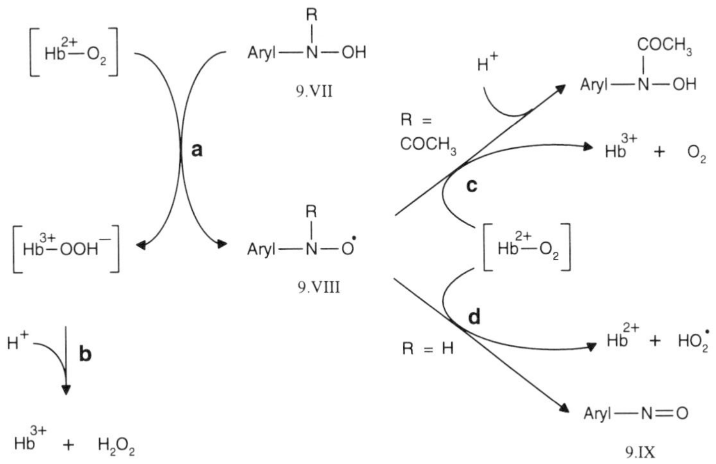

FIGURE 9.2 Interactions of arylhydroxylamines (**9.VII**; R = H) and N-hydroxy-N-arylacetamides (**9.VII**; R = acetyl) with oxyhemoglobin. The primary metabolite is a nitroxide radical (**9.VIII**) whose further fate depends on the chemical nature of the R substituent.

while elevating dopamine levels, thereby modulating sympathetic drive and permitting the treatment of some cardiovascular disorders.

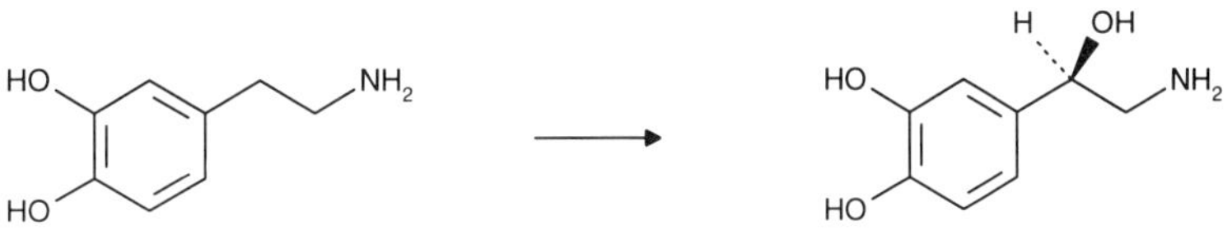

9.3.1 Enzymology and catalytic mechanism of DBM

Dopamine β-monooxygenase [3,4-dihydroxyphenethylamine, ascorbate:oxygen oxidoreductase (β-hydroxylating); EC 1.14.17.1] is a copper-containing monooxygenase expressed primarily in the sympathetic ganglia, the adrenal medulla and the brain nucleus locus ceruleus. The enzyme, which exists in both membranal and soluble forms, is a tetrameric glycoprotein whose subunits display apparent molecular weights of about 66 to 82 kDa (Klinman *et al.*, 1990; Lerch, 1981; Oyarce and Fleming, 1991). The tetramer (MW of about 290 kDa) has been termed **DBH-A**, but a dimer (**DBH-B**, MW 147 kDa) and a novel form (MW 125 kDa, designated as **DBH-C**) have been characterized and postulated to be the products of naturally occurring, tissue-specific degradation processes (Fraeyman *et al.*, 1988). Several studies have now established the primary amino acid sequence of bovine adrenal DBM (Lewis *et al.*, 1990; Robertson *et al.*, 1990; Taljanidisz *et al.*, 1989; Wang *et al.*, 1990; Wong and Bildstein, 1990).

   While large variations have been reported in the number of copper ions per subunit, maximal activity is found with 8 Cu(II) per tetramer, implying that the active site in each subunit of DBM contains two Cu(II) atoms. Each copper atom is believed to be equatorially coordinated to four nitrogen atoms, presumably four imidazole ligands of histidinyl side-chains in a planar square environment (Blumberg *et al.*, 1989; Scott *et al.*, 1988). Contradictory results have been presented

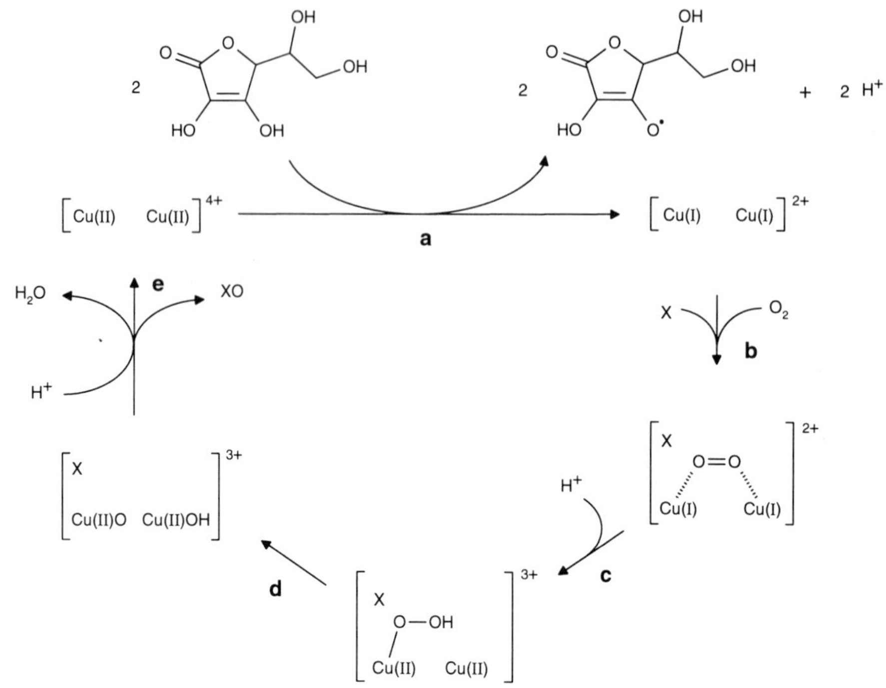

FIGURE 9.3 Postulated mechanism of oxygen activation and substrate monooxygenation by dopamine β-monooxygenase (symbolized by the two copper cations in its active site). The enzyme in its resting state is reduced by two molecules of ascorbate (reaction a). Binding of the substrate (X) and molecular oxygen leads to a ternary complex (reaction b); activation and cleavage of molecular oxygen (reactions c and d) is followed by substrate oxygenation and release of products (reaction e).

for the coordinated state of the Cu(I) atoms in the reduced, active form of the enzyme (see below); while one study concluded that there was a bicoordinated state plus a sulfur-containing ligand (Scott *et al.*, 1988), another indicated a tetracoordinated state closely resembling that of the oxidized form (Blumberg *et al.*, 1989).

DBM is a **genuine monooxygenase** in that, like cytochrome P450 and the FAD-containing monooxygenase, it cleaves molecular oxygen and transfers one oxygen atom to the substrate (X) while the other atom is released as H_2O:

$$X + O_2 + 2e^- + 2H^+ \rightarrow XO + H_2O \qquad \text{(Eq. 9.1)}$$

As in cytochrome P450, a catalytic role is played by the metal ion(s) to cleave O_2 and generate an active oxygen species. Further analogies between the catalytic mechanisms of the two monooxygenases can only be hypothesized in view of our preliminary understanding of the functioning of DBM.

Yet despite the many questions that remain, the available evidence is sufficient to postulate a fair if necessarily incomplete **catalytic cycle** (Fig. 9.3). The resting state of DBM is the oxidized one, and the enzymatic reaction begins with a double single-electron reduction to the reduced state (reaction **a** in Fig. 9.3). This reduction is mediated by two molecules of **ascorbate**, the electron donor in the reaction, which themselves are oxidized to semidehydroascorbate. In this one-electron oxidized form, vitamin C is recycled to reduced ascorbate by the vesicular cytochrome b_{561} system. High levels of ascorbate activate DBM, while fumarate and a number of other anions also stimulate the activity of DBM via complex kinetic effects (Huyghe and Klinman, 1991; Klinman *et al.*, 1990; Stewart and Klinman, 1991).

The reduced, catalytically competent form of DBM binds the substrate and molecular oxygen (reaction **b** in Fig. 9.3). Various kinetic mechanisms have been demonstrated depending on experimental conditions; at high pH values, the binding of oxygen and substrate seemingly occurs according to a random kinetic mechanism, while at low pH or in the presence of the activator fumarate an ordered mechanism exists with the substrate binding before oxygen (Kruse *et al.*, 1986a). Little is known of the substrate binding site, but evidence obtained with multisubstrate inhibitors (see Section 9.3.3) clearly shows that molecular oxygen binds to the two Cu(I) ions. Activation of oxygen then leads to a reactive copper–oxygen complex the nature of which has not been established. However, copper-to-oxygen transfer of two electrons to form an intermediate Cu(II)-hydroperoxide (reaction **c** in Fig. 9.3) appears as an attractive possibility (May *et al.*, 1981a; Padgette *et al.*, 1985; Wimalasena and May, 1987). This must be followed by oxygen cleavage (reaction **d** in Fig. 9.3) probably forming a copper–oxenoid complex $[CuO]^{2+}$ analogous to the iron–oxenoid complex $[FeO]^{3+}$ in cytochrome P450 and also exhibiting resonance forms. The second oxygen atom resulting from such a cleavage must appear as HO^- and yield H_2O (reaction **e** in Fig. 9.3).

To date, the best evidence for a copper–oxenoid complex comes from investigations on the **mechanism of substrate oxygenation** (reaction **e** in Fig. 9.3). Indeed, available data point to striking similarities with the iron–oxenoid complex in cytochrome P450 (see Chapters 3–7). Thus, hydroxylation of sp^3-hybridized carbons (next Section) is initiated by hydrogen radical abstraction—in other words it involves a typical **oxygen rebound mechanism** (see Section 4.2) (White, 1991). N-Demethylations and sulfoxidations (next Section) are initiated by one-electron oxidation of the heteroatom, another reaction typical of a metal–oxenoid complex (see Sections 6.2 and 7.7).

9.3.2 Reactions of oxygenation and oxidation

DBM is of considerable interest since it is able to catalyze several reactions of oxygenation or oxidation on carbon atoms or heteroatoms. The target sites attacked include sp^3- and sp^2-hybridized carbons, and nitrogen, sulfur and selenium atoms. Phenol oxidation (i.e. O–H homolytic cleavage) has also been recently characterized (see Section 9.3.3) (Kim and Klinman, 1991).

The oxygenation of **sp^3-hybridized carbons** is of course the best known reaction of DBM and is illustrated by the physiological function of this enzyme, i.e. the above-noted hydroxylation of **dopamine to noradrenaline**. This reaction occurs with apparently complete **product regioselectivity** for the benzylic position and **product enantioselectivity** to the *R*-configurated metabolite (which is the active enantiomer). This very high or complete product enantio-selectivity is much greater than is seen with cytochrome P450-catalyzed hydroxylations and suggests an even faster radical recombination (see Section 4.2).

Besides dopamine, a number of other derivatives of 2-phenylethylamine (**9.XII**; R = H) are substrates. Thus, the data in Table 9.2 show that **tyramine** (**9.XII**; R = OH) is as good a substrate as dopamine (**9.X**). The unfavourable influence of a number of substituents (e.g. *ortho*-hydroxy, *para*-methoxy, N-methyl, and 2-methyl) is also documented. A quantitative structure–metabolism relationship study concluded that an electron-withdrawing substituent in the *para*-position is unfavourable, as are bulky substituents on the aromatic ring in general, implying a constrained binding pocket (Miller and Klinman, 1985).

The high selectivity of DBM for the *pro-R* position allows this enzyme to hydroxylate phenylethylamines bearing a *2S*-OH group, e.g. (*S*)-octopamine (**9.XIII**) but not (*R*)-octopamine.

TABLE 9.2 *Relative activity of substrates of dopamine β-monooxygenase* (van der Schoot and Creveling, 1965)

Substrate	Relative activity
2-Phenylethylamine (**9.XII**; R = H)	63
2-(4-Hydroxyphenyl)ethylamine (tyramine)	100
2-(3-Hydroxyphenyl)ethylamine	77
2-(2-Hydroxyphenyl)ethylamine	0
2-(4-Methoxyphenyl)ethylamine	3
N-Methyl-2-(4-hydroxyphenyl)ethylamine	25
N,N-Dimethyl-2-(4-hydroxyphenyl)ethylamine	0
2-(4-Hydroxyphenyl)-1-methylethylamine	65
2-(4-Hydroxyphenyl)-2-methylethylamine	8
2-(3,4-Dihydroxyphenyl)ethylamine (**9.X**)	93
2-(4-Hydroxy-3-methoxyphenyl)ethylamine	70
2-(3-Hydroxy-4-methoxyphenyl)ethylamine	2
2-(3,4-Dimethoxyphenyl)ethylamine	2

The proximate metabolite of the reaction is the *gem*-diol **9.XIV** which rapidly dehydrates to 4-hydroxy-α-aminoacetophenone (**9.XV**), the actual product which can be isolated. Kinetic analysis gave $k_{cat} = 33\ s^{-1}$ and $K_m = 14\ mM$, while tyramine gave $80\ s^{-1}$ and $2.0\ mM$, respectively (May *et al.*, 1981b). Such a reaction of carbinol hydroxylation, which is termed an **oxygenative ketonization**, also occurs with cytochrome P450 (Section 7.6). Xenobiotic substrates of DBM undergoing this reaction include (S)-noradrenaline to give the potent agent noradrenalone, and the Khat alkaloid (+)-(1S; 2S)-norpseudoephedrine (**9.XVI**) whose ketonization results in bioactivation to (S)-cathinone (**9.XVII**) (Debnath *et al.*, 1992; May *et al.*, 1982). The oxygenative ketonization of β-chlorophenethylamine will be discussed in Section 9.3.3.

That **an aromatic ring is not a requisite** for DBM substrate activity is illustrated by the comparatively facile hydroxylation of 2-(1-cyclohexenyl)ethylamine (**9.XVIII**) ($k_{cat} = 90 \text{ s}^{-1}$, $K_m = 6.1$ mM) (Sirimanne and May, 1988). The reaction occurred with complete regioselectivity for the exocyclic allylic position, and complete enantioselectivity for the *pro-R* position; no epoxide or ring-hydroxylated metabolites were detected. It is therefore all the more interesting to compare the oxygenation of **9.XVIII** to the oxidation of 1-(2-aminoethyl)-1,4-cyclohexadiene (**9.XIX**) ($k_{cat} = 72 \text{ s}^{-1}$, $K_m = 1.3$ mM). Indeed, this highly informative substrate *did* undergo hydrogen radical abstraction from a ring methylene, more precisely from position 6, to the postulated intermediate **9.XX**. The next stage however was not oxygen rebound but seemingly abstraction of a second hydrogen radical, resulting in aromatization and formation of phenylethylamine (**9.XXI**), the isolated metabolite (Wimalasena and May, 1989). Compound **9.XIX** thus offers one of the very few known examples of **redirected regioselectivity** in a DBM-catalyzed reaction. Other possible pathways leading from **9.XIX** to **9.XXI** were ruled out by various experiments, and this cleverly chosen substrate afforded one of the most convincing proofs for hydrogen radical abstraction in the mechanism of DBM.

In the above examples, no ring epoxides were detected as products of olefin oxygenation, but there are a few examples to show that DBM can catalyze **sp²-carbon epoxidation** at catalytically accessible positions. Thus, 1-phenyl-1-(aminomethyl)ethene (**9.XXII**) is both a substrate of DBM (yielding the epoxide **9.XXIII** with $k_{cat} = 14 \text{ s}^{-1}$, $K_m = 6.7$ mM) and an inhibitor acting in an apparent mechanism-based manner (see Section 9.3.3). A common radical intermediate was postulated to account for substrate oxygenation and enzyme inactivation (Padgette *et al.*, 1985).

9.XVIII

9.XIX

9.XX

9.XXI

9.XXII

9.XXIII

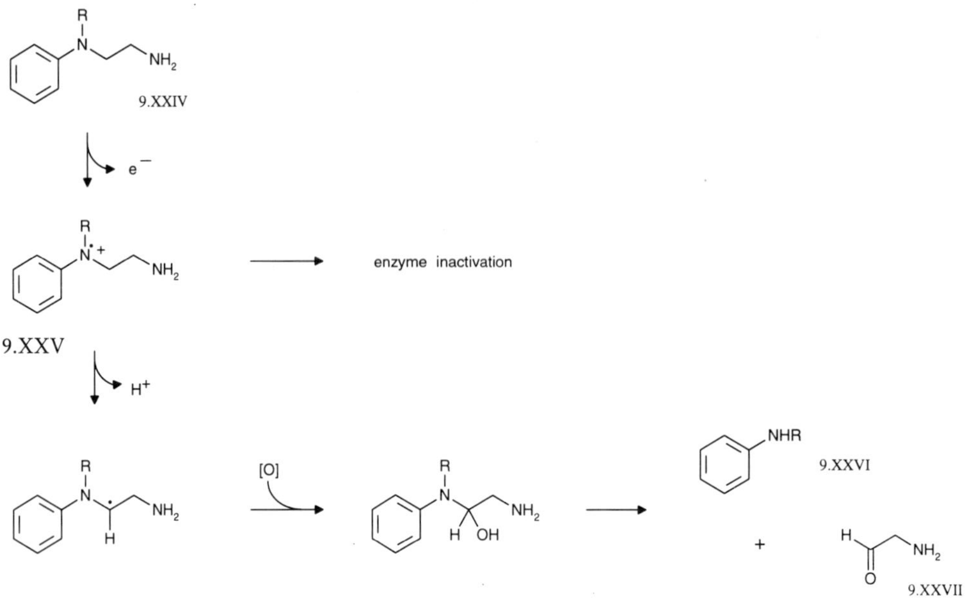

FIGURE 9.4 Postulated mechanism of DBM-mediated N-dealkylation of N-phenylethylenediamine (**9.XXIV**; R = H) and N-methyl-N-phenylethylenediamine (**9.XXIV**; R = methyl) via single-electron N-oxidation. The nitrogen cation radical **9.XXV** also binds covalently to the enzyme and inactivates it (Wimalasena and May, 1987).

The versatility of DBM is most eloquently demonstrated by its ability **to oxidize or oxygenate some heteroatoms** adjacent to the phenyl ring in analogues of phenylethylamine. Specifically, oxidation (i.e. one-electron abstraction) can occur for a nitrogen atom, while oxygenation is documented for a sulfur or selenium atom. Thus, **N-oxidation** was demonstrated for N-phenylethylenediamine (**9.XXIV** in Fig. 9.4; R = H) and its N-methyl derivative (**9.XXIV** in Fig. 9.4; R = methyl). The products of the reaction were characterized as aniline (**9.XXVI** in Fig. 9.4; R = H) or N-methylaniline (**9.XXVI** in Fig. 9.4; R = methyl), respectively, and 2-aminoacetaldehyde (**9.XXVII** in Fig. 9.4) (Wimalasena and May, 1987). Proof that this reaction of **N-dealkylation** occurs via single-electron oxidation of the nitrogen atom to yield the nitrogen cation radical **9.XXV** in Fig. 9.4 was given by the fact that the oxygen isostere (phenyl 2-aminoethyl ether) and other oxygenated analogues were not substrates but competitive inhibitors. In the postulated mechanism (Fig. 9.4), the cation radical **9.XXV** rearranges by proton expulsion to a C-centred radical that becomes the target of oxygen rebound to form a carbinolamine which will then hydrolyze to the amine **9.XXVI** and the aldehyde **9.XXVII**. The analogy with one of the mechanisms of cytochrome P450-catalyzed N-dealkylation is essentially complete (Section 6.2).

The nitrogen cation radical **9.XXV** in Fig. 9.4 is also directly responsible for **enzyme inactivation** by covalent attachment, with a kinetic partition ratio for N-phenylethylenediamine of 1750 turnovers per inactivation (Wimalasena and May, 1987). Interestingly, analogues lacking the basic side-chain, e.g. aniline, N-ethylaniline, and ring-substituted anilines, were found not to exhibit substrate activity but to be pure mechanism-based inactivators, again indicating oxidation of the nitrogen atom adjacent to the aromatic ring.

DBM also mediates **S-oxygenation**, as exemplified by the substrate phenyl 2-aminoethyl sulfide (**9.XXVIII**) (May and Phillips, 1980; May et al., 1981). The product was the sulfoxide with *S*-configuration (**9.XXIX**), i.e. the same spatial arrangement of oxygen, phenyl and side-chain as seen in the (*R*)-phenylethanolamines. The reaction was a facile process with kinetic constants comparable to those for the hydroxylation of phenylethylamines. As far as the catalytic mechanism is concerned, it was found to involve a nucleophilic attack with a much larger charge development in the transition state than in the hydroxylation reaction (as deduced from quantitative structure–metabolism relationships for *para*-substituted analogues). It has been suggested that S-oxygenation occurs concertedly with O–O cleavage (May *et al.*, 1981).

9.XXVIII   9.XXIX

9.XXX   9.XXXI

Phenyl 2-aminoethyl selenide (**9.XXX**) is also a substrate of DBM, undergoing **Se-oxygenation** to the selenoxide **9.XXXI** (May *et al.*, 1988). There is however a major difference between the sulfoxide and selenoxide metabolites in that the latter is non-enzymatically reduced back to the selenide by the cofactor ascorbate. In this reaction, ascorbate is fully oxidized to dehydroascorbate which, in contrast to semidehydroascorbate, cannot be regenerated by the cytochrome b_{561} recycling system. This leads *in vitro* to rapid termination of DBM-catalyzed turnover due to depletion of the essential reductant; a similar situation occurs *in vivo* due to compartmentalized cofactor depletion. This turnover-dependent cofactor depletion was shown to be accompanied in rats by marked antihypertensive effects (May *et al.*, 1988).

9.3.3 Multisubstrate and mechanism-based inactivators of DBM

Besides competitive inhibitors not considered here, cofactor depletors mentioned above, and mechanism-based inactivators discussed below, there exists a class of inhibitors particular to DBM. These compounds bind to the reduced enzyme at both the substrate and oxygen binding sites and thus behave simultaneously as substrate and O_2 mimics. They are thus called **multisubstrate inhibitors**, and their mode of binding, as illustrated in Fig. 9.5, sheds light on the topography of the DBM active site.

Such inhibitors include for example 1-benzylimidazole-2-thiones (Fig. 9.5B) where the phenyl ring is the dopamine mimic and the heterocycle the oxygen mimic (Kruse *et al.*, 1986a and 1986b). Other multisubstrate inhibitors have been described, e.g. analogues with the oxygen mimic being a triazole-thione, a tetrazole-thione, a pyridine-thione, or a pyrimidine-thione (Kruse *et al.*, 1990). Some of these compounds are quite active, with IC_{50} values in the micromolar range or even below (Kruse *et al.*, 1986b and 1990). The kinetics of inhibition are rather complex and condition-dependent and change with the sequence of substrate and oxygen binding (Kruse *et al.*, 1986a).

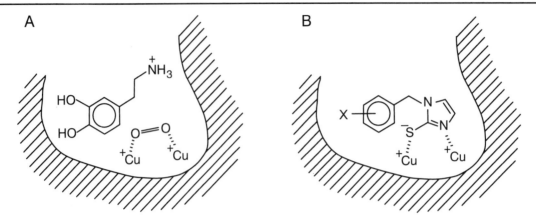

FIGURE 9.5 Comparison between postulated modes of binding to the active site of DBM. A: Dopamine and oxygen; B: multisubstrate inhibitors of the 1-benzylimidazole-2-thione type. (Reproduced from Kruse *et al.*, 1990, with the permission of the copyright holder.)

Mechanism-based inactivators are also of interest in the present context in that they afford valuable information on the catalytic mechanism of DBM. A few such inhibitors have been discussed in the previous section, e.g. 1-phenyl-1-(aminomethyl)ethene (**9.XXII**) and N-phenylethylenediamines (**9.XXIV**), inasmuch as they uniquely illustrate novel metabolic reactions of DBM to stable products. Most of the mechanism-based inhibitors to be examined now also **partition between turnover and inactivation**, but the stable metabolites they generate are not novel.

A first group of inhibitors to be considered are phenols (**9.XXXII** in Fig. 9.6). They undergo C-hydroxylation in the benzylic position to stable products (**9.XXXIV** in Fig. 9.6), but the intermediate C-centred radical (**9.XXXIII** in Fig. 9.6) partitions between oxygen rebound (reaction **a** in Fig. 9.6) and covalent binding to the enzyme either directly (reaction **b** in Fig. 9.6) or after rearrangement to a radical centred in a terminal position (reactions **c** and **d** in Fig. 9.6). The first case is that of *p*-cresol (**9.XXXII** in Fig. 9.6; R = R′ = H) and related alkylphenols (Goodhart *et al.*, 1987). DBM oxidizes *p*-cresol to 4-hydroxybenzyl alcohol (**9.XXXIV** in Fig. 9.6; R = H, R′ = OH), and this metabolite can be further oxidized by DBM to the aldehyde in an interesting reaction of oxygenative ketonization or rather **carbonylation**. The intermediate radical in the oxidation of *p*-cresol also binds covalently to the enzyme, its partition ratio (turnover/inactivation) being approximately 1300:1. The fact that cresols can be substrates of DBM indicates that binding to and oxidation by DBM do not require an aminoethyl side-chain.

Recent studies suggest that the mechanism of cresol oxidation by DBM might be more complex than shown in Fig. 9.6, with C–H cleavage leading to turnover, and O–H cleavage leading to inactivation (Kim and Klinman, 1991). The fact that phenol itself is also a mechanism-based inactivator of DBM confirms that an alkyl side-chain is not an obligatory component of enzyme inhibition. These findings indicate the ability of DBM also to catalyze **phenol oxidation**, when the structure of the substrate is such that it can bind with the hydroxyl group oriented towards the catalytic site.

Other irreversible inhibitors activated according to Fig. 9.6 include 3-phenylpropenes (**9.XXXII** in Fig. 9.6; R = –C(X)=CH$_2$, R′ = H) and β-ethynyltyramine. The former compounds (X = H, Cl, Br or CH$_3$) displayed partition ratios in the range 40–90, i.e. considerable efficiency in inactivating the enzyme (Flory and Villafranca, 1988). As for β-ethynyltyramine (**9.XXXII** in Fig. 9.6; R = ethynyl, R′ = –CH$_2$NH$_2$), the *R*-enantiomer was a reversible,

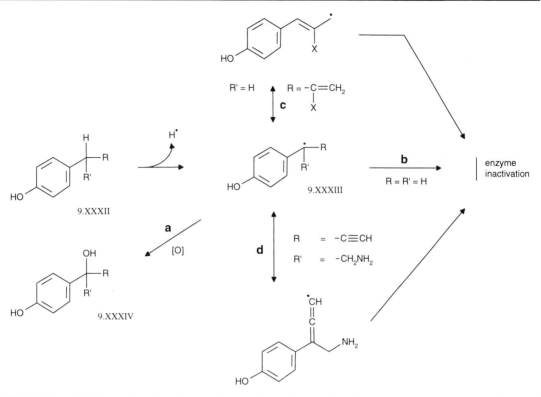

FIGURE 9.6 DBM-catalyzed oxidation of benzylic mechanism-based inactivators to reactive radicals and stable metabolites (compiled from DeWolf *et al.*, 1989; Flory and Villafranca, 1988; Goodhart *et al.*, 1987). In the case of *p*-cresol (**9.XXXII**; R = R′ = H), enzyme inactivation results (perhaps predominantly) from O–H cleavage (Kim and Klinman, 1991).

competitive inhibitor of DBM, while the *S*-enantiomer was both a competitive inhibitor (albeit less active than the *R*-enantiomer) and a mechanism-based inactivator with a very low partition ratio of about 2.5 (DeWolf *et al.*, 1989). Indeed, β-ethynyltyramine, while having a nearly 100-fold higher affinity for the enzyme than tyramine, is β-hydroxylated with 100-fold slower k_{cat}. It is also interesting that covalent binding was to a histidine residue.

   Ketones, aldehydes and amides form another group of irreversible inhibitors, the mechanisms of which show similarities in the last steps of activation, but differences in the first steps (Fig. 9.7). β-Chlorophenethylamine (**9.XXXV** in Fig. 9.7) is particularly interesting both as a substrate and an inactivator. Indeed, the compound reacts like a β-hydroxylated compound and undergoes oxygenative ketonization to α-aminoacetophenone (**9.XXXVI** in Fig. 9.7) (Bossard and Kliman, 1990). This metabolite can either dissociate from the enzyme, or, while remaining bound, be oxidized by DBM as the enol tautomer to a radical cation (**9.XXXIX** in Fig. 9.7) which inactivates the enzyme. The postulated mechanism of one-electron oxidation of the enol is believed to involve reduction of a Cu(II) atom in the active site. A similar mechanism occurs in the activation of aldehydes such phenylacetaldehyde (**9.XXXVII** in Fig. 9.7), which undergoes benzylic hydroxylation to the stable metabolite hydroxyphenylacetaldehyde (**9.XXXVIII** in Fig. 9.7). The latter can partition between release from the enzyme and one-electron oxidation (in the enolic form) to a protonated radical (**9.XXXIX** in Fig. 9.7) which inactivates the enzyme (Bossard and Klinman, 1986).

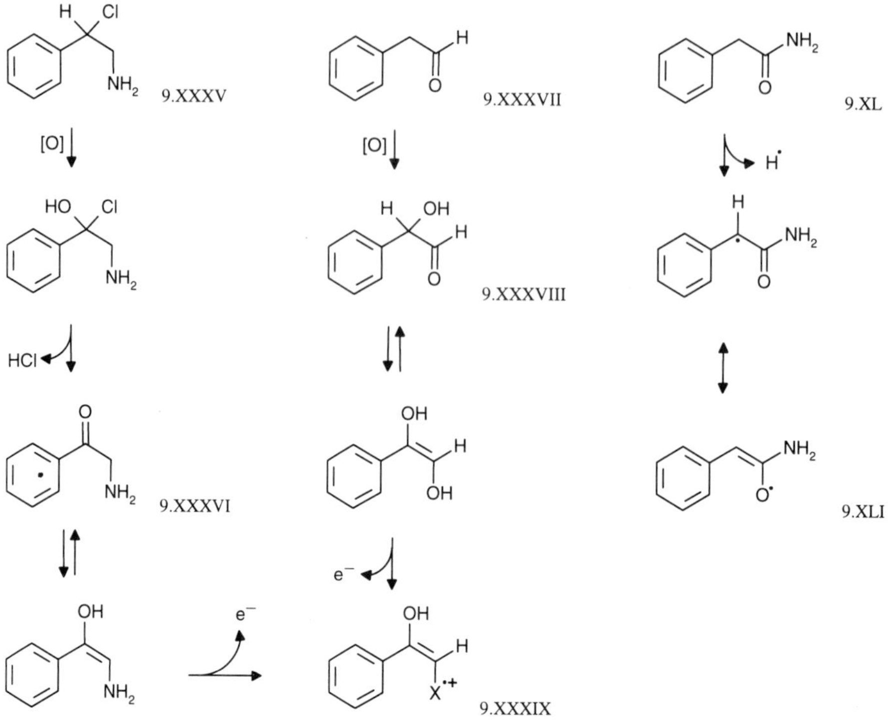

FIGURE 9.7 Postulated mechanisms in the DBM-catalyzed activation of ketones, aldehydes and amides to radicals which are the inactivating species. (Modified from Bossard and Klinman, 1986 and 1990.)

Amides such as phenylacetamide (**9.XL** in Fig. 9.7) are activated to similar radicals, but the reaction is simpler since the hydroxylation step does not occur. Abstraction of a hydrogen atom from the benzylic position forms a radical which delocalizes (as does **9.XXXIX** in Fig. 9.7) over several atoms (**9.XLI** in Fig. 9.7). This radical is again the form which inactivates the enzyme (Bossard and Klinman, 1986). Partition ratios of 2000, 1600 and 610 were reported for β-chlorophenethylamine, phenylacetaldehyde and p-hydroxyphenylacetamide, respectively.

Other mechanism-based inactivators of DBM have been characterized. Thus, **olefins** such as 1-phenyl-1-(aminomethylethene) (**9.XXII**, see Section 9.3.2) form a C-centred radical which can partition between epoxidation and enzyme inactivation, as do hydroxybenzofurans (Farrington *et al.*, 1989; Padgette *et al.*, 1985). Interestingly, **phenylhydrazine** (**9.IV** in Fig. 9.1; R = phenyl) which is discussed in Section 9.2.3 as an inactivator of hemoglobin is also a mechanism-based inhibitor of DBM. While the reactive intermediate is the phenyl radical in both cases, the mechanisms catalyzed by the two enzymes differ in that DBM oxidizes the nitrogen atom adjacent to the aromatic ring rather than the terminal one (Farrington *et al.*, 1990).

In conclusion, dopamine β-monooxygenase has in recent years been shown to have an unexpected versatility in terms of **chemospecificity** rather than regiospecificity and catalytic mechanisms. While these findings markedly increase the number of known and potential substrates of DBM, the quantitative involvement of this enzyme in xenobiotic metabolism is unlikely ever to reach the significance of cytochrome P450 and the FAD-containing mono-oxygenase, if only for its restricted localization. In contrast, the qualitative significance of DBM as a target of inhibitors of therapeutic interest justifies the comparative length of the above discussion.

9.4 REACTIONS CATALYZED BY MONOAMINE OXIDASE

Monoamine oxidase (MAO) has for decades interested medicinal chemists as a target for **irreversible inhibitors** used therapeutically as antidepressants. These agents are now considered obsolete due to side-effects such as the well-known "cheese effect", i.e. hypertensive crises due to inhibition of the degradation of alimentary tyramine. In contrast, modern investigations aimed at developing selective, **reversible inhibitors** of MAO have met with significant success (Kyburz, 1990; Youdim and Finberg, 1991). In addition to this therapeutic interest, MAO has gained considerable significance since the mid-eighties when its capacity to activate exogenous neurotoxins was discovered (e.g. Maret *et al.*, 1990a).

9.4.1 Enzymology and endogenous substrates of MAO

Monoamine oxidase [monoamine:oxygen oxidoreductase (deaminating) (flavin-containing); EC 1.4.3.4] is an FAD-containing enzyme which is widely distributed in most tissues of mammals and other animals (Singer, 1991; Tipton, 1980). The presence of MAO in brain is of particular importance in connection with the therapeutic profile of its inhibitors and its role as an activator of xenobiotics (Gerlach and Riederer, 1993; O'Carroll *et al.*, 1989).

   MAO is a membrane-bound enzyme mainly located in the mitochondria, although some activity has also been found in microsomes, in cytosol and even in the extracellular space (Gomez *et al.*, 1988; Sim and Lim, 1992; Tipton, 1986). The existence of two different forms of the enzyme (**MAO-A** and **MAO-B**) has been proven beyond doubt by protein sequencing and by cloning and sequencing cDNA coding for human, bovine and rat MAO-A and MAO-B (Hsu *et al.*, 1989; Powell, 1991; Shih, 1991 and 1993; Weyler *et al.*, 1990; Wu *et al.*, 1993). The **subunits** of MAO-A and MAO-B are composed of 527 and 520 amino acids, respectively, and are derived from separate genes. The overall structural homology between the two forms from the same species is about 70%, with highly conserved regions. One of these regions (residues 389–460 for MAO-A) near the C-terminal contains the cysteine residue (406 for MAO-A, 397 for MAO-B) which serves as the site of covalent attachment of flavine-adenine dinucleotide (FAD), as shown in Fig. 9.8. Another conserved region near the N-terminal includes an ADP-binding domain (residues 15–45 for MAO-A) and is presumably also involved in binding of FAD at the active site of the enzyme. A third highly conserved region (residues 187–230 for MAO-A) has also been postulated to be part of the active site. A hydrophobic region (residues 504–521 in MAO-A) flanked by positively charged residues might be involved in the targeting and anchoring of the protein. MAO enzymes are seemingly made up of two subunits, each of which carries its own FAD. It is not known with certainty at this time whether multiple subunits exist, but there are indications to this effect (Chen and Weyler, 1988; Hsu *et al.*, 1989; Kyburz, 1990; Obata *et al.*, 1990).

   Some studies suggest a complex interplay between the two enzyme forms, since MAO-A or a factor tightly bound to it was found to modify MAO-B. This resulted in the modified MAO-B preserving its immunospecificity but displaying both MAO-A and MAO-B substrate and inhibitor affinities (Szutowicz *et al.*, 1989).

   Selective **substrates** and selective **inhibitors** afforded the first evidence for the existence of two enzymatic forms. A number of inhibitors and physiological/endogenous substrates of MAO are shown in Fig. 9.9. Serotonin (5-hydroxytryptamine, **9.XLII** in Fig. 9.9) and phenylethylamine (**9.XXI** in Fig. 9.9) are traditionally cited as selective substrates of MAO-A and MAO-B, respectively (Glover and Sandler, 1987). To this list, one can add the secondary amine adrenaline as a non-selective substrate, and benzylamine as a selective MAO-B substrate. An interesting

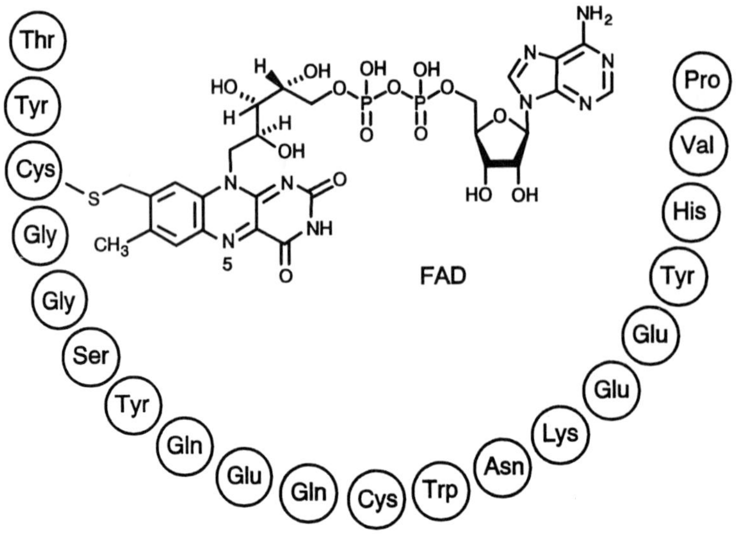

FIGURE 9.8 FAD and its site of covalent attachment to MAO-A (Cys-406) and MAO-B (Cys-397), together with a few residues in the highly conserved region. (Reproduced from Kyburz, 1990, with the permission of the copyright holder.)

rationalization derived from studies with both endogenous substrates and mechanism-based irreversible inactivators (suicide substrates, see Section 9.4.4) showed that MAO-A and MAO-B react with amines having a distance of 2–3 atoms and 1–2 atoms between the basic nitrogen and the aromatic ring, respectively (Kalir *et al.*, 1981).

9.4.2 Catalytic mechanism of MAO

The physiological substrates of MAO are predominantly primary amines which are oxidatively deaminated according to the following **reaction** (Tipton *et al.*, 1987; Weyler *et al.*, 1990):

$$RCH_2NR'R'' + O_2 + H_2O \rightarrow RCHO + NHR'R'' + H_2O_2 \qquad \text{(Eq. 9.2)}$$

This overall reaction is composed of **two half-reactions**, the first of which produces the aldehyde, the amine, and the enzyme in the reduced form:

$$[FAD] + RCH_2NR'R'' + H_2O \rightarrow [FADH_2] + RCHO + NHR'R'' \qquad \text{(Eq. 9.3)}$$

In the second half-reaction, reoxidation of the reduced enzyme by molecular oxygen occurs with production of hydrogen peroxide:

$$[FADH_2] + O_2 \rightarrow [FAD] + H_2O_2 \qquad \text{(Eq. 9.4)}$$

The hydrogen peroxide thus released may activate some neurotoxins such as 6-hydroxydopamine and 5,7-dihydroxytryptamine, a fact of potential toxicological significance (Cohen, 1986).

The detailed **catalytic mechanism** of MAO is now partly understood following ongoing studies of particular elegance with both substrates and mechanism-based inactivators (e.g. Kyburz, 1990; Ottoboni *et al.*, 1989; Ramsay *et al.*, 1987; Silverman and Zieske, 1985; Silverman

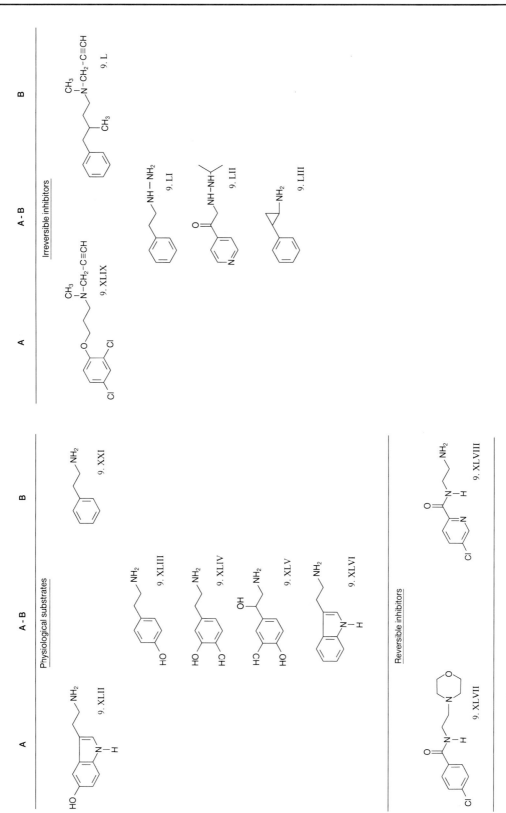

FIGURE 9.9 Chemical structures of a few selective or non-selective substrates, reversible inhibitors, and irreversible inhibitors of MAO. The compounds are: 5-hydroxytryptamine (**9.XLII**), phenylethylamine (**9.XXI**), *p*-tyramine (**9.XLIII**), dopamine (**9.XLIV**), noradrenaline (**9.XLV**), tryptamine (**9.XVI**), moclobemide (**9.XLVII**), lazabemide (**9.XLVIII**), clorgyline (**9.XLIX**), selegiline (**9.L**, (−)-deprenyl), phenelzine (**9.LI**), iproniazid (**9.LII**), and tranylcypromine (**9.LIII**).

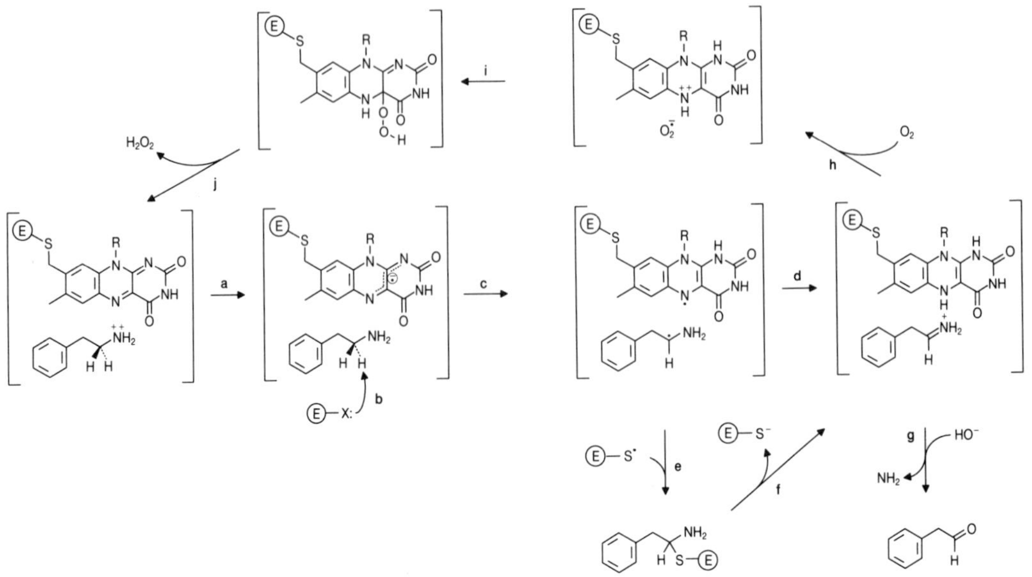

FIGURE 9.10 Postulated general mechanism of MAO-catalyzed oxidative deamination, phenylethylamine being taken as a representative substrate. Pathways of deamination follow reactions **a–g**, while flavin reoxidation follows reactions **h–j**. For further details see text.

et al., 1980; Simpson *et al.*, 1982; Tipton, 1986; Tipton *et al.*, 1987; Tullman and Hanzlik, 1984; Yu and Tipton, 1989). As shown in Fig. 9.10 for 2-phenylethylamine, the reaction begins with a **single electron oxidation** of the nitrogen atom (reaction **a** in Fig. 9.10). This reaction is either rate-determining or contributes significantly to rate limitation.

One-electron oxidation of the amine renders more acidic the alpha-protons in the amine radical cation and facilitates the next step of **proton abstraction** (or abstraction of a hydrogen atom followed by fast electron loss) (Silverman and Zelechonok, 1992). Specifically, the *pro-R* hydrogen is removed (reactions **b** and **c** in Fig. 9.10) as demonstrated for a variety of substrates such as benzylamine, dopamine and *n*-heptylamine (Battersby *et al.*, 1979; Yu and Davis, 1988; Yu *et al.*, 1986). This stereoselectivity implies that the reaction of proton removal is catalyzed, presumably by a nucleophilic group on the apoenzyme. Note that an alternative pathway, namely abstraction of a hydrogen radical, has also been discussed by some authors (see Section 9.4.3).

Following proton abstraction, a *second oxidation* step occurs to generate an imine or its iminium ion, while the enzyme reaches its two-electron reduced form (reaction **d** in Fig. 9.10). This FAD-mediated second oxidation step may well be restricted to substrates of relatively low oxidation potential. For substrates with a high second-electron oxidation potential, studies with mechanism-based inactivators have suggested an **alternative mechanism**, namely combination with an active-site residue, possibly a cysteinyl radical or another heteroatom in an amino acid side-chain, to give a covalent intermediate (reaction **e** in Fig. 9.10), followed by β-elimination to give the iminium ion (reaction **f** in Fig. 9.10) (Gates and Silverman, 1990; Silverman and Ding, 1993). However, insights obtained with time-dependent inhibitors (see Section 9.4.4) lead one to wonder which of the two pathways in Fig. 9.10, i.e. reactions **e–f** vs. reaction **d**, is the general mechanism of iminium formation. Note that, following reaction **f**, FAD can indeed reach the two-electron reduced form shown in Fig. 9.10 if electron transfer occurs within the active site.

The iminium ion undergoes **hydrolysis** to the corresponding aldehyde (reaction **g** in Fig.

9.10); kinetic evidence suggests that, at least in a number of cases, this reaction occurs on the enzyme surface without the imine being released. As for the reduced enzyme, it binds molecular oxygen and undergoes reoxidation with release of hydrogen peroxide (reactions **h**, **i** and **j** in Fig. 9.10).

The mechanism shown in Fig. 9.10 neglects some **subtle differences** that exist between the two forms of MAO in their mechanism and kinetics of deamination of various substrates (Tan and Ramsay, 1993). In the case of phenylethylamine and some other substrates of MAO-B, the release of products (i.e. the aldehyde and the amine) precedes oxygen binding, implying that deamination occurs exclusively via **binary complex** formation. In contrast, deamination of benzylamines by MAO-B involves the formation of a **ternary complex** with the reduced form of the enzyme (Edmondson *et al.*, 1993; Pearce and Roth, 1985; Ramsay, 1991; Tipton *et al.*, 1987). For MAO-A, formation of a ternary complex is also possible, but it involves oxygen plus substrate rather than product (Ramsay, 1991).

The above discussion shows clearly that MAO-catalyzed oxidative deamination differs fundamentally from the same reaction catalyzed by cytochrome P450 (Chapter 5). Not only do the mechanisms display essential differences, but one of the products is hydrogen peroxide with MAO and water with P450.

9.4.3 Exogenous substrates

A number of primary, secondary and tertiary amines of exogenous origin are known to be substrates of MAO. However, caution is necessary when examining published results as there is a danger of confusing cytochrome P450- and MAO-mediated deamination. For example, the oxidative deamination of amphetamine in highly purified rat liver mitochondria was ascribed to MAO, but without separating the potential activities of mitochondrial MAO and P450 (Blume, 1981). In fact, the effects of cofactors and inhibitors in this study are strongly suggestive of a significant contribution by mitochondrial cytochrome P450 activity. In a recent review, MAO involvement in xenobiotic metabolism is attributed to insufficiently documented cases (Strolin Benedetti *et al.*, 1988). Monitoring of hydrogen peroxide production, use of highly purified enzymes, high sensitivity to specific inhibitors, are some of the complementary ways of establishing the involvement of MAO.

Simple **primary n-alkylamines** of sufficient lipophilicity are good substrates of MAO-B (Yu, 1989). As shown in Table 9.3, activity increases from propylamine, reaches a maximum with octylamine, and drops dramatically beyond decylamine; methylamine and ethylamine are not metabolized, and nor are diamines such as putrescine (1,4-diaminobutane) and cadaverine (1,5-diaminopentane). Interestingly, N-acetylputrescine (a monoamine) is a substrate of MAO-B (Youdim and Finberg, 1991). The oxidation of ring-substituted benzylamines by MAO-B was shown to be markedly influenced by the position and electronic properties of the substituent (Walker and Edmondson, 1987). Another substrate of MAO-B is 2-propyl-1-aminopentane, whose deaminated product, 2-propyl-1-pentaldehyde, is a bioprecursor of the anticonvulsant valproic acid (Yu and Davis, 1991).

Among **secondary amines**, we may note the oxidation of the anticonvulsant **milacemide** (**9.LIV**), which is deaminated by MAO-B to pentanal (**9.LV**) and glycinamide (**9.LVI**), as well as to the products resulting from attack at the other alpha-carbon (Silverman *et al.*, 1993a; Youdim *et al.*, 1991). However, milacemide is also an inactivator of MAO-B; following its oxidation, the entire molecule partitions between deamination (reactions **d** and **g** in Fig. 9.10) and attachment to an amino acid residue (reaction **e** in Fig. 9.10) (Nishimura *et al.*, 1993; Silverman *et al.*, 1993a). As for the metabolite glycinamide (**9.LVI**), it is further hydrolyzed to glycine, the active metabolite, suggesting that milacemide could be a promising MAO-activated prodrug, although a direct

TABLE 9.3 *Deamination of aliphatic amines by rat liver MAO-B (Yu, 1989)*

Amine	V_{max}/K_m*
Methylamine	—†
Ethylamine	—
n-Propylamine	0.07
n-Butylamine	5.11
n-Pentylamine	37.40
n-Hexylamine	46.29
n-Heptylamine	51.85
n-Octylamine	61.80
n-Nonylamine	56.50
n-Decylamine	38.94
n-Dodecylamine	0.93
n-Octadecylamine	0.05
Putrescine	—
Cadaverine	—

*V_{max} in nmol min^{-1} mg^{-1}, K_m in 10^{-4} M.
†No detectable activity.

action cannot be excluded (Janssens de Varebeke *et al.*, 1989; O'Brien *et al.*, 1991). Another interesting drug is MD 780236 (**9.LVII**). Both enantiomers are deaminated by MAO-A, but the (*S*)-enantiomer is also an irreversible inactivator of MAO-B (see Section 9.4.4) (Strolin Benedetti *et al.*, 1983).

The discovery that MAO activates **MPTP** (N-methyl-4-phenyl-1,2,3,6-tetrahydropyridine; **9.LVIII** in Fig. 9.11) to a neurotoxin causing Parkinsonism in humans and monkeys has renewed interest in this enzyme and led to the characterization of many tertiary amines as exogenous substrates (Maret *et al.*, 1990a; Singer and Ramsay, 1991). The activation of MPTP is due mainly to MAO-B and to a lesser extent to MAO-A, the first steps of the reaction being identical to

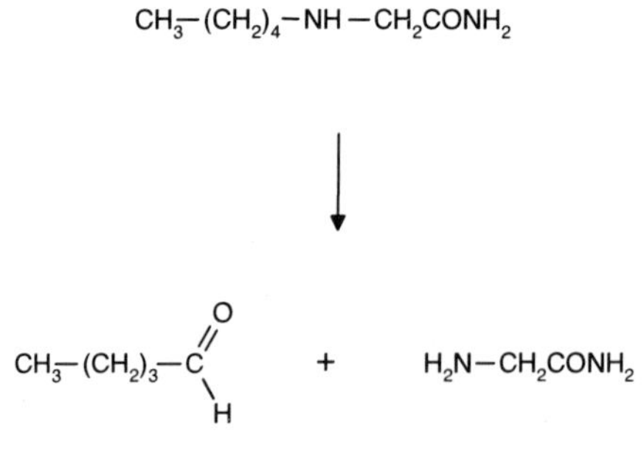

$$CH_3-(CH_2)_4-NH-CH_2CONH_2 \qquad 9.LIV$$

$$CH_3-(CH_2)_3-\overset{\overset{\displaystyle O}{\|}}{C}-H \quad + \quad H_2N-CH_2CONH_2$$

9.LV　　　　　　　　　　　9.LVI

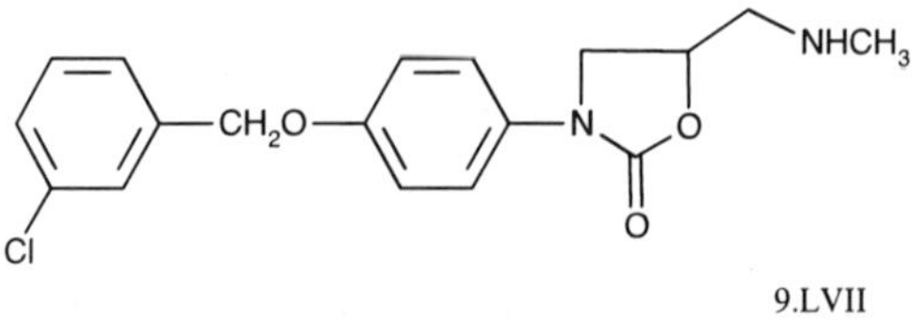

9.LVII

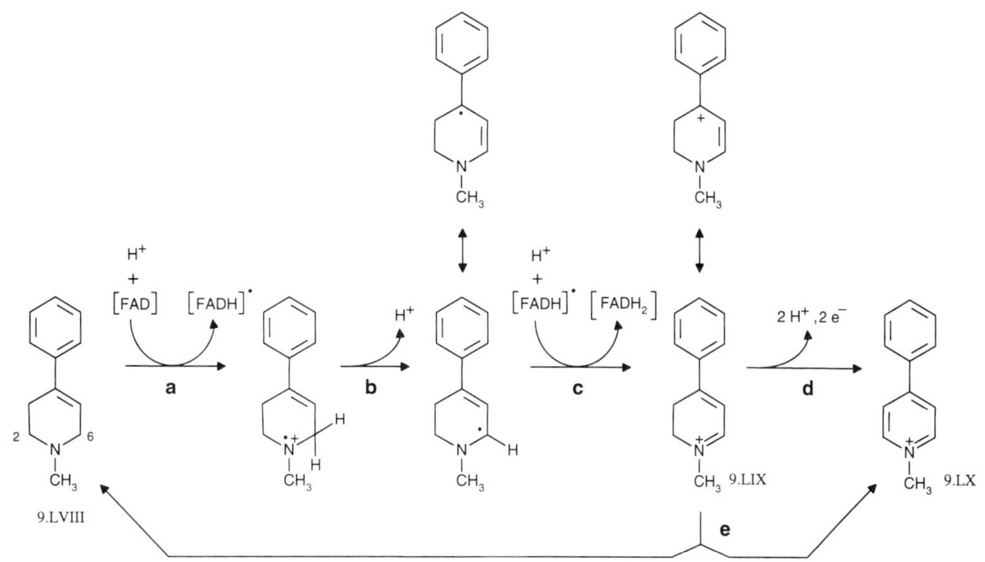

FIGURE 9.11 Main reactions postulated to describe the MAO-catalyzed toxication of 1-methyl-4-phenyl-1,2,3,6-tetrahydropyridine (MPTP, **9.LVIII**) to 1-methyl-4-phenylpyridinium (MPP$^+$, **9.LX**) via the intermediate 1-methyl-4-phenyl-2,3-dihydropyridinium (MPDP$^+$, **9.LIX**).

those outlined in Fig. 9.10 (Trevor *et al.*, 1987). Indeed, one-electron oxidation (reaction **a** in Fig. 9.11) followed by proton removal (reaction **b** in Fig. 9.11) forms a radical which is further oxidized (reaction **c** in Fig. 9.11) to the iminium analogue MPDP$^+$ (N-methyl-4-phenyl-2,3-dihydropyridinium; **9.LIX** in Fig. 9.11). Stabilization by delocalization possibly accounts for the particular reactivity of the radical intermediate and of MPDP$^+$ (Chacon *et al.*, 1987).

While the reaction sequence **a**, **b** and **c** in Fig. 9.11 is the one considered most likely by a number of authors, deuterium isotope effects of comparatively high magnitude have suggested that MPTP activation proceeds via **radical hydrogen abstraction** at the allylic position rather than aminium radical deprotonation (Ottoboni *et al.*, 1989); but whether this involves the amine or the aminium radical is not always clear. Interestingly, similar isotope effects were seen in the oxidation of benzylamine, suggesting that the MAO-B catalyzed oxidation of benzylic and allylic positions may proceed by an alternative pathway despite the fact that the abstracted hydrogen is always the *pro-R* one (see Section 9.4.2) (Ottoboni *et al.*, 1989).

MPDP$^+$, rather than undergoing extensive hydrolysis like imines formed from "normal" substrates, can be **further oxidized** (reaction **d** in Fig. 9.11) by unidentified membrane-bound enzymes to **MPP$^+$** (N-methyl-4-phenylpyridinium; **9.LX** in Fig. 9.11), the ultimate neurotoxin causing cell death. In addition, MPDP$^+$ can disproportionate to MPTP and MPP$^+$ (reaction **e** in Fig. 9.11), undergo autoxidation to generate reactive oxygen species, or be oxidized by MAO, but the role played by these reactions under physiological conditions is not well understood (Adams and Odunze, 1991; Wu *et al.*, 1988; Zang and Misra, 1992 and 1993).

Kinetically, the MAO-mediated oxidation of MPTP is more complex than schematized in Fig. 9.11. Indeed, with this substrate there are three pathways for the reoxidation of the reduced form of MAO-B: as the free reduced form, as the reduced enzyme–substrate complex, and as the reduced enzyme–product complex. For MAO-A on the contrary, only the free enzyme undergoes reoxidation (Ramsay *et al.*, 1987). To add to the complexity of the picture, MPTP is also both a competitive and a mechanism-based inactivator of MAO-A and MAO-B (Singer *et al.*, 1985). As far as competitive-reversible inhibition is concerned, the order of potency is

$MPDP^+ > MPP^+ > MPTP$ for MAO-A, and $MPTP > MPDP^+ > MPP^+$ for MAO-B. Of the two isozymes, MAO-B oxidizes MPTP faster and is also more sensitive to mechanism-based inactivation. MPTP, $MPDP^+$ and a number of analogues are also mechanism-based inactivators of MAO-A and/or MAO-B (Hall *et al.*, 1992; Krueger *et al.*, 1990). It appears that enzyme inactivation by MPTP must occur after $MPDP^+$ formation and involve C(2)–H cleavage, but the mechanism proposed is still hypothetical (Ottoboni *et al.*, 1989).

A very large number of **MPTP analogues** have been tested for MAO reactivity (Efange and Boudreau, 1991; Efange *et al.*, 1993; Harik *et al.*, 1993; Kalgutkar and Castagnoli, 1992; Krueger *et al.*, 1992; Maret *et al.*, 1990a; Singer and Ramsay, 1993; Singer *et al.*, 1993; Zhao *et al.*, 1992). Thus, 2'-methyl-MPTP (**9.LXI**) is an even better substrate of MAO than MPTP, and particularly of MAO-A (Kindt *et al.*, 1988). In contrast, the saturated analogue N-methyl-4-phenylpiperidine (**9.LXIV**) is not a substrate. Interestingly, the secondary amine 4-phenyl-1,2,3,6-tetrahydropyridine (PTP, **9.LXII**) is a substrate, albeit a poor one, as is ethyl N-methyl-1,2,3,6-tetrahydro-4-pyridinecarboxylate (**9.LXIII**; $R = COOC_2H_5$), an analogue without a second ring (Gibb *et al.*, 1987). The high substrate activity of N-methyl-4-cyclohexyl-1,2,3,6-tetrahydropyridine (**9.LXIII**; R = cyclohexyl), N-methyl-4-benzyl-1,2,3,6-tetrahydropyridine (**9.LXIII**; R = benzyl) and N-methyl-4-(phenylethyl)-1,2,3,6-tetrahydropyridine (**9.LXIII**; R = phenylethyl) indicates that electronic conjugation of the heterocycle with an aromatic ring (see Fig. 9.11) is not necessary for MAO-mediated oxidation (Efange *et al.*, 1990; Maret *et al.*, 1990a).

9.LXI   9.LXII   9.LXIII   9.LXIV

Three-dimensional quantitative structure–metabolism relationship (*3D-QSMR*) studies based on the MAO substrate activity of large series of analogues revealed some of the positions around the MPTP molecule where substitution increases (Fig. 9.12A) or decreases (Fig. 9.12B) MAO substrate activity (Altomare *et al.*, 1992; Maret *et al.*, 1990a, 1990b). In particular:

- N-alkyl substituents larger than a methyl decrease or abolish activity;
- 2'-substituents tend to increase activity;
- 3'-substituents have little influence;
- 4'-substituents tend to decrease or abolish activity, for MAO-B at least.

It has recently been proposed that the readiness to act upon tertiary amines may be a general feature of MAO-B (Blaschko, 1989). Many data indeed support this rationalization, but it should be not be forgotten that MAO-A is known also to play a marked role in the oxidation of some MPTP analogues (Efange *et al.*, 1990; Kindt *et al.*, 1988; Krueger *et al.*, 1992).

9.4.4 Mechanism-based inhibitors

Various N-containing moieties in a number of compounds are activated by MAO to reactive intermediates which **inactivate the enzyme irreversibly**, e.g. hydrazines, propargylamines, and

A   B

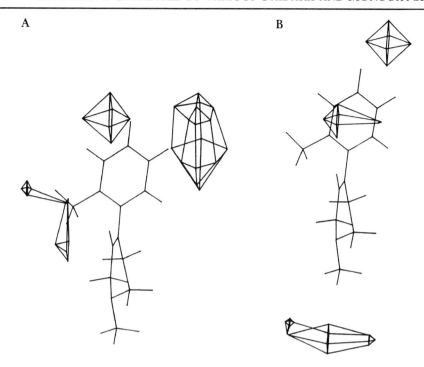

FIGURE 9.12 Results of a Comparative Molecular Field Analysis (CoMFA) of MPTP analogues as MAO substrates. Contour maps showing the major steric features around the MPTP molecule influencing MAO substrate reactivity. The molecule shown in the figure is 2'-methyl-MPTP. In **A** contours surround regions where a higher steric interaction increases reactivity, while in **B** contours represent regions where steric interactions decrease reactivity. (Reproduced from Maret *et al.*, 1990a, with the permission of the copyright holder.)

cyclopropylamines (see Fig. 9.9) (Silverman, 1991; Silverman *et al.*, 1993b). Such compounds are mechanism-based inactivators, also (not quite properly) known as suicide substrates. Their therapeutic interest falls outside the scope of this book, while their mechanism of activation allows insights into the catalytic mechanism(s) of MAO. **Phenelzine** (**9.LI** in Figs. 9.9 and 9.13) is a representative **hydrazine** which is oxidized by MAO to a **diazene**, i.e. phenylethyldiazene (**9.LXV** in Fig. 9.13). This metabolite may rearrange to a **hydrazone**, i.e. phenylethylidene hydrazine (**9.LXVI** in Fig. 9.13), which hydrolyzes to hydrazine and an aldehyde, in this case phenylacetaldehyde. The latter yields phenylacetic acid, the major urinary metabolite of phenelzine. But in addition to being an MAO substrate, phenelzine is a mechanism-based inactivator of the enzyme, a property explained by the facile breakdown of the diazene to N_2 and the phenylethyl radical. This radical forms covalent adducts with the enzyme, in particular at C(4a) of the flavin (Fig. 9.13) and at unknown residues of the apoenzyme (Kyburz, 1990; Yu and Tipton, 1989).

Effective **propargylamines** include **clorgyline** and **selegiline** (**9.XLIX** and **9.L** in Fig. 9.9), but also aliphatic derivatives (Kalir *et al.*, 1981; Yu *et al.*, 1992). Their mechanism of inactivation is schematized in Fig. 9.14 (Kyburz, 1990; Simpson *et al.*, 1982). The formation of a C(α)-centred radical (reaction **a** in Fig. 9.14) may occur by the usual pathway (one-electron oxidation followed by deprotonation, see Fig. 9.10) or more probably, the position being a propargylic one, by radical hydrogen abstraction (see Section 9.4.3). This C(α)-centred propargyl radical is in resonance with a C(γ)-centred allenic radical which binds covalently at N(5) of the one-electron reduced FAD (reaction **b** in Fig. 9.14). In addition, the radical intermediate may undergo the

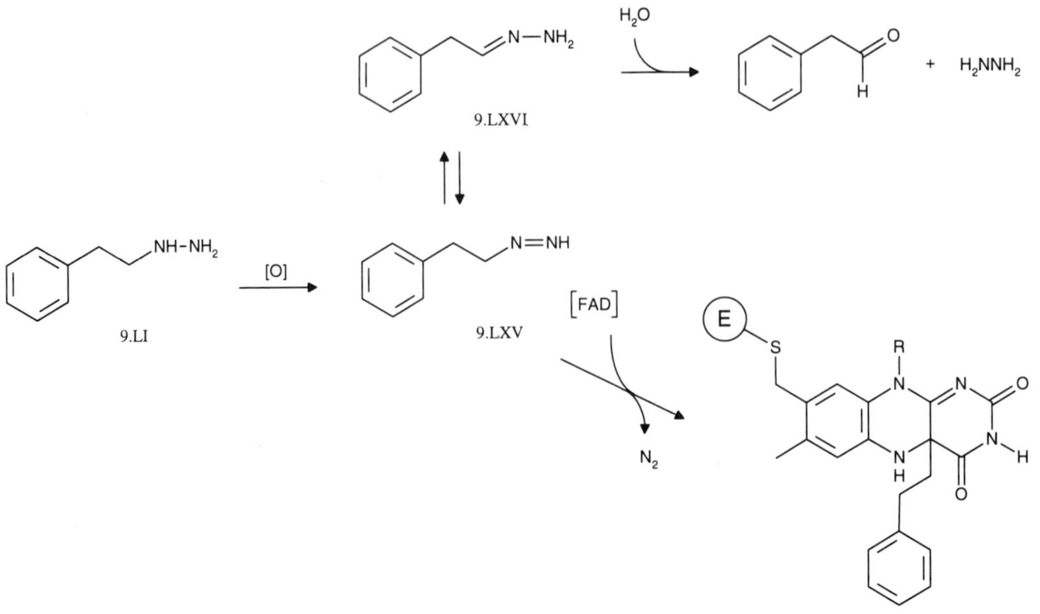

FIGURE 9.13 Mechanism of MAO-catalyzed oxidation of phenelzine (9.LI), resulting in deamination to phenylacetaldehyde via a hydrazone (9.LXVI) (substrate behaviour), and in enzyme inactivation by alkylation ("suicide substrate" behaviour).

usual second-electron oxidation to an iminium intermediate (reaction c in Fig. 9.14) which binds covalently to FADH$_2$ (reaction d in Fig. 9.14) or undergoes hydrolysis. The N(5)-adduct rearranges upon protonation as shown (reaction e in Fig. 9.14).

Another important group of mechanism-based inactivators of MAO are various **cyclopropylamines** as exemplified by **tranylcypromine** (9.LIII in Fig. 9.9) (Kyburz, 1990; Silverman and Zieske, 1985; Tullman and Hanzlik, 1984; Vazquez and Silverman, 1985). These compounds are primary or secondary amines (Fig. 9.15, e.g. R = benzyl, R' = H or methyl; R = H, R' = phenyl or benzyl) which undergo the usual one-electron oxidation to the aminium radical (reaction a in Fig. 9.15). In these cases, however, the aminium radical is highly unstable and rather than undergoing deprotonation rearranges by homolytic ring opening to a C(γ)-centred radical (reaction b in Fig. 9.15) (Silverman et al., 1993b). It is the latter which binds covalently to the apoenzyme (probably to a cysteinyl residue) or to N(5) of FAD. Note that with both propargylamines and cyclopropylamines the bound fragment contains an iminium functionality that may hydrolyze to a carbonyl and an amine.

Other mechanism-based inactivators of MAO include 3-amino-1-phenylprop-1-enes, 5-(aminomethyl)-3-aryl-2-oxazolidinones (e.g. MD 780236, 9.LVII) and (aminomethyl)trimethyl-silanes (Banik and Silverman, 1990; Gates and Silverman, 1990; Strolin Benedetti et al., 1983; Williams et al., 1992). Like the inhibitors discussed above, these compounds are MAO substrates which do not follow the usual reaction pathway due to the high reactivity of a metabolic intermediate.

In summary, there exist **two classes of time-dependent, mechanism-based inactivators of MAO,** depending whether covalent binding occurs to FAD (Figs. 9.13 and 9.14) or an amino acid side-chain in the active site (reaction e in Fig. 9.10). And in the latter class, a continuum of possibilities exists between very stable adducts (resulting in **irreversible inactivation**) and more labile covalent intermediates which break down according to reaction f (Fig. 9.10). In the latter

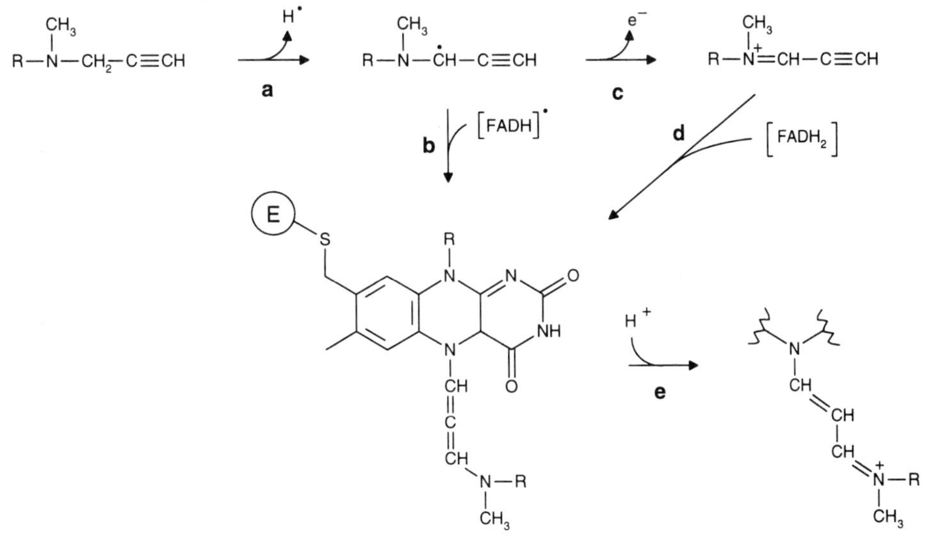

FIGURE 9.14 Mechanism of MAO-catalyzed oxidation of propargylamines resulting in enzyme inactivation.

case, a **time-dependent, reversible inhibition** is seen, e.g. with ethylenediamine derivatives such as lazabemide (**9.XLVIII**) and the active metabolite of moclobemide (**9.XLVII**). In fact, a number of time-dependent, reversible inhibitors are compounds having the general structure R–X–C–C–NH_2 (X = heteroatom), while their secondary and tertiary amino derivatives of structure R–X–C–C–NH-alkyl and R–X–C–C–NMe_2 are irreversible inactivators. This difference has been explained in terms of stereoelectronic effects on the stability of the covalent intermediate formed by reaction **e** in Fig. 9.10 (Ding and Silverman, 1993; Ding *et al.*, 1993).

9.5 REACTIONS CATALYZED BY XANTHINE OXIDASE AND ALDEHYDE OXIDASE

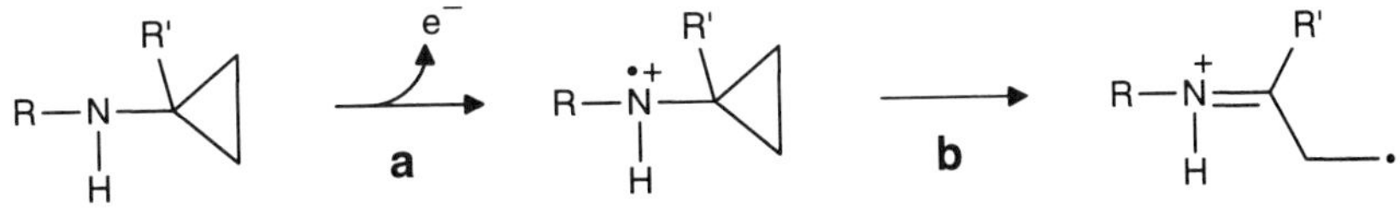

FIGURE 9.15 Mechanism of MAO-mediated activation of cyclopropylamines to a C(γ)-centred radical which binds covalently to the enzyme.

The enzymes to be discussed in this section are sometimes designated as the **molybdenum hydroxylases** and comprise:

- **xanthine oxidase** (XO) [xanthine:oxygen oxidoreductase; hypoxanthine oxidase; EC 1.1.3.22];
- **xanthine dehydrogenase** (XDH) [xanthine:NAD^+ oxidoreductase; EC 1.1.1.204];
- **aldehyde oxidase** (AO) [aldehyde:oxygen oxidoreductase; EC 1.2.3.1].

Note that aldehyde dehydrogenase (Section 2.3) is completely unrelated to the molybdenum hydroxylases despite a (misleading) parallel in names with XO and XDH. A few comprehensive reviews deal with the molybdenum hydroxylases and cover the most important literature (Beedham, 1985 and 1987; Rajagopalan, 1980; Wootton *et al.*, 1991).

9.5.1 Enzymology and catalytic mechanism of the molybdenum hydroxylases

XO, XDH and AO are widely distributed throughout the animal kingdom. They are cytosolic enzymes fulfilling roles complementary to those of the monooxygenases in the metabolism of both endogenous and exogenous compounds (Krenitsky, 1978). The molybdenum hydroxylases have a MW of about 300,000 and are composed of two subunits of equal size. Thus, the subunit of rat liver XDH contains 1319 amino acids with a calculated molecular mass of 145,034 Da (Amaya *et al.*, 1990). Human XO/XDH has also been extensively characterized (Wright *et al.*, 1993). Each subunit contains as **cofactors** (Beedham, 1985; Eagle *et al.*, 1992; Folkers *et al.*, 1987; Hille and Anderson, 1991; Howes *et al.*, 1991; Saito *et al.*, 1989):

- one FAD molecule;
- one atom of molybdenum in a core which is the essential component of a molybdopterin cofactor and whose oxidized form can be written as $[Mo^{VI}(=S)(=O)]^{2+}$;
- four non-heme iron atoms in the form of two Fe_2/S_2 clusters of the spinach ferredoxin type.

This combination of prosthetic groups is seemingly unique and explains why these enzymes are sometimes also grouped under the heading of molybdeno-flavoproteins.

The **reaction** catalyzed by these enzymes obeys the general equation:

$$RH + H_2O \rightarrow ROH + 2e^- + 2H^+ \tag{Eq. 9.5}$$

where RH is the substrate and ROH the hydroxylated metabolite. Eq. 9.5 means that (a) the oxygen atom transferred to the substrate is ultimately derived from water, and (b) the reaction formally liberates two electrons, hence an **electron acceptor** must also be present. In mechanistic terms, these enzymes function by being alternately reduced by the (reducing) substrate and reoxidized by an electron acceptor (sometimes called the oxidizing substrate). **Xanthine oxidase** uses molecular oxygen as an electron acceptor, and its reaction with xanthine generates uric acid (see Section 9.5.2) plus both hydrogen peroxide and superoxide, but not the hydroxyl radical, according to the following equations (Beedham, 1985; Britigan *et al.*, 1990):

$$Xanthine + H_2O + 2O_2 \rightarrow Urate + 2O_2^{\bullet-} + 2H^+ \tag{Eq. 9.6}$$

$$Xanthine + H_2O + O_2 \rightarrow Urate + H_2O_2 \tag{Eq. 9.7}$$

Of course it may well be that disproportionation of superoxide (Section 3.5) accounts for part or most of the hydrogen peroxide produced, since the *in vivo* validity of *in vitro* results is always difficult to assess. **Aldehyde oxidase** also uses molecular oxygen as an electron acceptor, as follows:

$$Aldehyde + H_2O + 2O_2 \rightarrow Acid + 2O_2^{\bullet-} + 2H^+ \tag{Eq. 9.8}$$

In contrast to XO and AO, **xanthine dehydrogenase** uses oxidized NAD^+ as the electron acceptor:

$$Xanthine + H_2O + NAD^+ \rightarrow Urate + NADH + H^+ \tag{Eq. 9.9}$$

In fact, xanthine oxidase and xanthine dehydrogenase are two different forms of the same enzyme (xanthine oxidoreductase), designated as **type O** and **type D**, respectively (Amaya *et al.*, 1990). Xanthine dehydrogenase is the native form in rat liver but is converted to the O_2-dependent type during extraction and purification (Reinke *et al.*, 1987). This change can be reversible (through oxidation–reduction of cysteinyl thiol groups) or irreversible (through proteolysis) depending upon experimental conditions (Sultatos, 1988). In contrast, chicken liver XDH does not appear to be convertible to type O, while in some other animal tissues the enzyme exists almost entirely as the type O. Bovine milk is also a convenient source of xanthine oxidase. One major difference between the two forms is found in the flavin binding site, which shows the presence of a strong negative charge in the dehydrogenase but not in the oxidase (Massey *et al.*, 1989; Walker *et al.*, 1991).

The conversion of xanthine dehydrogenase to xanthine oxidase occurs not only *in vitro*, but also *in vivo* under the influence of different metabolic states such as hypoxia and ischaemia. This may result in increased production of reactive oxygen species (Eqs. 9.6 and 9.7) and amplification of oxidative damage in cells. Interestingly, **aldehydes produced by lipid peroxidation** interact in different ways with the enzyme. As substrates of XO (see Section 9.5.2), they lead to the production of superoxide and this is one way by which they may contribute to oxidative damage (Bounds and Winston, 1991). As enzyme regulators, their feedback effects are more complex; malondialdehyde increases XDH activity and decrease XO activity, while another product of lipoperoxidation, 4-hydroxynonenal, activates XO but has no effect on XDH (Haberland *et al.*, 1992).

Besides O_2 and NAD^+, other compounds, both inorganic and organic, have been shown to function as electron acceptors *in vitro*, e.g. permanganate, iodine, ferricyanide, methylene blue,

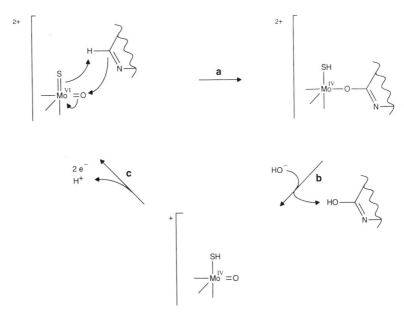

FIGURE 9.16 Postulated catalytic mechanism of the molybdenum hydroxylases. The oxidized molybdenum core provides the catalytic centre. Concerted deprotonation is believed to activate the substrate to a nucleophile attacking the oxygen ligand, with the Mo(VI) atom acting as an electron sink. This results in the formation (reaction **a**) of a covalent intermediate which may break down as shown (reaction **b**) by liberation of the metabolite and the 2-electron reduced molybdenum core. The latter is then reoxidized (reaction **c**) by transferring two electrons to the other cofactors (Hille and Sprecher, 1987; Oertling and Hille, 1990).

quinones, dinitrobenzene, tetrazolium salts, dichlorophenolindophenol and cytochrome c. In fact, the **reducing activity** of XO and AO towards a number of xenobiotics is well recognized (Chapter 12).

Our understanding of the **kinetics and catalytic mechanism** of molybdenum hydroxylases has progressed significantly in recent years, although much remains to be elucidated. Most published work deals with XDH and XO but appears transposable to AO. Thus, the cofactors in molybdenum hydroxylases have a capacity for holding a maximum of six electrons per subunit, i.e. two when FAD is reduced to $FADH_2$, two when the molybdenum atom is reduced from Mo(VI) to Mo(IV), and one electron per Fe_2/S_2 cluster. Since xanthine hydroxylation liberates two electrons (Eq. 9.5), there is the potential for oxidizing three equivalents of substrate. However, it was shown for XDH that binding of NAD^+ and substrate controls the end-point of the reaction, which stops at stages intermediate between the fully oxidized and the fully reduced enzyme (Schopfer et al., 1988). Major differences were seen in the redox and kinetic properties of XO and XDH (D'Ardenne and Edmondson, 1990; Saito and Nishino, 1989).

As discussed in the next section, the targets of these enzymes are sp^2-hybridized carbon atoms rendered electron-deficient by a nitrogen or oxygen atom to which they are linked by a double bond (i.e. –CH=X). The hydroxylation of such carbon atoms is thus a **nucleophilic oxidation** in contrast to the electrophilic oxidation mediated by monooxygenases. The postulated catalytic mechanism of molybdenum hydroxylases is presented in simplified form in Fig. 9.16 for aromatic azaheterocycles (Hille and Sprecher, 1987; Lee and Han, 1992).

It is now recognized that the oxidized molybdenum core provides the catalytic centre, and detailed molecular graphics studies have yielded insight into the docking mode of a substrate such as xanthine to the molybdopterin cofactor (Folkers et al., 1987). The reaction is believed to be initiated by concerted deprotonation of the target carbon, thus activating the substrate to a carbanion. The latter binds to the oxygen ligand, with the Mo(VI) atom acting as an electron sink. The covalent intermediate thus formed decomposes, perhaps as shown in Fig. 9.16, by liberating the metabolite and the 2-electron reduced molybdenum core (Oertling and Hille, 1990). The latter is then reoxidized by transferring two electrons to the other prosthetic groups, i.e. FAD and the two iron/sulfur clusters. During reduction by the substrate and reoxidation by NAD^+ or O_2, a number of resonance forms have been characterized and their rate constants of interconversion determined (Saito and Nishino, 1989; Schopfer et al., 1988).

9.5.2 Substrate specificity of the molybdenum hydroxylases

An important point to be established at the onset is that XO and AO have overlapping but not identical **substrate specificities** and **product regiospecificities**. This is illustrated with purine (**9.LXVII**, shown here as the N(9)-H tautomer), whose oxidation by XO occurs with high affinity and at C(6) to yield hypoxanthine, then at C(2) to yield xanthine (**9.LXVIII**, 2,6-dihydroxypurine), and finally at C(8) to yield uric acid (**9.LXIX**) as mentioned above (Krenitsky et al., 1972). In contrast, AO is more regiospecific, since it hydroxylates purines almost exclusively at the C(8) position. Also, its substrate specificity differs from that of XO (e.g. Table 9.4). Other examples illustrating these differences can be found below.

The **electron-deficient** sp^2-hybridized carbon atoms that are targets of molybdenum hydroxylases (i.e. carbon atoms in moieties of the type –CH=X, see previous section) can be found in substrates belonging to three chemical classes:

- aromatic azaheterocycles, be they monocyclic, bicyclic, or polycyclic (i.e. containing the moiety –CH=N–);

9.LXVII   9.LXVIII   9.LXIX

- aromatic or nonaromatic charged azaheterocycles (i.e. containing the moiety $-CH=N^+<$);
- aldehydes (i.e. containing the moiety $-CH=O$).

The above substrate specificity is now broadened by the discovery that xanthine oxidase is able to hydroxylate an **sp³-carbon adjacent to an azoxy moiety** ($-N(O)=N-CH_2-$), as seen with the azoxy metabolite of procarbazine (Tweedie *et al.*, 1991).

Formally, the reaction catalyzed by XO and AO is one of hydroxylation, and indeed aldehydes are oxidized to carboxylic acids. However, hydroxylated aromatic azaheterocycles are seldom isolated as such since they have a marked tendency to tautomerize to the **lactam form,** e.g. uric acid (**9.LXIX**).

The exclusive attack by molybdenum hydroxylases at electron-deficient carbons is well illustrated by the regioselective hydroxylation of **aromatic azaheterocycles**, and particularly **diazaheterocycles**, catalyzed by rabbit liver AO (Fig. 9.17) (McCormack *et al.*, 1978; Stubley *et al.*, 1977 and 1979). Thus, phthalazine (**9.LXX**) yielded 1-hydroxyphthalazine, while quinazoline (**9.LXXI**) and quinoxaline (**9.LXXII**) gave the 4-hydroxy and 2-hydroxy products, respectively; these metabolites were substrates for a second hydroxylation reaction to 2,4-dihydroxyquinazoline and 2,3-dihydroxyquinoxaline, respectively. As shown in Fig. 9.17, the positions of hydroxylation in the three substrates are the electron-deficient alpha-carbon atoms. Cinnoline (**9.LXXIII**) is one of the few exceptions to the rule of alpha-carbon hydroxylation since rabbit liver AO formed the 4-hydroxylated rather than the 3-hydroxylated metabolite. However, the discrepancy is merely apparent since C(4) is more electron-deficient than C(3) (see Fig. 9.17). The fact that these four compounds are very poor substrates of cytochrome P450 (Stubley *et al.*, 1977) is one of the many examples of the complementary roles of molybdenum hydroxylases and monooxygenases in the biotransformation of xenobiotics (see above).

Many other azaheterocycles have been examined as substrates of AO and/or XO. **Monoazanaphthalenes** (i.e. quinoline and isoquinoline) are relatively good substrates of AO, while **monocyclic azaheterocycles** (pyridine and the three diazabenzenes pyrazine, pyrimidine and pyridazine) are poor substrates (Stubley and Stell, 1977; Stubley *et al.*, 1979; see also Table 9.4). Following this trend, a **tricyclic azaheteroaromatic compound** such as phenanthridine is a very good substrate. It has been shown with various heterocyclic compounds that substituents can markedly affect the affinity, velocity and even regioselectivity of the reaction of hydroxyla-

TABLE 9.4 *Comparative substrate specificities of bovine milk xanthine oxidase (XO) and rabbit liver aldehyde oxidase (AO)*

Substrate	XO	AO
Pyridine	—	22
N^1-Methylnicotinamide	<14	755
Pyrimidine	<14	22
2-Hydroxypyrimidine	134	6220
4-Hydroxypyrimidine	623	2980
Quinoline	<14	200
N-Methylquinolinium	<14	1780
Purine (**9.LXVII**)	480	2220
2-Hydroxypurine	255	3110
6-Hydroxypurine (hypoxanthine)	625	67
8-Hydroxypurine	115	<22
2,6-Dihydroxypurine (**9.LXVIII**)	815	<22
2,8-Dihydroxypurine	14	22
6,8-Dihydroxypurine	575	<22
1-Methylhypoxanthine	600	755
3-Methylhypoxanthine	<14	15,800
7-Methylhypoxanthine	19	600
9-Methylhypoxanthine	<14	45
1-Methylxanthine	815	<22
3-Methylxanthine	<14	<22
7-Methylxanthine	19	22
Theophylline (1,3-dimethylxanthine)	574	<22
Theobromine (3,7-dimethylxanthine)	<14	<22
Caffeine (1,3,7-trimethylxanthine)	<14	<22
Allopurinol (**9.LXXIV**)	380	355
Alloxanthine (**9.LXXV**)	<14	<22
Allopurinol ribonucleoside	<14	488
Allopurinol ribonucleotide	<14	<22
8-Azapurine	29	710
Adenine	29	44
Guanine	<14	<22
Pteridine	270	5330

The values reported are turnover numbers as calculated by Rajagopalan (1980) from literature data, and expressed in mole substrate oxidized per minute per mole active site.

tion (Beedham, 1985 and 1987; Beedham *et al.*, 1990; Hall and Krenitsky, 1986) (see also Table 9.4). With a few exceptions, aromatic azaheterocycles containing an oxygen or sulfur as second heteroatom (i.e. oxaza- or thiazaheterocyclic compounds) are not substrates of molybdenum hydroxylases, but some are inhibitors, suggesting unproductive binding (Gristwood and Wilson, 1988).

Various azaheterocyclic compounds of **biological or medicinal interest** are substrates of the molybdenum hydroxylases. One such compound is allopurinol (**9.LXXIV**), which is oxidized by both XO and AO to alloxanthine (**9.LXXV**) (Table 9.4). The latter is a tight-binding, potent *in vitro* and *in vivo* inhibitor of XO but is devoid of inhibitory effects on AO (Moriwaki *et al.*, 1993).

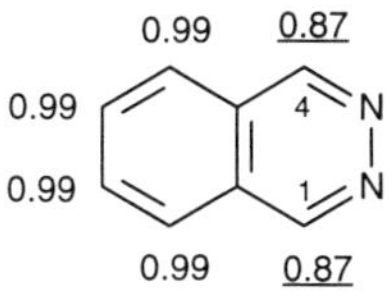

FIGURE 9.17 Some diazanaphthalenes and the electron density of their carbon atoms, as reported by Damani and Case (1984) and rounded to the second decimal: phthalazine (**9.LXX**), quinazoline (**9.LXXI**), quinoxaline (**9.LXXII**) and cinnoline (**9.LXXIII**). Underlined positions mark the electron-deficient carbon(s) that is/are hydroxylated by AO (McCormack *et al.*, 1978; Stubley *et al.*, 1977 and 1979).

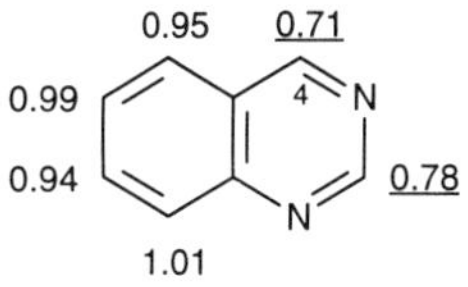

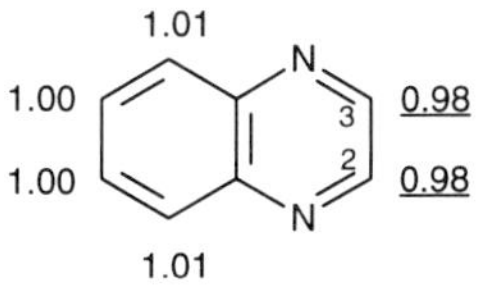

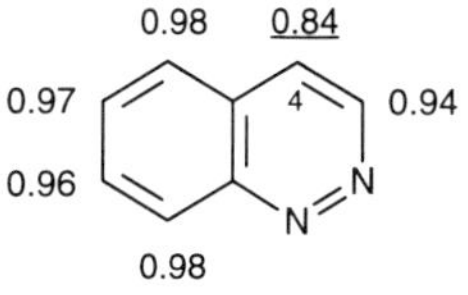

Xanthine oxidase has a role to play in the complex metabolism of **caffeine** (1,3,7-trimethylxanthine) (Kalow, 1985). While the 8-hydroxylation of caffeine itself is catalyzed by cytochrome P450, that of its metabolites theophylline and 1-methylxanthine is catalyzed by XO (in its dehydrogenase form as far as 1-methylxanthine is concerned) but not AO. In contrast, the other methylxanthine metabolites are poor substrates (Reinke *et al.*, 1987) (Table 9.4). Interestingly, methylhypoxanthines (which are not caffeine metabolites) display structure–metabolism relationships quite different from those of methylxanthines (Table 9.4).

Among representative **drugs**, the cardiac stimulant carbazeran (**9.LXXVI**) is rapidly deactivated in humans by AO-catalyzed 4-hydroxylation (Kaye *et al.*, 1985). Another interesting

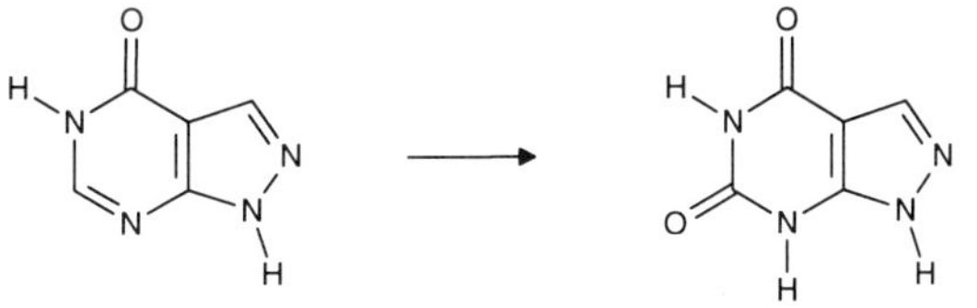

compound is 6-deoxyacyclovir (**9.LXXVII**), a 2-aminopurine nucleoside analogue that is efficiently converted by XO to acyclovir (**9.LXXVIII**) in a reaction strongly inhibited by allopurinol in the perfused rat liver (Jones *et al.*, 1987). Acyclovir is an antiviral agent with high activity against the herpes group of viruses, and its formation from 6-deoxyacyclovir offers a rare and promising example of XO-mediated prodrug activation. The fact that 6-deoxyacyclovir is a nucleoside analogue is not fortuitous since some nucleosides, but not nucleotides, are known to be substrates of molybdenum hydroxylases (Beedham, 1985 and 1987) (see also Table 9.4). Note that acyclovir is further oxidized by AO to the 8-hydroxy metabolite.

While **azabenzenes** as a rule are but poorly metabolized by the molybdenum hydroxylases if at all (see above), some exceptions do exist (see Table 9.4), including a few drugs, e.g. metyrapone (**9.LXXIX**) which is oxidized in rat liver cytosol to an α-pyridone metabolite (**9.LXXX**) (Damani *et al.*, 1981). Interestingly, the reaction appears regiospecific for the carbonyl-substituted pyridyl

9.LXXVI

9.LXXVII   9.LXXVIII

ring, and metyrapol (i.e. the analogue with the reduced keto group) is not a substrate for the reaction. Clearly much remains to be understood in the structure–metabolism relationships of oxidations catalyzed by XO and AO.

A very simple compound, Δ^1-pyrroline (**9.LXXXI**), was metabolized by rabbit liver cytosol to 2-pyrrolidinone (**9.LXXXII**) and γ-aminobutyric acid (**9.LXXXIII**, GABA) in a reaction inhibited by allopurinol (Callery *et al.*, 1982). Such a substrate, which is quite different chemically from all the compounds discussed above or shown in Table 9.4, is likely to be oxidized as the protonated iminium species. Indeed, **cationic azaheterocycles** are very good substrates of AO, yielding a lactam (Beedham, 1985 and 1987). In Section 6.4, the involvement of AO has been mentioned in connection with the formation of cotinine from the $\Delta^{1'(5')}$-iminium metabolite of nicotine (Fig. 6.5); convincing proof for a major role of AO in the reaction has been obtained (Brandänge and Lindblom, 1979). It was postulated that nicotine iminium ion is the molecular species serving as substrate (reaction **b** in Fig. 9.18), but another possibility cannot be excluded. By addition of the hydroxyl anion, iminium ions form the corresponding **pseudobases**

9.LXXIX   9.LXXX

9.LXXXI   9.LXXXII   9.LXXXIII

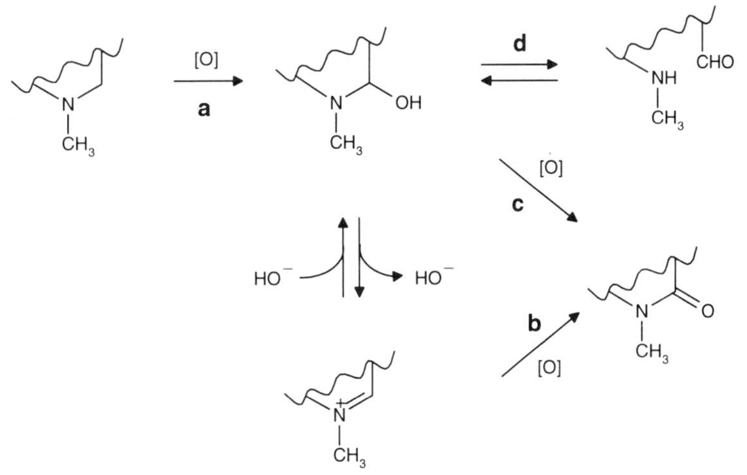

FIGURE 9.18 Partial view of the metabolism of saturated azaheterocycles. Cytochrome P450-catalyzed oxidation (reaction **a**) leads to a carbinolamine existing in equilibrium with an iminium ion. Both the carbinolamine and the iminium ion are potential substrates for the AO-catalyzed formation of a lactam (reactions **b** and **c**). The ring–chain tautomerism (reaction **d**) is a competitive reaction to lactam formation.

(i.e. the carbinolamines), a condition- and compound-dependent equilibrium existing between the two forms (Fig. 9.18). Since compounds existing predominantly as the pseudobase are also very good AO substrates, it is reasonable to assume that the enzyme can react with both iminium ions and their pseudobase. The reaction with pseudobases (reaction **c** in Fig. 9.18) is a dehydrogenation, implying that in the latter case aldehyde oxidase is functioning as a dehydrogenase (Beedham, 1985).

Fig. 9.18 can be assumed to have a general descriptive value extending well beyond nicotine and analogues (Beedham, 1985). In fact, it would be interesting to know whether the sequential actions of cytochrome P450 (to form a carbinolamine, reaction **a** in Fig. 9.18) and AO (to oxidize the carbinolamine to a lactam, reactions **b** and **c** in Fig. 9.18) occur for a large or limited variety of saturated azaheterocycles. Other factors influencing the action of AO are the relative contribution of dehydrogenases (reaction **c** in Fig. 9.18) and the ring–chain tautomerism of the carbinolamine (reaction **d** in Fig. 9.18) (see Section 6.4).

Aromatic azaheterocycles rendered cationic by N-alkylation form another group of AO substrates. As shown in Table 9.4 for N^1-methylnicotinamide and N-methylquinolinium, such cations are oxidized by AO rather than XO. The latter enzyme however is not completely devoid of activity towards nitrogen heteroaromatic cations, as documented for a variety of N-methylpyridinium cations bearing a carbonyl group in the 3-position, and for 6-substituted N-methylquinolinium cations (Bunting *et al.*, 1980).

In cationic azaheterocycles, the nitrogen atom shares much of its positive charge with neighbouring carbon atoms, particularly the alpha-carbons. Nucleophilic oxidation at the alpha-position is thus to be expected and this has been verified in a number of cases, e.g. N-methylphthalazinium (**9.LXXXIV**) oxidation to 2-methyl-1-(2H)-phthalazinone (**9.LXXXV**) (Beedham *et al.*, 1990). However, electronic and steric factors may direct hydroxylation to another electron-deficient position. For example, N-phenylquinolinium (**9.LXXXVI**) can be oxidized by AO in the 2- and 4-position, with a marked predominance for the latter position in the guinea-pig (Beedham *et al.*, 1989).

9.LXXXIV

9.LXXXV

9.LXXXVI

Although the molybdenum hydroxylases preferentially oxidize purines and other heterocyclic compounds as discussed above, **aldehydes** also represent an important group of substrates (Weiner, 1980). Both AO and XO catalyze the oxidation of aldehydes to the corresponding carboxylic acids, but their *in vivo* contribution appears usually less important than that of aldehyde dehydrogenase (ALDH, Section 2.3). Thus, most of the acetaldehyde-oxidizing activity in rat liver is due to ALDH. However, the activity of AO increases towards higher homologues up to an optimum of three carbons and decreases sharply beyond six carbons. The molybdenum hydroxylases are usually more active towards aromatic aldehydes and chemically complex endogenous aldehydes, e.g. retinal (Beedham, 1985). A good example of the complexity of the *in vivo* metabolic situation is offered by the hypoglycaemic drug tolbutamide, whose aldehyde metabolite (**9.LXXXVII**) (generated by the sequential action of cytochrome P450 and alcohol dehydrogenase) is oxidized to carboxytolbutamide by both XO and an NAD-linked aldehyde dehydrogenase (McDaniel *et al.*, 1969).

An interesting study has compared the substrate regioselectivity of XO towards *para-* and *ortho*-substituted benzaldehydes (**9.LXXXVIII** and **9.LXXXIX**, respectively) (Pelsy and Klibanov, 1983). In the *ortho* series, steric factors dominated the reactivity in that the rate of oxidation decreased sharply with increasing bulk of the substitutent. In contrast, the oxidation of *para*-substituted benzaldehydes was not detectably influenced by steric/lipophilic factors but was increased by electron-withdrawing substituents (halogens) and decreased by electron-donating alkyl and alkoxy substituents. As a result, the *para/ortho* ratio in reaction rates increased linearly with substituent bulk, but the effect was more pronounced for the electron-withdrawing than for the electron-donating substituents (Fig. 9.19).

9.LXXXVII

9.LXXXVIII

9.LXXXIX

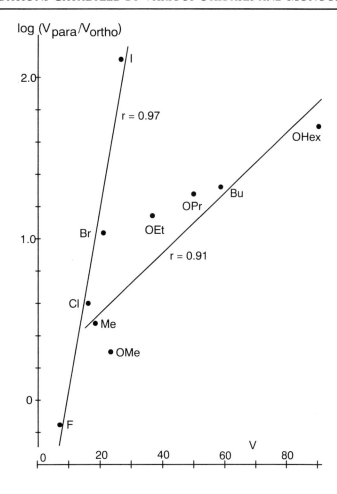

FIGURE 9.19 XO-catalyzed oxidation of *ortho-* and *para-*substituted benzaldehydes: *para/ortho* ratio in reaction rates (log scale) vs. volume of substituent (in ml mol^{-1}) (calculated from data published by Pelsy and Klibanov, 1983).

Several compounds are known to be **inhibitors** of molybdenum hydroxylases, acting either as competitive substrates, non-substrate ligands, or active site reagents (Rajagopalan, 1980). Cyanide, methanol and sulfhydryl reagents belong to the latter category, while a variety of poor substrates or non-substrates bind with high affinity but unproductively to the enzyme(s) and act as competitive inhibitors. Studies with 2- or 8-substituted hypoxanthines have revealed how the positioning of the ligand in the active site of XO determines the productivity or non-productivity of the complex (Biagi *et al.*, 1993). Unproductive binding is characteristic of a wide variety of purines, pteridines, and other heterocyclic molecules such as the oxaza- or thiazaheterocyclic compounds mentioned above (Gristwood and Wilson, 1988). While alloxanthine (**9.LXXV**) is a selective inhibitor of XO (see above), menadione (**9.XC**) is often used as a selective inhibitor of AO. Interestingly, a number of hydroxylated derivatives of anthraquinone (**9.XCI**) of natural or synthetic origin are inhibitors of XO (Noro *et al.*, 1987). Further investigations with competitive inhibitors may help unravel the compared topographies of the active site of AO and XO (Naeff *et al.*, 1991).

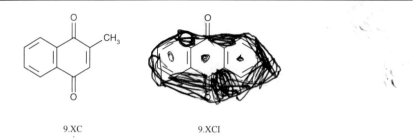

9.XC   9.XCI

As cogently discussed by Damani and Case (1984), the involvement of the molybdenum hydroxylases in the metabolism of endogenous compounds has been extensively studied, but their contribution to the biotransformation of foreign compounds is poorly understood. As this section has shown, this role may be more important than hitherto assumed considering the plethora of xenobiotics that contain potential target functions. This is all the more true considering the involvement of the molybdenum hydroxylases in reductive reactions (Chapter 12), as well as their potential to **oxidize compounds through release of superoxide** (Eq. 9.6). Thus, superoxide generated by XO/hypoxanthine or XO/xanthine was able to oxidize N-hydroxyphentermine to 2-methyl-2-nitro-1-phenylpropane and 1-naphthol to 1,4-naphthoquinone (Eastmond *et al.*, 1987: Maynard and Cho, 1981).

9.6 COPPER-CONTAINING AMINE OXIDASES, AND OTHER OXIDOREDUCTASES

Besides the oxidases and monooxygenases discussed above and in previous chapters, a few other enzymes are known to act on xenobiotics. In addition, a large number of such enzymes appear to have the potential capacity to do the same, although data are lacking. A comprehensive presentation of such oxidoreductases is beyond the scope of this work, and we shall restrict ourselves to discussing copper-containing amine oxidases and briefly mentioning three other enzymes of potential interest.

9.6.1 Copper-containing amine oxidases

The broad group of copper-containing amine oxidases [amine:oxygen oxidoreductase (deaminating; copper containing); diamine oxidase; histaminase; EC 1.4.3.6], also referred to as **semicarbazide-sensitive amine oxidase** (SSAO), comprises a variety of activities/enzymes including plasma amine oxidase and diamine oxidase (DAO) (Callingham *et al.*, 1990; McIntire and Hartmann, 1993). However, there are still ambiguities regarding the classification of these diverse enzymes. Here as elsewhere, molecular biology will bring clarification (Callingham *et al.*, 1991).

These enzymes are found in the plasma as well as in many tissues, with differences in distribution between species. They exist in soluble and membrane-bound form, but in contrast to MAO they are not mitochondrial enzymes (Strolin Benedetti, 1989). A number of them contain two subunits of molecular mass around 85–90 kDa and are associated with copper as an inorganic cofactor (two atoms per dimer), plus an organic cofactor to be discussed below. Their common substrate is benzylamine, and they catalyze the **oxidative deamination of primary amines** according to Eq. 9.10:

$$RCH_2NH_2 + H_2O + O_2 \rightarrow RCHO + NH_3 + H_2O_2 \qquad \text{(Eq. 9.10)}$$

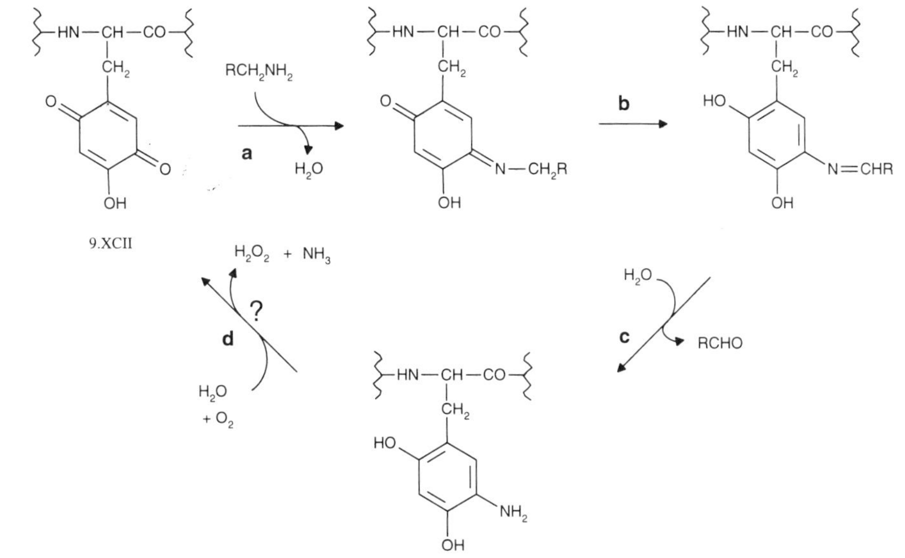

FIGURE 9.20 Simplified postulated catalytic mechanism of copper-containing amine oxidases in the deamination of primary amines (modified from Brown *et al.*, 1991; Hartmann and Klinman, 1991; Sayre *et al.*, 1991).

The covalently bound, **organic cofactor** at the catalytic site was first thought to be a pyridoxal derivative, then pyrroloquinoline quinone, and is now known to be **topa quinone** (6-hydroxydopa quinone; **9.XCII** in Fig. 9.20) (Brown *et al.*, 1991; Collison *et al.*, 1989; Janes *et al.*, 1990 and 1992; Klinman *et al.*, 1991; Mu *et al.*, 1992). The **catalytic mechanism** is now fairly understood and can be represented in simplified form as shown in Fig. 9.20, neglecting in particular the ionized states of the imino and phenolic groups (Brown *et al.*, 1991; Hartmann and Klinman, 1991; Hartmann *et al.*, 1993; Pedersen *et al.*, 1992; Sayre *et al.*, 1991). The substrate reacts with a carbonyl group in topa quinone to form a quinone imine (reaction **a** in Fig. 9.20) which isomerizes to an iminophenol (reaction **b** in Fig. 9.20). Hydrolysis of the latter (reaction **c** in Fig. 9.20) liberates the aldehyde (i.e. the deaminated metabolite) with the cofactor now an aminophenol. How the reduced cofactor is oxidized back to the quinone (reaction **d** in Fig. 9.20) is beginning to be understood, an overall aminotransferase mechanism being apparent (Janes and Klinman, 1991). The role of the copper cofactor is also unclear and is not made explicit in Fig. 9.20 (Greenaway *et al.*, 1991; Thomson, 1991).

What Fig. 9.20 does show, however, is the essential role of a carbonyl group in the quinone cofactor. This carbonyl group reacts with carbonyl reagents, in particular with phenylhydrazine and semicarbazide to form inactive hydrazones (Morpurgo *et al.*, 1988 and 1992). It is this specific and high sensitivity to semicarbazide with has led this group of amine oxidases to be known as SSAO (see above). Other **inactivators** of these enzymes include oximes which are believed to act by chelating the copper ions (Hiraoka *et al.*, 1988).

While the catalytic mechanism appears comparable for all copper-containing amine oxidases, subtle differences must exist in their active site to account for some opposite **stereospecificities** in the removal of the hydrogen on the alpha-carbon (reaction **b** in Fig. 9.20). Indeed, rat aorta benzylamine oxidase and hog kidney diamine oxidase were found to remove the *pro-S* hydrogen of benzylamine, while porcine plasma amine oxidase removed the *pro-R* hydrogen of dopamine and tyramine. In contrast, bovine plasma amine oxidase was non-stereospecific in the three reactions (Coleman *et al.*, 1989 and 1991; Scaman and Palcic, 1992; Yu and Davis, 1988).

According to the catalytic mechanism in Fig. 9.20, only **primary amines** (both monoamines and diamines) can be oxidatively deaminated by copper-containing amine oxidases, with large differences seen between tissues and animal species. Among **monoamines**, benzylamine has already been mentioned; it is for example a particularly good substrate (low K_m, high V_{max}) of some SSAOs (Lizcano *et al.*, 1991). Very high affinities were seen in the SSAO-catalyzed deamination of a homologous series of aliphatic amines of 1–18 straight-chain carbon atoms, the lowest K_m being seen with nonylamine. In contrast, diamines are poor substrates for SSAOs in human plasma, umbilical artery and rat aorta (Conforti *et al.*, 1993; Lyles *et al.*, 1990; Yu, 1990). The unsaturated primary amine allylamine (**9.XCIII**) is a cardiovascular toxin postulated to be deaminated by tissue-specific amine oxidase(s) to acrolein, a reactive aldehyde; pretreatment of rats with semicarbazide indeed protects animals against allylamine-induced cardiotoxicity (Callingham *et al.*, 1991; Strolin Benedetti, 1989).

While very few **drugs** have been investigated for their biotransformation by copper-containing amine oxidases, one interesting finding suggests that the phenomenon deserves better attention. The calcium channel blocker **amlodipine (9.XCIV)** is oxidatively deaminated in humans and dogs, but not in rats. This reaction was shown to occur on incubation of the drug in dog plasma but not in rat plasma, and the involvement of plasma amine oxidases was suggested (Beresford *et al.*, 1988). Deamination of 2-propyl-1-aminopentane by rat aorta SSAO lead to the aldehyde, a bioprecursor of valproic acid (Yu and Davis, 1991).

Oxidative deamination is also seen with **primary diamines** and involves **diamine oxidases** (DAOs) which as mentioned above also belong to the copper-containing amine oxidases. DAO catalyzes the oxidative loss of one amino group in endogenous substrates such as 1,4-diaminobutane (putrescine) and 1,5-diaminopentane (cadaverine). The dissymmetric substrate 2-methylputrescine (**9.XCV**) was deaminated selectively at the 4-amino group by pea seedling DAO, while no regioselectivity was seen with pig kidney DAO (i.e. deamination occurred at either end with equal efficiency). This indicates different structural requirements in the two

9.XCIII

9.XCIV

9.XCV

9.XCVI   9.XCVII

DAOs, which may affect the capacity of substrates to reorient into alternate binding conformations prior to catalytic attack (Callery *et al.*, 1992; Santaniello *et al.*, 1982).

An example of medicinal interest is that of **1,6-diaminohexane** (**9.XCVI**), a metabolite found in the urine of patients treated with the cell-differentiating agent hexamethylene bisacetamide. Incubation of 1,6-diaminohexane with DAO yielded 3,4,5,6-tetrahydro-2*H*-azepine (**9.XCVII**) as the sole metabolite. This product is the dehydrated form of the carbinolamine formed by tautomeric cyclization of 6-aminohexanal, the primary metabolite resulting from the deamination of 1,6-diaminohexane. 3,4,5,6-Tetrahydro-2*H*-azepine itself was converted by aldehyde oxidase to 6-aminohexanoic acid and caprolactam, two other urinary metabolites of hexamethylene bisacetamide. These findings give strong support to the involvement of DAO in the human metabolism of hexamethylene bisacetamide (Subramanyam *et al.*, 1989).

9.6.2 Other oxidoreductases

Polyamine oxidase [N^1-acetylspermidine:oxygen oxidoreductase (deaminating); EC 1.5.3.11] is a flavin- and iron-containing enzyme which splits N^1-acetylspermine and N^1-acetylspermidine into an aldehyde (3-acetamidopropanal) and an amine (spermidine and putrescine, respectively), with liberation of one molecule of H_2O_2 (Bolkenius and Seiler, 1989; Strolin Benedetti, 1989). This enzyme is also able to N-dealkylate a secondary amino group in xenobiotic di- and polyamines such as bis(benzyl)polyamines and N-alkyl-α,ω-diamines (Bitonti *et al.*, 1990; Bolkenius and Seiler, 1989). The latter example is particularly promising from a medicinal viewpoint since it suggests a method to accumulate diamines in the brain and to release intracellularly an aldehyde from a chemically stable prodrug. Interestingly, polyamine oxidase also appears able to deaminate a non-polyamine xenobiotic, namely milacemide (**9.LIV**) (see Section 9.4.3). But while MAO attack occurs at the two carbons adjacent to the basic nitrogen (see Section 9.4.3), polyamine oxidase apparently cleaves only the acetamido moiety to form glyoxylamide (HCO–CONH$_2$) (Strolin Benedetti *et al.*, 1992).

Human **ceruloplasmin** [Fe(II):oxygen oxidoreductase; ferroxidase; EC 1.16.3.1] is a serum enzyme belonging to the group of multicopper oxidases (Cole *et al.*, 1991). This oxidase was shown to transform vinblastin to catharinine and other metabolites. However, vinblastin was not a true substrate, its oxidation requiring the presence of a "shuttle oxidant" such as chlorpromazine (Elmarakby *et al.*, 1989).

Tyrosinase, a copper monooxygenase, has two activities both of which are of potential interest in xenobiotic metabolism. As a monophenol monooxygenase [monophenol,L-dopa:oxygen oxidoreductase; phenolase; EC 1.14.18.1] it oxidizes a monophenol (e.g. L-tyrosine) plus L-dopa to a catechol (e.g. L-dopa) plus dopaquinone. As a catechol oxidase [1,2-benzenediol:oxygen oxidoreductase; diphenol oxidase; EC 1.10.3.1] it oxidizes a catechol to a 1,2-benzoquinone (Lerch, 1981). The capacity of tyrosinase to act on xenobiotics is poorly assessed but it is tempting to hypothesize a "not too narrow" substrate specificity.

9.7 REFERENCES

Adams J.D. Jr and Odunze I.N. (1991). Biochemical mechanisms of 1-methyl-4-phenyl-1,2,3,6-tetrahydro-pyridine toxicity. Could oxidative stress be involved in the brain? *Biochem. Pharmacol.* **41**, 1099–1105.

Altomare C., Carrupt P.-A., Gaillard P., El Tayar N., Testa B. and Carotti A. (1992). Quantitative structure-metabolism relationship analyses of MAO-mediated toxication of 1-methyl-4-phenyl-1,2,3,6-tetrahydropyridine and analogues. *Chem. Res. Toxicol.* **5**, 366–375.

Amaya Y., Yamazaki K., Sato M., Noda K., Nishino T.

and Nishino T. (1990). Proteolytic conversion of xanthine dehydrogenase from the NAD-dependent type to the O_2-dependent type. *J. Biol. Chem.* **265**, 14,170–14,175.

Banik G.M. and Silverman R.B. (1990). Mechanism of inactivation of monoamine oxidase B by (aminomethyl)-trimethylsilane. *J. Amer. Chem. Soc.* **112**, 4499–4507.

Battersby A.R., Buckley D.G., Staunton J. and Williams P.J. (1979). Studies on enzyme-mediated reactions. Part 10. Stereochemical course of the dehydrogenation of stereo-specifically labelled 1-aminoheptanes by the amine oxidase from rat liver mitochondria (E.C. 1.4.3.4). *J. Chem. Soc.* **PTI**, 2550–2558.

Beedham C. (1985). Molybdenum hydroxylases as drug-metabolizing enzymes. *Drug Metab. Rev.* **16**, 119–156.

Beedham C. (1987). Molybdenum hydroxylases. Biological distribution and substrate-inhibitor specifity. In *Progress in Medicinal Chemistry*, Vol. 24 (eds Ellis G.P. and West G.B.). pp. 85–127. Elsevier, Amsterdam.

Beedham C., Padwick D.J., Al-Tayib Y. and Smith J.A. (1989). Diurnal variation and melatonin induction of hepatic molybdenum hydroxylase activity in the guinea-pig. *Biochem. Pharmacol.* **38**, 1459–1464.

Beedham C., Bruce S.E., Critchley D.J. and Rance D.J. (1990). 1-Substituted phthalazines as probes of the substrate-binding site of mammalian molybdenum hydroxylases. *Biochem. Pharmacol.* **39**, 1213–1221.

Belvedere G. and Tursi F. (1981). Styrene oxidation to styrene oxide in human blood erythrocytes and lymphocytes. *Res. Commun. Chem. Pathol. Pharmacol.* **33**, 273–282.

Beresford A.P., Macrae P.V. and Stopher D.A. (1988). Metabolism of amlodipine in the rat and dog: a species difference. *Xenobiotica* **18**, 169–182.

Biagi G., Giorgi R., Livi O., Scartoni V., Tonetti I. and Lucacchini A. (1993). Xanthine oxidase (XO): relative configuration of complexes formed by the enzyme, 2- or 8-n-alkyl-hypoxanthines and 2-n-alkyl-8- azahypoxanthines. XII. *Farmaco* **48**, 357–374.

Bitonti A.J., Dumont J.A., Bush T.L., Stemerick D.M., Edwards M.L. and McCann P.P. (1990). Bis(benzyl)-polyamine analogs as novel substrates for polyamine oxidase. *J. Biol. Chem.* **265**, 382–388.

Blaschko H. (1989). Oxidation of tertiary amines by monoamine oxidases. *J. Pharm. Pharmacol.* **41**, 664.

Blisard K.S. and Mieyal J.J. (1979). Characterization of the aniline hydroxylase activity of erythrocytes. *J. Biol. Chem.* **254**, 5104–5110.

Blumberg W.E., Desai P.R., Powers L., Freedman J.H. and Villafranca J.J. (1989). X-Ray absorption spectroscopic study of the active copper sites in dopamine β-hydroxylase. *J. Biol. Chem.* **264**, 6029–6032.

Blume H. (1981). Biotransformation von Amphetamin-Derivaten durch Rattenleber-Mitonchondrien. 2. Mitt.: Oxidative Deaminierung von Amphetamin und Reduktion von Phenylaceton. *Arzneim.-Forsch. (Drug Res.)* **31**, 994–997.

Bolkenius F.N. and Seiler N. (1989). New substrates of polyamine oxidase. Dealkylation of N-alkyl-α,ω-diamines. *Biol. Chem. Hoppe-Seyler* **370**, 525–531.

Bossard M.J. and Klinman J.P. (1986). Mechanism-based

inhibition of dopamine β-monooxygenase by aldehydes and amines. *J. Biol. Chem.* **261**, 16,421–16,427.

Bossard M.J. and Klinman J.P. (1990). Use of isotope effects to characterize intermediates in mechanism-based inactivation of dopamine β-monooxygenase by β-chlorophenethylamine. *J. Biol. Chem.* **265**, 5640–5647.

Bounds P.L. and Winston G.W. (1991). The reaction of xanthine oxidase with aldehydic products of lipid peroxidation. *Free Radical Biol. Med.* **11**, 447–453.

Brandänge S. and Lindblom L. (1979). The enzyme "aldehyde oxidase" is an iminium oxidase. Reaction with nicotine $\Delta^{1'(5')}$ iminium ion. *Biochem. Biophys. Res. Commun.* **91**, 991–996.

Britigan B.E., Pou S., Rosen G.M., Lilleg D.M. and Buettner G.R. (1990). Hydroxyl radical is not a product of the reaction of xanthine oxidase and xanthine. *J. Biol. Chem.* **265**, 17,533–17,538.

Brown D.E., McGuirl M.A., Dooley D.M., Janes S.M., Mu D. and Klinman J.P. (1991). The organic functional group in copper-containing amine oxidases. *J. Biol. Chem.* **266**, 4049–4051.

Bunting J.W., Laderoute K.R. and Norris D.J. (1980). Specificity of xanthine oxidase for nitrogen heteroaromatic cation substrates. *Can. J. Biochem.* **58**, 49–57.

Callery P.S., Geelhaar L.A., Nayar M.S.B., Stogniew M. and Rao K.G. (1982). Pyrrolines as prodrugs of gamma-aminobutyric acid analogs. *J. Neurochem.* **38**, 1063–1067.

Callery P.S., Subramanyam B., Yuan Z.M., Pou S., Geelhaar L.A. and Reynolds K.A. (1992). Isotopically sensitive regioselectivity in the oxidative deamination of a homologous series of diamines catalyzed by diamine oxidase. *Chem.-Biol. Interact.* **85**, 15–26.

Callingham B.A., Holt A. and Elliott J. (1990). Some aspects of the pharmacology of semicarbazide-sensitive amine oxidases. *J. Neural. Transm., Suppl.* **32**, 279–290.

Callingham B.A., Holt A. and Elliott J. (1991). Properties and functions of the semicarbazide sensitive amine oxidases. *Biochem. Soc. Transact.* **19**, 228–233.

Chacon J.N., Chedekel M.R., Land E.J. and Truscott T.G. (1987). Chemically induced Parkinson's disease: intermediates in the oxidation of 1-methyl-4-phenyl-1,2,3,6-tetrahydropyridine to the 1-methyl-4-phenyl-pyridinium ion. *Biochem. Biophys. Res. Commun.* **144**, 957–964.

Chen S. and Weyler W. (1988). Partial amino acid sequence analysis of human placenta monoamine oxidase A and bovine monoamine oxidase B. *Biochem. Biophys. Res. Commun.* **156**, 445–450.

Cohen G. (1986). Monoamine oxidase, hydrogen peroxide, and Parkinson's disease. *Adv. Neurol.* **45**, 119–125.

Cole J.L., Ballou D.P. and Solomon E.I. (1991). Spectroscopic characterization of the peroxide intermediate in the reduction of dioxygen catalyzed by the multicopper oxidases. *J. Amer. Chem. Soc.* **113**, 8544–8546.

Coleman A.A., Hindsgaul O. and Palcic M.M. (1989). Stereochemistry of copper amine oxidase reactions. *J. Biol. Chem.* **264**, 19,500–19,505.

Coleman A.A., Scaman C.H., Kang Y.J. and Palcic M.M.

(1991). Stereochemical trends in copper amine oxidase reactions. *J. Biol. Chem.* **266**, 6795–6800.

Collison D., Knowles P.F., Mabbs F.E., Rius F.X., Singh I., Dooley D.M., Cote C.E. and McGuirl M. (1989). Studies on the active site of pig plasma amine oxidase. *Biochem. J.* **264**, 663–669.

Conforti L., Raimondi L. and Lyles G.A. (1993). Metabolism of methylamine by semicarbazide-sensitive amine oxidase in white and brown adipose tissue of the rat. *Biochem. Pharmacol.* **46**, 603–607.

Cossum P.A. (1988). Role of the red blood cell in drug metabolism. *Biopharm. Drug Disposit.* **9**, 321–336.

Damani L.A. and Case D.E. (1984). Metabolism of heterocycles. In *Comprehensive Heterocyclic Chemistry*, Vol. 1 (ed. Meth-Cohn O). pp. 223–246. Pergamon Press, Oxford.

Damani L.A., Crooks P.A. and Cowan D.A. (1981). Metabolism of metyrapone. III. Formation of an α-pyridone metabolite by rat hepatic soluble enzymes. *Drug Metab. Disposit.* **9**, 270–273.

D'Ardenne S.C. and Edmondson D.E. (1990). Kinetic isotope effect studies on milk xanthine oxidase and on chicken liver xanthine dehydrogenase. *Biochemistry* **29**, 9046–9052.

Debnath J., Husain P.A. and May S.W. (1992). Activation of an adrenergic prodrug though sequential stereoselective action of tandem target enzymes. *Biochem. Biophys. Res. Commun.* **189**, 33–39.

Dewolf W.E. Jr, Chambers P.A., Southan C., Saunders D. and Kruse L.I. (1989). Inactivation of dopamine β-hydroxylase by β-ethynyltyramine: kinetic characterization and covalent modification of an active site peptide. *Biochemistry* **28**, 3833–3842.

Ding C.Z. and Silverman R.B. (1993). Transformation of heterocyclic reversible monoamine oxidase-B inactivators into irreversible inactivators by N-methylation. *J. Med. Chem.* **36**, 3606–3610.

Ding C.Z., Lu X., Nishimura K. and Silverman R.B. (1993). Transformation of monoamine oxidase-B primary amine substrates into time-dependent inhibitors. Tertiary amine homologues of primary amine substrates. *J. Med. Chem.* **36**, 1711–1715.

Duverger-van Bogaert M., Wiame D. and Stecca C. (1992). Oxidative activation of 2-aminofluorene by human red blood cell cytosol. *Biochem. Pharmacol.* **44**, 2422–2424.

Eagle A.A., Laughlin L.J., Young C.G. and Tiekink E.R.T. (1992). An oxothio-molybdenum(VI) complex stabilized by an intramolecular sulfur–sulfur interaction: Implications for the active site of oxidized xanthine oxidase and related enzymes. *J. Amer. Chem. Soc.* **114**, 9195–9197.

Eastmond D.A., French R.C., Ross D. and Smith M.T. (1987). Metabolic activation of 1-naphthol and phenol by a simple superoxide-generating system and human leukocytes. *Chem.-Biol. Interact.* **63**, 47–62.

Edmondson D.E., Battacharyya A.K. and Walker M.C. (1993). Spectral and kinetic studies of imine product formation in the oxidation of p-(N,N-dimethylamino)benzylamine analogues by monoamine oxidase B. *Biochemistry* **32**, 5196–5202.

Efange S.M.N. and Boudreau R.J. (1991). Molecular determinants in the bioactivation of the dopaminergic neurotoxin N-methyl-4-phenyl-1,2,3,6-tetrahydropyridine (MPTP). *J. Comput.-Aided Molec. Design* **5**, 405–417.

Efange S.M.N., Michelson R.H., Remmel R.P., Boudreau R.J., Dutta A.K. and Freshler A. (1990). Flexible N-methyl-4-phenyl-1,2,3,6-tetrahydropyridine analogues: synthesis and monoamine oxidase catalyzed bioactivation. *J. Med. Chem.* **33**, 3133–3138.

Efange S.M.N., Michelson R.H., Tan A.K., Krueger M.J. and Singer T.P. (1993). Molecular size and flexibility as determinants of selectivity in the oxidation of N-methyl-4-phenyl-1,2,3,6-tetrahydropyridine analogs by monoamine oxidase A. *J. Med. Chem.* **36**, 1278–1283.

Elmarakby S.A., Duffel M.W. and Rosazza J.P.N. (1989). In vitro metabolic transformation of vinblastine: oxidations catalyzed by human ceruloplasmin. *J. Med. Chem.* **32**, 2158–2162.

Farrington G.K., Kumar A. and Villafranca J.J. (1989). Benzofurans as mechanism-based inhibitors of dopamine β-hydroxylase. *J. Med. Chem.* **32**, 735–737.

Farrington G.K., Kumar A. and Villafranca J.J. (1990). Active site labeling of dopamine β-hydroxylase by two mechanism-based inhibitors: 6-hydroxybenzofuran and phenylhydrazine. *J. Biol. Chem.* **265**, 1036–1040.

Ferraiolo B.L. and Mieyal J.J. (1982). Subunit selectivity in the monooxygenase-like activity of tetrameric hemoglobin. *Molec. Pharmacol.* **21**, 1–4.

Flory D.R. Jr and Villafranca J.J. (1988). Characterization of 3-phenylpropenes as mechanism-based inhibitors of dopamine β-hydroxylase. *Bioorg. Chem.* **16**, 232–244.

Folkers G., Krug M. and Trumpp S. (1987). Computer graphic study on models of the molybdenum cofactor of xanthine oxidase. *J. Comput.-Aid. Molec. Design* **1**, 87–94.

Fraeyman N.H., Van de Velde E.J. and De Smet F.H. (1988). Molecular forms of dopamine beta-hydroxylase in rat superior cervical ganglion and adrenal gland. *Experientia* **44**, 746–749.

Gates K.S. and Silverman R.B. (1990). 5-(Aminomethyl)-3-aryl-2-oxazolidinones. A novel class of mechanism-based inactivators of monoamine oxidase B. *J. Amer. Chem. Soc.* **112**, 9364–9372.

Gerlach M. and Riederer P. (1993). Human brain MAO. In *Monoamine Oxidase: Basic and Clinical Aspects* (eds Yasuhara H., Parvez S.H., Oguchi K., Sandler M. and Nagatsu T.). pp. 147–158. VSP, Utrecht, The Netherlands.

Gibb C., Willoughby J., Glover V., Sandler M., Testa B., Jenner P. and Marsden C.D. (1987). Analogues of 1-methyl-4-phenyl-1,2,3,6-tetrahydropyridine as monoamine oxidase substrates: a second ring is not necessary. *Neurosci. Lett.* **76**, 316–322.

Glover V. and Sandler M. (1987). Monoamine oxidase and the brain. *Rev. Neurosci.* **1**, 145–156.

Gomez N., Balsa D. and Unzeta M. (1988). A comparative study of some kinetic and molecular properties of microsomal and mitochondrial monoamine oxidase. *Biochem. Pharmacol.* **37**, 3407–3413.

Goodhart P.J., DeWolf W.E. Jr and Kruse L.I. (1987). Mechanism-based inactivation of dopamine β-hydroxylase by *p*-cresol and related alkylphenols. *Biochemistry* **26**, 2576–2583.

Greenaway F.T., O'Gara C.Y., Marchena J.M., Poku J.W., Urtiaga J.G. and Zou Y. (1991). EPR Studies of spin-labeled bovine plasma amine oxidase: the nature of the substrate-binding site. *Arch. Biochem. Biophys.* **285**, 291–296.

Gristwood W. and Wilson K. (1988). Kinetics of some benzothiazoles, benzoxazoles, and quinolines as substrates and inhibitors of rabbit liver aldehyde oxidase. *Xenobiotica* **18**, 949–954.

Haberland A., Schütz A.K. and Schimke I. (1992). The influence of lipid peroxidation products (malondialdehyde, 4-hydroxynonenal) on xanthine oxidoreductase prepared from rat liver. *Biochem. Pharmacol.* **43**, 2117–2120.

Hall W.W. and Krenitsky T.A. (1986). Aldehyde oxidase from rabbit liver. Specificity toward purines and their analogs. *Arch. Biochem. Biophys.* **251**, 36–46.

Hall L., Murray S., Castagnoli K. and Castagnoli N. Jr (1992). Studies on 1,2,3,6-tetrahydropyridine derivatives as potential monoamine oxidase inactivators. *Chem. Res. Toxicol.* **5**, 625–633.

Harik S.I., Riachi N.J., Hritz M.A., Berridge M.S. and Sayre L.M. (1993). Development of fluorinated 1-methyl-4-phenyl-1,2,3,6-tetrahydropyridine analogs with potent nigrostriatal toxicity for potential use in positron emission tomography studies. *J. Pharmacol. Exp. Therap.* **266**, 790–795.

Harrison J.H. Jr and Jollow D.J. (1987). Contribution of aniline metabolites to aniline-induced methemoglobinemia. *Molec. Pharmacol.* **32**, 423–431.

Hartmann C. and Klinman J.P. (1991). Structure–function studies of substrate oxidation by bovine serum amine oxidase: relationship to cofactor structure and mechanism. *Biochemistry* **30**, 4605–4611.

Hartmann C., Brzovic P. and Klinman J.P. (1993). Spectroscopic detection of chemical intermediates in the reaction of *para*-substituted benzylamines with bovine serum amine oxidase. *Biochemistry* **32**, 2234–2241.

Heilmair R., Lenk W. and Sterzl H. (1987). N-Hydroxy-N-arylacetamides. IV. Differences in the mechanism of haemoglobin oxidation *in vitro* between N-hydroxy-N-arylacetamides and arylhydroxylamines. *Biochem. Pharmacol.* **36**, 2963–2972.

Heilmair R., Karreth S. and Lenk W. (1991). The metabolism of 4-aminobiphenyl in rat. II. Reaction of N-hydroxy-4-aminobiphenyl with rat blood *in vitro. Xenobiotica* **21**, 805–815.

Hille R. and Sprecher H. (1987). On the mechanism of action of xanthine oxidase. Evidence in support of an oxo transfer mechanism in the molybdenum-containing hydroxylases. *J. Biol. Chem.* **262**, 10,914–10,917.

Hille R. and Anderson R.F. (1991). Electron transfer in milk xanthine oxidase as studied by pulse radiolysis. *J. Biol. Chem.* **266**, 5608–5615.

Hiraoka A., Ohtaka J., Koike S., Tsuboi Y., Tsuchikawa S. and Miura I. (1988). Inhibition of copper-containing amine oxidase by oximes. *Chem. Pharm. Bull.* **36**, 3027–3031.

Howes B.D., Bennett B., Koppenhöfer A., Lowe D.J. and Bray R.C. (1991). ^{31}P ENDOR studies of xanthine oxidase: coupling of phosphorus of the pterin cofactor to molybdenum(V). *Biochemistry* **30**, 3969–3975.

Hsu Y.P.P., Powell J.F., Sims K.B. and Breakefield X.O. (1989). Molecular genetics of the monoamine oxidases. *J. Neurochem.* **53**, 12–18.

Huyghe B.G. and Klinman J.P. (1991). Activity of membranous dopamine β-monooxygenase within chromaffin granule ghosts. Interaction with ascorbate. *J. Biol. Chem.* **266**, 11,544–11,550.

Itano H.A. and Matteson J.L. (1982). Mechanism of initial reaction of phenylhydrazine with oxyhemoglobin and effect of ring substitutions on the bimolecular rate constant of this reaction. *Biochemistry* **21**, 2421–2426.

Janes S.M. and Klinman J.P. (1991). An investigation of bovine serum amine oxidase active site stoichiometry: Evidence for an aminotransferase mechanism involving two carbonyl cofactors per enzyme dimer. *Biochemistry* **30**, 4599–4605.

Janes S.M., Mu D., Wemmer D., Smith A.J., Kaur S., Maltby D., Burlingame A.L. and Klinman J.P. (1990). A new redox cofactor on eukaryotic enzymes: 6-hydroxydopa at the active site of bovine serum amine oxidase. *Science* **248**, 981–987.

Janes S.M., Palcic M.M., Scaman C.H., Smith A.J., Brown D.E., Dooley D.M., Mure M. and Klinman J.P. (1992). Identification of topaquinone and its consensus sequence in copper amine oxidases. *Biochemistry* **31**, 12,147–12,154.

Janssens de Varebeke P., Pauwels G., Buyse C., David-Remacle M., De Mey J., Roba J. and Youdim M.B.H. (1989). The novel neuropsychotropic agent milacemide is a specific enzyme-activated inhibitor of brain monoamine oxidase B. *J. Neurochem.* **53**, 1109–1116.

Jones D.B., Rustgi V.K., Kornhauser D.M., Woods A., Quinn R., Hoofnagle J.H. and Jones E.A. (1987). The disposition of 6-deoxyacyclovir, a xanthine oxidase-activated prodrug of acyclovir, in the isolated perfused rat liver. *Hepatology* **7**, 345–348.

Kalgutkar A.S. and Castagnoli Jr N. (1992). Synthesis of novel MPTP analogs as potential monoamine oxidase B (MAO-B) inhibitors. *J. Med. Chem.* **35**, 4165–4174.

Kalir A., Sabbagh A. and Youdim M.B.H. (1981). Selective acetylenic "suicide" and reversible inhibitors of monoamine oxidase types A and B. *Brit J. Pharmacol.* **73**, 55–64.

Kalow W. (1985). Variability of caffeine metabolism in humans. *Arzneim.-Forsch. (Drug Res.)* **35**, 319–324.

Kaye B., Rance D.J. and Waring L. (1985). Oxidative metabolism of carbazeran *in vitro* by liver cytosol of baboon and man. *Xenobiotica* **15**, 237–242.

Kim S.C. and Klinman J.P. (1991). Mechanism of inhibition of dopamine β-monooxygenase by quinol and phenol derivatives, as determined by solvent and substrate deuterium isotope effects. *Biochemistry* **30**, 8138–8144.

Kindt M.V., Youngster S.K., Sonsalla P.K., Duvoisin R.C. and Heikkila R.E. (1988). Role of monoamine oxidase-A (MAO-A) in the bioactivation and nigrostriatal dopaminergic neurotoxicity of the MPTP analog, 2'Me-MPTP. *Eur. J. Pharmacol.* **146**, 313–318.

Klinman J.P., Huyghe B., Stewart L. and Taljanidisz J. (1990). Structure–function studies of dopamine β-hydroxylase. *Biol. Oxid. Syst.* **1**, 329–346.

Klinman J.P., Dooley D.M., Duine J.A., Knowles P.F., Mondovi B. and Villafranca J.J. (1991). Status of the cofactor identity in copper oxidative enzymes. *FEBS Lett.* **282**, 1–4.

Krenitsky T.A. (1978). Aldehyde oxidase and xanthine oxidase—functional and evolutionary relationships. *Biochem. Pharmacol.* **27**, 2763–2764.

Krenitsky T.A., Neil S.M., Elion G.B. and Hitchings G.C. (1972). A comparison of the specificities of xanthine oxidase and aldehyde oxidase. *Arch Biochem. Biophys.* **150**, 585–599.

Krueger M.J., McKeown K., Ramsay R.R., Youngster S.K. and Singer T.P. (1990). Mechanism-based inactivation of monoamine oxidases A and B by tetrahydropyridines and dihydropyridines. *Biochem. J.* **268**, 219–224.

Krueger M.J., Efange S.M.N., Michelson R.H. and Singer T.P. (1992). Interaction of flexible analogs of N-methyl-4-phenyl-1,2,3,6-tetrahydropyridine and of N-methyl-4-phenylpyridinium with highly purified monoamine oxidase A and B. *Biochemistry* **31**, 5611–5615.

Kruse L.I., DeWolf W.E. Jr, Chambers P.A. and Goodhart P.J. (1986a). Design and kinetic characterization of multisubstrate inhibitors of dopamine β-hydroxylase. *Biochemistry* **25**, 7271–7278.

Kruse L.I., Kaiser C., DeWolf W.E. Jr, Frazee J.S., Garvey E., Hilbert E.L., Faulkner W.A., Flaim K.E., Sawyer J.L. and Berkowitz B.A. (1986b). Multisubstrate inhibitors of dopamine β-hydroxylase. 1. Some 1-phenyl and 1-phenyl-bridged derivatives of imidazole-2-thione. *J. Med. Chem.* **29**, 2465–2472.

Kruse L.I., Kaiser C., DeWolf W.E., Finkelstein J.A., Frazee J.S., Hilbert E.L., Ross S.T., Flaim K.E. and Sawyer J.L. (1990). Some benzyl-substituted imidazoles, triazoles, tetrazoles, pyridithiones, and structural relatives as multisubstrate inhibitors of dopamine β-hydroxylase. 4. Structure–activity relationships at the copper binding site. *J. Med. Chem.* **33**, 781–789.

Kyburz E. (1990). New developments in the field of MAO inhibitors. *Drug News Perspect.* **3**, 592–599.

Lee C.H. and Han I.S. (1992). Modified purines as mechanistic probes of substrates oxidation by xanthine oxidase. *J. Korean Chem. Soc.* **36**, 335–337.

Lenk W. and Riedl M. (1989). N-Hydroxy-N-arylacetamides. V. Differences in the mechanism of haemoglobin oxidation *in vitro* by N-hydroxy-4-chloroacetanilide and N-hydroxy-4-chloroaniline. *Xenobiotica* **19**, 453–475.

Lerch K. (1981). Copper monooxygenases: tyrosinase and dopamine β-monooxygenase. In *Metal Ions in Biological Systems*, Vol. 13 (ed. Sigel H.). pp. 143–186. Dekker, New York.

Lewis E.J., Allison S., Fader D., Claflin V. and Baizer L. (1990). Bovine dopamine β-hydroxylase cDNA. Complete coding sequence and expression in mammalian cells

with vaccinia virus vector. *J. Biol. Chem.* **265**, 1021–1028.

Lizcano J.M., Balsa D., Tipton K.F. and Unzeta M. (1991). The oxidation of dopamine by the semicarbazide-sensitive amine oxidase (SSAO) from the rat vas deferens. *Biochem. Pharmacol.* **41**, 1107–1110.

Lyles G.A., Holt A. and Marshall C.M.S. (1990). Further studies on the metabolism of methylamine by semicarbazide-sensitive amine oxidase activities in human plasma, umbilical artery and rat aorta. *J. Pharm. Pharmacol.* **42**, 322–338.

Maples K.R., Jordan S.J. and Mason R.P. (1988a). *In vivo* rat hemoglobin thiyl free radical formation following phenylhydrazine administration. *Molec. Pharmacol.* **33**, 344–350.

Maples K.R., Jordan S.J. and Mason R.P. (1988b). *In vivo* rat hemoglobin thiyl free radical formation following administration of phenylhydrazine and hydrazine-based drugs. *Drug Metab. Disposit.* **16**, 799–803.

Maret G., Testa B., Jenner P., El Tayar N. and Carrupt P.A. (1990a). The MPTP story: MAO activates tetrahydropyridine derivatives to toxins causing parkinsonism. *Drug Metab. Rev.* **22**, 291–332.

Maret G., El Tayar N., Carrupt P.A., Testa B., Jenner P. and Baird M. (1990b). Toxication of MPTP (1-methyl-4-phenyl-1,2,3,6-tetrahydro-pyridine) and analogs by monoamine oxidase. A structure–reactivity relationship study. *Biochem. Pharmacol.* **40**, 783–792.

Mason R.P. and Maples K.R. (1990). *In vivo* hemoglobin thiyl radical formation as a consequence of hydrazine-based drug metabolism. In *Sulfur-Centered Reactive Intermediates in Chemistry and Biology* (eds Chatgilialoglu C. and Asmus K.D.). pp. 429–434. Plenum Press, New York.

Massey V., Schopfer L.M., Nishino T. and Nishino T. (1989). Differences in protein structure of xanthine dehydrogenase and xanthine oxidase revealed by reconstitution with flavin active site probes. *J. Biol. Chem.* **264**, 10,567–10,573.

May S.W. and Phillips R.S. (1980). Asymmetric sulfoxidation by dopamine β-hydroxylase, an oxygenase heretofore considered specific for methylene hydroxylation. *J. Amer. Chem. Soc.* **102**, 5981–5983.

May S.W., Phillips R.S., Mueller P.W. and Herman H.H. (1981a). Dopamine β-hydroxylase. Comparative specificities and mechanisms of the oxygenation reactions. *J. Biol. Chem.* **256**, 8470–8475.

May S.W., Phillips R.S., Mueller P.W. and Herman H.H. (1981b). Dopamine β-hydroxylase. Demonstration of enzymatic ketonization of the product enantiomer, S-octopamine. *J. Biol. Chem.* **256**, 2258–2261.

May S.W., Phillips R.S., Herman H.H. and Mueller P.W. (1982). Bioactivation of catha edulis alkaloids: enzymatic ketonization of norpseudoephedrine. *Biochem. Biophys. Res. Commun.* **104**, 38–44.

May S.W., Wimalasena K., Herman H.H., Fowler L.C., Ciccarello M.C. and Pollock S.H. (1988). Novel antihypertensives targeted at dopamine β-monooxygenase: turnover-dependent cofactor depletion by phenyl aminoethyl selenide. *J. Med. Chem.* **31**, 1066–1068.

Maynard M.S. and Cho A.K. (1981). Oxidation of N-hydroxyphentermine to 2-methyl-2-nitro-1-phenyl-propane by liver microsomes. *Biochem. Pharmacol.* **30**, 1115–1119.

McCormack J.J., Allen B.A. and Hodnett C.N. (1978). Oxidation of quinazoline and quinoxaline by xanthine oxidase and aldehyde oxidase. *J. Heterocycl. Chem.* **15**, 1249–1254.

McDaniel H.G., Podgainy H. and Bressler R. (1969). The metabolism of tolbutamide in rat liver. *J. Pharmacol. Exp. Therap.* **167**, 91-97.

McIntire W.S. and Hartmann C. (1993). Copper-containing amine oxidases. In *Principles and Applications of Quinoproteins* (ed. Davidson V.I.). pp. 97–171. Dekker, New York.

Mieyal J.J. (1985). Monooxygenase activity of hemoglobin and myoglobin. In *Reviews in Biochemical Toxicology*, Vol. 7 (eds Hodgson E., Bend J.R. and Philpot R.M.). pp. 1–66. Elsevier, New York.

Mieyal J.J., Ackerman R.S., Blumer J.L. and Freeman L.S. (1976). Characterization of enzyme-like activity of human hemoglobin. Properties of the hemoglobin-P450 reductase-coupled aniline hydroxylase system. *J. Biol. Chem.* **251**, 3436–3441.

Miller S.M. and Klinman J.P. (1985). Secondary isotope effects and structure–reactivity correlations in the dopamine β-monooxygenase reaction. Evidence for a chemical mechanism. *Biochemistry* **24**, 2114–2127.

Moriwaki Y., Yamamoto T., Nasako Y., Takahashi S., Suda M., Hiroishi K., Hada T. and Higashino K. (1993). *In vitro* oxidation of pyrazinamide and allopurinol by rat liver aldehyde oxidase. *Biochem. Pharmacol.* **46**, 975–981.

Morpurgo L., Befani O., Sabatini S., Mondovi B., Artico M., Corelli F., Massa S., Stefancich G. and Avigliano L. (1988). Spectroscopic studies of the reaction between bovine serum amine oxidase (copper-containing) and some hydrazides and hydrazines. *Biochem. J.* **256**, 565–570.

Morpurgo L., Agostinelli E., Mondovi B., Avigliano L., Silvestri R., Stefancich G. and Artico M. (1992). Bovine serum amine oxidase: half-site reactivity with phenylhydrazine, semicarbazide, and aromatic hydrazides. *Biochemistry* **31**, 2615–2621.

Mu D., Janes S.M., Smith A.J., Brown D.E., Dooley D.M. and Klinman J.P. (1992). Tyrosine codon corresponds to topa quinone at the active site of copper amine oxidases. *J. Biol. Chem.* **267**, 7979–7982.

Naeff H.S.D., Franssen M.C.R. and Van der Plas H.C. (1991). Quantitative structure–activity relationship (QSAT) studies of the inhibition of xanthine oxidase by heterocyclic compounds. *Recl. Trav. Chim. Pays-Bas* **110**, 139–150.

Nishimura K., Lu X. and Silverman R.B. (1993). Inactivation of monoamine oxidase B by analogues of the anticonvulsant agent milacemide (2-(*n*-propylamino)-(acetamide). *J. Med. Chem.* **36**, 446–448.

Noro T., Noro K., Miyase T., Kuroyanagi M., Umehara

K., Ueno A. and Fukushima S. (1987). Inhibition of xanthine oxidase by anthraquinones. *Chem. Pharm. Bull.* **35**, 4314–4316.

Obata T., Egashira T. and Yamanaka Y. (1990). Isoelectric focusing of isoenzymes of monkey platelet monoamine oxidase. *Biochem. Pharmacol.* **40**, 1689–1693.

O'Brien E.M., Tipton K.F., Strolin Benedetti M., Bonsignori A., Marrari P. and Dostert P. (1991). Is the oxidation of milacemide by monoamine oxidase a major factor in its anticonvulsant actions? *Biochem. Pharmacol.* **41**, 1731–1737.

O'Carroll A.M., Anderson M.C., Tobbia I., Phillips J.P. and Tipton K.F. (1989). Determination of the absolute concentrations of monoamine oxidase A and B in human tissues. *Biochem. Pharmacol.* **38**, 901–905.

Oertling W.A. and Hille R. (1990). Resonance-enhanced Raman scattering from the molybdenum center of xanthine oxidase. *J. Biol. Chem.* **265**, 17,446–17,450.

Ottoboni S., Caldera P., Trevor A. and Castagnoli N. Jr (1989). Deuterium isotope effect measurement on the interaction of the neurotoxin 1-methyl-4-phenyl-1,2,3,6-tetrahydropyridine with monoamine oxidase B. *J. Biol. Chem.* **264**, 13,684–13,688. Correction **265**, 8345 (1990).

Oyarce A.M. and Fleming P.J. (1991). Multiple forms of human dopamine β-hydroxylase in SH-SY5Y neuroblastoma cells. *Arch Biochem. Biophys.* **290**, 503–510.

Padgette S.R., Wimalasena K., Herman H.H., Sirimanne S.R. and May S.W. (1985). Olefin oxygenation and N-dealkylation by dopamine β-monooxygenase: catalysis and mechanism-based inhibition. *Biochemistry* **24**, 5826–5839.

Pearce L.B. and Roth J.A. (1985). Human brain monoamine oxidase type B: mechanism of deamination as probed by steady-state methods. *Biochemistry* **24**, 1821–1826.

Pedersen J.Z., El-Sherbini S., Finazzi-Agrò A. and Rotilio G. (1992). A substrate-cofactor free radical intermediate in the reaction mechanism of copper amine oxidase. *Biochemistry* **31**, 8–12.

Pelsy G. and Klibanov A.M. (1983). Remarkable positional (regio)specificity of xanthine oxidase and some dehydrogenases in the reactions with substituted benzaldehydes. *Biochim. Biophys. Acta* **742**, 352–357.

Powell J.F. (1991). Molecular biological studies of monoamine oxidase: structure and function. *Biochem. Soc. Transact.* **19**, 199–201.

Rajagopalan K.V. (1980). Xanthine oxidase and aldehyde oxidase. In *Enzymatic Basis of Detoxication*, Vol. 1 (ed. Jakoby W.B.). pp. 295–309. Academic Press, New York.

Ramsay R.R. (1991). Kinetic mechanism of monoamine oxidase A. *Biochemistry* **30**, 4624–4629.

Ramsay R.R., Koerber S.C. and Singer T.P. (1987). Stopped-flow studies on the mechanism of N-methyl-4-phenyl-1,2,3,6-tetrahydropyridine (MPTP) by monoamine oxidase. In *Flavins and Flavoproteins 1987* (eds Edmondson D.E. and McCormick D.B.). pp. 705–708. De Gruyter, Berlin.

Reinke L.A., Nakamura M., Logan L., Christensen H.D. and Carney J.M. (1987). *In vivo* and *in vitro* 1-

methylxanthine metabolism in the rat. Evidence that the dehydrogenase form of xanthine oxidase predominates in intact perfused liver. *Drug Metab. Disposit.* **15**, 295–299.

Robertson J.G., Desai P.R., Kumar A., Farrington G.K., Fitzpatrick P.F. and Villafranca J.J. (1990). Primary amino acid sequence of bovine dopamine β-hydroxylase. *J. Biol. Chem.* **265**, 1029–1035.

Sabbioni G. (1992). Hemoglobin binding of monocyclic aromatic amines: molecular dosimetry and quantitative structure–activity relationships for the N-oxidation. *Chem.-Biol. Interact.* **81**, 91–117.

Saito T. and Nishino T. (1989). Differences in redox and kinetic properties between NAD-dependent and O$_2$-dependent types of rat liver xanthine dehydrogenase. *J. Biol. Chem.* **264**, 10,015–10,022.

Santaniello E., Manzocchi A., Biondi P.A. and Simonic T. (1982). Regioselectivity in the oxidative deamination of 2-methyl-1,4-diaminobutane catalyzed by diamine oxidase. *Experientia* **38**, 782–784.

Sayre L.M., Singh M.P., Kokil P.B. and Wang F. (1991). Non-electron-transfer quinone-mediated oxidative cleavage of cyclopropylamines. Implications regarding their utility as probes of enzyme mechanism. *J. Org. Chem.* **56**, 1353–1355.

Scaman C.H. and Palcic M.M. (1992). Stereochemical course of tyramine oxidation by semicarbazide-sensitive amine oxidase. *Biochemistry* **31**, 6829–6841.

Schopfer L.M., Massey V. and Nishino T. (1988). Rapid reaction studies on the reduction and oxidation of chicken liver xanthine dehydrogenase by the xanthine/urate and NAD/NADH couples. *J. Biol. Chem.* **263**, 13,528–13,538.

Scott R.A., Sullivan R.J., DeWolf W.E. Jr, Dolle R.E. and Kruse L.I. (1988). The copper sites of dopamine β-hydroxylase: an X-ray absorption spectroscopic study. *Biochemistry* **27**, 5411–5417.

Shih J.C. (1991). Molecular basis of human MAO A and B. *Neuropsychopharmacology* **4**, 1–7.

Shih J.C. (1993). cDNA cloning of human liver MAO-A and MAO-B. In *Monoamine Oxidase: Basic and Clinical Aspects* (eds Yasuhara H., Parvez S.H., Oguchi K., Sandler M. and Nagatsu T.). pp. 15–21. VSP, Utrecht, The Netherlands.

Silverman R.B. (1991). The use of mechanism-based inactivators to probe the mechanism of monoamine oxidase. *Biochem. Soc. Transact.* **19**, 201–206.

Silverman R.B. and Ding C.Z. (1993). Chemical model for a mechanism of inactivation of monoamine oxidase by heterocyclic compounds. Electronic effects on acetal hydrolysis. *J. Amer. Chem. Soc.* **115**, 4571–4576.

Silverman R.B. and Zelechonok Y. (1992). Evidence for a hydrogen atom transfer mechanism or a proton/fast electron transfer mechanism for monoamine oxidase. *J. Org. Chem.* **57**, 6373–6374.

Silverman R.B. and Zieske P.A. (1985). 1-Benzyl-cyclopropylamine and 1-(phenylcyclopropyl)methyl-amine: an inactivator and a substrate of monoamine oxidase. *J. Med. Chem.* **28**, 1953–1957.

Silverman R.B., Hoffman S.J. and Catus W.B. (1980). A mechanism for mitochondrial monoamine oxidase catalyzed amine oxidation. *J. Amer. Chem. Soc.* **102**, 7126–7128.

Silverman R.B., Nishimura K. and Lu X. (1993a). Mechanism of inactivation of monoamine oxidase-B by the anticonvulsant agent milacemide (2-(n-pentylamino)-acetamide). *J. Amer. Chem. Soc.* **115**, 4949–4954.

Silverman R.B., Cesarone J.M. and Lu X. (1993b). Stereoselective ring opening of 1-phenylcyclo-propylamine catalyzed by monoamine oxidase-B. *J. Amer. Chem. Soc.* **115**, 4955–4961.

Sim M.K. and Lim S.E. (1992). Discovery of a novel soluble form of monoamine oxidase in the rat brain. *Biochem. Pharmacol.* **1181–1184.V.**

Simpson J.T., Krantz A., Lewis F.D. and Kokel B. (1982). Photochemical and photophysical studies of amines with excited flavins. Relevance to the mechanism of action of the flavin-dependent monoamine oxidase. *J. Amer. Chem. Soc.* **104**, 7155–7161.

Singer T.P. (1991). Monoamine oxidases. In *Chemistry and Biochemistry of Flavoenzymes*, Vol. 2 (ed. Mueller F.). pp. 437–470. CRC, Boca Raton, FL.

Singer T.P. and Ramsay R.R. (1991). The interaction of monoamine oxidases with tertiary amines. *Biochem. Soc. Transact.* **19**, 211–215.

Singer T.P. and Ramsay R.R. (1993). New aspects of the substrate specificities, kinetic mechanisms and inhibition of monoamine oxidases. In *Monoamine Oxidase: Basic and Clinical Aspects* (eds. Yasuhara H., Parvez S.H., Oguchi K., Sandler M. and Nagatsu T.). pp. 23–43. VSP, Utrecht, The Netherlands.

Singer T.P., Salach J.I. and Crabtree D. (1985). Reversible inhibition and mechanism-based irreversible inactivation of monoamine oxidases by 1-methyl-4-phenyl-1,2,3,6-tetrahydropyridine (MPTP). *Biochem. Biophys. Res. Commun.* **127**, 707–712.

Singer T.P., Ramsay R.R., Sonsalla P.K., Nicklas W.J. and Heikkila R.E. (1993). Biochemical mechanisms underlying MPTP-induced and idiopathic Parkinsonism. New Vistas. *Adv. Neurol.* **60**, 300–305.

Sirimanne S.R. and May S.W. (1988). Facile stereoselective allylic hydroxylation by dopamine β-monooxygenase. *J. Amer. Chem. Soc.* **110**, 7560–7561.

Starke D.W. and Mieyal J.J. (1989). Hemoglobin catalysis of a monooxygenase-like aliphatic hydroxylation reaction. *Biochem. Pharmacol.* **38**, 201–208.

Starke D.W., Blisard K.S. and Mieyal J.J. (1984). Substrate specificity of the monooxygenase activity of hemoglobin. *Molec. Pharmacol.* **25**, 467–475.

Stecca C., Cumps J. and Duverger-Van Bogaert M. (1992). Enzymic N-demethylation reaction catalysed by red blood cell cytosol. *Biochem. Pharmacol.* **43**, 207–211.

Stewart L.C. and Klinman J.P. (1991). Cooperativity in the dopamine β-monooxygenase reaction. Evidence for ascorbate regulation of enzyme activity. *J. Biol. Chem.* **266**, 11,53–11,543.

Strolin Benedetti M. (1989). Oxidative drug metabolism not cytochrome P-450 dependent. In *Actualités de Chimie Thérapeutique*, Vol. 16 (ed. Combet Farnoux

C.). pp. 337–356. Société de Chimie Thérapeutique, Châtenay-Malabry, France.

Strolin Benedetti M., Dow J., Boucher T. and Dostert P. (1983). Metabolism of the monoamine oxidase-B inhibitor, MD 780236 and its enantiomers by the A and B forms of the enzyme in the rat. *J. Pharm. Pharmacol.* **35**, 837–840.

Strolin Benedetti M., Dostert P. and Tipton K.F. (1988). Contributions of monoamine oxidase to the metabolism of xenobiotics. In *Progress in Drug Metabolism*, Vol. 11 (ed. Gibson G.G.). pp. 149–174. Taylor and Francis, London.

Strolin Benedetti M., Allievi C., Cocchiara G., Pevarello P. and Dostert P. (1992). Involvement of FAD-dependent polyamine oxidase in the metabolism of milacemide in the rat. *Xenobiotica* **22**, 191–197.

Stubley C. and Stell J.G.P. (1980). Investigation of the substrate-binding site of aldehyde oxidase. *J. Pharm. Pharmacol.* **32**, 51P.

Stubley C., Subryan L., Stell J.G.P., Perrett R.H., Ingle P.B.H. and Mathieson D.W. (1977). The metabolism of N-heterocycles. *J. Pharm. Pharmacol.* **29**, 77P.

Stubley C., Stell J.G.P. and Mathieson D.W. (1979). The oxidation of azaheterocycles with mammalian liver aldehyde oxidase. *Xenobiotica* **9**, 475–484.

Subramanyam B., Callery P.S., Geelhaar L.A. and Egorin M.J. (1989). A cyclic intermediate in the *in vivo* metabolic conversion of 1,6-diaminohexane to 6-aminohexanoic acid and caprolactam. *Xenobiotica* **19**, 33–42.

Sultatos L.G. (1988). Effects of acute ethanol administration on the hepatic xanthine dehydrogenase/oxidase system in the rat. *J. Pharmacol. Exp. Therap.* **246**, 946–949.

Szutowicz A., Tomaszewicz M. and Orsulak P.J. (1989). Modifications of substrate-inhibitor affinities of human platelet monoamine oxidase B *in vitro*. *J. Biol. Chem.* **264**, 17,660–17,664.

Taljanidisz J., Stewart L., Smith A.J. and Klinman J.P. (1989). Structure of bovine adrenal dopamine β-monooxygenase, as deduced from cDNA and protein sequencing: evidence that the membrane-bound form of the enzyme is anchored by an uncleaved signal peptide. *Biochemistry* **28**, 10,054–10,061.

Tan A.K. and Ramsay R.R. (1993). Substrate-specific enhancement of the oxidative half-reaction of monoamine oxidase. *Biochemistry* **32**, 2137–2143.

Thomson A.J. (1991). Radical copper in oxidases. *Nature* **350**, 22–23.

Tipton K.F. (1980). Monoamine oxidase. In *Enzymatic Basis of Detoxication*, Volume 1 (ed. Jakoby W.B.). pp. 355–370. Academic Press, New York.

Tipton K.F. (1986). Enzymology of monoamine oxidase. *Cell Biochem. Funct.* **4**, 79–87.

Tipton K.F., O'Carroll A.M. and McCrodden J.M. (1987). The catalytic behaviour of monoamine oxidase. *J. Neural. Transm.* [Suppl.] **23**, 25–35.

Tomoda A., Yubisui T., Ida M., Kawachi N. and Yoneyama Y. (1977). Aniline hydroxylation in human red cells. *Experientia* **33**, 1276–1277.

Trevor A.J., Singer T.P., Ramsay R.R. and Castagnoli N. Jr (1987). Processing of MPTP by monoamine oxidases: implications for molecular toxicology. *J. Neural. Transm.* [Suppl.] **23**, 73–89.

Tullman R.H. and Hanzlik R.P. (1984). Inactivation of cytochrome P-450 and monoamine oxidase by cyclopropylamines. *Drug Metab. Rev.* **15**, 1163–1182.

Tweedie D.J., Fernandez D., Spearman M.E., Feldhoff R.C. and Prough R.A. (1991). Metabolism of azoxy derivatives of procarbazine by aldehyde dehydrogenase and xanthine oxidase. *Drug Metab. Disposit.* **19**, 793–803.

van der Schoot J.B. and Creveling C.R. (1965). Substrates and inhibitors of dopamine-β-hydroxylase (DBH). In *Advances in Drug Research*, Vol. 2 (eds Harper N.J. and Simmonds A.B.). pp. 47–88. Academic Press, London.

Vazquez M.L. and Silverman R.B. (1985). Revised mechanism for inactivation of mitochondrial monoamine oxidase by N-cyclopropylbenzylamine. *Biochemistry* **24**, 6538–6543.

Walker M.C. and Edmondson D.E. (1987). Kinetic probes of the proposed radical mechanism of monoamine oxidase. In *Flavins and Flavoproteins 1987* (eds Edmondson D.E. and McCormick D.B.). pp. 699–703. De Gruyter, Berlin.

Walker M.C., Hazzard J.T., Tollin G. and Edmondson D.E. (1991). Kinetic comparison of reduction and intramolecular electron transfer in milk xanthine oxidase and chicken liver xanthine dehydrogenase by laser flash photolysis. *Biochemistry* **30**, 5912–5917.

Wang N., Southan C., DeWolf W.E. Jr, Wells T.N.C., Kruse L.I. and Leatherbarrow R.J. (1990). Bovine dopamine β-hydroxylase, primary structure determined by cDNA cloning and amino acid sequencing. *Biochemistry* **29**, 6466–6474.

Weiner H. (1980). Aldehyde oxidizing enzymes. In *Enzymatic Basis of Detoxication*, Vol. 1 (ed. Jakoby W.B.). pp. 261–280. Academic Press, New York.

Weyler W., Hsu Y.P.P. and Breakefield X.O. (1990). Biochemistry and genetics of monoamine oxidase. *Pharmacol. Therap.* **47**, 391–417.

White R.E. (1991). The involvement of free radicals in the mechanisms of monooxygenases. *Pharmacol. Therap.* **49**, 21–42.

Williams C.H., Lawson J. and Backwell F.R.C. (1992). Inhibition and inactivation of monoamine oxidase by 3-amino-1-phenyl-pro-1-enes. *Biochim. Biophys. Acta* **1119**, 111–117.

Wimalasena K. and May S.W. (1987). Mechanistic studies on dopamine β-monooxygenase catalysis: N-dealkylation and mechanism-based inhibition by benzylic-nitrogen-containing compounds. Evidence for a single-electron-transfer mechanism. *J. Amer. Chem. Soc.* **109**, 4036–4046.

Wimalasena K. and May S.W. (1989). Dopamine β-monooxygenase catalyzed aromatization of 1-(2-aminoethyl)-1,4-cyclohexadiene: redirection of specificity and evidence for a hydrogen atom transfer mechanism. *J. Amer. Chem. Soc.* **111**, 2729–2731.

Wong D.L. and Bildstein C.L. (1990). Subunit characterization and primary structure of bovine adrenal
medullary dopamine β-hydroxylase. *Neuropsychopharmacology* **3**, 115–128.

Wootton J.C., Nicolson R.E., Cock J.M., Walters D.E.,
Burke J.F., Doyle W.A. and Bray R.C. (1991). Enzymes
depending on the pterin molybdenum cofactor—
Sequence families, spectroscopic properties of molybde-
num and possible cofactor-binding domains. *Biochim.
Biophys. Acta* **1057**, 157–185.

Wright R.M., Vaitaitis G.M., Wilson C.M., Repine T.B.,
Terada L.S. and Repine J.E. (1993). cDNA cloning,
characterization, and tissue-specific expression of human
xanthine dehydrogenase/xanthine oxidase. *Proc. Nat.
Acad. Sci. USA* **90**, 10,690–10,695.

Wu E., Shinka T., Caldera-Munoz P., Yoshizumi H.,
Trevor A. and Castagnoli N. Jr (1988). Metabolic studies
on the nigrostriatal toxin MPTP and its MAO B
generated dihydropyridinium metabolite MPDP+.
Chem. Res. Toxicol. **1**, 186–194.

Wu H.F., Chen K. and Shih J.C. (1993). Site-directed
mutagenesis of monoamine oxidase A and B: role of
cysteines. *Molec. Pharmacol.* **43**, 888–893.

Youdim M.B.H. and Finberg J.P.M. (1991). New directions in monoamine oxidase A and B selective inhibitors
and substrates. *Biochem. Pharmacol.* **41**, 155–162.

Youdim M.B.H., Harshak N., Yoshioka M., Araki H.,
Mukai Y. and Gotto G. (1991). Novel substrates and
products of amine oxidase-catalyzed reactions. *Biochem.
Soc. Transact.* **19**, 224–228.

Yu P.H. (1989). Deamination of aliphatic amines of
different chain lengths by rat liver monoamine oxidase A
and B. *J. Pharm. Pharmacol.* **41**, 205–208.

Yu P.H. (1990). Oxidative deamination of aliphatic amines
by rat aorta semicarbazide-sensitive amine oxidase. *J.
Pharm. Pharmacol.* **42**, 882–884.

Yu P.H. and Davis B.A. (1988). Stereospecific deamination
of benzylamine catalyzed by different amine oxidases.
Int. J. Biochem. **20**, 1197–1201.

Yu P.H. and Davis B.A. (1991). 2-Propyl-1-aminopentane,
its deamination by monoamine oxidase and
semicarbazide-sensitive amine oxidase, conversion to
valproic acid and behavioral effects. *Neuropharmacology*
30, 507–515.

Yu P.H. and Tipton K.F. (1989). Deuterium isotope effect
of phenelzine on the inhibition of rat liver mitochondrial
monoamine oxidase activity. *Biochem. Pharmacol.* **38**,
4245–4251.

Yu P.H., Bailey B.A., Durden D.A. and Boulton A.A.
(1986). Stereospecific deuterium substitution at the α-
carbon position of dopamine and its effect on oxidative
deamination catalyzed by MAO-A and MAO-B from
different tissues. *Biochem. Pharmacol.* **35**, 1027–1036.

Yu P.H., Davis B.A. and Boulton A.A. (1992). Aliphatic
propargylamines: potent, selective, irreversible
monoamine oxidase B inhibitors. *J. Med. Chem.* **35**,
3705–3713.

Zang L.Y. and Misra H.P. (1992). Superoxide radical
production during the autoxidation of 1-methyl-4-
phenyl-2,3-dihydropyridinium perchlorate. *J. Biol.
Chem.* **267**, 17,547–17,552.

Zang L.Y. and Misra H.P. (1993). Generation of reactive
oxygen species during the monoamine oxidase-catalyzed
oxidation of the neurotoxicant, 1-methyl-4-phenyl-
1,2,3,6-tetrahydropyridine. *J. Biol. Chem.* **268**, 16,504–
16,512.

Zhao Z., Dalvie D., Naiman N., Castagnoli K. and
Castagnoli Jr N. (1992). Design, synthesis and biological
evaluation of novel 4-substituted 1-methyl-1,2,3,6-
tetrahydropyridine analogs of MPTP. *J. Med. Chem.* **35**,
4473–4478.

chapter 10

REACTIONS CATALYZED BY PEROXIDASES

Contents

10.1 INTRODUCTION

In Chapters 3–8 we have discussed a large variety of reactions of monooxygenation which involve the cleavage of molecular oxygen with transfer of one oxygen atom to the substrate. Other types of substrate oxidation reactions have been presented in Chapters 2 (reactions catalyzed by dehydrogenases) and 9 (reactions catalyzed by various oxidases). The present chapter is mainly devoted to other important reactions of substrate oxidation, namely those mediated by peroxidases and enzymes displaying peroxidase-like activities.

The reaction mechanisms of such enzymes show analogies and differences with those of monooxygenases, as apparent below (Castro, 1980). A particularly significant difference concerns the origin of the active oxygen, which is not derived from molecular oxygen but from reduced forms thereof (i.e. hydrogen peroxide [H_2O_2] or organic hydroperoxides [ROOH]). The various enzymes that function solely or occasionally as peroxidases include cytochrome P450, prostaglandin-endoperoxide synthase and catalase, as well as other peroxidases such as chloroperoxidase and myeloperoxidase. The present chapter focuses mainly on these enzymes, and it ends with a brief section on reactions catalyzed by dioxygenases and reactions of dioxygenations.

The enzymes to be discussed in this chapter are mainly *hemoproteins*, i.e. they contain iron protoporphyrin IX (heme) as their prosthetic group. The many and marked differences in enzymatic activities, types of reaction, nature of substrates, and even catalytic mechanisms are largely accounted for by the nature of the protein component and the way it interacts with the prosthetic group. For example, cytochrome P450 and chloroperoxidase have their iron centre ligated with a **thiolate group** from a cysteinyl residue, whereas in prostaglandin-endoperoxide synthase, myeloperoxidase, lactoperoxidase and horseradish peroxidase the iron centre is ligated with an **imidazole group** from a histidinyl residue. The catalytic activity also requires the participation of other amino acid side-chains at the active site. For example, hydroperoxide oxygen–oxygen cleavage is postulated to occur by an electron "push" mechanism in thiolate-ligated systems, but by a "push-pull" mechanism (push by histidine, pull by histidine and/or arginine) in histidine-ligated systems (Dawson, 1988; McCarthy and White, 1983a; Marnett *et al.*, 1988; Ortiz de Montellano, 1987).

10.2 PEROXYGENASE ACTIVITY OF CYTOCHROME P450

It was discovered in the early 1970s that hydroperoxides or hydrogen peroxide can support the cytochrome P450-catalyzed hydroxylation of various substrates in a reaction that requires neither O_2, NADPH nor NADPH-cytochrome P450 reductase, and which is not inhibited by carbon monoxide (Rahimtula and O'Brien, 1977a; Thompson and Yumibe, 1989). This reaction, which was first viewed as a laboratory curiosity, has yielded many valuable insights into the catalytic mechanism of cytochrome P450 and is now believed to have physiological significance.

10.2.1 Catalytic mechanisms

In simplified form, the peroxidase activity of cytochrome P450 can be described by Eq. 10.1 where XH is the substrate and ROOH the hydroperoxide (see also Section 3.5):

$$XH + ROOH \rightarrow XOH + ROH \qquad \text{(Eq. 10.1)}$$

In this reaction, the enzyme functions as a "**peroxygenase**", a term sometimes used to draw a parallel with its monooxygenase activity and meaning that the oxygen atom transferred to the substrate comes from a hydroperoxide. Note that in the presence of NADPH, cytochrome P450 can also interact reductively with hydroperoxides, as discussed in Chapter 12.

The mechanism of cytochrome P450 peroxygenase activity is schematized in Fig. 10.1. The reaction begins with the formation of a ternary complex (reaction **a** in Fig. 10.1) having the two substrates (i.e. the hydroperoxide and the substrate undergoing hydroxylation) bound to the oxidized (ferric) form of cytochrome P450 (Koop and Hollenberg, 1980). Such a complex has been designated as Complex C by some authors; its formation can be monitored spectropho-

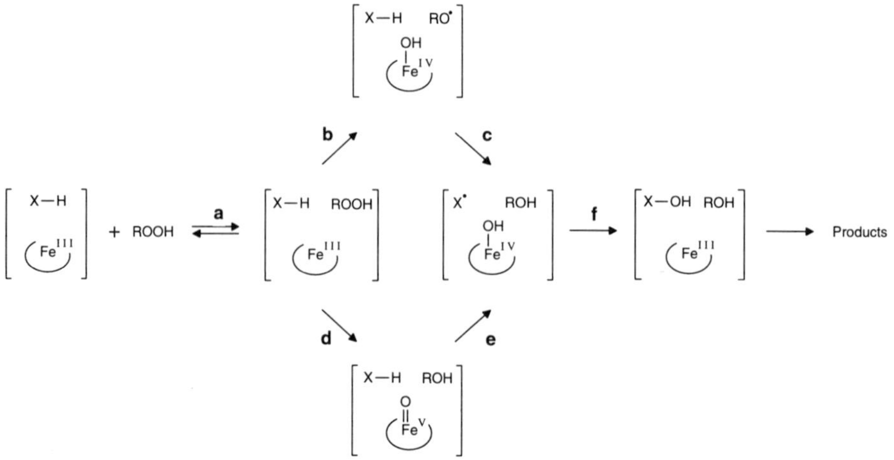

FIGURE 10.1 Reaction mechanisms of the peroxygenase activity of cytochrome P450 leading to substrate hydroxylation. Cleavage of the oxygen–oxygen bond occurs either by a homolytic pathway (reactions **b** and **c**) or a heterolytic pathway (reactions **d** and **e**).

tometrically, as can the formation of binary hydroperoxide–cytochrome P450 complexes (Blake and Coon, 1980, 1981a and 1981b; Rahimtula and O'Brien, 1977a). In a non-productive side-reaction, Complex C was shown to be reversibly converted to a form termed Complex D (Blake and Coon, 1980; 1981a and 1981b).

Cleavage of the oxygen–oxygen bond occurs following formation of this Complex C and involves either a *homolytic mechanism* (reaction **b** in Fig. 10.1) or a *heterolytic mechanism* (reaction **d** in Fig. 10.1). The former mechanism is a one-electron process which yields an alkoxyl $RO^\bullet$ radical and the $[FeOH]^{3+}$ form of the enzyme. In contrast, the heterolytic mechanism is a two-electron process in which the hydroperoxide is reduced to a hydroxylated derivative while the ferric cytochrome P450 is oxidized to the $[FeO]^{3+}$ state. Both these intermediate states rearrange to a common secondary intermediate, the reaction in both cases (either **c** or **e** in Fig. 10.1) involving hydrogen abstraction from the substrate XH. But while in reaction **c** (Fig. 10.1) the $RO^\bullet$ radical mediates hydrogen abstraction, reaction **e** in Fig. 10.1 is nothing else than the first step of the well-known **oxygen rebound mechanism** occurring during the monooxygenase reaction (see Section 4.2). The final step is reaction **f** in Fig. 10.1 during which the actual substrate hydroxylation takes place.

Varied evidence has been published regarding the occurrence of the homolytic and/or heterolytic pathways (Blake and Coon, 1981a and 1981b; Bruice, 1991; Bruice *et al.*, 1988; Groves and Watanabe, 1988; Hollenberg, 1992; Larroque *et al.*, 1990; Traylor and Xu, 1990; Wand and Thompson, 1986; White *et al.*, 1980). Both reactions do occur, their relative contribution depending on the chemical nature of the hydroperoxide used (Thompson and Yumibe, 1989). Among **alkyl hydroperoxides**, the frequently used cumene hydroperoxide (**10.I**) appears to be cleaved with slight predominance by the heterolytic pathway. In contrast, 2,6-di-*tert*-butyl-4-hydroperoxy-4-methyl-2,5-cyclohexadienone (**10.II**) appears to react homolytically and heterolytically with comparable ease.

Acyl hydroperoxides (peracids) such as phenylperacetic acid (**10.III**) act like alkyl hydroperoxides in supporting cytochrome P450-catalyzed hydroxylations, oxygen–oxygen cleavage being predominantly heterolytic (Bruice *et al.*, 1988; Traylor and Xu, 1990). Heterolytic cleavage of an acyl peroxyl bond at the catalytic site of cytochrome P450 has already been discussed in Section 3.5.

10.I   10.II   10.III

Hydrogen peroxide itself can also function as a donor of active oxygen to cytochrome P450. Traylor and colleagues (1989) have stressed the mechanistic unicity of the hemin-catalyzed heterolytic cleavage of alkyl hydroperoxides, acyl hydroperoxides, hydrogen peroxide, and iodosobenzenes (Section 3.5). This is the common mechanism of peroxidases and catalase (see also Sections 10.3 and 10.4), and cytochrome P450 appears to be unique among these enzyme systems in that it can act both heterolytically and homolytically (McCarthy and White, 1983a and 1983b). But only in the heterolytic cleavage mechanism can peroxides, iodosobenzenes and other oxidizing agents be considered to act as oxene donors.

10.2.2 Fate of the hydroperoxide substrate

While the heterolytic pathway transforms a hydroperoxide solely to the corresponding alcohol (reaction **d** in Fig. 10.1), the alkoxyl radical generated by homolytic cleavage can react intramolecularly to give various **rearrangement products**. Thus, cumene hydroperoxide is transformed in part to acetophenone (**10.IV**) by β-scission (in this case loss of a $^\bullet CH_3$ radical), while the hydroperoxide **10.II** and homologous 4-alkyl-1,4-peroxyquinols yield a variety of products resulting from β-scission, ring expansion and ring contraction (Thompson and Yumibe, 1989; Wand and Thompson, 1986; Yumibe and Thompson, 1988). Some hydroperoxides of unsaturated fatty acids can also be metabolized by cytochrome P450 to allene oxides as precursors of prostaglandin-like products. The reaction is believed to involve homolytic cleavage followed by hydrogen abstraction from the β-carbon and radical recombination (Song and Brash, 1991).

10.IV   10.V

The fact that peracids do not react exclusively via the heterolytic pathway is shown by their cytochrome P450-catalyzed **decarboxylation**. This reaction, which is strictly restricted to intact cytochrome P450 enzymes, yields an alcohol and CO_2, and it proceeds via the homolytic route by the postulated mechanism being shown in Fig. 10.2 (McCarthy and White, 1983a; Traylor and Xu, 1990). The importance of decarboxylation relative to the competing reaction of substrate hydroxylation via the heterolytic route depends on both the peracid and the nature of the substrate (McCarthy and White, 1983b).

In the heterolytic pathway, some hydroperoxides can serve as both **oxygen donor and acceptor**. This is seen for example with **10.II**, which following heterolytic cleavage is hydroxylated on the *tert*-butyl group, or in the metabolism of 20-hydroperoxycholesterol (**10.V**)

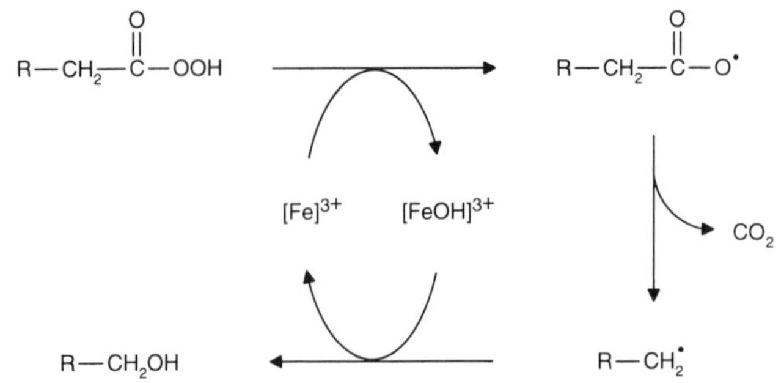

FIGURE 10.2 Postulated mechanism of the cytochrome P450-catalyzed decarboxylation of peracids via homolytic oxygen–oxygen bond cleavage. For example, phenylperacetic acid (R = phenyl) yields benzyl alcohol (McCarthy and White, 1983a).

with CYP11A1 (Yumibe and Thompson, 1988). Indeed, the (20R)-epimer of **10.V** forms (20R)-20,21-dihydroxycholesterol, while (20S)-**10.V** forms (20R,22R)-20,22-dihydroxycholesterol; here again, heterolytic cleavage was evidenced (Larroque et al., 1990).

Note that the interaction between cytochrome P450 and hydroperoxides is not limited to the mechanisms outlined in Fig. 10.1. In the presence of linoleate hydroperoxide only, rat liver microsomes exhibited a **consumption of molecular oxygen** approximately 100-fold greater than that for usual monooxygenase reactions (Wheeler, 1983). The products were not identified, but it was rightly speculated that the reaction may have a physiological significance in the metabolism of lipid hydroperoxides. Another reaction of probable physiological significance involves the **reductive cleavage** of lipid hydroperoxides and other hydroperoxides by cytochrome P450 in the presence of NADPH; this reaction is discussed in Section 12.2.

10.2.3 Reactions of xenobiotic oxidation mediated by the peroxygenase activity of cytochrome P450

Over the years, a large number of xenobiotics have been shown to be oxidized *in vitro* by the peroxygenase activity of cytochrome P450. How much these reactions have *in vivo* significance remains to be firmly established. Peroxides of cellular lipids have repeatedly been postulated to be oxygen donors towards cytochrome P450 *in vivo*, but the presence of O_2 and NADPH in tissues is expected to affect the nature of the reaction as discussed above. Clearly a better understanding of the *in vivo* relevance of the reactions discussed here is needed.

Representative examples covering a broad range of reactions, xenobiotic substrates and peroxides are assembled in Table 10.1, some of which warrant a brief discussion.

The **oxidation of aromatic substrates** by the hydroperoxide- and NADPH-dependent reactions proceed by similar mechanisms. Indeed, comparable NIH shifts (Section 4.3) were seen in the hydroxylation of acetanilide, while the primary metabolite of phenanthrene was the 9,10-oxide (Rahimtula et al., 1978). However, some differences in regioselectivity (and mechanism?) must occur since the major metabolites formed from benzo[a]pyrene (BP, **10.VI** in Fig. 10.3) were not the same; while the monooxygenase reaction yielded mainly phenols (3-, 6- and 9-hydroxy-BP) and less dihydrodiols and quinones, the hydroperoxide-dependent reaction produced mostly quinones (1,6-, 3,6- and 6,12-quinone) (Capdevila et al., 1980). These quinones are known to be formed readily by enzymatic (peroxygenase activity of cytochrome P450) or

TABLE 10.1 *Representative hydroperoxide-dependent oxidations catalyzed by cytochrome P450*

Reaction and substrate	Hydroperoxide[*]	Enzyme source[†]	Reference
Aromatic oxidation			
Acetanilide	CU–OOH	Rat or rabbit LM Purified P450s	Rahimtula *et al.*, 1978
Phenanthrene		Rat LM	
Aniline	H_2O_2	Rabbit LM	Mohr *et al.*, 1979
Benzo[*a*]pyrene (**10.VI**)	CU–OOH	Rat LM	Capdevila *et al.*, 1980
Propranolol		Human LM	Otton *et al.*, 1990
Aliphatic hydroxylation			
Cyclohexane	CU–OOH	Purified P450	Nordblom *et al.*, 1976
N-Dealkylation			
Benzphetamine	H_2O_2	Rabbit LM Purified P450	Mohr *et al.*, 1979 Nordblom *et al.*, 1976
	Sodium chlorite Peracids Alkyl hydroperoxides		
Aminopyrine	CU–OOH		
N-Methylaniline			
N,N-Dimethylaniline			
Diphenhydramine	H_2O_2	Rat LM	Estabrook *et al.*, 1984
Ethylmorphine			
Imipramine			
Ketamine			
Methamphetamine			
Mephentermine			
Morphine			
Phendimetrazine			
Pargyline (**10.VII**)			Weli and Lindeke, 1986
O-Dealkylation			
para-Nitroanisole	Alkyl hydroperoxides Peracids Peroxyesters	Rabbit LM	Koop and Hollenberg, 1980
7-Isopropoxycoumarin	H_2O_2 CU–OOH	P450 cam	Shinohara *et al.*, 1987
C-Denitrification			
2-Nitropropane	CU–OOH	Mouse LM	Marker and Kulkarni, 1986
N-Oxidation			
N,N-Dimethylaniline	CU–OOH H_2O_2	Rabbit LM CYP2B4	Hlavica and Kuenzel-Mulas, 1993
Pargyline (**10.VII**)	H_2O_2 CU–OOH	Rat LM	Weli and Lindeke, 1986
Felodipine			Bäärnhielm and Hansson, 1986
Phenylalkylamines	H_2O_2		Jönsson and Lindeke, 1990
O-Oxidation			
Alkanols	CU–OOH	Rat LM	Rahimtula and O'Brien, 1977b
Acetaminophen			Potter and Hinson, 1987

A blank means "same as above".
[*]CU–OOH = cumene hydroperoxide.
[†]LM = liver microsomes.

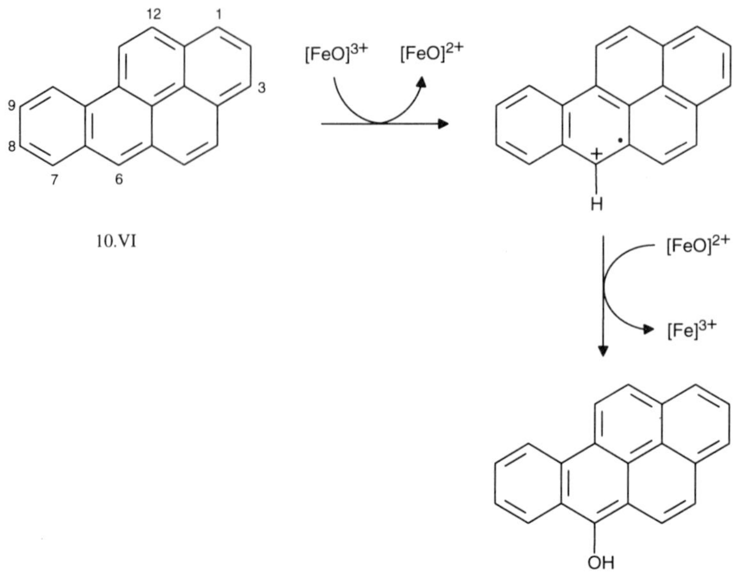

FIGURE 10.3 Postulated mechanism for the 6-hydroxylation of benzo[a]pyrene (**10.VI**) by cytochrome P450 (monooxygenase and peroxygenase activities), prostaglandin-endoperoxide synthase, and horseradish peroxidase. The radical-cation formed by enzymatic one-electron oxidation exists with the positive charge located on C(6), while the unpaired electron is delocalized to various positions, e.g. C(1), C(5a) and C(10b) (Cavalieri *et al.*, 1988a and 1988b).

non-enzymatic oxidation of 6-hydroxy-BP; formation of the latter was demonstrated to occur via a radical cation, as shown in Fig. 10.3 (Cavalieri *et al.*, 1988a).

The **N-dealkylations** listed in Table 10.1 are all N-demethylations apart from some reactions of pargyline (**10.VII**). Indeed, this MAO inhibitor was N-demethylated, N-debenzylated, N-depropargylated, and N-oxygenated with comparable ease in the presence of microsomes and H_2O_2 (or cumene hydroperoxide) (Weli and Lindeke, 1986). Thus there are similarities in the types of N–C cleavage supported by hydroperoxides and NADPH. A further analogy is seen in the denitrification of 2-nitropropane to acetone and nitrite (Marker and Kulkarni, 1986). The fact that this reaction is supported by cumene hydroperoxide confirms a mechanism of C(α)-hydroxylation for the monooxygenasic denitrification (see Section 6.5).

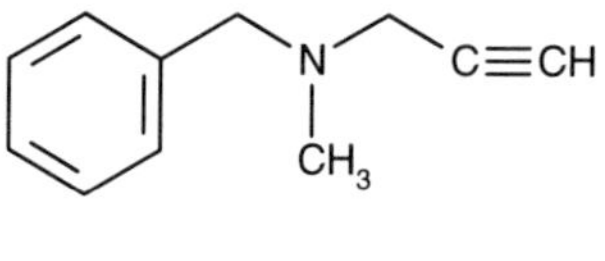

10.VII

The reactions of **N-oxidation** reported in Table 10.1 include two tertiary amines (dimethylaniline and pargyline), a secondary amine of the 1,4-dihydropyridine type (felodipine), and primary phenylalkylamines. The peroxidatic N-oxidation of felodipine yields a pyridine derivative as does cytochrome P450 acting as a monooxygenase (Section 5.4). As for the phenylalkylamines, different substrate selectivities were seen between the monooxygenase and peroxygenase N-oxygenations and the formation of cytochrome P450-nitroso complexes (Jönsson and Lindeke, 1990). This suggests that the presence of the hydroperoxide can affect the three-dimensional structure of the substrate binding site.

The alkanols mentioned in Table 10.1 are ethanol and a few higher homologues; their hydroperoxide-dependent **O-oxidation** yielded the corresponding aldehyde (compare with Section 7.6) (Rahimtula and O'Brien, 1977b). In contrast to its NADPH-dependent oxidation, the hydroperoxide-supported oxidation of acetaminophen was shown to be mainly a one-electron process yielding N-acetyl-p-benzosemiquinone imine as the metabolic intermediate; the latter then formed acetaminophen polymers (see Section 10.3.4) (Potter and Hinson, 1987a). Homolytic oxygen–oxygen cleavage presumably accounts for this one-electron oxidation.

10.3 COOXIDATIONS CATALYZED BY PROSTAGLANDIN-ENDOPEROXIDE SYNTHASE

Following the epoch-making discovery of prostaglandins (PGs) as physiologically active metabolites of arachidonic acid and other essential polyunsaturated fatty acids, it was reported in 1975 that various xenobiotics are oxidized during PG formation (Marnett et al., 1975). A considerable variety of organic substrates are now known to be metabolized by this route, and the mechanisms of the reaction are now comprehensible (Eling and Curits, 1992; Eling et al., 1983 and 1990; Smith et al., 1991 and 1992).

10.3.1 Enzymology and catalytic mechanisms of prostaglandin-endoperoxide synthase

Arachidonic acid (AA, also abbreviated 20:4 to indicate the number of its carbon atoms and carbon–carbon double bonds) is converted into an endoperoxide, prostaglandin H_2 (PGH_2), and thence to a number of active metabolites such as prostaglandins, prostacyclin, thromboxane and leukotrienes. The enzyme responsible for PGH_2 formation is prostaglandin-endoperoxide synthase (PES) [(5Z,8Z,11Z,14Z)-icosa-5,8,11,14-tetraenoate,hydrogen-donor:oxygen oxido-reductase; prostaglandin synthase; prostaglandin G/H synthase; EC 1.14.99.1]. The global reaction catalyzed by PES is:

$$AA + 2O_2 + 2H^+ + 2e^- \rightarrow PGH_2 + H_2O \qquad \text{(Eq. 10.2)}$$

As seen in Fig. 10.4, the first product of the reaction is prostaglandin G_2 (PGG_2), which is both an endoperoxide and a hydroperoxide; its formation results from a double reaction of **dioxygenation** for which no external source of electrons is required. In this reaction, PES acts as a dioxygenase, but the term most frequently used to describe this activity is a **cyclooxygenase**. The second activity of PES is that of a **hydroperoxidase** which reduces the hydroperoxide to an alcohol group, thereby producing PGH_2. Reducing substrates then restore the resting form of the enzyme (Eling et al., 1983 and 1990; Markey et al., 1987; Marnett and Eling, 1983).

PES is a single enzyme catalyzing both cyclooxygenase and hydroperoxidase activities. The enzyme is associated with the endoplasmic reticulum and nuclear membranes and is thus present in microsomal preparations. Ram seminal vesicles contain very high PES activity and are therefore the primary source for investigations. However, PES has been found in almost every mammalian tissue investigated, not to mention tissues of other vertebrates and invertebrates (Eling et al., 1990). The enzyme exists as a homodimer of 71 kDa subunits; amino acid sequences have been published (DeWitt et al., 1990). Both catalytic activities require the presence of one molecule of **ferriprotoporphyrin IX** per monomer (see Section 3.2); the two catalytic activities have distinct but interdependent binding sites for their lipid substrates (Kulmacz, 1989; Marnett et al., 1988; Marshall and Kulmacz, 1988).

The cyclooxygenase activity, which is inhibited by aspirin and numerous non-steroidal anti-inflammatory drugs (NSAIDs), requires specific polyunsaturated fatty acid substrates. The

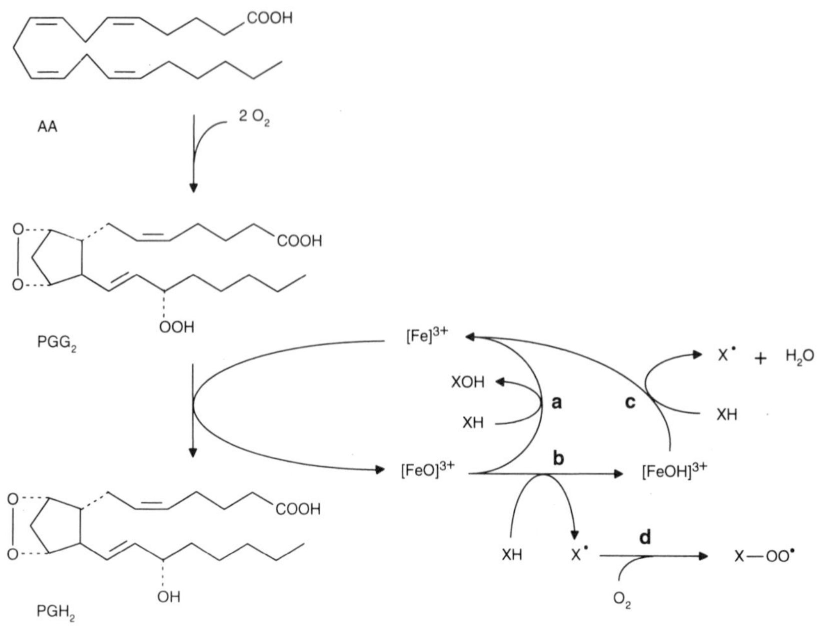

FIGURE 10.4 Formation of prostaglandin H_2 by the cyclooxygenase and peroxidase activities of PES, and postulated mechanisms of xenobiotic cooxidation by either oxygen transfer (reaction **a**) or two single-electron steps (reactions **b** and **c**). AA = arachidonic acid; PG = prostaglandin; $[Fe]^{3+}$ = ferriprotoporphyrin IX in PES; XH = electron donor/substrate to be oxidized.

minimum structural requirement for PES is a conjugated trienoic fatty acid in which the last double bond is located six carbons from the methyl terminus (ω–6) (Marnett, 1981).

In the peroxidase reaction, the hydroperoxide is cleaved heterolytically and the heme moiety is oxidized to a hypervalent iron-oxo form $[FeO]^{3+}$ analogous to or identical with the iron-oxene form of cytochrome P450 (Fig. 10.4). This form is analogous to Compound I of other peroxidases (see Section 10.4), while its one-electron reduced form $[FeOH]^{3+}$ resembles Compound II of other peroxidases (Eling *et al.*, 1990). Substrates of the peroxidase activity are mainly fatty acid hydroperoxides, but not compounds such as cumene hydroperoxide (Reed, 1987). These substrate hydroperoxides have an essential role to play in the oxygenation of AA since they are obligatory initiators of the cyclooxygenase reaction. Indeed, this reaction is initiated by intermediates of the peroxidase catalytic cycle, indicating a coordination between the two activities (Markey *et al.*, 1987; Marshall and Kulmacz, 1988). As a matter of fact, it may be postulated that the formation of AA radicals, which initiates the two reactions of dioxygenation, resembles the first step in the cooxidation of substrates such as 13-*cis*-retinoic acid (i.e. reactions **b** and **d** in Fig. 10.4, see below).

In addition to being the preferred substrate of PES, AA is also oxygenated by various **lipoxygenases** to yield hydroperoxides. Other unsaturated fatty acids are similarly metabolized to hydroperoxy-fatty acids, while lipid peroxidation also yields hydroperoxy-fatty acids. The role of these hydroperoxides as substrates of PES, cytochrome P450 and other peroxidases is beginning to be investigated, but very little is known about their (probable) interference with xenobiotic metabolism (see Section 10.5) (Moldéus *et al.*, 1985).

A large number and variety of **xenobiotics** have been found to act as cofactors for the enzymatic reduction of PGG$_2$ to PGH$_2$ and are therefore called **reducing substrates** (Eling and Curtis, 1992; Eling *et al.*, 1983, 1990; Marnett, 1981; Marnett and Eling, 1983; Markey *et al.*,

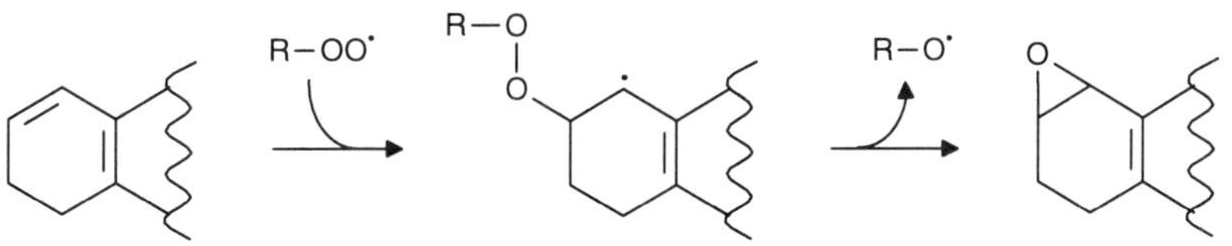

FIGURE 10.5 Postulated mechanism of PES-catalyzed xenobiotic epoxidation by means of a peroxyl radical, as exemplified with 7,8-dihydrobenzo[*a*]pyrene (partial structure shown) (Reed *et al.*, 1984).

1987). Two major mechanisms govern this **cooxidation**, namely direct oxygen transfer from the oxygenated heme (reaction **a** in Fig. 10.4, as exemplified by sulfides), or two single-electron transfers (reactions **b** and **c** in Fig. 10.4, as exemplified by phenols and aromatic amines). In addition to the two pathways shown in Fig. 10.4, other mechanisms are believed to exist based on the following evidence (Eling *et al.*, 1990; Marnett and Eling, 1983; Reed, 1987):

- Some xenobiotics are cooxidized without being good reducing cofactors (e.g. polycyclic aromatic hydrocarbons and aflatoxin).
- For some of these compounds, the source of the oxygen incorporated into the xenobiotic appears to be O_2 and not hydroperoxide oxygen.
- Furthermore, the cooxidation of these compounds is very sensitive to inhibition by antioxidants.

These additional mechanisms are hydroperoxide-derived and their involvement in the co-oxidation of xenobiotics that are not, or are poor, reducing cofactors will be discussed at the beginning of the next section (Reed, 1987).

An increasing number of drugs, differing greatly in their chemical structures, have been reported to be cooxidized by PES, although the resulting metabolites are not known in every case. In addition to the various drugs discussed below, we simply mention here diethylstilbestrol, 5-nitrofurans, and phenytoin (Eling *et al.*, 1990; Marnett, 1981; Marnett and Eling, 1983).

10.3.2 Reactions of carbon oxidation

A few **polycyclic aromatic hydrocarbons** (PAHs) have been investigated as (non-reducing) substrates of PES. Thus, benzo[*a*]pyrene (BP, **10.VI** in Fig. 10.3) is cooxidized to the 3,6-, 1,6- and 6,12-quinones, i.e. the same products as formed by the peroxidatic activity of cytochrome P450. As explained above, these quinones are generated via the intermediacy of a BP cation radical and 6-hydroxy-BP (Cavalieri *et al.*, 1988b). 6-Hydroxy-BP, being highly oxidizable, can either be non-enzymatically or peroxidatively activated to the 6-oxy radical which then oxidizes to the quinones (see also Section 10.2) (Cavalieri *et al.*, 1988a; Marnett, 1981). Despite BP being a very weak reducing substrate, it is clear that the mechanism of 6-hydroxylation documented by Cavalieri *et al.* (1988a and 1988b) is that of a reducing cofactor (reactions **b** and **c** in Fig. 10.4) (Eling *et al.*, 1990).

PES also catalyzes the oxidation of 7,8-dihydrobenzo[*a*]pyrene and that of 7,8-dihydroxy-7,8-dihydrobenzo[*a*]pyrene (i.e., BP-7,8-dihydrodiol) to the corresponding 9,10-epoxides (Marnett, 1981; Reed and Marnett, 1982). The mechanism of this **epoxidation** is different from that leading to quinones and could result from the action of a peroxyl radical, perhaps that of PGG_2 (i.e. the immediate precursor of PGG_2) or a fatty acid, as shown in Fig. 10.5 (Eling *et al.*, 1990). It is relevant that the 4-peroxyl radical of phenylbutazone (see below) is able to mediate the 9,10-epoxidation of BP-7,8-dihydrodiol (Reed *et al.*, 1984).

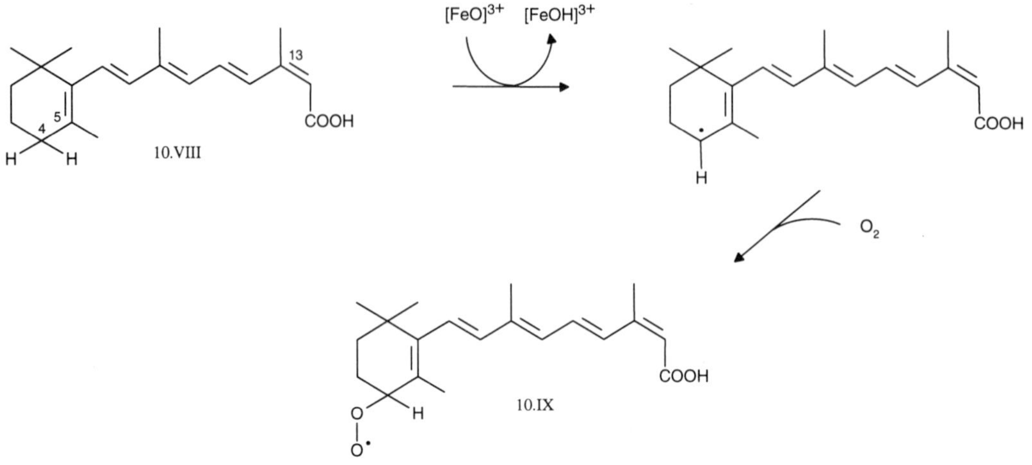

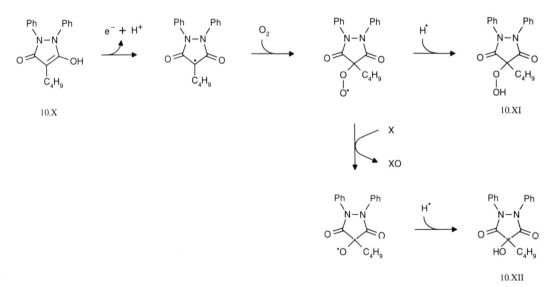

FIGURE 10.6 Postulated mechanism of the PES-mediated oxidation of 13-*cis*-retinoic acid (**10.VIII**) to the 4-peroxyl radical (Samokyszyn and Marnett, 1987).

Of particular interest is the metabolism of **13-*cis*-retinoic acid** (**10.VIII** in Fig. 10.6) catalyzed by PES, which again exemplifies a hydrocarbon moiety acting as reducing cofactor of PES (i.e. reaction **b** in Fig. 10.4). Several oxygenated metabolites were characterized including 4-hydroxy-, 5,6-epoxy-, and 5,8-oxy-13-*cis*-retinoic acid, their common precursor being the 4-peroxyl radical of 13-*cis*-retinoic acid (**10.IX** in Fig. 10.6) (Samokyszyn and Marnett, 1987). The mechanism of formation of this intermediate is shown in Fig. 10.6. It involves abstraction of a hydrogen atom from the allylic position by the iron-oxo form of the peroxidase to generate a C(4)-centred radical (i.e. reaction **b** in Fig. 10.4); peroxyl radicals were unable to mediate this hydrogen abstraction. The C(4)-centred radical then adds molecular oxygen (i.e. reaction **d** in Fig. 10.4) in analogy with a reaction that occurs twice in the oxygenation of AA to PGG_2. Such addition of molecular oxygen forms the highly reactive 4-peroxyl radical, which oxygenates a molecule of 13-*cis*-retinoic acid to the 5,6-epoxide and is itself reduced to the 4-hydroxyl

FIGURE 10.7 Postulated mechanism of phenylbutazone (**10.X**) cooxidation catalyzed by PES (Hughes *et al.*, 1988).

metabolite (in analogy with the reaction shown in Fig. 10.5). Under acid catalysis, the 5,6-epoxide isomerizes to 5,8-oxo-13-*cis*-retinoic acid. These results have recently been confirmed and extended using all-*trans*-retinoic as a reducing substrate (Samokyszyn, 1993).

Phenylbutazone (**10.X** in Fig. 10.7) is also a substrate of PES, but a difficult one to classify. As an enol of high acidity, it has some analogies with phenols although large differences exist in the respective metabolic pathways. Indeed, one-electron oxidation of phenylbutazone by PES generates a C-centred radical whose transient existence can be demonstrated, and which binds one molecule of oxygen (Fig. 10.7). The resulting peroxyl radical is a potent inhibitor of PES and may well be the active form of phenylbutazone. Two stable metabolites were isolated, namely 4-hydroperoxy- and 4-hydroxyphenylbutazone (**10.XI** and **10.XII** in Fig. 10.7, respectively); their formation is schematized in Fig. 10.7. Formation of 4-hydroxyphenylbutazone is particularly interesting because it results from the transfer of one atom of oxygen to a suitable acceptor such as 7,8-dihydroxy-7,8-dihydrobenzo[*a*]pyrene (see above). 4-Hydroxyphenyl-butazone has also been postulated to be formed from two interacting molecules of the peroxyl radical (Hughes *et al.*, 1988; Reed *et al.*, 1984). In addition to binding molecular oxygen, the C-centred radical of phenylbutazone may also bind covalently to form **conjugates**, a finding whose pharmacodynamic implications remain to be established (Lakshmi *et al.*, 1993).

Taken as a whole, the above examples show that PES is able to catalyze a variety of reactions of cooxidation of hydrocarbonated moieties, and to do so by a variety of mechanisms (Reed, 1987).

10.3.3 Oxidation and oxygenation of amines

An important group of reducing substrates of PES are amines, and particularly **aromatic amines**. These compounds can undergo two types of PES-catalyzed cooxidation, namely nitrogen oxidation or oxygenation, and N-dealkylation. **N-Oxidation** is of particular importance for a number of carcinogenic and mutagenic aromatic amines (Eling *et al.*, 1990; Zenser *et al.*, 1985). For example, **benzidine** (**10.XIII** in Fig. 10.8) is an excellent substrate of PES, being oxidized by two sequential one-electron steps to the cation radical **10.XIV** (Fig. 10.8) and then to the diimine **10.XV** (Fig. 10.8) which is in resonance with the nitrenium ion **10.XVI** (Fig. 10.8) (Eling *et al.*, 1985a). The only stable metabolite of benzidine identified is azobenzidine (**10.XVII** in Fig. 10.8), but the reactive intermediates bind covalently with high efficiency to nucleic acids and proteins and may account for the mutagenic activity of benzidine (Josephy, 1986).

Another primary aromatic amine of interest is **2-aminofluorene** (**10.XVIII**), whose metabolism shows analogies with that of benzidine. Again, N-oxidation leads to adduct-forming intermediates and to azofluorene. In addition, however, **N-oxygenation** has been documented by the formation of 2-nitrofluorene (Boyd *et al.*, 1983). Amongst **drugs**, the antibacterial sulfamethoxazole (**10.XIX**) was also shown to be oxygenated by PES on the primary aromatic group. The metabolites thus formed were the hydroxylamino and the nitro derivatives, and the pathway is postulated to be of toxicological relevance (Cribb *et al.*, 1990). *para*-Phenetidine (**10.XX** in Fig. 10.9), the N-deacetylated metabolite of phenacetin, is another primary amine of medicinal significance whose N-oxidation by PES results in covalent binding to proteins and nucleic acids (Moldéus *et al.*, 1984 and 1985). As shown in Fig. 10.9, one-electron oxidation and proton loss leads to a radical intermediate which dimerizes to *para*-phenetidine quinone imine (**10.XXI** in Fig. 10.9) and *para*-phenetidine quinone diimine (**10.XXII** in Fig. 10.9). These are the metabolites believed to bind covalently to biomacromolecules and elicit genotoxic effects (Larsson *et al.*, 1985). As with many electrophilic metabolites, conjugation with glutathione (see the volume in this series, *Biochemistry of Conjugation Reactions*) is a competitive route of detoxication.

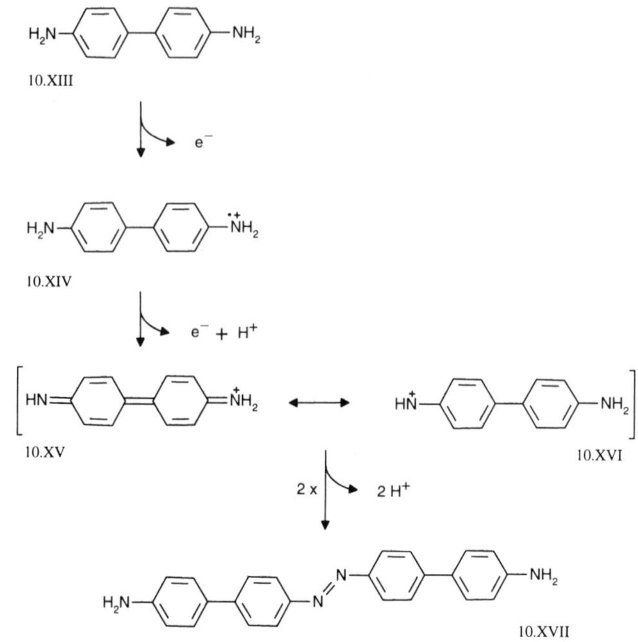

FIGURE 10.8 PES- and horseradish peroxidase-catalyzed oxidation of benzidine to azo-benzidine via reactive intermediates which bind covalently to nucleic acids and proteins (Eling *et al.*, 1985a).

One-electron N-oxidation is not restricted to primary aromatic amines, since a non-aromatic, secondary amine of the 1,4-dihydropyridine class can be substrate of PES. This is exemplified by the N-oxidation of felodipine (see Section 5.4) to yield the pyridine derivative (Bäärnhielm and Hansson, 1986). The reaction is initiated by one-electron oxidation as in the cytochrome P450-catalyzed aromatization supported by NADPH (Section 5.4) or hydroperoxide (Section 10.2).

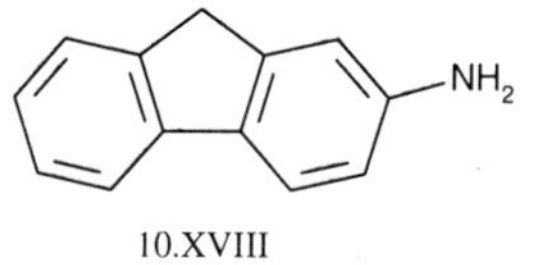

N-Dealkylation, and more specifically **N-demethylation**, can also be catalyzed by PES. A number of secondary and tertiary N-methylated aromatic amines were thus shown to be readily N-demethylated, e.g. N-methyl- and N,N-dimethylanilines (Sivarajah *et al.*, 1982). In contrast, a sterically hindered aliphatic amine such as pargyline (**10.VII**) is not a substrate of PES (Weli and Lindeke, 1986). One of the best and most investigated substrates is aminopyrine (**10.XXIII**), a tertiary amine comparable in its basicity to aromatic amines. Its PES-catalyzed N-demethylation liberates formaldehyde and was demonstrated to follow the pathway defined by reactions **d, f, g** and **c** in Fig. 6.1 (Chapter 6) (Eling *et al.*, 1985b; Lasker *et al.*, 1981). In other words, the initial step in the reaction is a one-electron oxidation of the basic nitrogen atom to form a cation radical. This transient species is then believed to disproportionate to an iminium cation and aminopyrine. The iminium cation is further hydrolyzed to the demethylated amine and formaldehyde. However, not every N-oxidation of an N-methyl tertiary amine leads to N-demethylation, as suggested by the PES-catalyzed formation of nicotine $\Delta^{4',5'}$-enamine (**10.XXV**) from nicotine

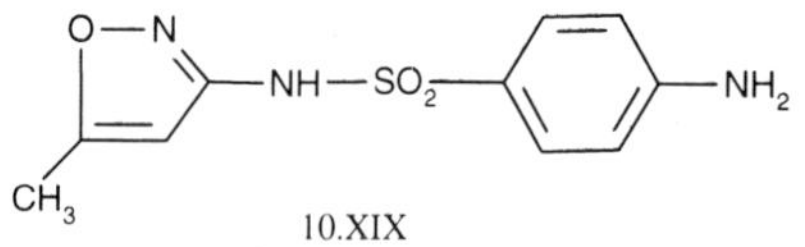

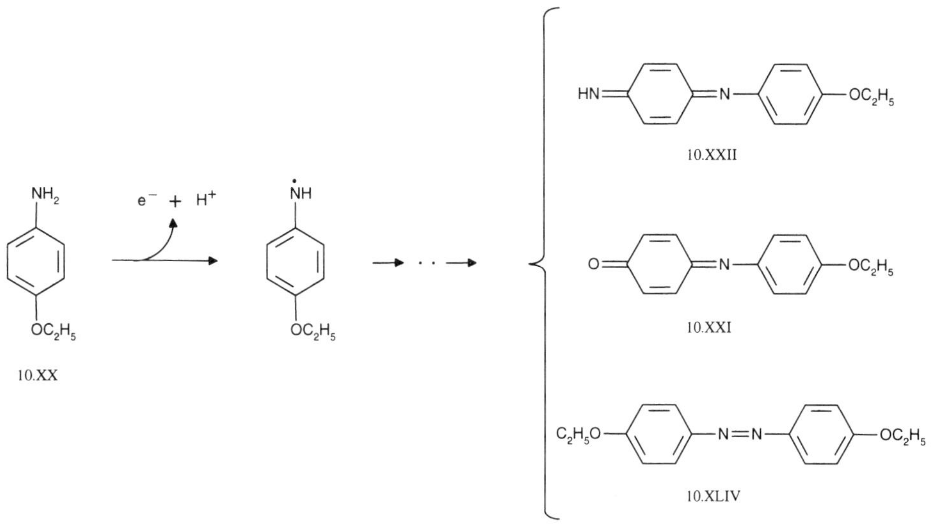

FIGURE 10.9 Postulated pathway of PES- and HRP-catalyzed toxication of *para*-phenetidine to quinoid metabolites binding covalently to biomacromolecules (Larsson *et al.*, 1985; Ross *et al.*, 1985). Also shown is 4,4′-diethoxyazobenzene (**10.XLIV**) formed by these enzymes (Lindquist *et al.*, 1985).

(**10.XXIV**) (Mattammal *et al.*, 1987). Rather than involving C(4′)- and/or C(5′)-oxidation as postulated, formation of **10.XXV** can also be explained by a favoured general acid–base-catalyzed isomerization of the $\Delta^{1',5'}$-iminium cation (Masumoto *et al.*, 1991, and references therein).

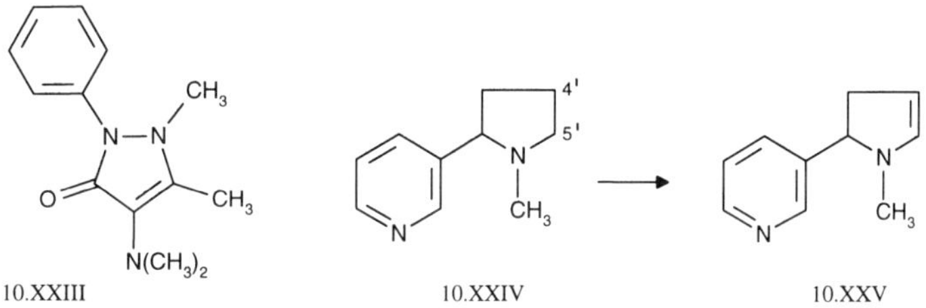

The above mechanism of N-demethylation via N-oxidation is consistent with the apparent inability of PES to catalyze O- and S-dealkylations (Sivarajah *et al.*, 1982), since these reactions occur by C(α)-hydroxylation rather than by heteroatom oxidation (Chapter 7).

Recent findings indicate that PES can also oxidize phenylhydrazones of the type C_6H_5–NH–N=R (Mahy *et al.*, 1993). Of particular interest is the fact that such phenylhydrazones are **substrates of the dioxygenase activity** of PES, in contrast to all reducing substrates discussed in the present Section 10.3. The dioxygenation of phenylhydrazones consumes O_2 and forms α-azo hydroperoxides as intermediates which are then reduced by the peroxidase reaction of PES and finally oxidized to the phenyl radical which binds to the heme and inhibits the enzyme.

10.3.4 Oxidation of phenols

In a very informative study, the efficiency of fifty reducing substrates of PES was compared, and the highest activity was found among **phenols** (Markey *et al.*, 1987). Indeed, a number of phenols have been examined as substrates of PES, the first intermediate in the reaction being a phenoxyl radical resulting from one-electron oxidation, as shown directly or indirectly. Thus, **hydroquinone (10.XXVI)** was cooxidized by PES to 1,4-benzoquinone and, in the presence of cysteine, to a thiol conjugate (see a subsequent volume) (Schlosser *et al.*, 1990). The mechanism of formation of these metabolites was investigated in greater detail using 2-bromohydroquinone as a substrate (Lau and Monks, 1987). Formation of the phenoxyl radical (i.e. the semiquinone) as the first intermediate can be followed by a number of enzymatic and non-enzymatic reactions. For example, the semiquinone can be (a) reduced back to the hydroquinone by glutathione acting as a one-electron reductant; (b) oxidized to the benzoquinone by O_2 (which is reduced to $O_2^{\bullet-}$); and (c) possibly oxidized to the benzoquinone by the peroxidase. In turn, the 1,4-benzoquinone can (a) bind covalently to macromolecules, forming adducts of potential toxicological significance; (b) be detoxified by forming conjugates with glutathione acting as a nucleophile; and (c) be reduced to the hydroquinone by glutathione (see a subsequent volume). For example, the toxication of hydroquinone to benzoquinone and protein-binding species is documented in macrophages, which are known to contain high PES activities (Schlosser and Kalf, 1989).

10.XXVI

Comparable reactions were seen in the PES-catalyzed activation of **butylated hydroxytoluene** (BHT, **7.XLVIII** in Section 7.6) and **butylated hydroxyanisole** (BHA) (Thompson *et al.*, 1989). Evidence for the formation of the phenoxyl radical was obtained in both cases, and there was extensive covalent binding to microsomal proteins. BHA, the better substrate, yielded dimers formed from the phenoxyl radical. As for the phenoxyl radical of BHT, it was further oxidized to the quinone methide (**7.XLIX** in Section 7.6) by direct chemical interaction with BHA-phenoxyl radical. This interesting result suggests a potential role for phenoxyl radicals in the toxication of xenobiotics (Thompson *et al.*, 1989).

The most extensively investigated phenol in the present context is **acetaminophen** (**10.XXVII** in Fig. 10.10). Its NADPH-supported, cytochrome P450-catalyzed oxidation has been presented in Section 7.6 (Fig. 7.12) and shown to be an overall two-electron reaction leading to N-acetyl-*p*-benzoquinone imine (NAPQI, **10.XXIX** in Fig. 10.10) via the semiquinone imine (**10.XXVIII** in Fig. 10.10). PES also catalyzes this reaction, and NAPQI can then (a) bind covalently to microsomal protein; (b) react with glutathione to form conjugates; or (c) be reduced back to acetaminophen (Ben-Zvi *et al.*, 1990; Boyd and Eling, 1981; Larsson *et al.*, 1985; Moldéus *et al.*, 1984 and 1985). In addition to forming NAPQI, the PES-catalyzed oxidation of acetaminophen also yields metabolites derived from the semiquinone imine, namely oligomers such as the dimer **10.XXX** (Fig. 10.10) (Harvison *et al.*, 1988; Potter and Hinson, 1987b). Formation of these oligomers does not occur in the NADPH-supported oxidation mediated by cytochrome P450, but is seen in the hydroperoxide-supported oxidation as noted in Section 10.2.3. This indicates that, during the NADPH-supported cycle, the semiquinone imine intermediate is not able to leave the active site of cytochrome P450 where it immediately undergoes the second oxidation step (Fig. 7.12 in Section 7.6). In contrast, it is able to do so during hydroperoxide-supported oxidations.

The fact that acetaminophen is both an inhibitor and a cosubstrate of PES is in itself an intriguing phenomenon. Careful investigations have revealed that at high concentrations (>10 mM under the conditions of the study), the drug indeed inhibits both the formation of PGG_2 and its own oxidation. At low concentrations (0.02–0.2 mM), however, acetaminophen stimulated PES

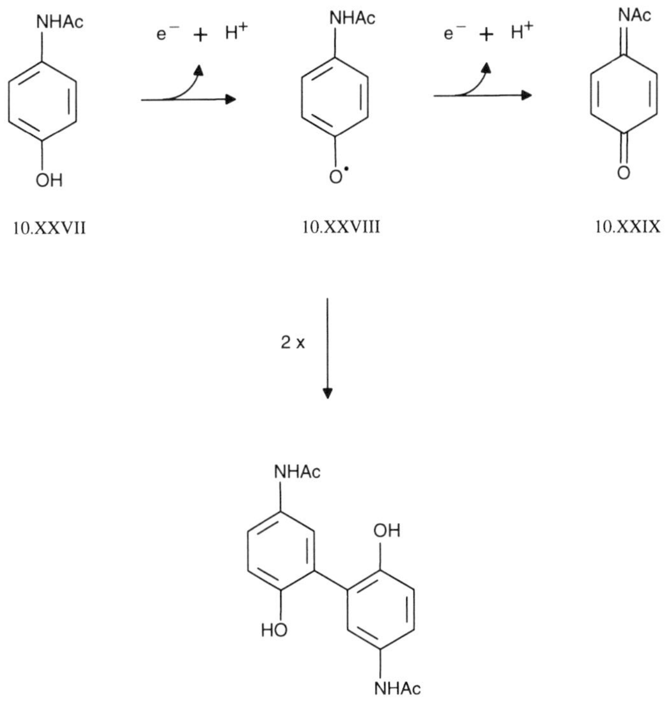

FIGURE 10.10 Prostaglandin synthase-catalyzed oxidation of acetaminophen (**10.XXVII**) to N-acetyl-*p*-benzo-semiquinone imine (**10.XXVIII**) and N-acetyl-*p*-benzoquinone imine (**10.XXIX**) by two single-electron steps. The possibility of interruption after the first step is evidenced by the formation of dimers and other oligomers, e.g. **10.XXX** (Harvison *et al.*, 1988; Potter and Hinson, 1987b).

activity, and interestingly also the chlorinating activity of myeloperoxidase (Harvison *et al.*, 1988; Marquez and Dunford, 1993).

10.3.5 Oxidation of sulfur-containing compounds

A number of sulfur-containing chemicals are oxidized and/or oxygenated by PES. Among **inorganic compounds**, we find bisulfite (HSO_3^-) or rather its deprotonated form SO_3^{2-} (pK_a 7.0), which undergoes one-electron oxidation by PES to a sulfur trioxide radical anion (i.e. $SO_3^{\bullet-}$). The latter can then disproportionate:

$$2SO_3^{\bullet-} \rightarrow SO_3 + SO_3^{2-} \qquad \text{(Eq. 10.3)}$$

or dimerize:

$$2SO_3^{\bullet-} \rightleftarrows S_2O_6^{2-} \qquad \text{(Eq. 10.4)}$$

or react with molecular oxygen:

$$SO_3^{\bullet-} + O_2 \rightarrow SO_3 + O_2^{\bullet-} \qquad \text{(Eq. 10.5)}$$

$$SO_3^{\bullet-} + O_2 \rightarrow SO_5^{\bullet-} \qquad \text{(Eq. 10.6)}$$

The superoxide radical and the peroxyl radical generated according to Eqs. 10.5 and 10.6, respectively, can form an additional sulfur trioxide radical anion:

$$O_2^{\bullet-} + SO_3^{2-} + 2H^+ \rightarrow SO_3^{\bullet-} + H_2O_2 \qquad \text{(Eq. 10.7)}$$

$$SO_5^{\bullet-} + SO_3^{2-} \rightarrow SO_3^{\bullet-} + SO_5^{2-} \qquad \text{(Eq. 10.8)}$$

Thus PES converts bisulfite to sulfur trioxide (which hydrates to sulfate) and other stable, highly oxidized anions such as peroxosulfate (SO_5^{2-}) (Mottley *et al.*, 1982). Some of the intermediates involved are very reactive and could attack various biological molecules in the absence of protection mechanisms. The peroxyl radical $SO_5^{\bullet-}$ can also oxidize dihydrodiols to diol epoxides in a reaction analogous to that shown in Fig. 10.5, thus offering a plausible explanation for the pulmonary cocarcinogenicity observed for sulfur dioxide and polycyclic aromatic hydrocarbons (Eling *et al.*, 1990).

Organic sulfur derivatives are variously oxidized by PES. For example, some **thiols** (i.e. R–SH) have been shown to be oxidized to the corresponding thiyl radical (i.e. R–S$^{\bullet}$). Two mechanisms have been postulated, the thiol acting either: (a) as a reducing substrate (reaction **b** in Fig. 10.4); or (b) reducing a radical ($X^{\bullet}$) formed from a better reducing substrate (Eling *et al.*, 1990), i.e.:

$$X^{\bullet} + R\text{–}SH \rightarrow XH + R\text{–}S^{\bullet} \qquad \text{(Eq. 10.9)}$$

A thiol compound whose PES-catalyzed oxidation has been repeatedly investigated is glutathione (L-glutamyl-L-cysteinylglycine, abbreviated GSH, see the volume in this series, *Biochemistry of Conjugation Reaction*), an endogenous tripeptide of immense biological significance. The thiyl radical of glutathione (GS$^{\bullet}$) can react with itself to form glutathione disulfide (also known as oxidized glutathione):

$$2GS^{\bullet} \rightarrow GSSG \qquad \text{(Eq. 10.10)}$$

The reactions described by Eqs. 10.9 and 10.10 are one of the most effective means available to biological systems for the detoxication of radicals and the termination of radical reactions (Eling *et al.*, 1990).

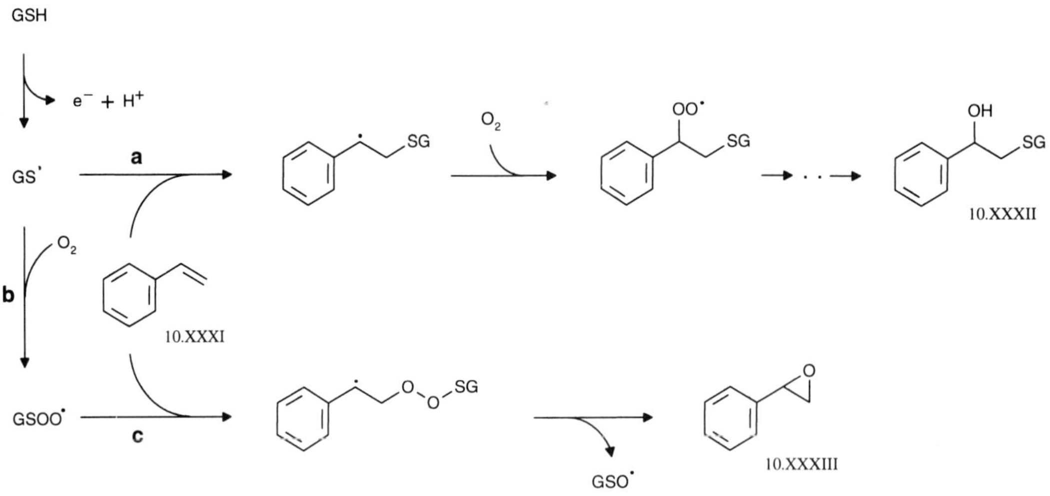

FIGURE 10.11 Some of the postulated mechanisms of formation of styrene–glutathione conjugates (**10.XXXII**) and styrene epoxide (**10.XXXIII**) catalyzed by peroxidases (Ortiz de Montellano and Grab, 1986; Stock *et al.*, 1986).

In addition to Eq. 10.10, the glutathionyl radical may also add directly to compounds, thereby forming **glutathione conjugates** by a route not requiring the glutathione S-transferases (see a subsequent volume). This pathway is exemplified by the formation of glutathione conjugates with styrene (**10.XXXI** in Fig. 10.11). Addition of the glutathionyl radical to styrene (reaction **a** in Fig. 10.11) occurs only on the terminal carbon and leads to the formation of a C-centred radical. The latter adds O_2 to form a peroxyl radical which is then reduced to a stable, hydroxylated styrene–glutathione conjugate (**10.XXXII** in Fig. 10.11) existing as a mixture of the (2S)- and (2R)-diastereomers (Eling *et al.*, 1990; Stock *et al.*, 1986). The alternative route for the formation of styrene–glutathione conjugates is by reaction with styrene epoxide, to which glutathione can bind either on C(1) or C(2).

A few **sulfides** have been shown to be oxygenated to their sulfoxide by PES, e.g. methyl phenyl sulfide and sulindac sulfide (Egan *et al.*, 1981). Both these substrates are aryl methyl sulfides, but too few data are available to derive structure–metabolism relationships (Marnett and Eling, 1983).

10.4 REACTIONS CATALYZED BY VARIOUS PEROXIDASES

10.4.1 Enzymes and reaction mechanisms

Various peroxidases (EC 1.11.1) have a role as xenobiotic-metabolizing enzymes. While horseradish peroxidase (HRP) is of interest here only as a model enzyme, other enzymes such as myeloperoxidase are of major toxicological significance. The peroxidases to be discussed in this section include:

- Catalase [hydrogen-peroxide:hydrogen-peroxide oxidoreductase; EC 1.11.1.6], a hemoprotein;
- Peroxidase [donor:hydrogen-peroxide oxidoreductase; EC 1.11.1.7], a hemoprotein; here are classified horseradish peroxidase (a non-mammalian enzyme), lactoperoxidase and myeloperoxidase;
- Iodide peroxidase [iodide:hydrogen-peroxide oxidoreductase; iodotyrosine deiodase; iodinase; thyroid peroxidase; EC 1.11.1.8], a hemoprotein;
- Glutathione peroxidase [glutathione:hydrogen-peroxide oxidoreductase; EC 1.11.1.9], a protein containing a selenocysteine residue;
- Chloroperoxidase [chloride:hydrogen-peroxide oxidoreductase; EC 1.11.1.10], a non-mammalian hemoprotein.

Other enzymes may also display peroxidatic activity without being classified as peroxidases, e.g. hemoglobin, serum albumin, liver alcohol dehydrogenase and indoleamine 2,3-dioxygenase (Cals *et al.*, 1991; Favilla *et al.*, 1988; Hayaishi *et al.*, 1990; Ignesti *et al.*, 1983; Leoncini *et al.*, 1991; Stadtman, 1991; Wendel, 1980).

The peroxidases exist in a large variety of tissues and cell types, of which **leukocytes** have received particular attention due to the potential toxicological relevance of some of the reactions of xenobiotic metabolism they catalyze (Uetrecht, 1992). The reader may find it useful to be reminded that leukocytes comprise monocytes, lymphocytes, polymorphonuclear leukocytes (neutrophils and eosinophils), and platelets.

In simplified form, the reaction of all these enzymes can be written as:

$$\text{Donor} + H_2O_2 \rightarrow \text{Oxidized donor} + 2H_2O$$ (Eq. 10.11)

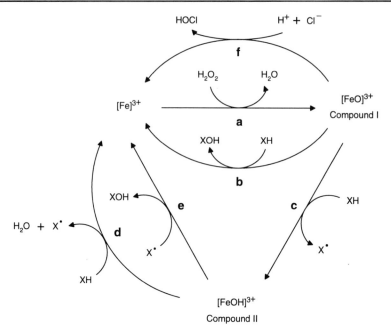

FIGURE 10.12 General reaction mechanism of peroxidases (here symbolized by [Fe]) which upon heterolytic cleavage of hydrogen peroxide (or an organic hydroperoxide) are oxidized to Compound I (reaction **a**). Compound I can donate its oxygen atom to a substrate XH (reaction **b**), or to a halide to form a weakly acidic hypohalous acid (reaction **f**). Compound I can also undergo two single-electron reduction steps (reactions **c** and **d**) via Compound II.

For the physiological reaction of catalase, this equation translates as:

$$H_2O_2 + H_2O_2 \rightarrow O_2 + 2H_2O \qquad \text{(Eq. 10.12)}$$

where the donor (i.e. the donor to be oxidized = the hydrogen donor) is a molecule of H_2O_2 and the oxidized donor is O_2. A more detailed view of the **reaction mechanisms** of hemoprotein peroxidases is given in Fig. 10.12 where the enzyme is symbolized by [Fe]. Following binding, hydrogen peroxide is cleaved heterolytically to yield H_2O and an oxygenated form of the enzyme known as Compound I (reaction **a** in Fig. 10.12) with the iron atom in a formal ferryl state, i.e. $[Fe(V)O^{2-}]^{3+}$ or $[Fe(V)=O]^{3+}$ or even more simply $[FeO]^{3+}$. Since one oxidation equivalent may reside either in the porphyrin or a nearby amino acid side-chain, Compound I can also be written as $[P^+Fe(IV)O^{2-}]^{3+}$. Many similarities exist between this oxidation/oxygenation state of hemoprotein peroxidases and the $[FeO]^{3+}$ state of cytochrome P450 (i.e. the oxene-binding state) formed upon heterolytic cleavage of a hydroperoxide (reaction **d** in Fig. 10.1) (Bruice *et al.*, 1988; Dawson, 1988; McCarthy and White, 1983; Ortiz de Montellano, 1987; Samokyszyn and Ortiz de Montellano, 1991; Traylor *et al.*, 1989). The same holds for the $[FeO]^{3+}$ state of PES (Fig. 10.4).

Compound I can react in two ways with reducing substrates, either by oxygen transfer (peroxygenation, reaction **b** in Fig. 10.12) or by two single-electron transfers (reactions **c** and **d** in Fig. 10.12), in close analogy with PES (reactions **a**, **b** and **c** in Fig. 10.4). The nature of both the substrate and of the enzyme itself influences the course of reaction of Compound I, as exemplified by the fact that the active site of horseradish peroxidase seemingly forbids transfer of the ferryl oxygen to substrates (Ortiz de Montellano, 1987). In fact, most of the reactions of xenobiotic oxidation to be discussed below involve single-electron steps. The first step of single-electron transfer (reaction **c** in Fig. 10.12) generates **Compound II** which can be written as $[Fe(IV)O^{2-}]^{2+}$, $[Fe(IV)=O]^{2+}$, $[Fe(IV)-OH]^{3+}$, or simply $[FeOH]^{3+}$. In addition to the architecture of the active site, another factor controlling the reactivity of Compounds I and II is the fifth iron ligand, i.e. a cysteinyl thiolate group in chloroperoxidase (and in cytochrome P450, see above), and a histidinyl imidazole group in myeloperoxidase, lactoperoxidase and horseradish peroxidase (and PES) (Dawson, 1988; Dugad *et al.*, 1992; Hu and Kincaid, 1993; Mohr *et al.*, 1979; Ortiz de Montellano, 1987 and 1992). The possibility that Compound II acts by transferring a hydroxyl moiety (reaction **e** in Fig. 10.12) will be discussed in connection with reactions of N-demethylation; at this stage, we can note that the sequence of reactions **c** and **e** in Fig. 10.12 is formally identical with the oxygen rebound mechanism discussed for cytochrome P450 (Section 4.2).

In the presence of excess H_2O_2, Compound II of lactoperoxidase forms another oxygenated derivative known as **Compound III**. This is a highly stable $Fe-O_2$ complex whose involvement in xenobiotic oxidation remains to be investigated (Hu and Kincaid, 1991).

While hydrogen peroxide is the most frequent oxygen donor for peroxidases, a number of **organic hydroperoxides**, in particular fatty acid hydroperoxides, are also active. The same is true of **peracids** (La Mar *et al.*, 1992). A compound of practical interest is 5-phenyl-4-pentenyl hydroperoxide (**10.XXXIV**) whose reduction to the corresponding alcohol affords a convenient means to monitor peroxidases and to evaluate reducing substrates (Weller *et al.*, 1985).

10.XXXIV

Xenobiotics oxidized by single-electron transfer reactions (reactions **c** and **d** in Fig. 10.12) form radical intermediates which can either react as discussed in the following sections, or catalyze the oxygenation of a cosubstrate. Thus, a great variety of xenobiotics have been tested for their ability to support the oxygenation of arachidonic acid following their own one-electron oxidation by Compound I (Lehmann *et al.*, 1989).

Some hemoprotein peroxidases display the ability **to oxidize halide anions**, namely the chloride, bromide and iodide anions. In mechanistic terms, Compound I of these peroxidases transfers its ferryl oxygen to the halide anion, thus forming the corresponding, weakly acidic hypohalous acid (reaction **f** in Fig. 10.12) (Kettle and Winterbourn, 1991; Lagorce *et al.*, 1991). Such a reaction is characteristic of myeloperoxidase (the only mammalian chloroperoxidase, showing a preference for Cl⁻) and eosinophil peroxidase (which shows a marked preference for Br⁻ over Cl⁻) (Harris *et al.*, 1993; Kanofsky *et al.*, 1988; O'Brien *et al.*, 1991; Weiss, 1991; Weiss *et al.*, 1986).

The **hypohalous acid** thus formed acts as an oxidizing agent towards a number of endogenous and exogenous compounds, as discussed below (Floris and Wever, 1992). This mechanism of oxidation may be direct, but indirect pathways should also exist since stimulated leukocytes liberate superoxide, which in turn can react with hypochlorous acid to produce a hydroxyl radical (Ramos *et al.*, 1992). It is of great potential significance that many non-steroidal anti-inflammatory drugs (NSAIDs, whose main mechanism of action is inhibition of PES) act as competitive **inhibitors of hypochlorous acid formation** by myeloperoxidase, e.g. aminopyrine and phenylbutazone; indomethacin, sulindac and ibuprofen; mefenamic acid; piroxicam; salicylate and aspirin (Kettle and Winterbourn, 1991; Kettle *et al.*, 1993; Shacter *et al.*, 1991). These inhibitors have been shown to act by converting Compound I to Compound II. The same property is shared by chemotherapeutic agents such as dapsone, quinacrine and primaquine. The best inhibitor was 4-bromoaniline, and the structure–activity relationship was rationalized in terms of an optimal redox potential allowing easy reduction of Compound I to Compound II but not reduction of the latter to the active enzyme (Kettle and Winterbourn, 1991). In contrast, the antileprotic agent clofazimine inhibits the effect of myeloperoxidase by scavenging the hypochlorous acid formed (van Zyl *et al.*, 1991).

10.4.2 Reactions of carbon oxidation

Relatively few xenobiotics have been investigated as substrates in peroxidase-catalyzed carbon oxidations. This could be the mechanism of dealkylation of **ethyl mercury** and **methyl mercury** to inorganic mercury (Hg^0), a reaction catalyzed by a hypohalous acid formed by **myeloperoxidase**/H_2O_2/X^- (X^- = Cl^-, Br^- or I^-), or by **chloroperoxidase**/H_2O_2/I^- (Suda and Takahashi, 1992). But most known cases of peroxidase-catalyzed carbon oxidations involve **sp^2-carbons**, e.g. 1,3-butadiene and **styrene** (**10.XXXI** in Fig. 10.13). The latter compound is directly oxidized by cytochrome P450 (see Section 4.4) and **chloroperoxidase** (i.e. hemoproteins with a thiolate-ligated iron), but seemingly not by horseradish peroxidase (which has an imidazole-ligated iron). The oxidation of styrene by chloroperoxidase or cytochrome P450 yields styrene oxide (**10.XXXIII** in Fig. 10.13) and phenylacetaldehyde (**10.XXXV** in Fig. 10.13), but not benzaldehyde (a product of cooxidation). The reaction mechanism was rationalized as shown in Fig. 10.13 and indicates that chloroperoxidase can function as a peroxygenase (like cytochrome P450) in addition to being a peroxidase. The much higher ratio of phenylacetaldehyde to styrene oxide produced by chloroperoxidase than by cytochrome P450 suggests that, despite their great analogy, the active sites of the two enzymes must differ to some extent (Ortiz de Montellano *et al.*, 1987). Analogous reactions were seen in the oxidation of 1,3-butadiene by chloroperoxidase and human myeloperoxidase (Duescher and Elfarra, 1992 and 1993). An example of medicinal relevance is **carbamazepine** whose double bond is chlorinated and oxidized by myeloperoxidase/H_2O_2/Cl^- to a reactive intermediate that undergoes ring contraction and forms adducts (Furst and Uetrecht, 1993).

The one-electron oxidation of **polycyclic aromatic hydrocarbons** (PAHs) has been seen with benzo[*a*]pyrene (**10.VI** in Fig. 10.3), which undergoes **horseradish peroxidase**-catalyzed

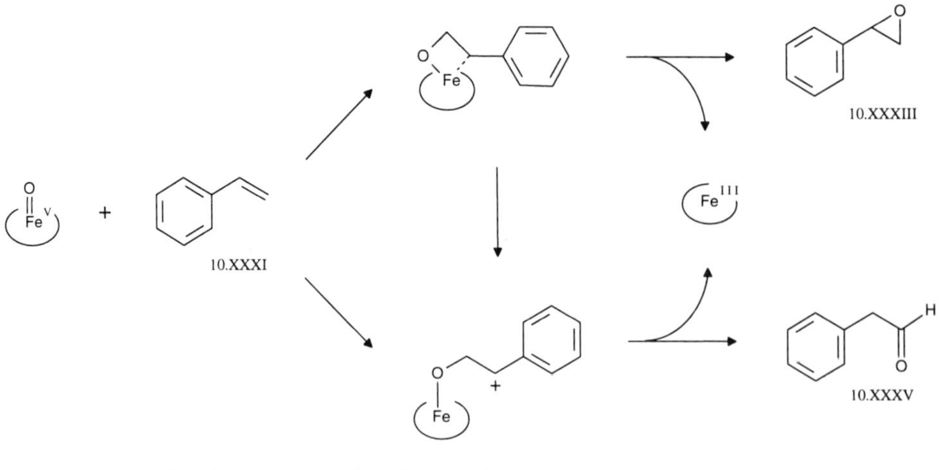

FIGURE 10.13 Postulated mechanism of oxidation of styrene (**10.XXXI**) to styrene oxide (**10.XXXIII**) and phenylacetaldehyde (**10.XXXV**) as catalyzed by the two thiolate-ligated hemoproteins chloroperoxidase and cytochrome P450 (Ortiz de Montellano *et al.*, 1987).

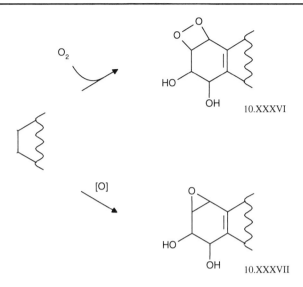

FIGURE 10.14 Reactions of oxygenation and dioxygenation of benzo[*a*]pyrene-7,8-dihydrodiol catalyzed by myeloperoxidase (Trush *et al.*, 1990).

formation of the 1,6-, 3,6- and 6,12-quinones (Cavalieri *et al.*, 1988b). The enzyme also catalyzes the covalent binding of BP to DNA. Thus PES (Section 10.3.2) and HRP oxidize and activate BP by the same mechanism (shown in Fig. 10.3) and to the same products.

In addition to this single-electron oxidation, oxygenation of benzo[*a*]pyrene-7,8-dihydrodiol has also been characterized (Fig. 10.14). This reaction is catalyzed by polymorphonuclear leukocytes and principally by their **myeloperoxidase** activity (Trush *et al.*, 1990). Two metabolites were formed, namely a chemiluminescent 9,10-dioxetane derivative (**10.XXXVI** in Fig. 10.14) and a 9,10-epoxide derivative (**10.XXXVII** in Fig. 10.14) responsible for covalent binding. Such a metabolic scheme is interesting on two accounts. First, it indicates that peroxidase-catalyzed toxication of PAHs can occur by more than one mechanism; and second, it affords a rare example of a reaction of dioxygenation (see Section 10.5).

Another recently uncovered example of carbon oxygenation mediated by myeloperoxidase is that of the aromatic amino acid **phenylalanine** (Fujimoto *et al.*, 1991). This compound was hydroxylated in the *para*, *meta* and *ortho* positions to the corresponding phenols, i.e. *p*-, *m*- and *o*-tyrosine. Addition of chloride in low concentrations increased, but higher concentrations decreased, the rate of reaction. The fact that hydroxyl radical scavengers (mannitol, benzoate or formate) or superoxide dismutase inhibited tyrosine formation provides evidence that the reaction mechanism(s) may be more complex than implied by Fig. 10.12 and that activated forms of oxygen participate in carbon hydroxylation (see end of previous section).

Phenylbutazone (**10.X** in Fig. 10.7) has been discussed in Section 10.3.2 as a substrate of PES. Here, we note that **horseradish peroxidase** catalyzes the same oxygenation to the 4-hydroxyl and 4-hydroperoxyl derivatives via a C(4)-centred radical (Fig. 10.7) (Hughes *et al.*, 1988). Phenylbutazone contains an acidic C–H group carrying two carbonyl functions, i.e. a β-dicarbonyl moiety OC–CH–CO, and is thus in tautomeric equilibrium with an enol. The same structural motif is displayed by anti-inflammatory **oxicams**, and indeed isoxicam (**10.XXXVIII**) is oxidized by HRP to the 3-hydroperoxyl intermediate which then decomposes to a variety of metabolites such as N-methylsaccharin (Woolf *et al.*, 1989a and 1992). That the same metabolites are formed *in vivo* suggests the capacity of mammalian peroxidases to catalyze the same reaction (Woolf *et al.*, 1989b).

Insights into the mechanism and pharmacological significance of peroxidase-catalyzed degradation of oxicams have been obtained from metabolic studies of tenoxicam (**10.XXXIX** in Fig. 10.15) in the presence of rat leukocyte **myeloperoxidase** (Ichihara *et al.*, 1989). Upon addition of H_2O_2 (reaction **a** in Fig. 10.15), four metabolites were formed, namely 2-carboxyl-3-thiophenesulfinic acid (**10.XL** in Fig. 10.15) which underwent oxidation to the corresponding sulfonic acid, and 4,5-dihydro-4-oxo-5-methyliminopyrido[1,2*a*]imidazole (**10.XLI** in Fig. 10.15) which was hydrolyzed to a ring-opened oxamide. The formation of these metabolites was explained by a one-electron oxidation at the carbon atom in the β-dicarbonyl moiety, as shown in Fig. 10.15. When chloride was added to the incubation medium (reaction **b** in Fig. 10.15), three other metabolites were formed which included the thiophene analogue of N-methylsaccharin (**10.XLII** in Fig. 10.15) and corresponded to the products of HRP-mediated oxidation of isoxicam (see above). These results demonstrate the capacity of oxicams to act as reducing cofactors of Compound I of peroxidases, an activity that may account for part of their anti-inflammatory effects.

10.XXXVIII

10.4.3 Oxidation of aromatic amines

Aromatic amines are readily oxidized by Compound I of peroxidases, as revealed by systematic studies using a large variety of such substrates (Lehmann *et al.*, 1989; Vasquez *et al.*, 1992; Weller *et al.*, 1985). In contrast, most **aliphatic amines** are not substrates of peroxidases, as exemplified by pargyline (**10.VII**) (Weli and Lindeke, 1986). A notable exception is vinblastine, as discussed below. The oxidation of aromatic amines can be initiated by three different reaction mechanisms, namely one-electron oxidation, N-chlorination, or N-oxygenation. The metabolites thus formed include azo compounds, quinone imines, quinone diimines, dimers and oligomers, N-chloroamines, hydroxylamines, nitrosoarenes and nitroarenes, and N-demethylated amines.

In some cases, the N-centred radical cation (i.e. the aminium cation radical) resulting from **one-electron oxidation** of an aromatic amine can be detected, e.g. by ESR spectroscopy (Fischer *et al.*, 1991; Van der Zee *et al.*, 1989). A number of drugs undergo this activation to reactive and potentially damaging intermediates, e.g. mianserin and primaquine (Roberts *et al.*, 1993; Sa Silva Morais and Augusto, 1993). A particularly telling example is that of the neuroleptic **chlorpromazine**, which is oxidized by various peroxidase systems to the N-centred radical **10.XLIII**, detectable by UV spectrophotometry. Thus, formation of this radical by **methemoglobin/H_2O_2** results in covalent binding to methemoglobin (Kelder *et al.*, 1991a). Human neutrophil **myeloperoxidase/H_2O_2** also forms **10.XLIII**, and does so faster in the presence of chloride, indicating that both Compound I and HOCl are active in oxidizing chlorpromazine (van Zyl *et al.*, 1990). Another example is that of **phenytoin**, which may be oxidized by **horseradish peroxidase, thyroid peroxidase**, and **PES** to a radical of unknown structure (possibly an N-centred one). The covalent binding of the phenytoin radical to proteins, and radical-induced lipid peroxidation, is of potential toxicological significance (Kubow and Wells, 1989).

In most studies, however, the occurrence of **aminium radical cations** in the one-electron oxidation of aromatic amines has been shown indirectly from the chemical nature of stable

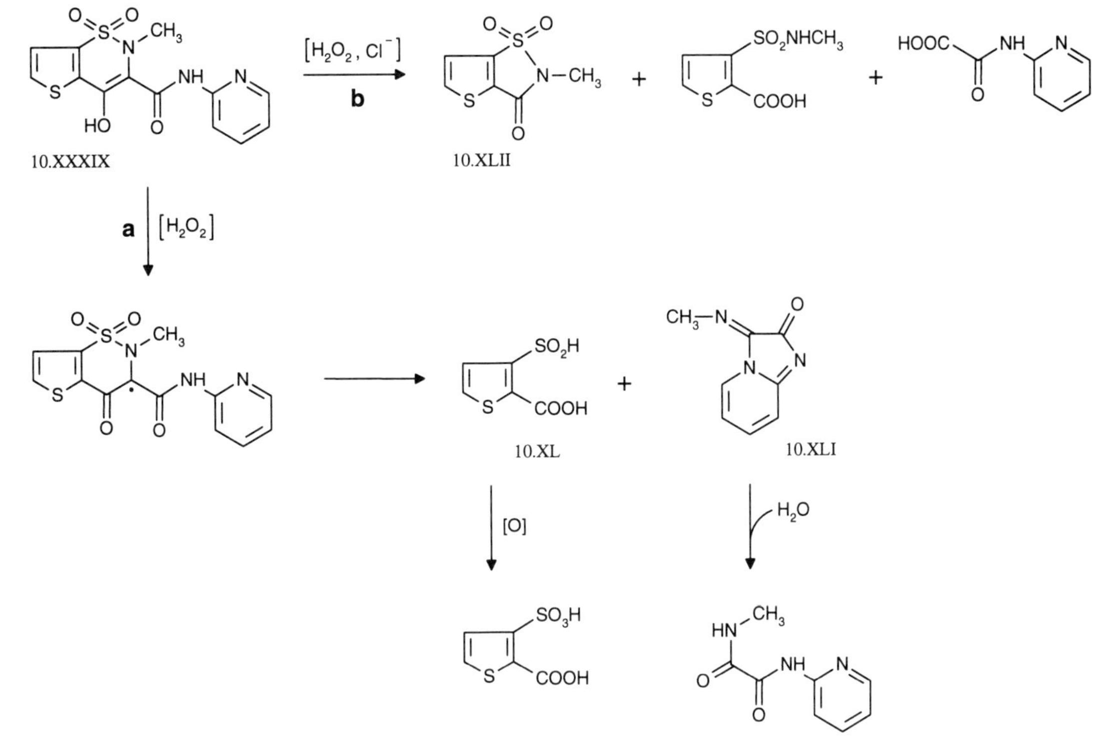

FIGURE 10.15 Oxidative metabolism of tenoxicam (**10.XXXIX**) by leukocyte myeloperoxidase in the absence (reaction **a**) and presence (reaction **b**) of chloride (Ichihara *et al.*, 1989).

rearrangement products derived from them, particularly dimers and oligomers. For example, *para*-phenetidine (**10.XX** in Fig. 10.9) was oxidized by **HRP** to the quinone imine, the quinone diimine, and the azo derivative (**10.XXI**, **10.XXII** and **10.XLIV** in Fig. 10.9, respectively) (Lindquist *et al.*, 1985; Ross *et al.*, 1985). The toxicological implication of these reactive metabolites has been discussed in Section 10.3. Recent studies on the HRP-catalyzed oxidation of *para*-anisidine (**10.XLV**), the lower homologue of *para*-phenetidine (**10.XX** in Fig. 10.9), and its *ortho* isomer (**10.XLVI**) have again proven the formation of quinone imines, quinone diimines, and azo dimers. In addition, a tetramer of *para*-anisidine has also been characterized, while substantial covalent binding to proteins and DNA was seen (Thompson and Eling, 1991). Another relevant example is that of 4-aminobiphenyl (Hughes *et al.*, 1992).

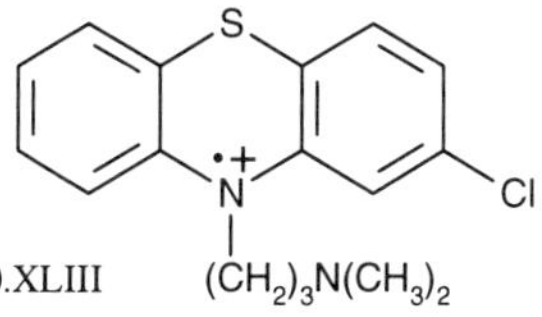

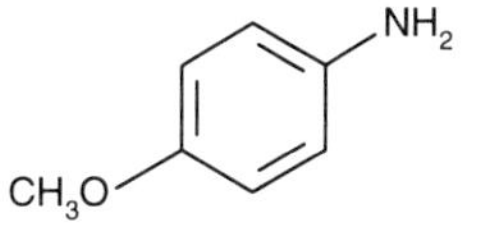

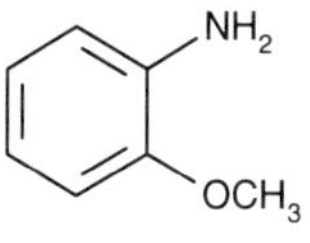

An unexpected product of cleavage and dimerization (presumably via N-oxidation) was recently seen in the metabolism of the anti-inflammatory agent **diclofenac (10.XLVII)**. This drug inhibited the chlorinating activity of **myeloperoxidase** isolated from human polymorphonuclear neutrophils, an activity which may add to its beneficial effects. In turn, diclofenac was oxidized by Compound I and Compound II of the enzyme to a dihydroxyazobenzene (**10.XLVIII**, in which the position of the hydroxyl groups is unknown) (Zuurbier *et al.*, 1990). Diclofenac is thus a reducing substrate of myeloperoxidase, by virtue of its competing with Cl⁻ for Compound I.

N-Chlorination of a number of aromatic amines has been observed upon incubation with chloroperoxidases (Uetrecht *et al.*, 1993). A typical drug in this respect is **procainamide (10.XLIX)** which was found to be oxidized by **myeloperoxidase/H$_2$O$_2$/Cl⁻** or activated leukocytes to N-chloroprocainamide. This metabolite (a) spontaneously rearranged to 3-chloroprocainamide; (b) reacted rapidly with reducing agents (e.g. ascorbate) or proteins (e.g. albumin) to form procainamide; or (c) was able to chlorinate other compounds such as phenylbutazone (Uetrecht and Sokoluk, 1992; Uetrecht and Zahid, 1991). N-Chloroprocainamide, and its N-oxygenated metabolites formed by myeloperoxidase in the absence of chloride (see below), have been suggested to be responsible for procainamide-induced agranulocytosis (Uetrecht, 1990). The tertiary amine **aminopyrine (10.XXIII)** was also oxidized by myeloperoxidase/H$_2$O$_2$/Cl⁻ to form an N-centred radical cation according to Eqs. 10.13–10.15 (Sayo and Saito, 1990):

$$R-NMe_2 + HOCl \rightarrow R-N^+(Cl)Me_2 + HO^- \qquad \text{(Eq. 10.13)}$$

$$R-N^+(Cl)Me_2 \rightarrow R-N^{+\bullet}Me_2 + Cl^\bullet \qquad \text{(Eq. 10.14)}$$

$$R-NMe_2 + Cl^\bullet \rightarrow R-N^{+\bullet}Me_2 + Cl^- \qquad \text{(Eq. 10.15)}$$

Interestingly, aminopyrine oxidation was much more rapid under the influence of HOBr when bromide replaced chloride in the incubation, and was much slower in the absence of chloride. Aminopyrine radical cation decomposed rapidly in aqueous solution, suggesting that it may be potentially damaging to biological systems.

A number of other aromatic amines have been shown to be oxidized by HOCl or HOBr generated by **myeloperoxidase** or **eosinophil peroxidase** (O'Brien *et al.*, 1991). The observation that **phenytoin** is chlorinated by myeloperoxidase to N,N'-dichlorophenytoin (**10.L**) is intriguing because the reaction involves lactam rather than amine functions (Uetrecht, 1990). Here again, N-chlorination was a reaction of toxication leading to increased covalent binding of the drug to proteins. In general terms, N-chlorination and N-bromination thus appear as effective routes of bioactivation, leading to chloroamines and bromoamines which can react with a variety of compounds such as amines, thiols, sulfides, disulfides, and aromatic rings (Weiss, 1991).

Direct N-oxygenation of primary aromatic amines under the influence of peroxidases has also been demonstrated in a few cases while in other cases N-oxygenated metabolites were not seen. Thus, *para*-phenetidine (**10.XX** in Fig. 10.9) did not form a hydroxylamino or a nitroso metabolite in the presence of PES or HRP (Lindquist *et al.*, 1985). In contrast, a careful study

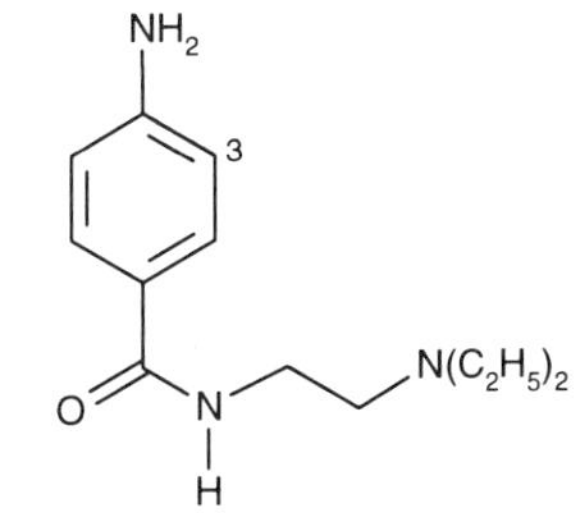

10.XLIX 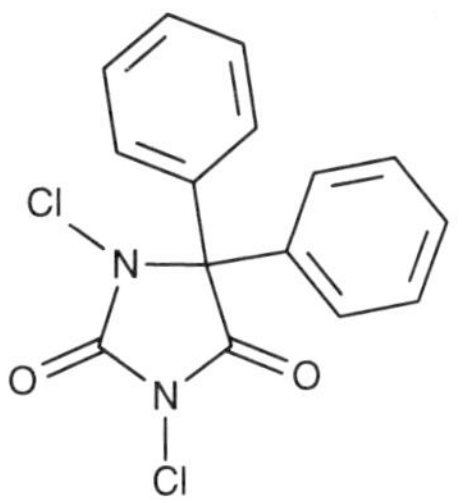   10.L

using **chloroperoxidase**/[^{18}O]H$_2$O$_2$ showed that the mechanism of N-oxygenation of *para*-toluidine, 4-chloroaniline and 3,4-dichloroaniline to the corresponding hydroxylamine involves transfer of the oxygen atom of Compound I to the amino nitrogen (Doerge and Corbett, 1991). Dehydrogenation of the hydroxylamines to the nitroso metabolites occurred without exchange of oxygen.

Examples of aromatic amines undergoing N-oxygenation include 2-aminofluorene (**10.XVIII**), whose metabolism to 2-nitrofluorene is catalyzed not only by PES as discussed in Section 10.3.3, but also by **horseradish peroxidase. Chloroperoxidase**/H$_2$O$_2$ is also active, but for unknown reasons the metabolite formed was 2-nitrosofluorene (Boyd *et al.*, 1983). Sulfamethoxazole (**10.XIX**) is similarly N-oxygenated to the hydroxylamino and nitro derivatives not only by PES (Section 10.3.3), but also by **myeloperoxidase** (Cribb *et al.*, 1990). As discussed above, procainamide (**10.XLIX**) is N-chlorinated by the system myeloperoxidase/H$_2$O$_2$/Cl$^-$. In the absence of Cl$^-$, however, N-oxygenation occurred to form the hydroxylamino and nitroso derivatives. The same reaction of N-oxygenation was seen in the presence of activated leukocytes (Uetrecht and Zahid, 1991). The toxicological consequences of these reactions have been discussed in detail (Uetrecht, 1990 and 1992).

A particularly interesting case of N-oxygenation can be found in the **catalase**-mediated bioactivation of the alcohol deterrent agent **cyanamide** (**10.LI** in Fig. 10.16) (Nagasawa *et al.*, 1990). This agent is not directly active but must undergo bioactivation prior to eliciting ethanol deterrence due to the side-effects associated with inhibition of aldehyde dehydrogenase. It has been demonstrated that catalase/H$_2$O$_2$ catalyzes this activation by forming the unstable intermediate N-hydroxycyanamide whose decomposition generates cyanide and nitroxyl (**10.LII** in Fig. 10.16, nitrosyl hydride), the putative inhibitor of aldehyde dehydrogenase. There is evidence that cytochrome P450 may also catalyze the same bioactivation reaction.

N-Demethylation is one of the metabolic pathways open to the radical species of **N-methylated and N,N-dimethylated aromatic amines**. Thus, aminopyrine (**10.XXIII**) was N-demethylated by the **catalase**/cumene hydroperoxide system via its transient free radical (see above) and with production of formaldehyde (Sayo and Hosokawa, 1980). From a study of the cumene hydroperoxide-supported N-demethylation of N,N-dimethylanilines catalyzed by cata-

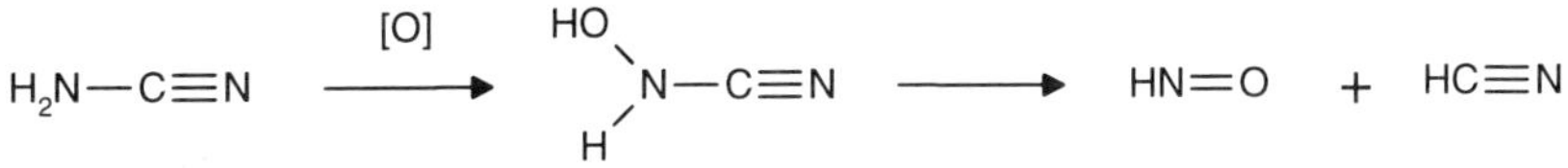

10.LI   10.LII

FIGURE 10.16 Mechanism of bioactivation of cyanamide (**10.LI**) to nitroxyl (**10.LII**) catalyzed by catalase/H$_2$O$_2$ (and possibly also by cytochrome P450) (Nagasawa *et al.*, 1990).

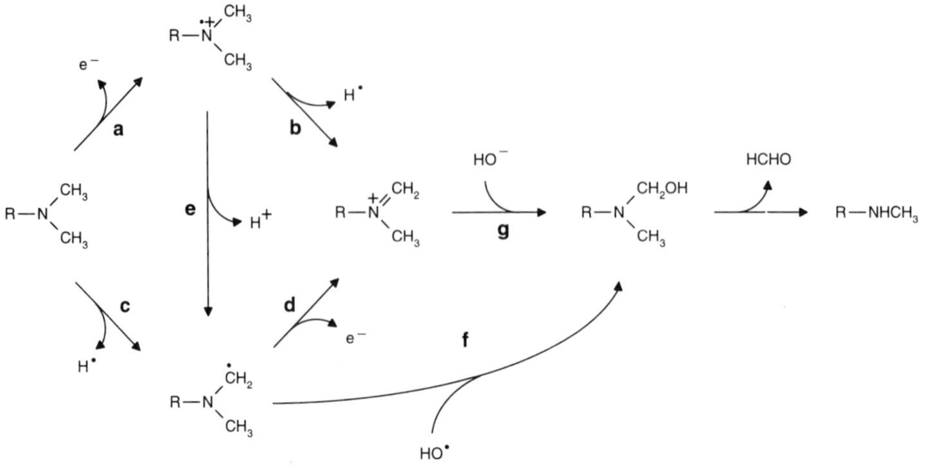

FIGURE 10.17 Postulated mechanism(s) of the peroxidase-catalyzed N-demethylation of aromatic amines. See text for further details.

lase, the same authors have concluded that the reaction occurs by one-electron oxidation to the aminium cation radical followed by proton abstraction (reactions **a** and **e** in Fig. 10.17). At low substrate concentrations of N,N-dimethylaniline, the neutral carbon-centred radical thus formed has been postulated to disproportionate to the original amine and to the iminium cation which then adds the hydroxyl anion (reaction **g** in Fig. 10.17) and breaks down to the N-demethylated amine and to formaldehyde (Section 6.2). At higher substrate concentrations, *para–para* dimerization of the neutral radical was observed and led to N,N,N′,N′-tetramethylbenzidine.

Intramolecular isotope kinetic effects have allowed an insight into the mechanisms of N-demethylation catalyzed by peroxidase/ROOH systems (Hollenberg *et al.*, 1985). Small kinetic effects (i.e. k_H/k_D values in the range 1–3) were exhibited by **chloroperoxidase** and some cytochrome P450 isozymes, implying one-electron oxidation of the amino group (reactions **a** and **e** in Fig. 10.17), while values in the range 8–10 were exhibited by the imidazole-ligated peroxidases (**HRP, lactoperoxidase, hemoglobin, myoglobin**), indicating a hydrogen abstraction mechanism (reaction **c** in Fig. 10.17). The predominance of radical recombination (reaction **f** in Fig. 10.17) over iminium hydration (reaction **g** in Fig. 10.17) was indicated by ^{18}O incorporation studies, suggesting the occurrence of reaction **e** in Fig. 10.12. In contradiction to these results, the formation of carbon-centred radicals and marked oxygen consumption did not occur during the N-demethylation of N,N-dimethylanilines by horseradish peroxidase, supporting the pathway of reactions **a**, **b** and **g** in Fig. 10.17 (Van der Zee *et al.*, 1989). We must conclude from such contradictory results that either experimental conditions determine the dominating mechanism, and/or current interpretations of experimental data are based on some invalid assumptions. An indication supporting the former possibility (but not disproving the latter) is given by the fact that antioxidants inhibit horseradish peroxidase-catalyzed but not hydroperoxide/cytochrome P450-catalyzed N-demethylation (O'Brien *et al.*, 1985).

All above examples pertain to aromatic amines. That the substrate selectivity of peroxidases may include other amino moieties is suggested by the oxidation of vinblastine to catharinine catalyzed by horseradish peroxidase/H_2O_2 (Elmarakby *et al.*, 1989). Indeed, this reaction involves oxidative N–C cleavage in a piperidine ring.

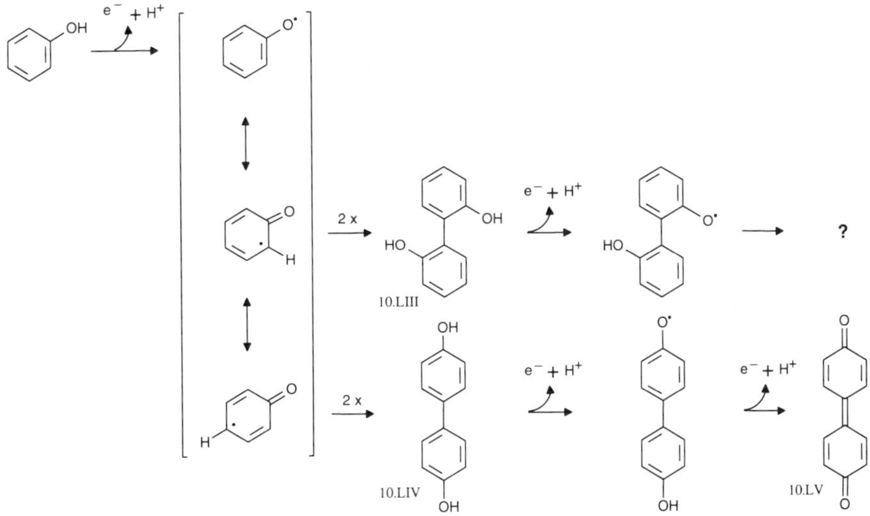

FIGURE 10.18 Metabolic activation of phenol by human myeloperoxidase and horseradish peroxidase to reactive metabolites, in particular diphenoquinone (**10.LV**) and the phenoxyl radicals of phenol, 2,2′-biphenol (**10.LIII**) and 4,4′-biphenol (**10.LIV**) (Eastmond *et al.*, 1986).

10.4.4 Oxidation of alcohols and phenols

The ability of peroxidases to oxidize **alcohols** appears restricted to cytochrome P450 (see Section 10.2.3 and Table 10.1) and **catalase**. Indeed, one molecule of H_2O_2 in the reaction catalyzed by the latter enzyme (i.e. the hydrogen donor, see Eq. 10.12) can be replaced by various alcohols such as methanol, ethanol and 1-propanol (Aragon *et al.*, 1992; Thurman and Handler, 1989).

In contrast to alcohols, **phenols** are good reducing substrates of all peroxidases discussed here, being for example oxidized as readily as aromatic amines by horseradish peroxidase (Chignell, 1985; Lehmann *et al.*, 1989; Weller *et al.*, 1985). The reaction is a one-electron oxidation to phenoxyl radicals, as discussed above for cytochrome P450 and PES (Brewster *et al.*, 1991; Kettle and Winterbourn, 1992).

Phenol and a number of congeners are activated by various peroxidases to reactive metabolites which can dimerize or bind covalently to proteins. Thus, human **myeloperoxidase** and **horseradish peroxidase** were found to oxidize phenol to two major metabolites, namely 4,4′-biphenol and diphenoquinone (**10.LIV** and **10.LV**, respectively, in Fig. 10.18); trace amounts of 2,2′-biphenol (**10.LIII** in Fig. 10.18) were also detected (Eastmond *et al.*, 1986). Extensive covalent binding to proteins occurred and was ascribed to the phenoxyl radicals of phenol, 2,2′-biphenol and 4,4′-biphenol, the structures of which are shown in Fig. 10.18. Diphenoquinone must also be adduct-forming as it reacted avidly with glutathione to form conjugates. Other monophenols shown to be oxidized by horseradish peroxidase to the corresponding phenoxyl radical and other more or less reactive species include 1-naphthol, 2,4,6-trimethylphenol, butylated hydroxyanisole (BHA), butylated hydroxytoluene (BHT, **7.XLVIII** in Section 7.6), 3-*t*-butyl-4-hydroxyanisole and Trolox (d'Arcy Doherty *et al.*, 1986; Metodiewa and Dunford, 1991; Ortiz de Montellano *et al.*, 1987; Tajima *et al.*, 1992; Thompson *et al.*, 1989). Interestingly, while both horseradish peroxidase and PES (see Section 10.3.4) formed the phenoxyl radical of BHA, subsequent reactions must have been different since three dimers were formed by the former enzyme and only two by the latter (Thompson *et al.*, 1989).

10.LVI   10.LVII

10.LVIII

Besides forming oligomers or adducts, resonance forms of some phenoxyl radicals can also add O_2 to form **hydroperoxyl radicals** (e.g. reaction **d** in Fig. 10.4) which then oxidize a second substrate (e.g. the reaction shown in Fig. 10.5). This is for example the mechanism by which the 4-methylphenoxyl radical, formed from 4-methylphenol by horseradish peroxidase, oxidizes styrene giving styrene oxide and benzaldehyde (Ortiz de Montellano and Grab, 1987).

A few drugs bearing phenolic groups have been shown to be activated by peroxidases. Thus, **acetaminophen** (**10.XXVII** in Fig. 10.10) is oxidized by horseradish peroxidase and other peroxidases to the highly reactive acetaminophen phenoxyl radical (**10.XXVIII** in Fig. 10.10) which can then bind covalently to proteins, oxidize glutathione to the thiyl radical or ascorbate to the ascorbyl radical, and form dimers and polymers (see Section 10.3.4) (Mason and Fischer, 1986; Nelson *et al.*, 1981; Rao *et al.*, 1990). A comparable fate is displayed by the antimalarial **amodiaquine** (**10.LVI**), a drug displaying structural similarities with acetaminophen and known to cause agranulocytosis and liver damage in humans (Maggs *et al.*, 1988). Under catalysis by horseradish peroxidase, amodiaquine formed a phenoxyl radical (i.e. the semiquinone imine) which was then oxidized to the quinone imine, leading to extensive covalent binding to proteins. In the presence of hypochlorous acid (i.e. a model of the myeloperoxidase/H_2O_2/Cl^- system), N-chloro-amodiaquine was formed and also reacted with proteins.

The synthetic estrogen and transplacental carcinogen **diethylstilbestrol** (**10.LVII**) was also oxidized by horseradish peroxidase or **mouse uterus peroxidases** in the presence of H_2O_2 to a large number of metabolites and to DNA-bound material (Metzler and Haaf, 1985). A major metabolite was Z,Z-dienestrol (**10.LVIII**) formed via the semiquinone and quinone intermediates which were also suspected to be responsible for covalent binding. Reactions of carbon–carbon cleavage were also catalyzed by the peroxidases and were particularly effective with large excesses of H_2O_2; they led to the formation of oxidized metabolites having either lost one of the aromatic rings or resulting from C(3)–C(4) cleavage in dienestrol.

Peroxidases display a marked activity towards **catechols**. Thus, **horseradish peroxidase** and **human leukocyte peroxidase** oxidize catechol (**10.LIX** in Fig. 10.19) to *o*-benzoquinone (**10.LX** in Fig. 10.19) (Sadler *et al.*, 1988). The mechanism of the reaction is a one-electron oxidation to *o*-benzosemiquinone, which then disproportionates to catechol and *o*-benzoquinone (Fig. 10.19); under physiological conditions, molecular oxygen did not appear to play a role in the oxidation

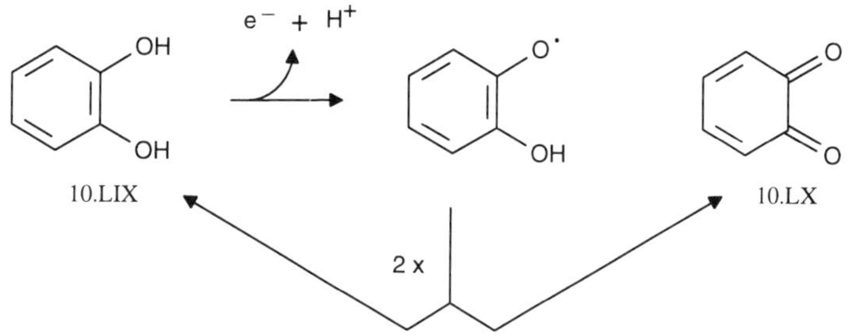

FIGURE 10.19 Mechanism of peroxidase-catalyzed bioactivation of catechol (**10.LIX**) to an *o*-benzo-semiquinone and *o*-benzoquinone (**10.LX**) (Sadler *et al.*, 1988).

of the semiquinone radical to the quinone. The formation of the semiquinone and quinone leads to covalent binding to proteins and was also shown to occur in rat and human bone marrow cells under the influence of myeloperoxidase (Bhat *et al.*, 1988). Since both catechol and trihydroxy-benzene are metabolites of benzene, their bioactivation to reactive products explains at least in part the myelotoxicity of benzene (Smart and Zannoni, 1984).

Other relevant examples include the oxidation of noradrenaline, DOPA methyl ester, and 6-hydroxy-DOPA by myeloperoxidase or lactoperoxidase (Metodiewa and Dunford, 1990; Metodiewa *et al.*, 1989). Here again, the first oxidation step is enzyme-catalyzed, while disproportionation and/or autoxidation generate quinones, which can then rearrange to dopachromes. The oxidation of **catechol estrogens** (e.g. 2-hydroxyestradiol **10.LXI** and 4-hydroxyestradiol) by peroxidases also generates *o*-semiquinones of particular toxicological significance (Kalyanaraman *et al.*, 1984).

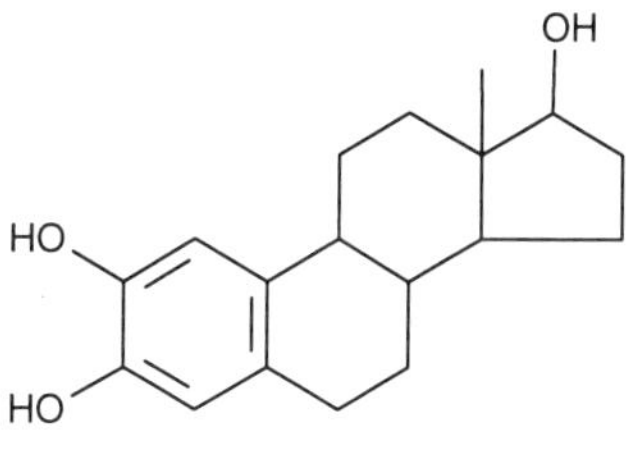

10.LXI

The various examples discussed above clearly indicate that a variety of phenolic compounds can be activated by peroxidases to reactive metabolites. Glutathione (see a subsequent volume) affords a major protection mechanism, but covalent binding may be difficult to suppress entirely and its consequences may be dramatic.

10.4.5 Oxidation of sulfur-containing compounds

Thiols are seemingly less effective reducing substrates of horseradish peroxidase than phenols and aromatic amines (Weller *et al.*, 1985). However, this observation cannot be generalized since there are conditions under which peroxidases oxidize thiols and other sulfur-containing compounds. Thus, the one-electron oxidation of *sulfite* (SO_3^{2-}) to the sulfur trioxide radical anion ($SO_3^{\bullet-}$) is mediated not only by PES as discussed in Section 10.3.5, but also by **horseradish peroxidase** (Mottley *et al.*, 1982).

Reactions of **thiol oxidation** are amply documented. Thus, the tripeptide **glutathione** (GSH, Section 10.3.5) is oxidized by horseradish peroxidase, the first product of the reaction being the free thiyl radical GS• also formed by PES (Section 10.3.5) (Harman *et al.*, 1986). This radical, besides (a) reacting with itself to form stable glutathione disulfide (Eq. 10.10), (b) can also react with molecular oxygen to form the glutathione-derived peroxyl radical (reaction **b** in Fig. 10.11); or (c) react with glutathione anion (GS$^-$) to form a disulfide anion radical in analogy with some other thiols (see below Fig. 10.20). Both the glutathione thiyl radical and the glutathione-derived peroxyl radical may react with other compounds, in particular certain xenobiotics. Formation of the hydroxylated styrene–GSH conjugate (**10.XXXII** in Fig. 10.11) is catalyzed not only by PES as discussed in Section 10.3.5 but also by horseradish peroxidase (Stock *et al.*, 1986). In addition,

10.LXII   10.LXIII

the cooxidation of styrene by horseradish peroxidase and glutathione led to styrene epoxide (**10.XXXIII** in Fig. 10.11), a postulated mechanism involving the glutathione-derived peroxyl radical being shown as reaction **c** in Fig. 10.11 (Ortiz de Montellano and Grab, 1986).

Beside undergoing one-electron oxidation by PES, HRP and possibly other peroxidases, glutathione is also oxidized by **glutathione peroxidase** (see Section 10.4.1) (Mason and Rao, 1990). The overall reaction involved is written as:

$$2GSH + ROOH \rightarrow GSSG + ROH \qquad \text{(Eq. 10.16)}$$

This reaction is of particular interest in connection with **futile redox cycles of quinones**. Indeed, such cycles involve the enzymatic reduction of quinones (Section 12.2), for example anticancer quinones, and their non-enzymatic reoxidation by O_2 (autoxidation, see Section 7.6). The superoxide anion radical thus formed yields H_2O_2 either by disproportionation (see Section 3.5) or under catalysis by superoxide dismutase; H_2O_2 is then destroyed by glutathione peroxidase according to Eq. 10.16 (Doroshow *et al.*, 1990; Koster, 1991). From a mechanistic viewpoint, the formation of GSSG catalyzed by glutathione peroxidase does not involve a thiyl radical intermediate and is thus different from the same reaction catalyzed by PES or HRP (Harman *et al.*, 1986).

A number of thiol-containing **endogenous compounds** such as cysteine, cysteamine, N-acetylcysteine and glutathione, and **drugs** such as penicillamine (**10.LXII**) and captopril (**10.LXIII**), were shown to be oxidized by the **lactoperoxidase/H_2O_2 system** under uptake of molecular oxygen (Mottley *et al.*, 1987). The main reactions occurring in this system are depicted in Fig. 10.20, again indicating formation of a thiyl radical as the first oxidative step. Reaction of this radical with the thiolate anion (reaction **a** in Fig. 10.20) produced a disulfide anion-radical which was oxidized by O_2 to the **disulfide** (reaction **b** in Fig. 10.20), thereby forming superoxide and then H_2O_2. Oxygen uptake was particularly marked with cysteine and penicillamine, but limited with N-acetylcysteine, glutathione and captopril. While coupling of two thiyl radicals to form a disulfide (reaction **c** in Fig. 10.20) was not investigated, its occurrence is likely (Mottley *et al.*, 1987). Clearly Figs. 10.11 and 10.20 and Eq. 10.10 demonstrate the variety of peroxidase-mediated reactions undergone by some thiols.

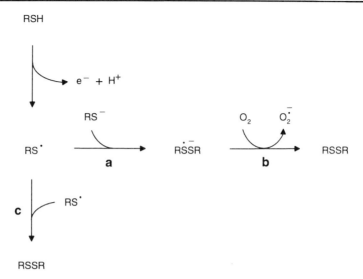

FIGURE 10.20 Main reactions of peroxidase-mediated oxidation undergone by some thiol drugs and biochemicals (Mottley *et al.*, 1987).

Activated neutrophils or the **myeloperoxidase**/H_2O_2/Cl^- system are also able to attack thiols, forming reactive intermediates of toxicological significance. The initial reaction, which results from the direct action of HOCl, is believed to be one of *s-chlorination* leading to a **sulfenyl chloride**, itself a precursor of a variety of more or less reactive metabolites. The reaction is particularly well documented for cyclic thioureas existing in a thione–thiol equilibrium (see Section 7.8 and Fig. 7.20).

For example, **propylthiouracil** (**10.LXIV**, thiol tautomer) reacts as shown in Fig. 10.21, forming first its sulfenyl chloride (reaction **a** and **10.LXV** in Fig. 10.21) (Lee *et al.*, 1988; Uetrecht, 1990; Waldhauser and Uetrecht, 1991). This sulfenyl chloride can react with thiols, e.g. with propylthiouracil itself to form propylthiouracil disulfide (reaction **b** in Fig. 10.21), or with a cysteinyl residue in proteins (reaction **c** in Fig. 10.21) to form a mixed disulfide (i.e. protein-propylthiouracil disulfide). As for the latter disulfide, it can be oxidized further (reaction **d** in Fig. 10.21) to the thiosulfinic ester (**10.LXVI** in Fig. 10.21) which leads to the sulfinic acid (**10.LXVII** in Fig. 10.21) and then to the sulfonic acid (**10.LXVIII** in Fig. 10.21). The latter can also react with nucleophiles, in particular cysteinyl residues in proteins (reaction **e** in Fig. 10.21), producing adducts. Propylthiouracil-protein adducts of the types shown in Fig. 10.21 have been postulated to be involved in hypersensitivity reactions associated with the drug, such as agranulocytosis (Waldhauser and Uetrecht, 1991). Similar reactions have been reported for

10.LXIV   10.LXIX   10.LXX

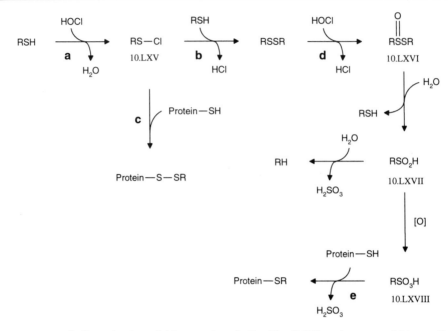

FIGURE 10.21 Metabolic activation of thioureas (symbolized by RSH) such as propylthiouracil (**10.LXIV**) by the myeloperoxidase/H_2O_2/Cl^- system to oxidized metabolites such as disulfides, sulfinic acids (**10.LXVII**) and sulfonic acids (**10.LXVIII**), and to protein adducts (Uetrecht, 1990; Waldhauser and Uetrecht, 1991).

methimazole (**10.LXIX**) (Sayo and Saito, 1991). There is a clear parallel with the reactions shown in Fig. 7.20.

Reactions of *s-oxygenation* have also been reported to be mediated by peroxidases other than chloroperoxidases, in a reaction occurring directly (reaction **b** in Fig. 10.12) rather than via a sulfenyl chloride (Doerge *et al.*, 1991). A simple example is that of thiocyanate ($^-$SCN) whose oxygenation by **lactoperoxidase**/H_2O_2 yields hypothiocyanite ($^-$OSCN), a potent non-specific bactericidal agent (Modi *et al.*, 1991). Goitrogenic thioureas such as methimazole (**10.LXIX**) are time-dependent and irreversible inactivators of lactoperoxidase in the presence of hydroperoxides, the **sulfenic acid** (R–SOH) or **sulfinic acid** (R–SO$_2$H) metabolites being postulated to be the reactive intermediates which bind covalently to the heme group of the enzyme (see **7.XC** and **7.XCI**, respectively, in Fig. 7.20) (Doerge, 1988). The formation of these intermediates was supported by the characterization of desulfurated imidazole metabolites resulting from hydrolysis (e.g. reaction 1 in Fig. 7.18), for example benzimidazole from 2-mercaptobenzimidazole (**10.LXX**).

Other examples of S-oxygenation involve the formation of **sulfoxides** from alkyl aryl sulfides as catalyzed by peroxidases in the presence of various hydroperoxides (but in the absence of chloride) (Casella *et al.*, 1992; Colonna *et al.*, 1990). Thus, chloroperoxidase afforded the sulfoxides having *R* absolute configuration in high enantiomeric excess, while horseradish peroxidase gave racemic products. This indicates differences in active sites and/or catalytic mechanisms which remain to be understood. S-Oxygenation is also a major reaction of chlorpromazine and other phenothiazine drugs in the presence of methemoglobin/H_2O_2 (Kelder *et al.*, 1991a and 1991b).

10.5 REACTIONS CATALYZED BY DIOXYGENASES AND REACTIONS OF DIOXYGENATION

In this last and short section, three additional types of reactions are mentioned and briefly illustrated. First, attention is given to dioxygenases and their potential to oxidize xenobiotics. Second, the role of lipid peroxidation is examined. And third, the dioxygenation of xenobiotics is shown to be a genuine if poorly documented metabolic pathway.

10.5.1 Reactions catalyzed by dioxygenases

Dioxygenases [EC 1.13.11] are an important group of enzymes which act by incorporating the two atoms of O_2 into the substrate oxidized (Naidu *et al.*, 1992). The primary products thus formed are usually quite reactive and rearrange enzymatically or chemically (postenzymatically) to stable compounds such as decyclized (ring-opened) metabolites. There is for example a genuine possibility that a mammalian enzyme such as the hemoprotein **tryptophan 2,3-dioxygenase** [L-tryptophan:oxygen 2,3-oxidoreductase (decyclizing); EC 1.13.11.11] could act on xenobiotic indolamines, but to the best of our knowledge this has not been investigated.

The N-demethylation of benzphetamine catalyzed by rabbit intestinal **indoleamine 2,3-dioxygenase** is also of potential interest. Indeed, this hemoprotein [indoleamine:oxygcn 2,3-oxidoreductase (indole-decyclizing); indoleamine-pyrrole 2,3-dioxygenase; EC 1.13.11.42] can demethylate benzphetamine by two mechanisms, i.e. as a monooxygenase (NADPH/O_2 dependence) or as a peroxygenase (H_2O_2 or organic hydroperoxide dependence) (Sun, 1989; Takikawa *et al.*, 1983). It is not known at present whether the reaction of N-demethylation is initiated by N-oxidation or by C-hydroxylation. The enzyme also catalyzes the *para*-hydroxylation of aniline in a reaction that requires both H_2O_2 and $O_2^{\bullet-}$, suggesting the involvement of a unique, unidentified oxygen species. This example indicates that a number of enzymes may well play as yet unrecognized roles in the metabolism of xenobiotics.

Lipoxygenases are a large family of non-heme, iron-containing dioxygenases, e.g. arachidonate 5-lipoxygenase [EC 1.13.11.34] and arachidonate 15-lipoxygenase [EC 1.13.11.33] (Schewe and Kühn, 1991). Their primary products are (*S*)-5- and (*S*)-15-hydroperoxyarachidonate, respectively, but these fairly reactive hydroperoxides are either rapidly reduced to the corresponding hydroxylated compounds or converted to secondary products such as keto and epoxyhydroxy compounds. During reduction of the hydroperoxide, lipoxygenases can mediate the cooxidation of xenobiotics, thereby demonstrating hydroperoxidase activity (Kulkarni and Cook, 1988). For example, **lipoxygenase** [linoleate:oxygen 13-oxidoreductase; lipoxidase; EC 1.13.11.12] in the presence of linoleic acid was very active in the epoxidation of the organochlorine insecticide aldrin to dieldrin (Naidu *et al.*, 1991).

Although the catalytic mechanisms must differ, if only because of the heme vs. non-heme nature of active sites, the hydroperoxidase reaction of lipoxygenases can be postulated to be comparable to that of cytochrome P450 (Fig. 10.1) and prostaglandin synthase (Fig. 10.4). In fact, the mechanism postulated for the epoxidation of aldrin is similar to that shown in Fig. 10.5 (Naidu *et al.*, 1991). Obviously much remains to be done to improve our understanding of the cooxidation of xenobiotics by lipoxygenases and its pharmacological significance.

10.5.2 Is there a role for lipid peroxidation in the metabolism of xenobiotics?

Lipid peroxidation is a manifold and complex phenomenon which in itself lies outside the scope of the present work. However, its pivotal position at the interface of endobiotic and xenobiotic metabolism calls for a brief introduction.

In strict terms, lipid peroxidation is a non-enzymatic or postenzymatic process by which highly reactive radicals (mainly the hydroxyl radical but also alkoxyl radicals or peroxyl radicals) abstract a hydrogen atom from unsaturated fatty acids present in membrane or free lipids and phospholipids (**initiation step**). The carbon-centred radical thus formed adds molecular oxygen to generate a fatty acid peroxyl radical ($ROO^\bullet$). This radical can either abstract a hydrogen atom from another lipid to give a fatty acid hydroperoxide and another peroxyl radical (**propagation step**), or decay to products of lipid peroxidation such as alkanes, aldehydes, ketones, and epoxyhydroxy compounds (Aikens and Dix, 1991; Buettner, 1993; Burton *et al.*, 1985; Chamulitrat *et al.*, 1991; Dix and Aikens, 1993; Iwahashi *et al.*, 1991; Ross, 1989; Wilcox and Marnett, 1993).

Alkoxyl radicals ($RO^\bullet$) acting as initiators of lipid peroxidation may be formed from hydroperoxides by the peroxidase activity of **cytochrome P450** (Section 10.2 and Fig. 10.1), **prostaglandin-endoperoxide synthase** (Section 10.3), or various **peroxidases** (Section 10.4) (Ohmori *et al.*, 1993; Sevanian *et al.*, 1990; Stelmaszynska *et al.*, 1992). Thus, cumene hydroperoxide-dependent lipid peroxidation may be catalyzed by cytochrome P450, which generates the cumyloxyl radical as the initiator (Weiss and Estabrook, 1986). Similarly, carbon tetrachloride is reduced by cytochrome P450 to the trichloromethyl radical (Section 12.3) which adds O_2, thereby generating a peroxyl radical which is a very potent initiator of lipid peroxidation (Battioni *et al.*, 1991). However, the more common origin of lipid peroxidation is now recognized as being the hydroxyl radical ($HO^\bullet$) (Dicker and Cederbaum, 1991; Kameda *et al.*, 1979).

In biological systems, the **hydroxyl radical** is not formed directly but as a product of decomposition of H_2O_2 and/or $O_2^{\bullet-}$ (Haber–Weiss and/or Fenton reactions, see Section 3.5). The Fenton reaction, which involves the transition metal-catalyzed breakdown of hydrogen peroxide to the hydroxyl radical, is of particular importance in initiating lipid peroxidation and explains the key role played by ferrous ions (Kameda *et al.*, 1979). As for H_2O_2 and $O_2^{\bullet-}$, they can be liberated during the catalytic cycle of various oxidoreductases (see sections 3.5, 9.2, 9.4 and 9.5), while $O_2^{\bullet-}$ is also a well-known product of O_2 reduction during the autoxidation of semiquinones and hydroquinones (Sections 7.6). Quinones such as menadione and quinonic cytostatic drugs (e.g. doxorubicinone and mitomycin C) are classical redox cycling agents, as is paraquat (Dicker and Cederbaum, 1991; Koster, 1991).

Lipid hydroperoxides can thus be formed as a result of xenobiotic metabolism (enzymatic or non-enzymatic). In addition, they may also be cofactors in xenobiotic oxidation by acting as oxygen donors in reactions catalyzed by the various peroxidases discussed above (see Section 10.3) (Reed, 1987). A single example serves to illustrate this phenomenon, namely that of benzo[*a*]pyrene-7,8-dihydrodiol (Dix and Marnett, 1983). In the presence of rat liver microsomes and under conditions favouring lipid peroxidation, this compound underwent epoxidation to yield the 9,10-epoxide (**10.XXXVII** in Fig. 10.14).

10.5.3 Reactions of dioxygenation

Dioxygenation means the transfer to a substrate molecule of the two atoms of O_2. This results in the formation of hydroperoxide or cyclic peroxide metabolites some of which may be fairly reactive and difficult to isolate and characterize.

6β-Hydroperoxyprogesterone (**10.LXXI**) appears to be a reasonably stable **hydroperoxide**. This compound was formed from progesterone or 5-pregnene-3,20-dione in the presence of rat liver microsomes, and is an intermediate in the formation of 6β-hydroxy- and 6-oxoprogesterone

10.LXXI   10.LXXII

(Tan *et al.*, 1982). The formation of steroid hydroperoxides may have physiological significance and suggests the possibility of analogous reactions in the metabolism of xenobiotic steroids.

Indirect evidence has also been presented that renal mitochondrial cytochrome P450 may act as a dioxygenase during the oxidation of 25-hydroxycholecalciferol (25-OH–D$_3$) (Warner, 1983). The 1-hydroperoxy-25-hydroxycholecalciferol thus formed was postulated to be the intermediate leading to the metabolites 1α,25-(OH)$_2$D$_3$ (reductive reaction) and 24,25-(OH)$_2$D$_3$ (peroxidase reaction).

One example of **cyclic peroxide** formation has been discussed in Section 10.4.2, namely the formation of a 9,10-dioxetane derivative (**10.XXXVI** in Fig. 10.14) during the myeloperoxidase-catalyzed oxidation of benzo[*a*]pyrene-7,8-dihydrodiol (Trush *et al.*, 1990). Another older but still interesting example is that of 7,10-dimethylbenz[*a*]anthracene, which was oxygenated by rat liver microsomes to the 7,12-epidioxide (**10.LXXII**) (Chen and Tu, 1976). This compound was reduced to the corresponding *cis*-7,12-dihydroxy compound, and also appeared able to bind covalently to cellular macromolecules. A few other cases of dioxygenation have been compiled by Marnett and Eling (1983).

In few if any of these examples of dioxygenation has a complete mechanistic picture been obtained. One likely general mechanism is the addition of O$_2$ to a C-centred radical formed by cytochrome P450 or another oxidase. Reactions of this type are depicted in Figs. 10.4, 10.6, 10.7, and 10.11. But whatever the mechanism(s) involved, the reactions of biooxidation and bio-oxygenation affecting both endogenous and exogenous substrates appear unendingly complex.

10.6 REFERENCES

Aikens J. and Dix T.A. (1991). Perhydroxyl radical (HOO•) initiated lipid peroxidation. The role of fatty acid hydroperoxides. *J. Biol. Chem.* **266**, 15,091–15,098.

Aragon C.M.G., Rogan F. and Amit Z. (1992). Ethanol metabolism in rat brain homogenates by a catalase-H$_2$O$_2$ system. *Biochem. Pharmacol.* **44**, 93–98.

Bäärnhielm C. and Hansson G. (1986). Oxidation of 1,4-dihydropyridines by prostaglandin synthase and the peroxidic function of cytochrome P-450. Demonstration of a free radical intermediate. *Biochem. Pharmacol.* **35**, 1419–1425.

Battioni J.P., Fontecave M., Jaouen M. and Mansuy D. (1991). Vitamin E derivatives as new potent inhibitors of microsomal lipid peroxidation. *Biochem. Biophys. Res. Commun.* **174**, 1103–1108.

Ben-Zvi Z., Weissman-Teitellman B., Katz S. and Danon A. (1990). Acetaminophen hepatotoxicity: is there a role for prostaglandin synthesis? *Arch. Toxicol.* **64**, 299–304.

Bhat R.V., Subrahmanyam V.V., Sadler A. and Ross D. (1988). Bioactivation of catechol in rat and human bone marrow cells. *Toxicol. Appl. Pharmacol.* **94**, 297–304.

Blake II R.C. and Coon M.J. (1980). On the mechanism of action of cytochrome P-450. Spectral intermediates in the reaction of P-450$_{LM2}$ with peroxy compounds. *J. Biol. Chem.* **255**, 4100–4111.

Blake II R.C. and Coon M.J. (1981a). On the mechanism of action of cytochrome P-450. Role of peroxy spectral intermediates in substrate hydroxylation. *J. Biol. Chem.* **256**, 5755–5763.

Blake II R.C. and Coon M.J. (1981b). On the mechanism of action of cytochrome P-450. Evaluation of homolytic and heterolytic mechanisms of oxygen–oxygen bond cleavage during substrate hydroxylation by peroxides. *J. Biol. Chem.* **256**, 12,127–12,133.

Boyd J.A. and Eling T.E. (1981). Prostaglandin endoperox-ide synthetase-dependent cooxidation of acetaminophen to intermediates which covalently bind *in vitro* to rabbit renal medullary microsomes. *J. Pharmacol. Exp. Therap.* **219**, 659–664.

Boyd J.A., Harvan D.J. and Eling T.E. (1983). The oxidation of 2-aminofluorene by prostaglandin endoperoxide synthetase. Comparison with other peroxidases. *J. Biol. Chem.* **258**, 8246–8254.

Brewster M.E., Doerge D.R., Huang M.J., Kaminski J.J., Pop E. and Bodor N. (1991). Application of semiempirical molecular orbital techniques to the study of peroxidase-mediated oxidation of phenols, anilines, sulphides and thiobenzamides. *Tetrahedron* **47**, 7525–7536.

Bruice T.C. (1991). Reactions of hydroperoxides with metallotetraphenylporphyrins in aqueous solutions. *Acc. Chem. Res.* **24**, 243–249.

Bruice T.C., Balasubramanian P.N., Lee R.W. and Lindsay Smith J.R. (1988). The mechanism of hydroperoxide O–O bond scission on reaction of hydroperoxides with iron(III) porphyrins. *J. Amer. Chem. Soc.* **110**, 7890–7892.

Buettner G.R. (1993). The pecking order of free radicals and antioxidants—Lipid peroxidation, α-tocopherol and ascorbate. *Arch. Biochem. Biophys.* **300**, 535–543.

Burton G.W., Foster D.O., Perly B., Slater T.F., Smith I.C.P. and Ingold K.U. (1985). Biological antioxidants. *Phil. Trans. Roy. Soc. London* **B 311**, 565–578.

Cals M.M., Mailliart P., Brignon G., Anglade P. and Dumas B.R. (1991). Primary structure of bovine lactoperoxidase, a fourth member of a mammalian heme peroxidase family. *Eur. J. Biochem.* **198**, 733–739.

Capdevila J., Estabrook R.W. and Prough R.A. (1980). Differences in the mechanism of NADPH- and cumene hydroperoxide-supported reactions of cytochrome P-450. *Arch. Biochem. Biophys.* **200**, 186–195.

Casella L., Gullotti M., Ghezzi R., Poli S., Beringhelli T., Colonna S. and Carrea G. (1992). Mechanism of enantioselective oxygenation of sulphides catalyzed by chloroperoxidase and horseradish peroxidase. Spectral studies and characterization of enzyme–substrate complexes. *Biochemistry* **31**, 9451–9459.

Castro C.E. (1980). Mechanisms of reaction of hemeproteins with oxygen and hydrogen peroxide in the oxidation of organic substrates. *Pharmacol. Therap.* **10**, 171–189.

Cavalieri E.L., Rogan E.G., Cremonesi P. and Devanesan P.D. (1988a). Radical cations as precursors in the metabolic formation of quinones from benzo[a]pyrene and 6-fluorobenzo[a]pyrene. *Biochem. Pharmacol.* **37**, 2173–2182.

Cavalieri E.L., Devanesan P.D. and Rogan E.G. (1988b). Radical cations in the horseradish peroxidase and prostaglandin H synthase mediated metabolism and binding of benzo[a]pyrene to deoxyribonucleic acid. *Biochem. Pharmacol.* **37**, 2183–2187.

Chamulitrat W., Hughes M.F., Eling T.E. and Mason R.P. (1991). Superoxide and peroxyl radical generation from the reduction of polyunsaturated fatty acid hydroperoxides by soybean lipoxygenase. *Arch. Biochem. Biophys.* **290**, 153–159.

Chen C. and Tu M.H. (1976). Transannular dioxygenation

of 9,10-dimethyl-1,2-benzanthracene by cytochrome P-450 oxygenase of rat liver. *Biochem. J.* **160**, 805–808.

Chignell C.F. (1985). Structure–activity relationships in the free-radical metabolism of xenobiotics. *Environm. Health Perspect.* **61**, 133–137.

Colonna S., Gaggero N., Manfredi A., Casella L., Gullotti M., Carrea G. and Pasta P. (1990). Enantioselective oxidations of sulfides catalyzed by chloroperoxidases. *Biochemistry* **29**, 10,465–10,468.

Cribb A.E., Miller M., Tesoro A. and Spielberg S.P. (1990). Peroxidase-dependent oxidation of sulfonamides by monocytes and neutrophils from humans and dogs. *Molec. Pharmacol.* **38**, 744–751.

d'Arcy Doherty M., Wilson I., Wardman P., Basra J., Patterson L.H. and Cohen G.M. (1986). Peroxidase activation of 1-naphthol to naphthoxy or naphthoxy-derived radicals and their reaction with glutathione. *Chem.-Biol. Interact.* **58**, 199–215.

Dawson J.H. (1988). Probing structure–function relations in heme-containing oxygenases and peroxidases. *Science* **240**, 433–439.

DeWitt D.L., El-Harith E.A., Kraemer S.A., Andrews M.J., Yao E.F., Armstrong R.L. and Smith W.L. (1990). The aspirin and heme-binding sites of ovine and murine prostaglandin endoperoxide synthases. *J. Biol. Chem.* **265**, 5192–5198.

Dicker E. and Cederbaum A.I. (1991). NADH-Dependent generation of reactive oxygen species by microsomes in the presence of iron and redox cycling agents. *Biochem. Pharmacol.* **42**, 529–535.

Dix T.A. and Aikens J. (1993). Mechanisms and biological relevance of lipid peroxidation initiation. *Chem. Res. Toxicol.* **6**, 2–18.

Dix T.A. and Marnett L.J. (1983). Metabolism of polycyclic aromatic hydrocarbon derivatives to ultimate carcinogens during lipid peroxidation. *Science* **221**, 77–79.

Doerge D.R. (1988). Hydroperoxide-dependent metabolism of goitrogenic thiocarbamides by lactoperoxidase. *Xenobiotica* **18**, 1291–1296.

Doerge D.R. and Corbett M.D. (1991). Peroxygenation mechanism for chloroperoxidase-catalyzed N-oxidation of arylamines. *Chem. Res. Toxicol.* **4**, 556–560.

Doerge D.R., Cooray N.M. and Brewster M.E. (1991). Peroxidase-catalyzed S-oxygenation: mechanism of oxygen transfer for lactoperoxidase. *Biochemistry* **30**, 8960–8964.

Doroshow J.H., Akman S., Chu F.F. and Esworthy S. (1990). Role of the glutathione–glutathione peroxidase cycle in the cytotoxicity of the anticancer quinones. *Pharmacol. Therap.* **47**, 359–370.

Duescher R.J. and Elfarra A.A. (1992). 1,3-Butadiene oxidation by human myeloperoxidase. Role of chloride ion in catalysis of divergent pathways. *J. Biol. Chem.* **267**, 19,859–19,865.

Duescher R.J. and Elfarra A.A. (1993). Chloroperoxidase-mediated oxidation of 1,3-butadiene to 3-butenal, a crotonaldehyde precursor. *Chem. Res. Toxicol.* **6**, 669–673.

Dugad L.B., Wang X., Wang C.C., Lukat G.S. and Goff H.M. (1992). Proton nuclear Overgauser effect study of the heme active site structure of chloroperoxidase. *Biochemistry* **31**, 1651–1655.

Eastmond D.A., Smith M.T., Ruzo L.O. and Ross D. (1986). Metabolic activation of phenol by human myeloperoxidase and horseradish peroxidase. *Molec. Pharmacol.* **30**, 674–679.

Egan R.W., Gale P.H., Baptista E.M., Kennicott K.L., VandenHeuvel W.J.A., Walker R.W., Fagerness P.E. and Kuehl F.A. Jr (1981). Oxidation reactions by prostaglandin cyclooxygenase-hydroperoxidase. *J. Biol. Chem.* **256**, 7352–7361.

Eling T.E. and Curtis J.F. (1992). Xenobiotic metabolism by prostaglandin H synthase. *Pharmacol. Therap.* **53**, 261–273.

Eling T., Boyd J., Reed G., Mason R. and Sivarajah K. (1983). Xenobiotic metabolism by prostaglandin endoperoxide synthetase. *Drug Metab. Rev.* **14**, 1023–1053.

Eling T.E., Boyd J.A., Ktrauss R.S. and Mason R.P. (1985a). Metabolism of aromatic amines by prostaglandin H synthetase. In *Biological Oxidation of Nitrogen in Organic Molecules* (eds Gorrod J.W. and Damani L.A.). pp. 313–319. Horwood, Chichester.

Eling T.E., Mason R.P. and Sivarajah K. (1985b). The formation of aminopyrine cation radical by the peroxidase activity of prostaglandin H synthase and subsequent reactions of the radical. *J. Biol. Chem.* **260**, 1601–1607.

Eling T.E., Thompson D.C., Foureman G.L., Curtis J.F. and Hughes M.F. (1990). Prostaglandin H synthase and xenobiotic oxidation. *Ann. Rev. Pharmacol. Toxicol.* **30**, 1–45.

Elmarakby S.A., Duffel M.W., Goswami A., Sariaslani F.S. and Rosazza J.P.N. (1989). *In vitro* metabolic transformations of vinblastine: oxidations catalyzed by peroxidase. *J. Med. Chem.* **32**, 674–679.

Estabrook R.W., Martin-Wixtrom C., Saeki Y., Renneberg R., Hildebrandt A. and Werringloer J. (1984). The peroxidatic function of liver microsomal cytochrome P-450: comparison of hydrogen peroxide and NADPH-catalysed N-demethylation reactions. *Xenobiotica* **14**, 87–104.

Favilla R., Giorani B. and Mazzini A. (1988). Fast kinetics analysis of the peroxidatic reaction catalysed by horse liver alcohol dehydrogenase. *Biochim. Biophys. Acta* **956**, 285–292.

Fischer V., Haar J.A., Greiner L., Lloyd R.V. and Mason R.P. (1991). Possible role or free radical formation in clozapine-induced agranulocytosis. *Molec. Pharmacol.* **40**, 846–853.

Floris R. and Wever R. (1992). Reaction of myeloperoxidase with its product HOCl. *Eur. J. Biochem.* **207**, 697–702.

Fujimoto S., Ishimitsu S., Hirayama S., Kawakami N. and Ohara A. (1991). Hydroxylation of phenylalanine by myeloperoxidase-hydrogen peroxide system. *Chem. Pharm. Bull.* **39**, 1598–1600.

Furst S.M. and Uetrecht J.P. (1993). Carbamazepine metabolism to a reactive intermediate by the myeloperoxidase system of activated neutrophils. *Biochem. Pharmacol.* **45**, 1267–1275.

Groves J.T. and Watanabe Y. (1988). Reactive iron porphyrin derivatives related to the catalytic cycles of cytochrome P-450 and peroxidase. Studies of the mechanism of oxygen activation. *J. Amer. Chem. Soc.* **110**, 8443–8452.

Harman L.S., Carver D.K., Schreiber J. and Mason R.P. (1986). One- and two-electron oxidation of reduced glutathione by peroxidases. *J. Biol. Chem.* **261**, 1642–1648.

Harris R.Z., Newmyer S.L. and Ortiz de Montellano P.R. (1993). Horseradish peroxidase-catalyzed 2-electron oxidations—oxidation of iodide, thioanisoles and phenols at distinct sites. *J. Biol. Chem.* **268**, 1637–1645.

Harvison P.J., Egan R.W., Gale P.H., Christian G.D., Hill B.S. and Nelson S.D. (1988). Acetaminophen and analogs as cosubstrates and inhibitors of prostaglandin H synthase. *Chem.-Biol. Interact.* **64**, 251–266.

Hayaishi O., Takikawa O. and Yoshida R. (1990). Indoleamine 2,3-dioxygenase: properties and functions of a superoxide utilizing enzyme. *Prog. Inorg. Chem.* **38**, 75–95.

Hlavica P. and Kuenzel-Mulas U. (1993). Metabolic N-oxide formation by rabbit-liver microsomal cytochrome P-4502B4: involvement of superoxide in the NADPH-dependent N-oxygenation of N,N-dimethylaniline. *Biochim. Biophys. Acta* **1158**, 83–90.

Hollenberg P.F. (1992). Mechanisms of cytochrome P450 and peroxidase-catalyzed xenobiotic metabolism. *FASEB J.* **6**, 686–694.

Hollenberg P.F., Miwa G.T., Walsh J.S., Dwyer L.A., Rickert D.E. and Ketteris G.L. (1985). Mechanisms of N-demethylation reactions catalyzed by cytochrome P-450 and peroxidases. *Drug Metab. Disposit.* **13**, 272–275.

Hu S. and Kincaid J.R. (1991). Resonance Raman structural characterization and the mechanism of formation of lactoperoxidase Compound III. *J. Amer. Chem. Soc.* **113**, 7189–7194.

Hu S.Z. and Kincaid J.R. (1993). Heme active-site structural characterization of chloroperoxidase by resonance Raman spectroscopy. *J. Biol. Chem.* **268**, 6189–6193.

Hughes M.F., Mason R.P. and Eling T.E. (1988). Prostaglandin hydroperoxide-dependent oxidation of phenylbutazone: relationship to inhibition of prostaglandin cyclooxygenase. *Molec. Pharmacol.* **34**, 186–193.

Hughes M.F., Smith B.L. and Eling T.E. (1992). The oxidation of 4-aminobiphenyl by horseradish peroxidase. *Chem. Res. Toxicol.* **5**, 340–345.

Ichihara S., Tomisawa H., Fukazawa H., Tateishi M., Joly R. and Heintz R. (1989). Oxidation of tenoxicam by leukocyte peroxidases and H_2O_2 produces novel products. *Drug Metab. Disposit.* **17**, 463–468.

Ignesti G., Banchelli M.G., Pirisino R., Raimondi L. and Buffoni F. (1983). Catalytic properties of serum albumin. *Pharmacol. Res. Commun.* **15**, 569–579.

Iwahashi H., Albro P.W., McGown S.R., Tomer K.B. and Mason R.P. (1991). Isolation and identification of α-(4-

pyridyl-1-oxide)-N-*tert*-butylnitrone radical adducts formed by the decomposition of the hydroperoxides of linoleic acid, linolenic acid, and arachidonic acid by soybean lipoxygenase. *Arch. Biochem. Biophys.* **285**, 172–180.

Jönsson K.H. and Lindeke B. (1990). Cytochrome P-455 nm complex formation in the metabolism of phenylalkylamines. XI. Peroxygenase versus monooxygenase function of cytochrome P-450 in rat liver microsomes. *Chem.-Biol. Interact.* **75**, 276–279.

Josephy P.D. (1986). Benzidine: mechanisms of oxidative activation and mutagenesis. *Fed. Proc.* **45**, 2465–2470.

Kalyanaraman B., Sealy R.C. and Siwarajah K. (1984). An electron spin resonance study of *o*-semiquinone formed during the enzymatic and autoxidation of catechol estrogens. *J. Biol. Chem.* **259**, 14,018–14,022.

Kameda K., Ono T. and Imai Y. (1979). Participation of superoxide, hydrogen peroxide and hydroxyl radicals in NADPH-cytochrome P-450 reductase-catalyzed peroxidation of methyl linolenate. *Biochim. Biophys. Acta* **572**, 77–82.

Kanofsky J.R., Hoogland H., Wever R. and Weiss S.J. (1988). Singlet oxygen production by human eosinophils. *J. Biol. Chem.* **263**, 9692–9696.

Kelder P.P., Fischer M.J.E., de Mol N.J. and Janssen L.H.M. (1991a). Oxidation of chlorpromazine by methemoglobin in the presence of hydrogen peroxide. Formation of chlorpromazine radical cation and its covalent binding to methemoglobin. *Arch. Biochem. Biophys.* **284**, 313–319.

Kelder P.P., de Mol N.J. and Janssen L.H.M. (1991b). Mechanistic aspects of the oxidation of phenothiazine derivatives by methemoglobin in the presence of hydrogen peroxide. *Biochem. Pharmacol.* **42**, 1551–1559.

Kettle A.J. and Winterbourn C.C. (1991). Mechanism of inhibition of myeloperoxidase by anti-inflammatory drugs. *Biochem. Pharmacol.* **41**, 1485–1492.

Kettle A.J. and Winterbourn C.C. (1992). Oxidation of hydroquinone by myeloperoxidase. Mechanism of stimulation by benzoquinone. *J. Biol. Chem.* **267**, 8319–8324.

Kettle A.J., Gedye C.A. and Winterbourn C.C. (1993). Superoxide is an antagonist of anti-inflammatory drugs that inhibit hypochlorous acid production by myeloperoxidase. *Biochem. Pharmacol.* **45**, 2003–2010.

Koop D.R. and Hollenberg P.F. (1980). Kinetics of the hydroperoxide-dependent dealkylation reactions catalyzed by rabbit liver microsomal cytochrome P-450. *J. Biol. Chem.* **255**, 9685–9692.

Koster A.S. (1991). Bioreductive activation of quinones: a mixed blessing. *Pharm. Weekbl. Sci. Ed.* **13**, 123–126.

Kubow S. and Wells P.G. (1989). *In vitro* bioactivation of phenytoin to a reactive free radical intermediate by prostaglandin synthetase, horseradish peroxidase, and thyroid peroxidase. *Molec. Pharmacol.* **35**, 504–511.

Kulkarni A.P. and Cook D.C. (1988). Hydroperoxysase activity of lipoxygenase: a potential pathway for xenobiotic metabolism in the presence of linoleic acid. *Res. Commun. Chem. Pathol. Pharmacol.* **61**, 305–314.

Kulmacz R.J. (1989). Topography of prostaglandin H synthase. *J. Biol. Chem.* **264**, 14,136–14,144.

Lagorce J.F., Thomes J.C., Catanzano G., Buxeraud J., Raby M. and Raby C. (1991). Formation of molecular iodine during oxidation of iodide by the peroxidase/ H_2O_2 system. *Biochem. Pharmacol.* **42**, S89–S92.

Lakshmi V.M., Zenser T.V., Mattammal M.B. and Davis B.B. (1993). Phenylbutazone peroxidatic metabolism and conjugation. *J. Pharmacol. Exp. Therap.* **266**, 81–88.

La Mar G.N., Hernández G. and de Ropp J.S. (1992). ^{1}H NMR investigation of the influence of interacting sites on the dynamics and thermodynamics of substrate and ligand binding to horseradish peroxidase. *Biochemistry* **31**, 9158–9168.

Larroque C., Lange R., Maurin L., Bienvenue A. and van Lier J.E. (1990). On the nature of the cytochrome P450scc "ultimate oxidant": Characterization of a productive radical intermediate. *Arch. Biochem. Biophys.* **282**, 198–201.

Larsson R., Ross D., Berlin T., Olsson L.I. and Moldéus P. (1985). Prostaglandin synthase catalyzed metabolic activation of *p*-phenetidine and acetaminophen by microsomes isolated from rabbit and human kidney. *J. Pharmacol. Exp. Therap.* **235**, 475–480.

Lasker J.M., Sivarajah K., Mason R.P., Kalyanaraman B., Abou-Donia M.H. and Eling T.E. (1981). A free radical mechanism of prostaglandin synthase-dependent aminopyrine demethylation. *J. Biol. Chem.* **256**, 7764–7767.

Lau S.S. and Monks T.J. (1987). Co-oxidation of 2-bromohydroquinone by renal prostaglandin synthase. *Drug Metab. Disposit.* **15**, 801–807.

Lee E., Miki Y., Hosokawa M., Sayo H. and Kariya K. (1988). Oxidative metabolism of propylthiouracil by peroxidases from rat bone marrow. *Xenobiotica* **18**, 1135–1142.

Lehmann F.M., Bretz N., von Bruchhausen F. and Wurm G. (1989). Substrates for arachidonic acid co-oxidation with peroxidase/hydrogen peroxide. *Biochem. Pharmacol.* **38**, 1209–1216.

Leoncini G., Maresca M. and Colao C. (1991). Oxidative metabolism of human platelets. *Biochem. Intern.* **25**, 647–655.

Lindquist T., Hillver S.E., Lindeke B., Moldéus P., Ross D. and Larsson R. (1985). On the chemistry of the peroxidative oxidation of *p*-phenetidine. In *Biological Oxidation of Nitrogen in Organic Molecules* (eds Gorrod J.W. and Damani L.A.). pp. 350–354. Horwood, Chichester.

Maggs J.L., Tingle M.D., Kitteringham N.R. and Park B.K. (1988). Drug-protein conjugates—XIV. Mechanisms of formation of protein arylating intermediates from amodiaquine, a myelotoxin and hepatotoxin in man. *Biochem. Pharmacol.* **37**, 303–311.

Mahy J.P., Gaspard S. and Mansuy D. (1993). Phenylhydrazones as new good substrates for the dioxygenase and peroxidase reactions of prostaglandin synthase: Formation of iron(III)-σ-phenyl complexes. *Biochemistry* **32**, 4012–4021.

Marker E.K. and Kulkarni A.P. (1986). Cumene

hydroperoxide-supported denitrification of 2-nitro-propane in uninduced mouse liver microsomes. *Int. J. Biochem.* **18**, 595–601.

Markey C.M., Alward A., Weller P.E. and Marnett L.J. (1987). Quantitative studies of hydroperoxide reduction by prostaglandin H synthase. Reducing substrate specificity and the relationship of peroxidase to cyclooxygenase activities. *J. Biol. Chem.* **262**, 6266–6279.

Marnett L.J. (1981). Polycyclic aromatic hydrocarbon oxidation during prostaglandin biosynthesis. *Life Sci.* **29**, 531–546.

Marnett L.J. (1983). Cooxidation during prostaglandin biosynthesis: A pathway for the metabolic activation of xenobiotics. In *Reviews in Biochemical Toxicology*, Vol. 5 (eds Hodgson E., Bend J.R. and Philpot R.M.). pp. 135–172. Elsevier Biomedical, New York.

Marnett L.J., Wlodawer P. and Samuelsson B. (1975). Cooxygenation of organic substrates by the prostaglandin synthetase of sheep vesicular gland. *J. Biol. Chem.* **250**, 8510–8517.

Marnett L.J., Pan Chen Y.N., Maddipati K.R., Plé P. and Labèque R. (1988). Functional differentiation of cyclooxygenase and peroxidase activities of prostaglandin synthase by trypsin treatment. *J. Biol. Chem.* **263**, 16,532–16,535.

Marquez L.A. and Dunford H.B. (1993). Interaction of acetaminophen with myeloperoxidase intermediates: optimum stimulation of enzyme activity. *Arch. Biochem. Biophys.* **305**, 414–420.

Marshall P.J. and Kulmacz R.J. (1988). Prostaglandin H synthase: distinct binding sites for cyclooxygenase and peroxidase substrates. *Arch. Biochem. Biophys.* **266**, 162–170.

Mason R.P. and Fischer V. (1986). Free radicals of acetaminophen: their subsequent reactions and toxicological significance. *Fed. Proc.* **45**, 2493–2499.

Mason R.P. and Rao D.N.R. (1990). Thiyl free radical metabolites of thiol drugs, glutathione, and proteins. *Methods Enzymol.* **186**, 318–329.

Masumoto H., Ohta S. and Hirobe M. (1991). Application of chemical cytochrome P-450 model systems to studies on drug metabolism. *Drug Metab. Disposit.* **19**, 768–780.

Mattammal M.B., Lakshmi V.M., Zenser T.V. and Davis B.B. (1987). Lung prostaglandin H synthase and mixed-function oxidase metabolism of nicotine. *J. Pharmacol. Exp. Therap.* **242**, 827–832.

McCarthy M.B. and White R.E. (1983a). Functional differences between peroxidase compound I and the cytochrome P-450 reactive oxygen intermediate. *J. Biol. Chem.* **258**, 9153–9158.

McCarthy M.B. and White R.E. (1983b). Competing modes of peroxyacid flux through cytochrome P-450. *J. Biol. Chem.* **258**, 11,610–11,616.

Metodiewa D. and Dunford H.B. (1990). The role of myeloperoxidase in the oxidation of biologically active polyhydroxyphenols (substituted catechols). *Eur. J. Biochem.* **193**, 445–448.

Metodiewa D. and Dunford H.B. (1991). On the ability of lactoperoxidase to catalyze the peroxidase-oxidase oxida-tion of a vitamin E water-soluble derivative (Trolox C). *Biochem. Intern.* **25**, 895–904.

Metodiewa D., Reszka K. and Dunford H.B. (1989). Oxidation of the substituted catechols dihydroxyphenylalanine methyl ester and trihydroxyphenylalanine by lactoperoxidase and its compounds. *Arch. Biochem. Biophys.* **274**, 601–608.

Metzler M. and Haaf H. (1985). Dearylation and other cleavage reactions of diethylstilbestrol: novel oxidative pathways mediated by peroxidases. *Xenobiotica* **15**, 41–49.

Modi S., Behere D.V. and Mitra S. (1991). Horseradish peroxidase catalyzed oxidation of thiocyanate by hydrogen peroxide: comparison with lactoperoxidase-catalyzed oxidation and role of distal histidine. *Biochim. Biophys. Acta* **1080**, 45–50.

Mohr P., Kühn M., Wesuls E., Renneberg R. and Scheller F. (1979). Comparison of the peroxidatic activity of cytochrome P-450 with other hemoproteins and model compounds. *Acta Biol. Med. Germ.* **38**, 495–501.

Moldéus P., Larsson R., Ross D. and Andersson B. (1984). Peroxidase-catalysed metabolism of drugs and carcinogens. *Biochem. Soc. Transact.* **12**, 20–23.

Moldéus P., Ross D. and Larsson R. (1985). Cooxidation of xenobiotics. *Biochem. Soc. Transact.* **13**, 847–850.

Mottley C., Mason R.P., Chignell C.F., Sivarajah K. and Eling T.E. (1982). The formation of sulfur trioxide radical anion during the prostaglandin hydroperoxidase-catalyzed oxidation of bisulfite (hydrated sulfur dioxide). *J. Biol. Chem.* **257**, 5050–5055.

Mottley C., Toy K. and Mason R.P. (1987). Oxidation of thiol drugs and biochemicals by the lactoperoxidase/hydrogen peroxide system. *Molec. Pharmacol.* **31**, 417–421.

Nagasawa H.T., DeMaster E.G., Redfern B., Shirota F.N. and Goon D.J.W. (1990). Evidence for nitroxyl in the catalase-mediated bioactivation of the alcohol deterrent agent cyanamide. *J. Med. Chem.* **33**, 3120–3122.

Naidu A.K., Naidu A.K. and Kulkarni A.P. (1991). Aldrin epoxidation. Catalytic potential of lipoxygenase coupled with linoleic acid oxidation. *Drug Metab. Disposit.* **19**, 758–763.

Naidu A.K., Naidu A.K. and Kulkarni A.P. (1992) Dioxygenase and hydroperoxidase activities of rat brain cytosolic lipoxygenase. *Res. Commun. Chem. Pathol. Pharmacol.* **75**, 347–356.

Nelson S.D., Dahlin D.C., Rauckman E.J. and Rosen G.M. (1981). Peroxidase-mediated formation of reactive metabolites of acetaminophen. *Molec. Pharmacol.* **20**, 195–199.

Nordblom G.D., White R.E. and Coon M.J. (1976). Studies on hydroperoxide-dependent substrate hydroxylation by purified liver microsomal cytochrome P-450. *Arch. Biochem. Biophys.* **175**, 524–533.

O'Brien P.J., Forbes S. and Slaughter D. (1985). Peroxidase versus cytochrome P-450 catalysed N-demethylation of N,N-dimethylaniline. In *Biological Oxidation of Nitrogen in Organic Molecules* (eds Gorrod J.W. and Damani L.A.). pp. 344–349. Horwood, Chichester.

O'Brien P.J., Zhu O. and Khan, S. (1991). Drug metabolism by activated neutrophils and eosinophils. *Acta Pharm. Nord.* **3**, 119–120.

Ohmori S., Misaizu T., Nakamura T., Takano N., Kitagawa H. and Kitada M. (1993). Differential role in lipid peroxidation between rat P450 1A1 and P450 1A2. *Biochem. Pharmacol.* **46**, 55–60.

Ortiz de Montellano P.R. (1987). Control of the catalytic activity of prosthetic heme by the structure of hemoproteins. *Acc. Chem. Res.* **20**, 289–294.

Ortiz de Montellano P.R. (1992). Catalytic sites of hemoprotein peroxidases. *Annu. Rev. Pharmacol. Toxicol.* **32**, 89–107.

Ortiz de Montellano P.R. and Grab L.A. (1986). Cooxidation of styrene by horseradish peroxidase and glutathione. *Molec. Pharmacol.* **30**, 666–669.

Ortiz de Montellano P.R. and Grab L.A. (1987). Cooxidation of styrene by horseradish peroxidase and phenols: a biochemical model for protein-mediated cooxidation. *Biochemistry* **26**, 5310–5314.

Ortiz de Montellano P.R., Choe Y.S., DePillis G. and Catalano C.E. (1987). Structure–mechanism relationships in hemoproteins. Oxygenations catalyzed by chloroperoxidase and horseradish peroxidase. *J. Biol. Chem.* **262**, 11,641–11,646.

Otton S.V., Gillam E.M.J., Lennard M.S., Tucker G.T. and Woods H.F. (1990). Propranolol oxidation by human liver microsomes—the use of cumene hydroperoxide to probe isoenzyme specificity and regio- and stereoselectivity. *Brit. J. Clin. Pharmacol.* **30**, 751–760.

Potter D.W. and Hinson J.A. (1987a). Mechanisms of acetaminophen oxidation to N-acetyl-p-benzoquinone imine by horseradish peroxidase and cytochrome P-450. *J. Biol. Chem.* **262**, 966–973.

Potter D.W. and Hinson J.A. (1987b). The 1- and 2-electron oxidation of acetaminophen catalyzed by prostaglandin H synthase. *J. Biol. Chem.* **262**, 974–980.

Rahimtula A.D. and O'Brien P.J. (1977a). The peroxidase nature of cytochrome P450. In *Microsomes and Drug Oxidations* (eds Ullrich V., Roots I., Hildebrandt A., Estabrook R.W. and Conney A.H.). pp. 210–217. Pergamon Press, Oxford.

Rahimtula A.D. and O'Brien P.J. (1977b). The role of cytochrome P-450 in the hydroperoxide-catalyzed oxidation of alcohols by rat-liver microsomes. *Eur. J. Biochem.* **77**, 201–208.

Rahimtula A.D., O'Brien P.J., Seifried H.E. and Jerina D.M. (1978). The mechanism of action of cytochrome P-450. Occurrence of the "NIH shift" during hydroperoxide-dependent aromatic hydroxylations. *Eur. J. Biochem.* **89**, 133–141.

Ramos C.L., Pou S., Britigan B.E., Cohen M.S. and Rosen G.M. (1992). Spin trapping evidence for myeloperoxidase-dependent hydroxyl radical formation by human neutrophils and monocytes. *J. Biol. Chem.* **267**, 8307–8312.

Rao D.N.R., Fischer V. and Mason R.P. (1990). Glutathione and ascorbate reduction of the acetaminophen radical formed by peroxidase. *J. Biol. Chem.* **265**, 844–847.

Reed G.A. (1987). Co-oxidation of xenobiotics: lipid peroxyl derivatives as mediators of metabolism. *Chem. Phys. Lipids* **44**, 127–148.

Reed G.A. and Marnett L.J. (1982). Metabolism and activation of 7,8-dihydrobenzo[a]pyrene during prostaglandin biosynthesis. Intermediacy of a bay-region epoxide. *J. Biol. Chem.* **257**, 11,368–11,376.

Reed G.A., Brooks E.A. and Eling T.E. (1984). Phenylbutazone-dependent epoxidation of 7,8-dihydroxy-7,8-dihydrobenzo[a]pyrene. A new mechanism for prostaglandin H synthase-catalyzed oxidations. *J. Biol. Chem.* **259**, 5591–5595.

Roberts P., Kitteringham N.R. and Park B.K. (1993). Elucidation of the structural requirements for the bioactivation of mianserin *in vitro. J. Pharm. Pharmacol.* **45**, 663–665.

Ross D. (1989). Mechanistic toxicology: a radical perspective. *J. Pharm. Pharmacol.* **41**, 505–511.

Ross D., Larsson R., Norbeck K., Ryhage R. and Moldéus P. (1985). Characterization and mechanism of formation of reactive products formed during peroxidase-catalyzed oxidation of p-phenetidine. *Molec. Pharmacol.* **27**, 277–286.

Sadler A., Subrahmanyam V.V. and Ross D. (1988). Oxidation of catechol by horseradish peroxidase and human leukocyte peroxidase: reactions of o-benzoquinone and o-benzosemiquinone. *Toxicol. Appl. Pharmacol.* **93**, 62–71.

Samokyszyn V.M. (1993). Oxidation of retinoic acid by prostaglandin H synthase. In *ISSX Proceedings*, Vol. 4. International Society for the Study of Xenobiotics, Bethesda, MD, USA, p. 134.

Samokyszyn V.M. and Marnett L.J. (1987). Hydroperoxide-dependent cooxidation of 13-cis-retinoic acid by prostaglandin H synthase. *J. Biol. Chem.* **262**, 14,119–14,133.

Samokyszyn V.M. and Ortiz de Montellano P.R. (1991). Topology of the chloroperoxidase active site: Regiospecificity of heme modification by phenylhydrazine and sodium azide. *Biochemistry* **30**, 11,646–11,653.

Sa Silva Morais M. and Augusto O. (1993). Peroxidation of the antimalarial drug primaquine: characterization of a benzidine-like metabolite with methaemoglobin-forming activity. *Xenobiotica* **23**, 133–139.

Sayo H. and Hosokawa M. (1980). Free radical intermediate in the N-demethylation of aminopyrine by catalase-cumene hydroperoxide system. *Chem. Pharm. Bull.* **28**, 683–685.

Sayo H. and Hosokawa M. (1985). Cumene hydroperoxide-supported N-demethylation of N,N-dimethylanilines catalyzed by catalase. *Chem. Pharm. Bull.* **33**, 4471–4477.

Sayo H. and Saito M. (1990). The mechanism of myeloperoxidase-catalysed oxidation of aminopyrine. *Xenobiotica* **20**, 957–965.

Sayo H. and Saito M. (1991). Hydrogen peroxide-dependent oxidative metabolism of 1-methyl-2-mercaptoimidazole (methimazole) catalysed by myeloperoxidase. *Xenobiotica* **21**, 1217–1224.

Schewe T. and Kühn H. (1991). Do 15-lipoxygenases have

a common biological role? *Trends Biochem. Sci.* **16**, 369–373.

Schlosser M.J. and Kalf G.F. (1989). Metabolic activation of hydroquinone by macrophage peroxidase. *Chem.-Biol. Interact.* **72**, 191–207.

Schlosser M.J., Shurina R.D. and Kalf G.F. (1990). Prostaglandin H synthase catalyzed oxidation of hydroquinone to a sufhydryl-binding and DNA-damaging metabolite. *Chem. Res. Toxicol.* **3**, 333–339.

Sevanian A., Nordenbrand K., Kim E., Ernster L. and Hochstein P. (1990). Microsomal lipid peroxidation: the role of NADPH-cytochrome P450 reductase and cytochrome P450. *Free Rad. Biol. Med.* **8**, 145–152.

Shacter E., Lopez R.L. and Pati S. (1991). Inhibition of the myeloperoxidase-H$_2$O$_2$-chloride system of neutrophils by indomethacin and other non-steroidal anti-inflammatory drugs. *Biochem. Pharmacol.* **41**, 975–984.

Shinohara A., Kamataki T., Iizuka T., Ishimura Y., Ogoshi H., Okuda K. and Kato R. (1987). Drug oxidation activities of horseradish peroxidase, myoglobin and cytochrome P-450$_{cam}$ reconstituted with synthetic hemes. *Jap. J. Pharmacol.* **45**, 107–114.

Sivarajah K., Lasker J.M., Eling T.E. and Abou-Donia M.B. (1982). Metabolism of N-alkyl compounds during the biosynthesis of prostaglandins. *Molec. Pharmacol.* **21**, 133–141.

Smart R.C. and Zannoni V.G. (1984). DT-Diaphorase and peroxidase influence the covalent binding of the metabolites of phenol, the major metabolite of benzene. *Molec. Pharmacol.* **26**, 105–111.

Smith B.J., Curtis J.F. and Eling T.E. (1991). Bioactivation of xenobiotics by prostaglandin H synthase. *Chem.-Biol. Interact.* **79**, 245–264.

Smith W.L., Eling T.E., Kulmacz R.J., Marnett L.J. and Tsai A.L. (1992). Tyrosyl radicals and their role in hydroperoxide-dependent activation and inactivation of prostaglandin endoperoxide synthase. *Biochemistry* **31**, 3–7.

Song W.C. and Brash A.R. (1991). Purification of an allene oxide synthase and identification of the enzyme as a cytochrome P-450. *Science* **253**, 781–784.

Stadtman T.C. (1991). Biosynthesis and function of selenocysteine-containing enzymes. *J. Biol. Chem.* **266**, 16,257–16,260.

Stelmaszynska T., Kukovetz E., Egger G. and Schaur R.J. (1992). Possible involvement of myeloperoxidase in lipid peroxidation. *Intern. J. Biochem.* **24**, 121–128.

Stock B.H., Schreiber J., Guenat C., Mason R.P., Bend J.R. and Eling T.E. (1986). Evidence for a free radical mechanism of styrene-glutathione conjugate formation catalyzed by prostaglandin H synthase and horseradish peroxidase. *J. Biol. Chem.* **261**, 15,915–15,922.

Suda I. and Takahashi H. (1992). Degradation of methyl and ethyl mercury into inorganic mercury by other reactive oxygen species besides hydroxyl radical. *Arch. Toxicol.* **66**, 34–39.

Sun Y. (1989). Indoleamine 2,3-dioxygenase—a new antioxidant enzyme. *Mater. Med. Pol. (Engl. Ed.)* **21**, 244–250.

Tajima K., Hashizaki M., Yamamoto K. and Mizutani T.

(1992). Metabolism of 3-tert-butyl-4-hydroxyanisole by horseradish peroxidase and hydrogen peroxide. *Drug Metab. Disposit.* **20**, 816–820.

Takikawa O., Yoshida R. and Hayaishi O. (1983). Monooxygenase activities of dioxygenases. Benzphetamine demethylation and aniline hydroxylation reactions catalyzed by indoleamine 2,3-dioxygenase. *J. Biol. Chem.* **258**, 6808–6815.

Tan L., Rao A.J. and Yu P.H. (1982). Formation of 6β-hydroperoxyprogesterone in rat liver microsomes. *J. Steroid. Biochem.* **17**, 89–94.

Thompson J.A. and Yumibe N.P. (1989). Mechanistic aspects of cytochrome P-450-hydroperoxide interactions: substituent effects on degradative pathways. *Drug Metab. Rev.* **20**, 365–378.

Thompson D.C. and Eling T.E. (1991). Reactive intermediates formed during the peroxidative oxidation of anisidine isomers. *Chem. Res. Toxicol.* **4**, 474–481.

Thompson D.C., Cha Y.N. and Trush M.A. (1989). The peroxidase-dependent activation of butylated hydroxyanisole and butylated hydroxytoluene to reactive intermediates. *J. Biol. Chem.* **264**, 357–3965.

Thurman R.G. and Handler J.A. (1989). New perspectives in catalase-dependent ethanol metabolism. *Drug Metab. Rev.* **20**, 679–688.

Traylor T.G. and Xu F. (1990). Mechanisms of reactions of iron(III) porphyrins with hydrogen peroxide and hydroperoxides: solvent and solvent isotope effects. *J. Amer. Chem. Soc.* **112**, 178–186.

Traylor T.G., Fann W.P. and Bandyopadhyay D. (1989). A common heterolytic mechanism for reactions of iodosobenzenes, peracids, hydroperoxides and hydrogen peroxide with iron(III) porphyrins. *J. Amer. Chem. Soc.* **111**, 8009–8010.

Trush M.A., Twerdok L.E. and Esterline R.L. (1990). Comparison of oxidant activities and the activation of benzo[*a*]pyrene-7,8-dihydrodiol by polymorphonuclear leucocytes from human, rat and mouse. *Xenobiotica* **20**, 925–932.

Uetrecht J.P. (1990). Drug metabolism by leukocytes and its role in drug-induced lupus and other idiosyncratic drug reactions. *Crit. Rev. Toxicol.* **20**, 213–235.

Uetrecht J.P. (1992). The role of leukocyte-generated reactive metabolites in the pathogenesis of idiosyncratic drug reactions. *Drug Metab. Rev.* **24**, 299–366.

Uetrecht J.P. and Zahid N. (1991). N-Chlorination and oxidation of procainamide by myeloperoxidase: toxicological implications. *Chem. Res. Toxicol.* **4**, 218–222.

Uetrecht J.P. and Sokoluk B. (1992). Comparative metabolism and covalent binding of procainamide by human leukocytes. *Drug Metab. Disposit.* **20**, 120–123.

Uetrecht J.P., Shear N.H. and Zahid N. (1993). N-Chlorination of sulfamethoxazole and dapsone by the myeloperoxidase system. *Drug Metab. Disposit.* **21**, 830–834.

Van der Zee J., Duling D.R., Mason R.P. and Eling T.E. (1989). The oxidation of N-substituted aromatic amines by horseradish peroxidase. *J. Biol. Chem.* **264**, 19,828–19,836.

van Zyl J.M., Basson K., Kriegler A. and van der Walt B.J.

(1991). Mechanisms by which clofazimine and dapsone inhibit the myeloperoxidase system. A possible correlation with their anti-inflammatory properties. *Biochem. Pharmacol.* **42**, 599–608.

van Zyl J.M., Basson K., Kriegler A. and van der Walt B.J. (1990). Activation of chlorpromazine by the myeloperoxidase system of the human neutrophil. *Biochem. Pharmacol.* **40**, 947–954.

Vasquez A., Tudela J., Varon R. and Garcia-Canovas F. (1992). A kinetic study of the generation and decomposition of some phenothiazine free radicals formed during enzymatic oxidation of phenothiazines by peroxidase-hydrogen peroxide. *Biochem. Pharmacol.* **44**, 889–894.

Waldhauser L. and Uetrecht J. (1991). Oxidation of propylthiouracyl to reactive metabolites by activated neutrophils. *Drug Metab. Disposit.* **19**, 354–359.

Wand M.D. and Thompson J.A. (1986). Cytochrome P-450-catalyzed rearrangement of a peroxyquinol derived from butylated hydroxytoluene. Involvement of radical and cationic intermediates. *J. Biol. Chem.* **261**, 14,049–14,057.

Warner M. (1983). 25-Hydroxyvitamin D hydroxylation. Evidence for a dioxygenase activity of solubilized renal mitochondrial cytochrome P-450. *J. Biol. Chem.* **258**, 11,590–11,593.

Weiss R.H. and Estabrook R.W. (1986). The mechanism of cumene hydroperoxide-dependent lipid peroxidation: the function of cytochrome P-450. *Arch. Biochem. Biophys.* **251**, 348–360.

Weiss S.J. (1991). Oxidative regulation of inflammatory proteases. *Acta Pharm. Nord.* **3**, 120.

Weiss S.J., Test S.T., Eckmann C.M., Ross D. and Regiani S. (1986). Brominating oxidants generated by human eosinophils. *Science* **234**, 200–203.

Weli A.M. and Lindeke B. (1986). Peroxidative N-oxidation and N-dealkylation reactions of pargyline. *Xenobiotica* **16**, 281–288.

Weller P.E., Markey C.M. and Marnett L.J. (1985). Enzymatic reduction of 5-phenyl-4-pentenyl-hydroperoxide: Detection of peroxidases and identification of peroxidase reducing substrates. *Arch. Biochem. Biophys.*

243, 633–643.

Wendel A. (1980). Glutathione peroxidase. In *Enzymatic Basis of Detoxication*, Volume 1 (ed. Jakoby W.B.). pp. 333–353. Academic Press, New York.

Wheeler E.L. (1983). Cytochrome P-450 mediated interaction between hydroperoxide and molecular oxygen. *Biochem. Biophys. Res. Commun.* **110**, 646–653.

White R.E., Sligar S.G. and Coon M.J. (1980). Evidence for a homolytic mechanism of peroxide oxygen–oxygen bond cleavage during substrate hydroxylation by cytochrome P-450. *J. Biol. Chem.* **255**, 11,108–11,111.

Wilcox A.L. and Marnett L.J. (1993). Polyunsaturated fatty acid alkoxyl radicals exist as carbon-centred epoxy-allylic radicals: a key step in hydroxyperoxide-amplified lipid peroxidation. *Chem. Res. Toxicol.*

Woolf T.F., Black A. and Chang T. (1989a). *In vitro* metabolism of isoxicam by horseradish peroxidase. *Xenobiotica* **19**, 1369–1377.

Woolf T.F., Black A., Hicks J.L., Lee H., Huang C.C. and Chang T. (1989b). *In vivo* metabolism of isoxicam in rats, dogs and monkeys. *Drug Metab. Disposit.* **17**, 662–668.

Woolf T.F., Black A., Sedman A. and Chang T. (1992). Metabolic disposition of the non-steroidal anti-inflammatory agent isoxicam in man. *Eur. J. Drug. Metab. Pharmacokin.* **17**, 21–27.

Yumibe N.P. and Thompson J.A. (1988). Fate of free radicals generated during one-electron reductions of 4-alkyl-1,4-peroxyquinols by cytochrome P-450. *Chem. Res. Toxicol.* **1**, 385–390.

Zenser T.V., Wise R.W. and Davis B.B. (1985). Involvement of prostaglandin H synthetase in aromatic amine-induced transitional cell carcinoma of urinary bladder. In *Biological Oxidation of Nitrogen in Organic Molecules* (eds Gorrod J.W. and Damani L.A.). pp. 327–333. Horwood, Chichester.

Zuurbier K.W.M., Bakkenist A.R.J., Fokkens R.H., Nibbering N.M.M., Wever R. and Muijsers A.O. (1990). Interaction of myeloperoxidase with diclofenac. *Biochem. Pharmacol.* **40**, 1801–1808.

chapter 11

OXIDATION OF MERCURY, SILICON, PHOSPHORUS, ARSENIC, SELENIUM AND HALOGENS

Contents

11.1 INTRODUCTION

Previous chapters have examined in detail the oxidation of the most common atoms in organic molecules, namely carbon (Chapters 2–4 and 6–10), nitrogen (Chapters 5, 6, 9 and 10), oxygen and sulfur (Chapters 7 and 10). To conclude the series of chapters dedicated to oxidation reactions, and before discussing reduction reactions in the next chapter, it remains only to mention and briefly exemplify the oxidation of a few other elements which play a role in the chemistry of inorganic or organic xenobiotics. The sections to follow will consider:

- Group IIB: mercury;
- Group IVA: silicon;
- Group VA: phosphorus and arsenic;
- Group VIA: selenium;
- Group VIIA: the halogens.

Such a list is by no means complete; witness for example the increasing interest given to metal ions in connection with redox reactions of toxication (Kasprzak, 1991).

11.2 OXIDATION OF MERCURY

While the dealkylation of organomercurials has been presented in Section 8.3, we have yet to mention the capacity of some biological systems to oxidize metallic mercury to divalent inorganic mercury (Eq. 11.1):

$$Hg^0 \rightarrow Hg^{2+} \qquad \text{(Eq. 11.1)}$$

This reaction is known to be fast in the blood, and it has also been demonstrated in, for example, rat brain homogenates challenged with mercury vapour. The most important enzyme responsible for the oxidation of Hg^0 appears to be catalase [EC 1.11.1.6] in its Compound I form, i.e. the $[FeO]^{3+}$ oxygenated species of the enzyme (see Section 10.4). However, catalase-independent pathways may also be operative (Sichak *et al.*, 1986). Cerebral oxidation of Hg^0 appears to be of particular toxicological significance, since mercuric ion may not readily cross the blood–brain barrier and thus remain trapped in the brain.

11.3 OXIDATION OF SILICON

Silicon has many similarities with carbon, its precursor in Group IVA, and is a component of a number of xenobiotic molecules (see also Section 8.3). In particular, the replacement of a specific carbon atom by a silicon atom has proved favourable for some drugs.

One of the few documented cases of silicon oxidation is that of the model compound **dimethylphenylsilane (11.I)**, which after administration to rats yielded dimethylphenylsilanol **(11.II)** (Fessenden and Hartman, 1970). The metabolite accounted for about 80% of the dose, and unlike its isostere isopropylbenzene no other products were seen, suggesting facilitated oxidation of the Si–H group relative to the C–H group. Note that a quaternary silicon atom, like a quaternary carbon atom, cannot undergo direct hydroxylation (Section 8.3).

11.I   11.II

11.4 OXIDATION OF PHOSPHORUS AND ARSENIC

Oxidation of the prototype Group VA element nitrogen in xenobiotic molecules is abundantly documented (Chapters 5, 6, 9 and 10). In contrast, only a limited number of studies have examined the oxidation of the next two elements, phosphorus and arsenic.

11.4.1 Oxidation of phosphorus

Phosphorothionates, phosphonothionates and their analogues are important organophosphorus xenobiotics, the metabolism of which has been presented in Section 7.9 rather than here for the simple reason that oxidative attack is considered to occur at the sulfur atom. However, it is of interest to note now that some **organic phosphates (11.III)** were found to undergo oxidative dearylation like the organic phosphorothionates discussed in Section 7.9 [i.e. (RO)(R′O)P=S(OR″)]. The reaction, which was catalyzed by monooxygenases, yielded *para*-nitrophenol **(11.IV)** and other products which remained unidentified but did not include the corresponding dialkyl phosphate (Cammer and Hollingworth, 1976). The catalytic mechanism was not unravelled but must have been different from that underlying the oxidative dearylation of

11.III   11.IV

thiophosphates. The fact that one of the alkyl groups had to be a three-carbon chain or its steric equivalent may or may not be catalytically relevant. Perhaps the mechanism was one of oxygenation of the P=O moiety to form a peroxide-type linkage, but carbon oxidation of an alkyl group could not be excluded.

Unambiguous evidence for phosphorus oxidation in organophosphates comes from several metabolic studies using **phosphines** like alkyldiphenyl- and dialkylphenylphosphines as substrates. Their analogy with tertiary amines is evident, and indeed formation of phosphine oxides is a known metabolic pathway. Thus, diethylphenylphosphine (**11.V**) is a good substrate of various FAD-containing monooxygenases, diethylphenylphosphine oxide (**11.VI**) being the major product of biotransformation (Smyser and Hodgson, 1985; Tynes and Hodgson, 1985). Phenobarbital-inducible cytochrome P450 isozymes catalyze the same reaction (Smyser et al., 1986), indicating the ability of tertiary amines and tertiary phosphines alike to be substrates of both the FAD-containing monooxygenase and cytochrome P450.

11.V

11.VI

11.VII   R = −CH₃

11.VIII   R = −(CH₂)₃N(CH₃)₂

Diphenylmethylphosphine   (**11.VII**)   and   3-dimethylaminopropyldiphenyl-phosphine (**11.VIII**, a CNS depressant) were also shown to be oxygenated to the corresponding phosphine oxide by rat liver microsomal cytochrome P450 (Wiley et al., 1972). Interestingly, compound **11.VIII** yielded the N,P-dioxide as the second metabolite, but no N-monooxide was seen. This suggested a marked **chemoselectivity** for the phosphine versus amine group, a finding explained by the highly localized electron density on the phosphorus atom.

11.4.2 Oxidation of arsenic

Oxidation of inorganic As^{3+} (**arsenite, 11.IX**) to As^{5+} (arsenate, **11.X**) is documented in a number of biological conditions (Aposhian, 1989; Bencko et al., 1976). The reaction is considered to be one of detoxication, and its increase with time in mice chronically exposed to sodium

$$O^- \!-\! \underset{\underset{O^-}{|}}{\overset{\overset{O^-}{|}}{As}} \!-\! O^- \quad \underset{[H]}{\overset{[O]}{\rightleftharpoons}} \quad O \!=\! \underset{\underset{O^-}{|}}{\overset{\overset{O^-}{|}}{As}} \!-\! O^-$$

11.IX   11.X

$$CH_3\!-\!\underset{\underset{CH_3}{|}}{\overset{\overset{CH_3}{|}}{As}} \quad \underset{[H]}{\overset{[O]}{\rightleftharpoons}} \quad CH_3\!-\!\underset{\underset{CH_3}{|}}{\overset{\overset{CH_3}{|}}{As}}\!=\!O$$

11.XI   11.XII

arsenite may be one of the factors involved in arsenic tolerance (Bencko *et al.*, 1976). Note that the reverse reaction (i.e. arsenate reduction) also occurs (Section 12.6).

Among **aliphatic arsenicals**, trimethylarsine (**11.XI**) has been shown to be extensively oxygenated in the guinea-pig to trimethylarsine oxide (**11.XII**) (Yamauchi *et al.*, 1990). This metabolite accounted for about 80% of a dose, while no demethylation occurred. A number of **aromatic arsenicals** have had or retain importance as chemotherapeutic agents in the treatment of parasitic diseases (Doak and Freedman, 1970). For such compounds, arsenic oxidation (and reduction; see Section 12.6) is known to occur in mammals and to play an activating or deactivating role. Thus, metabolic oxidation of **arseno compounds** (**11.XIII**; e.g. arsphenamine **11.XVI** and neoarsphenamine **11.XVII**) splits the As=As double bond to form the corresponding arsenoxide (**11.XIV**). This is an activation reaction since arsenoxides react with thiol groups in proteins, thereby inhibiting enzymes. Further oxidation of the **arsenoxide** to the arsonic acid

$$R\!-\!As\!=\!As\!-\!R \quad \overset{[O]}{\longrightarrow} \quad 2\ R\!-\!As\!=\!O \quad \underset{[H]}{\overset{[O]}{\rightleftharpoons}} \quad 2\ R\!-\!\underset{\underset{O^-}{|}}{\overset{\overset{O^-}{|}}{As}}\!=\!O$$

11.XIII   11.XIV   11.XV

R   =   -H   11.XVI

R   =   -CH$_2$SO$_2$Na   11.XVII

(11.XV) must be viewed as a reaction of deactivation, but it is a reversible one since phenylarsonic acids can be reduced back to phenylarsenoxides (Parke, 1968).

11.5 OXIDATION OF SELENIUM

Selenium follows oxygen and sulfur in Group VIA, and recent data indicate that both selenols (R–SeH) and selenides (R′–Se–R) can undergo metabolic oxidation. A number of **organoselenium compounds** are now receiving attention in medicinal chemistry, one such compound being **benzyl selenocyanate** (**11.XVIII**), an inhibitor of chemically induced tumours in various animal models (Wendel, 1989). The compound was metabolized by rats *in vivo* and *in vitro* (liver 9000 **g** supernatant) to a number of compounds including benzylseleninic acid (**11.XX**). This

metabolite is interesting in the present context because it must have arisen by enzymatic oxidation of benzylselenol (**11.XIX**), a reaction showing analogies with the oxidation of thiols (Section 7.7) (El-Bayoumy *et al.*, 1991). Another important metabolite was benzoic acid, indicating facile bond cleavage between the benzyl moiety and the selenium atom.

Another informative example is that of **ebselen** (**11.XXI** in Fig. 11.1), an *in vivo* anti-inflammatory agent which belongs to a promising group of organoselenium compounds exhibiting glutathione peroxidase-like activity by catalyzing the degradation of H_2O_2 and organic hydroperoxides (Cotgreave *et al.*, 1992; Haenen *et al.*, 1990; Sies, 1993). Ebselen is metabolized *in vivo* and *in vitro* to a number of compounds of particular interest in the present context. The **selenol** 2-selenylbenzanilide (**11.XXII** in Fig. 11.1) and the **selenide** 2-(methylseleno)benzanilide (**11.XXIV** in Fig. 11.1) are indeed oxidized in rat liver microsomes and by pig liver FAD-containing monooxygenase (FMO1) to the **selenenic acid** (**11.XXIII** and reaction **b** in Fig. 11.1) and to the **selenoxide** 2-(methylseleninyl)benzanilide (**11.XXV** and reaction **d** in Fig. 11.1), respectively (Fischer *et al.*, 1988; John *et al.*, 1990; Ziegler *et al.*, 1992). Reaction **d** in Fig. 11.1 was much faster than *para*-hydroxylation of the phenyl ring, and both reactions document the capacity of FMO to oxygenate selenols and selenides in analogy with thiols and sulfides.

However, an important difference in reactivity exists between sulfoxides and selenoxides in that the former are very stable while the latter readily rearrange to **selenenic esters**. This was seen with 2-(methylseleninyl)benzanilide (**11.XXV** in Fig. 11.1), which was rapidly transformed to ebselen (**11.XXI** in Fig. 11.1) via formation of the selenenic acid methyl ester (**11.XXVI** in Fig. 11.1) and liberation of methanol (reactions **e** and **f** in Fig. 11.1) (John *et al.*, 1990).

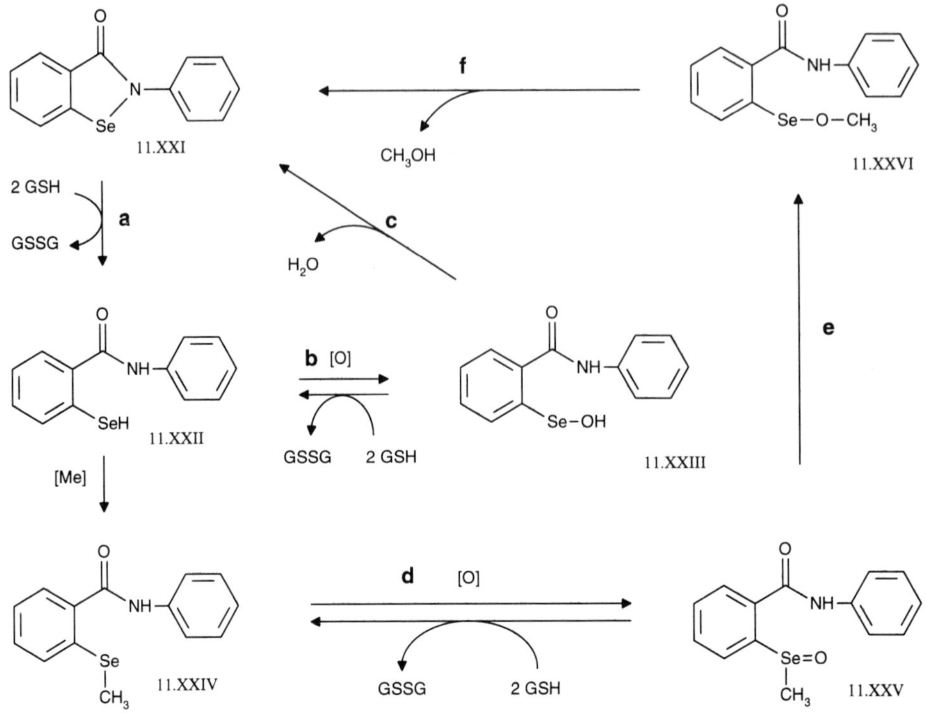

FIGURE 11.1 Reaction of selenium monooxygenation (reactions **b** and **d**) in the metabolism of ebselen (**11.XXI**), and rearrangement of the selenoxide **11.XXV** to a selenenic acid methyl ester (**11.XXVI**) and then to ebselen (reactions **e** and **f**, respectively) (John *et al.*, 1990; Ziegler *et al.*, 1992).

11.6 OXIDATION OF HALOGENS

In Section 10.4, we have seen the peroxidase-mediated oxidation of halide anions (Cl$^-$, Br$^-$ and I$^-$) to hypohalous acids. Other studies indicate that, for a number of organic substrates, cytochrome P450 has the capacity to oxidize **chlorine**, **bromine** or **iodine** atoms substituting alkyl or aryl groups. The reaction may be a one-electron oxidation or an oxygenation, the reactivity usually increasing in the series Cl < Br < I. In Section 8.2, we have discussed oxidative dehalogenation (alpha-carbon hydroxylation) of haloalkanes and have shown that this reaction may occur concurrently with one-electron oxidation or oxygenation of the halogen atom (Figs. 8.1 and 8.3) (Guengerich *et al.*, 1984; Tachizawa *et al.*, 1982).

A few other studies show that monooxygenase-catalyzed halogen oxidation is possible in some cases. For example, a work of particular elegance used [^{125}I]iodobenzene (**11.XXVII** in Fig. 11.2) as a substrate and unlabelled iodosobenzene (**11.XXVIII** in Fig. 11.2) as an oxene donor to investigate the capacity of cytochrome P450 to oxygenate **aromatic iodine** (Fig. 11.2) (Burka *et al.*, 1980). As seen in Sections 3.5 and 10.2, iodosobenzene can donate oxene to ferric cytochrome P450 to form directly the [FeO]$^{3+}$ state of the enzyme. The characterization of [^{125}I]iodosobenzene (**11.XXIX** in Fig. 11.2) and unlabelled iodobenzene (**11.XXX** in Fig. 11.2) in the incubation mixture clearly demonstrated the cytochrome P450-catalyzed oxygenation of aromatic iodine.

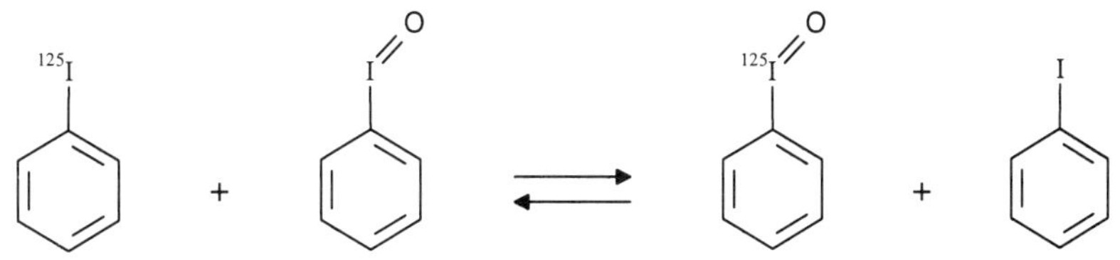

FIGURE 11.2 Demonstration of the cytochrome P450-catalyzed oxygenation of iodobenzene (**11.XXVII** and **11.XXX**) to iodosobenzene (**11.XXVIII** and **11.XXIX**) (Burka et al., 1980).

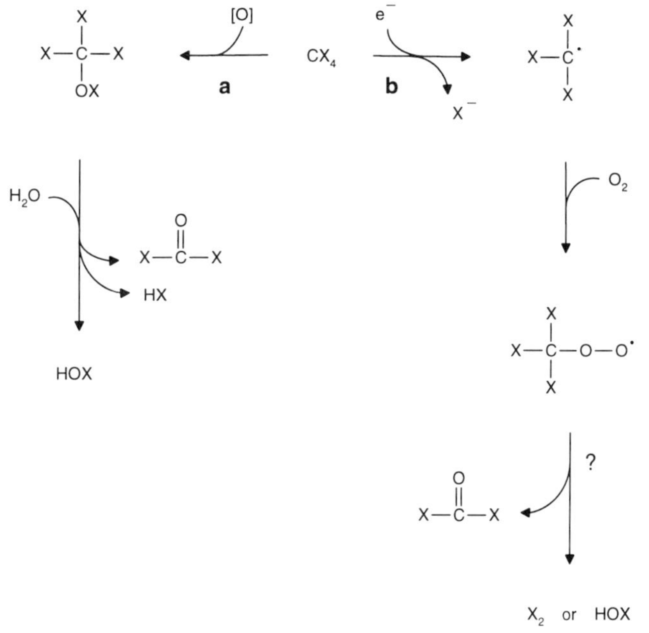

FIGURE 11.3 Postulated mechanisms in the cytochrome P450-catalyzed metabolism of tetrahalomethanes leading to the formation of electrophilic chlorine or bromine species (Mico et al., 1982 and 1983).

The cytochrome P450-catalyzed metabolism of halogenated sp^3-carbons carrying no hydrogen leads to dehalogenated products by a mechanism of **dehalogenation** distinct from that discussed in Section 8.2 for halogenated carbons carrying at least one hydrogen. The representative substrates to be discussed here are **tetrahalomethanes** (e.g. CCl_4, $CBrCl_3$, or CBr_4), whose oxidative metabolism can lead to the formation of electrophilic chlorine or bromine (in the case of CBr_4). While such a reaction is formally one of halogen oxidation, its mechanism and the exact nature of the electrophilic species do not appear to have been established unambiguously. The electrophilic halogen species may be a hypohalous acid (HOCl or HOBr) or molecular halogen (Cl_2 or Br_2), and its characterization was achieved by trapping it with 2,6-dimethylphenol to form the 4-chloro- or 4-bromo-2,6-dimethylphenol (Mico et al., 1982 and 1983). As for the postulated mechanisms, the two most likely ones are depicted in Fig. 11.3 and involve either initial oxidation (reaction **a** in Fig. 11.3) or one-electron reduction (reaction **b** in

Fig. 11.3, see Section 12.3) of the tetrahalomethane. In the case of carbon tetrachloride, reaction **a** would lead to trichloromethyl hypochloride which upon hydrolysis yields $COCl_2$, HCl and hypochlorous acid. In contrast, reaction **b** in Fig. 11.3 would form the trichloromethyl radical which adds oxygen to give the trichloromethylperoxyl radical. The latter decomposes to $COCl_2$ and an electrophilic species that may be molecular chlorine or hypochlorous acid (Mico *et al.*, 1982).

The above examples document the existence, variety and complexity of metabolic reactions of halogen oxidation. The complex interplay of enzymatic and postenzymatic steps in these reactions is particularly noteworthy.

11.7 REFERENCES

Aposhian H.V. (1989). Biochemical toxicology of arsenic. In *Reviews in Biochemical Toxicology*, Vol. 10 (eds Hodgson E., Bend J.R. and Philpot R.M.). pp. 265–299. Elsevier, New York.

Bencko V., Benes B. and Cikrt M. (1976). Biotransformation of As(III) to As(V) and arsenic tolerance. *Arch. Toxicol.* 36, 159–162.

Burka L.T., Thorsen A. and Guengerich F.P. (1980). Enzymatic monooxygenation of halogen atoms: cytochrome P-450 calalyzed oxidation of iodobenzene by iodosobenzene. *J. Amer. Chem. Soc.* 102, 7615–7616.

Cammer P.A. and Hollingworth R.M. (1976). Unusual substrate specificity in the oxidative dearylation of paraoxon analogs by mouse hepatic microsomal enzymes. *Biochem. Pharmacol.* 25, 1799–1807.

Cotgreave I.A., Moldéus P., Brattsand R., Hallberg A., Andersson C.M. and Engman L. (1992). α-(Phenylselenenyl)acetophenone derivatives with glutathione peroxidase-like activity. A comparison with ebselen. *Biochem. Pharmacol.* 43, 793–802.

Doak G.O. and Freedman L.D. (1970). Arsenicals, antimonials, and bismuthials. In *Medicinal Chemistry*, Part I, 3rd Edition (ed. Burger A). pp. 610–626. Wiley-Interscience, New York.

El-Bayoumy K., Upadhyaya P., Date V., Sohn O.S., Fiala E.S. and Reddy B. (1991). Metabolism of [^{14}C]benzyl selenocyanate in the F344 rat. *Chem. Res. Toxicol.* 4, 560–565.

Fessenden R.J. and Hartman R.A. (1970). Metabolic fate of phenyltrimethyl-silane and phenyldimethylsilane. *J. Med. Chem.* 13, 52–54.

Fischer H., Terlinden R., Löhr J.P. and Römer A. (1988). A novel biologically active selenoorganic compound. VIII. Biotransformation of ebselen. *Xenobiotica* 18, 1347–1359.

Guengerich F.P., Willard R.J., Shea J.P., Richards L.E. and Macdonald T.L. (1984). Mechanism-based inactivation of cytochrome P-450 by heteroatom-substituted cyclopropanes and formation of ring-openend products. *J. Amer. Chem. Soc.* 106, 6446–6447.

Haenen G.R.M.M., De Rooij B.M., Vermeulen N.P.E. and Bast A. (1990). Mechanism of the reaction of ebselen with endogenous thiols: dihydrolipoate is a better cofactor than glutathione in the peroxidase activity of ebselen.

Molec. Pharmacol. 37, 412–422.

John N.J., Terlinden R., Fischer H., Evers M. and Sies H. (1990). Microsomal metabolism of 2-(methylseleno)benzanilide. *Chem. Res. Toxicol.* 3, 199–203.

Kasprzak K.S. (1991). The role of oxidative damage in metal carcinogenicity. *Chem. Res. Toxicol.* 4, 604–615.

Mico B.A., Branchflower R.V., Pohl L.R., Pudzianowski A.T. and Loew G.H. (1982). Oxidation of carbon tetrachloride, bromotrichloromethane and carbon tetrabromide by rat liver microsomes to electrophilic halogens. *Life Sci.* 30, 131–137.

Mico B.A., Branchflower R.V. and Pohl L.R. (1983). Formation of electrophilic chlorine from carbon tetrachloride—involvement of cytochrome P-450. *Biochem. Pharmacol.* 32, 2357–2359.

Parke D.V. (1968). *The Biochemistry of Foreign Compounds.* 171, pp. 72–73. Pergamon Press, Oxford.

Sichak S.P., Mavis R.D., Finkelstein J.N. and Clarkson T.W. (1986). An examination of the oxidation of mercury vapor by rat brain homogenates. *J. Biochem. Toxicol.* 1, 53–68.

Sies H. (1993). Ebselen, a selenoorganic compound as glutathione peroxidase mimic. *Free Rad. Biol. Med.* 14, 313–323.

Smyser B.P. and Hodgson E. (1985). Metabolism of phosphorus-containing compounds by pig liver microsomal FAD-containing monooxygenase. *Biochem. Pharmacol.* 34, 1145–1150.

Smyser B.P., Levi P.E. and Hodgson E. (1986). Interactions of diethylphenyl-phosphine with purified, reconstituted mouse liver cytochrome P-450 monooxygenase systems. *Biochem. Pharmacol.* 35, 1719–1723.

Tachizawa H., Macdonald T.L. and Neal R.A. (1982). Rat liver microsomal metabolism of propyl halides. *Molec. Pharmacol.* 22, 745–751.

Tynes R.E. and Hodgson E. (1985). Catalytic activity and substrate specificity of the flavin-containing monooxygenase in microsomal systems: Characterization of the hepatic, pulmonary and renal enzymes of the mouse, rabbit, and rat. *Arch. Biochem. Biophys.* 240, 77–93.

Wendel A., ed. (1989). *Selenium in Biology and Medicine.* Springer, Heidelberg, FRG.

Wiley R.A., Sternson L.A., Sasame H.A. and Gillette J.R. (1972). Enzymatic oxidation of diphenylmethylphosphine and 3-dimethylaminopropyldiphenyl-phosphine by rat liver microsomes. *Biochem. Pharmacol.* **21**, 3235–3247.

Yamauchi H., Kaise T., Takahashi K. and Yamamura Y. (1990). Toxicity and metabolism of trimethylarsine in mice and hamsters. *Fund. Appl. Toxicol.* **14**, 399–407.

Ziegler D.M., Graf P., Poulsen L.L., Stahl W. and Sies H. (1992). NADPH-Dependent oxidation of reduced ebselen, 2-selenylbenzanilide and of 2-(methylseleno)benzanilide catalyzed by pig liver flavin-containing monooxygenase. *Chem. Res. Toxicol.* **5**, 163–166.

chapter 12

REDUCTIONS CATALYZED BY CYTOCHROME P450 AND OTHER OXIDOREDUCTASES

Contents

12.1 INTRODUCTION

The counterparts of the many reactions of oxidation discussed in previous chapters are obviously reactions of reduction. But while both types of reactions are comparable in terms of chemical and mechanistic variety, their quantitative importance in xenobiotic metabolism is vastly different (Mc Lane *et al.*, 1983).

As animals are aerobic organisms, the high redox potential of their cells generally (but by no means always) favours oxidative over reductive reactions. Such a situation is in sharp contrast to that existing in many bacteria, especially anaerobes, where metabolism is largely hydrolytic and reductive. As a result, the gut flora of humans and animals can contribute significantly to bioreduction of xenobiotics (Chadwick et al., 1992; Rowland, 1986; Shamat, 1993). In fact, **mammalian tissues** and **gut flora** can to some extent be seen as making opposite contributions to xenobiotic metabolism, i.e. **oxidation and conjugation** vs. **reduction and hydrolysis** (Renwick, 1991). This does not imply, of course, that the liver and other major organs of biotransformation will not mediate xenobiotic reduction, but their *in vivo* contribution is sometimes difficult to assess because *in vitro* investigations may not reflect physiological conditions of oxygen concentrations and redox equilibrium of cofactors (e.g. $NADPH/NADP^+$).

Frequent lack of information about the principal site(s) of *in vivo* reduction of a given xenobiotic is often mirrored by a comparable paucity of data on the nature of the enzyme(s) catalyzing the reaction. In contrast, *in vitro* studies can be more informative and have indeed revealed the large variety of enzymes mediating reductive reactions (Kappus, 1986; Mc Lane *et al.*, 1983). Some of these enzymes have already been presented in previous chapters and will be discussed here in their reductive role, namely:

- Alcohol dehydrogenase (Section 2.2) and aldo-keto reductases (Section 2.4);
- Dihydrodiol dehydrogenases (Section 2.5);
- Cytochrome P450 (Chapter 3);
- NADPH-cytochrome P450 reductase and NADH-cytochrome b_5 reductase (Chapter 3);
- Xanthine oxidase and aldehyde oxidase (Section 9.5);
- Peroxidases (Chapter 10).

In addition, a number of other enzymes have been proved or reported to reduce xenobiotics, e.g.:

- Glutathione reductase [NADPH:oxidized-glutathione oxidoreductase; EC 1.6.4.2], a dimeric flavoprotein (Garcia-Alfonso *et al.*, 1993);
- Thioredoxin reductase [NADPH:oxidized-thioredoxin oxidoreductase; EC 1.6.4.5], a flavoprotein;
- Quinone reductase [NAD(P)H:(quinone-acceptor) oxidoreductase; DT-diaphorase; menadione reductase; phylloquinone reductase; EC 1.6.99.2] (Ma *et al.*, 1992; Segura-Aguilar *et al.*, 1992);
- Mitochondrial NADH dehydrogenase [NADH:(acceptor) oxidoreductase; cytochrome *c* reductase; EC 1.6.99.3], an iron-containing flavoprotein present as a complex known as NADH dehydrogenase (ubiquinone) [NADH:ubiquinone oxidoreductase; EC 1.6.5.3];
- Ferredoxin reductase [ferredoxin:NADP$^+$ oxidoreductase; adrenodoxin reductase; EC 1.18.1.2], a flavoprotein.

Regrettably, a number of studies have been published which do not examine the nature of the reductase and either neglect the question or implicate "unspecific" or "poorly characterized" reductases.

12.2 REDUCTION OF CARBON ATOMS AND CARBON–OXYGEN MOIETIES

This section examines the reduction of carbon atoms in olefinic groups, and of carbon–oxygen moieties in arene oxides, quinones and hydroperoxides. Note that quinone reduction is closely related to carbonyl reduction, a pathway discussed in Chapter 2 rather than here because it cannot be separated from alcohol and aldehyde dehydrogenation.

12.2.1 Reduction of carbon–carbon double bonds

A number of xenobiotics have been found to undergo olefinic reduction in mammals both *in vitro* and *in vivo*. Most frequently, the group undergoing this reaction is an α,β-unsaturated ketonic function, and more generally an **α,β-unsaturated carbonyl**, while the enzymes involved are NAD(P)H oxidoreductases. A typical compound in this respect is the benzylidene derivative **LY 140091 (12.I)**, which was efficiently reduced to the dihydro metabolite (**12.II**) in the cytosol of various mammalian tissues and in human blood (Lindstrom and Whitaker, 1984). This saturation reaction was supported by NADPH and catalyzed by an enzyme which was not fully characterized but was found to utilize the *pro-R* hydrogen (i.e. the A side hydrogen) at C(4) of the coenzyme (see Section 2.4). In other words, this enzyme acted by transferring a hydride anion in analogy with carbonyl reductases.

A similar reaction is displayed by **digoxin**, whose reduction in humans yielded the urinary metabolite 20,22-dihydrodigoxin. Stereochemical investigations showed this active metabolite to have the 20R configuration (**12.III**), indicating product diastereoselectivity in the creation of the C(20) chiral centre (Reuning *et al.*, 1985). Another informative substrate is the catechol-O-methyltransferase inhibitor **nitecapone** (**12.IV**), which undergoes both olefinic and carbonyl reduction in humans (Taskinen *et al.*, 1991). The relative importance of the two routes was not assessed but they appear to be the main Phase I reactions of this agent.

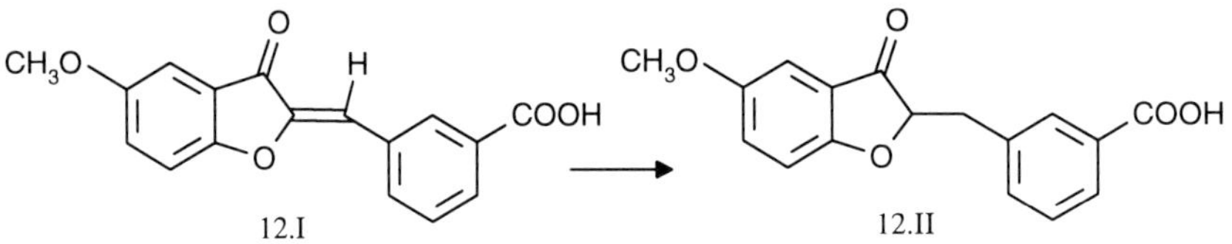

12.I   12.II

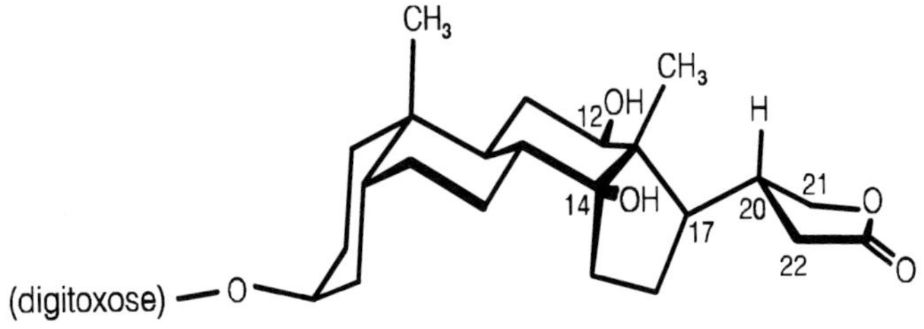

12.III

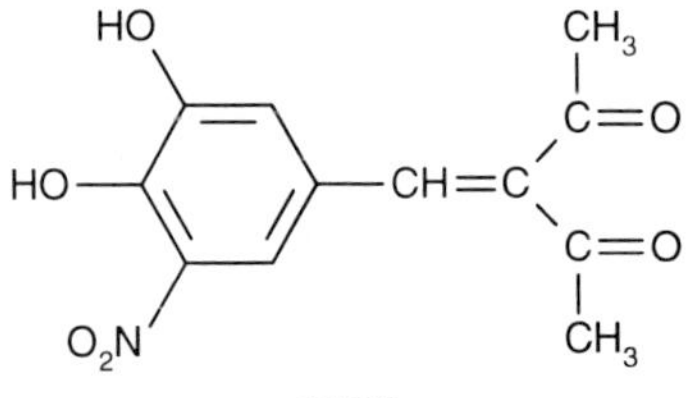

12.IV

A drug of particular interest in the present context is **5-fluorouracil (12.V)**. This major anticancer agent is activated by phosphorylation (see the volume in this series, *Biochemistry of Conjugation Reactions*) and catabolized by a sequence of metabolic reactions, the first of which is reduction of the olefinic bond to yield dihydrofluorouracil (**12.VI**). This latter is a major plasmatic metabolite in treated patients (Heggie *et al.*, 1987). The reaction is catalyzed by **dihydropyrimidine dehydrogenase** (NADP$^+$) [5,6-dihydrouracil:NADP$^+$ 5-oxidoreductase; EC 1.3.1.2], an enzyme whose physiological substrates are endogenous pyrimidines (Ho *et al.*, 1986; Lu *et al.*, 1993; Porter *et al.*, 1991). Note that the reduction of 5-fluorouracil displays some degree of reversibility when the same enzyme acts as a dehydrogenase on the reduced metabolite (Parker and Cheng, 1990).

All above substrates are **α,β-ketoalkenes**, which as stated represent the vast majority of documented cases of olefinic reduction. There are however a very few examples in the literature which suggest reduction of other types of **olefins**. Thus, the anti-inflammatory agent **S-H 766** (**12.VII**) was metabolized in humans to a number of metabolites several of which had undergone reduction of the carbon–carbon double bond (Jauch *et al.*, 1975). It is likely that the reaction is mediated by fatty acid-metabolizing enzymes following conjugation of the drug with coenzyme A (see the volume in this series, *Biochemistry of Conjugation Reactions*).

In contrast to olefinic bonds, there are no reports of the bioreduction of **carbon–carbon triple bonds**. To the best of our knowledge, the only exception is 4-ethynylbiphenyl, which under anaerobic conditions produced very small amounts of 4-vinylbiphenyl (**12.VIII**) in the presence of rat faecal contents (Wade *et al.*, 1980).

12.2.2 Deoxygenation of arene oxides

An intriguing reaction is the cytochrome P450-catalyzed reduction of arene oxides. In 1975, Sims and coworkers reported that a number of **epoxides of polycyclic aromatic hydrocarbons** (PAHs) were reduced back to the parent hydrocarbon by an "epoxide reductase" present in rat liver microsomes (Booth *et al.*, 1975). The reaction was NADPH-dependent, inhibited by molecular oxygen, and specific for both K-region epoxides (e.g. benzo[*a*]anthracene 5,6-oxide [**12.IX**], 3-methylcholanthrene 11,12-oxide, and benzo[*a*]pyrene 4,5-oxide) and non-K-region epoxides (e.g. benzo[*a*]anthracene 8,9-oxide). In contrast, the reaction was not observed for the corresponding cycloalkene oxides, e.g. 10,11-dihydrobenzo[*a*]anthracene 8,9-oxide.

12.IX

Evidence was soon published supporting the reduced form of **cytochrome P450**, i.e. ferrocytochrome P450, as the enzyme catalyzing the reaction. In addition, liver microsomes from 3-methylcholanthrene-pretreated rats exhibited the highest rate of reaction, implying the involvement of CYP1A (Kato *et al.*, 1976; Wrighton *et al.*, 1982; Yamazoe *et al.*, 1978).

The **mechanism** of this reaction of deoxygenation is not fully understood, but studies with a model compound of ferrocytochrome P450 have yielded valuable insights. Indeed, tetraphenyl-porphinato iron(II) (abbreviated Fe^{II}TPP) was found to abstract an oxygen atom directly from the oxide to form a ferryl oxide species [Fe(IV)=O] (which can also be written as [FeO]$^{2+}$) (Miyata *et al.*, 1984). The postulated mechanism is thus a direct oxene transfer from the oxide to iron(II). This is consistent with earlier findings which excluded a dihydromono-ol (i.e. a secondary alcohol obtained by dihydrogenation of the arene oxide) as a reduction intermediate (Booth *et al.*, 1975). The fact that simple epoxides (e.g. cyclohexene oxide and styrene oxide) were not deoxygenated by Fe^{II}TPP tells us that subtle electronic factors control the reaction, and is consistent with the lack of reduction of these epoxides by cytochrome P450.

12.2.3 Quinone reduction

Quinones are compounds of considerable significance in biology and toxicology (O'Brien, 1991; Monks *et al.*, 1992). As physiological compounds, a number of them fulfil essential functions in electron transfer (e.g. ubiquinone) and metabolic reactions (e.g. vitamin K) (Nohl *et al.*, 1986; Shigemura *et al.*, 1993). Quinones also represent an important group of metabolites resulting from the oxidation of aromatic rings in xenobiotics, as discussed in Chapters 4 and 10.

The reduction of quinones displays analogies with carbonyl reduction, as discussed in Chapter 2. From a chemical viewpoint, the reduction of a quinone can occur via two routes, namely: (a) a single, two-electron reduction step producing a hydroquinone (reaction **a** in Fig. 12.1); or (b) two consecutive single-electron reduction steps producing a semiquinone as intermediate (reactions **b** and **c** in Fig. 12.1). The two routes have biological significance, and both are mediated by enzymes.

Two enzymes are principally involved in the **two-electron reduction** of quinones; they are the carbonyl reductase [EC 1.1.1.184] discussed in Section 2.4, and quinone reductase (see above). Both enzymes utilize a reduced pyridine nucleotide as source of the two reducing equivalents, which take the form of a hydride anion. **Carbonyl reductase** is the predominant two-electron reductase for quinones in human liver, while quinone reductase is the major activity in rat liver (Wermuth *et al.*, 1986). The activity of human liver carbonyl reductase towards two quinones, toluquinone (2-methyl-*para*-benzoquinone) and menadione (2-methyl-1,4-naphthoquinone), is presented in Table 2.3 (Chapter 2) and is characterized by both high affinity and velocity. The substrate specificity of this enzyme preparation towards a broad variety of quinones has been systematically explored, revealing in particular the high affinity and rapid reduction of quinone metabolites of polycyclic aromatic hydrocarbons (e.g. benzo[*a*]pyrene-4,5-quinone) (Wermuth *et al.*, 1986). Many quinone metabolites of polycyclic aromatic hydrocarbons are also reduced by **dihydrodiol dehydrogenase/NADPH** (Klein *et al.*, 1992).

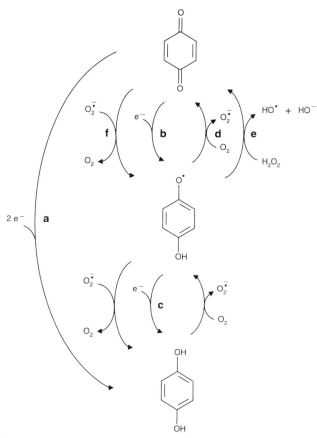

FIGURE 12.1 Redox reactions in the metabolism of quinones and semiquinones (represented by benzoquinone and benzosemiquinone). The figure shows two-electron and one-electron routes in the reduction of quinones (reactions **a**, **b** and **c**), and the interactions of quinones, semiquinones and hydroquinones with oxygen and oxygen metabolites (Hochstein, 1982; Kappus, 1986; Koster, 1991; Monks *et al.*, 1992; Nohl and Jordan, 1987; O'Brien, 1991).

The second major enzyme mediating the two-electron reductive formation of relatively stable hydroquinones is **quinone reductase** (DT-diaphorase), an enzyme strongly inhibited by dicoumarol. The bulk of the enzyme is cytosolic, although it is also found in liver microsomes, and it uses NADPH as well as NADH as cofactors (Lind *et al.*, 1982). The complete amino acid sequence of the enzyme isolated from rat liver has been established (Robertson *et al.*, 1986). Molecular biological investigations have revealed a wealth of information on this enzyme (e.g. Bayney *et al.*, 1989; Forrest *et al.*, 1990; Jaiswal *et al.*, 1990). Reduction of a number of quinones is documented, but it is of clear toxicological interest that the enzyme is also able to reduce quinone imines (see Section 4.3), e.g. N-acetyl-*para*-benzoquinone imine (**12.X**) and N,N-dimethylindoaniline (**12.XI**) (Chesis *et al.*, 1984; Lind *et al.*, 1982; Powis *et al.*, 1987). The activity of a rat liver enzyme towards four quinone imines is reported in Table 12.1. A number of 1,4-naphthoquinones were also found to be good substrates; so were glutathionyl-1,4-

TABLE 12.1 *Some kinetic parameters for rat liver quinone reductase activities* (data from Powis *et al.*, 1987)

Substrate	NADH		NADPH	
	K_m*	V_{max}†	K_m	V_{max}†
N-Acetyl-*p*-benzoquinone imine (**12.X**)	54.9	277.8	40.0	238.1
2-Amino-1,4-naphthoquinone imine	2.8	38.5	2.6	35.7
N,N-Dimethylindoaniline (**12.XI**)	1.7	22.2	0.9	14.3
2-Acetamido-N,N-dimethylindoaniline	0.4	9.1	0.5	12.5

*K_m values in μM.
†V_{max} values in μmol min^{-1} mg^{-1}.

naphthoquinones, a fact of particular relevance in the light of: (a) the glutathione conjugation of quinones to be discussed in the volume in this series, *Biochemistry of Conjugation Reactions*; and (b) the facile toxication of quinone thioethers (Buffinton *et al.*, 1989; Monks and Lau, 1992).

A number of quinones and quinone imines are toxic metabolites due to their ability to form covalent adducts with endogenous thiol groups in macromolecules (see the volume in this series, *Biochemistry of Conjugation Reactions*) (Flowers-Geary *et al.*, 1993). Perhaps more important is the toxication of quinones by another mechanism, namely their **one-electron reduction to semiquinones** (reaction **b** in Fig. 12.1). This reaction can be mediated by **cytochrome P450** or the three **flavoproteins** NADPH-cytochrome P450 reductase, NADH-cytochrome b_5 reductase, and mitochondrial NADH dehydrogenase (Capdevila *et al.*, 1978; Powis *et al.*, 1981). The first three among these four enzymes are essential constituents of the microsomal monooxygenase system and have been described at length in Chapter 3. It is of importance to note again that quinone reductase (see above) has a unique position among NAD(P)H-oxidizing flavoproteins in being a two-electron transfer enzyme.

Semiquinones and **semiquinone imines** are highly reactive intermediates which cannot be isolated, although their formation is detectable by electron paramagnetic resonance (EPR) spectroscopy. In the presence of molecular oxygen, they autoxidize rapidly to quinones or quinone imines with concomitant production of superoxide anion-radical ($O_2^{\bullet-}$) (reaction **d** in Fig. 12.1) (Nohl and Jordan, 1987). NADH consumption and $O_2^{\bullet-}$ formation have been shown to be maximal at a quinone one-electron reduction potential of -70 mV (Powis *et al.*, 1981). While semiquinones and semiquinone imines can elicit toxic effects in their own right by reacting with various biological nucleophiles, superoxide radicals also contribute significantly to semiquinone-mediated toxicity (e.g. cytotoxicity) (Bachur *et al.*, 1979; Chesis *et al.*, 1984; Smith *et al.*, 1985). In addition to forming superoxide radicals, semiquinones can also act as catalysts of the Haber–Weiss reaction in the biological generation of highly toxic hydroxyl radicals (reaction **e** in Fig. 12.1; see also Section 3.5) (Nohl and Jordan, 1987; van de Straat *et al.*, 1987). As shown in Fig. 12.1 (reaction **f**), semiquinones can also be formed by superoxide-mediated reduction of quinones, a reaction of synthetic and probably also biological significance (Nohl and Jordan, 1987).

Incubation of quinones with liver microsomes under conditions favouring NADPH-cytochrome P450 reductase leads to a steady-state level of the corresponding hydroquinones, suggesting that reaction **c** in Fig. 12.1 is either reductase-mediated or is due to **disproportionation** of the semiquinone (Bock *et al.*, 1980; Capdevila *et al.*, 1978; Ernster *et al.*, 1982). Taken together, these results lead to a complex picture (Fig. 12.1) of reactions of oxidation (Section 7.6) and reduction in the enzymatic and non-enzymatic metabolism of quinones and hydroquinones, coupled with the production or trapping of reactive metabolites of oxygen (Goeptar *et al.*, 1992; Hochstein, 1983). This **futile cycling**, as it is sometimes called, intertwines reactions of toxication and detoxication and is itself coupled to other reactions of formation or deactivation of reduced oxygen species, e.g. the disproportionation of superoxide to hydrogen peroxide and molecular oxygen (Section 3.5), and the reduction of hydrogen peroxide by peroxidases such as catalase and glutathione peroxidase (Section 10.4). Note in addition that xanthine oxidase and aldehyde oxidase (see Section 9.5) are also able to reduce quinones either directly or via superoxide, but the *in vivo* significance of this reaction appears unclear.

It is thus clear that depending on biological conditions and on their chemical structure, quinones may undergo reduction pathways of **detoxication** (two-electron reduction) or **toxication** (one-electron reduction) (Koster, 1991). Factors influencing this balance are important objects of study (e.g. Chesis *et al.*, 1984; Lind *et al.*, 1982). For example, the rate of reduction of various quinones by NADPH-cytochrome P450 reductase has been shown to be directly related to their one-electron reduction potential, when this was more negative than -165 mV (Butler and Hoey, 1993).

Quinone reduction is of significance in the metabolism of a number of **drugs and other xenobiotics**, some of which have been presented above. In Section 10.4, we have discussed the oxidation of diethylstilbestrol (**10.LVII**) to dienoestrol (**10.LVIII**) via the semiquinone and quinone intermediates. The latter metabolites have also been shown to undergo one-electron reduction catalyzed by rat liver microsomes, NADPH-cytochrome P450 reductase, NADH-cytochrome b_5 reductase, or xanthine oxidase. In addition, diethylstilbestrol quinone was directly reduced to diethylstilbestrol by quinone reductase (Roy *et al.*, 1991a and 1991b).

Reduction is an important reaction in the metabolism and activation of some **quinonic antitumour agents** (Bachur *et al.*, 1979; Mc Lane *et al.*, 1983; Riley and Workman, 1992a). These include the anthracycline glycosides to be discussed below, the mitosane antibiotics (e.g. mitomycin C) which act as bioreductive alkylating agents, and a range of other quinones (Bailey *et al.*, 1992; Begleiter and Leith, 1993; Begleiter *et al.*, 1992; Siegel *et al.*, 1992; Vromans *et al.*, 1990). A number of cases of bioactivation involve two-electron reduction by carbonyl reductase or quinone reductase (e.g. mitomycin C), while many studies in the literature report the one-electron reduction to semiquinones as catalyzed by xanthine oxidase, NADPH-cytochrome P450 reductase, NADH dehydrogenase, and ferredoxin reductase (Fisher *et al.*, 1992; Forrest *et al.*, 1991; Riley and Workman, 1992a; Ross *et al.*, 1991).

The **anthracycline glycosides** are exemplified by daunomycin (daunorubicine; **12.XII** in Fig. 12.2) and adriamycin (where the $-COCH_3$ group is replaced by a $-COCH_2OH$ group). The compounds undergo one-electron reduction to the semiquinone (reaction **a** in Fig. 12.2). The latter reacts readily with O_2 to form the superoxide anion-radical which has been proposed to produce DNA strand breaks and perhaps to be responsible for the well-known cardiotoxicity of anthracycline drugs, although the mechanism of this cardiotoxicity is not well understood (de Jong *et al.*, 1993). While xanthine oxidase is often used in *in vitro* studies to reduce anthracycline glycosides, NADPH-cytochrome P450 reductase may well be the major physiological reductant (Bartoszek and Wolf, 1992; Cummings *et al.*, 1992; Kalyanaraman *et al.*, 1991; Mc Lane *et al.*, 1983; Schreiber *et al.*, 1987). In addition to forming semiquinones, these drugs also undergo a specific metabolic reaction of **reductive cleavage** whereby they lose both the aminosugar moiety and the oxygen atom at C(7). The resulting 7-deoxy aglycones are considered to be inactive, and there are good indications to believe that the semiquinone is an intermediate in the reductive cleavage (reaction **b** in Fig. 12.2) (Bachur and Gee, 1976; Pan and Bachur, 1987).

12.2.4 Reduction of hydroperoxides

In Section 10.2, we have discussed the peroxidase activity of cytochrome P450 and shown how peroxides can act as oxygen donors to adequate substrates by homolytic or heterolytic cleavage of

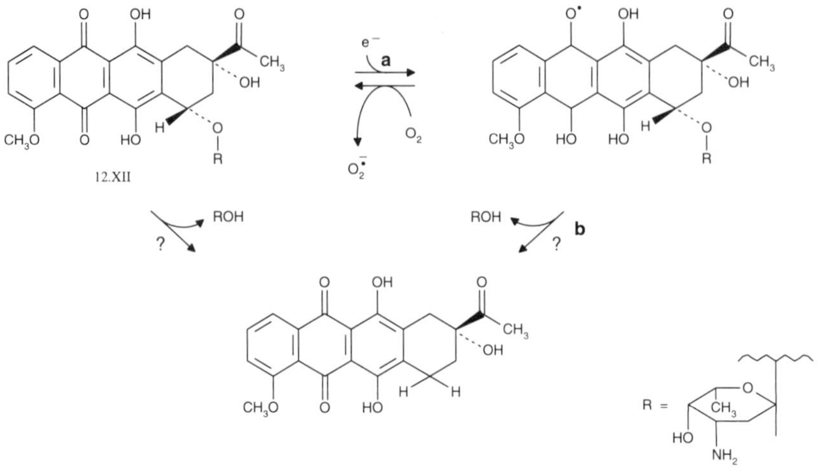

FIGURE 12.2 One-electron reduction of daunomycin (**12.XII**) to the semiquinone (reaction **a**) and to the 7-deoxy aglycone (probably via reaction **b**).

the O–O bond (Fig. 10.1). Such reactions thus involve the formation of ternary complexes between the enzyme, the substrate, and the hydroperoxide. This last component is reduced either to an alcohol (heterolytic cleavage) or to an alkoxyl radical (homolytic cleavage) which can react in a variety of ways (Section 10.2). In the present section, yet another reaction of hydroperoxides is examined, namely their **NADPH-dependent and cytochrome P450-catalyzed reductive cleavage**.

The reaction requires cytochrome P450, NADPH-cytochrome P450 reductase and NADPH, tolerates O_2, and is described by Eq. 12.1:

$$XRR'C\text{–}OOH + NADPH + H^+ \rightarrow XR'CO + RH + H_2O + NADPH^+ \qquad \text{(Eq. 12.1)}$$

where X is an alkyl or aryl group, and R and R' are hydrogen or alkyl groups. Thus, cumyl hydroperoxide (**12.XIII**) gave acetophenone (**12.XIV**) plus methane, α-methylbenzyl hydroperoxide (**12.XV**) gave acetophenone (**12.XIV**) plus benzaldehyde (**12.XVI**) plus methane, while *tert*-butyl hydroperoxide (**12.XVII**) formed acetone (**12.XVIII**) plus methane with stoichiometric consumption of NADPH (Vaz and Coon, 1987). It is noteworthy from a physiological viewpoint that **fatty acid hydroperoxides** are also good substrates. 13-Hydroperoxy-9,11-octadecadienoic acid (13-HOO–$C_{18:2}$) and 15-hydroperoxy-5,8,11,13-eicosatetraenoic acid (15-HOO–$C_{20:4}$) yielded an aldehyde acid and pentane. CYP2E1 was the most active of the isozymes tested (Vaz *et al.*, 1990).

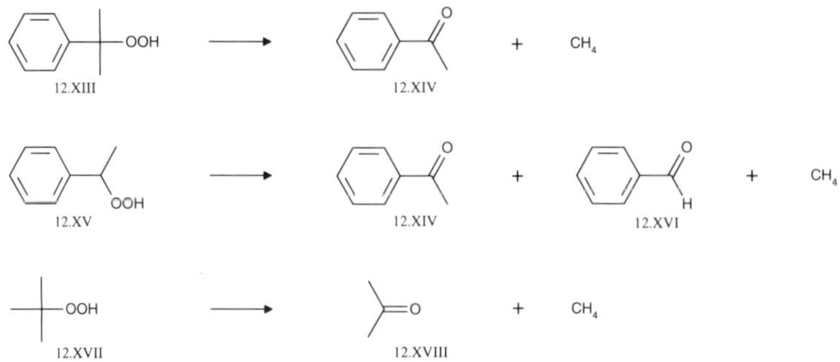

The **mechanism of the reaction** involves binding of the hydroperoxide to ferrocytochrome P450, transfer of one electron to the hydroperoxide, and homolytic cleavage of the O–O bond to form an **alkoxyl radical** (Vaz and Coon, 1987) (Eq. 12.2):

$$XRR'C–OOH + [Fe(II)] \rightarrow XRR'C–O^{\bullet} + HO^{-} + [Fe(III)] \qquad \text{(Eq. 12.2)}$$

The alkoxyl radical thus generated reacts by intramolecular β-scission to form the carbonyl metabolite and an alkyl radical (Eq. 12.3):

$$XRR'C–O^{\bullet} \rightarrow XR'C{=}O + R^{\bullet} \qquad \text{(Eq. 12.3)}$$

The alkyl radical forms the alkane metabolite probably by abstracting a hydrogen radical from a convenient source (e.g. a fatty acid).

Interestingly, the cytochrome P450-dependent lipid hydroperoxide reduction discussed here can also lead to the corresponding fatty alcohol, as seen with the formation of 13-hydroxy-9,11-octadecadienoic acid from 13-hydroperoxy-9,11-octadecadienoic acid (Lindstrom and Aust, 1984). The mechanism of this reaction has not been well explained, but it is conceivable that the alkoxyl radical does not react as per Eq. 12.3 but is either reduced enzymatically to the alcoholate anion, or leaves the active site and abstracts a hydrogen radical. These examples suggest that we have still much to learn about the metabolism of endogenous and exogenous hydroperoxides.

12.3 REDUCTIVE DEHALOGENATION

Reductive dehalogenation is a generic term for a number of reactions which result in the cleavage of a carbon–halogen bond, following the one-electron reduction of the substrate. As a rule, the halogen atom is replaced by a hydrogen atom, e.g. CCl_4 being reduced to $CHCl_3$, but the intricacies of the reaction mechanisms are such that a variety of additional metabolites are usually formed. As for the halogen atom, it is liberated as a **halide anion**, but here also exceptions do exist, e.g. the formation of "electrophilic" chlorine (Section 11.6).

Most of the functional groups involved in the reaction are haloalkyls, but the reductive dehalogenation of aromatic bonds is also documented. While **cytochrome P450** is the major enzyme catalyzing reductive dehalogenation, a few other systems may also be active (Anders, 1984).

Most studies discussed below were performed *in vitro* under conditions of anaerobiosis or low oxygen tension, and their *in vivo* relevance may therefore be questioned by some. In fact, low oxygen concentration (partial pressures of 1–10 mm Hg) does occur locally in the liver (mainly in the centrilobular region) and other tissues, and there are various examples of reductive dehalogenation being seen *in vivo* (De Groot and Sies, 1989).

12.3.1 Carbon tetrachloride

There are two major reasons why the reductive dehalogenation of carbon tetrachloride has been most actively investigated. First, it is an ideal model compound due to its chemical simplicity and absence of other metabolic reactions. And second, it is far more than a mere model compound, being a well-known and potent hepatotoxin whose chronic toxicity originates in its bioactivation. Indeed, carbon tetrachloride elicits such toxic effects as destruction of cytochrome P450, protein acylation, lipid peroxidation, and altered intracellular calcium distribution. These molecular and

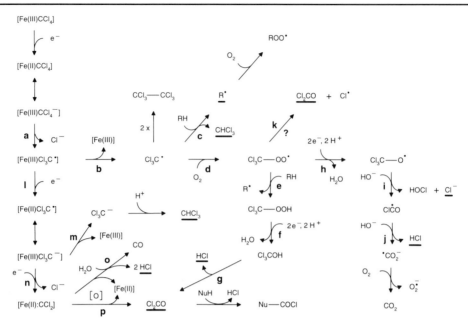

FIGURE 12.3 Cytochrome P450-catalyzed reductive metabolism of carbon tetrachloride. [Fe(III)X] are complexes of cytochrome P450 (in this case in its ferric state) with substrate and/or metabolic intermediate. RH symbolizes fatty acids undergoing lipid peroxidation; metabolites appearing more than once are underlined.

cellular effects can be followed *in vivo* by liver necrosis and death (Brattin *et al.*, 1985; Manno *et al.*, 1988).

The pivotal intermediate in the reduction of CCl_4 is the **trichloromethyl radical** $Cl_3C^{\bullet}$ whose formation is explained in Fig. 12.3 (Macdonald, 1983; McCay *et al.*, 1984). Following binding of CCl_4 to ferricytochrome P450 (type I difference spectrum), a one-electron reduction of the enzyme–substrate complex occurs, as is the case for all NADPH-supported cytochrome P450-catalyzed oxidations (Chapter 3). However, CCl_4 is not an ordinary substrate, and by virtue of its marked **electron-withdrawing character** it re-oxidizes the iron atom by forming a transient anion CCl_4^-, which in turn decomposes to $Cl_3C^{\bullet}$ by loss of a chloride anion (reaction **a** in Fig. 12.3). Carbon tetrachloride is exemplary in showing that it is principally the chemical nature of the substrate, rather than enzymatic or physiological factors, which causes cytochrome P450 to act as a reductase. Note that CCl_4 can also bind *in vitro* to ferrocytochrome P450 when this form predominates due to anaerobic or reducing conditions (Wolf *et al.*, 1977).

The trichloromethyl radical generated by reaction **a** in Fig. 12.3 can either remain bound in the active site of the enzyme and be further metabolized (see below), or be liberated (reaction **b** in Fig. 12.3) and enter a complex series of non-enzymatic reactions. While dimerization to hexachlorohexane appears minor, two reactions are significant, namely **chloroform** formation and oxygenation. The former is due to $Cl_3C^{\bullet}$ abstracting a hydrogen atom from a polyunsaturated fatty acid (e.g. **12.XIX**) in phospholipids (reaction **c** in Fig. 12.3). Fatty acid radicals formed by this mechanism have been observed repeatedly by electron paramagnetic resonance (EPR) spectroscopy, and there is evidence that they are pentadienyl free radicals (**12.XX**) (Calligaro and Vannini, 1978; McCay *et al.*, 1984). Such fatty acid free radicals are precursors of **lipid peroxidation**, as discussed in Section 10.5, leading to fatty acid peroxyl radicals, fatty acid hydroperoxides, alkoxyl radicals, and products of lipid peroxidation such as alkanes, aldehydes, ketones, and epoxyhydroxy compounds.

$$R—CH_2—CH=CH—CH_2—CH=CH—(CH_2)_3—COOH$$

12.XIX

H•

$$R—CH_2 \overline{\left[CH \cdots CH \cdots CH \cdots CH \cdots CH \right]} (CH_2)_3—COOH$$

12.XX

The fastest reaction of the trichloromethyl radical is with molecular oxygen to form the **trichloromethyl peroxyl radical** $Cl_3COO^\bullet$ (reaction **d** in Fig. 12.3) (Connor *et al.*, 1986; Mönig *et al.*, 1983; Pohl *et al.*, 1984). This highly reactive intermediate is itself at the crossroads of several reactions. By abstracting a hydrogen atom from fatty acids (reaction **e** in Fig. 12.3), it can, like $Cl_3C^\bullet$, induce fatty acid free radical formation and lipid peroxidation (McCay *et al.*, 1984). In addition, it has been postulated that the trichloromethyl hydroperoxide thus formed could be reduced to trichloromethanol (reaction **f** in Fig. 12.3) which would immediately eliminate HCl to yield **phosgene** (reaction **g** in Fig. 12.3) (Connor *et al.*, 1986; Macdonald, 1983; Mönig *et al.*, 1983; Pohl *et al.*, 1984).

Another reaction of $Cl_3COO^\bullet$ is formation of **carbon dioxide** via reduction to the trichloromethoxyl radical (reaction **h** in Fig. 12.3), hydrolysis to the chlorocarbonyl radical $^\bullet COCl$ (reaction **i** in Fig. 12.3), and hydrolysis to the carbon dioxide anion radical (reaction **j** in Fig. 12.3) whose formation has been proved unambiguously (Connor *et al.*, 1983; Mönig *et al.*, 1983).

An intriguing and incompletely understood reaction in the metabolism of carbon tetrachloride is the release of **electrophilic chlorine** from (most likely) the trichloromethyl peroxyl radical (reaction **k** in Fig. 12.3). Such an electrophilic species has been postulated to be a chlorine radical formed together with phosgene from the cleavage of a trichloromethyl peroxyl–iron complex, i.e. the trichloromethyl peroxyl radical bound to cytochrome P450 by a –O–O–Fe linkage (Mico and Pohl, 1983 and 1984). This electrophilic chlorine was not detected directly, but after having been trapped by 2,6-dimethylphenol to form 4-chloro-2,6-dimethylphenol.

As also shown in Fig. 12.3, the trichloromethyl radical may fail to dissociate from its complex with cytochrome P450 and thus undergo **further reductive metabolism** (reaction **l** in Fig. 12.3). This alternative route appears minor as compared to reaction **b** in Fig. 12.3, but low partial pressures of oxygen or phenobarbital induction may increase its importance (Kubic and Anders, 1981; Pohl *et al.*, 1984). Reduction of the trichloromethyl radical bound to cytochrome P450 yields the **trichloromethyl carbanion** (reaction **l** in Fig. 12.3) which, after dissociation from the enzyme, reacts with a proton to form chloroform (reaction **m** in Fig. 12.3) (Kubic and Anders, 1981). The trichloromethyl carbanion is of particular interest because loss of a chloride anion transforms it into **dichlorocarbene** (reaction **n** in Fig. 12.3), a strong ligand of the Fe^{2+} cation and hence a potent inhibitor of cytochrome P450. Liberation of dichlorocarbene results either in its hydrolysis to CO and HCl (reaction **o** in Fig. 12.3), or oxygenation to phosgene (reaction **p** in Fig. 12.3). The latter, a potent acylating agent, can react with nucleophilic groups of cell macromolecules leading to unstable Nu–COCl intermediates and stable Nu–CO–Nu adducts (Mansuy *et al.*, 1980). Together with radical formation and lipid peroxidation, the production of phosgene is one of the major chemical factors accounting for the marked hepatoxicity of carbon tetrachloride (Brattin *et al.*, 1985).

Carbon tetrachloride is also known to inhibit cytochrome P450 by another mechanism, namely destruction of its heme moiety. While the mechanism of the reaction is not fully elucidated, there is evidence that the step of heme destruction follows formation of the [Fe(II)Cl$_3$C$^\bullet$] complex (Manno $et\ al.$, 1988). In other words, carbon tetrachloride also behaves as a mechanism-based irreversible inhibitor.

Perhaps the most active cytochrome P450 reducing CCl$_4$ is the ethanol-inducible CYP2E1 (Koop, 1992; Persson $et\ al.$, 1990; Raucy $et\ al.$, 1993). In addition to microsomes, carbon tetrachloride has also been shown to be reduced in rat liver mitochondria under hypoxic conditions, leading to the formation of Cl$_3$C$^\bullet$ and to lipid peroxidation (Tomasi $et\ al.$, 1987). The reaction did not require NADPH, nor was it mediated by cytochrome P450. In fact, the mitochondrial electron transport chain was responsible for CCl$_4$ activation.

12.3.2 Polyhalogenated methanes and ethanes

In addition to carbon tetrachloride, a number of polyhalogenated methanes and ethanes are known to undergo reduction catalyzed by cytochrome P450 and particularly CYP2E1. Thus, the reactivity of **polyhalomethanes** was assessed by monitoring their binding spectra with reduced cytochrome P450 and the formation of carbon monoxide (reaction **o** in Fig. 12.3) (Wolf $et\ al.$, 1977). CYP101 was also able to reduce a number of halomethanes to the corresponding hydrogenohalomethane (i.e. reductive replacement of a chloro or bromo substituent by a hydrogen atom) (Castro $et\ al.$, 1985). Rats dosed with CCl$_4$ or CBr$_4$ reduced these compounds to radicals which reacted with a co-administered spin trapping compound, thus forming radical adducts which were detectable in the bile. In contrast, no radical adduct was detectable after CHCl$_3$ administration, while CHBr$_3$ was reduced only under hypoxic conditions (Knecht and Mason, 1991).

A number of studies have compared the metabolic reduction of polyhalomethanes to their **chemical reactivity**, for example as assessed by their half-wave reduction potential E$_{1/2}$ (i.e. ease of electrochemical reduction) or their electron-accepting ability calculated by quantum mechanical methods (Hanzlik, 1981; Luke $et\ al.$, 1988). It will not surprise chemists that the ease of reduction of these compounds decreases in the two series I > Br > Cl > F and CX$_4$ > CHX$_3$ > CH$_2$X$_2$ > CH$_3$X, where X is a halogen. Based on the above-cited studies, a tentative classification of polyhalomethanes and some analogues is presented in Table 12.2. As stressed by Hanzlik (1981), halomethanes that are reduced more easily than CCl$_4$ should all initiate lipid peroxidation and produce hepatotoxicity; in contrast, those analogues that are distinctly more difficult to reduce than CCl$_4$ or O$_2$ should not initiate lipid peroxidation and their hepatotoxicity, if any, must be explained by other mechanisms.

Polyhaloethanes are also able to undergo cytochrome P450-catalyzed reductive dehalogenation, as exemplified by the compounds discussed here and by halothane (Section 12.3.3). Unfortunately, the metabolism of polyhaloethanes has not received as much attention as that of polyhalomethanes, a situation that may well change with the search for non-ozone-depleting substitutes of chlorofluorocarbons (Olson $et\ al.$, 1991) (see Section 8.2 for their oxidative metabolism). While the mechanism of reductive dehalogenation does not differ in the two chemical groups, there is not yet enough evidence to indicate that polyhaloethanes form the wealth of reduced metabolites seen with CCl$_4$ and other polyhalomethanes.

One reaction that involves free radical intermediates (formed by halide loss) and is characteristic of polyhaloethanes (and presumably also of higher polyhaloalkanes) is known as ***vic*-bisdehalogenation**. This reaction, which is characterized by loss of two vicinal halogens and **formation of an olefinic bond**, is seen in the reductive metabolism of ethanes bearing three halogen atoms (often chlorine) on one carbon atom, and at least one halogen atom on the other (Town and Leibman, 1984). Thus, rat liver microsomes under anaerobic conditions metabolized

TABLE 12.2 *Tentative classification of some halomethanes and analogues as reducible substrates of cytochrome P450 (compiled from Castro et al., 1985; Hanzlik, 1981; Knecht and Mason, 1991; Luke et al., 1988)*

Very good substrates	
	$CCl_3(NO_2)$, CBr_4, CCl_3Br
	$CHCl_2(NO_2)$, CHI_3
Good substrates	
	CCl_4, $CFCl_3$
	$CHBr_3$
	$CH_2Cl(NO_2)$
Modestly or marginally reactive compounds	
	CF_2Cl_2
	$CHCl_3$
	CH_2Br_2, CH_2I_2
	CH_3I
Unreactive compounds	
	CF_3Cl, CF_4
	$CHFCl_2$, CHF_2Cl, CHF_3
	CH_2Br_2, CH_2Cl_2, CH_2FCl, CH_2F_2, CH_3Cl, CH_3F

hexachloroethane (**12.XXI**), pentachloroethane (**12.XXIII**) and 1,1,1,2-tetrachloroethane (**12.XXV**) to tetrachloroethylene (**12.XXII**), trichloroethylene (**12.XXIV**) and 1,1-dichloroethylene (**12.XXVI**), respectively. The mechanism of *vic*-bisdehalogenation consists of two single-electron reduction steps and loss of two halide anions (Fig. 12.4 in Section 12.3.3) (Nastainczyk *et al.*, 1982). Note that **polyhaloethylenes** formed as metabolites of polyhaloethanes can be further metabolized by epoxidation (Section 4.4) and as such are potentially toxic in their own right.

Two single-electron reduction steps and loss of two chloride anions (i.e. reactions **a**, **l** and **n** in Fig. 12.3) were also seen in the reductive metabolism of 1,1,1-trichloroethane in rats *in vivo* (hypoxia) and *in vitro*. Here, however, the resulting product was a carbene ($CH_3ClC:$) which immediately lost HCl to yield **acetylene** (Dürk *et al.*, 1992). Thus, given the proper substrates,

$$CCl_3\text{---}CCl_3 \longrightarrow Cl_2C\text{=}CCl_2$$

12.XXI   12.XXII

$$CCl_3\text{---}CHCl_2 \longrightarrow Cl_2C\text{=}CHCl$$

12.XXIII   12.XXIV

$$CCl_3\text{---}CH_2Cl \longrightarrow Cl_2C\text{=}CH_2$$

12.XXV   12.XXVI

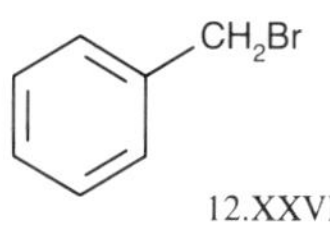

12.XXVII

reductive dehalogenation can generate not only olefinic bonds, but also **carbon–carbon triple bonds**.

Besides polyhalomethanes and polyhaloethanes, some other relatively simple chemicals can also undergo reductive dehalogenation, as exemplified by **benzyl halides**. Thus, benzyl bromide (**12.XXVII**) was reduced anaerobically to toluene by rat liver microsomes (Mansuy and Fontecave, 1983). The reaction was found to proceed by two mechanisms, one involving the C_6H_5–$CH_2^\bullet$ radical and the other the C_6H_5–CH_2^- anion. Some **perhalogenated** alkanes also appear to be substrates for reductive dehalogenation, as reported for poly(chlorotrifluoroethylene), a mixture of oligomers of chlorotrifluoroethene (Brashear *et al.*, 1992).

12.3.3 Halothane and other compounds of medicinal interest

The oxidative metabolism of the inhalation anaesthetic **halothane** (CF_3–CHClBr) has been presented in Section 8.2 where emphasis is given to the toxicological implications of highly reactive metabolites capable of acylating proteins. Here, we discuss the mechanism of reductive dehalogenation of halothane and its significant toxicological hazards (Baker *et al.*, 1983; Knecht *et al.*, 1992; Kubic and Anders, 1981; MacDonald, 1983; Manno *et al.*, 1991; Sipes *et al.*, 1980).

As shown in Fig. 12.4, the reductive metabolism of halothane displays many analogies with that of carbon tetrachloride. The main pathway leads to the formation of the **1-chloro-2,2,2-trifluoroethyl radical** (reactions **a** and **b** in Fig. 12.4) by a mechanism identical to the first step of CCl_4 reduction (Fig. 12.3). This radical intermediate can abstract a hydrogen atom from lipids or other biomolecules, resulting in the formation of **2-chloro-1,1,1-trifluoroethane** (reaction **c** in Fig. 12.4), a major metabolite formed by rat liver microsomes under conditions of low oxygen tension (Ahr *et al.*, 1982; Van Dyke *et al.*, 1988). More importantly, the 1-chloro-2,2,2-trifluoroethyl radical can bind covalently to proteins and (mainly) to unsaturated fatty acids in phospholipids (reaction **d** in Fig. 12.4) (Gandolfi *et al.*, 1980). The latter reaction first forms transient fatty acyl free radical adducts which pull a hydrogen atom from other lipids to yield stable adducts (**12.XXVIII** in Fig. 12.4), the chemical structure of which has been established unambiguously (Legler and Van Dyke, 1982; Trudell *et al.*, 1981 and 1982). Reactions **c** and **d** in Fig. 12.4 also form fatty acyl free radicals (shown as $R^\bullet$), thus initiating lipid peroxidation (van Iersel *et al.*, 1988). It is important to note again that the low oxygen tension under which halothane is reduced *in vitro* also occurs in the liver *in vivo*, indicating that adduct formation and lipid peroxidation are more than potential hazards.

Rather than dissociating from its complex with cytochrome P450, the 1-chloro-2,2,2-trifluoroethyl radical can undergo further reduction (reaction **e** in Fig. 12.4) to the 1-chloro-2,2,2-trifluoroethyl anion. The latter then rearranges to **2-chloro-1,1-difluoroethylene** (**12.XXIX** in Fig. 12.4), another major metabolite of halothane, with loss of a fluoride anion (reactions **f** and **g** in Fig. 12.4). The pathway leading from halothane to 2-chloro-1,1-difluoroethylene is the mechanism of *vic*-bisdehalogenation discussed in Section 12.3.2 (Ahr *et al.*, 1982; Baker *et al.*, 1983; Van Dyke *et al.*, 1988).

Much attention has been given to a Soret band at 470 nm appearing during the microsomal metabolism of halothane, but no agreement exists on the chemical nature of the complex showing this spectral absorption. A number of workers have postulated a complex between reduced cytochrome P450 and a **trifluoroethylcarbene** (i.e. the complex formed by reaction **h** in Fig. 12.4) (Loew and Goldblum, 1980). More recent studies have implicated the [Fe(III)CF_3CHCl$^-$] or [Fe(III)CF_2=CHCl] complexes (see Fig. 12.4) (Hildebrandt *et al.*, 1988; Ruf *et al.*, 1984). But whatever the chemical nature of this complex, its existence implies a **mechanism-based reversible inhibition** of cytochrome P450.

In addition, and like carbon tetrachloride, halothane is able to inhibit cytochrome P450

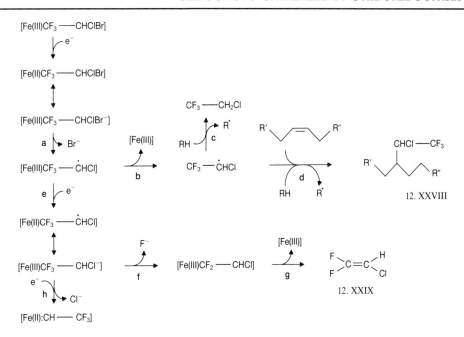

FIGURE 12.4 Cytochrome P450-catalyzed reductive metabolism of halothane. [Fe(III)X] are complexes of cytochrome P450 (in this case in its ferric state) with substrate and/or metabolic intermediate. RH symbolizes fatty acids undergoing lipid peroxidation.

irreversibly and does so by heme destruction. This reaction follows formation of the complex [Fe(II)CF$_3$C$^\bullet$HCl], but the chemical nature of the reactive intermediate is not known (Manno *et al.*, 1991).

A few other compounds of medicinal interest undergo reductive dehalogenation. One such compound is 1,1-*bis*(4-chlorophenyl)-2,2,2-trichloroethane (**DDT, 12.XXX**), which is reduced by cytochrome P450 to 1,1-*bis*(4-chlorophenyl)-2,2-dichloroethane (DDD, **12.XXXI**). The mechanism of the reaction involves one-electron reduction to the 1,1-*bis*(4-chlorophenyl)-2,2-dichloroethyl radical, followed by abstraction of a hydrogen atom from an unknown source (Kelner *et al.*, 1986). This is, in other words, the usual mechanism of reductive dehalogenation already discussed for carbon tetrachloride and halothane.

12.XXX   12.XXXI

One of the many metabolic pathways of the antibiotic **chloramphenicol (12.XXXII)** is reductive dehalogenation, albeit a rather unusual one in that it involves a haloacyl moiety (the dichloroacetyl group) rather than a haloalkyl moiety. Indeed, when incubated anaerobically with rat liver microsomes chloramphenicol was transformed to deschloro-chloramphenicol and products that became covalently bound to microsomal proteins (Morris *et al.*, 1983). These reactive products were postulated to be formed either after the first (i.e. the radical resulting from loss of the chloride anion) or second reduction steps (e.g. the carbene resulting from loss of a second chloride anion). Release of the monochloroacetyl moiety in the form of a molecule of monochloroketene (O=C=CHCl) was also postulated.

The last substrate to be discussed here is also a chemically peculiar one. **Nibroxane** (**12.XXXIII**) is a topically effective antimicrobial agent which in the rat was rapidly debrominated to 2-methyl-5-nitro-*m*-dioxane (**12.XXXIV**), a metabolite that underwent further extensive biotransformation (Sullivan *et al.*, 1978). In fact, the *in vivo* reaction of reductive debromination was so rapid that no parent compound was found in the plasma of rats even after high doses. Presumably the strong electron-withdrawing character of the two geminal groups markedly facilitates bioreduction.

12.XXXII

12.XXXIII

12.XXXIV

12.3.4 Halobenzenes

Reductive dehalogenation of halobenzenes is a little studied reaction whose importance is difficult to assess. The reaction has physiological significance in the catabolism of **thyroxine** (3,3',5,5'-tetraiodothyronine; T_4; **12.XXXV**) and lower substituted iodothyronines. Thus, the reductive 5'-deionidation of thyroxine and other iodinated thyronines is catalyzed in rat liver by a microsomal enzyme activated by thiol compounds such as glutathione (Fekkes *et al.*, 1982). Radiographic contrast agents are strong inhibitors of this activity *in vitro* but presumably not *in vivo* if they do not diffuse into cells.

12.XXXV

As far as xenobiotics are concerned, a few cases of reductive aromatic dechlorination have been reported which do not allow robust generalizations to be drawn. When administered to rats, *ortho*-**chlorinated phenols** (**12.XXXVI**) such as 2,6-dichlorophenol and 3-chloro-4-biphenylol gave the corresponding dechlorinated metabolite (**12.XXXVII**) in modest, but not negligible, amounts representing 5–15% of an oral dose (Tulp *et al.*, 1977). The presence of an *ortho*-hydroxyl group appeared to be necessary for reductive dechlorination to occur. However, this structural feature is not present in **hexachlorobenzene** (**12.XXXVIII**), another substrate for the reaction. When hexachlorobenzene was incubated with rat liver microsomes, pentachlorobenzene (**12.XXXIX**) appeared as the initial and major isolatable metabolite (Takazawa and Strobel, 1986). The reaction was shown to be mediated by cytochrome P450 and to be enhanced under

12.XXXVI   12.XXXVII

12.XXXVIII   12.XXXIX

anaerobic conditions. Reductive dechlorination of isolated aromatic chloro substituents has not been observed, and it would be of interest to know which other aromatic substituents render the reaction possible.

12.4 REDUCTION OF NITROGEN-CONTAINING FUNCTIONAL GROUPS

The oxidation of nitrogen-containing groups has been considered in Chapters 5, 6, 9 and 10, showing the chemical and enzymatic complexity of these reactions. Chapter 5 in general and Tables 5.1 and 5.2 in particular are indispensable for a proper understanding of what follows, and the reader is encouraged to commute as often as necessary between Chapter 5 and the present section.

The reactions of reduction discussed in this section are not simpler than reactions of N-oxidation but have been less extensively investigated. Chemically, it will be seen that some reactions of oxidation have a reductive counterpart and must thus be viewed as bioreversible. This is for example true of **N-oxides, nitroso compounds** and **hydroxylamines**, which are metabolites and substrates of oxidative and reductive pathways, respectively. In contrast, the metabolic capacity to reduce **nitro compounds, azo compounds, nitrosamines** and **azido compounds** is not mirrored by their oxidative formation (Lindeke, 1982).

The enzymology of nitrogen reduction is also complex and involves a large variety of enzymes (Mc Lane *et al.*, 1983). Many of these are listed in Section 12.1: e.g. cytochrome P450; NADPH-cytochrome P450 reductase; xanthine and aldehyde oxidases; and quinone reductase. In addition, the gut microflora appears to play a marked role in many reactions of nitrogen reduction (Rowland, 1986). The reactions discussed below cover the vast majority of nitrogen-containing functional groups undergoing metabolic reduction. Whether other groups share the same fate is a distinct possibility awaiting further studies, e.g. the (formally) reductive ring cleavage of benzothiazole (Wilson *et al.*, 1991).

12.4.1 N-Oxides

Reduction of N-oxides to the corresponding tertiary amine is well documented *in vitro* and has also been seen *in vivo* (Bickel, 1969; Mc Lane *et al.*, 1983). Thus, the **N-oxides of psychotropic**

drugs, e.g. chlorpromazine N-oxide (**12.XL**) and amitriptyline N-oxide were completely reduced in the rat, and extensively but not totally in the dog and humans. Reduction occurred in the intestine but also at other sites (Hawes *et al.*, 1991; Jaworski *et al.*, 1991).

A number of *in vitro* investigations have stressed the important but not unique role of **cytochrome P450**. Thus, imipramine N-oxide (**12.XLI**), tiaramide N-oxide and N,N-dimethylaniline N-oxide (**12.XLII**) were reduced anaerobically by rat liver microsomes. Reducers of cytochrome P450 such as flavins (FAD, FMN, or riboflavin) or viologens (methyl viologen or benzyl viologen) markedly stimulated the reaction, implying that the rate-limiting step in the reduction of N-oxides is the reduction of cytochrome P450 (Kato *et al.*, 1978; Sugiura *et al.*, 1976). Two **reaction mechanisms** have been proposed to explain the cytochrome P450-catalyzed reduction of N-oxides. According to the first mechanism, direct oxene transfer occurs from the N-oxide to Fe^{2+} in the reduced enzyme, which is thus oxidized to the ferryl oxide form [Fe(IV)=O] (see Section 12.2.2) (Miyata *et al.*, 1984). The reaction was fast for oxides of tertiary N,N-dimethylated amines, but much slower for aromatic azaheterocycle N-oxides (e.g. quinoline N-oxide).

12.XL   12.XLI   12.XLII

A second mechanism has been rationalized from the N-dealkylation of N-oxides. Here, oxene transfer has been postulated to occur from the N-oxide to Fe^{3+} in the oxidized form of the enzyme, which is thus oxygenated to the perferryl oxide form [Fe(V)=O]. The latter is immediately competent to catalyze N-demethylation either by electron abstraction from the nitrogen atom, or by abstraction of a hydrogen atom from the methyl group (Burka *et al.*, 1985; Heimbrook *et al.*, 1984) (see Section 6.2).

Horseradish peroxidase is another enzyme able to catalyze the deoxygenation of N-oxides (e.g. **12.XLI** and **12.XLII**). In fact, an activity was found in rat liver cytosol whose catalytic properties were modelled well by horseradish peroxidase (Gillespie and Duffel, 1989). Other cytosolic enzymes able to deoxygenate N-oxides are xanthine oxidase and aldehyde oxidase (see Section 9.5) (Beedham, 1985; Kitamura and Tatsumi, 1984). In addition, a reductase was found in the cytosol of rat tissues that was tetrameric, NADPH-specific, metal-free, and reduced N,N-dimethyl-*p*-aminoazobenzene N-oxide with high substrate selectivity (Lashmet Johnson and Ziegler, 1986).

Aryl N-oxides (i.e. N-oxides of aromatic azaheterocycles) have been mentioned above as being less readily reducible than the N-oxides of tertiary amines. More data are needed before this finding can be deemed general or exceptional, but examples do exist to suggest that N-oxides of pyridine-type amines are easily reducible under appropriate conditions. The simple compound nicotinamide N-oxide was not reduced by rabbit liver microsomes, NADPH-cytochrome P450 reductase or cytosolic aldehyde oxidase. However, when the microsomes were combined with the cytosolic enzyme, a significant reductase activity was observed in the presence of NADPH or NADH (Kitamura *et al.*, 1984). This finding led to the proposal of a new electron transport system consisting of liver microsomal NADPH-cytochrome P450 reductase and cytosolic aldehyde oxidase.

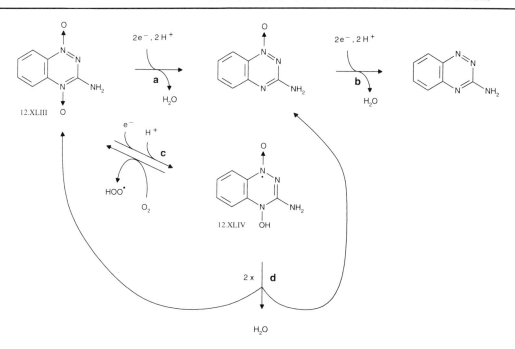

FIGURE 12.5 Postulated reductive metabolism of 3-amino-1,2,4-benzotriazine 1,4-dioxide (**12.XLIII**) by quinone reductase catalyzed two- and four-electron steps (reactions **a** and **b**), and by an NADPH-cytochrome P450 reductase catalyzed one-electron step to a nitroxide believed to be the cytotoxic species (Lloyd *et al.*, 1991; Riley and Workman, 1992b).

An example of particular interest is that of **3-amino-1,2,4-benzotriazine 1,4-dioxide** (**12.XLIII** in Fig. 12.5), a highly selective anticancer agent activated to a potent cytotoxin in hypoxic cells. The compound undergoes two- and four-electron reductions to the mono-N-oxide and to 3-amino-1,2,4-benzotriazine, respectively, in a sequential reaction (reactions **a** and **b** in Fig. 12.5) catalyzed by quinone reductase (Riley and Workman, 1992b). However, these metabolites are inactive and their formation may represent a bioprotection pathway. In contrast, microsomal reduction occurs by one-electron transfer (reaction **c** in Fig. 12.5) catalyzed by NADPH-cytochrome P450 reductase. The product, a radical best described as a nitroxide (**12.XLIV** in Fig. 12.5), is the active cytotoxic species; it is reoxidized by O_2 or appears to disproportionate non-enzymatically to the 1-oxide and the parent drug (reaction **d** in Fig. 12.5) (Lloyd *et al.*, 1991; Walton *et al.*, 1992).

12.4.2 Aromatic nitro compounds

A vast body of knowledge has accumulated on the reduction of aromatic nitro compounds, which have importance as industrial chemicals, drugs, and pollutants. The substrates for nitroreductases are characterized by their large number and structural variety which includes nitrobenzenes, polycyclic nitroarenes, nitroheterocycles, as well as aliphatic nitro compounds which will not receive special attention here (Linhart *et al.*, 1991; Mc Lane *et al.*, 1983).

The **sequential reduction** of aromatic nitro groups to the corresponding primary amine is shown in Fig. 12.6 (Biaglow *et al.*, 1986; Knox *et al.*, 1983; Minchin *et al.*, 1986). One-electron

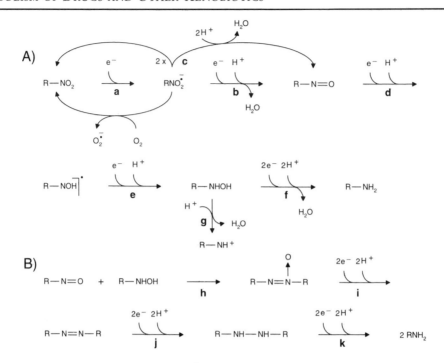

FIGURE 12.6 Steps in the reductive metabolism of aromatic nitro compounds to the corresponding primary amine. Pathway **A**: "direct" pathway; pathway **B**: "indirect" pathway via the azoxy metabolite.

reduction (reaction **a** in Fig. 12.6.A) yields a reactive **nitro anion-radical,** which can either undergo further reduction or be reoxidized by O_2 to the parent compound (futile cycling, see Section 12.2.3). One-electron reduction of the nitro anion-radical (reaction **b** in Fig. 12.6A) gives the stable nitroso metabolite, but it is interesting to note that the latter can also be produced by disproportionation of the former (reaction **c** in Fig. 12.6A). Further reductive steps yield an intermediate nitroxide (reaction **d** in Fig. 12.6A), a stable hydroxylamine (reaction **e** in Fig. 12.6A), and the ultimate primary amine (reaction **f** in Fig. 12.6A).

The **direct pathway** outlined in Fig. 12.6 is not the only one leading from a nitro to a primary amino group. Beside the **disproportionation** of nitro anion-radical, other bimolecular reactions also play a role which may well be more important *in vitro* than *in vivo*. As shown in Fig. 12.6B (reaction **h**), the reaction between a nitroso compound and a hydroxylamine yields an azoxy compound whose stepwise reduction also leads to the primary amine (see also Section 12.4.6). Another reaction occurs between a nitroxide and a protonated nitro radical to yield a hydroxylamine and a nitro compound (Eq. 12.4):

$$R\text{--}NOH^\bullet + R\text{--}NO_2H^\bullet \rightarrow R\text{--}NHOH + R\text{--}NO_2 \tag{Eq. 12.4}$$

As outlined above, the gut microflora also plays a marked role in the *in vivo* reduction of nitro compounds (Rowland, 1986). As for the **mammalian enzymes** able to catalyze nitro reduction, they are found:

- in mitochondria (a strictly NADH-dependent activity, e.g. Abou-Khalil *et al.*, 1985; Köchli *et al.*, 1980);
- in microsomes (cytochrome P450 and NADPH-cytochrome P450 reductase; e.g. Harada and Omura, 1980);

- in the cytosol (xanthine oxidase, aldehyde oxidase and other reductases; e.g. Nakao *et al.*, 1991).

Kinetic studies in rat liver microsomes have indicated that the initial step in the reduction of nitrobenzene is rate-limiting and catalyzed by both cytochrome P450 and NADPH-cytochrome P450 reductase, while nitrosobenzene and phenylhydroxylamine are substrates of the former enzyme only (Harada and Omura, 1980). Synergism between microsomes and cytosol was seen when rat liver preparations reduced the flukicidal agent nitroxynil (**12.XLV**) to the primary amine (Maffei Facino *et al.*, 1982), suggesting that cytochrome P450 and xanthine oxidase might not share the same rate-limiting steps. Indeed, there are indications that the hydroxylamine-to-amine step requires high concentrations of xanthine oxidase (Tatsumi *et al.*, 1981).

Numerous model compounds and simple industrial chemicals have been examined for nitro reduction (Rickert, 1987). In **nitrobenzenes**, the presence of a neutral, electron-withdrawing substituent facilitates reduction, the effect being maximal with *para*-substituents. Thus, the ease of reduction by a mitochondrial nitroreductase was found to decrease in the sequence 1,4-dinitrobenzene > niridazole (**12.LVII**, see below) > 4-nitrobenzaldehyde > 1,3-dinitrobenzene > 2-nitrobenzaldehyde > 4-nitrobenzyl alcohol > 4-nitroacetophenone > 3-nitrobenzaldehyde > nitrobenzene; 4-nitrobenzoate and 3-nitrophenol were not substrates (Köchli *et al.*, 1980). Using xanthine oxidase and a large number of model substrates, it was also found that electron-withdrawing *para*-substituents greatly facilitate reduction (e.g. $CO-C_6H_5$ > CHO > $CO-CH_3$ > NO_2 > $COOCH_3$ > $CONH_2$ > CN) (Tatsumi *et al.*, 1978). Electron-withdrawing *meta*- and *ortho*-substituents had less influence, but some electron-donating meta-substituents did facilitate reduction.

The same type of structure–metabolism relationship holds in isolated hepatocytes, with the additional observation that nitro reduction elicits cytotoxicity. Thus, the cytotoxicity of *para*-substituted nitrobenzenes was a function of their one-electron reduction potential, the more toxic compounds having the strongest electron-withdrawing substituents. It was concluded that aerobic toxicity is probably initiated by redox cycling of nitro anion-radicals and superoxide production, whereas hypoxic toxicity is probably due to alkylation of macromolecules by nitroso metabolites (O'Brien *et al.*, 1990).

12.XLV   12.XLVI   12.XLVII

Polycyclic aromatic nitro compounds (nitro-PAHs, e.g. **12.XLVI** and **12.XLVII**) have received considerable interest in recent years due to the marked genotoxicity displayed by many of these compounds, e.g. mutagenicity and carcinogenicity (Sera *et al.*, 1992). Nitro-PAHs are environmental pollutants produced by combustion and are found for example in diesel exhaust and urban aerosols. Carbon oxidation producing potent electrophiles such as diol-epoxides and quinones is one of the molecular mechanisms of their toxicity (Section 4.3) and is influenced by the presence of the nitro group(s) (Fu, 1990; Rickert, 1987). However, **nitro reduction** is also a route of toxication, and quantum mechanical calculations have revealed that the mutagenicity of these compounds is inversely correlated with the energy of their LUMO (lowest unoccupied molecular orbital) (Maynard *et al.*, 1986). In other words, the lower the energy of the LUMO and the greater its ease to accept an electron (thus reducing the nitro compound to an anion-radical), the greater the mutagenic activity. Interestingly, the energy of the LUMO is lowest when the nitro group is coplanar with the ring system, and it increases with increasing value of the dihedral angle. It has been verified experimentally that little or no mutagenic activity is displayed by nitroarenes in which steric hindrance forces the nitro group out of coplanarity (Fu, 1990).

The **mechanism of this genotoxicity** is not well understood but may involve the covalent binding to DNA of reduced metabolites, presumably the hydroxylamine or more likely the **nitrenium ion** (see Section 12.4.3). Covalent binding of nitroso metabolites to hemoglobin and other proteins by reaction with thiol groups to form **sulfinamides** is another biological hazard of nitroarenes (Suzuki *et al.*, 1989) (Eq. 12.5):

$$R'-SH + R-N=O \rightarrow R'-SO-NH-R \qquad \text{(Eq. 12.5)}$$

Probably the most studied nitro-PAH is **1-nitropyrene** (**12.XLVI**), a known carcinogen and mutagen whose DNA binding follows reduction. The compound is reduced *in vitro* by xanthine oxidase, aldehyde oxidase, cytochrome P450, or human intestinal microflora; *in vivo* reduction was seen for example in rabbits and newborn mice (El-Bayoumy *et al.*, 1988; Fu, 1990; Howard and Beland, 1982; Tatsumi and Amano, 1987). Another compound of interest is **6-nitrochrysene** (**12.XLVII**), one of the most active nitro-PAHs examined to date (Fu, 1990).

12.4.3 Aromatic nitro compounds of medicinal interest

The aromatic nitro group is of great importance in medicinal chemistry and is mainly found attached to benzene rings and aromatic five-membered heterocycles. In **medicinal nitrobenzenes**, the nitro group usually plays a favourable but not critical role, whereas in the chemotherapeutic nitroheterocycles discussed later the nitro group is essential for activity. **5-(aziridin-1-yl)-2,4-dinitrobenzamide** (CB1954; **12.XLVIII**) is a potential antitumour agent activated by reduction to a cytotoxic DNA interstrand cross-linking agent. This is achieved by reduction of the 4-nitro group to the corresponding hydroxylamine, a bioactivation observed in sensitive cell lines but which was very slow in insensitive cell lines (Boland *et al.*, 1991; Knox *et al.*, 1992). The reduction was mediated by rat quinone reductase but not by the human form of the enzyme, explaining why no sensitive cell lines of human origin were found.

While nitro reduction may account for the chemotherapeutic activity of CB1954, it seems to be related to unwanted side-effects in the case of the non-steroidal anti-androgen derivative

12.XLVIII   12.XLIX

nilutamide (**12.XLIX**). The compound was found to undergo *in vivo* reduction to the amino metabolite, and in rat liver microsomes was reduced by NADPH-cytochrome P450 reductase (Berson *et al.*, 1991). Under aerobic conditions, the nitro anion-radical was rapidly reoxidized by O_2 (futile cycling), forming reactive oxygen species. Under anaerobic conditions, reduction led to covalent binding, presumably of the nitroso and hydroxylamino metabolites. It was postulated that the hepatitis seen in some patients might be caused by oxygen stress and/or covalent binding.

In vivo reduction to the amino metabolite was observed as an important reaction of **acenocoumarol** (**12.L**) in humans (Dieterle *et al.*, 1977). Similarly, administration of **nimetazepam** (**12.LI**; R = CH_3) or **nitrazepam** (**12.LI**; R = H) to dogs resulted in the urinary and faecal excretion of sizeable amounts of the corresponding primary amine (Yanagi *et al.*, 1976). In contrast, no nitro reduction of nitecapone (**12.IV**) was seen in humans (Taskinen *et al.*, 1991).

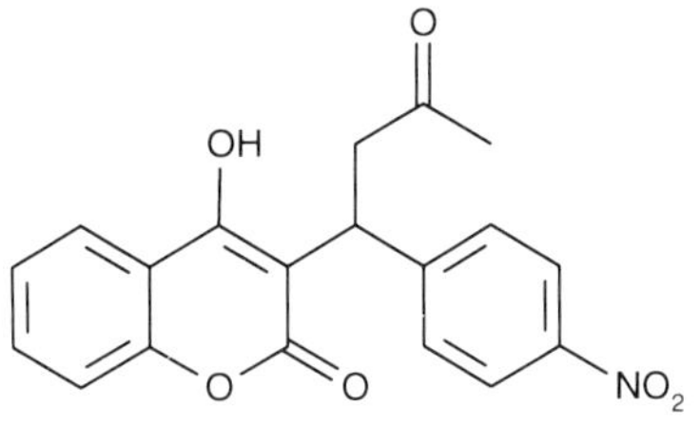

12.L

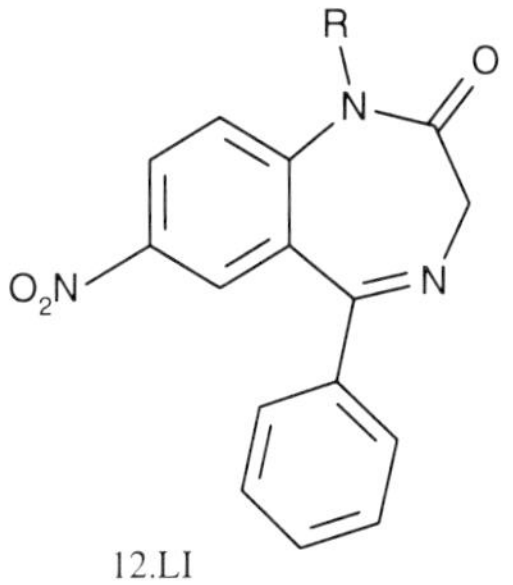

12.LI

Nitroheterocyclic compounds are an important group of chemotherapeutic agents activated by reduction (Biaglow *et al.*, 1986; Goldman *et al.*, 1986; Kedderis and Miwa, 1988). Noteworthy are **nitroimidazoles** such as benznidazole (**12.LII**), metronidazole (**12.LIII**) and misonidazole (**12.LIV**), **nitrothiazoles** such as niridazole (**12.LV**), and **nitrofurans** such as nitrofurantoin, nitrofurazone (**12.LVI**) and furazolidone (**12.LVII** in Fig. 12.7).

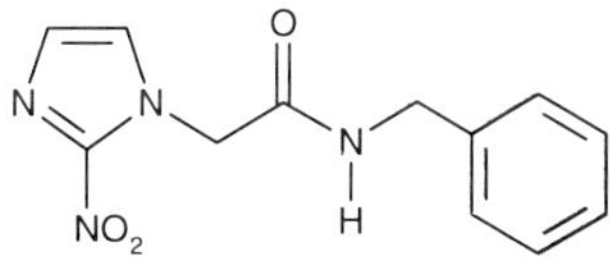

12.LII

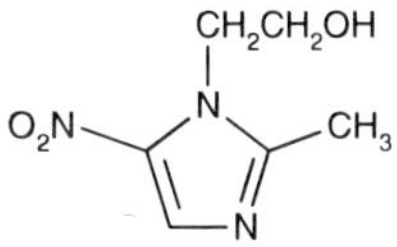

12.LIII

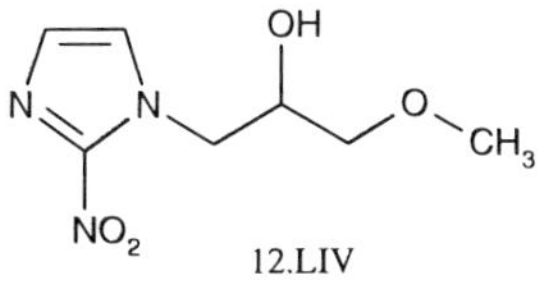

12.LIV

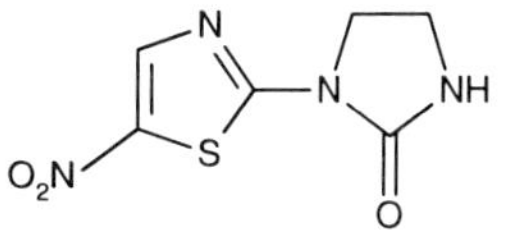

12.LV

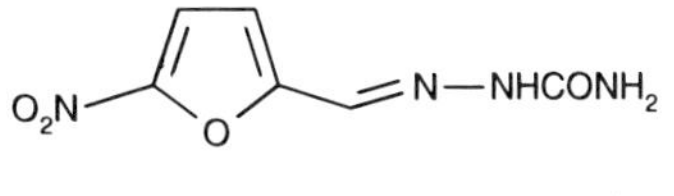

12.LVI

In heterocyclic as well as in carbocyclic nitro derivatives, the first reductive step appears rate-limiting and is related to the ease of acceptance of one electron. Thus, the proportion of reduced metabolites found in the urine of germ-free rats was large for **misonidazole (12.LIV)**, intermediate for **nitrofurazone (12.LVI)**, and small for **metronidazole (12.LIII)**, while the one-electron reduction potential of these drugs decreases in the same order (Yeung et al., 1983). Comparable relations were found for the one-electron reduction of various nitroheterocyclic drugs catalyzed by rat liver microsomes, xanthine oxidase, ferredoxin reductase, and NADPH-cytochrome P450 reductase (Clarke et al., 1982; Dubin et al., 1991; Orna and Mason, 1989).

The reductive metabolism of nitroheterocyclic drugs is usually complex and involves a variety of metabolites (Kedderis and Miwa, 1988). This appeared to be the case for **benznidazole (12.LII)** administered to mice, with the parent drug and its amino metabolite each accounting for only a few per cent of the dose (Walton and Workman, 1987). The complexity of nitroheterocycle metabolism is particularly well illustrated by **furazolidone (12.LVII in Fig. 12.7)**, which undergoes profound structural modifications following its metabolic reduction. The scheme presented in Fig. 12.7 summarizes results obtaining in rat liver microsomes but not restricted to this animal species (Tatsumi et al., 1984; Vroomen et al., 1987). A key metabolite appears to be the hydroxylamine, which can be further reduced to the primary amine (**12.LVIII in Fig. 12.7**) or rearranged by ring opening to a nitrile (**12.LIX in Fig. 12.7**) also seen in the urine of rabbits dosed orally. Hydrolysis of the nitrile **12.LIX in Fig. 12.7** and further degradation have been postulated to account for the formation of α-ketoglutaric acid (**12.LX in Fig. 12.7**). Not shown in Fig. 12.7 is a dimeric metabolite perhaps resulting from the coupling of the hydroxylamine with the parent drug.

Ring cleavage was also seen in the metabolism of **metronidazole (12.LIII)** in rats (Koch and Goldman, 1979). Indeed, reduction to the amine followed by hydrolytic steps led to the formation of N-(2-hydroxyethyl)oxamic acid, an open chain metabolite.

The above discussion leaves open the **nature of the active metabolite** of nitroheterocycles,

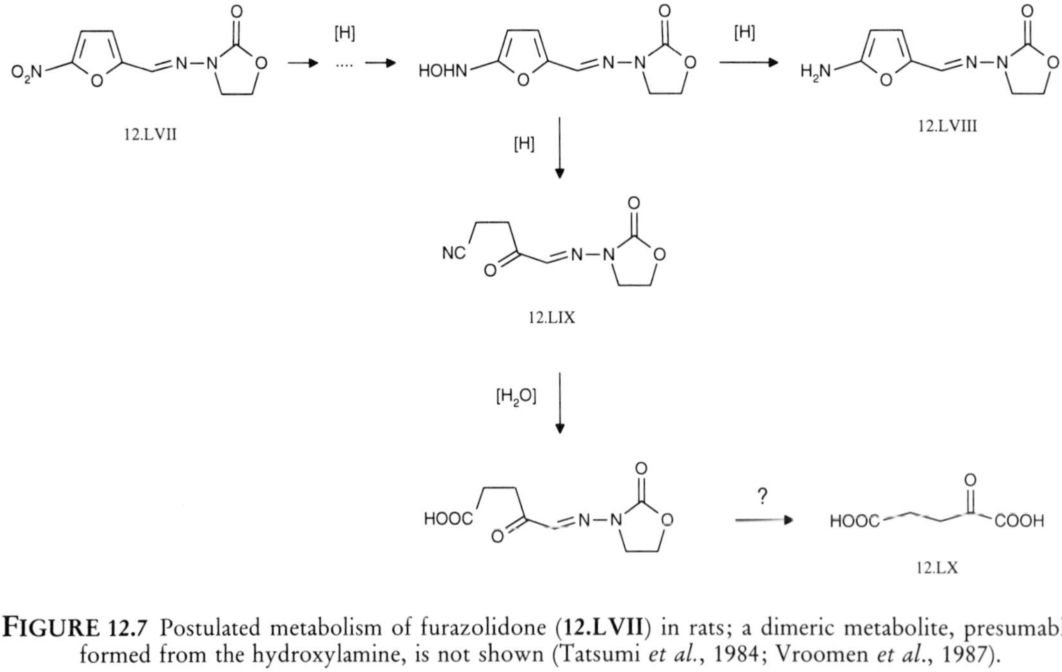

FIGURE 12.7 Postulated metabolism of furazolidone (**12.LVII**) in rats; a dimeric metabolite, presumably formed from the hydroxylamine, is not shown (Tatsumi et al., 1984; Vroomen et al., 1987).

i.e. the reactive species that acts as a bactericide and a parasiticide, and more generally as a cytotoxin. While the nitro anion-radical metabolites are long-lived enough to leak out of hepatocytes, they do not bind covalently to proteins, nucleic acids or thiol compounds such as glutathione (Polnaszek *et al.*, 1984; Rao *et al.*, 1988). Our current understanding is that nitroheterocycles, like other aromatic nitro compounds, undergo futile cycling under aerobic conditions (Fig. 12.6A) and are activated to their toxic metabolites only under hypoxic or anaerobic conditions. Because covalent binding is increased under mildly acidic conditions, there are good reasons to postulate that the active species is a **nitrenium ion** formed from the hydroxylamino metabolite (reaction **g** in Fig. 12.6A) (Streeter and Hoener, 1988).

12.4.4 Compounds containing other N–O moieties

The previous section discusses nitroso compounds, nitroxides and hydroxylamines as intermediate metabolites in the reduction of aromatic nitro compounds (Fig. 12.6). In addition, it is obvious that such intermediates may also undergo reduction when entering the body as xenobiotics. Among **nitrosoarenes**, 1-nitroso-2-naphthol and *p*-nitrosophenol were rapidly reduced by rat liver quinone reductase, while nitrosobenzene was a poor substrate. **N-Nitroso compounds** (nitrosamines, see Section 12.4.6) were not reduced (Hajos and Winston, 1992; Koga *et al.*, 1990).

12.LXI

But while nitroalkanes are absent from the previous section, it is of interest that the bioreduction of **nitrosoalkanes**, aliphatic nitroxides and aliphatic hydroxylamines is reasonably well documented. Consider for example **1-nitrosoadamantane (12.LXI)**, which was reduced aerobically to N-hydroxy-1-aminoadamantane but not to 1-aminoadamantane by an NADPH-dependent microsomal enzyme present in various animal tissues (Bélanger and Grech-Bélanger, 1978). This substrate is a tertiary C-nitrosoalkane, and like aromatic nitroso compounds it cannot isomerize to an oxime. Indeed, the nitroso–oxime isomerization (reaction **a** in Fig. 12.8) is what renders more complex the biochemistry of nitrosoalkanes having a hydrogen atom on the alpha-carbon. Such oximes may hydrolyze to a carbonyl compound and hydroxylamine (see Chapter 5). Oximes undergo reduction less readily than nitroso compounds, but the reaction is facilitated by a decrease in pH and yields the amine (reactions **b** and **c** in Fig. 12.8) (Lindeke, 1982). A few nitrosoalkanes, formed as metabolites of aliphatic amines (e.g. amphetamines) are known to be reduced (Coutts and Beckett, 1977; Lindeke, 1982).

In the absence of marked steric hindrance, nitroso compounds can also dimerize (reaction **d** in Fig. 12.8), or react with hydroxylamines to form azoxy compounds (reaction **h** in Fig. 12.7) (Lindeke, 1982). Reduction of the latter is documented (see Section 12.4.6), but it does not appear to be known whether nitroso dimers as such can be reduced.

Nitroxides formed as intermediate metabolites and nitroxides used as spin labels are also reduced in biological systems (Kappus, 1986). Thus, stable nitroxide radicals such as the spin labels 2,2,6,6-tetramethylpiperidine-1-oxyl (**12.LXII**) and di-*tert*-butyl nitroxide (**12.LXIV**) were

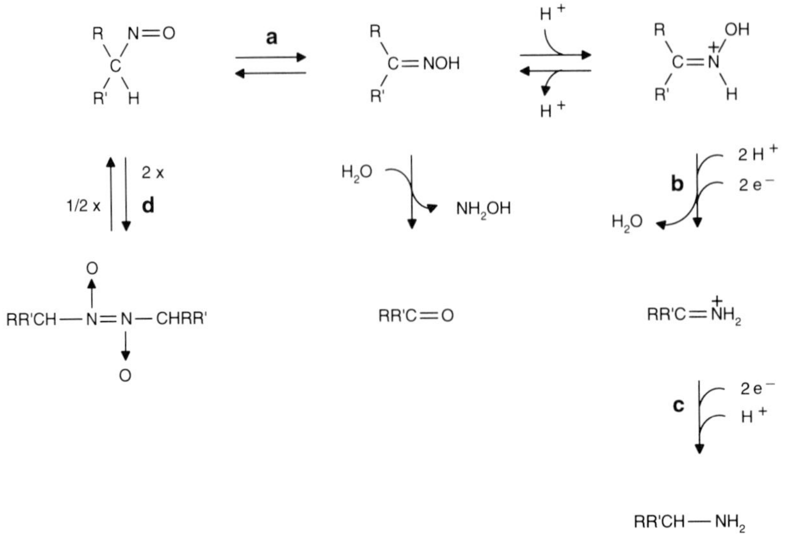

FIGURE 12.8 Chemical reactions of isomerization and hydrolysis, and enzymatic reactions of reduction, in the metabolism of primary and secondary nitrosoalkanes (Lindeke, 1982).

reduced by rat liver microsomal cytochrome P450 to the corresponding hydroxylamines (**12.LXIII** and **12.LXV**, respectively), while for unknown reasons 2-ethyl-2,4,4-trimethyl-3-oxazolidine-3-oxyl was not a substrate (Rosen *et al.*, 1977). This reaction is believed to involve a one-electron reduction to the hydroxylamine anion, followed by protonation.

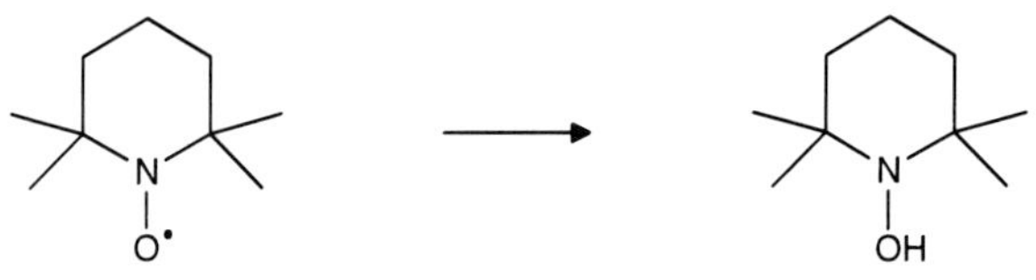

Interestingly, **non-enzymatic reductions of nitroxides** have also been reported (see also Section 13.2). A simple example is the reduction of a derivative of **12.LXII**, N-succinyl-4-amino-2,2,6,6-tetramethylpiperidine-1-oxyl, by ascorbic acid in rat liver and kidney ultrafiltrates and cytosol (Eriksson *et al.*, 1987). An even more complex non-enzymatic reaction has been uncovered in which nitroxides are reduced to hydroxylamines by superoxide in the presence of thiols under biomimetic conditions (Finkelstein *et al.*, 1984). The relevance of these findings for the *in vivo* metabolism of nitro compounds and amines may prove difficult to assess.

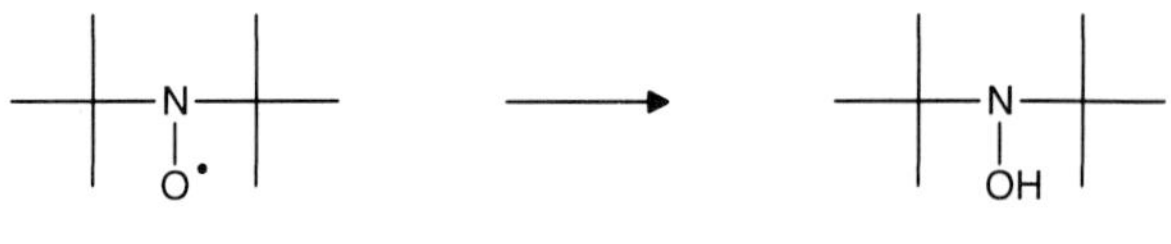

The reduction of aromatic and aliphatic **hydroxylamines** follows from what has been discussed at the beginning of this section. Numerous *in vitro* and *in vivo* examples document the formation of primary or secondary amines from the corresponding hydroxylamine (Clement and Kunze, 1992; Coutts and Beckett, 1977; Lindeke, 1982). Interestingly, the NADH-cytochrome b_5 reductase/cytochrome b_5 system was found to be readily active in reducing N-hydroxyamphetamine (**12.LXVI**) to amphetamine (**12.LXVII**) in NADH-fortified guinea-pig liver microsomes (Yamada *et al.*, 1988). These findings complement what has been discussed in Section 12.4.2 about the enzymology of hydroxylamine reduction.

12.LXVI   12.LXVII

Hydroxamic acids (hydroxylamides) represent a separate class of hydroxylamines with marked toxicological significance (Lindeke, 1982). N-Arylhydroxamic acids such as salicylhydroxamic acid (**12.LXVIII**) and nicotinylhydroxamic acid were reduced anaerobically by aldehyde oxidase to salicylamide (**12.LXIX**) and nicotinamide, respectively (Sugihara and Tatsumi, 1986). A number of other hydroxamic acids were similarly reduced, the rate of reaction being markedly dependent on the nature of the electron donor added to the preparations. Examples of good electron donors (reducing substrates; see Section 9.5) are 2-hydroxypyrimidine and benzaldehyde. Other reducible hydroxamic acids include N-hydroxyurethane (**12.LXX**) (Beedham, 1985).

12.LXVIII   12.LXIX

12.LXX

An intriguing metabolic pathway is the **reductive opening of the 1,2-isoxazole ring**, as seen in the metabolism of the anticonvulsant agent zonisamide (**12.LXXI** in Fig. 12.9). When administered to rats, a major pathway was reduction to an imino intermediate which was not excreted as such but underwent mainly hydrolysis to form a ketone (**12.LXXII** in Fig. 12.9) or further reduction to an amine (**12.LXXIII** in Fig. 12.9) (Stiff and Zemaitis, 1990). The reductive ring opening is a reaction of dihydrogenation and as such must involve transfer of two electrons. Microsomal **cytochrome P450** (preferably under anaerobic conditions) appears to mediate this reaction, while the intestinal microflora was inactive (Stiff *et al.*, 1992). Proof now exists that the reductive ring opening in zonisamide is catalyzed mainly by CYP3A enzymes in human and rat liver microsomes under anaerobic conditions (Nakasa *et al.*, 1993a and 1993b). Note that the same reaction was seen years ago in the metabolism of isoxathion, an insecticide which underwent extensive biotransformation in the rat via its primary metabolite 3-hydroxy-5-phenylisoxazole (**12.LXXIV**) (Ando *et al.*, 1975). This product was then reduced *in vivo* and *in vitro* (NADPH-fortified rat liver 9000 **g** supernatant) to benzoylacetamide (**12.LXXV**).

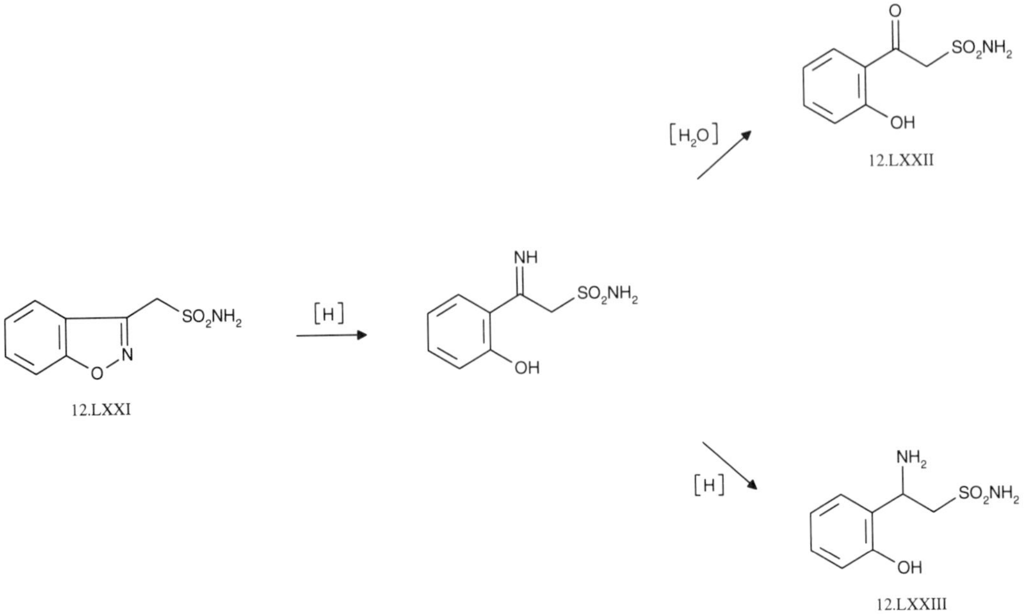

FIGURE 12.9 Reductive opening of the 1,2-isoxazole ring as a major route in the metabolism of zonisamide (**12.LXXI**) (Stiff and Zemaitis, 1990).

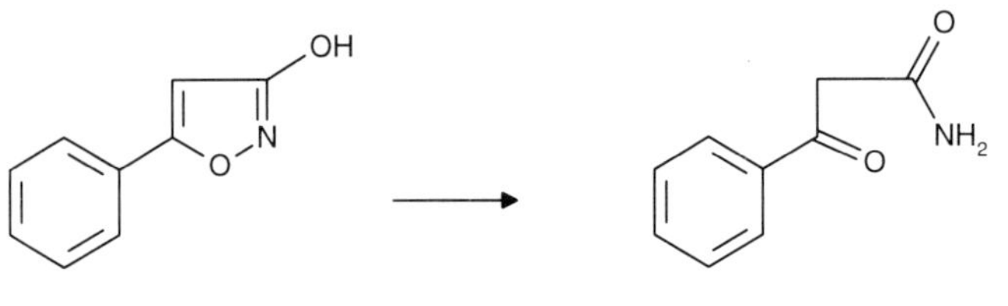

12.4.5 Medicinal bioprecursors of nitric oxide

Nitric oxide (NO, in fact the diatomic radical NO•) is currently a molecule of immense interest due to the discovery of its many physiological roles. One of the most important effects of NO is activation of guanylate cyclase, which underlies many of its cardiovascular and neural actions. The endothelium-derived relaxing factor (EDRF), a physiological regulator of blood vessel tone, has thus been identified as NO. In addition, nitric oxide is a central and peripheral neuronal messenger, it can elicit neuroprotective and neurodestructive effects, and it also contributes to immune function (Feldman *et al.*, 1993; Lipton *et al.*, 1993; McCall and Vallance, 1992).

Nitric oxide is synthetized from L-arginine via N^{ω}-hydroxy-L-arginine by a reaction whose mechanism is progressively being understood (Fukuto *et al.*, 1992). This reaction is catalyzed by NO synthase, an enzyme having close homology with NADPH-cytochrome P450 reductase and containing both FAD and FMN. In addition to opening a seemingly unlimited area of drug research, nitric oxide convincingly explains the mechanism of action of the well-known vasodilators discussed in this section, e.g. nitrate esters and nitrite esters. NO can also be produced as a metabolite of nitrosamines (see Section 12.4.6).

Glyceryl trinitrate (GTN, **12.LXXVI**) is the prototypal organic nitrate with potent vasodilating activity. In mammals, GTN is denitrated to two dinitrates and two mononitrates by the action of cytosolic **glutathione S-transferases** (see the volume in this series, *Biochemistry of Conjugation Reactions*) or **hemoglobin**, but simple thiols such as cysteine or N-acetylcysteine are also able to denitrate GTN to both nitric oxide and nitrite ions (Feelisch and Noack, 1987; Lau and Benet, 1990). In addition, hepatic and probably also vascular **cytochrome P450** has been shown to catalyze the denitration of GTN and other organic nitrates (Delaforge *et al.*, 1993; McDonald and Bennett, 1990; Schröder, 1992). Of special interest is the experimental proof that during the cytochrome P450-mediated reduction of GTN, nitric oxide is formed and binds to ferrocytochrome P450 (Servent *et al.*, 1989).

$$CH_2\!-\!ONO_2$$
$$|$$
$$CH\!-\!ONO_2$$
$$|$$
$$CH_2\!-\!ONO_2$$

12.LXXVI

$$CH_3$$
$$\diagdown$$
$$CH\!-\!CH_2\!-\!ONO$$
$$\diagup$$
$$CH_3$$

12.LXXVII

Evidence exists that both **organic nitrates** and **organic nitrites** are transformed into NO in vascular tissues, but the enzymes involved are still being debated and appear to be tissue-dependent (see above) and distinct for the two classes of drugs. Thus, isobutyl nitrite (**12.LXXVII**) and amyl nitrite are activated to NO in the cytosol and to a lesser extent in microsomes of vascular smooth muscles. In contrast, organic nitrates are activated in the plasma membrane of such tissues (Bennett *et al.*, 1992; Chung and Fung, 1992; Feelisch and Kelm, 1991; Kowaluk and Fung, 1991; Yeates, 1992).

Nitroprusside, $[Fe(CN)_5NO]^{2-}$, is also a potent hypotensive agent usually used as the sodium salt. This compound contains a nitrosonium ion (NO^+, the oxidized form of $NO^\bullet$), and acts by being a bioprecursor of nitric oxide. The biochemical reaction is only partly understood, but a number of reducing agents including thiols, ascorbic acid, ferrous chloride, hemoglobin, myoglobin, NADPH plus cytochrome P450, and NADPH-cytochrome P450 reductase can transfer electrons to nitroprusside and thus mediate the reduction of NO^+ and the release of $NO^\bullet$. Vascular tissues and human plasma are also active (Bates *et al.*, 1991; Rao *et al.*, 1991).

12.4.6 Compounds containing dinitrogen moieties

A variety of functional groups containing two or even three nitrogen atoms are of interest in the present context. This section will consider in turn nitrosamines, azo compounds and hydrazines, while triazenes and azido compounds will be discussed in the next section. The oxidative metabolism of some of these moieties has been discussed in previous chapters (see hydrazines and azo derivatives in Section 5.7).

Nitrosamines (N-nitroso compounds) have attracted much interest due to their carcinogenic and mutagenic potential. Besides oxidative metabolism (Section 6.5), a few of these compounds have also been shown to undergo reductive metabolism by either one-electron or two-electron mechanisms. Two consecutive two-electron steps reduce nitrosamines such as N-nitrosodiphenylamine (**12.LXXVIII** in Fig. 12.10; R = R′ = phenyl) to the corresponding 1,1-disubstituted hydrazine (reactions **a** and **b** in Fig. 12.10). This reaction is catalyzed by **aldehyde oxidase** and has been seen in guinea-pig liver 9000 **g** supernatant (anaerobic conditions) and in guinea-pigs *in vivo*. Cyclic nitrosamines such as N-nitrosomorpholine and N-nitrosopyrrolidine also formed the corresponding hydrazine (Tatsumi *et al.*, 1983a and 1983b).

The mechanism of aldehyde oxidase-catalyzed reduction of nitrosamines is not well elucidated, but there are indications that a 1-hydroxyhydrazine may be formed as an intermediate

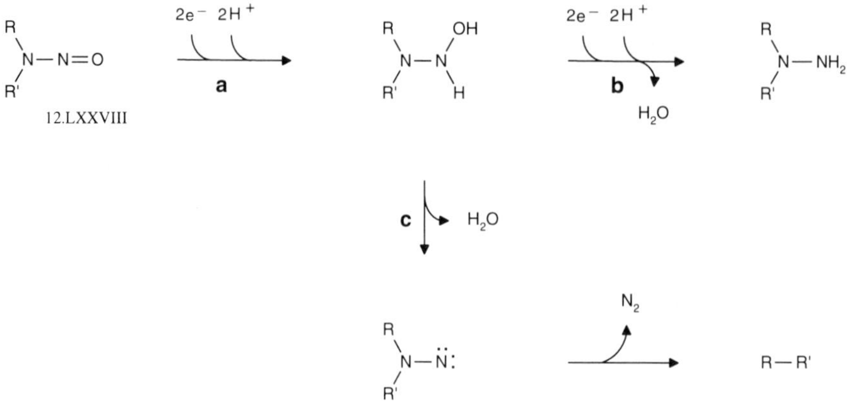

FIGURE 12.10 Postulated mechanisms in the two-electron reductive metabolism of nitrosamines to hydrazines or molecular nitrogen.

by reaction **a** in Fig. 12.10. Such 1-hydroxyhydrazines are unstable and break down to predictable products, and the sequence of reactions **a** and **c** in Fig. 12.10 nicely explains the formation of bibenzyl ($C_6H_5CH_2$–$CH_2C_6H_5$) from N-nitrosodibenzylamine (**12.LXXVIII** in Fig. 12.10; R = R′ = benzyl) in rabbit whole liver homogenates under anaerobic conditions (Gal *et al.*, 1978).

One-electron microsomal reduction of a few nitrosamines has been postulated to be catalyzed by **NADPH-cytochrome P450 reductase** and/or **cytochrome P450**. The reaction has been proposed to involve a reductive denitrosation whose mechanism closely resembles reductive dehalogenation (Section 12.3). Thus, N-nitroso-N-methylaniline was metabolized by mouse liver microsomes to nitric oxide and N-methylaniline as primary products (Scheper *et al.*, 1991). The involvement of NADPH-cytochrome P450 reductase was demonstrated in the reductive denitrosation of 1-(2-chloroethyl)-3-cyclohexyl-1-nitrosourea (**12.LXXIX**; CCNU), an anti-tumour agent (Potter and Reed, 1983).

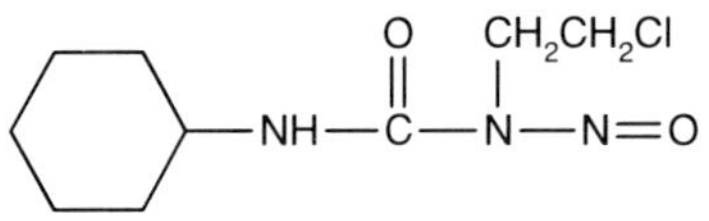

12.LXXIX

The little information available in the literature suggests that the reduction of **azoxy compounds** (reaction **i** in Fig. 12.6B) is markedly slower than that of N-oxides and azo compounds (Zbaida and Levine, 1992). In contrast, **aromatic azo compounds** and particularly azo dyes have received considerable attention in connection with the carcinogenicity of some congeners (Levine, 1991) (see below). Their reduction by two-electron steps to primary aromatic amines is shown in Fig. 12.6B (reactions **j** and **k**). Azo reduction has been seen *in vivo* and intestinal bacteria, microsomes (cytochrome P450 and NADPH-cytochrome P450 reductase), and cytosol (quinone reductase and aldehyde oxidase). The relative contribution of any one of these enzymes remains a poorly understood function of the substrate and of biological factors (Beedham, 1985; Mc Lane *et al.*, 1983; Rowland, 1986).

Azo dyes are exemplified by amaranth (**12.LXXX**), which was extensively reduced *in vivo* to highly polar and readily excretable aminonaphthalene sulfonic acids (Phillips *et al.*, 1987). In contrast, other azo dyes such as Congo red (**12.LXXXI**) liberate the carcinogen benzidine by reduction (Levine, 1991). An example of great historical interest is Prontosil (**12.LXXXII**), an antibacterial shown in 1935 to be inactive *per se* but to undergo *in vivo* activation by reduction to sulfanilamide (**12.LXXXIII**) (Tréfouël *et al.*, 1935). This epoch-making discovery opened the door to the discovery of antibacterial, hypoglycaemic and diuretic sulfonamides (Shepherd, 1970).

Some interesting studies have been published on the **structure–metabolism relationships** of azo reduction, be they catalyzed by intestinal microflora or liver azo reductases (Chung and Cerniglia, 1992). Thus, bacterial reductase was approximately two orders of magnitude more effective than liver reductase in reducing water-soluble, sulfonated azo dyes, while lipid-soluble azo dyes were not reduced by either enzyme system (Nambara and Yamaha, 1975). In another study, the reduction of azo dyes by rat liver 10,000 **g** supernatant was shown to be inversely correlated with partition coefficient, with the more lipophilic compounds being slowly but nevertheless detectably reduced. Recent studies using purified enzymes have been more informative, showing for example that water-soluble and charged azo dyes are good substrates of liver **aldehyde oxidase**, while lipophilic analogues are poor substrates of this enzyme but are

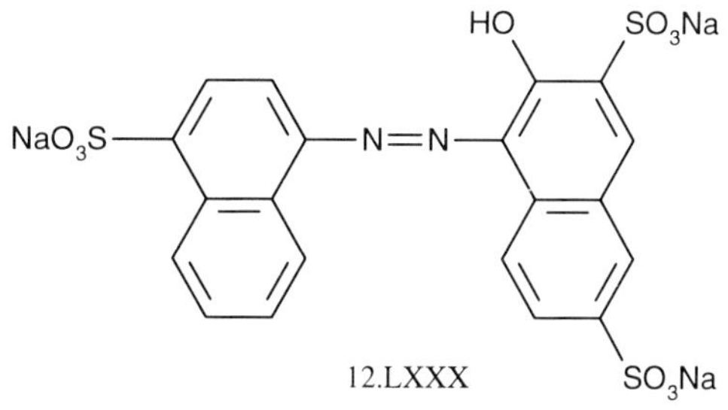

12.LXXX

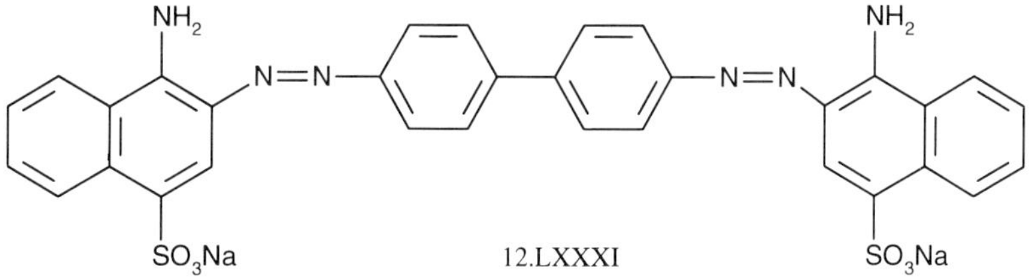

12.LXXXI

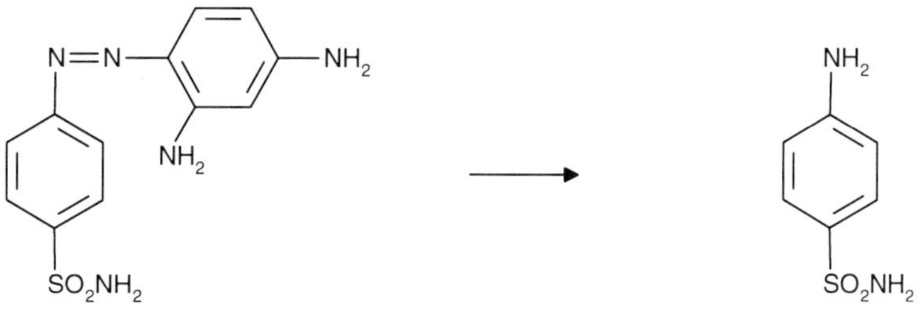

12.LXXXII

12.LXXXIII

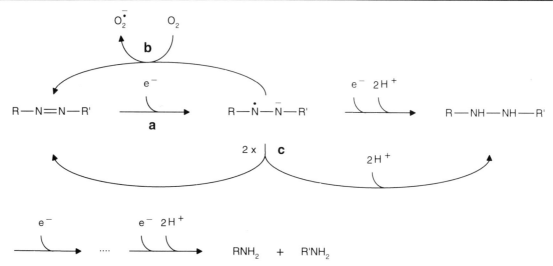

FIGURE 12.11 Postulated mechanism of the cytochrome P450-catalyzed reduction of aromatic azo compounds. Note the role of the azo anion-radical in futile redox cycling (reaction **b**) and disproportionation (reaction **c**).

readily reduced by **cytochrome P450** (Stoddart and Levine, 1992). Also and mechanistically more relevant, higher rates of reduction were observed for those dyes containing electron-withdrawing substituents, while in general azo compounds with the least negative charge on the nitrogens are the most easily reduced (Bragger *et al.*, 1993; Shargel *et al.*, 1984) (see also below).

The **cytochrome P450-catalyzed reduction** of azo compounds occurs by single-electron steps (Fig. 12.11; see also Fig. 12.6B). The first of these steps (reaction **a** in Fig. 12.11) yields the azo anion-radical intermediate which can either be reoxidized by O_2 to the parent azo compound (futile redox cycling; reaction **b** in Fig. 12.11), or disproportionate to the azo and hydrazino compounds (reaction **c** in Fig. 12.11), or undergo further reduction to the hydrazine and thence to the corresponding primary amines via an unknown intermediate (Mason *et al.*, 1978; Mc Lane *et al.*, 1983). Careful studies using liver microsomal preparations or reconstituted cytochrome P450 systems have revealed that derivatives of azobenzene can be classified into three groups (Levine, 1991; Levine *et al.*, 1992; Zbaida and Levine, 1990, 1991 and 1992; Zbaida *et al.*, 1992). The **non-substrates** lack a polar electron-donating substituent, e.g. azobenzene (**12.LXXXIV**; X = H) and its 4-isopropyl and 4-nitro derivatives (**12.LXXXIV**; X = isopropyl or nitro,

12.LXXXIV

respectively); the corresponding hydrazines are also non-substrates. The substrates are characterized by the presence of a relatively polar electron-donating substituent such as –OH or –N(CH$_3$)$_2$, and they exhibit a positive, irreversible potential which permits electron transfer to the dye. The substrates may be further subdivided into two groups:

- Those whose microsomal reduction is insensitive to carbon monoxide and oxygen. These **I substrates**, as they have been called, are exemplified by 4-dimethylaminoazobenzene (DAB, **12.LXXXIV**; X = N(CH$_3$)$_2$). Their microsomal reduction is catalyzed mainly by cytochrome P450;

- Those whose microsomal reduction is sensitive to CO and O_2. These so-called **S substrates** (e.g. 4'-carboxy-4-dimethylaminoazobenzene) are characterized by the presence on the second ring (i.e. the one not bearing the electron-donating substituent) of an additional substituent of high polarity and electron-withdrawing capacity (e.g. –COOH, –COOCH$_3$, –SO$_3$H). The microsomal reduction of S substrates appears to be catalyzed by both NADPH-cytochrome P450 reductase and cytochrome P450.

In addition to the positive potential, both I and S substrates also exhibit two negative potentials, which are less negative in S substrates. This fact is consistent with the faster reduction of S substrates by liver microsomes.

The connection between azo reduction and **toxicity** is not always fully understood. Liberation of a benzidine molecule by azo reduction must be considered as a reaction of toxication since benzidine may then be activated to carcinogenic products by N-oxidation (Section 5.5) and, possibly, by subsequent conjugations. For a number of other azo compounds, the primary amines liberated by reduction are not carcinogenic but may be mutagenic. This is particularly the case for carcinogenic azo compounds such as DAB (**12.LXXXIV**; X = N(CH$_3$)$_2$). Here, toxication is due to activation of the dimethylamino group, first by N-demethylation (Section 6.2), then by N-oxygenation (Section 5.5), and ultimately by conjugation, to electrophilic intermediates (e.g. nitrenium ions) that bind to DNA and other nucleophilic biomolecules. For DAB and analogues, the azo group appears to exert an electronic influence that facilitates these toxication reactions, and azo reduction must indeed be viewed as a reaction of detoxication because: (a) toxication of the dimethylamino group is no longer facilitated; and (b) the products of reductive cleavage are small primary amines of moderate toxicity. Two excellent reviews should be consulted for lucid and detailed discussions (Levine, 1991; Martin and Kennelly, 1985).

Our knowledge of the reduction of **hydrazines** is derived mainly from their involvement as metabolic intermediates between aromatic azo compounds and primary aromatic amines. Few studies have examined the reduction of hydrazines *per se*, and as a consequence only limited data are available on the reduction of hydrazides and aliphatic hydrazines. Hydrazine itself is metabolized in rats by a variety of pathways, one of which is reduction to NH$_3$ (Sanins *et al.*, 1992). A suggestion that hydrazides might undergo reductive cleavage can be found in the metabolism of iproclozide (**12.LXXXV**), a MAO inhibitor containing an aliphatic hydrazine function (de Sagher *et al.*, 1975). Indeed, humans receiving this drug were found to excrete a small fraction of the dose as *p*-chlorophenoxyacetamide (**12.LXXXVI**). While the mechanism of formation of this metabolite was not clarified, reductive cleavage can reasonably be assumed.

Cl—⟨benzene ring⟩—O—CH$_2$—CO—NHNH—CH(CH$_3$)$_2$

12.LXXXV

↓

Cl—⟨benzene ring⟩—O—CH$_2$—CONH$_2$

12.LXXXVI

12.4.7 Compounds containing trinitrogen moieties

Triazenes and azides are of interest as chemotherapeutic agents and deserve a brief discussion here in view of the metabolic reductive cleavage they can undergo. A **triazene** of interest in our context is the anticancer agent 1-(4-acetylphenyl)-3,3-dimethyltriazene (**12.LXXXVII**). *In vitro* metabolism (mouse liver 9000 g supernatant, aerobic conditions) yielded three metabolites, a major one being 4-aminoacetophenone (**12.LXXXVIII**) (Farina *et al.*, 1983). A reductive cleavage of the N=N moiety is clearly indicated. The other two metabolites resulted from N-demethylation and carbonyl reduction.

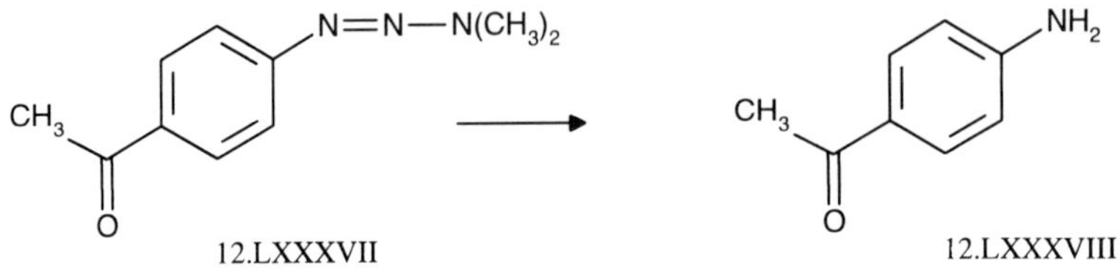

12.LXXXVII   12.LXXXVIII

While **azides** have been used extensively as photoaffinity labels for biochemical studies, the azido substituent ($-N_3$) has only recently attracted attention in drug design. It is represented as two resonance forms in **12.LXXXIX**, indicating the existence of a formal positive charge on the central nitrogen atom, and of partial negative charges on the two peripheral nitrogen atoms. Electrophilic reagents (e.g. H^+) attack at $N(\alpha)$, while nucleophilic attack occurs at $N(\gamma)$. The metabolism of model *p*-substituted phenyl azides (**12.XC**) by mouse liver microsomes or mouse hepatocytes under anaerobic conditions revealed their reduction to the corresponding primary aromatic amine (**12.XCI**) (Nicholls *et al.*, 1991). This was true of *p*-nitrophenyl azide (the best substrate), *p*-cyanophenyl azide, and *p*-chlorophenyl azide. In contrast, phenyl azide and its *p*-methoxy derivative were not reduced, nor was the aliphatic analogue phenethyl azide (**12.XCII**).

An investigational antineoplastic agent, **m-azidopyrimethamine (12.XCIII)**, was also reduced to the corresponding primary amine, *m*-aminopyrimethamine, in mouse tissue homogenates under anaerobic conditions (Kamali *et al.*, 1988). Hepatic microsomes, mitochondria and

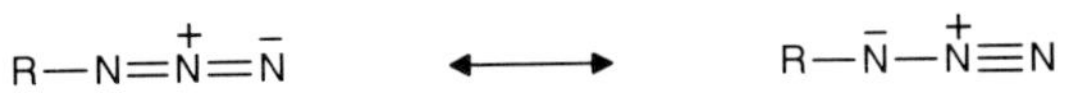

12.LXXXIX

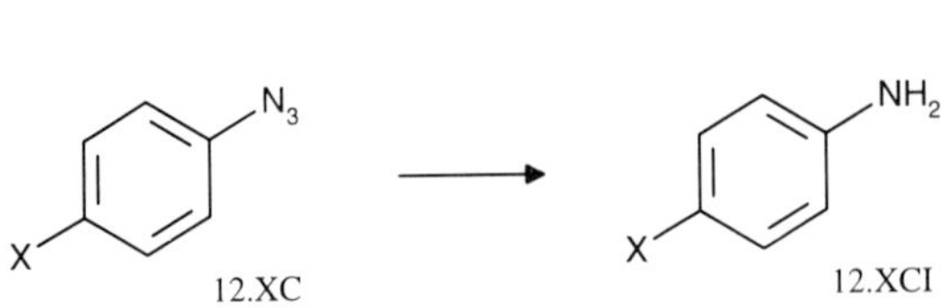

12.XC   12.XCI

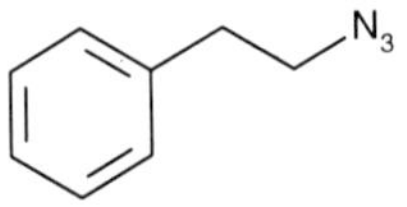

12.XCII

cytochrome P450 were all active. A non-enzymatic component was also seen which may be attributed to the action of thiols. In contrast, xanthine oxidase and aldehyde oxidase did not appear to be involved.

3'-Azido-3'-deoxythymidine (AZT, **12.XCIV**) is currently a major drug in the treatment of AIDS, and this compound also undergoes reduction to the primary amine, i.e. 3'-amino-3'-deoxythymidine (AMT). This was demonstrated under aerobic conditions for AZT and a number of 3'-azido analogues using rat or human liver microsomes, or rat hepatocytes (Cretton *et al.*, 1991 and 1992). The formation of AMT was greatly increased in the presence of NADPH, suggesting the involvement of an NADPH-dependent enzyme system, and indeed the involvement of **cytochrome P450** and **NADPH-cytochrome P450** reductase has subsequently been demonstrated (Cretton and Sommadossi, 1993). Of great importance is the fact that AMT proved to be five- to seven-fold more toxic than AZT to human bone marrow cells.

Future studies will reveal the catalytic mechanism(s) of azide reduction, which for the cytochrome P450 system should consist of two single-electron reduction steps to form the primary amine and N_2.

12.XCIII   12.XCIV

12.4.8 Quaternary nitrogen-containing delocalized compounds

In this short section, two reactions are presented which have in common the reduction of a quaternary nitrogen atom in a highly delocalized molecule. The first case is that of **paraquat** (**12.XCV** in Fig. 12.12) and other **bipyridylium cations** (e.g. diquat and benzyl viologen). Such compounds are non-selective contact herbicides, and the poisoning of plants and animals they elicit is believed to be due to the formation of oxygen-derived radicals. The mechanism of toxication of paraquat and analogues is now well understood and is related to their facile one-electron reduction to bipyridylium radical-cations (Fig. 12.12). This reaction is generally attributed to **NADPH-cytochrome P450 reductase**, although xanthine oxidase, glutathione reductase and ferredoxin reductase may also catalyze paraquat reduction (Degray *et al.*, 1991; Kappus, 1986). Once formed, the free radical-cations react very readily with O_2 to form superoxide, resulting in tissue damage to liver and lung in particular.

Triarylmethane dyes such as gentian violet (**12.XCVI** in Fig. 12.12) are reduced by liver preparations to colourless, two-electron reduction products known as leuko forms. **Cytochrome P450** catalyzes this reduction. Following anaerobic incubations with rat liver microsomes, the intermediate product resulting from the first one-electron reduction step has been characterized as the C-centred (but highly delocalized) radical shown in Fig. 12.12 (Harrelson and Mason, 1982). Such a radical can undergo a second reduction step to the leuko form, but it could also react with oxygen to form superoxide or a reactive peroxyl free radical (Chapter 10).

It thus appears that these delocalized, quaternary nitrogen-containing compounds are

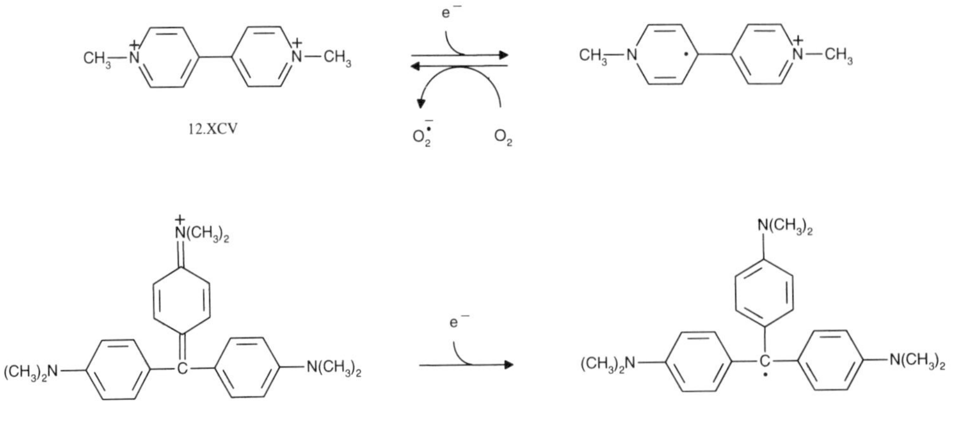

FIGURE 12.12 One-electron reduction of quaternary nitrogen-containing delocalized compounds, e.g. paraquat (**12.XCV**) and gentian violet (**12.XCVI**). Only one resonance form of the free radicals is shown.

reduced by a single-electron step to transient, reactive metabolites which are (mainly) C-centred radicals and contain a tertiary amino group. The toxicological significance of some of these metabolites is well established.

12.5 REDUCTION OF SULFUR- AND SELENIUM-CONTAINING GROUPS

The oxidation of sulfur-containing groups has been discussed in Chapters 7 and 10. For sulfur as for carbon and nitrogen, there exist reactions of bioreduction which mirror some but not all metabolic reactions of oxidation. Thus, disulfides can reversibly be converted to thiols and sulfoxides to sulfides, but the reduction of sulfones is not a known metabolic reaction in mammals. In fact, much remains to be studied about the possible reduction of a number of sulfur-containing groups listed in Table 7.1. Since selenium-containing groups have analogies with sulfur-containing groups, what little knowledge we have of their bioreduction will be briefly mentioned here.

Like the reactions discussed in the previous sections of this chapter, the reduction of sulfur-containing groups can be catalyzed by various enzymes among those listed in Section 12.1, e.g. glutathione reductase, aldehyde oxidase, thioredoxin reductase, cytochrome P450 and NADPH-cytochrome P450 reductase. In addition, the involvement of the gut microflora has been repeatedly documented.

In Section 7.7, we began the discussion of sulfur-containing groups with **inorganic sulfur**. It is therefore appropriate to mention here that one-electron reduction of sulfur dioxide (SO_2) or its hydrated form bisulfite (HSO_3^-) is catalyzed by **cytochrome P450**. The reaction produces the sulfur dioxide anion-radical (Eq. 12.6) which dimerizes to dithionite (Eq. 12.7).

$$[Fe^{2+}] + SO_2 \rightleftarrows [Fe^{3+}] + {}^{\bullet}SO_2^- \qquad \text{(Eq. 12.6)}$$

$$2\,{}^{\bullet}SO_2^- \rightleftarrows S_2O_4^{2-} \qquad \text{(Eq. 12.7)}$$

Dithionite is a well-known reducer of cytochrome P450 in microsomes, the actual reducing species being the sulfur dioxide anion-radical. Since cytochrome P450 reduces sulfur dioxide, it was concluded that its reduction by dithionite is reversible (Mottley *et al.*, 1985).

12.5.1 Disulfides

Section 7.7 has mentioned some examples of oxidation of exogenous thiols to disulfides, and it should not surprise the reader that the reduction of exogenous disulfides is also documented. Thus, **disulfiram** (**12.XCVII**) was rapidly cleaved by S–S reduction to diethyldithiocarbamate (**7.LI** in Section 7.7) (Cobby *et al.*, 1977). The reduction in dog and human blood was very rapid, being quantitative in about four minutes. The reaction is due to the **glutathione/glutathione reductase** system of erythrocytes, whose capacity to reduce disulfiram greatly exceeds therapeutic doses.

An example of an aromatic disulfide is provided by 2-mercaptobenzothiazole disulfide (**12.XCVIII**), an industrial chemical whose reduction in rats is again very rapid (El Dareer *et al.*, 1989). There are also indications that a cyclic disulfide such as asparagusic acid (**12.XCIX**) may be reduced in humans to dihydroasparagusic acid (**12.C**) prior to further metabolism to odorous urinary metabolites (Waring *et al.*, 1987).

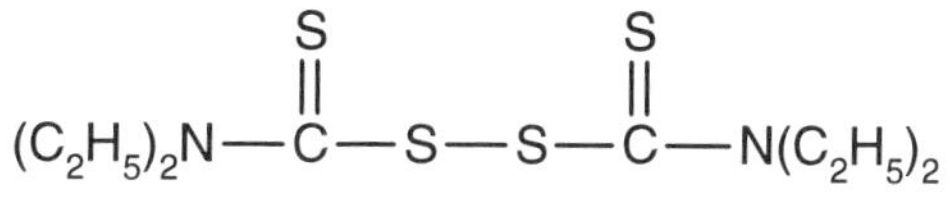

$$(C_2H_5)_2N-\overset{\overset{\displaystyle S}{\|}}{C}-S-S-\overset{\overset{\displaystyle S}{\|}}{C}-N(C_2H_5)_2$$

12.XCVII

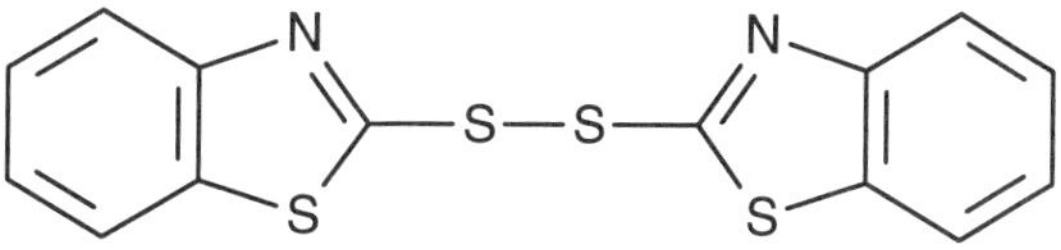

12.XCVIII

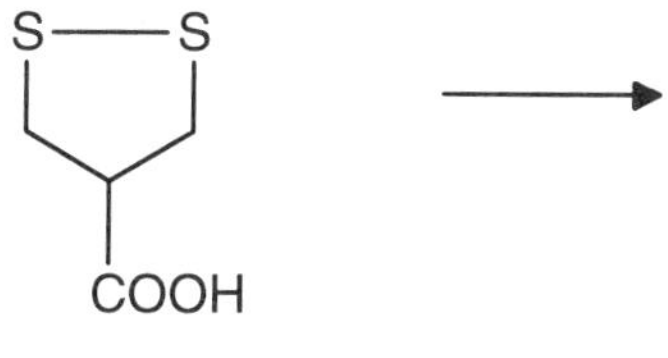

12.XCIX

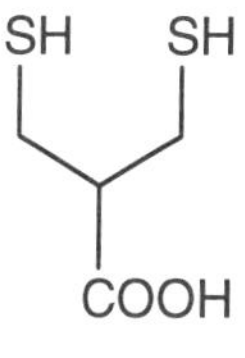

12.C

12.5.2 Sulfoxides

The two-electron reduction of sulfoxides to sulfides has not elicited much curiosity despite its biochemical and pharmacological interest (Mc Lane *et al.*, 1983). A number of sulfoxides are good substrates of liver **aldehyde oxidase**, e.g. diphenyl sulfoxide (**12.CI**), phenothiazine sulfoxide (**12.CII**), and sulindac (see later) (Tatsumi *et al.*, 1983c; Yoshihara and Tatsumi, 1990). The reaction was greatly accelerated by electron donors of aldehyde oxidase such as aldehydes (e.g.

propionaldehyde and benzaldehyde) and azaheterocyclic compounds (e.g. N^1-methylnicotinamide and 2-hydroxypyrimidine). In addition, the **xanthine/xanthine oxidase** system (but not xanthine alone) was found to act as an electron donor for aldehyde oxidase, suggesting a functional coupling between these two enzymes (Beedham, 1985).

12.CI   12.CII   12.CIII

Rat kidney was also found to contain two soluble sulfoxide reductases which might well be two forms of **thioredoxin reductase**. The enzyme has two thiol groups in its reduced form (thioredoxin-(SH)$_2$), and by reducing its substrates transforms the two thiols into a disulfide group (thioredoxin-S$_2$). The two soluble reductases displayed a marked substrate selectivity for **aryl (or alkyl) methyl sulfoxides**, e.g. 1-butyl methyl sulfoxide (**12.CIII**; R = n-butyl) or p-bromophenyl methyl sulfoxide (**12.CIII**; R = p-bromophenyl) (Anders *et al.*, 1981; Fukasawa *et al.*, 1987). Replacing the methyl group with higher alkyls drastically reduced substrate activity. These findings are of interest since they indicate an additional (and reversible) step in the long metabolic sequence of N-acetylcysteine conjugates (mercapturic acids, see a subsequent volume), i.e. C–S cleavage by renal β-lyase (Section 7.7), S-methylation, and S-oxygenation (Section 7.7).

Two drugs of particular significance in the present context are sulfinpyrazone and sulindac which both undergo sulfoxide reduction to an active sulfide metabolite, and sulfoxide oxidation to an inactive sulfone. **Sulfinpyrazone (12.CIV)**, a classical uricosuric drug, is reduced *in vivo* and *in vitro* to the sulfide, a metabolite considerably more potent than the parent compound as an inhibitor of arachidonate-induced platelet aggregation. In humans, the **gut microflora** has been shown to be the principal, possibly the sole, site of sulfinpyrazone reduction (Strong *et al.*, 1984 and 1987). The reduction of **sulindac (12.CV)** is even more important for therapeutic activity since the parent compound itself is inactive as a non-steroidal anti-inflammatory drug. Sulindac is therefore a prodrug, but a rather special one since it is in equilibrium with its active metabolite (Duggan, 1981). In the case of sulindac, reduction is effectively mediated by **aldehyde oxidase** and **thioredoxin reductase** in addition to the **gut microflora** (Anders *et al.*, 1981; Strong *et al.*, 1987; Tatsumi *et al.*, 1983c).

12.CIV   12.CV

12.5.3 Selenium-containing compounds

What little is known of the bioreduction of selenium-containing compounds suggests some analogies with sulfur-containing compounds, as do their oxidation reactions (Section 11.4). Selenious acid (H_2SeO_3) or its anion **selenite** (SeO_3^{2-}) is thus reduced to hydrogen selenide (H_2Se) in a complex reaction sequence involving glutathione (GSH) and glutathione reductase and having GS–Se–SG as an intermediate (Bopp *et al.*, 1982; Vadhanavikit *et al.*, 1993). The reduction of selenic acid (H_2SeO_4) or its anion **selenate** (SeO_4^{2-}) is also believed to occur *in vivo* and *in vitro* (Bopp *et al.*, 1982; Wilson *et al.*, 1992).

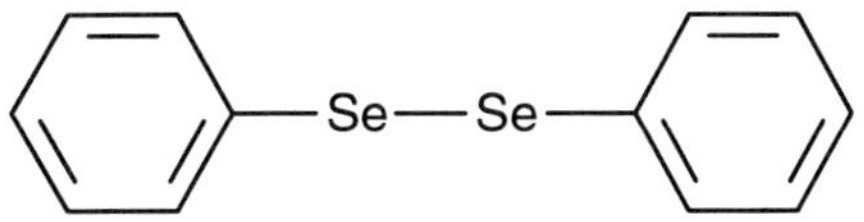

12.CVI

Reduction of **organoselenium compounds** is exemplified by diphenyl diselenide (**12.CVI**), which in mice underwent reductive Se–Se cleavage to phenylselenol (phenyl-SeH) and other metabolites (Adams *et al.*, 1989). Some monoxides of organoselenium compounds have also been shown to undergo fast **non-enzymatic reduction by glutathione**. This is the case for ebselen (**11.XXI** and reaction **a** in Fig. 11.1, Section 11.4), the selenenic acid **11.XXIII** in Fig. 11.1, and the selenoxide 2-(methylseleninyl)benzanilide (**11.XXV** in Fig. 11.1) (Ziegler *et al.*, 1992). Inactivation of FAD-containing monooxygenase by these monooxygenated metabolites of ebselen, suggests their marked capacity to oxidize thiol groups in proteins and implies that Se-oxygenation of selenides could in some cases be a route of toxication.

12.6 REDUCTION OF INORGANIC AND ORGANOMETALLIC COMPOUNDS

Some inorganic and organometallic compounds can be reduced in animals, as briefly illustrated here. **Mercury** (Group IIB), when administered to animals as mercuric ions (Hg^{2+}), can yield volatile mercury, i.e. Hg^0. This reduction reaction is considered to be a detoxication and was also characterized *in vitro*, e.g. in mouse liver cytosol (Dunn *et al.*, 1981). In this system, ethanol increased mercury reduction by inhibiting catalase, the enzyme responsible for Hg^0 oxidation (Section 11.2).

Arsenic (Group VA) is also an interesting element whose metabolic reactions of oxidation are in some cases mirrored by bioreduction of As(V) to As(III). The reduction of arsenate (**11.X** in Section 11.4) to arsenite (**11.IX** in Section 11.4) is well known in mammals (Aposhian, 1989). Among organoarsenic compounds, the reduction of trimethylarsine oxide (**11.XII** in Section 11.4) to trimethylarsine (**11.XI** in Section 11.4) has some formal analogy with amine oxide reduction. Aromatic arsonic acids (**11.XV** in Section 11.4) were the object of much interest several decades ago as chemotherapeutic agents; their reduction in mammalian tissues to arsenoxides (**11.XIV** in Section 11.4) is an essential reaction of activation (Doak and Freedman, 1970; Tomcufcik, 1970). Pentavalent **antimony compounds** (Group VA) are similarly reduced to a small extent to the highly toxic and active trivalent state.

The one-electron reduction of **vanadium(V)** (Group VB) by flavoenzymes has been reported (Shi and Dalal, 1993). A reduction of marked toxicological significance is that of **chromium** (Group VIB). Chromate (CrO_4^{2-}) is a known carcinogen which is readily transported into cells but must be reduced to produce deleterious effects such as DNA–protein cross-links (Mc Lane *et al.*, 1983). **Cytochrome P450** (and particularly CYP2E1) is the main but not sole enzyme catalyzing Cr(VI) reduction (Garcia and Jennette, 1981; Mikalsen *et al.*, 1989 and 1991). Other active enzymes include the mitochondrial electron-transport chain and other mitochondrial reducing systems (Rossi *et al.*, 1988). In addition, ascorbic acid reduces Cr(VI) non-enzymatically in aqueous solutions, and contributes to the reaction in human plasma (Capellmann and Bolt, 1992). The active form(s) of chromium do(es) not appear to be known with certainty and may be either the reactive intermediates Cr(V) and Cr(IV), or stable Cr(III) forms. While reduction ultimately leads to Cr(III), the formation of Cr(V) was seen in microsomes and mitochondria using electron paramagnetic resonance (EPR) spectroscopy (Jennette, 1982; Rossi *et al.*, 1988).

NADPH-dependent glutathione reductase also reduces chromate. The same is true of glutathione alone, which yields Cr(V), Cr(IV) and Cr(III) forms in complex reaction sequences involving various chromium–glutathione conjugates (Shi and Dalal, 1988 and 1990).

The last reduction to be discussed here involves an organometallic complex of **platinum** (Group VIII). The anticancer agent tetrachloro-*trans*-1,2-diaminocyclohexaneplatinum(IV) (tetraplatin, **12.CVII**) was reduced rapidly in rat plasma to dichloro-*trans*-1,2-diaminocyclohexaneplatinum(II) (**12.CVIII**) (Chaney et al., 1990). The reaction was dependent on the amount of thiol groups present in the incubation, suggesting a non-enzymatic pathway.

12.CVII   12.CVIII

12.7 REFERENCES

Abou-Khalil S., Abou-Khalil W.H. and Yunis A.A. (1985). Identification of a mitochondrial *p*-dinitrobenzene reductase activity in rat liver. *Pharmacology* **31**, 301–308.

Adams Jr W.J., Kocsis J.J. and Snyder R. (1989). Acute toxicity and urinary excretion of diphenyl diselenide. *Toxicol. Lett.* **48**, 301–310.

Ahr H.J., King L.J., Nastainczyk W. and Ullrich V. (1982). The mechanism of reductive dehalogenation of halothane by liver cytochrome P450. *Biochem. Pharmacol.* **31**, 383–390.

Anders M.W. (1984). Biotransformation of halogenated hydrocarbons. In *Drug Metabolism and Drug Toxicity* (eds. Mitchell J.R. and Horning M.G.). pp. 55–70. Raven Press, New York.

Anders M.W., Ratnayake J.H., Hanna P.E. and Fuchs J.A. (1981). Thioredoxin-dependent sulfoxide reduction by rat renal cytosol. *Drug Metab. Disposit.* **9**, 307–310.

Ando M., Nakagawa M., Nakamura T. and Tomita K. (1975). Metabolism of isoxathion, O,O-diethyl O-(5-phenyl-3-isoxazolyl)phosphorothioate in the rats. *Agric. Biol. Chem.* **39**, 803–809.

Aposhian H.V. (1989). Biochemical toxicology of arsenic. In *Reviews in Biochemical Toxicology*, Vol. **10** (eds

Hodgson E., Bend J.R. and Philpot R.M.). pp. 265–299. Elsevier, New York.

Bachur N.R. and Gee M. (1976). Microsomal reductive glycosidase. *J. Pharmacol. Exp. Therap.* **197**, 681–686.

Bachur N.R., Gordon S.L., Gee M.V. and Kon H. (1979). NADPH cytochrome P-450 reductase activation of quinone anticancer agents to free radicals. *Proc. Natl Acad. Sci. USA* **76**, 954–957.

Bailey S.M., Suggett N., Walton M.I. and Workman P. (1992). Structure–activity relationships for DT-diaphorase reduction of hypoxic cell directed agents: indoloquinones and diaziridinyl benzoquinones. *Int. J. Radiat. Oncol. Biol. Phys.* **22**, 649–653.

Baker M.T., Nelson R.M. and Van Dyke R.A. (1983). The release of inorganic fluoride from halothane and halothane metabolites by cytochrome P-450, hemin, and hemoglobin. *Drug Metab. Disposit.* **11**, 308–311.

Bartoszek A. and Wolf C.R. (1992). Enhancement of doxorubicin toxicity following activation by NADPH-cytochrome P450 reductase. *Biochem. Pharmacol.* **43**, 1449–1457.

Bates J.N., Baker M.T., Guerra Jr R. and Harrison D.G. (1991). Nitric oxide generation from nitroprusside by vascular tissue. *Biochem. Pharmacol.* **42**, S157–S165.

Bayney R.M., Morton M.R., Favreau L.V. and Pickett C.B. (1989). Rat liver NAD(P)H:quinone reductase. *J. Biol. Chem.* **264**, 21,793–21,797.

Beedham C. (1985). Molybdenum hydroxylases as drug-metabolizing enzymes. *Drug Metab. Rev.* **16**, 119–156.

Begleiter A. and Leith M.K. (1993). Role of NAD(P)H: (quinone acceptor) oxidoreductase (DT-diaphorase) in activation of mitomycin C under acidic conditions. *Molec. Pharmacol.* **44**, 210–215.

Begleiter A., Robotham E. and Leith M.K. (1992). Role of NAD(P)H: (quinone acceptor) oxidoreductase (DT-diaphorase) in activation of mitomycin C under hypoxia. *Molec. Pharmacol.* **41**, 677–682.

Bélanger P.M. and Grech-Bélanger O. (1978). Microsomal C-nitroso reductase activity. *Biochem. Biophys. Res. Commun.* **83**, 321–326.

Bennett B.M., McDonald B.J. and James M.J.S. (1992). Hepatic cytochrome P-450-mediated activation of rat aortic guanylyl cyclase by glyceryl trinitrate. *J. Pharmacol. Exp. Therap.* **261**, 716–723.

Berson A., Wolf C., Berger V., Fau D., Chachaty C., Fromenty B. and Pessayre D. (1991). Generation of free radicals during the reductive metabolism of the nitroaromatic compound, nilutamide. *J. Pharmacol. Exp. Therap.* **257**, 714–719.

Biaglow J.E., Varnes M.E., Roizen-Towle L., Clark E.P., Epp E.R., Astor M.B. and Hall E.J. (1986). Biochemistry of reduction of nitro heterocycles. *Biochem. Pharmacol.* **35**, 77–90.

Bickel M.H. (1969). The pharmacology and biochemistry of N-oxides. *Pharmacol. Rev.* **21**, 325–355.

Bock K.W., Lilienblum W. and Pfeil H. (1980). Conversion of benzo[a]pyrene-3,6-quinone to quinol glucuronides with rat liver microsomes or purified NADPH-cytochrome *c* reductase and UDP-glucuronosyl-transferase. *FEBS Lett.* **121**, 269–272.

Boland M.P., Knox R.J. and Roberts J.J. (1991). The differences in kinetics of rat and human DT diaphorase result in a differential sensitivity of derived cell lines to CB 1954 (5-(aziridin-1-yl)-2,4-dinitrobenzamide). *Biochem. Pharmacol.* **41**, 867–875.

Booth J., Hewer A., Keysell G.R. and Sims P. (1975). Enzymic reduction of aromatic hydrocarbon epoxides by the microsomal fraction of rat liver. *Xenobiotica* **5**, 197–203.

Bopp B.A., Sonders R.C. and Kesterson J.W. (1982). Metabolic fate of selected selenium compounds in laboratory animals and man. *Drug Metab. Rev.* **13**, 271–318.

Bragger J., Lloyd A.W., Barlow D., Martin G.P., Marriott C., Bloomfield S.F. and Phillips J. (1993). Application of molecular modelling to the design of azo compounds for the use in colon specific drug delivery. *J. Pharm. Pharmacol.* **45(S2)**, 1126.

Brashear W.T., Greene R.J. and Mahle D.A. (1992). Structural determination of the carboxylic acid metabolites of polychlorotrifluoroethylene. *Xenobiotica* **22**, 499–506.

Brattin W.J., Glende Jr E.A. and Recknagel R.O. (1985).

Pathological mechanisms in carbon tetrachloride hepatotoxicity. *J. Free Rad. Biol. Med.* **1**, 27–38.

Buffinton G.D., Öllinger K., Brunmark A. and Cadenas E. (1989). DT-Diaphorase-catalyzed reduction of 1,4-naphthoquinone derivatives and glutathionyl–quinone conjugates. Effect of substituents on autoxidation rates. *Biochem. J.* **257**, 561–571.

Burka L.T., Guengerich F.P., Willard R.J. and Macdonald T.L. (1985). Mechanism of cytochrome P-450 catalysis. Mechanism of N-dealkylation and amine oxide deoxygenation. *J. Amer. Chem. Soc.* **107**, 2549–2551.

Butler J. and Hoey B.M. (1993). The one-electron reduction potential of several substrates can be related to their reduction rates by cytochrome P-450 reductase. *Biochim. Biophys. Acta* **1161**, 73–78.

Calligaro A. and Vannini V. (1978). Electron spin resonance study of homolytic cleavage of carbon tetrachloride in rat liver: pentadienyl free radicals. *Pharmacol. Res. Commun.* **10**, 43–52.

Capdevila J., Estabrook R.W. and Prough R.A. (1978). The existence of a benzo(a)pyrene-3,6-quinone reductase in rat liver microsomal fractions. *Biochem. Biophys. Res. Comm.* **83**, 1291–1298.

Capellmann M. and Bolt H.M. (1992). Chromium(VI) reducing capacity of ascorbic acid and of human plasma *in vitro*. *Arch. Toxicol.* **6**, 45–50.

Castro C.E., Wade R.S. and Belser N.O. (1985). Biodehalogenation: Reactions of cytochrome P-450 with polyhalomethanes. *Biochemistry* **24**, 204–210.

Chadwick R.W., George S.E. and Claxton L.D. (1992). Role of the gastrointestinal mucosa and microflora in the bioactivation of dietary and environmental mutagens or carcinogens. *Drug Metab. Rev.* **24**, 425–492.

Chaney S.G., Wyrick S. and Till G.K. (1990). *In vitro* biotransformations of tetrachloro-(d,l-trans)-1,2-diaminocyclohexaneplatinum(IV) (Tetraplatin) in rat plasma. *Cancer Res.* **50**, 4539–4545.

Chesis P.L., Levin D.E., Smith M.T., Ernster L. and Ames B.N. (1984). Mutagenicity of quinones: pathways of metabolic activation and detoxication. *Proc. Natl Acad. Sci. USA* **81**, 1696–1700.

Chung S.J. and Fung H.L. (1992). A common enzyme may be responsible for the conversion of organic nitrates to nitric oxide in vascular microsomes. *Biochem. Biophys. Res. Commun.* **185**, 932–937.

Chung K.T. and Cerniglia C.E. (1992). Mutagenicity of azo dyes: structure–activity relationships. *Mutat. Res.* **277**, 201–210.

Clarke E.D., Goulding K.H. and Wardman P. (1982). Nitroimidazoles as anaerobic electron acceptors for xanthine oxidase. *Biochem. Pharmacol.* **31**, 3237–3242.

Clement B. and Kunze T. (1992). The reduction of 6-N-hydroxylaminopurine to adenine by xanthine oxidase. *Biochem. Pharmacol.* **44**, 1501–1509.

Cobby J., Mayersohn M. and Selliah S. (1977). The rapid reduction of disulfiram in blood and plasma. *J. Pharmacol. Exp. Therap.* **202**, 724–731.

Connor H.D., Thurman R.G., Galizi M.D. and Mason R.P. (1986). The formation of a novel free radical metabolite from CCl₄ in the perfused rat liver and in *vivo. J. Biol. Chem.* **261**, 4542–4548.

Coutts R.T. and Beckett A.H. (1977). Metabolic N-oxidation of primary and secondary aliphatic medicinal amines. *Drug Metab. Rev.* **6**, 51–104.

Cretton E.M., Xie M.Y., Bevan R.J., Goudgaon N.M., Schinazi R.F. and Sommadossi J.P. (1991). Catabolism of 3'-azido-3'-deoxythymidine in hepatocytes and liver microsomes, with evidence of formation of 3'-amino-3'-deoxythymidine, a highly toxic catabolite for human bone marrow cells. *Molec. Pharmacol.* **39**, 258–266.

Cretton E.M., Xie M.Y., Goudgaon N.M., Schinazi R.F., Chu C.K. and Sommadossi J.P. (1992). Catabolic disposition of 3'-azido-2',3'-dideoxyuridine in hepatocytes with evidence of azido reduction being a general catabolic pathway of 3'-azido-2',3'-dideoxynucleosides. *Biochem. Pharmacol* **44**, 973–980.

Cretton E.M. and Sommadossi J.P. (1993). Reduction of 3'-azido-2',3'-dideoxynucleosides to their 3'-amino metabolite is mediated by cytochrome P-450 and NADPH-cytochrome P-450 reductase in rat liver microsomes. *Drug Metab. Disposit.* **21**, 946–950.

Cummings J., Allan L., Willmott N., Riley R., Workman P. and Smyth J.F. (1992). The enzymology of doxorubicin quinone reduction in tumour tissue. *Biochem. Pharmacol.* **44**, 2175–2183.

DeGray J.A., Rao D.N.R. and Mason R.P. (1991). Reduction of paraquat and related bipyridylium compounds to free radical metabolites by rat hepatocytes. *Arch. Biochem. Biophys.* **289**, 145–152.

De Groot H. and Sies H. (1989). Cytochrome P-450, reductive metabolism, and cell injury. *Drug Metab. Rev.* **20**, 275–284.

de Jong J., Schoofs P.R., Snabilié A.M., Bast A. and van der Vijgh W.J.F. (1993). The role of biotransformation in anthracycline-induced cardiotoxicity in mice. *J. Pharmacol. Exp. Therap.* **266**, 1312–1320.

Delaforge M., Servent D., Wirsta P., Ducrocq C., Mansuy D. and Lenfant M. (1993). Particular ability of cytochrome P-450 CYP3A to reduce glyceryl trinitrate in rat liver microsomes: subsequent formation of nitric oxide. *Chem.-Biol. Interact.* **86**, 103–117.

de Sagher R.M., De Leenheer A.P., Cruyl A.A. and Claeys A.E. (1975). Identification and urinary excretion of *p*-chlorophenoxyacetamide, a metabolite of iproclozide, in humans. *Drug Metab. Disposit.* **3**, 423–429.

Dieterle W., Faigle J.W., Montigel C., Sulc M. and Theobald W. (1977). Biotransformation and pharmacokinetics of acenocoumarol (Sintrom[R]) in man. *Eur. J. Clin. Pharmacol.* **11**, 367–375.

Doak G.O. and Freedman L.D. (1970). Arsenicals, antimonials, and bismuthials. In *Medicinal Chemistry*, Part I, 3rd Edition (ed. Burger A). pp. 610–626. Wiley-Interscience, New York.

Dubin M., Fernandez Villamil S.H., Paulino de Blumemfeld M. and Stoppani A.O.M. (1991). Inhibition of microsomal lipid peroxidation and cytochrome P-450-catalyzed reactions by nitrofuran compounds. *Free Rad. Res. Commun.* **14**, 419–431.

Duggan D.E. (1981). Sulindac: therapeutic implications of the prodrug/pharmacophore equilibrium. *Drug Metab. Rev.* **12**, 325–337.

Dunn J.D., Clarkson T.W. and Magos L. (1981). Ethanol reveals novel mercury detoxification step in tissues. *Science* **213**, 1123–1125.

Dürk H., Poyer J.L., Klessen C. and Frank H. (1992). Acetylene, a mammalian metabolite of 1,1,1-trichloroethane. *Biochem. J.* **286**, 353–356.

El-Bayoumy K., Shiue G.H. and Hecht S.S. (1988). Metabolism and DNA binding of 1-nitropyrene and 1-nitrosopyrene in newborn mice. *Chem. Res. Toxicol.* **1**, 243–247.

El Dareer S.M., Kalin J.R., Tillery K.F., Hill D.L. and Barnett Jr J.W. (1989). Disposition of 2-mercaptobenzothiazole and 2-mercaptobenzothiazole disulphide in rats dosed intravenously, orally, and topically and in guinea-pigs dosed topically. *J. Toxicol. Environm. Health* **27**, 65–83.

Eriksson U.G., Brasch R.C. and Tozer T.N. (1987). Non-enzymatic bioreduction in rat liver and kidney of nitroxyl spin labels, potential contrast agents in magnetic resonance imaging. *Drug Metab. Disposit.* **15**, 155–160.

Ernster L., Lind C., Nordenbrand K., Thor H. and Orrenius S. (1982). In *Oxigenases and Oxygen Metabolism* (eds. Nozaki M., Yamamoto S., Ishimura Y., Coon M.J., Ernster L. and Estabrook R.W.). pp. 357–369. Academic Press, New York.

Farina P., Benfenati E., Reginato R., Torti L., D'Incalci M., Threadgill M.D. and Gescher A. (1983). Metabolism of the anticancer agent 1-(4-acetylphenyl)-3,3-dimethyltriazene. *Biomed. Mass Spectrom.* **10**, 485–488.

Feelisch M. and Noack E. (1987). Nitric oxide (NO) formation from vasodilators occurs independently of hemoglobin or non-heme iron. *Eur. J. Pharmacol.* **142**, 465–469.

Feelisch M. and Kelm M. (1991). Biotransformation of organic nitrates to nitric oxide by vascular smooth muscle and endothelial cells. *Biochem. Biophys. Res. Commun.* **180**, 286–293.

Fekkes D., Hennemann G. and Visser T.J. (1982). One enzyme for the 5'-deiodination of 3,3',5'-triiodothyronine and 3',5'-diiodothyronine in rat liver. *Biochem. Pharmacol.* **31**, 1705–1709.

Feldman P.L., Griffith O.W. and Stuehr D.J. (1993). The surprising life of nitric oxide. *Chem. Engin. News.* **71**(51), 26–38.

Finkelstein E., Rosen G.M. and Rauckman E.J. (1984). Superoxide-dependent reduction of nitroxides by thiols. *Biochim. Biophys. Acta* **802**, 90–98.

Fisher G.R., Gutierrez P.L., Oldcorne M.A. and Patterson L.H. (1992). NAD(P)H (quinone acceptor) oxidoreductase (DT-diaphorase)-mediated two-electron reduction of anthraquinone-based agents and generation of hydroxyl radicals. *Biochem. Pharmacol.* **43**, 575–585.

Flowers-Geary L., Harvey R.G. and Penning T.M. (1993). Cytotoxicity of polycyclic aromatic hydrocarbon o-quinones in rat and human hepatoma cells. *Chem. Res. Toxicol.* **6**, 252–260.

Forrest G.L., Qian J., Ma J.X., Kaplan W.D., Akman S.,

Doroshow J. and Chen S. (1990). Rat liver NAD(P)H: quinone oxidoreductase: cDNA expression and site-directed mutagenesis. *Biochem. Biophys. Res. Commun.* **169**, 1087–1093.

Forrest G.L., Akman S., Doroshow J., Rivera H. and Kaplan W.D. (1991). Genomic sequence and expression of a cloned human carbonyl reductase gene with daunorubicin reductase activity. *Molec. Pharmacol.* **40**, 502–507.

Fu P.P. (1990). Metabolism of nitro-polycyclic aromatic hydrocarbons. *Drug Metab. Rev.* **22**, 209–268.

Fukazawa H., Tomisawa H., Ichihara S. and Tateishi M. (1987). Purification and properties of methyl sulfoxide reductases from rat kidney. *Arch. Biochem. Biophys.* **256**, 48–489.

Fukuto J.M., Wallace G.C., Hszieh R. and Chaudhuri G. (1992). Chemical oxidation of N-hydroxyguanidine compounds. Release of nitric oxide, nitroxyl and possible relationship to the mechanism of biological nitric oxide generation. *Biochem. Pharmacol.* **43**, 607–613.

Gal J., Estin C.D. and Moon B.J. (1978). *In vitro* reductive metabolism of N-nitrosodibenzylamine: evidence for new reactive intermediates. *Biochem. Biophys. Res. Commun.* **85**, 1466–1471.

Gandolfi A.J., White R.D., Sipes I.G. and Pohl L.R. (1980). Bioactivation and covalent binding of halothane *in vitro*: studies with [^{3}H]- and [^{14}C]halothane. *J. Pharmacol. Exp. Therap.* **214**, 721–725.

Garcia J.D. and Jennette K.W. (1981). Electron-transport cytochrome P-450 system is involved in the microsomal metabolism of the carcinogen chromate. *J. Inorg. Biochem.* **14**, 281–295.

Garcia-Alfonso C., Martinez-Galisteo E., Llobell A., Barcena J.A. and Lopez-Barea J. (1993). Horse-liver glutathione reductase—purification and characterization. *Int. J. Biochem.* **25**, 61–68.

Gillespie S.G. and Duffel M.W. (1989). Peroxidase as a model for reduction of tertiary amine oxides catalyzed by rat hepatic supernatant and microsomal fractions. *Biochem. Pharmacol.* **38**, 573–579.

Goeptar A.R., te Koppele J.M., Neve E.P.A. and Vermeulen N.P.E. (1992). Reductase and oxidase activity of rat liver cytochrome P450 with 2,3,5,6-tetramethylbenzoquinone as substrate. *Chem.-Biol. Interact.* **83**, 249–269.

Goldman P., Koch R.L., Yeung T.C., Chrystal E.J.T., Beaulieu Jr B.B., McLafferty M.A. and Sudlow G. (1986). Comparing the reduction of nitroimidazoles in bacteria and mammalian tissues and relating it to biological activity. *Biochem. Pharmacol.* **35**, 43–51.

Hajos A.K.D. and Winston G.W. (1992). Role of cytosolic NAD(P)H-quinone oxidoreductase and alcohol dehydrogenase in the reduction of *para*-nitrosophenol following chronic ethanol ingestion. *Arch. Biochem. Biophys.* **295**, 223–229.

Hanzlik R.P. (1981). Reactivity and toxicity among halogenated methanes and related compounds. A physicochemical correlate with predictive value. *Biochem. Pharmacol.* **30**, 3027–3030.

Harada N. and Omura T. (1980). Participation of cytochrome P-450 in the reduction of nitro compounds by rat liver microsomes. *J. Biochem.* **87**, 1539–1554.

Harrelson Jr W.G. and Mason R.P. (1982). Microsomal reduction of gentian violet. Evidence for cytochrome P-450-catalyzed free radical formation. *Molec. Pharmacol.* **22**, 239–242.

Hawes E.M., Jaworski T.J., Midha K.K., McKay G., Hubbard J.W. and Korchinski E.D. (1991). *In vivo* metabolism of N-oxides. In *N-Oxidation of Drugs: Biochemistry, Pharmacology, Toxicology* (eds Hlavida H. and Damani L.A.). pp. 263–286. Chapman and Hall, London.

Heggie G.D., Sommadossi J.P., Cross D.S., Huster W.J. and Diasio R.B. (1987). Clinical pharmacokinetics of 5-fluorouracil and its metabolites in plasma, urine, and bile. *Cancer Res.* **47**, 2203–2206.

Heimbrook D.C., Murray R.I., Egeberg K.D., Sligar S.G., Nee M.W. and Bruice T.C. (1984). Demethylation of N,N-dimethylaniline and *p*-cyano-N,N-dimethylaniline and their N-oxides by cytochromes P450$_{LM2}$ and P450$_{CAM}$. *J. Amer. Chem. Soc.* **106**, 1514–1515.

Hildebrandt P., Garda H., Stier A., Stockburger M. and Van Dyke R.A. (1988). Resonance Raman study of the cytochrome P-450 LM2-halothane intermediate complex. *FEBS Lett.* **237**, 15–20.

Ho D.H., Townsend L., Luna M.A. and Bodey G.P. (1986). Distribution and inhibition of dihydrouracil dehydrogenase activities in human tissues using 5-fluorouracil as a substrate. *Anticancer Res.* **6**, 781–784.

Hochstein P. (1983). Futile redox cycling: implications for oxygen radical toxicity. *Fund. Appl. Toxicol.* **3**, 215–217.

Howard P.C. and Beland F.A. (1982). Xanthine oxidase catalyzed binding of 1-nitropyrene to DNA. *Biochem. Biophys. Res. Commun.* **104**, 727–732.

Jaiswal A.K., Burnett P., Adesnik M. and McBride O.W. (1990). Nucleotide and deduced amino acid sequence of a human cDNA (NQO$_2$) corresponding to a second member of the NAD(P)H:quinone oxidoreductase gene family. Extensive polymorphism at the NQO$_2$ gene locus on chromosome 6. *Biochemistry* **29**, 1899–1906.

Jauch R., Kopitar Z., Hammer R., Prox A. and Fricke R. (1975). Pharmakokinetik und Metabolismus des Antiphlogistikums S-H 766 beim Menschen. *Arzneim-Forsch. (Drug Res.)* **25**, 1947–1954.

Jaworski T.J., Hawes E.M., Hubbard J.W., McKay G. and Midha K.K. (1991). The metabolites of chlorpromazine N-oxide in rat bile. *Xenobiotica* **21**, 1451–1459.

Jennette K.W. (1982). Microsomal reduction of the carcinogen chromate produces chromium(V). *J. Amer. Chem. Soc.* **104**, 874–875.

Kalyanaraman B., Morehouse K.M. and Mason R.P. (1991). An electron paramagnetic resonance study of the interactions between the adriamycin semiquinone, hydrogen peroxide, iron-chelators, and radical scavengers. *Arch. Biochem. Biophys.* **286**, 164–170.

Kamali F., Gescher A. and Slack J.A. (1988). Medicinal azides. Part 3. The metabolism of the investigational antitumour agent *m*-azidopyrimethamine in mouse tissue *in vitro*. *Xenobiotica* **18**, 1157–1164.

Kappus H. (1986). Overview of enzyme systems involved in bio-reduction of drugs and in redox cycling. *Biochem. Pharmacol.* **35**, 1–6.

Kato R., Iwasaki K., Shiraga T. and Noguchi H. (1976). Evidence for the involvement of cytochrome P-450 in reduction of benzo[*a*]pyrene 4,5-oxide by rat liver microsomes. *Biochem. Biophys. Res. Commun.* **70**, 681–687.

Kato R., Iwasaki K. and Noguchi H. (1978). Reduction of tertiary amine N-oxides by cytochrome P-450. Mechanism of the stimulatory effect of flavins and methyl viologen. *Molec. Pharmacol.* **14**, 654–664.

Kedderis G.L. and Miwa G.T. (1988). The metabolic activation of nitroheterocyclic therapeutic agents. *Drug Metab. Rev.* **19**, 33–62.

Kelner M.J., McLenithan J.C. and Anders M.W. (1986). Thiol stimulation of the cytochrome P-450-dependent reduction of 1,1,1-trichloro-2,2-bis(*p*-chlorophenyl)-ethane (DDT) to 1,1-dichloro-2,2-bis(*p*-chlorophenyl)-ethane (DDD). *Biochem. Pharmacol.* **35**, 1805–1807.

Klein J., Post K., Seidel A., Frank H., Oesch F. and Platt K.L. (1992). Quinone reduction and redox cycling catalysed by purified rat liver dihydrodiol/3α-hydroxysteroid dehydrogenase. *Biochem. Pharmacol.* **44**, 341–349.

Kitamura S. and Tatsumi K. (1984). Reduction of tertiary amine N-oxides by liver preparations: function of aldehyde oxidase as a major N-oxide reductase. *Biochem. Biophys. Res. Commun.* **121**, 749–754.

Kitamura S., Wada Y. and Tatsumi K. (1984). NAD(P)H-Dependent reduction of nicotinamide N-oxide by an unique enzyme system consisting of liver microsomal NADPH-cytochrome c reductase and cytosolic aldehyde oxidase. *Biochem. Biophys. Res. Commun.* **125**, 1117–1122.

Knecht K.T. and Mason R.P. (1991). The detection of halothane-derived radical adducts in bile and liver of rats. *Drug Metab. Disposit.* **19**, 325–331.

Knecht K.T., DeGray J.A. and Mason R.P. (1992). Free radical metabolism of halothane *in vivo*: radical adducts detected in bile. *Molec. Pharmacol.* **41**, 943–949.

Knox R.J., Knight R.C. and Edwards D.I. (1983). Studies on the action of nitroimidazole drugs. The products of nitroimidazole reduction. *Biochem. Pharmacol.* **32**, 2149–2156.

Koch R.J., Friedlos F., Sherwood R.F., Melton R.G. and Anlezark G.M. (1992). The bioactivation of 5-(aziridin1-yl)-2,4-dinitrobenzamide (CB 1954). II. A comparison of an *Escherichia coli* nitroreductase and Walker DT-diaphorase. *Biochem. Pharmacol.* **44**, 2297–2301.

Koch R.L. and Goldman P. (1979). The anaerobic metabolism of metronidazole forms N-(2-hydroxyethyl)-oxamic acid. *J. Pharmacol. Exp. Therap.* **208**, 406–410.

Köchli H.W., Wermuth B. and von Wartburg J.P. (1980). Characterization of a mitochondrial NADH-dependent nitro reductase from rat brain. *Biochim. Biophys. Acta* **616**, 133–142.

Koga N., Hokama-Kuroki Y. and Yoshimura H. (1990). Rat liver DT-diaphorase as a nitroso-reductase. *Chem. Pharm. Bull.* **38**, 1096–1097.

Koop D.R. (1992). Oxidative and reductive metabolism by cytochrome P450 2E1. *FASEB J.* **6**, 724–730.

Koster A.S. (1991). Bioreductive activation of quinones: a mixed blessing. *Pharm. Weekbl. Sci. Ed.* **13**, 123–126.

Kowaluk E.A. and Fung H.L. (1991). Vascular nitric oxide-generating activities for organic nitrites and organic nitrates are distinct. *J. Pharmacol. Exp. Therap.* **259**, 519–525.

Kubic V.L. and Anders M.W. (1981). Mechanism of the microsomal reduction of carbon tetrachloride and halothane. *Chem.-Biol. Interact.* **34**, 201–207.

Lashmet Johnson P.R. and Ziegler D.M. (1986). Properties of an N,N-dimethyl-*p*-aminoazobenzene oxide reductase purified from rat liver cytosol. *J. Biochem. Toxicol.* **1**, 15–27.

Lau D.T.W. and Benet L.Z. (1990). Nitroglycerin metabolism in subcellular fractions of rabbit liver. Dose dependency of glyceryl dinitrate formation and possible involvement of multiple isozymes of glutathione S-transferases. *Drug Metab. Disposit.* **18**, 292–297.

Legler D. and Van Dyke R.A. (1982). Microsomal lipids as targets for halothane metabolites. *Res. Commun. Chem. Pathol. Pharmacol.* **37**, 395–402.

Levine W.G. (1991). Metabolism of azo dyes: implication for detoxication and activation. *Drug Metab. Rev.* **23**, 253–309.

Levine W.G., Stoddart A. and Zbaida S. (1992). Multiple mechanisms in hepatic microsomal azoreduction. *Xenobiotica* **22**, 1111–1120.

Lind C., Hochstein P. and Ernster L. (1982). DT-Diaphorase as a quinone reductase: a cellular control device against semi-quinone and superoxide radical formation. *Arch. Biochem. Biophys.* **216**, 178–185.

Lindeke B. (1982). The non- and postenzymatic chemistry of N-oxygenated molecules. *Drug Metab. Rev.* **13**, 71–121.

Lindstrom T.D. and Aust S.D. (1984). Studies on cytochrome P-450-dependent lipid hydroperoxide reduction. *Arch. Biochem. Biophys.* **233**, 80–87.

Lindstrom T.D. and Whitacker G.W. (1984). Saturation of an α,β-unsaturated ketone: a novel xenobiotic biotransformation in mammals. *Xenobiotica* **14**, 503–508.

Linhart I., Gescher A. and Goodwin B. (1991). Investigation of the chemical basis of nitroalkane toxicity: tautomerism and decomposition of propane 1- and 2-nitronate under physiological conditions. *Chem.-Biol. Interact.* **80**, 187–201.

Lipton S.A., Choi Y.B., Pan Z.H., Lei S.Z., Chen H.S.V., Sucher N.J., Loscalzo J., Singel D.J. and Stamler J.S. (1993). A redox-based mechanism for the neuroprotective and neurodestructive effects of nitric oxide and related nitroso-compounds. *Nature* **364**, 626–632 (see also **364**, 577 and **367**, 28).

Lloyd R.V., Duling D.R., Rumyantseva G.V., Mason R.P. and Bridson P.K. (1991). Microsomal reduction of 3-amino-1,2,4-benzotriazine 1,4-dioxide to a free radical. *Molec. Pharmacol.* **40**, 440–445.

Loew G. and Goldblum A. (1980). Electronic spectrum of model cytochrome P450 complex with postulated carbene metabolite of halothane. *J. Amer. Chem. Soc.* **102**,

3657–3659.

Lu Z.H., Zhang R. and Diasio R.B. (1993). Comparison of dihydropyrimidine dehydrogenase from human, rat, pig and cow liver. *Biochem. Pharmacol.* **46**, 945–952.

Luke B.T., Loew G.H. and McLean A.D. (1988). Theoretical investigation of the anaerobic reduction of halogenated alkanes by cytochrome P-450. 2. Vertical electron affinities of chlorofluoromethanes as a measure of their activity. *J. Amer. Chem. Soc.* **110**, 3396–3400.

Macdonald T.L. (1983). Chemical mechanisms of halocarbon metabolism. *CRC Crit. Rev. Toxicol.* **11**, 85–120.

McDonald B.L. and Bennett B.M. (1990). Cytochrome P-450 mediated biotransformation of organic nitrates. *Can. J. Physiol. Pharmacol.* **68**, 1552–1557.

Ma Q., Cui K., Wang R.W., Lu A.Y.H. and Yang C.S. (1992). Site-directed mutagenesis of rat liver NAD(P)H: quinone oxidoreductase: roles of lysine 76 and cysteine 179. *Arch. Biochem. Biophys.* **294**, 434–439.

Maffei facino R., Pitrè D. and Carini M. (1982). The reductive metabolism of the nitroaromatic flukicidal agent nitroxynil by liver microsomal cytochrome P-450. *Farmaco. Ed. Sci.* **37**, 463–474.

Manno M., De Matteis F. and King L.J. (1988). The mechanism of the suicidal, reductive inactivation of microsomal cytochrome P-450 by carbon tetrachloride. *Biochem. Pharmacol.* **37**, 1981–1990.

Manno M., Cazzaro S. and Rezzadore M. (1991). The mechanism of the suicidal reductive inactivation of microsomal cytochrome P-450 by halothane. *Arch. Toxicol.* **65**, 191–198.

Mansuy D. and Fontecave M. (1983). Reduction of benzyl halides by liver microsomes. *Biochem. Pharmacol.* **32**, 1871–1879.

Mansuy D., Fontecave M. and Chottard J.C. (1980). A heme model study of carbon tetrachloride metabolism: mechanisms of phosgene and carbon dioxide formation. *Biochem. Biophys. Res. Commun.* **95**, 1536–1542.

Martin C.N. and Kennelly J.C. (1985). Metabolism, mutagenicity, and DNA binding of biphenyl-based azodyes. *Drug Metab. Rev.* **16**, 89–117.

Mason R.P., Peterson F.J. and Holtzman J.L. (1978). Inhibition of azoreductase by oxygen. The role of the azo anion free radical metabolite in the reduction of oxygen to superoxide. *Molec. Pharmacol.* **14**, 665–671.

Maynard A.T., Pedersen L.G., Posner H.S. and McKinney J.D. (1986). An *ab initio* study of the relationship between nitroarene mutagenicity and electon affinity. *Molec. Pharmacol.* **29**, 629–636.

McCall T. and Vallance P. (1992). Nitric oxide takes centre-stage with newly defined roles. *Trends Pharmacol. Sci.* **13**, 1–6.

McCay P.B., Lai E.K., Poyer J.L., DuBose C.M. and Janzen E.G. (1984). Oxygen- and carbon-centered free radical formation during carbon tetrachloride metabolism. *J. Biol. Chem.* **259**, 2135–2143.

Mc Lane K.E., Fisher J. and Ramakrishnan K. (1983). Reductive drug metabolism. *Drug Metab. Rev.* **14**, 741–799.

Mico B.A. and Pohl L.R. (1983). Reductive oxygenation of carbon tetrachloride: trichloromethylperoxyl radical as a possible intermediate in the conversion of carbon tetrachloride to electrophilic chlorine. *Arch. Biochem. Biophys.* **225**, 596–609.

Mikalsen A., Alexander J. and Ryberg D. (1989). Microsomal metabolism of hexavalent chromium. Inhibitory effect of oxygen and involvement of cytochrome P-450. *Chem.-Biol. Interact.* **69**, 175–192.

Mikalsen A., Alexander J., Andersen R.A. and Ingelman-Sundberg M. (1991). Effect of *in vivo* chromate, acetone and combined treatment on rat liver *in vitro* microsomal chromium(VI) reductive activity and on cytochrome P450 expression. *Pharmacol. Toxicol.* **68**, 456–463.

Minchin R.F., Ho P.C. and Boyd M.R. (1986). Reductive metabolism of nitrofurantoin by rat lung and liver *in vitro*. *Biochem. Pharmacol.* **35**, 575–580.

Miyata N., Santa T. and Hirobe M. (1984). Deoxygenation of tertiary amine N-oxides and arene oxides by iron(II) porphyrin as a model of cytochrome P-450 dependent reduction. *Chem. Pharm. Bull.* **32**, 377–380.

Mönig J., Bahnemann D. and Asmus K.D. (1983). One-electron reduction of CCl$_4$ in oxygenated aqueous solutions: a CCl$_3$O$_2$-free radical mediated formation of Cl$^-$ and CO$_2$. *Chem.-Biol. Interact.* **47**, 15–27.

Monks T.J. and Lau S.S. (1992). Toxicology of quinonethioethers. *Crit. Rev. Toxicol.* **22**, 243–270.

Monks T.J., Hanzlik R.P., Cohen G.M., Ross D. and Graham D.G. (1992). Quinone chemistry and toxicity. *Toxicol. Appl. Pharmacol.* **112**, 2–16.

Morris P.L., Burke Jr T.R. and Pohl L.R. (1983). Reductive dechlorination of chloramphenicol by rat liver microsomes. *Drug Metab. Disposit.* **11**, 126–130.

Mottley C., Harman L.S. and Mason R.P. (1985). Microsomal reduction of bisulfide (aqueous sulfur dioxide)—Sulfur dioxide anion free radical formation by cytochrome P-450. *Biochem. Pharmacol.* **34**, 305–3008.

Nakao M., Goto Y., Hiratsuka A. and Watabe T. (1991). Reductive metabolism of nitro-*p*-phenylenediamine by rat liver. *Chem. Pharm. Bull.* **39**, 177–180.

Nakasa H., Komiya M., Ohmori S., Rikihisa T., Kiuchi M. and Kitada M. (1993a). Characterization of human liver microsomal cytochrome P450 involved in the reductive metabolism of zonisamide. *Molec. Pharmacol.* **44**, 216–221.

Nakasa H., Komiya M., Ohmori S., Rikihisa T. and Kitada M. (1993b). Rat liver microsomal cytochrome P-450 responsible for reductive metabolism of zonisamide. *Drug Metab. Disposit.* **21**, 777–801.

Nambara S. and Yamaha T. (1975). Comparison of bacterial and microsomal azo- and nitro-reductases. *Yakugaku Zasshi (J. Pharm. Soc. Jap.)* **95**, 1302–1306.

Nastainczyk W., Ahr H.J. and Ullrich V. (1982). The reductive metabolism of halogenated alkanes by liver microsomal cytochrome P-450. *Biochem. Pharmacol.* **31**, 391–396.

Nicholls D., Gescher A. and Griffin R.J. (1991). Medicinal azides. Part 8. The *in vitro* metabolism of *p*-substituted phenyl azides. *Xenobiotica* **21**, 935–943.

Nohl H. and Jordan W. (1987). The involvement of

biological quinones in the formation of hydroxyl radicals via the Haber–Weiss reaction. *BioOrg. Chem.* **15**, 374–382.

O'Brien P.J. (1991). Molecular mechanisms of quinone cytotoxicity. *Chem.-Biol. Interact.* **80**, 1–41.

O'Brien P.J., Wong W.C., Silva J. and Khan S. (1990). Toxicity of nitrobenzene compounds towards isolated hepatocytes: dependence on reduction potential. *Xenobiotica* **20**, 945–955.

Olson M.J., Johnson J.T., O'Gara J.F. and Surbrook Jr S.E. (1991). Metabolism *in vivo* and *in vitro* of the refrigerant substitute 1,1,1,2-tetrafluoro-2-chloroethane. *Drug Metab. Disposit.* **19**, 1004–1011.

Orna M.V. and Mason R.P. (1989). Correlation of kinetic parameters of nitroreductase enzymes with redox properties of nitroaromatic compounds. *J. Biol. Chem.* **264**, 12,379–12,384.

Pan S.S. and Bachur N.R. (1980). Xanthine oxidase catalyzed reductive cleavage of anthracycline antibiotics and free radical formation. *Molec. Pharmacol.* **17**, 95–99.

Parker W.B. and Cheng Y.C. (1990). Metabolism and mechanism of action of 5-fluorouracil. *Pharmacol. Therap.* **48**, 381–395.

Persson J.O., Terelius Y. and Ingelman-Sundberg M. (1990). Cytochrome P-450-dependent formation of reactive oxygen radicals: isozyme-specific inhibition of P-450-mediated reduction of oxygen and carbon tetrachloride. *Xenobiotica* **20**, 887–900.

Phillips J.C., Bex C.S., Mendis D., Walters D.G. and Gaunt I.F. (1987). Metabolic disposition of ^{14}C-labelled amaranth in the rat, mouse and guinea-pig. *Food Chem. Toxicol.* **25**, 947–953.

Pohl L.R. and Mico B.A. (1984). Electrophilic halogens as potentially toxic metabolites of halogenated compounds. *Trends Pharmacol. Sci.* **5**, 61–64.

Pohl L.R., Schulick R.D., Highet R.J. and George J.W. (1984). Reductive-oxygenation mechanism of metabolism of carbon tetrachloride to phosgene by cytochrome P-450. *Molec. Pharmacol.* **25**, 318–321.

Polnaszek C.F., Peterson F.J., Holtzman J.L. and Mason R.P. (1984). No detectable reaction of the anion metabolite of nitrofurans with reduced glutathione or macromolecules. *Chem.-Biol. Interact.* **51**, 263–271.

Porter D.J.T., Chestnut W.G., Taylor L.C.E., Merrill B.M. and Spector T. (1991). Inactivation of dihydropyrimidine dehydrogenase by 5-iodouracil. *J. Biol. Chem.* **266**, 19,988–19,994.

Potter D.W. and Reed D.J. (1983). Involvement of FMN and phenobarbital cytochrome P-450 in stimulating a one-electron reductive denitrosation of 1-(2-chloroethyl)-3-(cyclohexyl)-1-nitrosourea catalyzed by NADPH-cytochrome P-450 reductase. *J. Biol. Chem.* **258**, 6906–6911.

Powis G., Svingen B.A. and Appel P. (1981). Quinone-stimulated superoxide formation by subcellular fractions, isolated hepatocytes, and other cells. *Molec. Pharmacol.* **20**, 387–394.

Powis G., Lee See K., Santone K.S., Melder D.C. and Hodnett E.M. (1987). Quinoneimines as substrates for quinone reductase and the effect of dicumarol on their

cytotoxicity. *Biochem. Pharmacol.* **36**, 2473–2479.

Rao D.N.R., Jordan S. and Mason R.P. (1988). Generation of nitro radical anions of some 5-nitrofurans, and 2- and 5-nitroimidazoles by rat hepatocytes. *Biochem. Pharmacol.* **37**, 2907–2913.

Rao D.N.R., Elguindi S. and O'Brien P.J. (1991). Reductive metabolism of nitroprusside in rat hepatocytes and human erythrocytes. *Arch. Biochem. Biophys.* **286**, 30–37.

Raucy J.L., Kraner J.C. and Lasker J.M. (1993). Bioactivation of halogenated hydrocarbons by cytochrome P4502E1. *Crit. Rev. Toxicol.* **23**, 1–20.

Renwick A.G. (1991). Metabolism in the intestinal tract. *Acta Pharm. Nord.* **3**, 106–107.

Reuning R.H., Shepard T.A., Morrison B.E. and Bockbrader H.N. (1985). Formation of [20*R*]-dihydrodigoxin from digoxin in humans. *Drug Metab. Disposit.* **13**, 51–57.

Rickert D.E. (1987). Metabolism of nitroaromatic compounds. *Drug Metab. Rev.* **18**, 23–53.

Riley R.J. and Workman P. (1992a). DT-Diaphorase and cancer chemotherapy. *Biochem. Pharmacol.* **43**, 1657–1669.

Riley R.J. and Workman P. (1992b). Enzymology of the reduction of the potent benzotriazine-di-N-oxide hypoxic cell cytotoxin SR 4233 (WIN 59075) by NAD(P)H: (quinone acceptor) oxidoreductase (EC 1.6.99.2) purified from Walker 256 rat tumour cells. *Biochem. Pharmacol.* **43**, 167–174.

Robertson J.A., Chen H. and Nebert D.W. (1986). NAD-(P)H:menadione oxidoreductase. Novel purification of enzyme, cDNA and complete amino acid sequence, and gene regulation. *J. Biol. Chem.* **261**, 15,794–15,799.

Rosen G.M., Rauckman E.J. and Hanck K.W. (1977). Selective bioreduction of nitroxides by rat liver microsomes. *Toxicol. Lett.* **1**, 71–74.

Ross D., Siegel D. and Gibson N.W. (1991). Metabolism and bioreductive activation of mitomycin C by DT-diaphorase. In *Abstracts of the Third International ISSX Meeting*, Amsterdam, p. 277.

Rossi S.C., Gorman N. and Wetterhahn K.E. (1988). Mitochondrial reduction of the carcinogen chromate: formation of chromium(V). *Chem. Res. Toxicol.* **1**, 101–107.

Rowland I.R. (1986). Reduction by the gut microflora of animals and man. *Biochem. Pharmacol.* **35**, 27–32.

Roy D., Strobel H.W. and Liehr J.G. (1991a). Cytochrome b_5-mediated redox cycling of estrogen. *Arch. Biochem. Biophys.* **285**, 331–338.

Roy D., Kalyanaraman B. and Liehr J.G. (1991b). Xanthine oxidase-catalyzed reduction of estrogen quinones to semiquinones and hydroquinones. *Biochem. Pharmacol.* **42**, 1627–1631.

Ruf H.H., Ahr H., Nastainczyk W., Ullrich V., Mansuy D., Battioni J.P., Montiel-Montoya R. and Trautwein A. (1984). Formation of a ferric carbanion complex from halothane and cytochrome P-450: electron spin resonance, electronic spectra, and model complexes. *Biochemistry* **23**, 5300–5306.

Sanins S.M., Timbrell J.A., Elcombe C. and Nicholson

J.K. (1992). Proton NMR spectroscopic studies on the metabolism and biochemical effects of hydrazine *in vivo*. Arch. Toxicol. **66**, 489–495.

Scheper T., Appel K.E., Schunack W., Somogyi A. and Hildebrandt A.G. (1991). Metabolic denitrosation of N-nitroso-N-methylaniline: detection of amine-metabolites. *Chem.-Biol. Interact.* **77**, 81–96.

Schreiber J., Mottley C., Sinha B.K., Kalyanaraman B. and Mason R.P. (1987). One-electron reduction of daunomycin, daunomycinone and 7-deoxy-daunomycinone by the xanthine/xanthine oxidase system: detection of semiquinone free radicals by electron spin resonance. *J. Amer. Chem. Soc.* **109**, 348–351.

Schröder H. (1992). Cytochrome P-450 mediates bioactivation of organic nitrates. *J. Pharmacol. Exp. Therap.* **262**, 298–302.

Segura-Aguilar J., Keiser R. and Lind C. (1992). Separation and characterization of isoforms of DT-diaphorase from rat liver cytosol. *Biochim. Biophys. Acta* **1120**, 33–42.

Sera N., Fukuhara K., Miyata N., Horikawa K. and Tokiwa H. (1992). Mutagenicity of nitroazabenzo[*a*]pyrene and its related compounds. *Mutat. Res.* **280**, 81–85.

Servent D., Delaforge M., Ducrocq C., Mansuy D. and Lenfant M. (1989). Nitric oxide formation during microsomal hepatic denitration of glyceryl trinitrate: involvement of cytochrome P-450. *Biochem. Biophys. Res. Commun.* **163**, 1210–1216.

Shamat M.A. (1993). The role of the gastrointestinal microflora in the metabolism of drugs. *Int. J. Pharmaceut.* **97**, 1–13.

Shargel L., Banijamali A.R. and Kuttab S.H. (1984). Relationship between azo dye structure and rat hepatic azoreductase activity. *J. Pharm. Sci.* **73**, 161–164.

Shepherd R.G. (1970). Sulfanilamines and other *p*-aminobenzoic acid antagonists. In *Medicinal Chemistry*, Part I, 3rd Edition (ed. Burger A.). pp. 255–304. Wiley, New York.

Shi X. and Dalal N.S. (1988) On the mechanism of the chromate reduction by glutathione: ESR evidence for the glutathionyl radical and an isolable Cr(V) intermediate. *Biochem. Biophys. Res. Commun.* **156**, 137–142.

Shi X. and Dalal N.S. (1990). One-electron reduction of chromate by NADPH-dependent glutathione reductase. *J. Inorg. Biochem.* **40**, 1–12.

Shi X.L. and Dalal N.S. (1993). One-reduction of vanadium(V) by flavoenzymes/NADPH. *Arch. Biochem. Biophys.* **302**, 300–303.

Shigemura T., Kang D., Nagata-Kuno K., Takeshige K. and Hamasaki N. (1993). Characterization of NAD(P)H-dependent ubiquinone reductase activities in rat liver microsomes. *Biochim. Biophys. Acta* **1141**, 213–220.

Siegel D., Beall H., Senekowitsch C., Kasai M., Arai H., Gibson N.W. and Ross D. (1992). Bioreductive activation of mitomycin C by DT-diaphorase. *Biochemistry* **31**, 7879–7885.

Sipes I.G., Gandolfi A.J., Pohl L.R., Krishna G. and Brown Jr B.R. (1980). Comparison of the biotransformation and hepatotoxicity of halothane and deuter-ated halothane. *J. Pharmacol. Exp. Therap.* **214**, 716–720.

Smith M.T., Evans C.G., Thor H. and Orrenius S. (1985). Quinone-induced oxidative injury to cells and tissues. In *Oxidative Stress* (ed. Sies H.). pp. 91–113. Academic Press, London.

Stiff D.D. and Zemaitis M.A. (1990). Metabolism of the anticonvulsant agent zonisamide in the rat. *Drug Metab. Disposit.* **18**, 888–894.

Stiff D.D., Robicheau J.T. and Zemaitis M.A. (1992). Reductive metabolism of the anticonvulsant agent zonisamide, a 1,2-benzisoxazole derivative. *Xenobiotica* **22**, 1–11.

Stoddart A.M. and Levine W.G. (1992). Azoreductase activity by purified rabbit liver aldehyde oxidase. *Biochem. Pharmacol.* **43**, 2227–2235.

Streeter A.J. and Hoener B. (1988). Evidence for the involvement of a nitrenium ion in the covalent binding of nitrofurazone to DNA. *Pharm. Res.* **5**, 434–436.

Strong H.A., Oates J., Sembi J., Renwick A.G. and George C.F. (1984). Role of the gut flora in the reduction of sulfinpyrazone in humans. *J. Pharmacol. Exp. Therap.* **230**, 726–732.

Strong H.A., Renwick A.G., George C.F., Liu Y.F. and Hill M.J. (1987). The reduction of sulphinpyrazone and sulindac by intestinal bacteria. *Xenobiotica* **17**, 685–696.

Sugihara K. and Tatsumi K. (1986). Participation of liver aldehyde oxidase in reductive metabolism of hydroxamic acids to amides. *Arch. Biochem. Biophys.* **247**, 289–293.

Sugiura M., Iwasaki K. and Kato R. (1976). Reduction of tertiary amine N-oxides by liver microsomal cytochrome P-450. *Molec. Pharmacol.* **12**, 322–334.

Sullivan H.R., Marshall F.J. and Bopp R.J. (1978). Metabolism of the antimicrobial agent nibroxane, 5-bromo-2-methyl-5-nitro-*m*-dioxane, in the rat. *Xenobiotica* **8**, 495–502.

Suzuki J., Meguro S.I., Morita O., Hirayama S. and Suzuki S. (1989). Comparison of *in vivo* binding of aromatic nitro and amino compounds to rat hemoglobin. *Biochem. Pharmacol.* **38**, 3511–3519.

Takazawa R.S. and Strobel H.W. (1986). Cytochrome P-450 mediated reductive dehalogenation of the perhalogenated aromatic compound hexachlorobenzene. *Biochemistry* **25**, 4804–4809.

Taskinen J., Wikberg T., Ottoila P., Kanner L., Lotta T., Pippuri A. and Bäckström R. (1991). Identification of major metabolites of the catechol-O-methyltransferase-inhibitor nitecapone in human urine. *Drug Metab. Disposit.* **19**, 178–183.

Tatsumi K. and Amano H. (1987). Biotransformation of 1-nitropyrene and 2-nitrofluorene to novel metabolites, the corresponding formylamino compounds, in animal bodies. *Biochem. Biophys. Res. Commun.* **142**, 376–382.

Tatsumi K., Kitamura S., Yoshimura H. and Kawazoe Y. (1978). Susceptibility of aromatic nitro compounds to xanthine oxidase-catalyzed reduction. *Chem. Pharm. Bull.* **26**, 1713–1717.

Tatsumi K., Inoue A. and Yoshimura H. (1981). Mode of reactions between xanthine oxidase and aromatic nitro compounds. *J. Pharmacobio.-Dyn.* **4**, 101–108.

Tatsumi K., Yamada H. and Kitamura S. (1983a). Reductive metabolism of N-nitrosodiphenylamine to the corresponding hydrazine derivative. *Arch. Biochem. Biophys.* **226**, 174–181.

Tatsumi K., Yamada H. and Kitamura S. (1983b). Evidence for involvement of liver aldehyde oxidase in reduction of nitrosamines to the corresponding hydrazine. *Chem. Pharm. Bull.* **31**, 764–767.

Tatsumi K., Kitamura S. and Yamada H. (1983c). Sulfoxide reductase activity of liver aldehyde oxidase. *Biochim. Biophys. Acta* **747**, 86–92.

Tatsumi K., Nakabeppu H., Takahashi Y. and Kitamura S. (1984). Metabolism *in vivo* of furazolidone: Evidence for the formation of an open-chain carboxylic acid and α-ketoglutaric acid from the nitrofuran in rats. *Arch. Biochem. Biophys.* **234**, 112–116.

Tomasi A., Albano E., Banni S., Botti B., Corongiu F., Dessi M.A., Iannone A., Vannini V. and Dianzani M.U. (1987). Free-radical metabolism of carbon tetrachloride in rat liver mitochondria. A study of the mechanism of activation. *Biochem. J.* **246**, 313–317.

Tomcufcik A.S. (1970). Chemotherapy of trypanosomiasis and other protozoan diseases. In *Medicinal Chemistry*, Part I, 3rd Edition (ed. Burger A.). pp. 562–582. Wiley-Interscience, New York.

Town C. and Leibman K.C. (1984). The *in vitro* dechlorination of some polychlorinated ethanes. *Drug Metab. Disposit.* **12**, 4–8.

Tréfouël J., Tréfouël J., Nitti F. and Bovet D. (1935). Activité du *p*-aminophénylsulfamide sur les infections streptococciques. *Comptes. Rend. Séanc. Soc. Biol.* **120**, 756–762.

Trudell J.R., Bösterling B. and Trevor A.J. (1981). 1-Chloro-2,2,2-trifluoro-ethyl radical: formation from halothane by human cytochrome P-450 in reconstituted vesicles and binding to phospholipids. *Biochem. Biophys. Res. Commun.* **102**, 372–377.

Trudell J.R., Bösterling B. and Trevor A.J. (1982). Reductive metabolism of halothane by human and rabbit cytochrome P-450. Binding of 1-chloro-2,2,2-trifluoroethyl radical to phospholipids. *Molec. Pharmacol.* **21**, 710–717.

Tulp M.T.M., Bruggeman W.A. and Hutzinger O. (1977). Reductive dechlorination of chlorobiphenylols by rats. *Experientia* **33**, 1134–1136.

Vadhanavikit S., Ip C. and Ganther H.E. (1993). Metabolites of sodium selenite and methylated selenium compounds administered at cancer chemoprevention levels in the rat. *Xenobiotica* **23**, 731–745.

van de Straat R., de Vries J. and Vermeulen N.P.E. (1987). Role of hepatic microsomal and purified cytochrome P-450 in one-electron reduction of two quinone imines and concomitant reduction of molecular oxygen. *Biochem. Pharmacol.* **36**, 613–619.

Van Dyke R.A., Baker M.T., Jansson I. and Schenkman J. (1988). Reductive metabolism of halothane by purified cytochrome P-450. *Biochem. Pharmacol.* **37**, 2357–2361.

van Iersel A.A.J., de Boer A.J., van Holsteijn C.W.M. and Blaauboer B.J. (1988). The cytotoxicity of halothane in isolated hepatocytes: evidence for two different mechanisms. *Toxicol in vitro* **2**, 75–81.

Vaz A.D.N. and Coon M.J. (1987). Hydrocarbon formation in the reductive cleavage of hydroperoxides by cytochrome P-450. *Proc. Natl Acad. Sci. USA* **84**, 1172–1176.

Vaz A.D.N., Roberts E.S. and Coon M.J. (1990). Reductive β-scission of the hydroperoxide of fatty acids and xenobiotics: role of alcohol-inducible cytochrome P-450. *Proc. Natl Acad. Sci. USA* **87**, 5499–5503.

Vromans R.M., van de Straat R., Groeneveld M. and Vermeulen N.P.E. (1990). One-electron reduction of mitomycin *c* by rat liver: role of cytochrome P-450 and NADPH-cytochrome P-450 reductase. *Xenobiotica* **20**, 967–978.

Vroomen L.H.M., van Ommen B. and van Bladeren P.J. (1987). Quantitative studies of the metabolism of furazolidone by rat liver microsomes. *Toxicol. in vitro* **1**, 97–107.

Wade A., Symons A.M., Martin L. and Parke D.V. (1980). The metabolic oxidation of the ethynyl group in 4-ethynylbiphenyl *in vitro*. *Biochem. J.* **188**, 867–872.

Walton M.I. and Workman P. (1987). Nitroimidazole bioreductive metabolism. *Biochem. Pharmacol.* **36**, 887–896.

Walton M.I., Wolf C.R. and Workman P. (1992). The role of cytochrome P450 and cytochrome P450 reductase in the reductive bioactivation of the novel benzotriazine di-N-oxide hypoxic cytotoxin 3-amino-1,2,4-benzotriazine-1,4-dioxide by mouse liver. *Biochem. Pharmacol.* **44**, 251–259.

Waring R.H., Mitchell S.C. and Fenwick G.R. (1987). The chemical nature of the urinary odour produced by man after asparagus ingestion. *Xenobiotica* **17**, 1363–1371.

Wermuth B., Platts K.L., Seidel A. and Oesch F. (1986). Carbonyl reductase provides the enzymatic basis of quinone detoxication in man. *Biochem. Pharmacol.* **35**, 1277–1282.

Wilson K., Chissick H., Fowler A.M., Frearson F.J., Gittins M. and Swinbourne F.J. (1991). Metabolism of benzothiazole. I. Identification of ring-cleavage products. *Xenobiotica* **21**, 1179–1183.

Wilson A.C., Thompson H.J., Schedin P.J., Gibson N.W. and Ganther H.E. (1992). Effect of methylated forms of selenium on cell viability and the induction of DNA strand breakage. *Biochem. Pharmacol.* **43**, 1137–1141.

Wolf C.R., Mansuy D., Nastainczyk W., Deutschmann G. and Ullrich V. (1977). The reduction of polyhalogenated methanes by liver microsomal cytochrome P-450. *Molec. Pharmacol.* **13**, 698–705.

Wrighton S.A., Fahl W.E., Shinnick Jr F.L. and Jefcoate C.R. (1982). Characteristics of microsomal reduction of benzo[*a*]pyrene 4,5-oxide. *Chem.-Biol. Interact.* **40**, 345–356.

Yamada H., Baba T., Oguri K. and Yoshimura H. (1988). Enzymic reduction of N-hydroxyamphetamine: the role of electron transfer system containing cytochrome b_5. *Biochem. Pharmacol.* **37**, 368–370.

Yamazoe Y., Sugiura M., Kamataki T. and Kato R. (1978). Reconstitution of benzo[*a*]pyrene 4,5-oxide reductase activity by purified cytochrome P-450. *FEBS Lett.* **88**, 337–340.

Yanagi Y., Haga F., Endo M. and Kitagawa S. (1976). Comparative metabolic study of nimetazepam and its desmethyl derivative (nitrazepam) in dogs. *Xenobiotica* **6**, 101–112.

Yeates R.A. (1992). Possible mechanisms of activation of soluble guanylate cyclase by organic nitrates. *Arzneim-Forsch. (Drug Res.)* **42**, 1314–1317.

Yeung T.C., Sudlow G., Koch R.L. and Goldman P. (1983). Reduction of nitroheterocyclic compounds by mammalian tissues *in vivo*. *Biochem. Pharmacol.* **32**, 2249–2253.

Yoshihara S. and Tatsumi K. (1990). Metabolism of diphenyl sulfoxide in perfused guinea pig liver. Involvement of aldehyde oxidase as a sulfoxide reductase. *Drug Metab. Disposit.* **18**, 876–881.

Zbaida S. and Levine W.G. (1990). Characteristics of two classes of azo dye reductase activity associated with rat liver microsomal cytochrome P450. *Biochem. Pharmacol.* **40**, 2415–2423.

Zbaida S. and Levine W.G. (1991). A novel application of cyclic voltammetry for direct investigation of metabolic intermediates in microsomal azo reduction. *Chem. Res. Toxicol.* **4**, 82–88.

Zbaida S. and Levine W.G. (1992). Role of electronic factors in binding and reduction of azo dyes by hepatic microsomes. *J. Pharmacol. Exp. Therap.* **260**, 554–561.

Zbaida S., Brewer C.F. and Levine W.G. (1992). Substrates for microsomal azoreductase. Hammett substituent effects, NMR studies and response to inhibitors. *Drug Metab. Disposit.* **20**, 902–908.

Ziegler D.M., Graf P., Poulsen L.L., Stahl W. and Sies H. (1992). NADPH-Dependent oxidation of reduced ebselen, 2-selenylbenzanilide, and of 2-(methylseleno)-benzanilide catalyzed by pig liver flavin-containing monooxygenase. *Chem. Res. Toxicol.* **5**, 163–166.

chapter 13

VARIOUS ENZYMATIC AND NON-ENZYMATIC REACTIONS

Contents

13.1 INTRODUCTION

Every attempt to classify a large number of items into a limited number of hierarchical categories is bound to end up with some leftovers which defy classification for either of two reasons. First, an item may be recognized to be extraordinary in the true sense and to possess specific properties incompatible with existing categories. The problem is solved by creating a new category at the appropriate hierarchical level. And second, failure to categorize may simply be temporary, additional information on the item's properties being required.

Both types of problems were encountered in the preparation of the present volume. Furthermore, selections had to be made since so-called novel and/or unclassifiable metabolic reactions have been published in large numbers and in sometimes inconspicuous form (Jenner and Testa, 1978; Testa, 1987; Testa and Jenner, 1978). The present chapter is thus devoted to a few metabolic reactions, mostly but not exclusively of a redox nature, that were not classifiable in previous chapters either because of their specific characteristics or due to lack of information, and which have been selected here for their recognized or potential significance.

While some reactions discussed below are enzymatic, others are either non-enzymatic or involve postenzymatic steps (Hathway, 1980; Testa, 1982 and 1983). In fact, most of the previous chapters have already described some postenzymatic redox reactions (e.g. oxidations by superoxide) and a very few non-enzymatic reactions (e.g. reductions by glutathione). This is not to suggest that non-enzymatic metabolic reactions are rare, but experience shows that most of them pertain to hydrolysis or dehydration, and as such they will be discussed in the next volume.

13.2 NON-ENZYMATIC REDUCTIONS

Reduction by ascorbate and mainly by reduced glutathione have been mentioned earlier (see Sections 10.3, 12.4 and 12.5). The role of **glutathione** in reducing a number of xenobiotics and

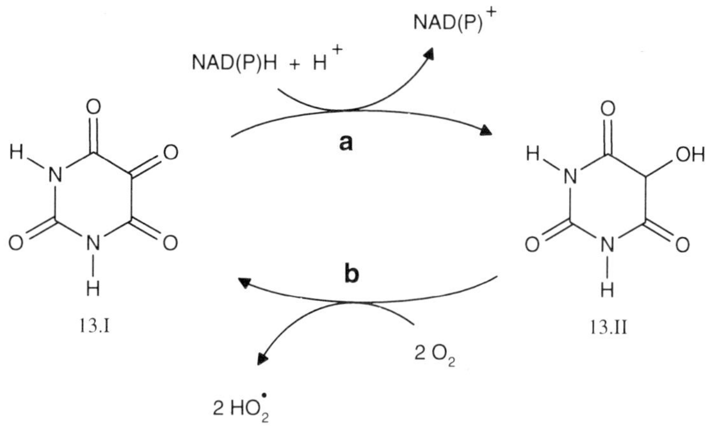

FIGURE 13.1 Non-enzymatic reduction of alloxan **13.I** to dialuric acid **13.II** (reaction **a**), and reoxidation of the latter by molecular oxygen (reaction **b**). This futile redox cycling generates cytoxic oxygen radicals, protonated superoxide being shown here.

metabolites thereof, not to mention endogenous compounds, is of considerable and actively investigated significance. Particular mention must be made of the capacity of reduced glutathione to reduce, and thereby to deactivate, a large variety of **free radicals** as described by Eq. 10.9 and 10.10 in Section 10.3. The free radicals thus reduced and inactivated include the superoxide anion, and radicals formed from halogenated hydrocarbons and many other xenobiotics. Other compounds reduced non-enzymatically by glutathione include selenoxides and some metal ions. But because glutathione-catalyzed reductions are but one aspect of the very rich biochemistry of glutathione, they will be considered in more detail in a subsequent volume together with the reactions of conjugation involving this peptide.

A few studies indicate that **reduced nicotinamide nucleotides** (NADH and NADPH) may also react non-enzymatically with some xenobiotics and mediate their reduction. Thus, nitrosobenzene was reduced to phenylhydroxylamine by NADH and NADPH in neutral aqueous solutions. The rate constants of the reaction were identical for the two reductants (about 150 M^{-1} s^{-1} at 25°C) (Becker and Sternson, 1980). While this reaction may affect *in vitro* results, its *in vivo* significance remains to be assessed.

Another reduction mediated by NAD(P)H is that of **alloxan** (**13.I** in Fig. 13.1). This compound is a well-known diabetogenic agent which acts by destroying pancreatic β-cells. The mechanism of this action is poorly understood, one attractive hypothesis being linked to futile redox cycling of alloxan. Indeed, this compound is reduced non-enzymatically by NADPH or NADH (reaction **a** in Fig. 13.1) and under biomimetic conditions (concentration, pH, temperature) to yield dialuric acid (5-hydroxybarbituric acid, **13.II** in Fig. 13.1) (Miwa and Okuda, 1982). Rapid autoxidation of dialuric acid occurs (reaction **b** in Fig. 13.1) with production of reduced oxygen species which have been postulated to be the cytotoxic agents. This appears particularly true for the hydroxyl radical (HO•) whose formation was demonstrated and which is likely to arise from superoxide (see Section 3.5).

13.3 THE OXIDATION OF DIHYDROPYRIDINE-BASED CHEMICAL DELIVERY SYSTEMS (BRAIN-TARGETED PRODRUGS)

In Section 5.4 we discussed the oxidation of 1,4-dihydropyridines catalyzed by cytochrome P450. Here, we examine the **4-dehydrogenation of N-alkyl-1,4-dihydronicotinic acid derivatives**, as

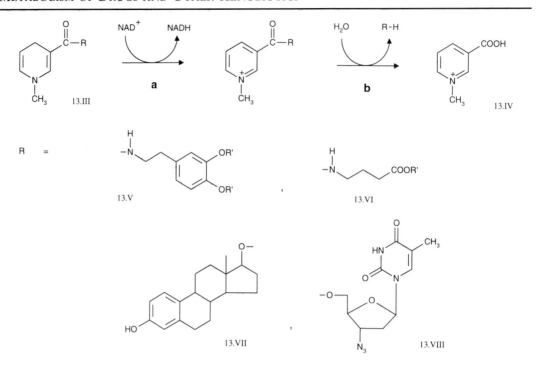

FIGURE 13.2 Mechanism of activation of N-methyl-1,4-dihydropyridine carrier systems for brain-specific delivery of drugs (Bodor, 1984; Bodor and Brewster, 1983).

intensively investigated by Bodor and associates (Bodor, 1984 and 1987; Bodor and AbdelAlim, 1985; Bodor and Brewster, 1983; Bodor *et al.*, 1988; Brewster *et al.*, 1986 and 1991; Woodard *et al.*, 1990). These compounds have been developed as chemical carrier systems for the brain-specific delivery of drugs. In many but not all published examples, the carrier system is an N-methyl-1,4-dihydronicotinoyl moiety (**13.III** in Fig. 13.2) coupled via an amide or ester link to a drug featuring an amino or hydroxyl function, respectively.

These delivery systems function as follows. After administration, the prodrug **13.III** (Fig. 13.2) distributes throughout the body and undergoes 4-dehydrogenation (reaction **a** in Fig. 13.2) in a number of tissues such as liver, blood and brain. The resulting metabolite is a charged pyridinium–drug complex which by virtue of its polarity is rapidly cleared from the peripheral circulation by renal and biliary excretion. Only in the brain does it remain trapped, allowing time for hydrolytic enzymes to act (reaction **b** in Fig. 13.2) by cleaving the active drug from the oxidized carrier (i.e. trigonelline, **13.IV** in Fig. 13.2). Examples of active agents which have been shown to be delivered selectively to the brain include L-DOPA esters (**13.V** in Fig. 13.2), GABA esters (**13.VI** in Fig. 13.2), testosterone (**13.VII** in Fig. 13.2) and other steroids, azidothymidine (**13.VIII** in Fig. 13.2) and 2′,3′-dideoxynucleosides (Bodor, 1984; Brewster *et al.*, 1986 and 1991; Palomino *et al.*, 1989; Woodard *et al.*, 1990).

No detailed study seems to have been undertaken to define thoroughly the nature of the enzymes catalyzing the oxidation of the dihydronicotinamide moiety. Available evidence points to membrane-bound **NADH dehydrogenases** whose catalytic mechanism involves hydride transfer (Chapter 2) (Bodor and Brewster, 1983; Bodor *et al.*, 1988).

13.4 REACTIONS OF DEAMINATION AND AMINATION

Several xenobiotics are known or suspected substrates of enzymes whose physiological function is the deamination or amination of endogenous compounds, e.g. cytidine deaminase [cytidine aminohydrolase; EC 3.5.4.5], L-amino-acid oxidase [L-amino-acid:oxygen oxidoreductase (deaminating); EC 1.4.3.2], or various transaminases [L-amino acid:2-oxoacid aminotransferases; EC 2.6.1].

A number of **synthetic cytosine nucleotides** are substrates of **cytidine deaminase**. Compounds of this type have been prepared as potential antitumour agents, and hydrolytic deamination results in loss of activity for a number of them. The relative velocity of deamination of over 30 analogues has been reported, revealing structural requirements for high and low reactivity (Kreis *et al.*, 1978). A few results are compiled in Table 13.1 to illustrate the large differences in velocities (two orders of magnitude), and the fact that some synthetic analogues are better substrates than cytidine itself.

Other cytidine analogues are activated by cytidine aminohydrolase, as exemplified by 5'-deoxy-5-fluorocytidine (**13.IX**) whose deamination yields 5'-deoxy-5-fluorouridine (**13.X**). This latter is itself a prodrug of the antitumour drug 5-fluorouracil, into which it is converted by pyrimidine nucleoside phosphorylases in tumour cells and intestinal tissues (Ninomiya *et al.*, 1990). In analogy, some adenine nucleoside derivatives are substrates of **adenosine deaminase** (Maury *et al.*, 1991).

TABLE 13.1 *Relative velocity of deamination of cytidine and certain analogues by mouse kidney cytidine aminohydrolase* (Kreis *et al.*, 1978)

Nucleoside*	Relative velocity
Cytidine (ribo-C)	1.00
Ribo-5-fluoro-C	8.20
Ribo-5-methyl-C	0.32
2'-Deoxy-ribo-C	0.72
2'-Chloro-ribo-C	0.23
2'-Chloro-ribo-5-fluoro-C	6.42
Ara-C	0.70
Ara-5-fluoro-C	1.11
Ara-5-methyl-C	0.10
5'-Deoxy-ara-C	0.59
3'-Deoxy-ara-C	0.09
3'-Amino-ara-C	0.05
2'-Fluoro-ara-C	0.40
2'-Fluoro-ara-5-fluoro-C	2.45
Xylo-C	0.07
Xylo-5-methyl-C	0.06
3'-Fluoro-xylo-C	<0.05
3'-Chloro-xylo-C	0.06
3'-Bromo-xylo-C	0.57

*C = cytosine; ara = 1-β-D-arabinofuranosyl; ribo = 1-β-D-ribofuranosyl; xylo = 1-β-D-xylofuranosyl.

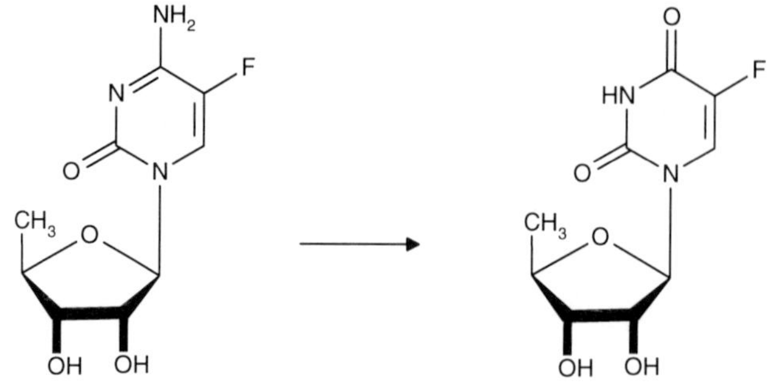

13.IX   13.X

Xenobiotic amino acid analogues are informative compounds whose biotransformation may involve a number of physiological pathways. The mucolytic drug **carbocysteine** (S-carboxymethyl-L-cysteine, **13.XI** in Fig. 13.3) is of particular interest in this context. Two metabolites, thiodiglycolic acid (**13.XIII** in Fig. 13.3) and thiodiglycolic acid sulfoxide (**13.XIV** in Fig. 13.3) were found to account for 1/3 of a dose of the drug in 24 h human urine (Hofmann *et al.*, 1991). These major metabolites were reasonably postulated to arise from 3-(carboxy-methylthio)pyruvic acid (**13.XII** in Fig. 13.3), the product of carbocysteine deamination (reaction **a** in Fig. 13.3). This hypothesis is strengthened by the fact that 3-(carboxymethylthio)lactic acid (the product of dihydrogenation of 3-(carboxymethylthio)pyruvic acid) is a minor human urinary metabolite of carbocysteine.

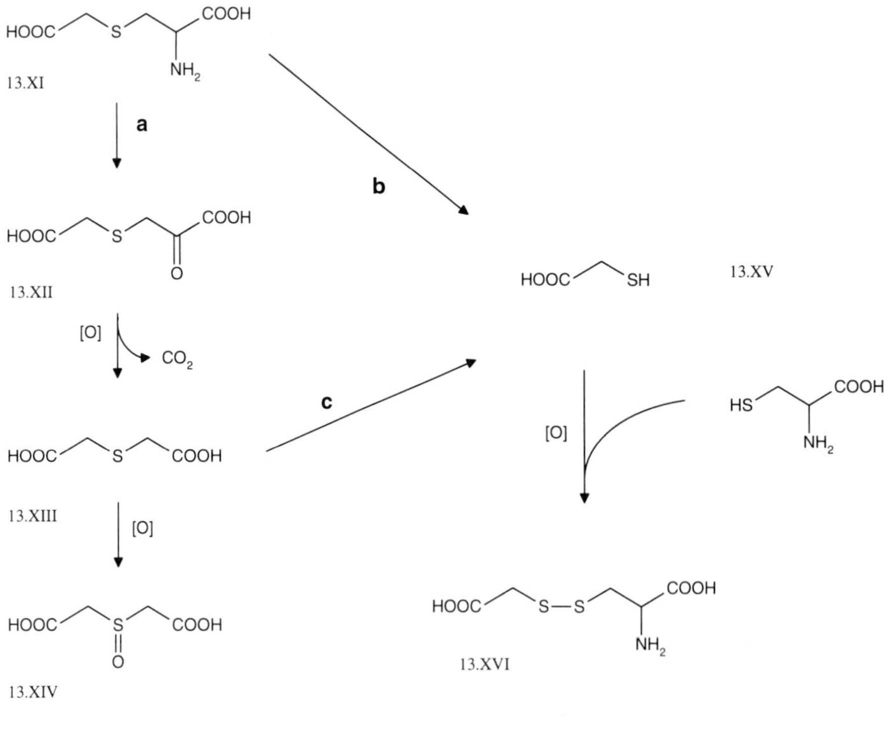

FIGURE 13.3 Postulated pathways of metabolism of carbocysteine (**13.XI**) in humans (Hofmann *et al.*, 1991; Meese *et al.*, 1991).

What does not appear to be known is the enzyme (an L-**amino acid oxidase** or an **aminotransferase**) catalyzing the deamination of carbocysteine. Additional but partial evidence for deamination comes from the identification of S-(carboxymethylthio)-L-cysteine (**13.XVI** in Fig. 13.3) as a novel but minor human metabolite of carboxycysteine. Compound **13.XVI** in Fig. 13.3 is believed to result from the conjugation of endogenous L-cysteine with thioglycolic acid (**13.XV** in Fig. 13.3), an intermediate in the metabolism of carbocysteine. Thioglycolic acid itself could be formed either by β-lyases (see Section 7.7) acting on carbocysteine (reaction **b** in Fig. 13.3), or by hydrolysis of thiodiglycolic acid (reaction **c** in Fig. 13.3) catalyzed by **β-thionase** [L-serine hydro-lyase (adding homocysteine); cystathionine β-synthase; EC 4.2.1.22] (Meese *et al.*, 1991).

Even more intriguing from an enzymatic viewpoint is the metabolism of the industrial chemical **n-butyl glycidyl ether** (**13.XVII**). Rats dosed with the compound excreted 3-butoxy-2-acetylaminopropionic acid (**13.XIX**) as the major urinary metabolite (Eadsforth *et al.*, 1985). One reasonable pathway to account for the formation of **13.XIX** involves hydrolytic cleavage of the oxirane ring by epoxide hydrolase (next volume) followed by oxidation of the resulting 1,2-diol to 3-butoxypyruvic acid (**13.XVIII**). Transamination of the latter by an aminotransferase should be a straightforward reaction in view of the resemblance of **13.XVIII** with endogenous 2-oxoacids. The same reasoning applies to N-acetylation (see a subsequent volume), the final reaction in the sequence. But whatever the mechanisms and enzymes forming 3-butoxy-2-acetylaminopropionic acid, this example shows that amination can involve xenobiotics, and its occurrence in the metabolism of other aliphatic oxiranes should be investigated.

13.XVII   13.XVIII

13.XIX

13.5 OXIDATIVE REACTIONS OF RING OPENING AND RING CLOSURE. FORMATION OF ENDOGENOUS ALKALOIDS

Oxidative opening of saturated heterocycles is reasonably well understood and has been discussed in Chapters 6 (N–C cleavage) and 7 (O–C and S–C cleavage). In contrast, perplexing examples of **oxidative opening** have been reported for some aromatic rings. Thus, **benzene** (**13.XX**) is metabolized in mammals to variable amounts of the ring-opened metabolite (E,E)-muconic acid (**13.XXI**) (McMahon and Birnbaum, 1991; Parke, 1968). While (E,E)-muconic acid has been repeatedly characterized as an *in vivo* metabolite, *in vitro* studies with mouse, rat and human liver slices failed to detect this metabolite, suggesting that its formation may involve a variety of factors (Brodfuehrer *et al.*, 1990). A possible pathway for the formation of muconic acid involves the benzene oxide–oxepin tautomeric equilibrium, followed by formation of epoxyoxepin which rearranges by ring opening to (Z,Z)-muconaldehyde. The latter isomerizes and is dehydrogenated to the final product (Greenberg *et al.*, 1993).

Various aromatic heterocycles are also known to undergo oxidative ring opening, as exemplified by some **2-acetamidothiazole derivatives** (**13.XXII**; R = H, methyl or phenyl) which yielded the corresponding 5-acetylthiohydantoic acid (**13.XXIII**) as a main metabolite in rats (Chatfield and Hunter, 1973). Interestingly, the ring of 2-acetamido-4-chloromethylthiazole (**13.XXII**; R = CH$_2$Cl) was not opened, due to metabolic shift towards the reactive chloromethyl moiety. Comparable observations have been made with **imidazole-containing compounds** which, depending on the nature of the chemical environment, undergo little or extensive ring opening. For example, the imidazole ring is resistant to opening in the drugs nafimidone and econazole. In contrast, the fungicide prochloraz (**13.XXIV**) is extensively metabolized in the rat, most of the dose being recovered as metabolites which had lost the imidazole ring (Needham and Challis, 1991). Compound **13.XXV** was postulated to be the intermediate resulting from oxidative opening of the imidazole ring, and which then underwent further degradation of the side-chain by hydrolysis, deamination and other reactions.

These results suggest that many unknown metabolites of heterocyclic compounds await discovery, and that much remains to be done to understand the enzymatic and mechanistic aspects of their formation.

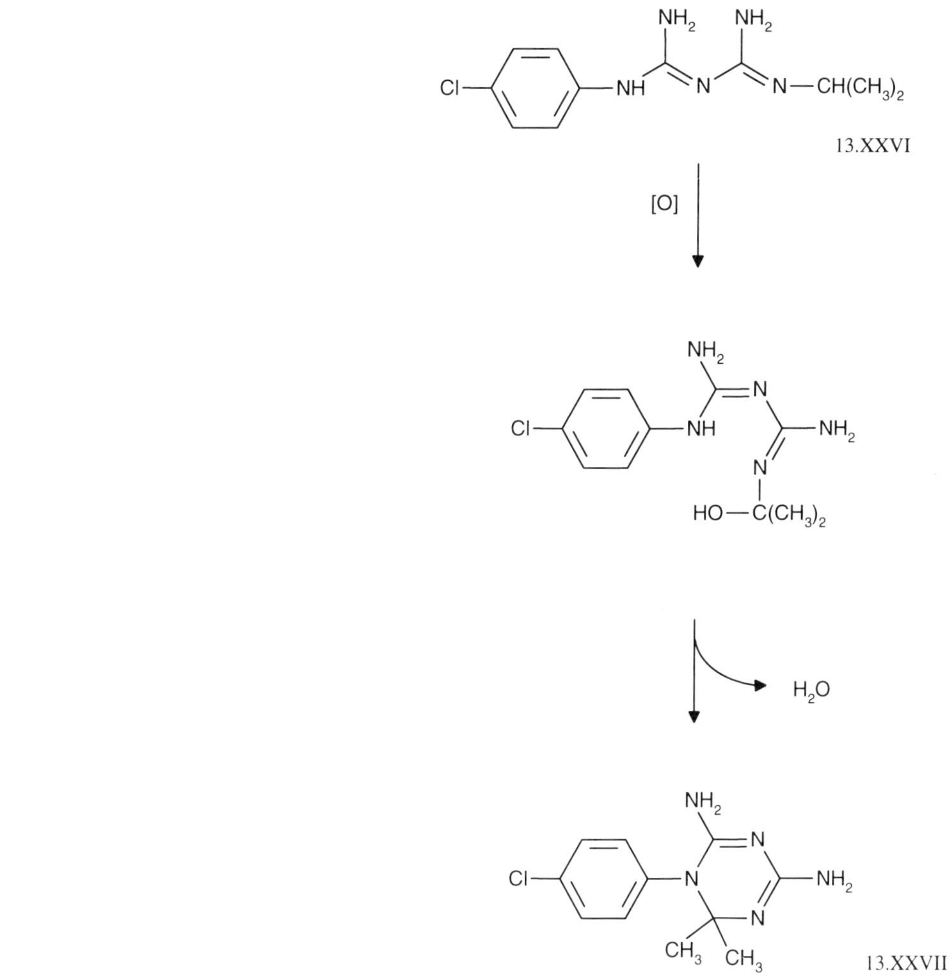

FIGURE 13.4 Simplified, formal mechanism for the oxidative ring closure of proguanil (**13.XXVI**) to cycloguanil (**13.XXVII**).

Perhaps even more intriguing and pharmacodynamically significant are **oxidative reactions of ring closure**. A classical example is that of **proguanil** (**13.XXVI** in Fig. 13.4), an antimalarial prodrug that is metabolized by oxidative ring closure to the active compound cycloguanil (**13.XXVII** in Fig. 13.4) (Hathway, 1980; Ward *et al.*, 1989). All available evidence indicates that the first step is a C(α)-oxidation of the isopropyl N-substituent, a reaction most likely catalyzed by cytochrome P450. The postenzymatic cyclization step that follows can be pictured as a reaction of dehydration (Fig. 13.4), although its actual mechanism is not known (Hathway, 1980).

Oxidative ring closure has gained particular significance in recent years with the discovery that mammals are capable of synthesizing **endogenous alkaloids** such as tetrahydroisoquinolines (e.g. salsolinol and tetrahydropapaveroline) and tetrahydro-β-carbolines (Bringmann *et al.*, 1991; Brossi, 1991; Mesnil *et al.*, 1984; Moser and Kömpf, 1992; Niwa *et al.*, 1993). The synthesis of endogenous opiate alkaloids will be discussed here as an example of particular significance. In the opium poppy (*Papaver somniferum*), tetrahydropapaveroline (THP, **13.XXIX** in Fig. 13.5) is biosynthesized from tyrosine-derived units. Methylation yields reticuline (**13.XXX** in Fig. 13.5) which forms salutaridine (**13.XXXI** in Fig. 13.5) by **intramolecular phenol oxidative coupling**

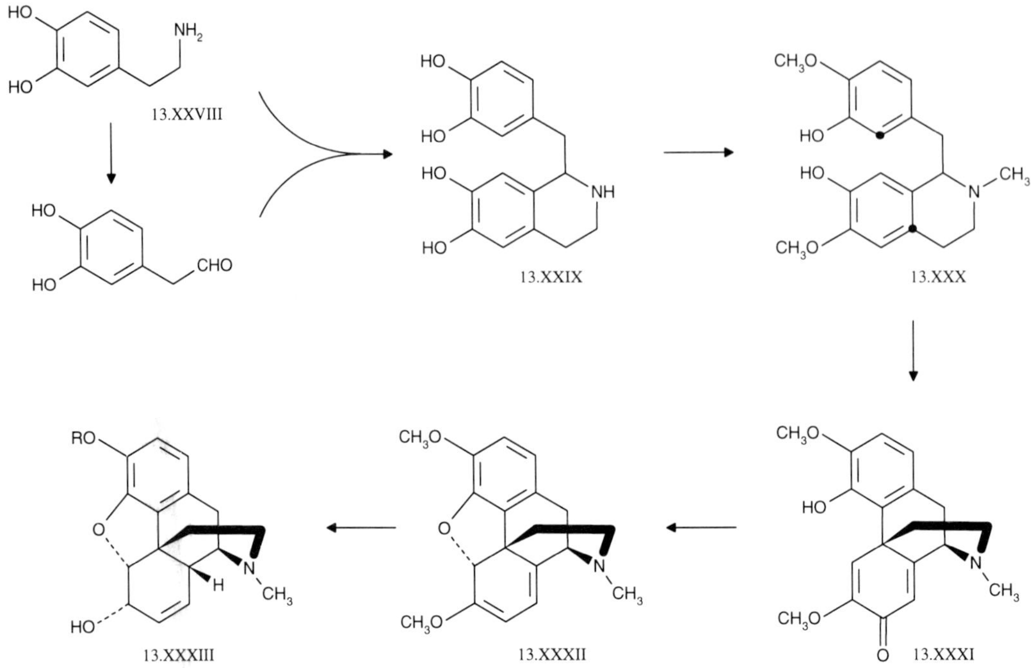

FIGURE 13.5 Postulated pathway for the formation of morphine (**13.XXXIII**; R = H) from dopamine (**13.XXVIII**) in mammals. The critical step in the generation of the morphine skeleton is an intramolecular oxidative coupling of reticuline (**13.XXX**) to form salutaridine (**13.XXXI**). The two carbon atoms to be linked are shown as dots in **13.XXX**.

(Section 7.6). This is the critical step that generates the morphine skeleton and is followed by the formation of thebaine (**13.XXXII** in Fig. 13.5), codeine (**13.XXXIII**; R = CH$_3$ in Fig. 13.5), and morphine (**13.XXXIII**; R = H in Fig. 13.5).

The **formation of opiate alkaloids** in mammals has been recognized for some years (Bringmann *et al.*, 1991; Brossi, 1991). Like other amines, dopamine (**13.XXVIII** in Fig. 13.5) can react with carbonyl compounds (for example its product of deamination 3,4-dihydroxyphenyl-acetaldehyde shown in Fig. 13.5), to form a Schiff's base which undergoes an acid-catalyzed cyclization (Pictet–Spengler condensation) (Mesnil *et al.*, 1984). However, only recently has the critical step in the formation of morphine been demonstrated conclusively in mammals. Indeed, reticuline (**13.XXX** in Fig. 13.5) can be converted to salutaridine (**13.XXXI** in Fig. 13.5) by rat liver *in vitro* and *in vivo* (Weitz *et al.*, 1987). The involvement of cytochrome P450 or peroxidases can be postulated but remains to be demonstrated conclusively (see also Section 7.6 and Chapter 10).

Another demonstration of the metabolic pathway in Fig. 13.5 comes from monitoring the urinary excretion of endogenous morphine, codeine and THP in humans, showing nanomolar concentrations in control subjects (Matsubara *et al.*, 1992). In contrast, Parkinsonian patients undergoing L-DOPA therapy excreted these three alkaloids in severalfold higher concentrations. These results confirm that opiates are endogenous alkaloids in mammals and particularly in humans, and that they are formed from dopamine.

13.6 NON-ENZYMATIC AND UNCLASSIFIABLE REACTIONS OF STEREOISOMERIZATION

Two types of reactions of stereoisomerization have significance in biochemistry, namely **cis–trans isomerization** about double bonds, and **inversion at chiral centres**. That some endogenous compounds undergo isomerization is a well-known phenomenon illustrated by 13-*cis*-retinoic acid. For example, rats dosed with this physiologically important retinoid converted it into a number of major tissue metabolites with the all-*trans*-configuration (McCormick *et al.*, 1983).

Much more intriguing are some reactions of isomerization involving xenobiotics. One case appears in Chapter 2, namely the dehydrogenation of secondary alcohols and subsequent hydrogenation of the resulting ketones. In this sequence, inversion of configuration of the secondary alcohol is a possibility. Other cases will be presented in a subsequent volume, namely the unidirectional chiral inversion of anti-inflammatory profens via their coenzyme A conjugates.

In the following paragraphs, one case of *cis–trans* isomerization and three of chiral inversion will be presented as peculiar reactions of xenobiotic biotransformation.

The compound (E)-5-(2-bromovinyl-2,2'-anhydrouridine (**13.XXXIV**; R = Br, R' = H) appears to be a potent antiviral agent which, in contrast to most analogues, is resistant to phosphorolytic N-glycosidic bond cleavage mediated by pyrimidine nucleoside phosphorylases such as uridine phosphorylase [EC 2.4.2.3] and thymidine phosphorylase [EC 2.4.2.4]. As a result, compound **13.XXXIV** (R = Br, R' = H) was found to be very stable in rats, the only metabolite (accounting for a few per cent of the dose) being its diastereoisomer (Z)-5-(2-bromovinyl-2,2'-anhydrouridine (**13.XXXIV**, R = H, R' = Br) (Szinai *et al.*, 1991). Nothing is known about the mechanism of the reaction or whether it is enzymatic, but it should be noted that the same reaction is catalyzed by light (photoisomerization), suggesting a radical intermediate.

13.XXXIV   13.XXXV

Also poorly understood is the reaction of **epimerization** seen in the metabolism of the synthetic estrogen STS 267 (**13.XXXV**; 16α-azido-3-methoxyestra-1,3,5(10)-trien-17-one). When perfused in the isolated rat liver, the compound was found to undergo three major biotransformations, namely O-demethylation, carbonyl reduction, and epimerization of the C(16) chiral centre to 16β-azido metabolites. Thus, the product resulting from all these three reactions was found to account for about 2/3 of all metabolites (Schumann, 1988). 16-Epimerization has also been reported for the 16α-chloro analogue. No clue was given as to the enzymatic or non-enzymatic nature of the reaction, but we note here that the latter possibility is more likely due to the presence of a vicinal carbonyl function (see below).

Indeed, a few drugs possessing a chiral centre adjacent to a carbonyl group (e.g. ketone or ester) are known to undergo **chemical racemization** under biomimetic conditions of pH and temperature. Consider for example the anorectic drug amfepramone (**13.XXXVI**), whose rate of racemization ($t_{1/2}$ of about 15 h at 37°C and pH 7.4) is slow when compared to the half-life of the drug in humans (1.5–2 h) but still fast enough to be of pharmacological relevance (Testa, 1973). An extreme example is that of oxazepam (**13.XXXVII**) whose rate of racemization is extremely fast (rate constant of about 0.05 min^{-1} at 20°C in the pH range 6–8, i.e. a $t_{1/2}$ of about 14 min) (Aso *et al.*, 1988). A constant feature of these drugs is the possibility of a keto–enol equilibrium involving the chiral centre and accounting for non-enzymatic racemization or epimerization. The topic has been reviewed and preliminary structure–reactivity relationships presented (Testa *et al.*, 1993).

13.XXXVI   13.XXXVII

13.7 REFERENCES

Aso Y., Yoshioka S., Shibazaki T., and Uchiyama M. (1988). The kinetics of the racemization of oxazepam in aqueous solution. *Chem. Pharm. Bull.* **36**, 1834–1840.

Becker A.R. and Sternson L.A. (1980). Nonenzymatic reduction of nitrosobenzene to phenylhydroxylamine by NAD(P)H. *BioOrg. Chem.* **9**, 305–312.

Bodor N. (1984). Novel approaches to the design of safer drugs: Soft drugs and site-specific chemical delivery systems. In *Advances in Drug Research*, Vol. 13 (ed. Testa B.). pp. 255–331. Academic Press, London.

Bodor N. (1987). Redox drug delivery systems for targeting drugs to the brain. *Ann. NY Acad. Sci.* **507**, 289–306.

Bodor N. and AbdelAlim A.M. (1985). Improved delivery through biological membranes XIX: Novel redox carriers for brain-specific chemical delivery systems. *J. Pharm. Sci.* **74**, 241–245.

Bodor N. and Brewster M.E. (1983). Problems of delivery of drugs to the brain. *Pharmacol. Therap.* **19**, 337–386.

Bodor N., Brewster M.E. and Kaminski J.J. (1988). Theoretical studies on the hydride transfer between 1-methyl-1,4-dihydronicotinamide and its corresponding pyridinium salt. *Tetrahedron* **44**, 7601–7610.

Brewster M.E., Estes K.S. and Bodor N. (1986). Improved delivery through biological membranes. XXIV. Synthesis, *in vitro* studies, and *in vivo* characterization of brain-specific and sustained progestin delivery systems. *Pharm. Res.* **3**, 278–285.

Brewster M.E., Anderson W. and Bodor N. (1991). Brain, blood, and cerebrospinal fluid distribution of a zidovurine chemical delivery system in rabbits. *J. Pharm. Sci.* **80**, 843–846.

Bringmann G., Feineis D., Friedrich H. and Hille A. (1991). Endogenous alkaloids in man—Synthesis, analytics, *in vivo* identification, and medicinal importance. *Planta Med.* **57**, S73–S84.

Brodfuehrer J.I., Chapman D.E., Wilke T.J. and Powis G. (1990). Comparative studies of the *in vitro* metabolism and covalent binding of [^{14}C]benzene by liver slices and microsomal fraction of mouse, rat and human. *Drug Metab. Disposit.* **18**, 20–27.

Brossi A. (1991). Mammalian alkaloids: Conversions of tetrahydroisoquinoline-1-carboxylic acids derived from dopamine. *Planta Med.* **57**, S93–S100.

Chatfield D.H. and Hunter W.H. (1973). The metabolism of acetamidothiazoles in the rat. *Biochem. J.* **134**, 869–878, 879–884.

Eadsforth C.V., Logan C.J., Page J.A. and Regan P.D. (1985). *n*-Butylglycidyl ether: the formation of a novel metabolite of an epoxide. *Drug Metab. Disposit.* **13**, 263–264.

Greenberg A., Bock C.W., George P. and Glusker J.P. (1993). Energetics of the metabolic production of (*E,E*)-muconaldehyde from benzene via the intermediates 2,3-epoxyoxepin and (*Z,Z*)- and (*E,Z*)-muconaldehyde: *ab initio* molecular orbital calculations. *Chem. Res. Toxicol.* **6**, 701–710.

Hathway D.E. (1980). The importance of (non-enzymic) chemical reaction processes to the fate of foreign compounds in mammals. *Chem. Soc. Rev.* **9**, 63–89.

Hofmann U., Eichelbaum M., Seefried S. and Meese C.O. (1991). Identification of thiodiglycolic acid, thiodiglycolic acid sulfoxide, and (3-carboxymethylthio)lactic acid as major human biotransformation products of S-carboxymethylcysteine. *Drug Metab. Disposit.* **19**, 222–226.

Jenner P. and Testa B. (1978). Novel pathways in drug metabolism. *Xenobiotica* **8**, 1–25.

Kreis W., Watanabe K.A. and Fox J.J. (1978). Structural requirements for the enzymatic deamination of cytosine nucleosides. *Helv. Chim. Acta* **61**, 1011–1016.

Matsubara K., Fukushima S., Akane A., Kobayashi S. and Shiono H. (1992). Increased urinary morphine, codeine and tetrahydropapaveroline in Parkinsonian patients undergoing L-dopa therapy: a possible biosynthetic pathway of morphine from L-dopa in humans. *J. Pharmacol. Exp. Therap.* **260**, 974–978.

Maury G., Daiboun T., Elalaoui A., Genu-Dellac C., Perigaud C., Bergogne C., Gosselin G. and Imbach J.L. (1991). Inhibition and substrate specificity of adenosine deaminase. Interactions with 2′,3′- and/or 5′-substituted adenine nucleoside derivatives. *Nucleosides Nucleotides* **10**, 1677–1692.

McCormick A.M., D'Ortona Kroll K. and Napoli J.L. (1983). 13-*cis*-Retinoic acid metabolism *in vivo*. The major tissue metabolites in the rat have the all-*trans*-configuration. *Biochemistry* **22**, 3933–3940.

McMahon T.F. and Birnbaum L.S. (1991). Age-related changes in disposition and metabolism of benzene in male C57BL/6N mice. *Drug Metab. Disposit.* **19**, 1052–1057.

Meese C.O., Fischer C., Küpfer A., Wisser H. and Eichelbaum M. (1991). Identification of the "major" polymorphic carbocysteine metabolite as S-(carboxymethylthio)-L-cysteine. *Biochem. Pharmacol.* **42**, R13–R16.

Mesnil M., Testa B. and Jenner P. (1984). Xenobiotic metabolism by brain monooxygenases and other cerebral enzymes. In *Advances in Drug Research*, Vol. 13 (ed. Testa B.). pp. 95–207. Academic Press, London.

Miwa I. and Okuda J. (1982). Non-enzymatic reduction of alloxan by reduced nicotinamide nucleotide. *Biochem. Pharmacol.* **31**, 921–925.

Moser A. and Kömpf D. (1992). Presence of methyl-6,7-dihydroxy-1,2,3,4-tetrahydroisoquinolines, derivatives of the neurotoxin isoquinoline, in Parkinsonian lumbar CSF. *Life Sci.* **50**, 1885–1891.

Needham D. and Challis I.R. (1991). The metabolism and excretion of prochloraz, an imidazole-based fungicide, in the rat. *Xenobiotica* **21**, 1473–1482.

Ninomiya Y., Miwa M., Eda H., Sahara H., Fujimoto K., Ishida M., Umeda I., Yokose K. and Ishitsuka H. (1990). Comparative antitumor activity and intestinal toxicity of 5′-deoxy-5-fluorouridine and its prodrug trimethoxy-benzoyl-5′-deoxy-5-fluorocytidine. *Jpn. J. Cancer. Res.* **81**, 188–195.

Niwa T., Takeda N., Yoshizumi H., Tatematsu A., Yoshida M., Dostert P., Naoi M. and Nagatsu T. (1993). Presence of tetrahydroisoquinoline-related compounds, possible MPTP-like neurotoxins, in Parkinsonian brain. *Adv. Neurol.* **60**, 234–237.

Palomino E., Kessel D. and Horwitz J.P. (1989). A dihydropyridine carrier system for sustained delivery of 2′,3′-dideoxynucleosides to the brain. *J. Med. Chem.* **32**, 622–625.

Parke D.V. (1968). *The Biochemistry of Foreign Compounds*, p. 71. Pergamon Press, Oxford.

Schumann W. (1988). Zur Biotransformation von STS 267 [16α - Azido - 3 - methoxyestra - 1,3,5(10) - trien - 17on]. Epimerizierung einer 16a-Azidogruppe—eine neue Stoffwechselreaktion in der Rattenleber. *Pharmazie* **43**, 329–332.

Szinai I., Veres Zs., Szabolcs A., Gács-Baitz E., Ujszászy K. and Dénes G. (1991). *Cis–trans* Isomerization of [*E*]-5-(2-bromovinyl)-2,2′-anhydrouridine *in vivo* in rats. *Xenobiotica* **21**, 359–369.

Testa B. (1973). Some chemical and stereochemical aspects of diethylpropion metabolism in man. *Acta Pharm. Suec.* **10**, 441–454.

Testa B. (1982). Non-enzymatic contributions to xenobiotic metabolism. *Drug Metab. Rev.* **13**, 25–50.

Testa B. (1983). Nonenzymatic biotransformation. In *Biological Basis of Detoxication* (eds Caldwell J. and Jakoby W.B.). pp. 137–150. Academic Press, New York.

Testa B. (1987). Recently discovered routes of metabolism. In *Drug Metabolism—from Molecules to Man* (eds Benford D.J., Bridges J.W. and Gibson G.G.). pp. 563–580. Taylor and Francis, London.

Testa B. and Jenner P. (1978). Novel drug metabolites produced by functionalization reactions: Chemistry and toxicology. *Drug Metab. Rev.* **7**, 325–369.

Testa B., Carrupt P.A. and Gal J. (1993). The so-called "interconversion" of stereoisomeric drugs: an attempt at clarification. *Chirality* **5**, 105–111.

Ward S.A., Watkins W.M., Mberu E., Saunders J.E., Koech D.K., Gilles H.M., Howells R.E. and Breckenridge A.M. (1989). Inter-subject variability in the metabolism of proguanil to the active metabolite cycloguanil in man. *Br. J. Clin. Pharmacol.* **27**, 781–787.

Weitz C.J., Faull K.F. and Goldstein A. (1987). Synthesis of the skeleton of the morphine molecule by mammalian liver. *Nature* **330**, 674–677.

Woodard P.A., Winwood D., Brewster M.E., Estes K.S. and Bodor N. (1990). Improved delivery through biological membranes. XXI. Brain-targeted anti-convulsant agents. *Drug Design Deliv.* **6**, 15–28.

chapter 14

CONCLUSION AND OUTLOOK

Contents

14.1 CONCLUDING REMARKS

The thirteen chapters which form the main part of this volume have much information to offer, and hopefully, also provide structure and knowledge. As the readers can now appreciate, the book intertwines analytical and synthetic approaches: an **analytical approach**, because the many metabolic reactions are examined separately, and a **synthetic approach**, because as often as possible cross-reference is made: (a) to other reactions of the same substrate; (b) to preceding and subsequent reactions in a metabolic sequence; and (c) more generally to related data.

Such a dual approach may both help and hinder the readers. It should help the maximum number of readers by facilitating the transformation of information into knowledge, but it also could prove a confusing handicap, hopefully a temporary one. As discussed in Section 1.2, a work such as the present one must be **read creatively**, meaning that it should be studied and understood, ultimately allowing it to support a creative act of synthesis in the reader's mind. Far from a modest endeavour, this is a demanding and time-consuming one.

This brings us to the impact time will have on this book. How fast will its content age and become outdated? The answer will unfold as the years pass, but already now we can be certain that some chapters (those devoted to the "hottest" fields) will age faster than others. This is unavoidable, and if this did not occur it would mean that all advances in the science of xenobiotic metabolism had stopped. But no writer is totally helpless. First, ageing can be delayed by offering a book as up-to-date as possible at publication. As explained in the Preface, this was done to the greatest possible extent by incorporating material published until the end of 1993. Second, and more significantly, information and knowledge do not senesce at the same rate. This is the writer's best consolatory argument, and the justification of many efforts.

14.2 OUTLOOK TO THE FORTHCOMING VOLUMES

The present volume is the first in the Series. Having come so far, the reader must wonder legitimately at the contents of the next volumes now in preparation. It is only fit, therefore, to end the present volume with an outlook to the forthcoming volumes, keeping in mind that the outlines opposite are indicative and far from final:

The Metabolism of Drugs and Other Xenobiotics: Biochemistry of Hydration Reactions

- Introduction to the volume
- The nature and functioning of hydrolytic enzymes
- Classification and roles of hydrolases
- Hydrolysis of amides and peptides
- Hydrolysis of esters
- Epoxide hydrolase and epoxide hydration
- Various reactions of hydration and dehydration

The Metabolism of Drugs and Other Xenobiotics: Biochemistry of Conjugation Reactions

- An overview of conjugation reactions
- Reactions of methylation
- Sulfoconjugation
- Glucuronidation
- Acetylation and other reactions of acylation
- Metabolic routes of xenobiotic acids via their acyl-coenzyme A thioesters
- Conjugation with glutathione and other thiols
- Other reactions of conjugation

The Metabolism of Drugs and Other Xenobiotics: Biological Regulation and Consequences

Part A: The Life Cycle of a Xenobiotic in the Organism
- The fate of xenobiotics in the organism

Part B: Anatomical Distribution of Metabolizing Capacity
- Subcellular distribution
- Tissue distribution

Part C: Regulation of Metabolism
- Molecular biology of enzyme induction
- Assessment of enzyme induction and inhibition *in vivo*
- Physiological influences
- Pathological influences
- Pharmacogenetics
- Species differences

Part D: The Consequences of Metabolism
- Influence of dose size on the fate of xenobiotics
- Pharmacological implications of metabolism
- Toxicological implications of metabolism
- Future perspectives on the continued importance of metabolic studies of xenobiotics

INDEX

THE BONDS THAT TIE

Blood
Bonds

Books by J Bree

The Mounts Bay Saga

The Butcher of the Bay: Part I
The Butcher of the Bay: Part II
*

Just Drop Out: Hannaford Prep Year One
Make Your Move: Hannaford Prep Year Two
Play the Game: Hannaford Prep Year Three
To the End: Hannaford Prep Year Four
Make My Move: Alternate POV of Year Two
*

All Hail
The Ruthless
Queen Crow
*

Angel Unseen

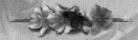

The Bonds That Tie Series

Broken Bonds
Savage Bonds
Blood Bonds
Forced Bonds

THE BONDS THAT TIE

Blood
Bonds

J BREE

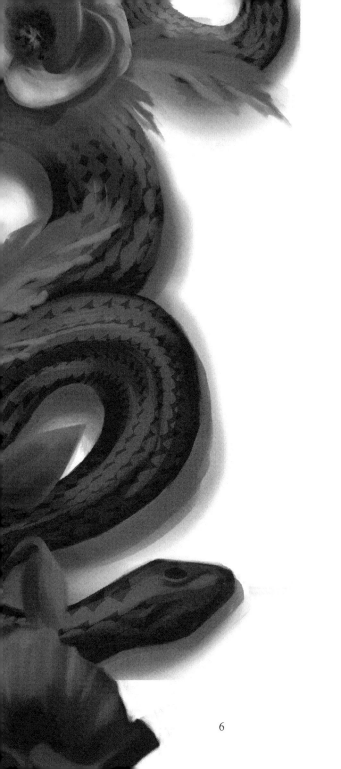

Prologue

OLI

The hospital is loud and cold.

My bond is quiet in my chest, as though the surge of it coming out to protect me has sated the constant thirst for blood it seems to have for now, but I already know it won't last long. The craving, the wanting, the overwhelming need to consume… it never goes away for long.

"Oleander? Oleander Fallows? God, you look like a pretty little thing sitting up there in that big bed. All of that long, blonde hair, your Bonds are going to be so happy to know that you made it out of that car wreck unharmed."

I can't look up at the nurse who is speaking to me, her tone warm and kind, and instead, my eyes focus on the long tendrils of my hair that are over my face. Blonde, it's not though. It's silver now, but yesterday it was black. Whatever happened in that car, it had bleached the color from my hair.

I struggle not to let the tears brimming in my eyes fall.

The nurse clicks her tongue, perching on the bed beside me and gently patting the back of my hand. "It's okay, I spoke to the head nurse, and she said your Bonds are on their way here. It's all very secret and hush-hush around here, so they must be important. I know that at least one of them is old enough to sign for your care, he's the one who got you moved into this big, private room, so he must be from one of the upper society families. Don't be scared, with a Bond like that, you're going to be okay."

The more she talks, the more furious my bond gets.

I didn't understand it then, but the woman is trying to get me to talk to her, to figure out who it was that I belong

8

to, so she could sell me out. My bond knew it, and so it urged me to keep my mouth shut, and even though I hate it most of the time, I listen when it tells me something like that.

"Belinda? What are you doing in here? Leave Oleander alone!"

I glance up to see Nurse June scowling in the doorway, one fist propped on her hip like she's ready to drag the other woman out of here at a moment's notice. When I woke up in the emergency room, she was the first person I'd seen, and she had been the person to tell me that my parents were killed in the accident. I'd already known, but the way that she had broken the news and treated me ever since, it made me like her and, more importantly, trust her.

Her eyes soften a fraction when they land on me and she says, "Your lunch is on its way up now, and the counselor will come in to speak with you as soon as you're done eating. He took a little while to get here, but he's the best in the city. Your Bond made sure of that."

Belinda's eyes snap over to me again but when she opens her mouth, Nurse June steps into the room and cuts her off. "I will be writing you up with a warning, now get out of this room, and stop sticking your nose in where it doesn't belong!"

With a huff and mumbled complaints, Belinda gets up from the bed and stalks out of the room with a sneer at Nurse June, who barely bothers to glance her way.

I tip my head back finally and look at the older woman, my words stilted and faltering, "I don't want to talk about my Bonds."

She nods and pulls the curtains open a little wider, the midday sun bright as it streams into the room, "It's for the best if you don't, not until they get here. Too many prying ears and eyes in this place. All you need to remember is that everything is going to be okay once they get here."

I nod and watch her fuss with things a little more, hoping she'll stay here until the food arrives. I want to speak to her, to tell her what the hell is going on right now, but my tongue is frozen in my mouth. After another moment of checking over my paperwork, she smiles at me and leaves without another word.

My eyes squeeze shut the moment the door closes, terror racing through my veins when the voice in the corner starts to speak again, "I thought they'd be in here forever, deadly little Soul Render. Now, where were we?

Ah, of course… I was telling you about all of the things you'll do to your Bonds if you stay here with them. All of that pain and suffering, all of the destruction, just for being with you. It's much safer for you all if you come with me."

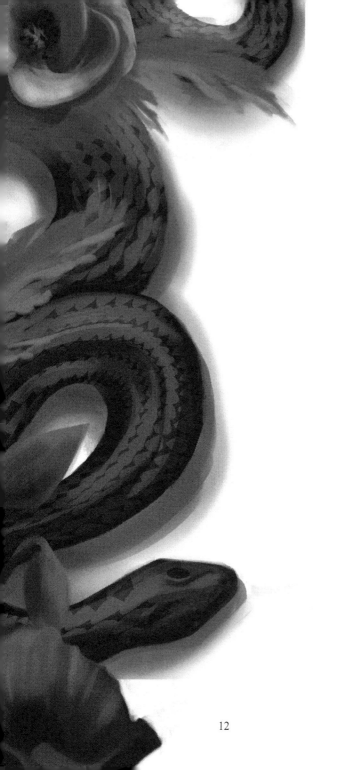

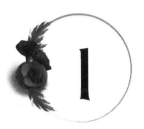

NORTH

Bodies fall to the dirt around us in unceremonious heaps, limbs torn away and chunks missing from their torsos, thanks to the hundreds of nightmare creatures roaming the camp.

All three of the TacTeams working with us today are forming a perimeter, careful not to move in while the carnage is taking place because the infamous Draven nightmares don't distinguish friend from foe when they're in a feeding frenzy like this. No, there's only bodies to consume and tear apart until blood and gore is dripping from their jaws as their eyes shine with an eerie and unnatural light.

The camp is an older one, more established and full of heavily brainwashed Gifted who'll take months to process and deprogram. I want to be noble and say that we're here to save them, that we've watched this camp for months and planned out this rescue to bring these people home to their families, and on paper, that's all true.

But as an older camp, it's also full of records, and Gryphon has become obsessed with sifting through Resistance data. It's not hard to figure out his motives. There's something he knows about our Bond that he's choosing not to share, but when he finds whatever he's looking for…

We might all finally get some answers.

There's a static sound in my earpiece and then Gryphon's voice comes through, "Prisoners are in the biggest tent on the east side. Bravo team, move out."

I unholster one of my guns and then hold my palm out to call my nightmare creatures back into myself now that the majority of the Resistance here have been dealt with. There's still a chance that we've missed some, thus the gun, but the risk of killing innocents is too high to keep them out and consuming.

Most of the creatures melt away back into me as though they're obedient, others go back in snarling and screaming. The biggest of them all, the one that I *refuse* to call August, stops short to stare at me with its glowing void eyes.

It stares at me like it is the docile puppy Oleander seems so intent on it being. It stares at me like it's pissed off she's not here, dropping to her knees to shower it with love and affection.

It stares at me like it knows something is wrong.

"Is he still giving you shit thanks to Oli?" Gryphon says as he walks up behind me, bolder and less cautious now that he's seen the creature heel to our little Bond.

"*It* is, yes. There's something… off about the camp. Keep your eyes peeled, and stick close."

He smirks at my distinction of the creature, enjoying riling me up on Oleander's behalf, which is both new and completely typical of him.

He's going to be a nightmare going forward, especially if he stays the only Bonded of us all.

I have to wrench my mind away from that particular path, something that could occupy me for days if I really wanted to follow that thought process. Maybe being stuck in council meetings has been a blessing in disguise, keeping me distracted and busy so that I don't have to think about our little mysterious Bond, who might just have had a real reason to run from us after all.

I hold my hand out to the creature again, a battle of wills and mental strength, until finally, with a soundless huff and snort, there's a pop sound as he disappears back into me. My bond rears its head in my chest, not so eager at being forced to heel, and I take a deep breath as Gryphon calls out again to get everyone moving.

Nox doesn't call his creatures into himself at all, but they've always been completely obedient to their master. Once he starts moving through the tents and clearing them, the other members of the Alpha team are happy enough to follow his lead. They're still cautious but no longer stuck standing rigidly like statues, like they are around mine. Something about the size difference, or the very obvious way that mine are rabid, reinforces the general rules of staying the fuck away from them nicely without any of our Bond Group having to say a word.

Gryphon takes his backup second with him to scout out a cluster of smaller tents that we already know from intel are the lodgings of the higher members of the

Resistance. His second, Harrison, is Arthur Rockelle's son, and a highly trained Flame who has always been loyal. He's the easy choice to back Gryphon while Kieran is on Oleander's protection detail.

I follow Nox to the torture camp.

He always goes to the questioning and processing areas first. He finds the men and women working there himself, just to make sure that they die a very messy and painful death at his hands, because the idea of a bullet between the eyes for their kind just doesn't sit well with him.

Or me.

I'm just a little less zealous about it.

Sure enough, we find an Empath and two Neuros in there, huddled together. Their panicked, whispered plans are useless and redundant, and I watch with a cold sort of interest as Nox stalks towards them with his palm outstretched, the black stains of our curse darkening his skin as their screams fill our ears.

He always does play with his food before he lets his nightmares eat them.

An hour later, we're climbing into the back of the truck with the knowledge that every Resistance member here is now dead. Gryphon calls out to the driver to get us back onto the road and headed back to the rendezvous point, blood covering us all from the knees down.

The Bravo team will stay behind and move the recovered Gifted to our version of the processing camps, only instead of poking and prodding at them to figure out what use they'll be to our manic mission, we'll be starting the long process of undoing all of the programming and torture they've endured since they were taken.

Some of them will die there.

It doesn't sit well with me, it never has, but sometimes they're too far gone, the damage is too much to come back from.

I blow out a breath and tip my head back against the seat, enjoying the quiet moment without having to think about council meetings or political moves. As much as I didn't want to leave my Bond behind, definitely not after the revelation of more Resistance interference, there's something about getting away from all of the trappings of being North Draven the Councilman that I desperately needed.

It all feels like bullshit, like sand slipping through my fingers while the world burns around us all anyway.

William would've known what to do, more than I ever have.

There were fifty captive Gifted here and we got thirty-eight out alive. It sounds like a terrible amount of casualties, and in other situations, heads would be rolling about losing twelve Gifted, but these sorts of recon missions… twelve is right about average.

We've never gotten everyone out alive before. We're outnumbered and always running on the defensive, our greatest weakness as a society, and with that comes far too much blood being spilled. It's easier to digest the numbers here on the ground, watching the TacTeams work their asses off to get the worst of the brainwashed victims restrained before they become a danger to themselves or others, but in my office back home when I get reports, those numbers burn a hole into my deepest marrow. It's never enough. Nothing we do ever is.

With those morose thoughts, I almost miss it.

It starts with Gryphon's fingers thrumming against the leather seats, a small outlet for his frustration. The calm over Nox's face, something I've barely seen before and that had only taken place when his own bloodlust had been sated, slowly melts away until the furrow in his brow is firmly back in place.

Blood and pain.

My bond hasn't stopped whispering to me all morning, telling me all about the darkest and most blood-soaked things it wants to do to every member of the Resistance we come across today. It makes it harder for me to notice that same tension entering me that has taken hold of the other two, but once I see the scowl on Gryphon's face, I take stock of myself.

My skin feels tight with irritation, as though it's pulled tighter over my frame now than it was ten minutes ago, and my entire body feels restless. There's a tension in me that wasn't there before. Something is happening within our Bond.

Oleander.

I don't have my phone with me, protocol on this sort of mission, and I try not to sound panicked or desperate when I murmur to Gryphon, "Contact Oleander. Tell me where she is right now."

His eyes flick to mine, the frown still firmly in place, and there's the slightest pause before he curses and his eyes flash white as he calls on his gift for an extra boost.

It's all I need to see to know that I'm not wrong,

that something is happening right now that even with hundreds of miles between us, I can feel her there under my skin. We might be Unbonded but it doesn't matter, she's there in my blood and the deepest, darkest corners of my soul.

The panic gets worse.

Nox is watching us both keenly, not faking his usual indifference when it's only the three of us, and when Gryphon curses again, he drawls, "Where is she? Are we about to go running after our little poisonous Bond again?"

Gryphon ignores him as he grabs out his comms, a feat because even I want to snarl at his jabs and I'm sure being Bonded only makes this feeling a million times worse. When he doesn't get an answer on the comms, he unbuckles his seatbelt and lurches into the front of the truck, coming back with his phone and a vaguely sick look on his face.

I take a deep breath and count down from ten to keep myself in line, forcing my bond back from lashing out.

"Kieran isn't answering me," Gryphon says as his scowl deepens, and I want to reach across the backseat and choke the answer out of him, another sign that something has gone wrong in the hours since we left the mansion.

My bond is *writhing* with bloodlust.

"She's not answering me either. Get Gabe on the phone, call Bassinger too," Gryphon snaps, throwing the phone to me as he presses both of his palms against his temples like he's in pain.

Nox's eyes meet mine, but he looks as though he's about to tear the driver out of the seat and turn this truck around. "What's wrong? Why do you look like you're about to puke?"

"Because I pushed to get her to answer and she's not… there. She's not ignoring me, there's something in the way. Something is wrong, get Gabe on the line *now*."

Except we left a lot more than just the other Bonds behind to keep an eye on her.

As I start dialing, Nox's eyes shift to black and Gryphon watches him check in with the… *Brutus*, like it's the only lifeline in the middle of the ocean while we're all drowning.

"She's alive. She's breathing, I can't see much else, but he's with her, so no one will get within spitting distance without him consuming them. Take a breath,

Gryph, she's alive."

He doesn't look any better at that news. "Well then, where the fuck is she? Don't tell me to calm down when she's gone again."

When the phone finally clicks as Gabe answers, I hear Bassinger snarling down the line, "So *now* you lot want to call us? Well, you're too fucking late!"

Gryphon's eyes snap to mine, too wide and glassy, thanks to the push he'd given his connection with his Bonded.

I snarl into the phone, "What the fuck has happened? We've been gone less than twelve hours—"

Gryphon cuts me off, snarling, "Where the fuck is she, Bassinger? I will come back there and tear your fucking spine out of your throat, if you had anything to do with this!"

Bassinger scoffs at him, a savage sort of sound, and snarls back, "Your useless, fucking asshole second took her, and they haven't come back! I will fucking kill you all if she's hurt. I'll gut that fucking dickhead Black too."

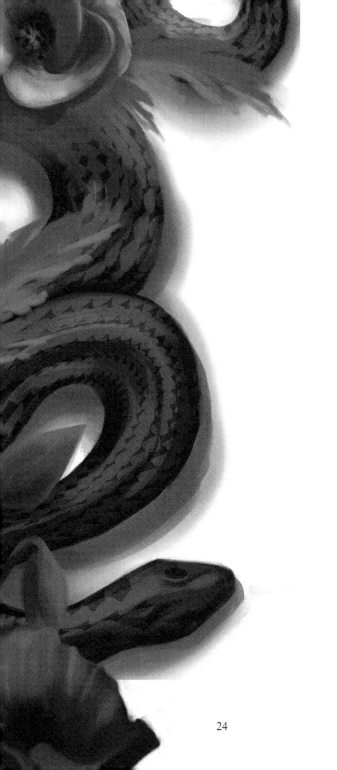

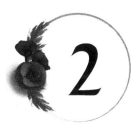

OLI

I wake up strapped to a chair, the smells of smoke, body odor, and despair hitting my nostrils, and my stomach turns as I squeeze my eyes shut tighter. There's rustling and quiet murmuring of two women in here, the noises a sign of them cleaning something here in the tent up, and I don't want them to know I'm awake yet.

It's hard to keep the disgust off of my face.

The stench here is familiar, a particular blend of gross that I'd been hoping to never come across again, and I have to choke back the bile that creeps up the back of my throat. Kieran and I were separated right away but not before I'd been forced to watch three guards beat the shit out of him.

No one lifted a finger against me, but I already knew they wouldn't.

Once he was bleeding from about ten different places and there was a rattle in his chest that suggested some serious internal injuries, Kieran had been dragged away to one of the holding tents unceremoniously by a couple of low-level thugs.

I had been escorted to the priority tent, somewhere I've spent way too much time.

"Why the fuck are we waiting on some sheep-bitch? It's demeaning, she should be eating slop in the cages with the rest of them."

There's a quiet grunt and then the other woman replies, quietly but in a rougher, aged voice, "She's a VIP. Her gift means she gets real food, a bath when she needs it, and she's off-limits to the men for a bit of fun. Don't worry about it, she'll be torn up good by Davies just the same as they all are."

Gross.

For one, I do *not* want to hear his name, but there's also something about the women talking so casually about the horrors that happen here, like it doesn't even matter to them what happens here after dark and in tight quarters, that makes my blood run cold. I guess I don't have to feel guilty about killing them all when the time comes. Does that make me just as bad as them?

I hope not, but I'll also accept it if it does.

"VIP... what does that even mean? Is she a Neuro? Davies doesn't usually keep those around for long."

Of course not, they're competition for him. Okay, they're not at all, because I've never heard of another Neuro who can do the shit he can, except Gryphon. As strong as my Bonded is, he's no match for *that man*.

I'm no match for him either.

It's terrifying.

I know how much power is pumping through my veins, so much that my body still can't use it without taking a three day nap to recover, and he could end my world without a second thought. Our gifts might be eons apart in ability but there's too many parallels with the destruction we're both capable of.

The woman with the rough voice mutters, reluctantly and somewhat reverently, "This girl, this little white-haired bitch who looks like nothing special, she's the

Infinite Weapon. They're going to use her to end the war and finally let us Gifted take control of this country like we deserve. No more making nice with the non-Gifted. No more living shackled to laws that shouldn't apply to us because we're above them. No more sheep in control, living in their mansions while the rest of us struggle to survive."

Fucking hell.

I'd almost forgotten how delusional they all sound, as though they're going to love living in the Wild West Dystopia that they're all gunning for when really... they'll all probably die for the cause. That man wouldn't hesitate to sacrifice them all to get what he wants.

Ultimate power.

There's more movement and then I hear one of the women walk away, rustling the tent flap, and then the smell of hot chicken and gravy hits my nose. My stomach rumbles and a wave of nausea hits me, the same as it always does when I wake up from one of these power-use naps.

I blink my eyes a few times as they stream against the harsh lighting and I get a look at both of the women. I don't recognize either of them, but I catalog their features anyway, storing away as much information as I can, in case I need it later.

Doing that has saved my life many times before.

The older woman is holding out the plate of food and with a downturned mouth, she says, "I'm not going to free your arms to eat, but if you try to stop me from feeding you, I have orders to force it down your throat with any means necessary."

I shrug and open my mouth. As obedient as it may look like I'm being, the eyes she gives me says she doesn't believe it one bit.

Hilarious, because I'm too hungry to bite the bitch or attempt to mess with her.

The other woman, who only looks a few years older than I am, watches us both with her hands fisted at her side as though she's ready to fly over and break my jaw the second I prove myself to be the unruly 'sheep' they think I am.

They really have no idea.

I eat the entire plate without a word or complaint, chewing the delicious chicken and gravy while keeping my face blank. I don't want them to know how much I'm enjoying it, how much I wish I could have seconds. Once the plate is clean, the woman holds a bottle of water to my lips and lets me down the entire thing. It feels like the elixir of life to my dry tongue and chapped lips.

Then the women both leave without another word.

I take a second to look around, but the tent is bare, completely empty, other than me and the chair I'm chained to. It feels a little too familiar. I wouldn't put it past these assholes to have brought in the exact one I'd spent two years parked on just to mess with my damn head a little more.

That's kind of *ugh*, Silas Davies' thing.

As if my thoughts conjured him, the tent flap parts and the man, the nightmare, himself steps into the space with me.

After so long of forcing myself to not think about him, to not even acknowledge that he exists in the world, it's weirdly uneventful to see him standing there in his carefully put together outfit. I know for sure that he puts in a lot of thought about how he dresses, a lot of thought on what color he'll be donning for the day, because I never wanted to see him on days where he'd wear white.

He enjoys the patterns of blood spatters, and there was always a sense of pride in him when he would leave the torture tents covered in the fruits of his labor. I think it also helped keep the other Resistance members in line because between that and the manic grin on his face, he definitely looks like the crazed torturer you wouldn't want to mess with.

"Little Soul Render… not so little now though, are you? You've grown up a lot since you ran off on me."

His voice is low and melodic. I keep my eyes on his boots for now while I focus on getting my heart rate back down to normal levels and not where it's currently sitting… which is pounding out of my chest.

I hope Gryphon can't feel this.

It's too dangerous to so much as think about him and my Bonds right now, even though I can feel him trying to contact me at the edges of my mind. Of course I know that he'd attempt it, the quickest and easiest way for him to find me is to just ask, but to speak to him now, with Silas in the room? That's a huge no.

It's also hard to block Gryphon out without making it too obvious.

Everything is a freaking mess.

"Are we really going to go back to the silent treatment, Weapon? I thought you might have grown out of this."

I smother the shiver that runs down my spine, forcing my shoulders not to move and give away just how much the mere sound of his voice scares me. I hate this man, sure, but I'm also completely aware of just how terrifying he truly is.

I need to keep my head together.

At my continued silence, Davies steps further into the tent, his footsteps slow and measured. He's an expert at drawing out the terror in the room, and I'm not entirely sure if it's a natural talent or the copious amount of experience he's had ruining people. I can't help but tense when he steps behind me, but then he steps back into my eyeline with another chair, carefully shrugging out of his jacket and slinging it over the back as he takes a seat.

He has this very careful and measured way of folding himself into it that makes my skin crawl. Ever the gentleman, but it's only a mask, a ruse he wears to cover the sadistic creature he really is.

I know I'm a monster, and I hate myself for it, but this man loves being this way with every fiber of his being... and that's why he scares the absolute fucking shit out of me.

Finally, I meet his eyes.

He smirks at me, enjoying just how much I hate looking at him, but it's actually easier to stay a blank canvas when I'm staring into the deep, evil abyss that are his eyes. There's nothing normal or human in them, nothing but the cold-blooded, sadistic man that he is shining there.

He doesn't say another word to me for a full minute, and then he leans back in the seat again, crossing his arms. There must be a camera in here, because the action triggers more people to enter the tent.

Two heavily armed men, to be precise, dragging a bleeding Kieran behind them, one of his legs jutting out at a very *wrong* angle.

Well, *fuck*.

The men drop him at my feet so that he's wedged between Davies and I and then walk out. I take a very slow, and hopefully discreet, breath.

Davies sighs and tuts at me again. "I have to say, it hurt my feelings, you know?"

I keep my eyes trained on his, because I *cannot* look at Kieran. You don't last here in the camps if you show your weaknesses, and all they know about the two of us so far is that we came here together.

That's already too much.

Davies drawls on, "You never spoke to any of the Gifted here, not the loyal or the sheep, and yet you came right back to us with some weakling Transporter? It cuts me deeply."

I am an expert at blocking this man out though. I think I would've gone crazy in the two years I'd spent stuck in the camps if I hadn't learned how to just tune his honeyed, poisonous monologues out. I hope Kieran is doing the same down there in the dirt, otherwise he's going to die a thousand slow and crazed deaths listening to it all.

"I guess we'll have to do something about him... something extreme. The punishment should fit the crime. How dare a lower-tiered Gifted befriend our Little Soul Render when she's spat on the rest of us, time and time again? How about the rack?"

Oh, fuck.

My eyes flick down to Kieran's bloodied and bruised form on the ground without meaning to, a reflex at hearing Silas' favorite torture machine mentioned. You'd think with all of the power pumping through his veins that he'd torture people with his gift, but no... he prefers machines that belong in the Middle Ages, you know, when they were invented.

No one survives the rack, not a single person in the two years I was here, and if I don't do something, Gryphon's second is about to die, all because I asked him to bring me here.

My voice cracks, "You can't."

I finally look down at Kieran but he's glaring at me, a soundless command to shut my mouth and let him take the pain and suffering for us both. He probably knows he's about to die, but typical macho man shit says he wants to do it honorably.

I'm not built like that. He should know that by now.

Silas turns and smirks at me, his handsome face curling into a ghoulish mask. "And why is that, Little Render? Give me one good reason why I should change my plans for the Transporter."

He really thinks he has this over me, he really thinks he's going to use Kieran's death to mess with my head… Well, trump card, asshole.

"He's my Bond."

The best thing about my bond is that it understands a life or death sort of situation and toes the goddamned line when I need it to, so when I look down at Kieran again and see the horror in his eyes, my own don't shift in retaliation. It's a win.

How the hell am I going to get him to play along here?

"You stood there and watched him get beaten. You expect me to believe you're Bonded to him?" Davies' voice drips with derision but when I glance back at him, he's tense, his body practically vibrating at the carrot I'm dangling in front of him.

How long had they tortured me for the names of my Bonds?

How many times had he promised me things, evil and glorious and kind things, if only I'd tell them who my Bonds were?

It's another piece of the puzzle that makes no sense to me, especially now that I know that someone in the Resistance has been messing with the labs and the Bonded groups, but it's clear that they still don't know about my Bonds.

I wonder why that traitorous bitch Giovanna hasn't told them? And how could Atlas' dad be here, very obviously a part of the Resistance, but hasn't told them?

Too fucking confusing.

Davies snaps his fingers in front of my face, and I shift my eyes away from the scowl on Kieran's face to mutter, "You said it yourself, you have to be cold-hearted to rip the souls out of people and watch them die. Besides, we're not Bonded yet, and you weren't killing him. My bond was happy to watch you test him out a little. The rack is too much. If you break him, you'll break me, and I'm not signing up for that."

I watch as the feverish glee fills his body. Me, his beloved weapon, back in his grasp and now with one more round of ammunition with me. A Bond.

He straightens up and turns on his heel to stalk towards the entrance of the tent, his usually fluid movements jerkier with his excitement, and I take the moment to do something incredibly risky. Risky but necessary, because Kieran looks like he's a second away from chewing me out for lying about him like this just to save his freaking life.

My eyes shift to black, and I send up the tiniest of

prayers that Davies really is too busy having his world rocked by getting me and one of my Bonds that he won't notice what the hell I'm doing.

I need you to tell Kieran to play along.

Gryphon's response is immediate and desperate sounding, *WHERE ARE YOU?*

I take a good, hard look at Davies as he turns back to us, my breath catching in my throat, but he's too busy eyeballing Kieran like he'll find my name branded on his skin if only he looks hard enough at him, so I take the chance to keep the conversation going for a moment longer. *Life or death situation here, Bonded. I need you to hack into Kieran's brain RIGHT NOW and tell him to play along, or your second is dead. Do it. I'll contact you again the moment it's safe. I swear on our Bond.*

There's a slight pause and then Gryphon says again, his blinding rage at me and this situation we've found ourselves in making my ears ring, *How did you know I can reach him? How did you know my Gift had grown that much?*

I want to slump in the chair against my restraints in relief but that would be too obvious, so instead, I send one last message before I block him out entirely again.

A lucky guess. I'll keep him safe, Kyrie too. I'll let you know the moment it's safe for you to come get us. I'll come back to you all, I promise. Tell North I didn't run.

I don't know why it's so important to me to tack that onto the end there, but I do, stupidly thinking that at least if Silas loses his mind and kills me off, at least North might… believe that I wasn't the worst choice for a Bond.

God, what a depressing thought.

I see the exact moment Gryphon gets through to Kieran. His shoulders square up, ever the obedient second in command. It's a much better look on him than the pissed off, bloodied TacTeam member who wants to murder me, that's for damn sure.

Davies finally decides to actually do something and walks over to Kieran, grabbing him by both arms and pulling him onto his feet. His bad leg doesn't support any of his weight, lolling out, and he grunts a little as he's probably blinded by the pain. I wish so badly that I could heal him, or take his pain away from him, but he's not actually my Bond, no matter what I tell Davies, so there is nothing I can offer him.

Davies doesn't notice his leg, or doesn't care, and starts one of his usual honeyed monologues. "A Transporter.

I'm a little disappointed at how mediocre that is. I was expecting something *magnificent*, to be paired with a beauty like you. I suppose I'm stuck with a Healer, so it makes sense that we can't all be once-in-a-lifetime powers. Still, I can't say I wasn't hoping for more."

My bond flashes to the forefront of my mind again, not liking the way he's speaking about our Bonds, even if he's got the wrong guy. It doesn't throw a tantrum or act spoiled the way it has for weeks back at the Draven mansion, and for once, I feel *safer* with it taking the reins for a bit. It always did do whatever was required to keep me alive, whole, and sane.

Kieran stares at Davies blankly, nothing showing on his face now that he's playing the good soldier and following Gryphon's orders. I feel oddly proud of him for not cowering in the face of this terrible man… but he also probably doesn't know the extent of his evil.

Not the way I do, anyway.

Davies shoves him to his knees at my feet again and though he grimaces, Kieran doesn't make a noise at the pain that's very obviously shooting through his body. I look at him now that my bond is at the helm, safer now that Davies can see the cold and aloof look of my void eyes because he's never seen the hungry look in them before... he's never seen me look at my Bonds and make demands of them.

Mine.

God, I miss them all already. What I wouldn't give to be sitting in a stupid Gifted 101 class with Nox snarling up at me, or sitting in the dining room with North making demands and Gryphon ignoring my existence. I'd take all of their bullshit right now to be back there with them.

I really have fallen.

Davies stares at me, watching my bond peruse Kieran and deciding it's not just a show put on for him, and the victory in his grin makes me feel sick. "Little Render... you're going to Bond with him, and then we're going to test you out all over again. God, how I've missed your screaming."

And then he leaves the tent, leaves Kieran on the ground at my feet, and me chained to my chair with cold, black, void eyes.

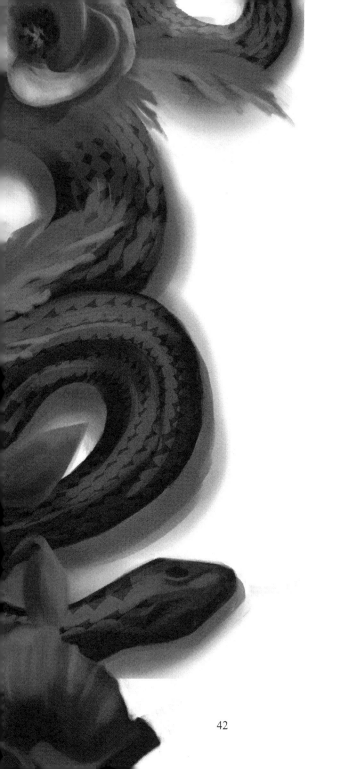

OLI

Kieran has tech handcuffs on, the type that will send volts of electricity tearing through your body if you step out of line to kill you, so I'm not surprised that Davies has just left him behind with me. I'm also aware that there's a camera on us. While I'm confident that it won't have a mic, I still don't want to be sitting here chatting about what's really going on.

When he looks up at me with a glare, I shush him and then I cast out my gift to feel who is around us, whether anyone will overhear his pissed off tirade that I'm sure is just bursting to get out.

Davies is over in the main tents with a handful of his strongest and most trusted men. None of them can hear shit from this far away though, so I'm safe there. There's a lot of new people here, but I can't sense any Neuros or Telekinetic-type gifts, so I decide it's worth the risk and call my gift back into myself, meeting Kieran's eye and giving him the go-ahead to speak.

I shouldn't have bothered.

"I'm not having sex with you."

I snort at him and snap back, remembering in the last second to keep my voice down and my head ducked despite my outrage, "That's never been the plan, Black! Get your head out of the gutter."

He huffs at me like *I'm* being the unreasonable one, and then winces as he jolts his leg, shifting slightly to attempt to relieve some of the pain he's obviously in. I hope it's not broken. I'm not sure how long it's going to take me to get the hell out of here, and Franklin is still here for some unknown reason, so the thought of having to drag Kieran out on my back is just too much.

"So what is your grand plan then? You heard Silas Davies, he's going to expect us to '*Bond*'."

I roll my eyes at him, extra petulant because I'm stuck

in the chair with a numb ass, but also to hide the thrill of terror that jolts through my veins at him saying the name. "I know exactly what the next few days are going to look like, so calm down. We just need to be patient, and then I'll get us out."

He blinks at me for a second and then curses under his breath, shaking his head. "Contact Shore. Tell him where we are and get an evac, because there's no way you're going to get us out of here."

My bond floods me at the sound of his name, and I have no control of my body as it takes over and my eyes shift to black, leaning down to hiss at Kieran, "I have endured too much for you to speak his name here. Don't *ever* speak of *any* of them."

He pauses for a second and then he gulps.

He honest-to-God gulps like I'm terrifying, which my bond loves, but it releases its grip on me, and I slump back in the seat with a gasp.

"You're a crazy fucking kid, you know that?"

I shrug and let out a quiet, slightly shaky, laugh. "I thought you were looking forward to watching me ruin everyone's lives? Come on now, don't give up on me over something so small. My bond barely spoke to you!"

He shakes his head and me and looks away. "And I'll do my best to never speak to it again, thank you very much."

I scoff at him, giggling a little, which is stupid, but there's also this weird sense of relief in me that we're trapped here together... that I have someone with me this time, and I'm not going to be completely alone. Plus, if it had to be anyone, I'm sort of glad it's him.

I'd be beside myself if it were Sage again. I'd be too worried about her getting hurt or assaulted to concentrate on my plans, and if it were truly one of my Bonds? Jesus, the bloodshed my own bond would have over them being in danger is just too much to even think about. A Technokinetic is no help, and Sawyer's smart mouth would get him in way too much trouble.

Felix would've also been helpful but, again, I'd be too worried about my bestie's Bonded getting himself killed to focus, so Kieran Black is the best goddamn choice here.

If only Kyrie wasn't also in the freaking camps with us.

There is a moment of silence between us while I try to figure out how the hell to get Kyrie in this tent with us before Kieran speaks again, his voice barely more than breath. "You're protecting them."

It feels so obvious to me, but I guess he assumed the same as the rest of them, that I'd hated my Bonds and run from them all rather than have them.

I duck my head again so whoever is watching that camera can't read my lips. "Always. Everything I've done has been to protect them. Every action, every word I've bitten back, every minute I spent running from them. If you're not terrified of that man, then you don't have good enough intel… or you haven't been paying attention to it. He's evil incarnate."

He doesn't answer for a second, his breathing even and slow, and then he murmurs back, "He tortured you. The IW… I read what they did to you. They tortured you. You didn't give them your Bonds' names. You didn't break."

I swallow and desperately want to change the subject. "I did break. I let my bond take the pain for me. I let it become the monster instead of me."

I refuse to speak about anything else with Kieran after that, too much honesty freaking me all the way out until I'm a jittery mess. I spend the time talking quietly with my bond to see if we can actually do something about how much pain Kieran is in but I'm not a Healer, no matter how well I can repair the men who belong to me, and my bond has nothing to give.

I wonder if I can convince someone else here to heal him for me?

There's a rustling and more noises outside, and then the tent flaps open again as the older woman from before bustles in again, this time with two plates filled to the brim with more of the same food. I'm not surprised to be getting a second helping. It's well known that I need the extra calories post-gift usage, but I'm guessing he's been given the slop they serve the so-called sheep. The steaming plate of roast chicken with all of the sides, smothered in gravy, is a sight for sore eyes.

Or growling belly.

She walks over to us both but ignores Kieran, instead meeting my eyes with an authoritative look and says, "I've been told to loosen your restraints so you can eat. If you attempt to move in any way, I will zap your ass into next year."

Ah.

So she hasn't been told that her gift won't work on me thanks to my bond being the second biggest monster in this camp? Poor woman. I play along nonetheless, mostly because I know it irritates that man when I do.

He never understood why I wouldn't just kill everyone he sent my way, and I'm sure he picks them all carefully. Choosing the most annoying, the sleaziest, or the most arrogant of his underlings that he can get his hands on.

Once my hands are bound in front of my body and I can feed myself, the woman hands me my plate and then finally turns to Kieran, shoving his plate at him as though he's dirt beneath her shoes, and walks back out.

"What the fuck is this? Are we being poisoned?"

I shake my head at him and shove a forkful into my mouth. "Welcome to VIP life in the camps, Black. As my Bond, you'll be fed three hot meals a day. You won't be beaten or attacked in the showers, and if anyone attempts to incapacitate you, they'll answer straight to the top man himself. All it will cost you is daily torture sessions and being forced to put up with lines of questioning that will have you considering suicide just to get it to end."

He blinks at me and then when he's watched me shove half my plate into my mouth, he finally picks up his own fork and gets to work on the chicken.

"It's flavorless," he gripes, and I scoff at him.

"It's the Resistance, were you really expecting something different? Who knew you were so spoiled?"

He shakes his head at me and keeps eating, with far more decorum than I have, goddamn him. There's a lot of noise in the camp around us, they're preparing for something big, some mission they're about to set out on to tear Gifted families and Bonded groups apart.

I loathe the lot of them.

We eat in silence for a few minutes longer, right until Kieran is using the last of his bread roll to sop up the gravy, and then I finally ask the question I've been working my way up to, afraid of the answer. "Have you seen Kyrie?"

He sets his empty plate down beside himself and stretches out his bad leg, wincing again. I curse under my breath, but he shrugs it off. I'm sure it's incredibly painful... I wonder if there's Tac training for learning how to ignore that level of pain or if he's just built like that?

I learned after many, many torture sessions.

Kieran grunts and then murmurs softly, "She's in the cages with the other women. They haven't sorted them or tested any of them yet. Davies has been too focused on having you back. He was positively gleeful about it."

I nod and look around the tent again as though a key or weapon is going to jump out at me to get me the hell out of these frustrating restraints. The forks are both plastic, and the tech in the restraints would just melt them if we tried.

Maybe Sawyer would be useful to me right about now.

I try to ignore Kieran's eyes on me, but they bore into my skin until finally he says, his voice low, "You're too calm. If this is the place you were tortured as a kid, for two years, you should be more... worried. What's your plan? Why are you so calm?"

I shove the last of my potatoes into my mouth so that I don't have to answer him for a minute, chewing slowly. How do I answer him without giving away too much? Is there such a thing anymore?

There's not really any secrets left... except one, and there's no amount of torture that could pry that out of me.

"I'm not calm… I'm sure. There's enough happening here that's the same as last time, so I know how this is going to go. I know what has to happen to get us out. We just have to be patient and, probably, take a little pain. I'm sorry about that part, but there's no avoiding it. Does your bond help out with that stuff? I'm not really sure how other people's bonds work."

He turns to keep his eyes trained on the opening of the tent like he's keeping watch, but I know all too well that we'll hear the woman coming. There's no mistaking it.

"My bond doesn't protect me like that. Mine is more… placid compared to yours. I'm the one in control, not it."

I hand him my plate so that he can set it down, because my restraints won't let me do it myself. "I'd love to think I'm in control, but I'm pretty sure my bond is just humoring me. I think it lets me run the show, but the second I'm in danger, it takes over. It's handy until some little jealous bitch starts throwing perfume around."

I shouldn't bring it up, not here, but there aren't enough details to tell the Resistance anything.

Obviously Gryphon didn't give his second all of the details, but he knows enough to smirk at me and shrug.

"Could be worse, Fallows. Could've been your arch-nemesis. Or his brother."

I snort at him and mutter, "I'm not actually sure which one you're referring to, but yeah, I guess you're right. It could've been *much* worse."

The smirk slowly melts from his mouth and he glances at the camera one last time before he turns his body into mine a little more, covering his mouth from sight as he murmurs, "You need to warn them… about who we saw here. You need to tell them sooner rather than later that there's a potential sleeper cell."

Atlas.

He's talking about Atlas, because we'd seen his father here. The likeness between them both was striking, absolutely no doubt of their relation, but then Davies had turned to him and called him 'Bassinger' and sealed the freaking deal.

I still don't know what to think of it.

I don't know why I didn't tell Gryphon while I was speaking to him.

I hope to God that I haven't fucked up royally by not saying something, but I just… I couldn't. I can't believe that he'd betray me like that.

My spiraling thoughts are interrupted by the woman coming back to collect our plates. She grumbles under her breath about the waste of good resources on us sheep, and I roll my eyes at her. They're all the same here. The more I can cultivate a spoiled brat persona with them, the more that they'll underestimate me.

It's how I got out last time.

I wait until her back is to us both, scraping off the plates into a scraps bin, before I cast out my gift to find Kyrie. I need to find my way over to her sooner rather than later, and when I find her in the showers tent, I try not to shiver in disgust.

It's the worst place in the entire damned camp.

I pitch my tone to be whiny and demanding. "I need a shower."

Kieran scowls and glances up at me, but the woman doesn't react to him. I'm sure he just looks like an overprotective Bond, so it's probably a good thing he's acting up.

"The others are in there now, you'll have to wait."

My eyes shift to black and I watch the color drain from her face as I smirk at her, letting my bond take over to snark back at her, "I'm not going to wait."

Her mouth opens and shuts soundlessly for a second before my eyes flash back to their usual violet hue and she recovers enough to croak, "I need to get more men here. I can't take you both over there by myself."

I shrug and make a dismissive noise. "I don't need my Bond to hold my hand in there, leave him here. I smell, and I need to get some of this filth off before I puke at my own stench."

I'm hamming it up because I barely smell, only a little bit of the clean sweat scent of sitting around in a hot tent for days while I slept off my gift usage.

The woman glances down at Kieran, unsure at what the hell our dynamic is because we're obviously not acting like the Bonds she knows. Of course, she's probably totally submissive to her own Bond, the good little Bonded woman following orders, and for a fleeting second, I think about being sorry for her.

"You're going to just let her leave like that?"

Kieran grits his teeth at us both and then snarks back at the woman, "I'm not worried about my Bond's safety. You should ask yourself why that is."

She doesn't question either of us again.

The showers are in another smaller, darker tent on the other side of the camp. I'm sure they're not lit up with appropriate lighting like the rest of the camp for nefarious and disgusting reasons, but I already know that the women are alone in there.

For now.

"Clear out of the far stall! There's a VIP here." Sarcasm drips from her words, and I roll my eyes.

The women all look over at us both and shuffle away from the stall, and I turn to get my restraints loosened. I still can't do all that much with my hands, but in theory, I'll be able to undress my lower half and wash off. My shirt won't come off, but I'm not going to go over the semantics with this woman right now.

All I care about is that, by some insane stroke of luck, Kyrie is in the next stall over.

I walk into the tiny space and snap the curtain closed as though I'm actually going to shower. The Resistance woman stands so close to the stall that I can see her feet poking through underneath the curtain. I want to punch her through the fabric, just to catch her unaware and serve the bitch a little justice, but I'm sure she'll get what's coming to her soon.

Patience, Oli.

I have to repeat that word over and over again until this is all over with.

I don't bother undressing or tuning the water on. I'm not even going to bother with that sort of farce here. Instead, I walk over to the far end of the stall and crouch down to wave my hand under the small wall until Kyrie notices it and crouches down as well. I stick enough of my arm under there so that she can see the clothes I'm in and can hopefully tell it's me. The gap is big enough that I can see that she's still in her underwear, just rinsing off the same way I did for two freaking years. It's smart.

You don't want to get caught completely unaware in here… by anyone. The women are just as bad as the men, jumping each other in the showers in power plays. It's stupid, and they shouldn't bother fighting amongst themselves like that, but they do. Something about desperation and fearing this place brings out the worst in them all. I can't really talk. If I were in their places, I'd be the same.

Once again, my bond saved me from that. Now I'm going to use the knowledge and the resources I have to keep Kyrie safe from it all too.

I pull Brutus down from my shoulder; his form is more smoke than solid. He doesn't attempt to play or nuzzle me, completely subdued from the boisterous puppy that he usually is.

I wonder if Nox is watching me through his eyes right now?

He mustn't have seen anything that would lead them to me, because there's no doubt in my mind that Nox would be first in line to drag me back, if for no other reason than to have his favorite verbal target back.

It occurs to me that I'm just squatting here in the showers, silently staring at a nightmare creature while Kyrie is probably assuming I'm having a breakdown of some kind.

Hell, I might be.

I bring him up to my lips and whisper softly, "Keep her safe. No one touches her, jumps her, without your protection. Leave no evidence behind."

When I drop my hand back down to usher him over to Kyrie, I see her startle and hesitate, her hand slow to come out and accept the little bundle of smoke, but Brutus moves to her without question. I have to believe that if Nox is watching, he'd be happy to know that I'm trying to keep Gryphon's sister alive and safe while we're stuck here.

I wait for a moment, and then I let our fingers grasp together for a second, squeezing them in the only reassurance I can give her right now, before I pull away and stand back up, rubbing my hands over my legs to brush away the soap suds and dirt from the muddy ground of the shower.

When I snap the curtain back, the woman is waiting there for me, her ear pressed close to the fabric like she was trying to figure out what I was doing in there without the shower on.

Good luck with that, bitch.

"I'm ready to go," I drawl, and she scowls at me.

"You didn't even wash anything. What's the point in me getting you over here?"

I shrug at her and enjoy the huff of frustration I get back, not even caring when she's rough about tightening my restraints and jerking me around to get me moving again.

Kieran is safe because of my lie.

Kyrie is safe with Brutus.

I'm as safe as I've ever been thanks to the bond growing angrier and more savage by the hour in my chest.

We'll survive until I can get us out.

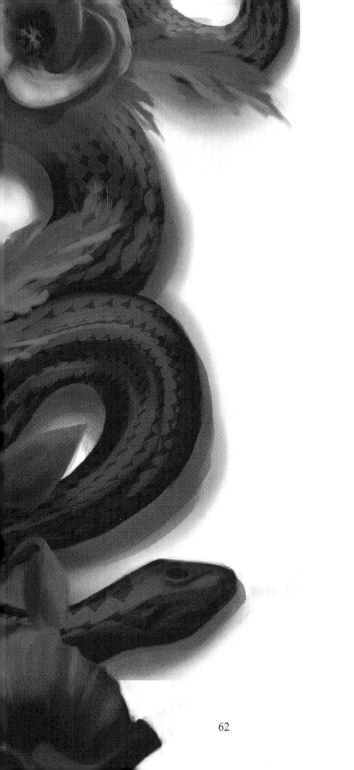

GRYPHON

It's getting harder by the day to keep my face passive and the contempt off of it while dealing with Gifted that we know are members of the Resistance. Daniella Jordan is no exception.

I've never trusted the slimy lawyer, and though North has always said I was just being difficult for the sake of it, it feels good to know that I was right. She doesn't like me standing in on their meetings, especially when I stand on North's side of the desk in his home office, behind his seat like I'm preparing to take a bullet for him as though he's not the most dangerous man in our entire community. She doesn't like the advantage it gives me, or that I'm looking down on her.

Well, I've never been looking down quite so hard before because this fucking bitch knows where my Bonded is. I know it. North knows it, and while she's sitting there talking about asinine Council bullshit, she knows it too. We're all just playing our parts and pretending the giant elephant isn't in the room. It's making my skin itch.

There's no way her sister was working alone to mess with Bond Groups. There's no way that Daniella has wormed her way into the good graces of North Draven for innocent reasons, and how much confidential information has she gotten directly from him in the last five years?

I'm going to call dibs on killing her, no matter how badly Nox wants it. There's a reason he's not here today. He's terrible at keeping a poker face in this kind of situation.

Daniella paints a frown onto her face, the picture of a concerned lawyer worried for her boss' Bond, but there's something about the very careful way that she speaks around me that's always flagged on my radar. Now we know why.

It takes everything inside of me to stop myself from

reaching across the desk and choking the life out of her, at least until some useful intel falls from that sharp tongue of hers.

The way she smiles at me, she knows it too.

"I'll get these documents drafted up for you, North. The Alpha and Bravo Teams will find her. They found her last time. I'm sure they have her scent already, it's only a matter of time," she says as she collects the papers in front of her and slips them into her briefcase.

North stands and runs a hand down his suit jacket as though he actually gives a shit about looking professional in this moment, just another part of the act, and then walks her out to Rafe, who will see her all the way out of the mansion.

I count to five after the door locks behind her before I murmur, "I have no idea how you put up with her. I would have killed her long before we figured her out."

North shrugs and shakes out his hand, the one with the thin black ring of smoke circling it, one of the many little warning signs that he's riding the edge of his control. "Being on the Council is exclusively dealing with people I don't like. It's that or I give up the seat, which I couldn't do while we were looking for Oleander. Now I need to keep it so we can find her every time she disappears on us."

It's the first time he's mentioned it without putting his fist through something, so I'll call it progress.

He moves back to the desk and unlocks the drawer to collect his own stack of papers, all of it relating to Oli and her code name.

The code name that Atlas Bassinger conveniently knew without her telling him.

North checks his watch. "It's dinner time. We both skipped breakfast and lunch today. With what we're doing tonight, we'll need the fuel."

No argument from me there, though I don't really want to deal with half the people coming to the table anymore.

The Benson kids and Felix Davenport have moved into Draven mansion with us. While there's a part of me that takes great pride in caring for my Bonded's closest friends in her absence, there's a part of me who resents having them here while she's gone. Salt in the wounds of her being taken from me again while we're stuck here, sitting on our goddamned hands, because they're not in any of the known camps.

When Atlas handed me her GPS chip, I wanted to strangle the life out of him with my bare hands. That feeling had only gotten worse when Gabe had debriefed us fully on how much Atlas really knew about her... right up until Gabe got to the part about Noakes' treachery.

North also didn't take it well.

He hasn't taken any of this well, and the more information we get about Oli's time with the Resistance, the closer to losing control I see him getting. It's been a very long time since I've seen him this close to the edge. The last thing that set him off, well, no one blamed him for losing it on his brother's behalf like that.

I certainly didn't.

With every day that she's gone, we're all starting to unravel. I'd thought it was bad the first time around, but back then, we'd lost the idea of a Bond. The hopes and dreams we'd all had about her, not the girl herself.

Losing the real, flesh and blood Oleander Fallows is like dying a death of a thousand tiny cuts.

Hearing her voice in my head had almost brought me to my goddamned knees in the middle of a debrief with the TacTeam we'd left behind, Team Delta, who had one fucking job. That was to keep her safe. The fact that she'd given me absolutely nothing to go on is both infuriating and completely expected. I'd had to point out to North that she survived in those camps as a fourteen-year-old for two years. We need to stop with the bullshit and just… trust her. For a few days, while we use every goddamned resource at our disposal to find her and bring her the fuck home.

We don't really have much choice about it. The moment I'd done what she'd asked and spoken directly to Kieran, Oli had blocked me back out. I'd been frustrated until North had pointed out the obvious.

"There are a lot of Gifted who can pick up on that sort of communication. She's keeping herself safe. She's keeping you both safe."

It's the only level-headed thing I've heard him say about this entire fucking mess, and it gives me just a little bit of hope for the two of them, that maybe they'll figure their shit out when we have her back.

When.

There are no ifs here.

When we get to the dining room, Nox is already there. His nose is still buried in a textbook as old as the Draven bloodline itself, the way it has been since he found out about Oli's gift. I knew he'd be this way, that he'd research and track every little part of her power until he's absolutely sure of what we're dealing with.

I wish him good luck, because I've never heard of a Soul Render like her before.

We take our usual seats and start to fill our plates, the usual spread laid out with fish and lobster as though my Bonded were still here to enjoy it. I fill my plate with it just to feel some sort of connection to her, like a fucking sap, but no one says a word to me about it.

When the doors open again and Gabe joins us, he looks as though he's been dragged through the mud. There are dark circles under his eyes and some streaks of blood down his throat and chest, peeking through the holes in his shirt. He's been down at the shifter fight clubs again, biding his time and working some of the frustration out, but he's obviously getting sloppy with his wins.

I don't mince my words. "You look like shit."

He shrugs and slides into his usual seat, his brows tugging together as he glances at Oli's empty seat. When he scrubs a hand over his face, his knuckles are bloodied and dirty too. "I don't give a shit."

There isn't a whole lot of information that can be

found at the shifter fight club, but if it's keeping him out of trouble and getting some of the aggression out of his system, then I'm all for it. There's not a huge amount he can do for the search here until we have a location.

Then, we'll all be going after our Bond and killing anyone responsible for keeping her away from us.

As the door to the kitchen opens, the others arrive for dinner. Sawyer walks into the room with a laptop open in his hands, his eyes glowing white as he works through the very classified and incredibly above his clearance-level data that North has him working through. Sage and Felix follow behind him, both of them looking exhausted and frazzled. It seems no one in the house is sleeping well. That's also soothing somehow, that we're all a little lost without my Soul Render Bonded.

Felix gets one look at Gabe and reaches out to heal him, until Gabe stops him with a curt, "Don't."

Felix gives him a wry look back, his hand still hovering in the air between them. "Punishing yourself with bleeding knuckles and scratches is just stupid, Ardern."

Gabe shakes his head at him, his eyes on his plate still. "Oli doesn't like us being healed by anyone but her.

If it's not life threatening, just leave it."

Felix's face drops and he glances over at Sage ruefully, obviously regretting saying anything, but she just takes a breath and says, "Oli always let Felix heal her. She wouldn't mind it if it were him doing it, Gabe. We both know it."

He just shrugs and tucks back into his plate without another word. The table falls silent again, only the sounds of cutlery scraping on plates and the clicking of keys on the laptop to be heard. It's stupid, and I know I shouldn't, but I try to reach out to Oli again, not to speak to her but just to feel that she's okay. I can tell she's alive. We'd all know if she died, but there's a lot of bad shit that can be happening to a girl without killing her.

I try not to think too much about that because my bond starts acting up about it otherwise.

Sage clears her throat and then steels herself to speak to North, "Is someone going to let Atlas out of his cell sometime soon? We all know he's not a Resistance member."

Nox scoffs and lifts his glass of whiskey to his lips. "Do we? Because he's a Bassinger. Nothing here makes more sense than him being part of that scum."

It's like watching Sage grow a spine in front of my very eyes. I'm careful to take in every second of it so I can share it with Oli later. Soon. I'll share it with her soon.

"I watched him dote on her for months. If I was going to believe anyone in her Bond was trying to hurt her, it would be you, *Draven*."

Oof.

I share a look with North, expecting him to come running to Nox's defense, but he just looks back down at the transcripts we've found of the experiments on the IW.

The Resistance records of the torture sessions of my Bonded.

Nox smirks back at Sage, oblivious to the nightmare that his brother is sifting through, and says, "And that's how the Resistance keeps winning, by putting on a kind and loving face to win simpering women over."

Gabe slams his knife and fork back down onto the table, and Sawyer shoves his laptop away from himself with a snarl. There's clearly about to be a brawl. Nox just smirks and his eyes flash black as he prepares to get them all off of his back with his creatures but instead, he stiffens for a second, and then he snaps at North, "She's given the creature to Kyrie. He's not hers to just give away."

North's eyes snap up at him, but then Nox curses under his breath and mutters, "She handed him off… for protection in the camps. She knows what happens to the women there."

There's quiet for a moment and then Sage throws a hand at him in a cutting gesture, snapping, "What a terrible, 'simpering' woman she is, running off to save people! Even when she's trapped in one of those fucking camps, she's thinking about others. So you go right ahead and tell me what idiots we both are for believing Atlas, because your word means nothing to me. Nothing, Draven! You're just a bitter, twisted man who needs a fucking therapist and to sober the hell up."

Still, North does nothing to intervene.

Whatever is going on between the brothers, I've never seen them act this way before. Never. North has protected, cared for, coveted, and coddled Nox through his teenage years. He has never let him fight his own battles like this without stepping in and throwing his gift into the mix.

Gabe ignores Nox and turns instead to North to snap,

"Are you going to speak to him or are we just… leaving him in there to rot until we get Oli back? Is there a plan here, or are we just hoping he disappears?"

Nox shoots me look from the other end of the table, but I don't want to talk too much about it in front of the others. Sawyer glances around at all of us and leans back in his seat as he waits for an answer, shifting closer to his sister protectively.

North chooses his words carefully but doesn't back down. "He's proven that he has knowledge that only someone with connections in the Resistance would have. He's lied to us, or at the very least, omitted the truth."

Gabe shrugs in that very youthful way of his. "Oli did too. None of you are suggesting we lock her up when she gets home."

North's eyes narrow back at him. "Oleander is not a part of this discussion, and she was *taken* by the Resistance. She's a victim, not a possible conspirator."

Sage stares at him and then lets out a breath and butts in, "Oli would be pissed, and you all know it. There's nothing I can do to get you guys to let him go, but I'm warning you, she'll go eight different levels of terrifying Bond on you all when she finds out—"

North interrupts her, "He's in isolation. He's in his own room, being fed three square meals a day, with access to all of his usual amenities, except for his phone and the internet. He is in no way suffering, and I can assure you that *when* Oli is home, I will speak directly to her about it. I've taken her thoughts and feelings into consideration, don't doubt it."

After saving her from the burning building and covering for her, North has clearly won some brownie points from Sage, and even though she gives him a stern once-over, she nods and gets back to her food.

It's the worst dinner since Nox stopped dragging women in here to antagonize our Bond. I finish my plate as quickly as I can choke it all down. The moment I'm done, North packs away his files, his own plate still half filled as he abandons it without another thought.

We leave through the kitchens and into the service hallways that run through the building for the staff to use. As I move to follow North, Nox grabs my arm to stop me, his eyes dark in the muted lighting. I urge North on without me and then turn back to Nox.

He's not drunk, but he's definitely drinking more at the moment. We're going to have to cut him off soon.

"North told me about your gift, the extra that you can do now that you've Bonded with her."

Her.

He says it like even just her name is poison on his tongue. It never bothered me before, I know all of the reasons why he's like that, but right now it's like a thrill of acid in my blood, burning everything it touches.

I give him a nod, not trusting my voice, and he takes it as a cue to go on.

"Don't *ever* practice that on me. I say this as your oldest friend. I will kill you if you look inside my head, even for a second."

I don't have to look at him to know that he's telling the truth. I also didn't have to be warned by him.

I know what horrors are hiding in there.

I shrug and murmur, "I won't. I've spoken to North about it, and I'll work my way up to getting into his. You'll be let out of this."

There's only one elevator that goes downstairs in the house, for good reason.

You don't want house guests stumbling on the work we've done down here, or the captives we've brought back from the council offices. And we definitely don't want any visiting council members to see Noakes chained to the floor, covered in blood, and trying to free the traitorous, despicable piece of shit.

He's looking in particularly bad shape tonight. I suppose three days down here without food or water will do that to a man. When he hears the elevator and the sounds of our footsteps on the concrete, he jerks against his chains.

"I have nothing else to say!" he mumbles, thready and weak, and North scoffs at him.

"We're not here to question you. We're past all of that now."

What little blood is left in Noakes' face drains away, and he scrambles up onto his knees. His voice is barely more than a croak as he rushes out with, "I had one job. Find your Bond and get her tracked. That's it! They were going to kill my children! What was I supposed to do?"

North's eyes don't even bother flicking to me. We've done this type of interrogation more than a thousand times by now. He knows how I move when I'm hearing lies. I shift on my feet, exactly how I am right now, because they taste wrong in the air to me.

North blows out a breath and straightens his tie, the picture of calm and control. "You should really know better than to lie in front of Gryphon. You were on the committee that picked him for the TacTeams. You put forward the recommendation for him to become the Lead. Have you forgotten this in your betrayal of us all?"

Noakes' nose scrunches up and he simpers, "He's got it wrong, I'm telling the truth. They've only asked me to track the girl. I didn't give him anything else!"

I crouch down so that I'm at eye level with him. "You knew about the explosive though, didn't you? You knew you were putting my Bonded's life in danger."

He whimpers and sputters out, "I thought they were lying about that! I didn't think they'd be crazy enough to do that to some girl. They're not complete monsters."

North scoffs and holds out his hand, his palm slowly turning black. "No, but we are. Isn't that right, old friend? You were happy to help cultivate the rumors of the Monster Bond."

North's gift feels a lot like Oli's does, a tightness in your chest as he calls on it, and a slow smirk stretches over my face. He usually disposes of prisoners once we're done with them by using his death touch. Quick, efficient, and clean. That's him down to a T. Oli disappearing again has snapped his control, and I, for one, am glad to see it.

Glad that she's dug her way as deeply under his skin as she's burrowed under mine.

Noakes sputters and coughs in response and mumbles, "I did no such thing!"… lie, "The community was worried about what you were capable of, all of you! There was nothing I could do to stop the spread of misinformation,"… lie, "You can't blame all of that on me without credible evidence! I don't deserve to die like this!"… the biggest lie yet.

I scoff and meet his eyes one last time as August pops out of North's palm, salivating and snarling already, to say, "A monster sticks an explosive in a nineteen-year-old girl's head just to save his own skin. A monster walks into a fourteen-year-old girl's hospital room after her entire family was killed in an accident to threaten her into captivity. You think we've been monsters so far? You haven't seen what we're truly capable of yet… but now you will."

When his scream finally dies out, the crunching of his bones follow us out of the basement.

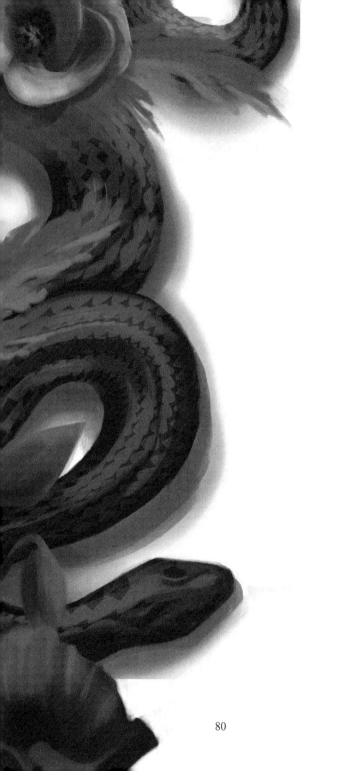

OLI

I wake up with a stiff neck and an aching ass from the chair. It's frustrating that my body has already forgotten how to sleep sitting up like this, especially since I slept in my car a lot while I was on the run as well, but months at the Draven mansion have spoiled me, apparently.

I groan under my breath and shift as much as the restraints will let me, wiggling my legs out to attempt to get some feeling back with little success.

"How the fuck did you actually sleep like that? And how has no one killed you yet for how badly you snore?" Kieran snarks from the ground at my feet where he's still huddled up, his hands resting awkwardly on his chest.

I yawn as I shrug. "I don't usually snore, this is extenuating circumstances, and you learn to do a lot of shit in this place. How long have you been awake?"

He rolls his eyes at me. "Long enough to know that the sun rose at least two hours ago, and we've missed the breakfast round. It smelled like bacon. I thought about waking you just to get some."

I scoff at him with a grin, rolling my shoulders back and staring right at the camera so they can see I'm awake. Being a VIP here has its perks, and I'll take the sleep in. Gryphon never let me have them, and hopefully it'll mean less time with that man today.

Doubt it, but a girl can hope, right?

"Stop grumping, they'll bring us something."

He pulls himself up into a sitting position without using his hands at all, like he's doing a crunch in hard mode, and it makes me miss Gabe and Gryphon like a hole in my chest. I've drooled over the both of them doing that about a million times in TT and training. Shirtless too, which I really shouldn't think about or my bond will start whining about getting them back.

"If they bring us slop, I'll remember it and get you

back once we're home. Mark my words. Tell me why they leave you to sleep and feed you so well? Just because you're a Render? That seems like an even better reason to deprive and torture you."

I wiggle my toes in my shoes, trying not to think about how stinky my socks will be in there, and my ass starts to get some feeling back. "They want me whole, undamaged, and at peak performance. I get tortured here plenty, just not like that. I'm sure you'll get to see it so just, like… prepare yourself for that. It's going to suck."

He stares at me and then says slowly, like I'm dense, "Suck… That's the best descriptive word you can come up with for actual torture? Is this a coping mechanism or something?"

"I compartmentalize like a pro and, well, you'll see once it happens. Davies won't make us wait for it for long. He never could keep his hands off of me."

I'm saved from having to explain much more than that to him by breakfast arriving. Both of the women I'd seen when I'd first woken up bring the plates in, except this time, the younger one is more subdued. She doesn't speak to either of us. When she leans down to hand Kieran his plate, I see the scratches and bruises forming on her cheek.

Once she's loosened my restraints and hands me my plate, I jerk my head at her and ask, "Fighting in the camps? Or did someone smack you around for your smart mouth? You should probably learn to keep it shut."

Her lip curls at me, but the older woman butts in, "Don't answer her, Zarah. We're not supposed to talk to her. She's just fishing for information. We'll leave them to eat our food that we're being so kind as to share with them."

I scoff at her and Zarah looks as though she's going to snarl something at me again, but the older woman snaps her fingers and they both walk out.

Kieran, who hadn't spoken but watched the entire interaction keenly, breaks off a piece of bread to dip into the egg yolks and then mumbles around his mouthful, "Something happened last night. It was a long time before dawn, probably closer to midnight. Lots of yelling and screaming. I was surprised you slept through it all. There were enough footsteps that whatever happened, they called in for backup. I didn't hear Davies specifically, but Franklin was there to stop any gifts in the mix."

I nod and get to work on my own plate of eggs,

dipping the bacon in the yolks because I wasn't given any cutlery to eat with so I'm making do.

Kieran grunts and says, "Are there fights here a lot? Have you ever been in them? I thought you were green when you started at TT."

I huff at him, because of course he wants to talk about it and not just stuff our faces. "There's usually beatings and ambushes in the shower stalls, all sorts of shit you don't want to hear. Fighting where the Resistance gets hurt? I've only seen it happen once before, and the guy who managed to get the hit in was put on the rack... publicly. They're really good at making you watch people die in terrible ways here."

He nods slowly, scraping up the rest of his eggs with the last little hunk of bread, and then says, "We're getting you in therapy when we get back. I'll make sure they all know how much you need it."

Over my dead body.

I don't know why I feel so adamant about that. Talking through my issues would probably be for the best, but my bond in my chest instantly rejects the very idea of it.

"And what about you? Are you going to go talk to someone about getting the shit kicked out of you by

Resistance assholes?" I mumble. To my surprise, he nods.

"All TacTeam operatives have mandated counseling sessions. Every last person who serves has to go to debriefs with their higher-ups and then a minimum of monthly sessions with an appointed psychologist."

What the fuck?

North and Nox both work in Teams when there's a need. Do they both go as well? Why do I suddenly want to burst into inappropriate giggles at the very thought of Nox sitting there talking about his feelings? I mean, if any of my Bonds needs therapy, it's that one.

I actually do giggle as the image of North lying on a couch, talking about his day, filters into my brain. How the hell would that go? The greatest control freak I've ever encountered just... spilling his guts to some suit.

I wonder if his psychologist is a man?

Oh my God. North has without a doubt fucked his female psychologist. He totally would. He'd bone her so he didn't have to talk about shit.

"What the fuck are you thinking about, Fallows? Rein it in!" Kieran hisses, breaking me out of my spiraling descent into madness. My eyes haven't shifted, but when I glance down at him, I can see the hair on his arms standing up and the whites of his eyes are bright as he freaks the hell out.

I blow out a breath and slow my racing heartbeat down as best as I can, murmuring, "Sorry. Shit, *sorry*. I just... I'm starting to lose it, being away from... being here. Fuck, I'll stop doing that."

He watches me carefully, almost gently, like he's handling a bomb with a hair-trigger, and that's the exact moment that the women decide to come back for our plates. Neither of them say a word as they grab them but when they stalk out, it's only a minute before they're back, carrying a bucket of soapy water and a pile of clothes each.

Ugh.

Wash time.

Zarah puts the bucket down in the center of the tent and snaps, "The showers are out of commission for a few days, but since you're both our *important guests* here, you're getting access to water and clean clothes. Strip and get to it, you both have places to be."

Another piece of the puzzle for us both to stew on; the fight happened in the showers. It's warm enough wherever the hell we are that it's going to be a sweaty, stinking nightmare here soon if they don't get it repaired and back in action in the next few days.

"Wash him first, I'm happy enough to wait," I say, jerking my head at where Kieran is at my feet.

I need to get him a chair.

Or a Healer.

"Why can't you both just do it together? You're Bonds, right?"

I roll my eyes at her and gesture between us. "You really want my bond getting an eyeful of what he's offering and wanting to complete the Bond? You know what? Hell yeah! I'll probably end up strong enough to pull your souls out through your nostrils, even with Franklin here. Go on, Bond. Get your pants off for me."

Kieran smirks, putting on the cockiest demeanor as he pushes himself up onto his knees and reaches for his pants zipper. I give him serious kudos in my head for playing along with me without question.

The older woman darts in front of me, getting the closest to touching me as she has this entire time, and waves her hands around. "No! No, turn around. Both of you face the opposite directions. Zarah, get the Render another bucket."

Thank God that one worked.

I mean, I'm not scared of seeing Kieran naked, but I don't know how to explain that to Gryphon and I've had just enough of a taste of his jealousy before to know that he wouldn't take it well. Even if it was his second-in-command and for a really good reason.

I'm surprised at how much I truly care. Me, not my bond. I don't want to upset Gryphon or any of the rest of them by looking at another naked man. Jesus, this Bond shit is unbelievable because six months ago, I would've gone to an all-male strip club just to mess with them, and now the very thought of that gives me hives.

The guys all better feel like this or I'm going to castrate the lot of them.

After my restraints are loosened, I get up and let Zarah cut my shirt away from my body, but I lose my pants myself. I refuse to let them take my underwear off and I use the washcloth to scrub around them.

I can hear Kieran washing up behind me, but there's no other sounds from outside the tent to alarm me, so I just focus on my scrubbing.

"If she's been here before, where's her scars? You said she got the same," Zarah murmurs, and the older woman grunts under her breath.

I can't help but play with her, but it also works in my favor for this stupid woman to be unsure of me, so I let my eyes shift to black and snark out, "You ask too many questions. No wonder you got smacked around. Too bad they didn't do a decent job of it."

The older woman slowly lowers her bucket to the ground and then fumbles at her waistband until she pulls a coms handpiece out, pressing a button and murmuring, "Her eyes have gone black again. How should we proceed?"

I grin slowly, showing off my teeth in a very predatory way, and Kieran turns his head, not enough to see me, but just so he can get a bit more of an idea of what's happening behind him.

There's a static sound down the handpiece and then Davies' voice comes through loud and clear.

"Get them dressed and bring them to my work space. If her bond wants to play, then I'm ready for her."

Six heavily armored guards escort me through the camps

while Kieran is dragged between two others, his leg still not holding any of his weight. I'm going to have to get crafty about finding him a Healer and getting it patched up, or at the very least, in working order again.

He's kind of a dead weight right now, and dead weights just become plain old dead in this hellhole. I've worked too damn hard to keep him alive for the asshole to die because of a snapped freaking leg.

This camp is bigger than the last one I'd been in with Sage and Gabe, but from what I can see, it's smaller than the one I was held in for the longest time during my two year stay with Davies. When we walk past the shower block, I count eight different guards standing around the perimeter. Two of them are using their gifts to study the grass and canvas like they are about to find a giant sign spelling out what happened there overnight.

I have a few guesses on what actually happened, but I'm still sort of hoping I'm wrong.

There is an entire section of smaller tents that the guards and grunt workers all camp in. They separate Davies from the sheep. It's very strategic of him to make sure that he's never going to be caught unaware overnight by an escapee, but I'm surprised he's keeping Kieran and me so far away.

I used to sleep in the tent over from him.

It was literally my worst nightmare, and it took a full year on the run before I stopped waking up in a puddle of sweat and panic. Thank God I was past it before I had to start sharing my bed with my Bonds. I couldn't have hidden that from Gryphon's gift. He would absolutely have 'tripped' over those feelings with his Neuro-snooping ways.

God, I miss him.

I miss North's caring and domineering ways, Atlas' complete acceptance and love for me, and Gabe's loyalty to me, kind and savage and sure.

I even miss worrying about Nox's loathing and his dream-like bed with a hundred nightmares keeping watch over us both, and I fucking miss Brutus like a hole in my heart.

"For the infamous IW, you look kind of pathetic," the guy holding my arm says. I shrug at him, because if I'm going to be stuck dealing with these assholes, then I might as well have some fun with it.

"It doesn't really matter how I look though, does it? You'll still be the first to die when I take this camp. Next will be mouthy Zarah. Then, whoever the fuck broke my Bond's leg will go next. He kinda needs it to keep up with me."

The guy scoffs, but the older, bigger guard beside him smacks him on the back of his head and snaps, "For a Neuro, you're pretty stupid, Cam. She was taking out more people than an atomic bomb at fourteen. Shut your mouth before it gets you killed the minute Franklin gets sent out."

Cam scoffs some more, puffing his chest out and putting some extra swagger in his step like he's a big man, but he doesn't say anything else. No one else tries to speak, and they all clutch at their weapons as we walk through the busy camp. There's a lot of people bustling around but they scatter away from us with either looks of concern or outright fear.

This is how I know that I really am a monster, no matter what my Bonds have to say otherwise.

When we reach Davies' tent, we stop outside while the older guard steps in first, probably to announce our arrival and get orders on where to put us, and I take a second to glance back at Kieran and check out how he's faring with all of the movement.

The answer to that is not well at all.

His usually tanned skin is sallow looking. There's a fine sheen of sweat over his forehead, and even with his mouth in a firmly controlled line, he looks like he's about to pass out.

I turn back to face the mouthy young guard again and say in a quiet, low tone, "If he dies from that broken leg, I will trigger every last one of your darkest nightmares until your brain breaks down inside your skull. I'll use every single trick that Davies tortured into me to prolong your death until you die *writhing*."

He gulps.

I'm starting to get addicted to that response.

I hear the tent flap pull back again and then I hear his voice say, "Who would've known that all it would take to bring out the darkness in you would be to have your Bonds here too? You delight me, little Render."

Don't react to him, Oli. Don't give him the satisfaction of knowing how much you hate having his approval.

The young guard snaps to attention and jerks me forward, acting as though he wasn't just shitting himself over my words, and he directs me into Davies' work space. We should count our blessings that it's this one and not his actual torture tent, but now isn't the time to point that out to Kieran.

It's easily five times bigger than the tent we were being kept in and there's lights hanging from the higher ceiling, making the space bright and inviting. It's all a farce, the careful way that Davies plans out everything to seem as though he's a good and decent man and not the utter freaking sadist he is.

There's a wooden desk at one end of the space near an operating table, complete with restraints and stirrups. I glance over to see Kieran scowling at it. When he meets my eyes, there's a question there that I can't really answer right now. He's probably coming up with all sorts of ideas about what happens on that table, and I'm sure that at least half of them will be correct.

Davies steps back up to his tool desk and then sweeps a dramatic hand towards the table. "Help our guest up onto the table, and leave her broken Bond over at the restraint point where he can observe all of my hard work."

I walk over myself, not giving the guards the satisfaction of dragging me, and even though it's awkward with my restraints, I climb up onto the table. They're extra cautious when they tie me down, securing the new straps on before they remove the old ones, and I want to scream at them because *of course* I'm not going to do anything.

Davies is without a doubt stronger than I am. I'm not a freaking idiot.

"No, you're not. They're all going to underestimate you, little Render. They're all going to look at you and see some pretty little girl forever. The only reason they look so worried is because I've missed you, you know? When you ran from me... the things I did to the men and women who let you escape, well, it's become a bit of a legend around here. They don't understand your power, what you can do... You really will be my weapon, just as soon as I've collected all of your Bonds. How many were there again?"

Nothing.

I think of nothing and I pray Kieran is smart enough to think of nothing as well. We might be screwed here, but I can keep—no, don't let him in, Oli, fuck—nothing.

There's nothing.

Davies tuts at me, lifting off the top of his desk to reveal what he keeps inside it. I can't see it from the angle I'm lying at, but I don't need to. I already know what's in there, and if he's brought in anything new… I don't need to freak myself out over it.

"I have acquired some new tools. I can't wait to show them to you, but we have time. No matter what your Bond is thinking about getting you out of here, we both know you can't. I've made better plans. Franklin is staying here with you from now on. Did you tell your Transporter that Franklin is also stronger than you are? For now. I'm sure that once I find all of your Bonds, you'll be stronger than him. I have so many plans for you, but let's stop talking and start with the fun, shall we?"

He snaps his fingers and the guards all finally clear out, leaving Kieran chained to the restraint point at the other end of the tent where he can see everything that Davies is about to do to me.

Fuck, I hope he has a strong stomach, because shit is about to get rough.

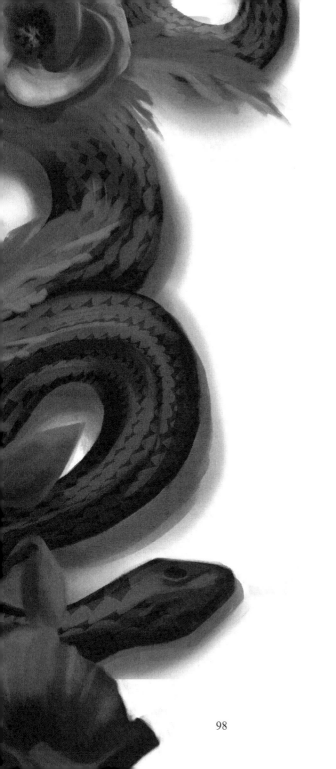

98

OLI

The obsession that Davies has with his set of knives is disturbing. I have to remind myself that he's absolutely getting off on prolonging his fondling of them in the tool desk. The sounds they make as he runs his fingers along the handles are like the world's most twisted and macabre bells, warning me of all of the pain he's about to put me through.

"There's something I need to discuss with you before we start, something that you gave to one of the women in the shower block yesterday. The cameras can see you both interact but not what you handed her. Tell me what it is, and I'll refrain from killing the girl."

I think of nothing.

Blackness.

Inky nothingness in a desolate and barren wasteland of oblivion.

Nothing makes Davies angrier than my faultless ability to empty my brain out. He had no idea that one of my fathers, Vincenzo, had been a Neuro. He was the stay-at-home father with whom I'd spent the most time with, and even as a small child, he'd played this simple game with me—how many different ways can we empty our minds to utter blankness? Even as a very little girl, I'd be quizzed and tested until I could become a calm, blank canvas.

I wonder often if he'd known that someday I'd be facing this man, if my mother's dreams of oleander flower-filled cribs also showed a madman obsessed with breaking inside my mind to destroy my life, and that's why Vincenzo had been the one chosen to primarily raise me.

It makes more sense than I want to admit.

Davies picks a knife, the long carving knife that's sharper than a surgeon's blade, and steps towards me.

"These games grow so tiresome, little Render. Must we always play them? The woman is strong enough that we were planning on keeping her, but that's not all. Her brother is a leading Tac operative, a pain in my ass."

Her brother is nothing.

Her brother is absolutely nothing.

Nothing.

I am a blank slate of zero thoughts about him.

"Did you meet him in your time away? Is he the reason you gave her something? She's not going to escape, you know. If you're hoping Shore will come after you, I can assure you that he might be strong and have tricks up his sleeve, but he's no match for me."

I need a subject change, and fast. "I didn't give her anything. She gave me a job, and I went to check she was okay. I came here in an apron and work sneakers, it's pretty obvious I'm not lying."

He grins at me and waves the knife. "Then why is it that a simple, Neuro-gifted woman could make three fully grown men disappear into thin air? Two of them were Shifters and at least twice her size, and when they approached her in the shower block for a little fun... gone."

It's easier to be blank about this. I'd already guessed what had happened in the shower stalls, and I'm incredibly glad that I'd been able to get to Kyrie before it happened.

I shrug and roll my head on my shoulders to look back up at the fabric panels of the ceiling. "I'm a little confused about why you're bringing this up with me. All of that chaos is outside of my skill set, and you know it."

He grins at me, his eyes wandering around the room before he snaps, leaning over me on the table and snarling in my face, "And we both know a little Neuro sheep couldn't *devour* grown men alive and leave nothing but a little DNA matter behind! So what *did* you do, Render? You know better than to make me angry."

I know better than to end up here again, and yet I walked right in here after that woman, so I'll be damned if I'm going to sell her out to save myself a little pain. "I know nothing. I'm still the same little stupid girl you had here last time, so you really shouldn't bother with all of this. It's a waste of time."

The first press of the knife to my skin doesn't actually break it, it's more of a warning that he doesn't appreciate my tone, and he snaps, "I saw you hand her something in the showers. The camera didn't pick up on what it was that you gave her, but you *will* tell me. Whatever you've done while you've been gone, whatever you've become, you'll never be stronger than I am. If you don't tell me what it was that you gave her, I will bring her here, and I will do everything to her that I've done to you, little Render. You'll repay that woman's kindness with pain and a slow death."

Nothingness.

Hold on to the nothingness because it's much harder to stay blank when there are other people in this stupid fucking hellhole who I want to protect, but if he brings Kyrie here, then I'll find a new plan.

There's always a way through this.

He clicks his tongue at me like he's disappointed and pulls the knife away from my skin. His favorite form of torture is edging, and I loathe him for it. I'd rather he just freaking stabbed me already.

He steps back over to his tools and puts the carving knife down, fussing with the handles again as he says, "Cold little Render, I should've known you wouldn't care that much about some useless woman. But what about your Bond, hm? I can heal him. Let your bond out to play with me now, answer the questions I have, and I'll heal your Bond. He's starting to look a little green over there. Linda and Zarah said the wound over the break is looking infected too. Blood infections can move quickly, you know."

I can go back to ignoring him, because there's no way he'll let Kieran die right now. He's spent too long trying to find my Bonds. He'd never let one die without experimentation first. It's the whole reason I lied in the first place.

Davies sighs, making a big show of it, as though I'm an unruly school child he's being forced to deal with. Then he straightens back up, finally selecting a new knife from his tool desk as he runs a hand down the side of it lovingly.

My heart starts to beat a little faster, panic slowly working its way down my spine, and I have to start focusing on my breathing to stop myself from hyperventilating.

Be blank, Oli. Be nothing.

He leans over me again to murmur right in my face, "I already know you won't break so easily, Render. I'm just making sure your Bond knows it too. Let's see how long it takes me to break him though, shall we?"

The moment the knife touches my skin, I start to

disassociate. My bond creeps up to the forefront of my brain, ever watching what's happening and waiting for the right moment to step in for me, but simple cuts are easy enough to block out. When Davies really starts to get creative with his slicing, my leg begins to shake involuntarily and a pool of sweat starts on my lower back. I can almost keep it blocked out, almost, until he starts cutting off my pants and working his way up the sensitive skin of my thighs.

My control slips for a second and my body is instantly flooding with Gryphon, his bond reaching out to me and breaking down the last of my barriers in a single sweep, and his voice is booming in my head.

WHAT IS HAPPENING?!

I watch as Davies' eyes flash wide and I slam my barriers back up, cursing myself a thousand times over for slipping and letting my Bonded in. One split second and I've ruined *everything* that I've spent five years guarding and protecting with my goddamn life.

Fingers as cold as ice and spattered with droplets of my blood trail over my cheek, leaving behind a red trail as Davies leans down to whisper to me, his lips touching the rim of my ear, "And who was that, my precious little

Soul Render?"

Two years.

I was a prisoner in one of these camps for two whole years, and not once did I so much as *think* their names. I knew them, *oh my God* did I know their names. The moment I'd woken up in that hospital with Nurse June standing over my bed with teary eyes and a file tucked under her arm, I'd memorized their names. I remember thinking how scary it was that North was almost a decade older than I was. The five years between me and Gryphon and Nox seemed like so much as well. I wanted so badly to know Gabe and Atlas because they were only a few months older than me, and I wanted friendship until we were old enough to Bond.

I spent a few short hours in that hospital planning and hoping and wishing that they'd hurry up and take me away from the horror of what had happened to my family.

And then I never thought of them again.

I never let myself.

And with three desperate words sent through our

Bonded link, Gryphon has revealed himself to the biggest threat our Bond Group will ever know.

On instinct, I think of nothingness. I let the panic ride me even as I force myself not to think of the details, the exact reasons why I'm panicking so badly. I triple check my barrier to my Bonded, and then I check on my bond because I might have to let it take over to distract Davies from what he'd heard.

My bond is ready and eager to be let out.

I'll take the pain for as long as I can and then I'll let my bond take over to finish this session off. If Davies forces me to kill innocent people then… well, I'm a monster, because if it keeps my Bonds and our loved ones safe, then I'll fucking loathe it but accept it.

I hate myself, but it's the line I've drawn here.

"Fine. Fine, insist on being a stubborn little shit. I have more than enough tools to bleed it out of you. If I need to have you screaming to find out who he is, then I guess we're going to need a bigger, *blunter* knife. How do you feel about being hacked to pieces with a butter knife, little Render? It'll be hard work for me but, oh, the satisfaction."

Deep breaths.

Deep, long breaths—in through the nose, hold for two counts, out through the mouth.

I can survive it.

I manage to convince myself of it too, right up until he actually starts hacking at my thigh, and then a scream rips out of my mouth, ragged and hoarse. Gryphon is pounding at my barrier, my head thumping with it, and I need to puke.

This is also when the entire scene becomes too much for Kieran and he shouts at Davies, startling me because I'd almost forgotten he was in here with us thanks to all of the pain, "Get your hands off of her, and I'll tell you where he is."

The knife buried in my thigh stops moving, but Davies doesn't take it out entirely. The muscle clenches around it like my body is trying to force it out, but his hand is firm on the handle.

I blink my eyes open finally, but Davies is focused on Kieran. When I glance over to where he's chained, he still looks like he's halfway to his grave, but there's a determined gleam in his eyes as he says, "Her other Bond, the one in her head, you'll want him. He's stronger than I am. If she Bonds with him, she'll get the kick of power you want from her. He's a Neuro, like you… he's a lot like you, actually. From the moment they met, he's been in her head. If anyone will be able to help you control her bond, it's him. Just stop fucking cutting her up, and I'll tell you where he is."

I want to scream at him to shut the fuck up, but I can't speak around the lump in the back of my throat caused by all of the pain and the moment I think that I see the triumph in Davies eyes. He knows that Kieran is about to give him another piece of the puzzle, another toy to play with to make me the weapon he so desperately wants. After years of getting nothing from me, there's no way he's going to even question Kieran about it.

He'll just take it and find my Bond, drag him back here to live through all of this right alongside me.

Davies decides to prove a point and presses the knife down harder, slicing through the muscle there, and my bond finally kicks in, taking over for me to spare my mind from the agony, and then I finally feel nothing. My bond soaks it all up for me like the greatest sponge in the world.

My eyes don't shift though. My bond knows better than doing that here.

Kieran has no idea that the pain just ended for me though and snaps, "Massachusetts. He's in Massachusetts. Give me a pen. I'll write down where, just stop cutting her."

There's a horrific spurt of blood that comes out of my leg when Davies finally pulls the knife out. Kieran's brow furrows at the sight of it, but Davies grabs a cloth and one of his tourniquets to staunch the bleeding. He's an expert at directing blood flow, but usually he uses it to keep me conscious for as long as possible during this process.

He wipes his hands off on a cloth and then he steps over to where Kieran is restrained on the other side of the tent, staring him down as though he'll be able to tell if he's being lied to.

He doesn't have that ability though.

Kieran plays his part well, staring back at him with no signs of deception as he lists off an address and even coordinates of a place that I've never heard of.

Davies smirks slowly, deciding he's been victorious, and steps back to his work desk. "If you're lying to me about this Bond and where he is, I'll come back here and I'll really torture her. This? This is just a warm up, but if you send me away for no good reason and I don't come back with this Neuro? I'll amputate her leg. No pain relief either, she doesn't need both legs to be my weapon. It was my next course of action when I last had her to get her to talk. I'm excited to give it a try."

I want to pass out at the very sound of that, but then he's back at the table and pushing a needle into my neck, injecting me with something that kicks in immediately, my brain fuzzing out.

"Extra insurance to keep you here, little Render. I'll be back with your next Bond soon. Be a good girl and wait here for me."

Then he walks out, and I lose track of what the actual fuck is going on here. I don't know up from down, the table feels as though it's spinning into space, and my skin begins to crawl as though a thousand fire ants have just been injected into my veins.

I lose my shit entirely.

There's a cracking sound and a muffled scream, like someone biting down on fabric to stop themselves from making noise but failing kind of miserably, and then there's some retching. My stomach doesn't like that sound one bit, protesting immediately, and I turn my head to vomit. My restraints are too tight to move much and I'm sure there's vomit running down my chin, but I can't feel anything, nothing but the sensations that the drug fills me with.

I think I'm crying.

Not that I want to, not that the tiny slivers of my sane brain are feeling that sort of emotion, but my breath is sawing out of my chest and I start to taste salt.

There's grunting and the sound of a heavy sack dragging along the dirt, and then somehow Kieran's face appears in front of mine. I have no idea how the hell he's here—it's probably a hallucination—and I think the sobbing gets worse.

He's trying to speak to me but his words are distorted, because even though I can see his mouth is moving, the words are all coming through wrong.

"Kill… just him… get help… Oli, please… kill… know you can…"

I scowl at him and finally take a gasping breath, but whatever the fuck Davies shot me up with turns my stomach again and bile rushes up my throat.

There's a moment of darkness, nothingness I want to climb into and stay in forever, and then there's Kieran's face again. There's vomit on his shirt and pants, my vomit, I think, but he's not angry or disgusted.

He's desperate.

"Kill him, Oli… kill Franklin…"

I don't understand what he's saying.

But my bond does.

And then there's nothing but death and pain, blood and destruction. I might be utterly fucked from the drugs, but my bond has always been stronger than *anyone* will ever comprehend, and *no one* threatens me without facing the dark god living inside me.

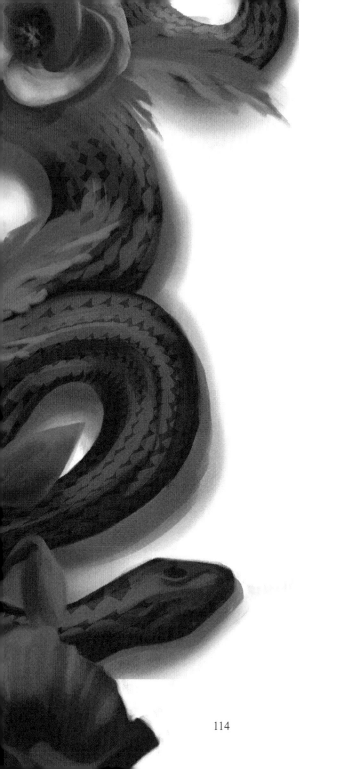

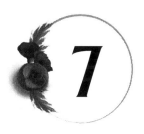

NOX

Three nights.

She's only been gone this time for three nights, and yet the chaos she's left behind is insane. Gryphon's foul moods and obsessive behavior makes sense to me because the idiot was stupid enough to fully Bond with her, but the rest of them?

Pathetic.

We all knew she'd run the moment she had a chance. Gabe and Bassinger were the ones without a shared coherent thought between them that wouldn't have possibly strung together the idea that maybe they should leave the GPS tracker in her.

Then there's the small fact that I think North's bond is going to take over and wipe out the entire country to get her back, and after decades of playing the gentile councilman, cultivating the sedate and moral man that he is, he's about to ruin it all for her.

Fucking Bonds.

Of course there's no sign of her or the other dozens of Gifted who were taken. The moment we'd gotten back here from the aborted mission, we found Gabe shifted into the biggest wolf form I've ever seen him in, snarling and snapping at Atlas like he was hoping to rip his throat out.

After we'd split them up, it had taken a good hour before Gabe calmed the fuck down enough to shift back, and then he'd told us all about Atlas' extensive knowledge of Fallows' time in the Resistance.

And what they named her.

I never liked him, and I've made my thoughts on his situation widely known because we've already lost one Draven to a Resistance sleeper cell this year. Keeping him around for the sake of a Bond who never wanted any of them in the first place is just plain stupidity.

North doesn't listen.

He never listens anymore, another strike against her.

But even after Bassinger is locked away, we've spent three entire days sitting around, trying to find where they're all being held, with no luck. All of the monitored campsites and residences are running business as usual, and there is no new intel. Zero. They know we're listening, so the moment they have Fallows, the lines all go dead silent.

So we're back to working through the old intel and searching for some clue or little sign that we might have missed about where they are. Gryphon is better at strategy than paperwork, and he spends his time keeping his Teams on standby for the moment we have something, so it's up to North and I to sift through it all with a fine-tooth comb.

There's only two things that pop out, and neither of them are enough to go on.

Alaska, in the highest and coldest area that would be an absolute logistical nightmare to attempt an extraction.

Or possibly in the middle of the Sahara desert, which would also require a lot of communication with the local authorities and Gifted community to go in and get them back, so either way, we need to be sure about it before we move in.

It doesn't come down to that.

At dinner on day three of her being gone, while we're all arguing viciously about what to do next because Gabe is furious that we're not going to just traipse around in a desert or a frozen tundra until we trip over her, Gryph lurches away from the table with a bark, his chair crashing to the ground.

The blood drains from his face as he feels *it*. The ghost of Fallows' pain as if it's his own. My bond begins writhing in my chest, that terrible thing it does now around her, but whatever is happening in the Resistance camps, Gryph can sense it stronger, thanks to their connection.

Then he lets out a roar and goes down to his knees as his legs buckle underneath his weight. I haven't heard a sound like that out of him since the last time he was shot while on duty, and North almost loses control of his own bond in response as he bolts over to him with a snarl. Gabe shoves away from the table, but his hands are shaking and his face is unnaturally pale.

Someone is hurting their Bond.

I know it because I can feel the echo as well, the sensation of pain that isn't my own, and my palms immediately break out in a sweat. My bond wants to find her, to save her, to take the pain for her and tear apart whoever dared lay a hand on her.

She's not mine. I shouldn't feel this way about her.

I should feel this way about anyone. I know better than to fall for these tricks, and there's no way I'm ever putting myself back in that situation.

Never.

"What is it? What's happening to her?" North snaps as his phone starts ringing on the table. We all ignore it but the moment it stops, Gabe's starts up, and he grunts at it.

"It's Bassinger. He must feel it too."

Gryphon takes a gasping sort of breath. "She's being tortured. I got into her head, but she shoved me back out. Someone is carving her up."

Kill them all. Filthy heathens, touching what's ours.

I shake my head as though it'll clear the sound of my bond away. My creatures don't like sharing, not even with the others, and no matter how much I tell them that I won't have her, they don't want someone touching her either.

Gabe shoves up to his feet and snaps, "Where the

fuck is she then? We're going to the desert, send a team to the snow. We can't just sit the fuck around anymore—"

He's cut off by the audible *pop* of a Transporter arriving, and then Kieran Black is groaning on the ground at Gryph's feet, looking as though he's been beaten by the entire population of the Resistance. From the look on both North and Gryph's faces, he'd better have been.

Because Fallows isn't with him.

"Get me a Healer. Now," he says through clenched teeth, and Gryph drops to his knees to grab at his vest, pulling him up into his face.

North is already on the phone and calling Felix Davenport down, his second phone in his hand as he starts calling in the TacTeams to be ready to move out.

"Where the fuck is my Bonded, Black?"

Kieran turns green, his teeth clenching in pain as Gryph manhandles him, and he chokes out, "Get me a Healer and I'll go back for her."

I check in with Azrael, the shadow that stays with her that she's doing her best to domesticate, to figure out what the hell is happening there. Kyrie is still in one of the cages, unharmed, but trapped nonetheless. There's no sign of danger or trouble yet. I tell Azrael to be on high alert and he whines a little at being away from Fallows if there's danger, his soft spot for her a mile wide.

"You left her behind?!"

Gryph snarl makes it clear that he might actually kill Black for this, but anyone with eyes can see what the hell is happening here. Black is good enough about laying it out there for him though.

He snaps out in a pain-filled growl, "I have two breaks in my leg and a raging blood infection. I didn't have enough power to bring her back with me. The second a Healer is done with me, I can take you to her. Just get me one *now,* because she's on her own."

Felix bursts through the door with both of the Bensons and rushes straight towards Black, not waiting for an order to heal him. He curses under his breath at the state of Keiran, but his gift is strong enough to do this. He's the top of his class and a prodigy amongst his peers, not that you can tell from how humble he is. He's one of a select handful of Healers that I'm willing to let touch me.

Gryph moves aside to let Black be tended to, stalking back over to the table and grabbing the weapons that he'd unstrapped from himself to eat. Gabe moves to stand with the Bensons, murmuring to catch them up on what's happened, and North is practically vibrating with his phone to his ear as he snaps out orders to mobilize the Alpha and Bravo teams. I can feel his relief that both of them are already on standby, because we've been waiting for this moment.

"You can talk while he heals you. Tell me what the fuck was happening to her," Gryphon snarls as he does one last check that his weapons are secure, and Black grits his teeth while the thigh bone is reset.

"Silas Davies is what happened to her. Silas Davies is what happened to her last time as well. He's fucking obsessed with her. He was… butchering her, that's when he heard you in her head. I had to think quick to stop her from getting herself murdered just to keep you all away from him."

Silas fucking Davies.

Only the fabled super villain of the Resistance, the boogeyman whose exploits are whispered about in the darkest corners of the Gifted world.

North looks over at me and I know that it's game over for him. That's the last puzzle piece in the mystery that is his Bond. Now he knows everything he ever needed to know about her. He's done for; hook, line, and sinker. He belongs to her now, whether he's admitting it to himself yet or not.

The Healer lifts his hand away from Black's chest and moves to roll up the leg of his pants to get a better look at his mangled ankle. It looks as though there's no bone structure left in there, like someone took a mallet to it and ground it to dust. Felix grimaces as he braces his hands on either side to start the reconstructive healing there too.

I have to swallow the bile down at the echoes of trauma in the back of my mind at the sight of it. I need to distract myself, to remind myself that this is something very different to what happened to me. I have to work at it to make sure my voice comes out bored. "What happened to you?"

North and Gryph both see through my attempt, but everyone else sends dark glares my way, as though their disapproval means anything to me.

Black glances at me, sweat still pouring down his face even as he's looking less sickly, and snaps, "The thigh break happened when we arrived. The blood infection is because they wouldn't treat it. I snapped my own ankle about a half hour ago to get out of the restraints to get Oli to take out John Franklin, the Resistance's strongest

Shield, so I could get back here. She did, by the way, her bond finally kicked in, and I got her off the torture table before I came here. I checked her bleeding and made sure all of the tourniquets on her were secure. She'll be fine there as long as Davies doesn't get back before we get her out. Not to be an asshole, Davenport, but you need to get a move on."

The Healer shoots him a rueful look and says, "You had sepsis, your kidneys were shutting down, and you were about twelve hours away from complete organ failure. Sorry it's taking a minute to stop your impending death."

Sage makes a little gasping sound in the back of her throat, lifting a hand to cover her mouth and muffle any other sounds of horror that she might have.

North curses and snaps, "Just tell us where Oleander is. You can stay here and receive treatment, there's no need for you to be going back out there. We have enough Transporters to get to her and take control of the situation safely."

Black grunts and lets out a low groan as the crunching sound of his bone resetting bounces around the room, panting to answer, "I can't... I don't know exactly where it is... I just followed the insurgents back there. I can map back, but I... don't have coordinates or a location."

I curse under my breath, because of course it couldn't be that easy for us, and snap, "How much longer until Davies is back at the camp then? We're running out of time while you're being pieced back together."

Black grunts again as there's another crunching of his bones, and snarls at me, "I sent him to the Hail Mary to buy time. I'm not a fucking idiot."

Fuck.

That'll just about do it.

I watch as half the room takes a breath, because Black is right, he's definitely not an idiot if he sent Davies there. The Hail Mary is the safe house in Massachusetts, and it's a rabbit warren of traps, barbed wires, and security surveillance. I know the place intimately, thanks to my uncle William dropping North and I both off there when I was a teenager over a security issue. Even with all of my nightmare creatures, I couldn't make my way out.

North meets my eye across the room as he pulls his suit jacket off, revealing just how many different weapons can be hidden under a Tom Ford, and then says, "If you're coming with us, then you need to be in full Tac gear. You too, Gabe. We leave the second Felix is done and Kieran can move."

The moment our feet hit the ground at the camps, it's very clear that things have changed dramatically since Black left here. I pull the gaiter up over my face and let my nightmare creatures out, checking in with Azrael, but Kyrie is still in the cages. Except now the tent's guards are all dead in a heap on the ground and the other women are shaking and sobbing at the trauma of what is happening around them.

Kyrie isn't.

A typical Shore reaction to this. She's sitting on her haunches, waiting for an opening to get the fuck out of there and take out whichever Resistance she comes across.

I lean towards Gryph and murmur, "Tell Kyrie we're here and heading to her. The prisoners are all looking shaken up."

He turns to look at me and scoffs, flinging out a hand. "We've just walked into a massacre and our Bond is lying injured in here somewhere… you're not even going to attempt to find her first?"

I look over at the piles of bodies, dozens of them lying wherever they've fallen in death, and then back at him. "I'm not an idiot. This? This is our little poisonous Bond. She's doing *just fine.* There are other Gifted here who can't kill people at will."

North pushes past us both, his own creatures coming out in full force, and he snaps, "Find our Bond first, then we'll take in the prisoners and any survivors."

Gabe stalks after him, looking a little shell-shocked, even though he's the only one of us to see her death powers up close, but he's also unwavering as he hunts for her. Gryph barks out commands to his team before he goes after the two of them, completing the triad of lovesick idiots going after a girl who does not need to be rescued.

Taken from here before Silas Davies gets back? Sure.

Rescued from the Resistance thugs he left her behind with? No. Anyone with eyes and two brain cells knocking around in their skulls can see she's got it handled. The only part of me desperate to get back to her is currently standing guard in the women's prisoner tents, so I'll be heading there to check that nothing has actually happened to Azrael or Kyrie before I trip over myself after some Bond.

Rahab, Procel, and Mephis follow closely after me as we work our way through the tents, all of them taking on their savage Doberman forms. The other creatures are all scouting in various shapes and sizes, checking for the moment Davies arrives back here so they can devour the piece of shit. There's no real need for concern about the Resistance left behind though.

Everyone is already dead.

She's good, I'll give her that, and to be able to kill this many without burning out? She's more powerful than any of us had given her credit for. The small amount of reading I've been able to do, around the intel-sifting North and I were elbows deep in, was entirely focused on what little we know about Soul Renders, and nothing I read comes close to this scale of destruction.

The void eyes make a lot more sense now.

Mine.

I curse and pull the gaiter up further, obscuring my face so that none of the Alpha team freak out at how furious I look when it's just my bond and the creatures

I'm dealing with. Bonds are dangerous, I'm not leaving myself open like that, and even if every last one of my creatures fall into obsession with her like Azrael has, I still won't have her.

Not even for a taste of that power.

Kyrie jumps onto her feet the moment she sees my outline, and I see her deflate a fraction when she realizes it's me and not her brother. I'm not going to be offended. They were close growing up and losing their parents only made them lean on each other even more.

She slumps back against the bars and groans, "Thank God. Please tell me you've gotten Oli out already?"

Why is everyone so single-mindedly focused on getting her out when she's strong enough to hold her own here?

"The others went to get her. I thought you'd be more worried about getting out of this little cage you've found yourself in?"

She scoffs at me and reaches up to pull her honey-colored hair away from her shoulder, revealing where Azrael is hiding in his smallest form. "She gave me this, even though I'm sure he would've been helpful to her. He saved me from being gang-raped in the showers by

Resistance scum, so excuse me for worrying about the kid."

Jesus fucking Christ.

I step up to the cage and motion for Rahab to get the door open. He's the most brutal of my creatures and with one yank, he breaks the lock and gets Kyrie free. The moment she steps out, Azrael jumps down from her shoulder and lands at my feet in his full-grown Doberman form. The others all snap at him, their own way of greeting him, but he sniffs at my feet like he's scenting everything that's happened since we were last together.

Which is nothing but a ton of frustration and Resistance intelligence records.

Kyrie does a little shiver, like she's shaking off a bad case of the creeps, and drawls, "No offense, but I'm glad to not have it anymore. Gimme a gun and a switchblade over a nightmare any day of the week."

I scoff at her and then I unstrap a Glock from my shoulder holster to hand over. She was a TacTeam operative for five years, only quitting to take over her mother's cafe when it was clear that Gloria was out to undercut it and drive them out, so she'll be more than up to scratch to cover my back as we get the others out.

I glance up at the other women, all still huddling and eyeing me like I'm a monster. Kyrie glances over her shoulder and scowls, snapping, "This is Nox Draven, here to rescue us, so you had all better treat him with respect, or I'll assume you're Resistance sympathizers and put you down."

I shoot her a look, but she just shrugs. "Gryph taught me how to deal with that monster bullshit early on. Nip it in the bud and move the fuck on. We don't have the time or energy to baby them through this."

She stalks over to frisk the corpse of one of the guards for keys and then gets to freeing the now-sheepish and quiet women. There's still a tent here of men to get out, and then the clusterfuck of getting everyone transported to deal with. I have no idea how long it's actually been since Davies went to the Hail Mary, but we must be running low on time.

We need to get a move on.

Azrael looks up at me with soft eyes, ones he should not be so open about showing in mixed company, and whines like a pup. She's ruining him. The more time he spends with her, the more he craves the gentle and loving tones she gives him. All of the belly scratches and soft pets… he'll be useless in a fight soon.

He whines again and I roll my eyes. "Fine, you can go find her. Don't eat anyone on the way."

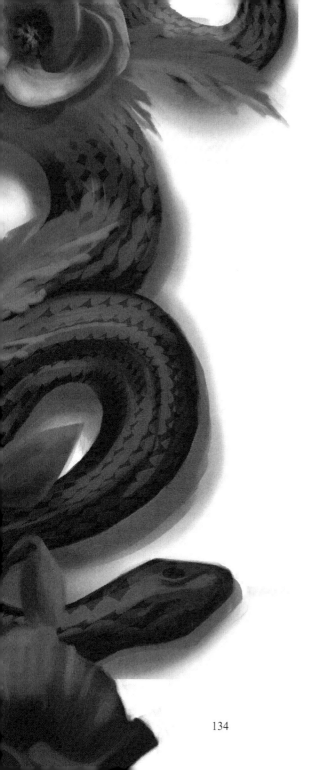

134

OLEANDER'S BOND

It's too easy to wipe out the camp.

Too easy and unsatisfying. I wish there were more challenges or people to torture but, aside from Franklin, there's only the women who were talking shit about me and the few guards.

Triggering their nightmares gives me a little something, a small thrill, but not enough, and I find myself eager to just tear their souls out and be done with it. Unsatisfying.

The little girl who is usually in control, she's there somewhere at the back of my consciousness, but the best way to do what needs to be done is to keep her out of it completely. She's too sweet for this amount of destruction.

I relish it.

I feel when they come for me, the edges of where I've cast out my senses tingling as they appear in the camp, but I'm too focused on the three Resistance idiots in front of me to go after those Bonds of mine.

I already know they'll come to me. Even when their petty, human differences were getting in the way, they were still coming after me and the girl I live within.

Zarah, Linda, and the mouthy guard, Cam, are all strung up on the tent poles by their wrists, their feet dangling a little off of the ground. I have to say, they sure do make these structures strong. It had been an absolute bitch to get the three of them up there but worth every moment of that pain.

Linda and Zarah are both dead already, their minds breaking far too quickly, which was honestly predictable for the type who would believe the Resistance propaganda. The moment they'd become blubbering shells, nothing left but a heart still pumping in their chests, I'd finished the job. There's nothing satisfying about a body going through the motions in a slow decay.

But Cam is holding out, a real sport.

He's jerking about as he slowly chokes on the blood pouring out of his eye sockets and into his open mouth. It's gory. I make a note to hide this memory from the girl, to tuck it so far back into the deepest recesses of her mind that she'll never feel that useless spike of guilt over it. She will, she always does over the things I do to protect us both, but I don't. They dared lay hands on us, so they're dead.

I hear the tent rustle behind me but I don't turn to look, because I don't want to miss a second of Cam dying. I can sense something entering the enclosed space with us, but it's not a Gifted, not even a human, and I finally force my eyes away from my prey to get a look at what is here, disturbing my work.

The serpent is as black as the darkest, starless night, though his scales still shine. It's unnatural and dangerous and *mine*. I stare at him, transfixed at his beauty, with my feet rooted to the grass underfoot. A dark god in his own right.

He rears up until his eyes—void perfection—are level with mine. We stare at each other for a moment, a moment of recognition because we were made for each other, made out of each other before we were separated and put on this Earth, only to seek each other out eternally.

And then he strikes.

Not me, obviously. He'd never harm me or the girl. No, he strikes and tears Cam from where he's hanging. Blood sprays over the tent walls, and I enjoy the sight of watching the Dark One's creature devour those who dared to touch me.

The tent flap rustles again and they arrive. Three pieces of my soul, only one who has given me what I want, the other two just as resistant as the girl is. A ripple of irritation runs down my spine, but I step forward to stroke a hand over the shining body of the serpent, reveling at the gleam of its unnatural scales against the blood-spattered ruin of my hands.

My Bonds and their abilities are magnificent.

"What the hell is she doing?" the Shifter whispers, and the Dark One hushes him, his footsteps rustling as he approaches me. I don't turn to face them. Instead, I watch as the last pieces of Cam are consumed in a bloody, fleshy mess. The way that he just disappears is comforting, because he deserves to be wiped from this earthly plane entirely.

The snake turns to stare at me again, its eyes taking in every inch of me but they get stuck on my leg, where the damage that Davies had done to the girl is soaking through my pants. It's not a concern to me, nothing to get in the way of the destruction this place needs that I *finally* get to wage.

I've waited a long time inside of the girl for this moment. No injury would stop me from getting what I'm due.

When the snake slides past me, bumping along my side and back over to his master, I stand and finally turn to face my Bonds. They all stare at me with very different expressions on their faces. Shock, horror, contempt, concern, disgust. I know most of it is for the men and women here that I've killed, but still, I preen a little at the awe. It doesn't matter if it's a horrified awe, they still look at me like they know I'm a god.

Finally, the Dark One speaks, "Oleander, you're bleeding."

I look down and see that the tourniquet has indeed shifted, but the pain is nothing. The blood loss might affect me, but we're not there yet.

My Bonded stops the Shifter from darting forward

to me with a palm to his chest, his eyes shifting to bright white as he says, "Bonded. Let me fix it."

I don't really want it fixed. I want them all naked and writhing here with me, my blood covering us all and marking them; to stop playing these childish, fearful games.

His head tips back a little as his breathing deepens, his chest expanding as he reacts to my lust, and this is exactly what I want.

The Dark One steps forward past the other two without hesitation and offers me a hand, his own eyes staying the deep blue color as he keeps his own bond under control.

I want to break it.

I want to break him open and pry my Bond out of his careful casing, get the power that belongs to me unleashed and revel in our shared Bond.

He reads me a little too well and speaks slowly, measuring every word as he lets it out of his mouth, "Let us get you home and then you can have whatever you want. Whatever you need, whatever whim you have, it's all yours. You'll die if we don't get the bleeding under control soon."

I curse the useless meat casing I'm trapped in, and

then take his hand. I let him move me over to the desk and lift me gently onto it to assess the damage and make adjustments to the tourniquet.

The Shifter comes back over and, hesitating just a little, he takes my other hand, threading our fingers together like he's trying to… comfort me. I won't break it to him that I do not need comfort.

I need to complete my Bonds and destroy *everything*.

My Bonded clicks his tongue at me and murmurs, "And I'd wager that's the exact reason Oli doesn't want to. Maybe you should calm down with the murder plans, and then you might just get what you want."

I give him a look, but he just shrugs back at me. Infuriating. The Shifter glances back at him with a confused look, but I move my focus back on the Dark One. His fingers are firm and sure as he looks at the mess my leg is in, his body shielding the other two from the sight of it. When he notices me watching him, he murmurs, "We need to get you to a Healer. The cuts are close to the artery, and you've been walking on it too much. Let one of us carry you to a Transporter, and we can get you to someone."

I cock my head at him and sigh. "The Fire girl's

Bonded. No one else."

The Dark One nods, reaching out to stroke a hand down my cheek. "We'll take you to Kieran, and he'll get you to Felix. We're only trusting our inner circle right now. I'll get you out to him now."

I want him, but I need strength right now and it flows through my Bonded and into me easier, thanks to our connection, so I say, "No. I want him."

The Dark One nods without hesitation, stepping back, and my Bonded steps in to lift me up into his arms. He's careful about the wound, one arm cradling my thigh protectively to his side, and he tucks my chest into his closely.

There are far too many layers of clothing between us for the power shift I need, but we're moving out of the tent before I can demand he strip down and give me what I need.

The moment we're out in the open, there are too many eyes on us.

The survivors and the cavalry alike, they all stare as we move through the camp. It's obvious why we're having to step over dozens of bodies to pick our way back over to the Transporter, but all of it is irrelevant to me. I don't care about their thoughts on what I've done here, but from the shuttered look on my Bonds' faces, they do.

I feel like I should point out that I'm a merciful god and I only kill those who torture, maim, and murder for their own nefarious gains. The little beings living quietly mean nothing to me.

"Jesus fucking Christ, be glad none of you can hear what's happening in her head right now. A lot more shit about our Bond and her fear of *this* is making sense," my Bonded says, and I fight the urge to reach into his chest and pull his heart out.

"You wouldn't. You need me and we both know it."

Still. It would be fun to do.

When we get to the edges of the tents and the small clearing, we find the Transporter waiting there for us with the other Dark One, the *damaged* one.

He doesn't react to our arrival, barely looks my way, but the Transporter fumbles over himself in his relief. "Oli! Thank God! I thought—Jesus, Gryph, what happened to her?"

"She needs to get out of here, and now isn't a great time to talk to her."

"Oli isn't really in right now, and her bond is trying

to plan how to take over the world, so maybe give her a minute," the Shifter says with a smirk, cocky and confident now that he knows what's going on.

I turn my face against my Bonded's chest to meet the Transporter's eye, acknowledging that his words have pulled me out of the girl and wrought this destruction, and he looks back at me with such relief, like he really was sitting here with bated breath, waiting for them to find me.

I decide to keep him alive. The Fire girl, her Bonded, and this one. Maybe the mouthy Techno boy, maybe. But I'd choose them to die last, right before my Bonds and I, if it were to come down to that.

"I'll be sure to let Sage know that too, Bonded."

I give him a withering glare that does nothing to remove the smirk on his lips. "Get out of my head, nosy Bonded, or maybe I'll rethink my plans of tearing your heart out."

He chuckles under his breath. "I have to admit, it's fun seeing this side of you. I can't help it. Besides, you ran off into danger again without any of your Bonds. You owe me a little fun."

There's no time to tell him exactly how that is not

the case, that I owe all of them nothing and they should all be worshipping me for merely existing, because the Transporter walks back over to us and with a steady, bloodied hand offered to me, he says, "Let's get the fuck out of here before anyone else gets cut up."

I'm expecting to go back to the Draven mansion, but instead we *pop* back into existence in a large warehouse full of men dressed in Tac gear and Healers wearing white coats to make them easily distinguishable. There are already freed prisoners being looked at by Healers and when they notice our arrival, a group of them come rushing at us.

I don't like that.

Even knowing they're not Resistance, I don't like being rushed, and especially not with four of my Bonds standing here with me. The moment I tense, my Bonded turns on his heel, putting his back between us and the Healers, and he snaps, "Back up! You're about to get fried."

"Or eaten," the other Dark One drawls, three of his

creatures baring their teeth at the approaching men, and though they look like perfect beings to me, all three men gulp from where I can see over my Bonded's shoulder.

Pathetic.

The Dark One steps out in front. "We need Felix Davenport. We brought him with us specifically to see to our Bond."

One of the men sputters indignantly and snaps, "He's a third year student! A councilman's Bond should be seen by—"

"She will be seen by Davenport and no one else. It's not your decision to make, Payne."

A Healer called Payne? I feel like the girl would enjoy that greatly. There's a lightness in my head and I rest my forehead back down onto my Bonded's chest, taking slow breaths to stop the swirling there. His arms tighten again and then he snaps, "Get the fuck out of the way before I hack into your brain and dredge up enough information to bury you."

There's more murmuring but then the Healer calls out, "I'm here! I was just getting Kyrie settled with some fluids, where's Oli—Jesus fucking Christ. Put her down; that's enough blood to kill a man, and that position is just making it worse."

My Bonded steps over to one of the stretchers, but instead of putting me down, he takes a seat, moving my legs around so that the Healer will have access to them. One of his big palms slides under my shirt to flatten over my spine, holding me securely against his chest, and it heats up as his gift spreads through my body.

The pain I know is there but don't actually *feel* disappears.

I sigh and turn to look at the Healer who is eyeing me carefully. My Bonded's arms tighten around me protectively, the palm almost scalding on my bare skin. He's very sensitive about everything in this room, the eyes and the words, everything is getting him ready for war.

I wonder what he's hearing that our ears can't.

"Watch yourself, Davenport. I'm not in the mood for excusing disrespect after everything we've been through today," he snaps, and the Healer throws his hands up like he's anticipating a fist to the jaw.

"This isn't being disrespectful. I've healed her enough to know exactly what she can do and how much power she has. I'm being cautious in case she's having some problems with control. We both know that's been an issue."

This makes him pause a little, just to look at me, but my void eyes give him nothing back. I feel my power winding down, the threat taken care of and none of the Gifted here a concern to any of us. Any one of my Bonds could crush these people like wet paper.

The Dark One glances down at me and then crouches down until he's back at my level, his voice firm as he says, "Give Oleander back so we can heal you."

I scowl at him. "No. I'm not giving her back while there's still pain. I don't let her feel it."

The arms tighten again, and then the Healer crouches down next to the Dark One. "If you can promise you'll be in control while I do what I need to, I'll do it. I'll take your word for it, because Gryphon will have to stop blocking the pain while I do."

My Bonded answers for me without hesitation, "No. You're not healing her while she can feel it."

The Healer shakes his head. "I can't pinpoint all of the damage if she can't feel the pain, I'm sorry. If I miss something, it could kill her later. I'm not willing to take that chance. Other Healers might, I won't. There's too much at stake here, and I'm not losing Oli because you're concerned about her feeling pain. I get it, but there's nothing I can do about it. I'm sorry."

I lean forward to be sure that I have his full attention, which I perhaps didn't need to do because I think I have the entire room's full attention right now, and say, "I won't harm you so long as you don't harm me or mine. Not now, not ever. The pain is nothing, only the girl feels it and she's sleeping right now. Do what you need to."

He nods, taking me at my word, and then he pulls up a seat next to the stretcher and gets to work. He explains where he's putting his hands and why he's touching me each time he moves and he gets my consent, the ultimate professional, and some of the tension leaves the space as my body slowly knits itself back together with his gift's guidance.

When he shifts again to press a palm over one side of my neck to check for brain injuries and any damage the drugs might have done to me, he drawls to my Bonded, "I don't know what you're fussing over her for. She's taking this better than anyone I've ever healed. Ease up a little, Shore. She still needs to breathe."

"I saw your face when you showed up to Draven's the

day Benson set a building on fire for you, don't pretend like you're above Bonded behavior," he snaps back.

After another few minutes of work, the Healer pulls his palm away from me and shifts in his seat, glancing over his shoulder at the audience of Healers and TacTeam still crowded around our perimeter before he shrugs out of his jacket.

"Gabe, give me a hand. I'll cover her and shut my eyes, so *don't* break my arm, but she needs skin-on-skin to finish the healing. Get her shirt off. Gryphon, you strip down too. Just to your waist."

The Dark One steps forward as well, taking his own jacket off and moving the Healer aside to take his place. Then the three of my Bonds all move me and fuss until I'm half naked and straddling my Bonded's thighs, our naked chests pressed together, with a jacket thrown over my back and my Bonded's strength flowing easily into me, thanks to our connection. I can feel my body breathing him in, taking everything I need from his vitality while he takes the same from me, a sharing of our resources, until I have everything I could ever need from him.

I finally take a deep, fulfilling breath.

"Holy shit, is it supposed to look like that?" the Shifter

mutters, and the Healer side-eyes him with a small shrug. I let my eyes flutter shut as I soak in the power, the girl's body slowly shutting down after the use of power. It always does, not used to channeling so much because she never lets me out.

The Healer's murmured words drift into my head slowly. "It's not usually so dramatic but yes, they're sharing power. It looks more… bright because she's so strong."

I drift off into unconsciousness, my hold on the girl still strong because I don't want her waking up while the healing is still underway, and I lose track of time. I only become aware of things happening around me when my Bonded speaks again, the sound loud in my ear that's pressed against his chest.

"Take your shirt off. She's scenting again and needs more. We need to get Bassinger to be ready for us back at the house as well. She's going to need us all."

The stretcher moves as someone else sits down, and then I'm moved over into the Shifter's arms, pressed firmly against his bare chest next. He smells warm, goosebumps exploding along his skin as I bury my nose into the crook of his neck.

I squeeze my eyes shut tighter, knowing that when they open again, it will no longer be me in charge and the girl will be back to deal with the consequences of my actions to save us.

But we're alive, mostly unscathed, and she won't remember the brunt of it. That has to be enough.

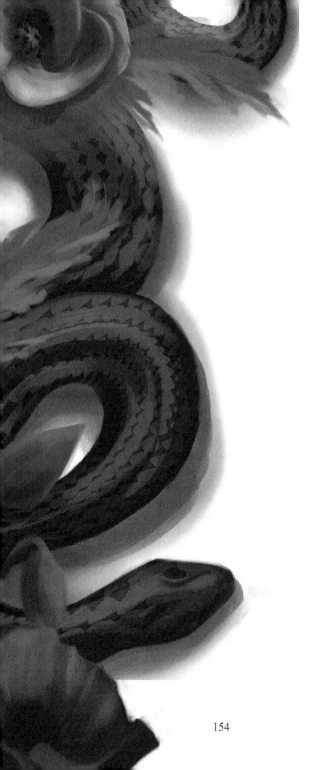

OLI

I wake up surrounded by delicious Bond scents, my nose buried in warm skin and with arms tight around me. I'm naked from the waist up, and so is North where we're pressed tightly together, though there's something thrown over my shoulders to cover me up, and my legs are wrapped around his waist.

When I sigh, totally content with how I've found myself because my brain isn't processing at all the 'what the fuck' of this moment, his arms tighten around me and he turns his head into mine a little more to murmur into my ear, "Ten more minutes, Bond. Then I'll get you to a bed."

Goosebumps explode over my skin and I shiver, my nipples tightening until they're pebbled where they're pressed into his chest, and his hand drops back down to grip my thigh, pulling me in closer to his body. My bond purrs in my chest, humming with pleasure at having him desperate to keep me close, because there's no other way to describe the grip of his hand.

There's voices around us, some I don't recognize, but I let my face stay buried in his neck as I ignore it all. I'm sure if there were danger, he would have shared that information with me already, and I doubt he'd have me half naked if there were.

The longer we sit there together, the more my brain begins to work and information filters in. This man doesn't trust me, sitting here on top of him is going to cost me big time the moment I get up, and I'm going to have to move soon because nature calls.

There's also a lot of talk happening about whether or not the Resistance is going to retaliate against us in the next seventy-two hours that has me tensing and an icy bead of sweat rolling down my spine.

What if I've led them here, to my Bonds and my

friends, and we're about to be wiped out?

My panic must be obvious because the chatter stops around me and then there's movement. I turn my head just as Gryphon reaches us, bending until he's at eye level with me, his gaze sharp on my face as he assesses me. "What's wrong, what do you need? Anything, Bonded."

I can't say it out loud. I can't admit what it is that's tearing me in half right now, so I take the coward's way out and send the words directly to him as I squeeze my eyes shut. *I don't want to leave him, but I need the bathroom. I don't want to lose this.*

There's a moment of quiet and then I hear rustling, the tight arms around me gently falling away. I have to swallow the whimper that creeps up my throat, and I keep my eyes shut until Gryphon's hands tug me away from the warmth and security I'm clinging to.

The air in the room is cold against my exposed skin, and he's quick to get a sweater over my head that smells like Nox. I take a deep lungful of that scent and finally open my eyes, just in time to see the furious look on North's face as Gryphon slides my arms into the sweater. His body acts as a shield from the rest of the room so that no one can see me. This time I'm choking down tears at the next round of rejection I'm going to face from my Bond.

Don't think like that. He's pissed that Hannity and Rockelle are insisting on the debrief happening now so that he can't just tend to you like he wants to. No one is rejecting you, Bonded. Not now, not ever.

I don't even argue with Gryphon for reading my mind. I can't let myself believe what he's saying. I can't afford to open myself up to that kind of pain, but then North's eyes flick back down to mine and I watch them soften.

Soften.

He leans forward until my breath catches in my throat. It feels like he's about to kiss me, right here for the first time, in front of God knows who, and my cheeks heat, but instead he murmurs to me quietly, "Go with Gryphon. I'll get this wrapped up as soon as I can."

His hands hold onto my hips as I stand, keeping me steady until I'm sure my legs won't give out, and the second I wince at my first step, Gryphon wraps an arm around my waist. I allow myself one last glance at North's face before we leave him behind, and if I thought his hands felt desperate on me earlier, they had nothing on the dark possession in his eyes now.

He's staring at me like I'm prey.

I glance quickly away and let Gryphon lead me out of the room slowly. I keep my eyes on the ground so that no one can see the shock I'm experiencing. When I curse at the pain in my freshly healed thigh, Gryphon murmurs, "Felix said you need to stretch the muscles out, otherwise I'd just carry you. He's told me not to take the pain away so that he can check up on it again and get more accurate in the healing, but if it's too bad, I'll just carry you. Fuck what he says."

I shake my head and grit my teeth. "He's a Healer, we should do what he says. It's not so bad, more of an old ache than pain anyway. Please tell me there's a toilet nearby though, because it's about to get awkward as hell if we have to make it back to my room."

He shakes his head at my stupid attempts at humor, walking me over to a bathroom only two doors down, and then I spend way too long convincing him to leave me alone to pee. He tries to talk me into letting him stay in there with his back to me, but there's no freaking way I could pee like that. No way, and he's crazy for even suggesting it.

Brutus pops out from behind my ear and jumps

down onto the tiles in front of my feet. Tears fill my eyes because I'm tired, emotional, and so fucking relieved to have him back. Seriously, the few hours we'd been apart were too much for me now, and it occurs to me that Nox now holds a massive trump card over me.

If he takes this puppy away from me, I will break in half.

The moment Gryphon hears the toilet flush, he's rushing back into the room, his eyes raking over me like he's checking for any damage I might have taken while sitting on the goddamned toilet, and I huff at him.

"Stop being ridiculous. I'm healed up and perfectly safe here. I have Brutus with me and, I'm not sure if you know, but my gift is to literally rip people's souls out, killing them instantly. I think I can handle a toilet break without you having a complete meltdown over it."

His eyes narrow at me but I turn my back on him as I wash up. Brutus curls around my ankles and supports me like he knows that the ache in my thigh is now more of a burning sensation that has my knee buckling a little.

"At least I know you've woken up as yourself again, no mistaking that sass."

I turn to grab a hand towel and flash him a grin. "You

missed it though, right? You hate to admit it, but you missed my smart mouth."

He steps forward and grabs my wrist, pulling me into his arms and ignoring Brutus snapping his jaws in irritation. "I'll admit to every part of what I'm feeling. You left here again, but this time it was worse because you weren't just the idea of a Bond to me anymore. You're *you*. You're mine, and you walked away from us again."

I snap, "I went after your—"

"I know. You went after my sister for me, and I can both love you for it and be fucking furious at you for doing it. I'm never leaving you behind again. I'm never trusting anyone, not even our own Bond Group, to watch you *ever* again."

I'm just going to skip over the usage of the L word, because I'm sure it's just a little slip up, so instead I nod to him. "I like that plan. The feeling of you leaving was… let's not do it again. There's no real reason we can't just stay here together from now on, right?"

His eyes narrow like he doesn't trust what I'm saying, which is ridiculous because he can literally sense my lies and I've never been so honest with him in all of the months we've known each other. But after a minute, he gets over whatever it is that's bothering him and pulls me back into his arms to get out of the bathroom and back into... whatever the hell the room we just left is called.

Hell, maybe?

Purgatory, or maybe even Limbo because I'm stuck there not knowing what the ever-loving-fuck is going on with North Draven and the soft eyes he just gave me.

Soft.

I wouldn't believe it if I hadn't been inches away from them and staring up at him like he was the goddamn sun. Hope that maybe he believes me now blooms like a weed inside of me, impossible to kill off, even though it could choke the life out of me if it turns out to not be the case.

I need to stop myself from thinking about it.

Embarrassingly, as we step into the hallway, we bump into none other but Kieran and Kyrie, my Bonded's sister.

Kyrie smirks at us both wobbling along together, or maybe the fact we just walked out of a bathroom together, which is a little bit cringe-worthy.

When Gryphon just stares at them both, a slow grin stretching across his face at the sight of his very alive and unharmed sister, she huffs at him and snaps, "Let your Bonded go so I can hug you. It's also creepy seeing you smile like that, tone it down a little."

Gryphon helps me brace myself against the wall and then tugs her into his arms, squeezing his eyes shut as he sighs a little in relief. "How about you never let yourself be taken again so my goddamned Bonded doesn't go charging after you? Such a pain in my ass, Ky."

She makes a watery sound and then shoves at him. "I didn't ask her to! Although, she's handy to have around. You should hear how they all talk about her, like she's the harbinger of death or something. It was freaking weird… until I saw people dropping dead everywhere. It made a little more sense then."

Gryphon makes a dismissive noise under his breath and snaps, "They deserved a much slower death after everything they did, but at least, for once, there were no survivors."

Kieran makes an equally pissed off sound, butting into their little tirade, and says, "Yeah, except that the asshole who is responsible for all of this got away. He's still out there and still obsessed with your little murderous Bonded, Shore."

Then the three of them turn to look at me, where I'm slowly shuffling down the hall away from this conversation, and I grimace. "Listen, I wasn't going to be able to kill that man anyway, so it was leave him alive or die trying, and I know that I, for one, am happy with how it turned out."

Kyrie steps over to me and is a little bit faltering and cautious as she gives me a hug, but it's clear she's more worried about hurting me than touching a Soul Render. "Thank you. The little beast at your feet saved me instead of stopping you from being carved open, and I'll never be able to repay you for that."

I have no idea what to do with someone's thanks.

Awkward.

So I deflect like a pro instead. "I knew I was safe from certain things in those camps that you weren't, it wasn't a hard choice to make. Besides, who hasn't been sliced and diced a little in their spare time?"

None of them so much as crack a smile at my lame attempt at a joke, but it seems they're all falling flat today. I glance at Gryphon and say, "Not to be a pain in the ass, but I need to sit down."

He's immediately hauling me up into his arms, and when I try to protest, he snaps, "You've been walking for long enough. Davenport can come at me over it; I'll deal with it."

Kyrie starts cackling behind us, but Gryphon ignores her, stalking back into the room that I now see is North's office. I slide out of Gryphon's arms as we step through the door, not wanting to be inappropriate around people I don't know, even though Gryphon mutters a protest about it.

North is still sitting where we left him, his dress shirt only half buttoned, with a thunderous look on his face as he faces two older men that I vaguely recognize from that cursed dinner we'd attended a lifetime ago.

The moment we step into the room, one of them glances back at me and says, "Well, she's here now—"

North cuts him off with acid dripping from his words, "Attempt to address my Bond right now, Hannity, and I'll not be held responsible for what happens."

I freeze, but Gryphon just slides in front of me, his arm tucking behind his back to hold me close to his body but clearly shielding me from sight of anyone in the room who might want something from me.

Hannity clears his throat and then chooses his words carefully. "I'm just trying to say that only one person knows exactly what happened. If we could hear it directly from your Bond—"

"No. You will hear *nothing* from her, and neither will any of the rest of the council. You're sitting here because Gryphon has vetted you. If that status changes, if he finds even the slightest whiff of deception from any of you, you'll be dealt with."

"And how are you planning on achieving that, North? You're strong, but you're not a god."

I should just let it go, but them questioning him like that? My bond isn't happy about it. Gryphon's arms tighten around me as he feels my bond take over and my eyes shift. I lean in his arms just enough that Hannity and Rockelle can get a look at me and say, "Me. He won't get the chance to set August and his creatures on you, because I'll have you dead on the ground before they get the chance."

I watch as two fully grown, Top Tier, Gifted men gulp at the sight of my void-like eyes. The look of exaltation in North's eyes only draws me into him even more.

It feels too damn good; my bond preens in my chest.

The moment Hannity and Rockelle finally give up on their questioning of North and leave us behind, he grabs his phone and demands that Felix comes to have another look at me. I want to protest, but I'm now sweating over the very sharp pains in my thigh and there's no hiding that from either of my Bonds. Gryphon directs me into a seat while we wait for my only trusted Healer friend.

Felix arrives in under a minute, looking harried and completely fried, but gets straight into healing me. When our eyes meet, there's a very clear look of relief in him that has me cringing.

"You met my bond, huh?"

He huffs out a laugh as he presses a palm to my bare ankle and his gift floods me. "Sure did. Wouldn't have thought something that terrifying lived inside of you."

I roll my eyes back at him as the door opens again and the room becomes very crowded with my Bonds, our friends, and some more people I don't know. "I tried to warn you all, but no one believed me. It's a cantankerous bitch at the best of times."

Gabe comes straight over to me and cups my cheek, ignoring Felix's disapproving protests, and he kisses me softly. "Thank fuck you're awake."

I swipe my tongue over my bottom lip, chasing the taste of him absentmindedly. "I didn't really… sleep the way I need to. I give it maybe another hour or two, and I'll be out for a few days. I did sleep the first three days at the camp away as well, that helped get me through the boredom."

He nods and then steps away to get out of Felix's way as he finishes up on whatever repairs my thigh needs. Sawyer has an arm over Sage's shoulders, and I can see the effort it's taking him to keep her away from me. I give her a smile anyway, knowing I'll be throwing myself at her for that hug the second I can.

She looks freaking exhausted.

Kieran scoffs at me and takes the seat next to me, waiting his turn to be looked over by Felix, and snaps, "You slept most of the time away. Slept like a fucking baby, even strapped to a chair."

"Are you still complaining about that? At least you could lie down and I got you decent food, you could say thank you, you know."

He stares at me for a second and then says sullenly, "The chicken was shit."

I laugh back at him. "The chicken is always shit. The

slops are worse though, so, again, you're welcome."

Felix finally removes his hand from me and when he shuffles over to Kieran, there's a wobble in his gift that wasn't there before, and he's clearly nearing the end of his power source for the day.

Sage senses it too, of course, they're Bonded after all. She eyes him, her brows drawn together in a frown, and then I watch as her bond bursts out of her and into him in a wave. He grunts a little and rocks back on his heels, but the lines of tension melt away almost instantly.

"Shit, sorry! I'm still figuring out how to do that!" Sage stutters, and Felix steps back over to reassure her, but my attention is drawn elsewhere.

Mainly over to where Kieran is staring at Sage with something close to… wonder.

What the fuck is that?!

He notices the daggers I'm staring into the side of his head. When his eyes swing in my direction, my own eyes drop down to his leg, where his Tac gear is still cut up. Where the long gash that had only been partially healed in a rush job before they came for me should be, there's now nothing but freshly healed skin.

My jaw almost hits the goddamn ground, but then

Kieran glares at me savagely and my brain kicks back in. Of course it isn't my place to freak the fuck out about this, in a crowded room full of people we definitely don't trust, because there are TacTeam people here, waiting on orders from North, and some other men in suits.

North's assistant, who I hadn't noticed had arrived and who is hovering in the corner, is watching him obsessively, and nothing about my time away has lessened my urge to gouge her eyeballs out.

I've just been pulled off of him while I needed him, to pee and be healed, but having this bitch staring him down is unacceptable to me.

"Pen, you should head home now that we have this all under control," Gryphon says as he pulls me back out of the seat and plants himself in front of me, his arms crossed over his chest and his tone very firm. He's a lot less friendly with her, a very welcome change, and my bond settles a little in my chest at his loyalty.

Gabe steps in, flanking me as though he's prepared for this to all go very badly, but I like having him close to me again.

She makes a disgruntled noise, like she's pissed at him, but then North cuts her off with a no-bullshit sort of tone, "Go home, and don't come in tomorrow either. I'll arrange a time for us to meet at the council offices. The manor is going down to minimal contact, and you're not on the security list."

Oh.

Oh, I like that *a lot.*

I try to keep the smug look off of my face at his words, but Gabe snorts at me and shakes his head, so I'm obviously failing. Well, who cares really, because she was more than okay with walking into his room with me in his bed. With a key. Picking out his clothes.

His underwear.

"Take a deep breath. Another one, Bonded," Gryphon murmurs, his head turned slightly my way but his body is still between me and the room. I'm now not entirely sure if he's doing it for my protection or theirs.

I should do the right thing and get the fuck out of here.

I fumble around until I get a hold of Gabe's hand, sidestepping until I'm tucked into his body. He accepts me without question or hesitation, turning towards me and wrapping his free arm around me protectively.

When I rise up onto my tiptoes, he bends down to

meet me halfway, tilting his head so I can whisper into his ear, "Take me somewhere, please. Somewhere on this level where we can be alone but still close. I can't... I can't handle—"

He looks at me like he's expecting me to burst into tears, with a vague sort of panic, and then he murmurs in a placating tone, "Okay, I can do that. C'mon, Bond. I know where to go."

He leads me down a hallway I've never seen before—the place is ridiculous—and then we duck into a small alcove that is carved out of one of the walls. There's a large potted plant in the entrance that partially covers the loveseat built into the wall, and there's a small bookcase with old tomes on it.

The Dravens really love their books.

Gabe tugs me over to the loveseat, which is the size of a double bed really, and covered in European cushions, and when he sits on it, I glance around the space a little more. It's too open, more open than what I was hoping for, and my bond starts getting pissy in my chest all over again.

I make an unhappy sound in the back of my throat, and Gabe grins lazily at me, even if it feels a little forced, and says, "There's not a lot of options here, Bond. I'm working with what we have."

When my eyes flash back to black, the grins falters and he gulps, but I move to tug his shirt back over his head and shove him down on the chair. I want to strip and press our bodies together. Hell, what I really want to do is fuck him against the wall until his scent is all over me and his cum drips down my legs in the most brutal and obvious branding, but my senses are still too aware of all of the extra bodies in the house and the giant opening to this little alcove he's brought me to.

I don't want anyone to see what's mine.

So instead, I curl up on his chest, pressing my ear against the steady beat of his heart, and burrow into his warmth. He moves slowly to wrap his arms around me and hold me, as though he's worried he'll trigger some animalistic response from me that loses him a limb. My bond enjoys that sort of respect from him.

The fact that he's so sure of how dangerous I really am is comforting somehow.

I huff, frustrated at the layers still between us, and lean back to pull the sweater off of myself. Gabe swallows roughly, color bright and high on his cheeks as he sees me bare to the waist, but he doesn't attempt to stop me. When I press myself in tight against him again, he grabs the sweater and covers my back up. Another point in his favor. My bond likes him coveting me just as hard as I covet him.

"Can you change back? If I promise not to move away or cover either of us up? Gryph's going to kill me if he sees you like this again," Gabe mutters, and I wrestle my bond back into the background of my mind again.

He takes a deep breath when he feels my bond ease away, his hand rubbing down my spine in one long stroke that almost has me melting all over him. Weeks of sitting in a Resistance camp has every inch of my body tense and sore.

"Ugh, I probably smell. How can you stand me being this close to you right now?" I mumble, and he shrugs.

"Maybe if I shifted you'd be bad, but the need to have you here is greater than your stink so far. Besides, keeping your bond happy is more important than a bit of dirt and sweat."

He chuckles quietly at me grumbling under my breath, but when I attempt to pull away, he just tightens his arms and gets back to stroking my spine until I turn into putty right there on top of him. I might be desperate for a shower and a proper sleep in a comfortable bed, but this little moment between us? It feels like pure magic, and I know the moment my bond starts pulling from his energy.

"You're glowing again. Shit, I think I am too."

My eyes feel as though they weigh about a million pounds as I murmur, my voice slurring with fatigue, "Sorry about that. I think I'm stealing your energy."

His answer comes through to my brain like a dream, whispered but still meaningful. "Take it. Take whatever you want, just don't fucking leave me again."

I startle awake to two very terse Bonds speaking over each other at us both some unknown amount of time later.

"What the hell is going on?"

"You're in the open. Where the fuck is her shirt?"

Gabe's chest moves underneath me like he's motioning with his arm, but my eyes stay glued shut. I'm tired, too tired to deal with any of them, and he's so warm and comfortable.

He whispers, "Her bond came out again. I did whatever I had to, just like we all agreed, to stop her from a full-blown reign of bond terror on everyone in the house who isn't her Bond. She's still healing, maybe, or—is this nesting? Or something like it? She needs skin and scent, and her bond does *not* want to be argued with."

It's quiet for a moment, and then Gryphon says, "Good work. Everyone else has left now, and it's only a skeleton staff on, so we can get her upstairs without bumping into anyone."

I hear movement again and then Gabe says, "If you're going to take her, you need to get your shirt off. She's not interested in clothes right now."

Smart boy, I definitely do want skin.

Horny, tantrum-throwing bond. I huff a little, and Gabe stiffens again like he's afraid my bond is about to wreck their shit, and his hand strokes down my spine again. He's very good at this whole calming, petting thing he has going on for me right now. I could honestly start purring.

"I'll take her up, Gabe. You go ahead and make sure no one uses this hallway or the elevator."

"Is she staying in your room? She's been very vocal about not doing that."

North's arms are tight around me as he lifts me up, and Gabe rolls up onto his feet, immediately grabbing the sweater to cover my back up. I tuck my face into the column of North's neck and breathe him in, taking in everything I could ever need from him as well.

I just need Atlas back, and then maybe I'll be whole again.

"I'll kill my assistant if I have to, no one is going to burst into *any* room in this house going forward. We're on a security lockdown, and if Oleander wants to sleep somewhere else, she can when she wakes up. Until then, she's staying with me."

Oh, I like that too. I like that a lot.

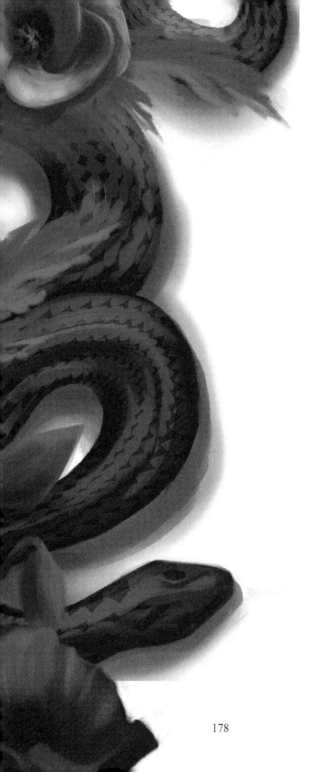

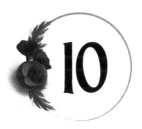

OLI

My eyes flutter open at the sound of the shower turning on, and North's arms tense around me as he readjusts his hold to stick his hand under the stream of water, checking the temperature. I'm still wearing Nox's sweater but my pants have been stripped off, leaving me in my underwear, and my face is pressed into his neck so that I'm surrounded by his scent once again.

I clear my throat and try not to sound like an embarrassed child as I say, "I'm awake. You can just put me down."

He doesn't answer me as he steps fully into the

shower stall and then sits down on the built-in marble bench that runs along one of the walls, still holding me close to his chest. I really should get my face out of the crook of his shoulder and face the man, but we're in a *shower stall* together and I feel a little light-headed at what's happening here right now.

Especially the part where I have *no fucking idea* of what that is.

I clear my throat again and finally he says, "Do you need something to drink? When did you last have something? Your bond wouldn't accept anything from us while it was in control."

Holy shit.

How long was my bond in control, and what the hell did it do if he's in here cuddling up to me and pulling me into a shower?

"This morning... or how long was I asleep? Maybe yesterday."

He nods and starts to tug at the sweater to get it off of my body. "This morning. You've only been asleep for an hour. I thought you might sleep through the shower."

The moment he gets the sweater over my head, I realize I have nothing on underneath the damned thing. I finally sit up a little in his lap to unwind myself from him and freak out about this, wrapping my arms around my chest and shooting him a very scandalized look.

His face doesn't change, and his tone is kind but also very matter-of-fact as he says, "There isn't a single one of your Bonds who hasn't seen you bare to the waist, Oleander. We all held you while you healed."

I groan and shove my face into my hands, desperate to pass out again and forget that the conversation is even happening. "Is there anything else entirely shameful I did? Did my bond attempt to assault any of you again, or am I going to be spared that particular horror this time around?"

"Whatever you need, it's our duty and honor to provide."

I have no words to even attempt to answer that, and it doesn't really answer anything for me anyway. "What the hell happened while I was gone? Where is all of this coming from? The last I knew, you didn't trust me. Now, you're in here with soft words and offering me whatever I want... I'm so fucking confused right now. Which one of us has a head injury I need to freak out about right now?"

He's way too calm about my rambled word vomit.

So calm that he doesn't react at all, except to shift his grip on me to my hips to hold me steady, and once he has a good grip, he opens his mouth and all of my secrets come out of it. "You were kidnapped from the hospital. You were held in a Resistance camp for two years while they tortured you for information about your gift and your Bonds. You gave them nothing. You escaped when Silas Davies left, and your bond took over to get you out. You then spent three years on the run to lead them away from us. You slept in halfway homes, sublets, and the streets while you were barely more than a kid because you didn't want them to get access to us... or your gift. That's what's changed."

My mouth opens and then closes with a snap, because that's a whole lot more information than I was expecting him to have. That's a lot more than knowing my Resistance code name would have gotten him, but I guess it was a good enough starting point for him to hunt down the rest.

My cheeks heat again, and when I slide off of his legs, this time he lets me, though his hands stay over my hips to brace me and hold me up. "You're making it sound heroic. It was mostly me being terrified and trying to flee."

He stares up at me with those same broody eyes he's been giving me throughout this entire conversation. "You were sixteen when you escaped them, of course you were terrified. How you endured what they did to you without murmuring a single word is beyond me, but it was more than the *something* I asked from you before you left."

I swallow roughly, trying not to feel self-conscious about my basically naked state, and mutter, "I didn't give it to you though. Atlas told you, and you've figured it all out from there."

He shrugs and then his fingers hook around the elastic waistband of my underwear, drawing them down my legs without a single word, and my dumb ass just stands there and lets him. I'm kind of stunned at his presumption, that it's just totally fine for him to undress me completely and I'll just... be fine with it.

I guess this is the most North action I've seen out of him since I returned, and that's why my brain hasn't caught up with the situation fully.

He stands up and motions to the marble bench. "Sit down. Davenport has had to fix your leg in stages, and you still have one last session before it's fully healed."

Again, I just do it because I think the information

dump has broken the small, sassy part of my brain that woke up with me, and now I'm on autopilot while shit reconfigures in there.

Then, with a rapt sort of focus, I watch as he strips down, peeling off his Tac gear and dropping it on the ground outside of the shower stall. He doesn't hesitate or pause until he's standing there completely naked in front of me.

I force my eyes to stay very firmly above his waist, a feat that I'll go to the grave being proud of considering that I'm sitting down and my eyeline is, of course, dick level.

I can't speak, my voice has dried up, and he either doesn't notice my meltdown at the magnificent sight of his chest, or he's choosing to leave me in the puddle he's made of me as he turns his back on me to test out the water again. Then he ducks his head under and gives himself a quick scrub down.

Blood and dirt I hadn't noticed before muddy the water, and the strong, masculine scent of his soap fills the air until he's practically glowing with cleanliness.

Then he turns back to me and holds out a hand.

I take it, and a deep breath, and let him pull me up

and under the blissfully hot stream of water. Because he doesn't make a comment or even a sound while he works, I manage to get through him cleaning me without too much awkwardness.

He uses all of his own supplies, his soaps, and then he massages his shampoo into my hair with fingers that might just be magic. I have to hold in a moan of pure pleasure as goosebumps explode over my skin.

When he takes the handheld showerhead down to wash out the shampoo, I get self-conscious again, though this time it has more to do with the fact that my nipples are pebbled up and betraying just how much I'm enjoying this little moment of his ministrations, and I try to grab the showerhead from him. "My leg should be okay, I can do the rest."

He's at least a foot taller than I am and easily moves it out of my reach. "No, stay right where you are. Just shut your eyes and enjoy it."

Goddammit. His fingers slip easily into my hair, massaging my scalp again as he rinses out the shampoo, and I just give in. I'm still tired, and I'll use that as my excuse later when this all inevitably bites me in the ass.

Is it going to?

It has to, right? There's no way that hearing the sad little story of what they did to me would have him changing his tune this drastically... right?

Once my hair is clean, he goes over my body one last time with the soap, which I'm sure it doesn't need, but I do what he told me to and just keep my eyes shut for it all. When he shuts the water off and opens the door again to grab a towel, I stay where he left me, my arms wrapped around my waist and his scent overwhelming me.

I feel safe and secure and loved for the first time since my parents died.

I have to take some very long and deep breaths to stop myself from bursting into tears. I'm sure I could pass them off as exhaustion or some sort of bond reaction, but I think North has seen more than enough of me for one day. If I haven't scared him off so far, then I'm sure it'll be me weeping over a fucking shower that'll do it.

His feet are almost silent on the wet tiles but not quite so when a huge, luxurious towel wraps around me, completely enveloping my small frame in its sheer magnificence, I'm not startled and I keep my eyes shut for another moment.

Then his lips brush over my bare shoulder and I let a

single tear roll down my cheek unchecked.

No matter what else happens between us, I'll remember this small gift of kindness he's given me for the rest of my life. This will go down as the moment I let myself admit how much I want North Draven. How much I crave his domineering and assertive nature, how much I need him, even if he does act on my behalf without ever asking me what it is that I want.

That even while I was determined to hate him, he's worked his way under my skin and I don't want to dig him out.

"Turn around on your good leg. I'll get you out of here."

I do as he asks and let him scoop me up into his chest. There's another towel wrapped around his waist, but without the styling he usually puts into his hair, I can see the same tight, dark curls as his brother falling over his forehead. His eyes were always striking, the deep blue depths of them against his tanned skin, but there's something about the way he's looking at me tonight that has my breath catching in my throat dangerously.

Am I about to fall in love with a Draven, over a shower of all things?

He sets me down on the bathroom countertop and carefully dries me off without another word, his hands reverent and gentle over the miles of soft skin on display. I watch as he catalogs every last one of my injuries, every bruise and broken patch of skin that Felix hasn't bothered to heal up yet, thanks to the more devastating thigh injury. If I wasn't so sure about him right now, I'd assume the murder in his eyes was a warning to me.

It's not.

It's a plan he's putting together to go after any Gifted who might have touched me and is still breathing. There's plenty from my first time in the camps, but only Davies made it out this time around.

I don't want to think about that man anymore. I force my eyes to follow the droplets of water cascading down his chest instead, the way that there's the smallest of dimples on his cheek that I've never been close enough to notice before, and the strong muscles of his throat that flex as he works so diligently to getting me dry. He's fucking gorgeous, always has been, only now I'm letting myself take note of it.

The problem with looking at all of those details is that it wakes my bond up and, my God, does it want him to push me back and fuck me until my legs don't work. The exhaustion that was filling me up moments ago in the shower burns away, and my pussy throbs between my legs. I have to swallow a whimper that creeps up the back of my throat, and my body feels as though it's on fire.

North's nostrils flare and he drops the towel, bracing his hands on either side of my thighs as he leans into me, careful not to touch me, but taking up every inch of my personal space nonetheless.

"You can stop the Bond, can't you?"

It takes my brain a second to process his words, the lust and sex thickening the air around us taking over me completely, and when I finally make sense of him, I swallow roughly all over again.

He doesn't mention how he knows that I've done it before, because bringing up his brother's actions right now probably isn't for the best. I lick my lips, watching in awe as his eyes get stuck on the action and his pupils blow out and swallow his irises, almost looking like the void eyes we share.

It's a heady feeling, to have this power over him, and when I arch my back a little, stretching out on the bathroom counter, his teeth grind together as he holds himself back.

I could get addicted to this feeling.

"I can. It… hurts, but I can do it."

When I meet his eyes, he pins me there with a smoldering look, trapping my gaze so that I can't bear to look away. "Tell me how it hurts. Which parts and how bad?"

Fuck. Me. "After. It hurts when I come and I stop my bond from coming out to… claim you as my Bonded. I feel like I'm burning up from the inside out. It lasts a few minutes, and it's bad but not unbearable."

A scowl tugs his brows together and he pushes back from me, leaning until I'm sure he's about to step away from me and leave me to get dressed. I curse myself under my breath, but then one of his hands comes up to run a thumb over my bottom lip, pushing against the plump curve of it as he watches the movement obsessively.

His words catch me by surprise. "So if I edge you for the next couple of hours, you can enjoy it and only feel the pain at the end? Not ideal, but I'll take it."

Edging? Jesus. Do I want that? The rough feel of his palms over my body, his lips on my soft skin, hours of pleasure that never truly reaches its peak?

Wait, that sounds fucking amazing. A little frustrating, but if that isn't our relationship so far down to a T, nothing is. I want so badly to say yes to him and just spend the night getting lost in him, but there's still something there.

Something holding me back.

My legs can't help but part as he slides in closer, his eyelids dropping down a little so that he's practically smoldering at me. "Do you want this? Stop overthinking it and answer me."

"Of course I want it—"

"Then Bond or don't. I'm not waiting to taste you any longer. If you're hesitating about the power exchange, then just don't do it. I'm not waiting."

I open my mouth to argue with him, because it's not that easy, but he tugs my thighs forward until I'm balancing somewhere between my elbows and his shoulders. He moves like he's about to eat me out, and I have one last stupid thing rushing around my head that won't let me enjoy this moment.

"Wait! Wait one second. I need something first, just one thing."

He scowls at me, stopping the second I'd spoken, but not moving away from where he's got me balanced.

"Whatever it is, you're sure it can't wait? I'm not entirely above begging, Bond."

Interesting.

I attempt to sound confident. "Your bond is like mine, right? It's... more than the others. It's not just a force inside you. It's a living thing, right?"

The scowl grows on his face and he gives me the tiniest of nods, the smallest gesture, and I plow onwards like this is all fine and I'm not freaking out about even asking this. "Let me talk to it. There's something I want to ask it, and then we can... I mean, I think I want to Bond after. Properly. We can save the edging for later."

I think it's the mention of actually Bonding that gets him to agree because he's already shaking his head until that part slips out of me. I'm not bribing him, not exactly, because if he says no, I think I might still be Bonding with him tonight, but I have to at least try.

He carefully moves me back onto the countertop, gently and mindful of my thigh, and then he takes a step away, as if putting distance between us again will stop his bond from hurting me or attempting to approach me.

As if a single step away is all it will take to keep me safe.

"If it tries to bond with you, kill me. Or get Gryphon to knock me out. You can still contact him, can't you?"

I pull a face at him. "I think I'll lead with knocking you out. No need to kill you over a little bit of sex, North."

He raises an eyebrow at my sass and blows out a breath, muttering about how much of a bad idea this is, but after a minute, his eyes shift into the voids.

All emotions and humanness wipes clean from his face until there's nothing but the bond left behind.

It might happen to me on occasion, but it's still weird to see it like this. It's kind of hot though, especially the way it immediately fixates on me and rakes over every inch of my bare skin like a branding possession.

I like that a whole lot.

It takes a step forward, and I hold up a palm to stop it, surprised when that's all it takes to slow it down. Fuck, if only *my* bond were that obedient.

"One second! I need to ask you something, really quickly. I promise."

I sound like an idiot, but it doesn't notice, or care, and it just continues to stare at me like I'm so freaking fascinating.

"The creatures, they come from you, don't they?"

He nods and lifts a palm up as though he's about to summon them, and while I'd love nothing more than to check in with my baby August again, I know North will have a freaking aneurysm over it, so I reach out and cover his palm with mine.

The bond stills and takes in a breath before pulling my hand up to his nose and taking another big ol' whiff of my newly scrubbed skin. I wonder if it sees the soap and shampoo as its scent the way North does, or if he's about to throw a bond tantrum over how foreign I smell.

So I keep talking, hoping to distract him. "Are they going to hurt me? North is worried they will. He's worried about losing control of them around me, and I need to know if that's actually possible. If it's not, I want to keep August... ahh, the puppy. The Doberman-looking one. You know which one, right? Of course you do."

He takes in another lungful of my scent, and I start to think maybe he's getting high from it or something because he's not really keen on letting me go, but then he speaks.

His voice is sort of terrifying.

It sounds otherworldly. There's no other way to describe it. It sounds as though I'm speaking to something that does not belong here. Not in this room with me or on this planet, in this timeline, none of it. He doesn't belong here at all, and yet the pull in my chest that aches for him says he's *supposed* to be with me. No matter where that is.

"*Mine*. You're mine. No one will hurt you again. Not me, not the others, not anyone. The shadows cannot harm you, they belong to you, as I do. We all do."

My heart starts thumping wildly in my chest.

I look into those beautiful voids, as dark and beautiful as a starless sky, and murmur, "Can he hear me? Is he listening to us? I can hear it sometimes. Not always."

North's bond tilts his head like it's considering. "What secrets do you want just between us?"

I smile, because the bond talks just like mine does and it makes it easier to speak to it. "None. I just think he'll be upset at me for asking why he's so worried about you being around me. If you're this ready to protect me then… Why is he scared?"

The bond leans down until his nose bumps against mine softly, like it's afraid even now of hurting me. "The lie. He believes the lie because the truth is too painful. Even now that it's started to unravel around him, he can't let it go."

The lie?

Whether he sees my confusion or just chooses to keep going, I don't know, but the words keep coming out of him nonetheless. "Bonds cannot hurt each other. They cannot kill each other, not with intent or by accident. But if he believes the truth, then everything he has held on to for all of this time will be meaningless."

My eyebrows bunch together, but then the bond pushes forward again, sealing our lips together, and I'm kissing North for the first time. Only he's not the one kissing me. His bond is pushing me backward on the countertop and his tongue is sweeping into my mouth, taking over me and branding my very soul with his mark.

I panic a little, only because of what North will think of this, but he breaks away from me without pushing for more.

His palm takes hold of my chin, and he speaks to me one last time. "No more running."

The moment the bond slips away from North, he's

grabbing me, pulling me up and into his arms desperately, and hauling ass into his bedroom as though he can leave his bond and everything said between us behind. For a second, I think he's going to throw me out of the room for talking to his bond and accidentally uncovering a family secret.

One I'm still wrapping my head around.

But when he spreads me out on his bed, his body immediately covers my own, and this time when his lips touch mine, I know that it's all him in there and not his bond taking over.

They kiss differently.

Is that a weird thing to notice? Probably. Where the bond was a dark possession, North is a consuming force. He wants me, there's no doubting it, but he wants everything. I can barely stop myself from getting swept up in him, losing myself when we've barely even started.

"What did it say to you? What did it do?"

I blink up at him, and then a slow smile stretches over my cheeks. "It's devoted to me. It's not going to hurt me. North? I believe it. I know that neither of you will hurt me."

He stares at me, his eyes locked onto mine, and there's

a need inside of him that I can see so clearly, a need for me to trust him and believe exactly what he's capable of.

I already know it.

He moves slowly to pull the towel away from my body, as though he's still giving me time to change my mind and put a stop to this. I'm not going to, even with the impending freak out over my power growing, I know that this is exactly what I need right now.

I can worry about the consequences later.

When he kisses me again, shoving the towel off of the bed as though he's worried about it jumping back onto my body and covering me up once again, I forget about everything except his lips on mine. I forget about the Bonding and the beings who live inside us, even now straining towards each other. I forget that we're anything more than humans who want each other.

Then North's gift joins the party and shatters any chances of pretending that we're anything but Gifted Bonds.

The lights are on in the bedroom and bright through the open doorway to the bathroom, but the moment his gift bursts out of him, there's nothing but darkness around us both. I expect to be surrounded by his creatures, to find

August staring at me and waiting for pets, but instead there's only darkness.

A surprise but not a bad one. I can totally handle Bonding in his shadows.

His eyes stay blue, his level of control even in this situation is completely insane to me, but it's as though this is the small part of his bond he's willing to share me with right now, and I can get on board.

The tug on my ankle takes me by surprise.

I glance at North's hands first just to check that he's not messing with me, but then I feel the thing slide up my calf to circle my thigh and spread my legs out even further.

Before I have to chance to freak the fuck out, more of the shadows come out to grab me, one over each limb and splaying me out for North's viewing pleasure. He watches it all with rapt attention, an air of smug male surrounding him.

This is all at his command.

The shadow limbs might as well be restraints for how firmly they hold me down. Living ropes that move at North's every whim. I should have guessed he'd be full of these sorts of surprises in the bedroom.

When he moves to lick and suck his way across my chest, one of his hands slipping down between my thighs, I want to move my arms to bury my hands in his hair but the tendrils of smoke tighten around my wrists, pulling until my back arches off of the bed. North's lips close over my nipple as his teeth nip at the sensitive nub.

I'm in sensation overload.

How the hell he thought I could handle this without ever reaching my peak and Bonding with him is baffling, because his fingers barely graze over my clit and my entire soul begins to shake.

Then he moves his freaking hand.

"Not yet. We're coming together too, Bond. Be patient."

The sullen child inside of me, the one I've been so careful about hiding from him, wants to kick him and cuss him out.

"I've been patient. How you ever thought I could survive edging is stupid. Fuck me or make me come some other way. I don't care, just do it."

He huffs out a breath at me, and then he *ignores my demands*. Ignores them. Just goes back to his very slow and methodical exploration of my body until every inch is cataloged inside that impossible brain of his.

I might resort to murder, no matter what his bond just told me otherwise.

The worst part is that I can feel his cock, hard and hot against my thigh, a tease of what's to come, and yet he's still perfectly happy to be taking his time.

I attempt to tug my wrists free, but the shadows only tighten their hold, sliding down to wrap around my forearms as well so I lose even more of my mobility as a punishment for trying to rush him.

I might die if he doesn't hurry up.

Finally, with one last swipe of his rough tongue over my nipple, he pushes up and away from my body to sit on his heels between my legs. I try not to think about how obscene his view is, how my pussy is spread wide open for his eyes, thanks to the shadows. As if spurred on by my thoughts, another tendril appears out of the darkness and moves to slide through my slick pussy lips. I tense a little, half terrified and half hoping that it will push inside of me. The adrenaline rush it gives me is like a shot of heroine straight to the brain, my entire body shaking with pent-up desire.

I can feel my juices gush out onto the bed between us.

His nostrils flare as he fists himself, stroking his cock leisurely as he watches his shadow play with me. I feel my clit begin to pulse every time the shadow brushes against it in a cruel tease, just a whisper of friction, but nowhere near enough to give me what I want.

I whimper, a pathetic sound from deep in the back of my throat, and finally he shifts forward, adding his cock into the torturous teasing. There's a thin line of black over his irises that I know is his bond, watching over me while its host slowly drags his cock over my clit, teasing me with the hot flesh I desperately crave. I find that I also might not be above begging.

What a glorious thing to share.

"If you don't fuck me soon, my bond is going to come out. It's already right on the edge."

He smirks and pumps his hips, still teasing my most sensitive parts. "I think our bonds want to meet, but I'm not letting them have this before we do. You deserve to fuck each of your Bonds yourself before your bond takes her turn."

I reach down and take a hold of his cock, thick and hot in my palm, giving it a squeeze before pushing my hips up. His shadows wrap around my wrists but he doesn't pull me away, just a reminder that I'm touching him because he's allowing it. Goosebumps break out over my body at the thought of him shifting them again, pulling me apart and spreading me out on this bed and starting his torture all over again.

I like this side of his control issues.

"Stop telling me what I deserve and give it to me instead. I'm just about ready to cuss you out and find someone else to make me come."

His eyebrow rises at the taunt, but when I grin at him, enjoying the hell out of this, the shadow over my wrist finally tugs my hand away from him. Before I have a chance to pout about it, his hips finally pull back fully and then he's slamming into me; no gentle easing into it.

I never really wanted gentle.

I want desperate and raw. I want to know that they've been craving me just as badly as I've needed them. I want to know that the great councilman North Draven has been dreaming of what my pussy would feel like and that having it now is everything he's ever wanted.

I want to be the center of his fucking world, the only thing that matters to him.

He feels bigger inside of me, the girth of him

stretching me almost to the point of pain but riding the line instead until I'm sure I'm about to feel him between my legs for days. That feels right to me. It feels as though that's exactly how things should be between us.

If only I could make him feel the same way.

The long tendrils of smoke around my body move me until I have my thighs wrapped around North, his arms braced over me and my arms splayed out wide. His eyes can't stop moving between the pleasure on my face, my lips bitten raw and my hooded eyes, and the enticing way that my tits move with every one of his thrusts.

One of the shadows slips over my clit as it moves my hips, adjusting me so that North's strokes can go even deeper until I feel as though he's about to come out of my throat. How the fuck did I survive without this? How did I go so long sleeping with this man wrapped around me and not inside of me?

How could I have ever been scared of this?

His strokes are even and deep, his hips are sure in their movement, and with every minute, I can feel my body climbing higher and higher. I can't even attempt to bite back the whimpers of pleasure, the sounds of the almost-pain I'm in with overstimulation.

I need more.

I pull my wrist against the shadow, sharp enough that North's eyebrows drop down as he frees my hand. Before he has the chance to do something insane, like stop, I grab the back of his neck to drag his lips down to mine, tilting my hips more to meet his thrusts as I hitch my legs higher on his waist.

He groans into my mouth, his eyes squeezing shut as his movements get more frenzied and rough. I dig my nails into his nape, and the tendrils of smoke tighten around my thighs until I'm sure I'll be waking up bruised with his marks.

When his hips slam into me one last time, locking us together as we both finally break apart, the *relief* and euphoria flood me. His eyes shift, but the ecstasy stays on his face as he stays in control.

My own bond reaches out to touch his, but not the same rough claiming it had done with Gryphon. It feels more like two halves of a soul coming together again.

Like my bond has known about him forever and been waiting to feel whole again. Like the shadows have gone feral waiting for me and now that we're together again, maybe the storm in North's heart will calm.

I hope he can finally have some peace.

He leans down to press our foreheads together, and then his voice sounds in my head. *I have been waiting for you forever, little Bonded.*

My pussy tightens around him because there's nothing so arousing as a sex-drenched confession straight into your very consciousness.

I waited for you too. I waited for all of you.

I know there's a good chance that Gryphon is listening to us both right now as well. I haven't figured out how to shield my inner thoughts from him yet without blocking him out entirely, and I think he'd have an aneurysm if I pulled that on him again right now, but he's good about leaving this moment alone.

There's no stampede of Bonds arriving outside the door either, no one trying to interrupt this moment, which makes me think that maybe they were all expecting for this to happen. Whether through placating my bond or if North's revelation about what my motives were made it obvious that he was going to do whatever he had to to tie himself to me once I returned home.

Now I just have to deal with whatever power surge I end up with and try not to fry any poor, unsuspecting people who don't deserve it.

North turns to lie down on the sheets next to me, not caring at all that they're a bit gross now. "You won't. Stop thinking about it. If there's anything that I'm sure about, Oleander, it's that you're not going to hurt anyone. You're not a monster."

I'm not sure I agree with him. It's a testament to how much has shifted between us that I answer him without second-guessing myself. "I can barely control the power I have now. If it gets stronger... I don't think I can handle anything else."

He brushes a hand over my forehead, moving the silver strands away from my face. "We'll see what happens when you wake up again and face whatever it is together. You're not leaving here for the time being anyway, not until we're sure it's safe again. We can keep your contact with people outside of our Bond to a minimum. We can do this, Oleander."

He sounds so sure of that, so sure of me, and I want to believe him. I want to, but I'm not sure how yet. Baby steps, I guess.

What will the others think about us Bonding? Especially if I say that I'm still not comfortable Bonding with anyone else… at least not right now.

Once again, I find myself in a mess of my own making.

I should just pass the hell out and lose the next three days like I know I'm going to, but I feel wired after the Bonding. I roll onto my side to face him and grin when his eyes track my every movement even in the dark safety of his room. "I feel like I need another shower after that."

He stretches one hand up behind his head, his chest flexing deliciously like a private seduction. "Anything you want, Bonded. You should enjoy having me at your disposal while it lasts."

I don't want to think about the real world, all of the death and horror that we're going to have to deal with when we leave here, so I keep it light. "You really want to lug me around all over again? Because my legs are out of action and not because of the healing."

He smirks at me and scoops me up without another word.

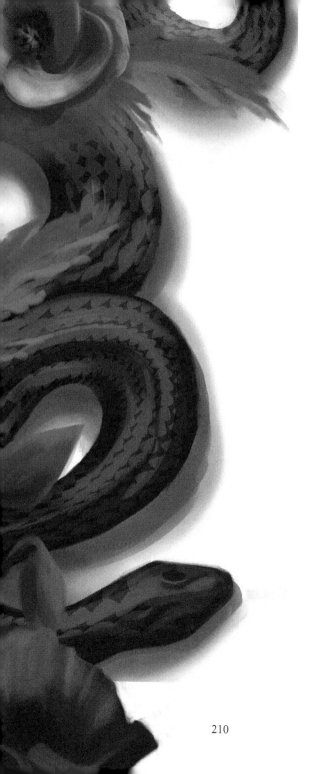

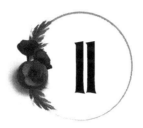

ATLAS

Staring at the same four walls for days on end is enough to drive me insane, especially in a room as barren and poorly designed as the sedate spare room the Dravens shoved me in when I arrived here. There's too much blue, terrible fucking shades of it, and the bed is uncomfortable as shit. If I manage to fix things with Oli, I'll be buying a new mattress.

I don't want to think about what I'll be doing if I can't fix it.

There's nothing to do in here except stare at walls, do homework for classes I'm repeating anyway, or jerking off at the thought of the perfect Bond I've managed to alienate, even though I tried everything to avoid it.

It might be wrong, but I go with jerking off.

There's two ways we could look at this; either I'm a creep for doing it while thinking about a girl who probably thinks I betrayed her in the worst fucking way, or I'm a devoted Bond who couldn't even get it up for anyone else at this point. Both of those things are true. I'm done trying to make sense of this.

I feel her the moment she pops into my head.

How can you feel an out-of-body experience when it's not happening to you? Fuck knows, but one minute I'm lying there with my dick in my hand by myself, and the next I can sense Oli's shock and confusion about where the hell she is and what she's seeing. It's as though I've summoned her here with the sheer force of my longing for her.

The spike of lust that comes from her is a great ego boost, not that I needed any help.

How the hell did I end up here?

I grin, hoping she can feel that I'm doing it even if she can't see it. *I'd guess you got a little power bump, Sweetness. But however it happened, I'm glad you're here.*

There's a throb of longing there in my chest, a sign she's been missing me just as bad as I've missed her, and it makes me angry.

If you need me, I'll break down this door to come find you. I've been toeing the line because I didn't want to start an argument and put you in the middle of it but, baby, if you need me, I'm coming to find you.

She glows inside my chest, preening about my need to be with her, and sends back, *It's okay. I've mostly been sleeping. I'll come find you when I'm awake properly again… if I can get back out of your head, that is.*

The grin turns into a smirk. *Well, while you're here, I guess I better finish what I started, Sweetness.*

She sends through a feeling of fake outrage that has me roaring with laughter like a crazy man, but then she moves my hand, stroking my dick for me, and the mechanics of it don't mean a fucking thing. I don't care that it's my hand, I nearly blow my load knowing she's a part of this.

Don't you dare make me come so fast and shame me, Sweetness.

Her answering giggle is fucking perfection, and I

want to lock the memory of it down forever.

I don't like to be kept waiting, Bond. If you want to show me how good you can be, then get a move on.

Who thought having a wank could be this erotic, but the emotions and little threads of lust she sends to me only stoke the fire as my fist slides up and down my cock. I can feel her testing me, checking what I'm doing and how I'm moving, like she's taking notes for later. Fuck, I hope she is. I need her to come find me and take over because this might be the best fucking experience of my life, but having the real deal here?

I'd take that over this a million times over.

I hold out for long enough that she's not going to have doubts about my stamina and not a second longer, her presence watching as I spill out all over my fist, grunting and trying to hold back a roar that would have Gabe banging on the wall.

It's the best fucking orgasm of my life, a small taste of what I'll have if I ever get to have my Bond.

The moment the lust clears, I can feel her hesitance and awkwardness creep in. She's here, in the possible traitor's head, while no one else in the house knows it.

I leap to reassure her.

You can see everything here. Whatever you need to believe me, take it.

She hesitates and my heart breaks a little. I don't blame her. I don't blame her for a fucking thing, but I'm so fucking desperate for her to believe me that the chance that she doesn't want to look into my memories breaks me.

I try again, trying to keep the desperation out of my tone. *There is nothing in my life that I want to keep from you. There's a lot of ugly, a lot of bad shit, and shit I'm ashamed of. But I would never hide it from you, not even if I thought you might think less of me. I'd rather you hate those parts of me and never doubt what I'm saying, than for us to live with this thing between us. Not having you and your trust isn't an option for me, Bond. It's not an option.*

She grows even more quiet in my chest, and I leave her alone. I can't push her, no matter how much I want to, because if she doesn't come to the decision herself, then what's the fucking point of it?

I grab a towel off of the ground next to the bed and wipe myself down. I get up and walk into the bathroom, avoiding the mirrors because I don't really feel like staring into my father's face right now. He's the entire fucking reason I'm in this mess, and the fact that I could be his slightly-younger-looking twin grates on me.

Oli stays quiet through the entire shower, her mind just sitting with me while I get myself clean. After I'm dried and back in a pair of clean boxers, I put a movie on, something mindless that I've seen a thousand times, and climb back into bed.

Once I'm settled, it's clear that Oli has something she wants to say, but she stays quiet throughout the movie. I don't want to fall asleep and miss out on her being here, but there's something so comforting about her presence that the fatigue of countless shitty sleepless nights slowly creeps up on me.

Right before I pass out, she finally speaks.

I don't want to look. I want you to tell me yourself. I want to hear it from you.

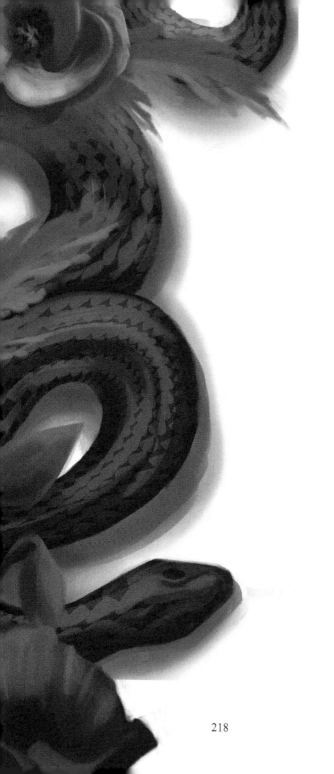

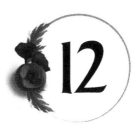

OLI

The bed is too toasty warm to want to wake up, but I instantly know that I've made it back into my own body once again. I don't want to open my eyes or exist today, every bone in my body aches, but there's an oddly temperature-less weight against my back. It takes me a second to realize that Brutus is back in the bed with me.

Which means that North is both awake and no longer in here with me because last night he'd been very firm on the 'no puppies in the bed' rule, no matter how hard I'd pushed it.

My senses are dulled thanks to how deep I was

sleeping, but I know that some of my Bonds are here with me. I can't tell which ones, which is frustrating, but I'll take what I can get.

There's a rustling sound next to me and then Gryphon murmurs into my ear, "Stop frowning, Bonded. It makes me want to murder something for you."

I squint one eye open in his direction. "What time is it, and do you have food?"

He smirks, his eyes shining at me like I'm being so damn amusing. I hear more movement on the other side of the room, and then North starts ordering food from the kitchens. My stomach rumbles at the list of things he asks for.

I want those goddamn scrambled eggs and waffles, extra bacon, and some hash browns, fuck yes. And coffee, a whole jug of it, with extra whip and sugar.

I move to get up and then realize I went to sleep naked after North had fucked me in his shower. I squint around the room, and while I could totally handle being naked in front of both of my Bonded at the same time, Gabe is sitting in one of the ornate chairs with his phone in his hands, and Nox is arguing with North over building schematics at a desk that has suddenly appeared while I was out cold.

I clutch at the duvet like some scandalized maiden, only to realize that I'm once again wearing silky pinstripe pajamas. North Draven is a sneaky asshole who takes the weirdest liberties while I'm passed out.

Gryphon starts cackling like an asshole and I shove my pillow in his face as I stomp off to the bathroom to pee. No one fusses over me walking, but they all watch me carefully, even Nox, though he's got his usual, distasteful look on his face.

When I wash up, I take a good look at myself in the mirror, checking my color and the general look of my skin and hair. The silver is even lighter. I swear the color drain there is getting worse. I do a very gentle check-in with my bond, just to see how we're tracking along there, and though it has a lot of feelings about missing Gabe and *Nox*, dammit, it doesn't seem to be getting any new weird tricks or power surges.

Small mercies for now.

I rummage through the drawers until I find one full of very girl-specific shit. I'm very proud of myself when I stay calm, sending him a quick, *Whose stuff is this?*

His answer is instant and amused, *Yours. If you want*

something that isn't there, just tell me.

I will not swoon over such basic kindness, dammit. *This is enough. Thank you.*

I brush out my hair so I no longer look as though North and his shadow tentacles fucked the life out of me and then I throw it into a high ponytail. I feel breathless already from such a small amount of movement, and when I head back into North's room, I beeline for the bed. Gryphon helps me in, tucking the blankets around me and shooing the shadow puppy away from me until I'm settled in. I'm a little surprised he lets him but the moment he steps back, Brutus covers me again.

Gryphon hands me a glass of water and snaps, "I will get him sent home right the fuck now if he's too heavy. Davenport will be up later to look at your leg and finish off the healing; let's not injure it all over again because you're spoiling the creature."

I shrug at him and eye Gabe from across the room. He's wearing a sweater that I want to steal, and when he glances up at me and notices me staring, he grins back at me.

Gryphon waves a hand in front of my face as the knock at the door interrupts us all and I snap, "He's made out of shadows and smoke, which weighs *nothing*. Brutus is just fussing with me like you are. Leave him alone."

He scowls at me as North opens the door, and then his attention is pulled to that situation.

The food smells incredible, but I feel bad for the kitchen staff bringing it in. Every last one of my Bonds that are here turn to watch her every move. When she's got it set out on the table for North, she turns to the door, only to be stopped by Gryphon.

I open my mouth, ready to defend the poor woman, when he says, "Has anyone but you and the chef touched any of this food?"

She answers straight away, "No, sir."

"Did you do anything to this food, add anything, or slip anything into it?"

"No, sir. No one has touched or tampered with any of it."

Jesus freaking Christ. Is this where we're at now? Questioning everything, even in the damn manor?

As the door swings shut behind the woman, Gryphon answers my very private thoughts, "Yes, that's exactly where we are now. No one in or out without speaking to me first. No one but your Bonds and select friends are allowed in a room alone with you. No one but the chef is touching your food."

I have no words, none except, "Get out of my head."

"Stop thinking so loudly."

I snap back, "Well, if I knew how I was doing it, I would stop. Buy some earplugs or something!"

I don't bother trying to get up or picking out what I want. North gets there first and picks everything out for me. He still glares at everything like he's not so sure that Gryphon's questioning did enough. It's crazy, but my heart does a super weird thumping motion over it anyway.

I pull myself up to sit propped up against the pillows and when he hands me the plate, he moves to pour out coffee. There's two cups, so one must be for me, right? He wouldn't withhold it from me after that huge glass of water I just gulped down.

Thank the fucking stars, North hands me a coffee and then heads back over to where Nox is still scowling at the papers. They start the same argument as before about security holes and how to ensure occupancy survival. It doesn't make a whole lot of sense to me, because it sounds as though they're arguing over a bomb shelter and that doesn't seem like the right sort of priority for us all right now.

Gryphon pulls a chair up to sit next to me with a plate of his own, and I get back to the more important questions. "Why are we staying here if we're so sure there's about to be another attack? Can we... evacuate? Jesus, what would that even look like?"

North nods and shares a look with Nox. "It's something we're looking into. We can't just leave the lower families behind to be picked off though, and there is a lot that would go into relocating this many Gifted at once, but it has been done before. We can do it again if things continue to get worse."

It's been done before? I didn't know that, but there's a lot about this community that I don't know about, so I just nod and nibble at my toast some more, avoiding Gryphon's grumpy looks because he's clearly in a *mood* today. One that has absolutely nothing to do with me because I've been asleep for... wait.

"How long did I sleep this time?"

North answers without looking up from the paperwork, "Fourteen hours. We weren't expecting you to wake up. You seem to be getting better at handling the power usage."

Huh.

I'll be happy if I don't need to use my gift again any time soon, but I guess it's good to know the three-day naps might be phasing out. The moment that his plate is clean, Gryphon takes my plate to refill it with more fruit and then leans down to kiss me soundly on the lips.

I'll be in the gym training with some Tac guys. Call me if you need me.

I don't know why he's talking just to me, but I nod and let him give me one last peck before he's out the door without another word. Whatever the hell is going on with him, I hope he beats it out of one of the guys downstairs.

I pick through the fruit and then put the empty plate on the bedside table, settling back down against the pillows to enjoy the last of my coffee with my Bonds around me. Gabe finishes off his plate and then collects mine, putting them back on the food tray and pushing the whole lot back out the door for someone to pick up.

North checks his phone and then walks over to me, kissing me soundly on the lips right here in front of everyone. I mean, Gryphon did too, but it still feels infinitely fucking weird for North to be doing it.

"We'll be downstairs. Just stay here, or in your room.

If you want something, call me. Don't go wandering."

I quirk an eyebrow at him but he gives me a very don't-fuck-with-me look, and I roll my eyes at him. "Fine. But you can't keep me trapped up here forever. Once I'm back to full health, I'll get bored and become a nightmare."

Nox scoffs as he heads for the door. "You're already there, Poison."

North's eyes narrow at his back, and I grab his chin to tilt his head back toward me. "Stay out of it. I can fight my own wars with him."

He gives me a look that says he definitely won't be doing that, then straightens up to follow Nox downstairs. I'm sure they're about to have a lovely trip down in the elevator, but I ignore it.

I have Gabe to myself.

He smirks at me and drawls, "Thank God, I thought we were going to be stuck in a full-blown Draven war for a second. I'd rather go to the gym and have Gryph kill me there instead."

I giggle at him. "Come here and lie with me. If I'm going to be trapped here, I should at least get a cuddle out of it."

Gabe stares at me for a second and then climbs up onto the bed carefully, moving as though he's expecting me to fall apart underneath him or something, and when I scowl and tug him down on top of me, he grumbles back at me. With my legs bracketing either side of his body and his head cradled on my belly, he's barely even on me. The small amount of weight that is there is comforting rather than… smothering.

I take a long, deep breath and feel whole again.

"No more running off," Gabe says, his tone almost sulky, and I thread my fingers through his hair.

"I didn't want to. I knew where Kyrie was going, and I couldn't leave her to that. I survived. I'm fine, and Keiran will heal. I feel guilty about dragging him along, but we're all going to be fine, because I went there too."

Gabe huffs and his hand spans over the side of my thigh, gently brushing it through the duvet like he's imagining all of the damage that has been wiped away thanks to Felix's care. There's still a small ache there, but it's nothing compared to the blinding pain I'd succumbed to, letting my bond take over and wreak its blood-soaked vengeance on the camps.

Gabe's fingers are gentle as he strokes over the duvet.

"Black is going to wish he'd never woken up that morning by the time Gryphon and North are done with him. They both have some very *creative* plans of punishment for him."

Jesus freaking Christ.

Gabe falls asleep on me and we spend most of the afternoon napping with Brutus between us, after he'd slowly inched Gabe away from me and taken his place. I doze off and on, watching the shadows cross the room as we waste away the day. Sometime in the late afternoon, I fall into a much deeper sleep, only to wake and find Gabe missing.

North is sitting at the desk, reading more of his endless paperwork with a glass of whiskey in front of him.

"There's a sandwich on the nightstand. If you want something more substantial, I'll call the chef for you."

I stretch out and struggle to sit up, pushing up until I'm once again drowning in the pillows. I've never met a man who enjoyed sleeping with a hundred pillows like a princess, but then there's no one quite like North out there.

"The sandwich is good. I feel horrible, the napping is only making it worse."

He glances up to frown at me. "Do you need Felix now? He checked in on you earlier but when he saw you were sleeping, he left you to it. He said sleep is more important right now."

I shake my head and grab the plate. "No, I just feel like I'm lazing around here, doing nothing, while everyone else is busy... doing things to keep us safe. I'm a liability and I hate that."

He huffs at me, draining the last of the whiskey in the glass and moving more papers around. "Do you know how many survivors we recover on average from the camps?"

I shake my head, taking another bite of the sandwich. It's cheese and ham, with the perfect amount of mayonnaise, and I want to marry the chef for it.

North ignores the sandwich-gasm I'm having and continues, "If we can get to the camps in the first twenty-four hours, it's twenty-two percent. After forty-eight hours, that drops to fifteen. After four days, as in the case of what happened when you went after them?

Three percent. Do you know how many survivors you brought home? Because it was all on you, we just came and picked you all up."

The door opens and Gryphon steps through, not bothering to knock. He's in his training gear, the full coverage stuff he wears around his team and not the teeny tiny shorts he saves for me. He doesn't blink at North's monologue, just comes over to get a look at me and take a seat back at my side.

"Thirty-three people were taken. Thirty-three came home. Only one was injured, and the reports said that thanks to Nox's creature protecting Kyrie and shutting down the showers, only one woman was assaulted in that time. That has *never* happened before, Oleander. You're the farthest thing from a liability."

Gryphon turns to give me a look, and I shove the last of the sandwich into my mouth to avoid speaking to him about it. There's a lot I need to say to him and fighting my position on being useless to them all right now isn't it.

He turns to share a look with North that spells trouble for me.

It finally occurs to me that I don't know how to do relationships. I barely know how to function as a Central

Bond, and having both of my Bonded, very alpha men here together is literally overwhelming for my poor brain. It was fine this morning with Nox and Gabe here too because they felt a little bit like a buffer, stopping any of this stuff from happening.

Now I'm at their mercy, and I already know they're both more than happy ganging up on me.

But I have to at least try, because if I shut my eyes and think about it hard enough, I can still hear the cracking sound of Kieran snapping his own ankle to save my life and the lives of my Bonds.

So once I swallow, I clear my throat and plead for Black's life. "Please... don't take everything that happened out on Kieran. I was the idiot who thought we'd get in and out without Franklin being there. I should've known better."

Gryphon's eyes narrow at me in a way that I'm so not used to being pointed in my direction. I gulp a little, mostly because he looks like he's about to give me the same punishment as his second is going to get. I was kind of hoping the leg injury would get me out of the pre-dawn training for at least a week. Two would be better. I guess his terrible mood is still around, which is just great news.

I don't look in North's direction.

I'd wager he's less reasonable about this shit than Gryphon is, so the longer I can keep him out of this, the better.

Gryphon snaps, "Wrong. North has only ever been unreasonable about you. Now that you're Bonded, he's probably going to go back to being the good councilman again."

My cheeks heat but my temper also flares and gets my mouth running. "Get out of my head! I will start avoiding you if you can't stay out of it."

He leans forward in his chair and says in a low and dangerous tone, "Try it. I'm about to chip you all over again just to make sure you don't fucking disappear on me."

I make a very embarrassing squeaking noise of outrage and snap back at him, "I went after your sister. I didn't run away. I went after someone you love, because I couldn't bear the thought of you losing her. Don't stand there and act like I'm a liability when I was doing it for you. I don't care about that man or what he did—"

He snarls to interrupt me, "You can't even say his name! I can see it now. I can see the trauma spots in your mind—"

"Then get. The. Fuck. Out. Of. My. Head. I don't want you in there. I deserve some goddamn privacy!"

He smirks but before he can open his mouth and ruin me even more, a solid body slides between the bed and the seat, in the tiny amount of space there, and North snaps, "She's still healing. Walk it off before you say something you regret. Get out of here. *Go*."

Gryphon leaves without another word, shutting the door a little harder than required, and I roll my eyes at the sound. North doesn't move. He just stands there with his back to me and legs pressed against the bed like he's expecting Gryphon to stomp back in for round two.

It makes me feel like an absolute asshole. "I'm sorry I thought you'd be unreasonable."

He makes a dismissive noise. "I deserve it. I told your bond I'd regain your trust, and now I'm saying it to you too. I'm under no illusions that Bonding with you was a magic cure, it'll take some time for me to prove myself to you. Gryphon is… he's feeling guilty. It's making him lash out, and he's going to be sore about it later. I was trying to stop him from really digging himself into his own grave."

I frown and lean back on the bed, exhaustion still creeping up inside my body even though I've barely been awake. Maybe I'm not past the sleeping forever phase like we were hoping. "What does he have to be guilty about? Jesus, he's got a savior complex, doesn't he? Typical."

North carefully rolls his sleeves back up his arms and then starts to loosen the top few buttons, revealing the tanned and smooth skin there. He's a fucking tease, and thank God Gryphon is no longer here to read all of the dirty thoughts running through my head, because I'm ready to spread out on the bed for him all over again.

"He's feeling guilty because it was the first time he had to think about the choice between his family and his Bonded. If he had to choose between saving the two of you… He's never had to think about it before and, like most men in his position, he always assumed he'd be able to stop there ever being a choice. You running after Kyrie made him aware that he'd rather you be safe here. That wasn't such a terrible thing until she told him about Brutus saving her in the showers. If you weren't there, she would have been assaulted."

That cuts into my dirty thoughts a bit. "Well, that's just stupid. Why worry about 'what-ifs' and made-up scenarios when there's only one situation that did happen? We're fine. Kyrie is safe and I just… I need a little more rest, but I'm fine."

He flicks a hand at my leg with a raised eyebrow. "You were hurt badly. You were much closer to death than any of us ever wanted to think about."

I roll my eyes. Men. *Bonds*. Bonded men with their heads up their asses. The list goes on. Honestly, my life will never be carefree again, and that has nothing to do with the Resistance chasing me and everything to do with five hot-blooded men that are fated to be tied to me for all of our lives.

North walks around the bed to shove the paperwork into a file and switch off the lamp over on that side of the room. "Do you need anything else? Hungry, thirsty? If you want another shower, I could be persuaded."

I can't cope with caring and attentive North Draven. Domineering and commanding North, sure. Asshole North? Not my favorite, but I've got him sorted.

This one?

Nope.

I could definitely go for another shower with him, and round three of playtime with his shadows, but the haze in my head still hasn't lifted. "I think I need more rest, but I'm bored of lying around. Why don't you have a TV in here so I can distract myself with something stupid on there?"

He looks over at me where I'm splayed out on the bed dramatically and then comes back over over to press a button underneath the lip of the marble-top, very luxurious looking bedside table.

The end of the bed *opens* and a TV slowly rises up out of freaking nowhere.

"You have too much money. Seriously, that is ridiculous! Why not just have it on the wall like the rest of the bedrooms?"

He shrugs and goes about meticulously stripping out of his suit, firmly distracting me from my outrage. "It would ruin the room. Besides, it's fun to watch you freak out about simple things."

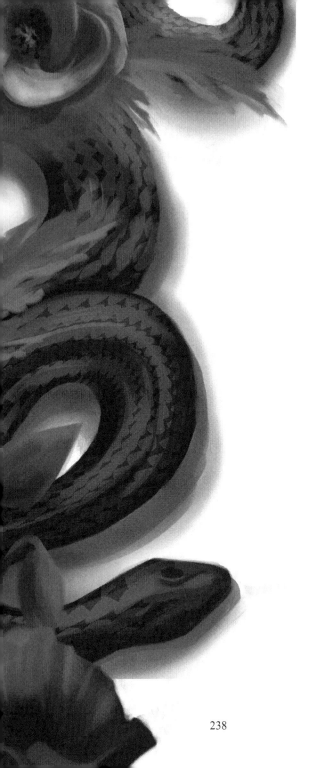

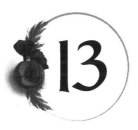

OLI

I fall asleep watching the world's most boring documentary because North refuses to watch trashy reality TV with me. I only suggested it in the first place to test just how far I could push his kindness. His retaliation of an old man droning on about deforestation was brutal.

I wake hours later in total darkness, and at first I think that I've jumped into another of my Bond's minds without intending to. It takes me a minute to realize that I'm not dreaming, that there's a warm body lying against my back with hands wandering over my body and a hard dick rubbing against my ass.

Is it strange that I can already tell which one of my Bonded it is? Because it's definitely Gryphon. The way he moves is like night and day to North. My brain takes a little longer to process what's happening and so instead of pointing out to him that this is someone else's bed and he for sure cannot be teasing me like that, I arch back against him, enjoying the grunt he lets out as my ass grinds down on his dick.

Then his fingers slip into the front of the silky pajama shorts North had dressed me in and plunge straight into my pussy, barely checking to see if I was actually wet or not.

I am dripping, just for the record.

My bond seems to think that merely being around my Bonded is enough of an aphrodisiac. I'm finding myself permanently ready for either one of them, which feels like it's going to be a problem for me. I can't spend my whole life panting after these men.

I need some autonomy again, dammit.

"Don't think about it," he murmurs, and before I can snap at him and point out how freaking impossible that is, he kisses me again until my bond floods my head with a chant of *yes, yes, yes* like the needy bitch it is. If he wants to get me off in front of North as some sort of apology, I guess that's fine. It's not like they haven't both seen me come, or heard the sounds I make. It's dark enough that neither of them should be able to see the mess I am.

I let him say everything he needs to say to me in the way that he worships my body.

It's probably not a good thing, and something I should not let slide in the future because it's me coming up against five strong-minded, alpha men. They'll walk all over me if I let them, but for tonight, I'm still recovering from the power surge, and I just want to feel something.

I just want to feel how much my Bonded needs me.

So I let him kiss me until I forget where we are and who else is here. I forget my own damn name, and I let our bonds come up to the surface to be with each other again.

It strikes me somewhere in the back of my mind that I'll have to think about later, that this feels different than when my bond was with North's.

But the moment I think about anything that might draw me out of this moment, Gryphon changes things up, the pace or the position or how far down my body his hands are working. When he turns me over to start kissing down my back, I'm forced back into the present and the fact that there is, in fact, a third person in this bed.

I should *not* enjoy the feel of North's eyes on my body this much, watching everything that Gryphon is doing, but when our eyes collide, a whimper tumbles out of my lips at the flare of heat I find there. He's enjoying the show we're putting on for him, not an ounce of jealousy in him, but a need that's building up instead. A need to have me under him as well.

Gryphon moves us both, just enough that he can look at the expression on my face, and his eyes twinkle as he grins. "You wanna be watched? You want him seeing you come all over my cock, gushing down my legs and screaming my name, baby? I thought I was pushing your boundaries here, but you need it... Don't you, Bonded?"

My eyes roll up into the back of my head and his lips wrap around my earlobe, his teeth sharp as they tug on it, and if this is how I die, then I will gladly go.

"Don't be so dramatic, Bonded. Like we'd ever let you leave us again. You'll have one of us with you at all times from now on."

Fuck.

I really need to figure out how the hell to keep him

out of my head, but as his fingers slip into the front of my silky sleep shorts again, it doesn't seem like much of a priority anymore.

The darkness in the room intensifies, deepens, and becomes a living thing, and I tip my head back to watch the changes in North as his bond fills the room. I'm addicted to it already, addicted to the way that his lust and need visibly clouding the room makes me feel.

Gryphon uses my distraction to switch positions again, pushing the silky shorts down and hovering over me as he peels them off of my legs. He leans down to bite at the soft skin of my belly where my shirt has ridden up until I squirm underneath the weight of him.

I want more. I'm in luck, because so do they.

Neither of them stop to think about condoms or birth control, something I really freaking need to figure out for myself or we'll have a whole new problem to deal with, and when Gryphon hitches my legs up a little higher to get me right where he wants me, I smile up at him. This is my favorite part, the stretch and pressure of his big cock filling me up. It feels like fucking heaven.

We both groan as he pushes in.

One of the black tendrils catches my thigh and tugs

my legs open wide so that North can see better, see every thrust of Gryphon into my dripping pussy, and his eyes shift to black.

Gryphon's hips falter a little, but when North's eyes meet mine, I'm not worried about his bond coming out to play. Not after his declaration to me earlier. I want him just as badly as I want the man he lives inside. The bond doesn't look angry or jealous, he looks hungry while he waits for his turn to have me.

More, more, more.

His fingers lift to push between my lips, stroking over my tongue. I've never sucked anyone off before but now feels like a great time to start.

"Good girl. Good fucking girl with this pretty Bonded pussy."

It tips me over the edge and I shudder out my orgasm at his dirty mouth, his lips brushing the curve of my ear as he whispers pure filth to me.

I'm going to die like this.

Five of them doing this to me? I won't survive it.

I whimper as Gryphon moves me, positioning me until I'm on my hands and knees between them, groaning as he pushes back into me.

North's bond strokes my hair away from my face, his fingers gentle until he grabs a fistful and tugs my head back to look up at him. The black voids of his eyes are addictive to stare into, so easy to get lost in the depths of them, and my pussy clenches around Gryphon instinctively.

I want to come again. I want to take him down my throat and taste him; I want to swallow every last drop of his cum and—

"If you don't fuck her throat right now, she's going to come without you just thinking about it, so hurry the fuck up before you miss out."

North's bond smiles at me, a dark and dangerous thing with his eyes still dark, unnatural voids, and he fists himself to direct his cock between my lips. Probably best to be doing this for the first time with my Bonded who enjoys being in control because he directs my every move. When he finally lets his dick go to rock his hips further into the wet heat of my mouth, he cups my jaw possessively. Even his bond treats me with a desperate sort of possession that has me whimpering around his cock.

Gryphon's hands are tight around my hips as he holds

me still while he drives into me, so all I have to do is focus on not using my teeth and ruining the whole damn night. My jaw aches a little with how wide my mouth needs to be to fit North's cock in, but the sounds he makes have me wanting to do more, be more, just to please him.

I want him to want this as much as I do.

And I think he does. He acts like he does as he takes what he wants from me without question. He pushes further and further, testing my limits and then pushing them out for me, until I'm having to concentrate on my breathing as I'm deep throating him just like I wanted to. I thought it would take longer to pick this skill up, but North's bond knows exactly how to direct me into giving him what he wants.

His fingers squeeze my jaw in warning right before he slams into me one last time, coming with a roar down my throat so that I have no choice but to swallow everything he's giving me. As my throat flexes, his cock pushes down even further and my nose bumps softly against his pubic bone. I didn't think it was possible to get him all the way down, but I did it.

The moment the bond pulls away, Gryphon's arm snakes around my chest and pulls me up, until I'm kneeling in front of him, his cock still buried inside of me. He bites down on my shoulder and comes, his hips still pumping inside of me as I come with him one last time. It almost hurts, my pussy is so sensitive, and I whimper when he pulls out.

He grabs his shirt from beside the bed to clean me up, wiping away his cum from my legs, and then gently moving me to lie back down between them both. North's bond watches us both carefully, still naked and half-hard, and I smile at him softly. I'm not sure I could take any more, but I'm definitely not opposed to sucking him off again if that's what he wants.

He leans over me, ignoring the careful way that Gryphon is watching him, and his fingers trace over my face carefully before he kisses me, deep and sure, like he's chasing the taste of himself. It's hot as fuck and my hands drift into his hair as I kiss him back with as much fire as I can muster after having the life fucked out of me by them both.

I feel the moment the bond slips away and leaves North behind, but he doesn't break away from my lips until he's had his own turn. I sigh when he finally pulls away, stretching out next to me and curling an arm behind his head.

It's quiet for one blissful moment between the three of us, I'm completely content, and then North and his big, bossy mouth ruin it.

"Get up and go to the bathroom."

I huff at him and turn towards Gryphon, giving him the cold shoulder in the most literal sense of the term. "Stop worrying about your sheets, they're already ruined. I just wanna sleep; leave me alone."

He slides a palm under my arm and levers me into a sitting position like I'm made out of air, not at all listening to my demands. "You'll regret it when you get a UTI. Just go pee, and then you can spread out all you want."

I huff at him and throw a pillow at his head while my face heats up. "Never say the word 'pee' to me again, Draven, or I'll go find somewhere else to sleep."

Gryphon chuckles as he bends down to pull his boxers back on. "You should be glad he's not insisting on following you in there to watch."

I immediately regret fucking the both of them, both separately and together.

Once I've peed and washed up, trying not to wince at just how abused my pussy is feeling after coming that many times and taking Gryphon's dick until I was goddamned rubbed raw, I take a small moment to breathe before stepping back out into the dark bedroom. I want to leave the bathroom light on so I don't bump into every piece of furniture between here and the bed, but then North raises his palm and August appears, trotting over to me in his full Doberman size.

I make an embarrassing squeaking noise as I drop down onto my knees to give him all of the love he deserves.

"Dogs do not belong on the bed, even ones made out of shadows," Gryphon grumbles, and I scoff at him.

I speak in my puppy-love voice as I reply, "And for that, August can sleep on your side and you can cuddle with him instead of me. You love cuddles, don't you, baby? Yes, you do. Let's get your brother out too, let him have some snugs too."

When I lift Brutus out of my hair, he doesn't snap or fight with August for my attention, both of them now very secure in my love because they know I'll give it equally to both of them.

I turn the bathroom light off and let the puppies lead me over to the bed safely, their heads butting into me when I get too close to sharp edges and Gryphon's boots. Neither North or Gryphon argue about me having the creatures wrapped around my legs, and August even rests his head against North's thigh in the most affectionate gesture I've ever seen between the two of them.

Maybe I can fix whatever issue North has with his creatures.

I fall asleep with Gryphon warm against my back and North's hand resting under my cheek, his thumb tracing over my face in rhythmic strokes that send me off to a peaceful and dreamless slumber.

I wake up after the threesome of my wildest dreams feeling like myself again, finally.

So much so that I spend a good twenty minutes staring at North's sleeping face and trying to figure out how the hell he went from barely tolerating me to being all in on the Bonded front. I mean, that's not even the strangest thing that's happened in the last few days of the recovery fog but staring at his long, sooty eyelashes as they rest against his high cheekbones I can forget about it for now.

I've never really let myself look at him for this long and never this close before, so the image distracts me for a good three seconds before the rest of the 'what the fuck' situations filter into my head.

Like the whole waking up in Atlas' head mess. I really need to figure out what the fuck happened there without actually telling anyone about it because they will freak—

"What the hell do you mean you woke up in Bassinger's head?"

Fuck.

A frown appears between North's eyebrows the moment he wakes up, and I elbow Gryphon in the ribs, both for doing that and for meddling in my head again.

He grunts and catches my elbow, turning me slightly to face him more fully. "It's not meddling, you're practically screaming in my ear with your thoughts. It woke me up. I'm not doing it on purpose."

I roll my eyes and murmur back to him, hoping North will go back to sleep, "Well then, teach me how to stop mind yelling at you. I should be allowed a little privacy, right?"

He raises an eyebrow back. "I would say yes, but I just found out you've somehow managed to astral project and weren't going to tell me, so maybe we'll keep you like this until you learn to trust me a little more."

"Did he just say 'astral project'? I need a coffee," North says in a sleepy rasp that does things to my body. He shouldn't be able to do these things to me without even trying, that's not fair at all. I watch as he rolls out of the bed in one smooth movement and walks into the bathroom, the tiny boxer briefs he's wearing doing nothing to help with calming my raging hormones.

This has to be a Bonded thing, right? I'm not going to be this horny forever... right?!

I glance at Gryphon and shove a pillow in his smug face when I find him smirking at me. "Shut up. Shut up and tell me how to get you out of my head. My brain has been shitty the last few days and... well, if I had've ended up in Gabe's head or Nox's, I probably would have told you about it, but you're all on Team Atlas-Is-A-Spy, so I thought maybe we should figure that out first."

Gryphon glances towards the bathroom door and then murmurs back to me quietly, "If you have any control over the ability at all, don't ever try it with Nox. If you never listen to another word I say, Bonded, just listen to this; stay out of Nox Draven's head."

Even with the quiet, gentle tone he's using, a chill takes over me as I nod back at him, swallowing roughly. "I didn't do anything to end up in Atlas' head in the first place. I just went to sleep and then woke up staring at his bedroom wall feeling so goddamned bored my skin was crawling. It took me a full minute to realize where I was and… I just spoke with him for a minute. That's it."

Gryphon nods slowly and North reappears from the bathroom, still looking tired and frowning over being conscious. It's weird to see him like this because even when he slept in my bed before I went to the camps, I would always wake up first and head down to the gym before he woke up. I don't even know what time he usually wakes.

Except for that one time that Penelope showed up—

Gryphon nips that thought spiral right in the bud and interrupts me. "Nope, we're not thinking about her right now, and you're definitely not going to get out of this conversation by thinking about things that make your bond murderous and send you both on a rampage."

North moves a panel on the wall and a coffee machine appears, Rich Man Syndrome at its finest, and I make grabby hands at him just so that he's clear on whether or not I want some. I highly doubt he has any decent flavors or creamers in there, but I'd take a black coffee at this point.

That's how I really know that the power fog has lifted.

"It probably didn't help that you Bonded in the middle of healing, that would've slowed things down. What extra powers do you have? Can you feel anything yet?"

I struggle to sit up, careful not to disturb August from where he's lying on his back with his paws in the air and snuffling in his sleep. Brutus is tucked into his side and even though he's awake, he's not moving or disturbing his brother. It's very sweet, and I fish around under my pillow until I can grab my phone and attempt to take a photo of them both.

The photo comes out black.

Like, completely black, as though I was holding my finger over the lens. I frown at it and try again, but the image still comes out with nothing. What the hell is that?

"Oli, this is important."

I huff at Gryphon and take the cup of coffee that North holds out to me, juggling my phone around a bit. "Nothing. Nothing except waking up in Atlas' head. Like, fully inside his mind. I could hear everything he was thinking and, if I wanted to, I could've seen any of his memories. Before you ask, I didn't look at anything. That's a gross invasion of privacy, and even though he told me to, I didn't. I believe he's on our side. I might not know all of his story yet, but I'll hear it from him, not by rustling through his mind like a freaking psycho."

North shares a look with Gryphon and then takes a long gulp of his own coffee, stalking back over to the bathroom with the cup still in his hand. When the shower starts up, I have to sigh at the sound of it, hot water and a coffee. He's living my dream right now.

"You could live your dream too, you know. You'd probably be making a bunch of his dreams come true too," Gryphon murmurs, and I shove another pillow in his face.

Then I take my coffee and do exactly what he suggested.

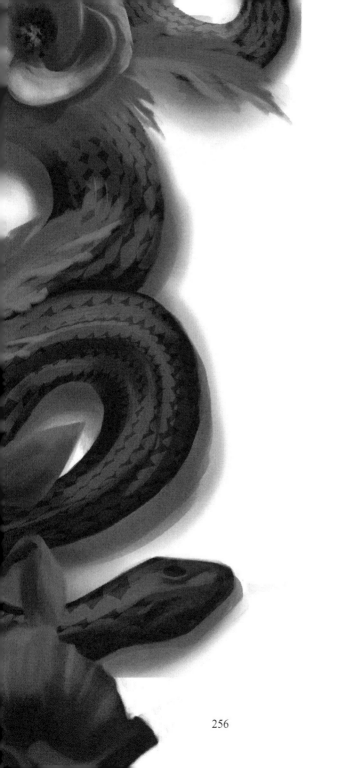

GABE

Pulling my bike up to my parents' house gets weirder and weirder the longer I live at the Draven's mansion.

It's not home anymore.

I feel guilty even thinking that, because my parents did everything to give me the best possible childhood. You only have to look at half the kids around me in my classes at Draven to know that I'm lucky. Half of them were brought up by parents so traumatized by what happened in the riots that they became overprotective to the point of smothering.

Grey can barely breathe without his dad's permission,

even at twenty years old he lives under their rules.

My parents were protective but wanted me to experience a normal childhood. They took me to football games and let me go out with my friends. Once I shifted for the first time, they'd relaxed the rules even more, because they knew I could defend myself better than most.

They were great parents... until they weren't.

Home, for me, is always going to be wherever Oli is.

I send a text to North to let him know that I've gotten here without incident and try not to feel like a child about it. I have to remind myself that we're all checking in with him at the moment. He's staying at the mansion, and everyone is answering to him so that we're all accounted for, but it still prickles at my skin a little.

I have to remind myself that it's for Oli, because that makes it worth it. She's the reason we're all staying close, staying connected, and staying vigilant, because there aren't just people out there who could hurt her, there are people specifically targeting her, which is a whole different beast.

Losing her is *not* an option.

So I'll toe all of the lines without question, the texting

and checking in and all of the extra security shit, because if it's keeping her safe, then it's worth every fucking second.

The front garden of the house is perfectly manicured and maintained; the gardener is doing his usual exemplary job. There's nothing out here that would suggest that anything had gone wrong inside over the last four years. There's no sign of the breakdown I'm about to face head on and hope to come out without feeling like having one of my own.

I fuss around with my keys until I get the door unlocked, wiping my feet on the mat and glancing around as though there's any chance of something being different here, as though maybe there was some life in the place again. Nothing. Of course.

I sigh and call out, "Mom? Are you home?"

It's a stupid question. She never leaves the house now. The housekeeper, Nina, spends her time keeping my mom fed and alive more than she actually cleans anymore. There's only really dusting to be done now that mom has taken to her bed.

I'm not being dramatic there. She's literally taken to her fucking bed.

I grab the pile of mail in the basket where Nina leaves it for me. It's tough to admit to myself that it's the only real reason I came here today. If I don't stay on top of shit around here, it's not getting done.

There's a fresh bunch of flowers in front of the family portrait in the foyer, the shrine that Nina keeps so that mom doesn't lose her shit on the off chance she walks down here. It's a good photo of the three of us, taken a few weeks before Oli's disappearance, and we're all genuinely happy in it. Fuck.

I let my eyes drop away and take the stairs two at a time, avoiding the creaks out of pure habit because there's no real need to be sneaking my way up here. I did that enough as a stupid teenager, coming in from parties and football tailgates that went on a little too long. Back before this shit.

I knock softly on my parents' bedroom door, pushing it open a little because there's no chance of catching mom in an awkward situation. She'd have to exist for that to happen. "Mom? How are you feeling today?"

The curtains are pulled shut and the room is only lit up by a soft lamp. I'd guess Nina turned it on this morning to attempt to get her up, but even the tray of food at her side has barely been touched.

"Mom? It's Gabriel. I'm home to see how you're doing."

There's a sigh from the lump on the bed, and I try not to let it dig under my skin. That tiny sound makes my skin shrivel in shame, like I'm a burden to her for being here to see her. Like she just wants to be left here to waste away to nothing and I'm forcing her to stay.

Am I?

Probably.

"Gabe, Mommy is tired. I'll come and play with you after a nap."

My stomach sinks even lower, practically in hell now. She does this sometimes, loses track of where and *when* she is. Like her mind is reverting back to when her life meant something and it wasn't this endless hell without either of her Bonded.

I fight to keep my tone even but, fuck, it's hard. "I don't need you to play with me, mom. I just need to know that you've eaten something today. Nina called me to say you were refusing food again."

She huffs and throws out a hand, but it's so frail that it barely makes a sound against the soft duvet. "She's meddling again! I need to let her go and find someone who will just leave me."

I shouldn't, I really fucking shouldn't, but my temper is shorter than ever at the moment. I have real shit to be thinking about, not this endless state of grief she refuses to leave. "To die, mom? You need to find someone who will let you waste away until you actually die? Because you're not far off. You can't fire Nina. I have power of attorney over you, remember? I hired her. I pay her. I take care of everything around here, because you can't!"

I stop myself, biting my lip until the words stay trapped on my tongue. I feel the moment she shuts down again, my anger sending her back into the empty space of her grief-stricken mind.

When she doesn't answer, or even move, I stalk back out of the room. She's alive, that's all I really needed to see, and I make it the entire way down the stairs before it hits me. Mostly because my father's portrait is still hanging there, staring at me like he can see me and knows exactly what I'm thinking.

The guilt might eat me alive.

Because if dad were here and mom was gone, he'd be mourning her just as hard, but at least he'd take care of himself.

Sometimes I wish it was her who died.

When I get back to the Draven mansion, I head straight up to Oli's room to find my Bond. I need to get the hell out of my own head and back to reality, where we all function and work on our shit instead of running from it in our own goddamn heads.

I take a breath before I knock on the door.

She calls out to me straight away and when I try the door handle, I find it unlocked. That's new. That feels big too, because she's always been extra jumpy about keeping it locked at all times. Whatever went down with North before they Bonded, it's definitely got her trusting us all a little more.

I'm not sure we *all* deserve that trust.

When I step in, I find schoolwork all over her floor, and Oli's wearing the tiniest pair of shorts I've ever seen as she's sprawled out in front of it all. She's alone, except for the two creatures, and there's a scowl on her face that means I know exactly what she's working on.

I don't get why she ties herself in knots over her Gifted 101 shit when North would pass her no matter what, just for being his Bonded, and Nox will never pass her for the exact same twisted reason.

They're both beyond fucked up over her, but I'll take North's brand over Nox's any day of the week. I don't need to know the exact reasons for it to know that whatever the hell happened in the Draven house messed with him in a very particular way.

She looks up at me with a soft smile, one that reaches her eyes, and I attempt to not trip over my own feet at the sight of it. She's fucking gorgeous, made perfectly just for me, and the more she opens up, the more of her perfection I find.

She props her chin up on one of her hands and tilts it to one side at me as she looks me over. "How was your mom? Did you get what you needed?"

I nod and drop my own bag by the door, toeing out of my shoes and coming over to sit with her. I definitely don't want to talk about my mom or the trip over there, so I focus on the good shit instead. Like how fucking gorgeous she looks today.

I trail a hand over the swell of her ass and she hums

under her breath happily at the touch. The waiting to Bond might mess with us all, but there's something about the anticipation that makes me enjoy the fuck out of it.

Knowing she's just as desperate for me as I am for her is everything I ever needed.

She heaves herself off of the floor with a grumble, but when she tucks herself into my side, I sling an arm around her shoulders to pull her closer into me and she hums happily. I dig my nose into the soft, silvery locks of her hair and something eases in my chest that had wound up tight over at my parents' place. Something that would have taken me weeks to undo myself, she does without even trying.

I love this girl already.

She mumbles quietly to me, her eyes on the shadows, "August is being pouty. I told him I'm sleeping in with Gryphon tonight, and he won't let the creatures on the bed."

I chuckle under my breath and lean into her. "You can always come back to my room. I might not love them like you do, but they're always welcome."

The grin she gives me is like looking directly into the sun, brilliant and bright, and August turns to sniff at me like he's checking to see if I'm being honest. It's still a little bit jarring being this close to North's meanest and most vicious creature, but I'm adjusting well enough.

Then the grin falters a little and she sighs under her breath. "If I didn't need a power up from him, I might've taken you up on that. I'm… struggling. Not having the pups makes it harder."

I scowl and lean back into her, pressing our foreheads together how she likes. Something about our noses being pressed together makes her grin like a child, so I do it as often as I can.

"What's wrong, Bond? What can I do?"

She sighs again and mumbles, "You all keep trying to help, but it's… a lot has happened and I'm trying to figure it all out. How to get through this next stage without completely losing it that you're all in danger. I got through the camps because it meant you were all safe. Now—now you're not. And it's hard to not feel responsible for that because if I had just stayed away—"

"No. No, this life of knowing we're all in danger is a million times better than the life without you."

Her lip quivers. "I feel selfish for thinking the same thing."

I shake my head, our noses almost colliding thanks to how closely we're pressed together, and murmur back to her, "Never. We need you as much as you need us. We all need you, Bond."

She swallows and nods, looking demure for half a second before her sass kicks in and she rolls her eyes at me. "I'm blaming Gryphon for this. I didn't give a shit until he started in on me with his guilt trip, and now I'm wallowing in it."

I pull her into my chest, damn near preening when she just moves into my lap to wrap herself around me and rest her head over my heart. She's tiny there, I can barely feel the weight of her, but when I bury my nose in her hair, I get a lungful of her scent that calms my bond inside me.

I'll do whatever it takes to keep her right the fuck there.

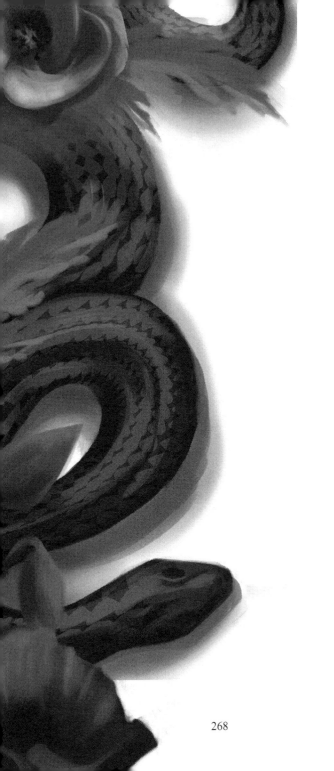

OLI

I bully Gabe into grabbing his own homework to get through his assignments with me. He tried to argue that we're not going back to Draven any time soon, but I need the distraction from everything going on around us, and I don't want to be caught slacking by Nox, so there's no real downside to keeping up with it.

Gabe cracks his back as he gets up to grab his bag from where he'd left it by the door, kicking his shoes out of his way in that very *boy* way of his. When he stalks back over to me with his arms full of books, he swoops down to give me a kiss. Brutus huffs at him but August moves over to sit between us, scooting Gabe away from me, and then turns his back on him to ignore him entirely.

It's cute.

Gabe shoots me a look and I giggle, burying my face in August's neck and taking a breath. It's been a very long, confusing, ever-changing week.

"You're sure you're okay now? You don't need anything?" Gabe murmurs, and I shake my head, pulling away from August and clearing my throat.

"Just you and the pups... and, well, I also need to find Sage and see how she's doing. Plus, I need to speak to Atlas, but I have no idea how North is going to react when I tell him I want to speak to him alone."

He smirks and shakes his head. "You mean more alone than projecting into Bassinger's head? I'm not sure that's possible, Bond."

Ah. So word has gotten out about that then. I desperately try not to think about that moment again as my cheeks heat up a little. "I want to stand in front of him and hear what he has to say. I don't want to be in his head for it."

He nods and slides down to join me on the floor. "You're better than me. I would've looked through every fucking second of his life to make sure he's not a spy."

He shrugs and scowls at August. "Any chance you can get him to move over a little so that I can get back to comforting my Bond? I've barely been able to see you since you got back, and now you're being guarded by these grumpy jailers."

I give August one last kiss and then snap my fingers to get him to swap sides, watching as he huffs about the move. He likes being between me and anyone else in the room, even North. He prefers to be a wall in front of me. It's cute and I adore him for it.

The moment August is out of the way, Gabe slings his arm around my shoulders and pulls me into his side. I tuck my face into his shoulder and get a good lungful of his scent—clean and masculine. I've missed him. I've missed Atlas too; the ache in my chest at the distance North has put between us is like a wound.

"It's all going to be okay. Once you're back on your feet, we'll figure something out for you to do. Gryph is already working with some operatives about... something big. Things aren't going to stay like this for long."

I clear my throat. "Have you been in to see Atlas? Is he okay?"

Gabe nods against my cheek. "He's fine. He's made it clear that he'll do anything he has to do to prove that he's not here to harm you. I believe him. I'm pretty sure Gryph does too, thanks to his lie detector, but the Dravens need more than that. They always have. He did… give North something that's bought him some favor though, so you'll be back with him in no time."

"What's that?"

"A list. A list of everyone Atlas has ever known in the Resistance and what he knows of their gifts. There's a lot of names on it. He proved that it's real by telling North how they got you out of the hospital in the first place. The invisible guy? Turns out he's a scout for the Resistance, and now that North knows how to look for him, they've found him in a lot of meetings and intel spots. Atlas might have just moved the needle in our favor."

I nod and rub a palm over my chest. "I get that he's helping, and I'm glad he is, but—"

I break it off there, but Gabe nods. "But he's betraying his family, and you feel terrible for him? You should speak to him about it. I did and… I understand his reasoning. He's wanted to talk to you about it since he got here, but he was scared you'd hate him the second he opened his mouth about it."

I give him a watery chuckle. "I'm surprised you didn't! You've been fighting with him since he got here."

He shrugs and says, "I knew he was too good to be true. No man, Bond or not, takes being run away from like it's nothing. I didn't trust him one bit. When I realized he knew, he knew your code name in the Resistance intel and he knew what your gift was, I beat the shit out of him. Not that it did all that much, he's indestructible, but it helped get some of my anger about it all out. Then once I heard Gryph interrogate him, had it confirmed as the honest truth… he's in this Bond Group. He belongs to you as much as I do. It would be a pretty shitty thing for me to cause shit just for my own feelings about it. I'm not going to do that to you."

I want to burst into tears.

I don't deserve him or any of them. I don't deserve that amount of consideration and care. He just pulls me into his body tighter and tucks his face into my shoulder.

"You smell like North."

Ugh.

My cheeks heat up because this is the first time anyone has mentioned it. "Sleeping in his bed and using his shower will do that."

Gabe grins at me and murmurs into my ear, his voice a tease, "Bonding with him would too. Have you changed your mind about it yet, or is North just *that* good at convincing you he's all in now?"

He doesn't sound like he's pushing or anything, just curious and clearing the air, so I'm happy enough to answer him. "He had some good points. My bond was also pretty strongly in favor and his bond was too. I'm... less worried about what it means to stay here. It's just the power boosts that are still a problem."

He nods and kisses my cheek again, not worried or concerned about it at all. I would feel insecure about it, except his hands are all over me, pulling me into his body closer, like he's trying to get under my skin, so there's no chance of me thinking he doesn't actually want me. I think he's just so sure that we'll figure it out that he's willing to wait.

There's a buzzing in his pocket and he moves me a little to pull it out, rolling his eyes at the screen and cursing under his breath. My stomach drops a little but he drawls, "It's just Sawyer, blowing my shit up for more help with moving Grey's shit in. I told him I was coming to see you first, and he's being a dick about it."

I glance up at him, surprised, and he nods. "Yeah, North is moving them all in here with us. Anyone we trust is being brought in so that we're not targeted separately. More power under one roof is a good thing right now, and Grey's parents are all about the move."

Relief floods me. "Did they come too?"

He shakes his head, scowling a little. "They've taken Briony to Switzerland. They were taking Grey as well, but North stepped in. There's a safe house there that only three people know the location of. They're leaving in the dead of the night, so they're going to be safe. Sawyer lost his shit about it and when the retesting of their bloods came back, Grey's dad finally broke and let him stay."

My jaw drops. "They're Bonds?!"

Gabe grins at my excited squeal and shakes his head. "No, but they're in the same Bonded group. They haven't found their Central yet, but the new testing is still going through the old samples. Sawyer has become *very* motivated to help with it."

I chuckle. "I'm sure he has. Nothing like a little skin in the game to get you working. God, I wish there was something I could do to help. Instead, I'm trapped up here like a princess in a tower. Stupid."

Gabe's phone buzzes again in his hand and I kiss him. "Go help him. I'll find Sage and see her, and then I'll come sleep in your bed tomorrow night. We'll be the masters of patience by the end of all of this."

Sage shows up at my door, Felix trailing behind her, three minutes after I message her.

How she can navigate this place so freaking seamlessly is beyond me, but apparently I'm the only one who struggles with that.

She takes one look at me with a frazzled sort of look in her eyes and throws her arms around my shoulders, squeezing me tight as she mumbles, "Never do any of this shit again, Oli. Not running off, or going full terminator, or coming home and being holed up for days where I couldn't come and see for myself that you were alive. I thought I was going to have to burn the place down around North to get him to budge. He was not having it."

I giggle, feeling oddly teary about the ragged tone of her voice, and when we pull away from each other, Felix leans in to give me a very sedate side hug as well. I'm not sure if he's worried about upsetting his Bonded or the many overprotective Bonds of mine in this house, but I can respect it.

I usher them both into my room, and Sage carefully steps around the pups to take a seat on the floor with me while Felix takes a seat at the small, never-used desk that's covered in books I've already used for my studies today, as well as all of Gabe's stuff. The small stack of Atlas' books acts like a little beacon to me, pointing out how badly I need to go find my Bond and hear from him.

I clear my throat, looking back at Sage and say, "So catch me up on what's been happening since the world as we knew it ended. What's been going on?"

I'm expecting to hear about everyone officially moving into the mansion, but that's not quite what I get.

Sage shoots me a look. "Oh, nothing much. Except that I'm definitely a Central Bond. Kieran is one of my Bonds, and I have *four* that flagged in my dad's very secure, very secret retest. So, you know. Business as usual around here."

Four.

Holy shit.

I suddenly care about nothing more than finding out about her Bonds. My own bullshit just evaporates out of my brain. "So, Kieran, Felix, Riley, and... some other guy? Do you know him?"

She huffs and leans herself back against the bed, tipping her head back dramatically, which I can totally get behind, and says, "Yeah, I know him. He already graduated from Draven a year ago and moved interstate for work. He's from one of the lower families, but he came to Draven on a scholarship because his gift was so strong. Gryphon tried to get him to join a TacTeam, but he wanted something that paid more."

Understandable. When you come from nothing, you're going to go for your best option. "So... are you going to contact him now or later?"

She groans and props herself up on her elbows to look back at me. "My dad and North are discussing it, as though I'm a child who can't make her own decisions on these things. They're also monitoring the Riley and Giovanna situation from a distance until it's safe to get him out of there even though I'm dying inside thinking about what is happening to him right now but my opinion on that matter is also very low on the list of priorities."

From the corner of my eye, I see Felix pulling a face, chewing on his lips like he's keeping himself from butting in, and I point at him. "Don't you even think about talking rationally about this right now, Davenport. We're here to hate on the controlling men in our lives, not their very sound and good reasoning for it."

He grins and shakes his head at me while Sage groans again. "I know it's a security risk thing and nothing to do with how they see me, but why does it always have to be this way? Why can't something, *anything*, be easy or normal for me?"

I stack up my homework to make more room for us to spread out on the floor, and August uses the opportunity to wedge himself more fully between Sage and I. I give him a scratch and he settles onto his belly, tucking his face into my legs as he watches the room keenly.

Brutus is on his back, fast asleep by my feet with zero cares.

Sage prods at the paperwork, drawling, "You'd think a near death experience would get us out of assignments, wouldn't you? I doubt your Bond will allow it though. We're going to be forced to hand shit in for him at least."

There's a pang in my chest as I think about Nox, a

craving for him that is going to mess with my plans to sleep in with Gabe tomorrow night. I know that North said I'd been 'tended to' by all of them after my bond went on its killing spree, but I wouldn't be surprised if Nox wasn't actually on that list.

Or if he did the bare minimum possible.

Felix looks over at me again, and I raise an eyebrow at him until he says, "I can't help but notice that there's two creatures in here with you now."

Sage glances over and shrugs at him. "That's August, one of North's creatures. We met when Oli came to grab me from The Great Fire Incident. You really think after Oli was captured and hurt he wasn't going to add his own little spy to the mix? I'm surprised he only gave you one."

August looks up at the sound of his name and I give him a scratch to settle him back down. Brutus wakes up and immediately asks for some love too, which he gets like the precious baby he is. "I might ask for the snake as well. My bond liked that one a *lot*."

Sage fumbles with her phone a little, gulping as she nods at me. She's clearly got a phobia but doesn't argue with my hopes because she's the best.

Felix does though. "You can't complain about being

stuck here and in the same breath, say you want a fucking snake following you around. Jesus Christ, Oli, that's pushing it. Even for you."

I giggle at the strain in his voice. "Scared of a widdle snakey? This changes everything I thought of you, Felix. Seriously. He's cute, and he ripped some guys' arms off for me. If that isn't the most precious thing I've ever seen, I don't know what is."

The memory floods me without warning and, though my hands shake a little at the ferocity of the moment, I don't feel guilty for all of the death and pain. They came for innocent people. They trapped a monster instead and that's their own stupid fault. I tried to warn them.

Where are you? What's upsetting you?

What's happened?

Gryphon and North speak over each other in my head, and I try not to roll my eyes at them both fussing. It still feels weird to have them in there like that, let alone having North being so... sweet.

Oleander, if you don't answer, I'll leave this meeting and come up there after you.

Ah, that's much more North-like.

I had a flashback to what my bond was doing in the

camp, not a big deal. Can you guys stop freaking out about me, especially while I'm safe in the mansion?

I'm careful about my tone, trying to tamp down my inner bitch so I don't start a fight, but I need to establish some boundaries with them, and fast, or they'll be walking all over me in no time.

My uncle was murdered in his bed. I'm not going to trust any households with your safety. Come downstairs so I can see you're okay.

Ridiculous.

Okay, he has a point about William's death, but I'm busy studying. So instead, I concentrate so hard I almost burst my brain wide open, but I manage to send him the image of Brutus lying over my legs and August sitting where I'm leaning against him, watching over me while I pretend I'm studying.

I'm safe with these two. Also, Sage has been known to set entire billion-year-old buildings on fire when provoked, so I'd put money on her in a fight.

Gryphon, who can also hear all of this because what is privacy, adds in, *We both know she wouldn't get the chance because your bond would deal with the danger. North is just trying to get out of his meeting. Go back to studying, Bonded.*

"Are you flirting with your Bonded right now? The carpet should not have you grinning like that, it's not interesting or funny," Sage grumbles, and I shoot her a rueful look.

"They're mother-henning me. Honestly, remember when we thought Bonds were bad? Bonded men are infinitely worse."

Felix shoots me a look. "You mean we want our Bonded safe, secure, and happy at all times? Terrible. The worst. Monsters."

Sage throws a pencil at him. "Don't say the 'm' word. Brutus will eat you."

"Now who's flirting? Gross, keep that out of my room," I say in an exaggerated tone, and Sage rolls her eyes at me with a grin.

Felix flicks the pencil at me and says, "We're all going to have to sit through dinner with you and your Bonds, so don't try for the higher ground here, Fallows. I'm expecting someone to attempt to fuck you over the potatoes the moment they get a chance."

I hold a hand up to my chest, feigning horror, and Sage cackles at me. It's stupid and ridiculous and everything I needed after all of the weird in my life right now.

Sage gives me a sly sort of look and murmurs, "We should take bets on which one. My bet is North, I've never seen him like this before. It's sort of… weird."

Felix opens his mouth, probably to place his own bet and embarrass the life out of me with some quip, but I'm saved by his phone buzzing. There's a lot of that going on today.

He barely looks at it, shooting Sage a look, before he says to me, "My parents are video calling in five, so we need to go. They've been extra freaked out since I refused to come home and North won't let them over here. Not that I blame him."

I don't even have to ask why, because it's very clear to me that it'll be about Gracie. After her perfume stunt provoked my bond to come out and Bond with Gryphon, they were both swift in their actions to get rid of the girl. I feel slightly bad about it, only because that's Felix's sister, but she also made me lose my v-card in a pretty animalistic and brutal way.

So fuck her and her silly little games.

I give him a look and he shrugs, packing away the last of his supplies. "I'm not mad about it. She's an adult and made choices; she can live with them. My parents, too. As long as Sage is safe and we're together, I'm happy with wherever that puts me."

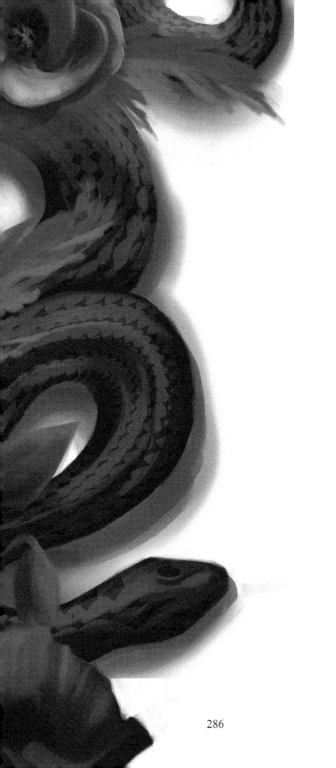

OLI

The moment Sage and Felix leave, I decide to put my big girl panties on and go see Atlas finally. I can't deal with the ache in my chest for Nox, but I can definitely do something about the mess in my head over my confined Bond.

I take the coward's way out and speak to North directly through our minds so that I don't have to argue with him face-to-face. *Is Atlas in his room? I want to see him. Without a guard or whatever, I want to see my Bond.*

I'm met with a very charged form of silence, one where I know he's hating this idea but wants to have a good argument on why I can't go see my own Bond. I stay quiet for a minute, but when I feel him hesitate, I push it a little further. *I don't... feel good and I need him.*

It's the truth, but it still feels like I'm being manipulative saying it because North immediately relents, agreeing for my own good to get over his concerns and fears of Atlas' motives if it means I'll feel better.

Take the creatures with you. I'll tell Nox to stay out of his, so long as you're not asking for help. Know that I'm only okay with this because Gryphon is sure about him, even if we're not. If he showed any deception so far, I wouldn't be doing this, Bonded.

The words sound controlling, but I'm seeing him clearer now. He's attempting to reassure me and tell me how much I mean to him, he's just not the best at wording it.

If anything feels wrong to me, I'll tell you. Is Gryphon close too? My bond isn't entirely opposed to killing Bonds if I'm in danger, so don't worry about that either, I send back, aiming for my own personal brand of reassurance, but he's not a huge fan of it either.

I change into pants and pull on one of Nox's sweaters to help push back the longing there for a little longer. I usually avoid Nox's things around Atlas if I can, but my skin is extra tight on my bones today.

I sigh and talk to Gryphon on my way down to Atlas' room, the puppies walking alongside me nicely with each other. *I think I need to sleep in Atlas' room tonight and not yours. Is that… okay? I also need to sleep in with Nox again, tomorrow if I can. Is it possible or will he get mad about it?*

When I get out of the elevator and attempt to take a wrong turn, August bumps my thigh to get me back on to the right path, the perfect guide through this ridiculous house.

I'll sort it out. Don't worry about him, Bonded. Just focus on Bassinger for now. I want to know what he says to you, so come see me after.

When I get to Atlas' door, I take a second to collect myself. It's stupid. I was in his damn head yesterday, but it still feels like there's something between us now. Something that's changed him from the Bond I was closest to, could rely on without question, to now being someone with secrets and a very questionable past.

It also makes him more real to me.

Gabe wasn't wrong, there was always something

about Atlas that put me a little on edge. Something about how all in he was that was a little disconcerting. It just didn't add up, but now that there's a reason for it all, I feel like it makes sense. It's still an issue, but I feel better about getting past it together.

Just as soon as I can knock on this door.

I lift my hand up right as it opens and Atlas drawls, "Do you need another minute, Bond, or do you wanna come in?"

I roll my eyes and step into him, scooting the puppies around him while I give my Bond a bone-crushing hug. Well, my bones feel crushed, but I'm sure his super strong and indestructible self is breathing just fine.

I tuck my face into his chest as he takes a step back, pulling me into his room with him and kicking the door shut behind us both. The puppies both sniff around in the space, though August stays within touching distance of me at all times. I know North promised not to spy on us both, but his creature is just as surly and overprotective as the Bonded, and I refuse to admit how endearing that is to me.

"I missed you so fucking much. I used to think sleeping separately four nights out of five was bad but, *fuck*, Sweetness. I can't go that long without you again."

I nod into his chest and rub my nose against the soft fabric of his shirt. He smells clean and warm and *mine,* which is my favorite combination, and when he tugs us both towards the bed to sit down together, I don't fight him.

When we finally pull away from each other, I look around the room a bit and blush, which is stupid, but the last time I saw his bed, I was in his head with him, jerking that glorious dick of his off until he came all over his fist.

"Wanna go again, little Bond?" he drawls, and I duck my head.

"Don't tempt me. It's been—it's a lot. All of this. It's a lot to process and go through. I also don't want to get stronger still, and everything is sort of messy."

He pulls a face, reminded of exactly what I'm here for, and I nod my head with a sigh. "I came here to hear it all. To hear from you about your family and... how you've decided to not be a part of the Resistance with them."

He swallows and nods, clearing his throat nervously. "I've been planning how I'd do this for months and now that it's time to do it, I feel like I'm about to fuck it up.

Please just… hear me out. It's not all wonderful and virtuous. I'm a shitty human for big chunks of it, but I came home to you. That's what counts, right?"

I refuse to nod, mostly because I can't agree to it until I have the details.

"I grew up in Resistance propaganda. My family is pretty high up in the ranks. My dad is even close personal friends with Silas Davies."

I nod. "I know. I saw him when I got to the camps with Kieran."

He grimaces and nods. "He was always leaving to check in on various different camps and going through the Gifted who had been taken. He knew they were after you for years before Silas took you. There had been rumors about your gift, but your parents moved you around a lot to keep you hidden. They were smart but outmatched by Silas' arsenal."

This isn't new to me.

Silas had told me all about this, about how I'm responsible in every way that counts for my parents' deaths. About how we moved constantly because I couldn't stop using my gift or showing off my void eyes at the worst of times. I know it, but it still hurts that he knows it too.

I swallow and nod so he'll continue, to get this story out faster, as though he's ripping a band-aid off of my soul.

"When we were called about my blood flagging in the same Bond Group as the Dravens, there was an entire family meeting. My dad was cagey as hell about it and Aurelia's Bonds all had opinions to throw into the mix, but my mom just got wasted. I've never seen her drink like that before, but she just downed glass after glass of wine as though it were water."

He takes another breath, shifting on the bed and scratching at the back of his neck like he's uncomfortable before he continues, "This is the part that I'm ashamed to tell you about, and the part I didn't tell the others, because it's none of their business. So, I found out right after that you'd gone missing. My dad made a fuss about it, but he was actually happy that I wouldn't be coming here and being around the Dravens. I... thought the same as the rest of the Bonds, that you didn't want us, and I acted like a fucking idiot. I went out with my friends a lot, drinking and partying, and I... slept around a lot. I thought I was getting back at you for leaving me behind before you'd even met me. I was a stupid, selfish dickhead."

I mean, I knew that all of my Bonds hadn't waited for me. Even the two closest to my age had very obviously chosen to sleep around before they'd met me, but I don't really want to hear about it, and knowing that he ramped it up in retaliation for something I'd never done... yeah, this isn't my favorite moment for us to share.

He looks at me closely and when I don't say anything, he continues, his voice a little stronger now that he's gotten that part over with, "This went on for a couple of years. Right up until about six months before North and Gryphon found you while you were on the run, actually. My parents were all out of town for a Resistance function. Yeah, the Top Tier families in the Resistance throw galas and shit to raise money for the cause. It's a whole different world on the East Coast than it is here. It's... really different than it is here, actually. So, anyway, they were out of town and my mom changed the password to the butler's cellar. It's a passcode thing, and she did it so I couldn't drink while they were gone, so I went snooping through her shit with one of my friends who knew enough about coding and hacking to be useful... On her computer, I found videos. I got my friend out before he saw anything really, but then I sat for two days while my parents were gone and watched the recordings of Silas Davies torturing you. My fourteen-year-old Bond being carved open as though you were nothing but a slab of meat to a butcher."

My heart stutters to a stop in my chest.

I never knew there were recordings. I knew there were cameras, so of course there was a chance that there were tapes but, fuck, I hadn't even thought it through that far.

I swallow roughly and he takes my hand, carefully so I can pull away from him if I want to. I don't want to though. I want him to hold me because… I don't even remember half of what was done to me thanks to my bond. To think that he's seen it all—nope.

What's happening? Oleander, I'm coming up.

I blink back the useless tears in my eyes and answer North immediately. *Don't. We're just talking and he told me about the tapes. I'm guessing he's told you already?*

He is slower to answer but the urgency is out of his tone. *I've seen them. Take a break and come see me. Leave this alone until later.*

But I can't. I need to know everything so that I can have my Bond back and know exactly what else he has on me that I didn't know about. Fuck, North's seen the tapes now too?

"You have them here, with you? Have they all seen them?" My voice is more of a croak, and when some of the tears spill out of my eyes, I hastily wipe them away.

He looks devastated when I pull my hand away from him but shakes his head. "No. Just North and Gryphon. I wouldn't let them keep the footage because I didn't want Nox seeing them. I know that you're still on the fence with him at least, and I wasn't letting him... see you like that. The other two had to see them to understand why I won't ever side with my family. *Ever*, Oli. I would never side with people who did that to you."

I can believe that, even without Gryphon's lie detecting ability, because I can feel just how badly he needs me to believe him pouring out of his soul in my direction. He's being very careful about keeping his bond away from mine, obviously so that I don't assume he's using it against me, but I can still read him like a book right now.

He means every word.

He also told me about sleeping around when I'm sure he'd rather not have talked about that but he's being completely transparent.

So I nod again and murmur, "What happened then?"

He takes a deep breath and tips his head back to stare at the ceiling. "I confronted my mom about it. She didn't want to tell me anything, but when I told her I was going to the Dravens to help look for you, she broke and admitted that she knew about them taking you. She'd lied to me about you so I wouldn't go looking for you, and she 'forbade' me from finding you because of what Silas wants from you. The problem with her plan was that I was already nineteen at that point and had access to my trust fund. There was nothing she could do to stop me, not without telling my dad or the others what I was doing. So I planned out how I was going to find you and be with you on the run, and when I say that I had everything planned out, I mean *everything*, Sweetness. From moving my trust fund into an offshore account so that my dad couldn't trace the money to knowing the exact whereabouts of all of the Resistance camps and having them mapped out so we could stay away from them."

My jaw drops, but he just smiles ruefully at me. "Getting you a passport without it flagging with Silas was hard, but I did it. I was going to try to talk you into going to Singapore with me. They have really strong anti-Resistance measures there, lots of security and surveillance. While I didn't love the idea of being monitored all of the time, I'm all about keeping you *out* of those fucking camps."

Tears start up in my eyes again, but this time it's because my heart is pounding in my chest like he's just declared his undying love to me. Well, I guess he sort of has. Running away together? To a whole other country just to keep us both safe which, in turn, would have kept the other Bonds safe as well?

As much as I need them all, I sort of wish it had gone that way.

"Except then Shore and his TacTeam found you. I have no fucking clue how they managed it when Silas couldn't, but they did. All of my planning went down the drain. I had to pivot to being here with you and hoping you'd want to run away with me. The GPS chip was in the way, and the sheer amount of security North has on you makes it really fucking hard, but I could've made it work... but then you started scenting and nesting. You Bonded with Shore thanks to that Davenport bitch. I knew we couldn't run without taking everyone. That would have been impossible, so now I'm working on giving the Dravens as much information as I can to keep you safe. Dad and Silas haven't figured out that I'm the one giving it to you all yet so, for now, it's useful."

I give him a look because this is all part of the story that has never made sense to me.

How did they not know that I was his Bond? They had all of the pieces and information and yet—they just didn't know? It's the one part that makes the story seem... like a story and not the complete truth.

Atlas nods slowly without me saying a word and answers the unasked question without hesitating, "My mom. That's how. She knew that Silas and my dad would both sacrifice me for their goals without second thought. My mom might be a part of the Resistance, but she's my mom first. She hates you, hates the Dravens, hates every part of this situation, but she loves me more than she hates. So, the day you escaped, the reason Silas finally left the camp? My mom. The reason you stayed a step ahead of them all the way? My mom. Every time something went your way that shouldn't have, my mom was behind it. She manipulated security footage, organized holes for you to slip through, and used her own gift to take out lower Resistance members to keep an eye on you. Then, once you were captured by the Dravens, she had the coordinates for the GPS chip sent to her as well so that she could keep an eye on you easier. Before you ask, I didn't know about it until Sawyer mentioned it. I knew it had to be her, and I called her to ream her about it. She just won't give up."

I blow out a breath and nod to him, looking away as I process that.

Well, it does neatly fix all of the holes in my story. Too neatly? Only time will tell, but when I think about it, I really did have too many close calls and lucky moments in my time on the run from them all. Holy shit. A reluctant and hateful guardian angel. Just my freaking luck.

I hum under my breath as I think, and he stands up from the bed, stretching out his back and stalking over to the closet, bringing back bottles of water for us both. I shoot him a look as I take the cold bottle and he grins. "I decided that if I'm going to be stuck in here, then I'm going to make the place more comfortable. I got a mini bar and some other shit so that I could stop calling the kitchens and dealing with the chef's attitude."

I drink some of the water and then put the bottle on

the bedside table before I finally bridge the gap between us. I'm sure there's more to talk about. I'm sure more shit will come up between us in the future, but for now, I'm satisfied. For now, I just want my goddamned Bond.

I lean forward to press my face back into his chest, and I can feel the instant relief in his as he pulls me into his arms. The buzzing feeling under my skin settles a little. It's strange the different ways that my bond protests being separated from each of them. Gryphon and North are different now that we've Bonded, but my need for Nox is a slow itch, Gabe is an ache in my chest, and Atlas is this energy that won't leave me, egging me on to find him and wrap myself around him.

He takes my hands as though he can read my mind as well and rubs his thumbs over my pulse points where my blood is thrumming with excess energy. "You Bonded with North."

Just like Gabe, he's not saying it as an accusation. He's just putting it out there into the air, and I nod. "I did. It was my choice this time and... I don't regret it."

He nods back. "I don't want you to regret it. I'd kill any of them for pushing you. But what did it do to your power? Did you have a surge or anything new pop up?"

I tilt my head to the side as I consider it. I've thought about it, of course I have, but the only answer I've come up with seems fake and like wishful thinking.

"I feel stronger. Not more powerful or anything, I just feel more sure of myself and what I can do."

He nods and squeezes my hands. "I'm not just saying this because I want you. I do want you, nothing will ever change that, but after you and Gryphon Bonded, I'd been watching for some big change that never happened. Oli, have you ever considered that maybe your bond won't grow in power because it's already at full capacity?"

I frown and he scoots back on the bed, tugging me until I'm straddling his thighs. My bond purrs in my chest at having him this close again. The distance between us has been the hardest part of all of the changes we've been going through. He lets go of my hands only to span his palms over my hips, pulling me down into his core a little more. He's hard underneath me, his dick reacting to having me this close to him, but he just continues on like this is all business as usual for him.

"You're the strongest Soul Render in recorded history. I know, I spent a long time researching it. What if Bonding with us is just going to make your bond more settled and secure? You were tortured. You were so young when Silas got his hands on you, your bond came out to protect you. I think that has changed the way things are happening. That and… the color of your eyes. That isn't Soul Render specific. The Dravens are the only other family I've found with black bond eyes. There's something there that we're missing too. I hope now that we're all on the same page about things, that maybe we can figure it out. Together."

He kisses me softly, slowly, but not pushing for more. "Just think about it, Sweetness. Just think about it, and we can talk more later. I'm not pushing you, but if you can think of anything that means I'm wrong, I want to know about it. This is all I care about right now, getting you settled and secure in your gift and your bond. You shouldn't be running scared anymore. I won't have it, Sweetness. I can't stand the thought of how long you've been doing this by yourself."

I nod and lean forward to press my face into his shoulder, something settling inside of me now that I've had my fill of them all. Nox is the only one I haven't spent any time with, but my constant connection to him thanks to Brutus means it takes longer for the cravings to hit me when it comes to him.

"Everything is going to be okay."

I scoff. "Why does everyone keep saying that to me?"

He chuckles at me and rubs a hand over my spine. "Because you're going to worry about every little part of this. You care about us all, you miss your freedom, everything seems terrible. Of course we're all going to try to reassure you, because it *will* get better."

I quiet down and enjoy the safety of his arms for a little longer, our heartbeats syncing up because we were made for each other. Maybe—maybe someday I will be able to Bond with him. Maybe he's right and we'll get this forever, this safety and security and *love*.

Eventually, he moves me over into his bed properly. He helps me strip off the sweater I'm wearing, and the yoga pants because I prefer to sleep in my underwear or shorts, and then he stalks over to his own side of the bed, shedding clothes as he goes. He's still hard, his dick not getting the 'no Bonding' memo at all, but after spending a morning in his head while he jerked off, it doesn't seem like a big deal to me anymore.

I have more experience handling men and their desires now, so much so in such a small amount of time that my head is still spinning from it.

I curl up in his arms and let him fuss with our position until he's happy with how we're lying. August stays on the floor next to the bed, watching me carefully until it's clear Atlas has fallen asleep, and then he lies down to sleep there. I know that he's here for North's peace of mind, but there's still something comforting about having him with us and I let myself drift off to sleep.

God knows how much later, I wake up at the sound of the door, but August doesn't move from where he's curled up on the floor by my side of the bed. Of course not, it's North coming in to check on us. When I lift my head, he steps over to give me a soft kiss, stroking my hair, as he pulls up another chair to sit in.

"You're going to watch us sleep?" I mumble.

He unbuttons his sleeves and rolls them up. "You. I'm going to watch over you."

I wake up with my bond feeling far more content in my chest about the proximity to Atlas. I try to convince North to let him out of his room for the day so we can go watch something in the giant home theater. When he doesn't budge, we lie around in bed and watch the normal-sized TV instead. It's less showy, but Atlas calls the kitchens and orders up a feast for us, telling them it's for me so that no one dares to question him about it, and we eat fish tacos and chicken quesadillas in bed like the best of heathens.

It's a little bit magical.

Gabe comes looking for me sometime after lunch to drag me away, and Atlas makes a big show of kissing me senseless at the door. Gabe barely bats an eyelid at the display, just waits until I pull away from him, red-faced and breathing a little too hard, before he slings an arm over my shoulders and directs me back down the hallway to head up to my own room.

I send Sage a text message and we agree to meet up at dinner, then I climb into the shower in an attempt to straighten myself out a bit.

I feel like I'm stuck in a time loop.

Like the days are stretching on and I'm just... lying around in a fucking bed all day with one of my Bonds, being absolutely useless while people like Davies are out there hurting, torturing, and murdering innocent people.

I'm a monster.

I try not to sound shrill and a bit psycho when I step out of the bathroom and say to Gabe, "I'm going to go crazy in this house if I'm not allowed out of it soon. I'm not trying to be a pain but seriously, Gabe, I can't stay in here like this forever."

I leave out the part where I have, indeed, already gone a little crazy.

He nods and takes my hand, threading our fingers together as he tugs me towards the door. "There's a plan for that. North is working pretty much nonstop on it, but I'll leave it to him to tell you. I'm not going to steal his thunder there. You just focus on getting better—"

I cut him off. "I am better! I'm all healed up and ready to use my gift and my terrifying bond on whoever I need to. Let's get out of here for the night. Go hunt something."

His eyebrows shoot all the way up his forehead and he blinks at me. "Go... hunt something? I thought you didn't want to use your gift? You change your mind too much for me to keep up with, Bond."

I huff and roll my shoulders back, the jitters taking over with how stir crazy I feel. "I don't want to go around killing people but… I guess it felt good to get a lot of people out of that camp. I'd just sort of run away from it all and tried to forget about it, but being back there and seeing what's happening to people there… I can't keep my head in the sand over it. I need to get off my spoiled ass and go help out."

He tugs me into his chest and reaches down with one hand to give said ass a firm squeeze. "It doesn't feel spoiled to me. It feels fucking perfect, and maybe you should just slow your roll a little. You have no real Tac training, only the few classes that you were giftless for, mostly anyway, and Gryph will knock you back the second you attempt to bring it up. Don't even think about running off. North has extra security on you, and there's no chance that Black will take you anywhere again. He will be killed if he tries, and that's not an exaggeration. North has made it clear that he'll face the shadow creatures if he ever transports you without one of them again."

Huh.

That seems a bit extreme, and I groan dramatically until Gabe grins down at me again and says, "Let's go down for dinner. That'll keep your mind away from *hunting* and wiping out the Resistance."

He's not wrong.

Dinner is a lot louder with this many people sitting around the table. Sawyer and Grey both attempt to butter up the creatures by feeding them pieces of steak, and I'm shocked when it works. Brutus is sitting at their feet with big, round eyes while he waits for his next piece. August stays at my side but happily takes the pieces Sawyer throws over to him.

"They don't really have taste buds or stomachs. You're just wasting food," drawls North, cutting his own steak up like an aristocrat.

I roll my eyes at him and snark, "You have a magic TV in your room that appears out of thin air. We can feed the babies steaks without worrying about the food bill."

Gabe smothers back a laugh, choking a little on it, and Gryphon grins at me from across the table. August rests his head on my thigh and licks at my fingers, enjoying the lobster juices even if it's not really doing anything nutritionally for him.

I wait until they all look happy enough with their meals before I very carefully say, "So what are the plans here, long term? I'm about ready to start tearing walls down if I'm holed up for much longer."

Gryphon raises an eyebrow at me. "Training starts again at five a.m. tomorrow. Do you still need me to come get you, or can you make it to the gym on your own now?"

Oh, that's definitely not what I was after.

Gabe roars with laughter at the horrified look on my face while I struggle to think of a good reason to get out of it.

If you're healed enough to fuck North and I at once, then you can train, Gryphon says. Although I want to murder the asshole for saying it, I can acknowledge that at least he didn't make it public.

The tiniest amount of brownie points to him.

Nothing that will strain her legs. Go easy on her.

My cheeks heat, because of course they're both happy to run free in my head while I'm trying to eat my goddamned seafood.

"Why are you the exact shade of tomato soup right now, Bond?" Gabe murmurs, and I startle back into myself, looking around the table like a criminal who's been caught with her hand in the cookie jar.

"Gryphon has no table manners, and that's all I'm saying. He's dragging me to training. You'll come too, right? Save me from his sadistic ways."

Atlas' hand is gentle on my thigh under the table, stroking reverently over the perfectly healed skin there. They all keep fussing with it. North wanting me to go easy on it makes no sense. I've healed up fully, so well that there's no scar, but I also won't argue about it. I don't want to do squats and burpees.

Running is taking it easy though, right?

Totally.

Kieran looks at me over the table and shakes his head slowly. "She needs to see a Tac Psych. You should put off the training until she has."

I poke a fork in his direction. "Shut your mouth, narc. I'm fine. I've healed, and there's nothing I need to talk about."

He cocks an eyebrow at me, the bastard, and says, "That man knew exactly where to cut you to get your bond out. You knew what was coming before he even opened the tool box. None of that comes without a lot of sessions. If your Bonds give a shit about you, they'll get you in therapy."

North looks over at me and I feel everyone's eyes on my skin, but I talk directly to him because I already know that it'll be him forcing me into it. "My bond is the one who deals with that shit. If you send me to therapy, it'll have to be the one to talk. Do you really want to do that to some poor woman?"

Shit.

Don't think about it being a woman, don't go down that thought spiral again, Oli.

What thought spiral?

I roll my eyes at Gryphon. *Are you ever going to get out of my head? Why am I even asking? Of course you won't. The spiral about thinking of how many people you lot have all fucked.*

He raises an eyebrow at me. *Why would thinking about a psych do that to you? Why exactly are you so convinced that North has fucked every woman he comes across? And why don't you feel the same way about the rest of us?*

Stupid Bonds.

I turn away from him and back to Kieran. "I don't need therapy. I need a nap and for everyone to leave my bond alone so it doesn't go on another soul-eating binge again. That's it. So just drop it."

Sage meets my eye across the table and nibbles on her

bottom lip a little, looking guilty.

"Don't do this to me, Sage. Don't throw me to the wolves like this. We're supposed to have each other's backs here!"

She scrunches her nose up with a smile and says, "I love my psych. Maybe you can see him?"

North cuts in before I can whine about my bestie's betrayal. "Who do you see? I'll arrange for him to come here once he's been through the security measures."

Sage opens her mouth but I cut her off, snapping at North, "I definitely do not need another man in my life trawling through my head. I have enough of that shit happening right here!"

All of the other chatter at the table stops at my outburst, and one of the kitchen staff who was putting out extra plates scurries back into the kitchens as though she's worried about what's going to happen to me for being so rude.

I'm not.

Sort of. Okay, I'm sure there's still plenty of shit that North will be more than willing to do to me as punishment for not just happily going along with his plans, but I draw the line here. I don't want to speak to someone. I don't want to pour my heart out to some stranger. I'm not ready for that sort of thing yet.

I barely want to talk about it with my Bonds, who are supposed to love me and accept me no matter what.

Sawyer leans into his sister's side and mock whispers, "Are we about to see them fuck over the potatoes? Because while I didn't ask for that on the menu, I'm down to have a front row seat."

The look that North levels at him makes me want to die on his behalf. I shove a spoonful of vegetables in my mouth so I look too busy to get involved, as though I can ignore this entire mess of a conversation and it'll just disappear. Grey just groans and covers his eyes with his hands like he's preparing himself for what shitstorm Sawyer has brought on him by default.

Sawyer excuses himself from the table shortly after, apparently too chicken-shit to deal with North now that he's pissed him off. Grey leaves with him, and shortly after, Sage gives me an apologetic sort of smile of her own as she heads out with her Bonds as well. I was hoping to actually speak to her but the tension in the room is thick, and I don't blame her for wanting to get the hell outta Dodge.

It's quiet for a minute, and then Nox opens his fat mouth.

I should've seen his attitude coming from a mile away because it's been too peaceful around here lately, so of course he wants to ruin it for us all.

"So Bassinger failed to convince you to Bond with him as well? Or are you only interested in Bonding with the more powerful Bonds in the group? You're a lot more calculating than I was expecting, Poison."

I roll my eyes and shake my head at North when he death stares his brother down the long expanse of the table. I don't need him fighting this war for me. If I let them all fight over me right here at the start, it'll never end.

Instead, I sigh and turn to face Nox. He's not drinking for once, but there's also a focus in him that hasn't been there for weeks, like whatever it was that knocked him off-kilter has passed and he's back to being the stable professor again.

I fight back all the same. "I'm not going to sit around and let you talk shit about me or try to make me feel bad about Bonding with North. Not now and not ever, Draven. So you can just give up on it. And not that it's anyone's business what I choose to do with my own goddamned body, but I'm going to see what my gift does now. If it gets stronger, then we'll make decisions from there. But again, it's none of your business or anyone else's. Being one of my Bonds doesn't mean I owe you shit, Nox."

Gabe's hand slips onto my thigh and squeezes gently, a silent show of support, but naturally Nox picks up on it anyway and sneers at us both. "Picking favorites? It appears panting after her like a lovesick puppy isn't doing you any favors, Gabe. You should really change tactics if you want her that badly."

Gabe turns to stone next to me and my eyes narrow in Nox's direction. I'm mostly fine with him taking swipes in my direction, but I'm learning that there's nothing that pisses me off faster than him taking a swipe at one of my other Bonds.

Especially the one who has accepted me and my reasons for wanting to take things extra slow.

"The only person around here who needs to change anything is you. I don't know what the hell has happened between us that makes you this twisted about me, but I don't owe you anything. Gabe doesn't owe you shit."

"So you've just been lying and manipulating all of

your Bonds to get what you want? I tried to warn my brother that this is what would happen—"

I cut him off before I have to hear anymore of his twisted version of things. "Oh yeah? What if I bond with you all and suddenly my power gets even stronger? What about if I sneeze and kill everyone in our town? Fuck you, Nox. Fuck you and your *unbelievably* privileged life. At least your shadows heel when you tell them to. You can stop whenever you want. I don't have that option."

His lip curls at me, but North has obviously had enough of listening to us tear into one another and says in a cold tone, "Nox, walk it off. You're not doing yourself any favors right now."

He stares North down for a minute and then grabs one of the linen napkins and wipes his hands, shoving his plate away from himself and pushing his chair back without another word.

I reach for the chocolate cheesecake that's sitting in front of me, because I'm done eating real food and now is the time for a sugar coma to kick in. I throw all of my sass into my tone, just to cut him down a little more as I snark, "Such a good little boy, doing just what you're told."

The reaction is instant and severe.

An emotion that I can't believe flashes across Nox's face right before his bond kicks in and his eyes flash into the voids as it takes over. Shadows begin pouring out of his body in a slow, ominous stream.

Stop.

North's voice echoes in my head, but I don't know what the hell I've done to trigger Nox's bond. The black curls wrap around his wrists and the creature that has come out of his chest to stare at me has its jaw wide open, its teeth glistening as he snarls soundlessly in my direction.

What did I do?

North answers immediately, firmly and with a no-bullshit air that helps the panic in my chest ease a little. *Nothing. This is just a problem for him, and you need to leave it alone. He can't control his reactions to… this sort of thing.*

I try to meet his eye across the table but he's focused entirely on Nox, his own eyes shifting to black as well.

"Fuck," Gabe mutters. He braces a hand on the table across me like he's preparing to cover me entirely. I want to think that it's just overprotective Bond shit, but Gryphon is moving slowly on the other side of the table, clearly trying not to provoke either of the brothers, but he's moving towards me as well.

What did I do?

There's a cold press of a wet nose on my ankle and I look down at Brutus. He looks miserable, sadness pouring out of him, but he's still checking in on me to see if I'm okay while his Gifted is having a very man-version of a meltdown at the dinner table.

Thank God Sage and the others aren't here for it as well.

Gryphon answers me. *You didn't do it on purpose, but don't talk to him like that, Oli. I know that's not fair because he was crossing the line already, but you just hit a trip line inside him and he can't stop himself from this sort of reaction.*

I barely even remember what I'd said.

When Gryphon finally makes it over to me, he continues to move slowly as he pulls me up out of the chair and into his body, shifting until he's covering me entirely. The problem is that what North's bond said to me in the bathroom keeps swirling around in my head. I don't want him between me and the shadows, even when they're snarling.

But when I try to step around him, Gryphon's arm tightens around me and Gabe moves to begin pulling me towards the door as well. I don't want to leave either of them, not when it's my fault this is happening. I'm not going to beat myself up about it but, fuck, I should help, right?

You'll only make things worse. You're his Bond. That's enough to break what shred of control he has left.

They both bully me out of the dining room, but I hold firm about staying in the hallway, listening to the murmuring of North attempting to firmly talk his brother down from whatever the fuck I've caused here.

When Gryphon tries one last time to get me moving, I stand my ground. "I'm staying here until they're done in there. I'm sleeping in Nox's bed tonight anyway. I have to wait for them."

Gryphon gives me a look but nods, sliding his hulking form down the wall until he's sitting with me, and Gabe folds himself into a pile on the other side of me. I don't feel tired but as the minutes stretch into an hour, I let my head drop down onto Gryphon's shoulder and my eyes drift shut.

I wake up to North murmuring quietly, "He's fine.

He's gone down to the gym. Maybe you should go and keep an eye on him."

I blink to try to clear the sleep from my eyes, but North is good about helping me up and getting me back over to the elevator without much effort on my part. With a gentle hand, he directs me the whole way there, opening Nox's bedroom door for me and then holding my hand up the stairs. He perches on the couch while I climb into the bed.

"I'll stay until you're asleep, Bonded. Just rest, and Gryphon will be here for you in the morning."

It shouldn't be that easy, but my bond trusts him implicitly, so I'm drifting off in minutes. Nox is on the couch instead of North when I wake a few hours later, his creatures surrounding me except for the one who had snarled at me at the table who looked as though he'd rip my throat out at the drop of a hat. No, that one is sleeping across Nox's chest in a savage looking smoke form that is still more teeth than anything else. I get the feeling he's there to make sure I don't get close to his master.

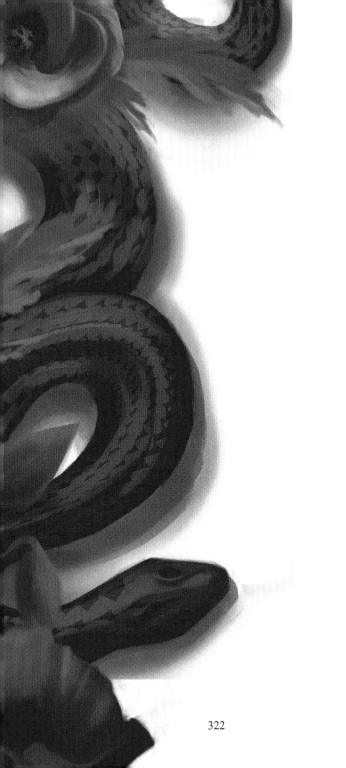

322

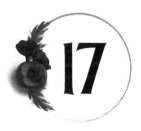

NORTH

I should leave them both alone.

I already know that. I know that they have their own Bond to work out for themselves, but when I leave Nox's room for my own, there's a dull fog of dread clouding up my brain. The moment I lie down in my own bed and shut my eyes, all I can see is the haunted look in my brother's eyes right before they void out.

I can't sleep like this.

So instead of even trying, I get up and throw on one of the sweatshirts my Bonded left behind in my room that smells like her. She has a good point about the scents calming bonds down. Then I make my way over to Nox's room. The door is unlocked, it always is, and I don't bother knocking. His creatures will tell him that I'm coming up and, sure enough, when I make it to the top of the stairs, he's blinking up at me from the couch.

Oleander is asleep on the bed, alone and looking safe enough.

"You really don't trust me, do you?"

I glance at him and step over the sleeping pile of shadows by the landing to join him on the couch. The biggest of his shadows, the meanest one now that Oleander has tamed Brutus, lifts his head from Nox's chest to growl in my direction. It's always been protective but what happened at dinner has opened up old wounds.

"I'm here for you both. I'm here because, while you might not ever want it, I want to help you. No matter what you need. I said that to you and I meant it."

He huffs and runs his fingers through his hair, tugging at the ends of it like he's really trying to tear it from his head. He's usually better about keeping up the front, acting like the put together professor he's emulating, and I attempt to take it as a sign of progress that he's allowing himself to crack a little with our Bond so close to him.

Even asleep, she's still within touching distance of him, which is a trigger of its own.

"You're here for her, don't lie to me. It's okay. I knew when Gryph brought her back here that you'd fall over yourself for her. A little thing like that who needs all sorts of your help? She's built to break you, Baba."

It's been years since he called me that, and my chest tightens at the sound of it. Baba Yaga, the boogeyman, the old tale of protection I'd given him as a child that he'd held on to for years.

He's not wrong about Oleander, but he is wrong about himself. I gave him my word that I would stand by him, protect him, provide for him if he couldn't do it for himself. I swore that I would do everything I could to… fix him.

I know now that I can't, but I will *never* leave him behind.

"She was made for you too. You're not there yet, and that's okay, but maybe you should stop hating her for things she hasn't done. Maybe you should think about finding level ground with her."

He sneers at me. "And how can I do that when she's in my fucking bed every week? I can't forget about her for five minutes with my sheets stinking of my Bond."

I take a deep breath, breathing in her scent on the sweatshirt, and his eyes flick down to the fabric because he can read me like an open book. He always could. We're two sides of the same coin and always have been.

I cut him off before he can start a new rant all about my weakness for her. It's nothing new, and I'm not ashamed of it. She's my Bonded, and she's proven that she's more than worthy. I'm the one who needs to prove myself here, not her. "Just leave it. If having her sleep in here isn't working out, then we can make changes. There's always another solution. I went with this one because I thought it would be the least... *invasive* for you. If you have any other ideas, just tell me."

He snorts and pets at the creature on his chest, scratching behind his ear. He's not usually affectionate with them around me. I've known that he has a better, stronger connection with his creatures, but I've never actually seen that affection in action before.

More of Oleander's influence.

My own bond itches under my skin, August wanting out to be with her, but with all of Nox's arsenal around us, this isn't the place for him right now. Brutus might tolerate him but the others won't. They know a rabid shadow when they see it, and while he might have tamed a little, I don't trust August fully. I still keep a very tight leash on him, especially when Oleander isn't awake.

No matter what my bond told her, I can't take that chance. Not with her.

"Go to bed, brother. You look like shit, and now you've seen that your little poisonous Bonded is alive and well, you should get some rest."

I roll my eyes at his jabs at her, the little barbs that do nothing to *me* but dig under her skin, exactly the way he wants them to.

I rub a hand over my face and try to stifle the yawn threatening to take over me. "I'll never sleep well again. Not with the sheer amount of threats we're facing. The Sanctuary isn't going to be ready in time."

Because we both know the biggest of my concerns is getting us all out of the path of the Resistance, to stop them from being able to just pop into our community and pick us off one-by-one. Though I've been working on a solution for *years*, now is the time to move.

He glances at me, stroking a hand down the creature's back. "You'll get it done. The problem is going to be convincing people to move into it."

I might be the monster that everyone thinks I am, because when it comes down to it, I don't care about whether or not we get the Top Tier families out there. I care about the vulnerable and the poor, those who can't get themselves out of the Resistance's path.

I care about my brother and the rest of the Bonded Group.

And, more than anything else, I care about making sure that Silas fucking Davies never lays his sadistic cunt eyes on my Bonded again.

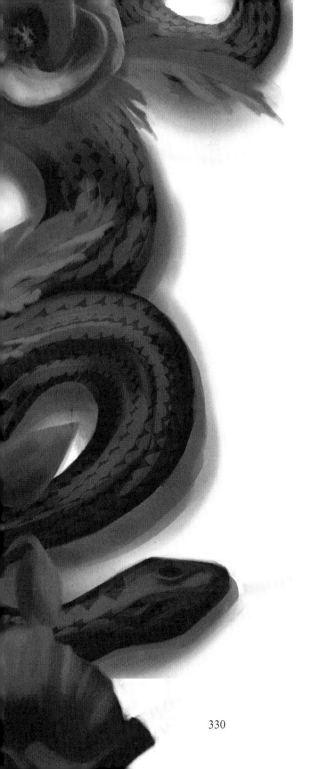

OLI

I not-so-slowly but very surely lose my mind being stuck in the Draven mansion.

I mean, I knew it was coming, but with every day that I'm feeling better and needing less sleep, the itch to go and do things gets worse. Gryphon tries to tamp it down by thoroughly destroying me in the gym, but that only pisses me off. North's attempts are more about coaxing more information about the five years I spent alone, firsthand accounts, because he wants to know everything in case we've overlooked some vital information.

That only makes me feel useless and morose about

leading the enemy to my Bonds.

Gabe does the best job of distracting me, but only because he offers to chaperone for Atlas and I to hang out, and the three of us spend hours trying to figure out how the hell to get out of this place. Atlas is good at this game, mostly because he has so much experience in escaping from well-connected people, and some of his suggestions astound Gabe and me.

Nox disappears again.

I'm not surprised, but I am a little envious that he's allowed to just come and go freely. I have the ability to literally rip people's souls out, and yet I'm the most protected person on the freaking planet at this point, I'm sure.

One incredibly slow and boring week after I come home, the Resistance finally make their next move against us.

I find out mid-training session at the gym a little before dawn while I'm sweating my ass off on the treadmill. Gabe and Grey are on the weight machines while Gryphon is sparring with Sawyer, Felix, and Sage. Well, Sage is mostly trying to get out of the sparring, but every time she inches towards me, Gryphon sends her a look that terrifies her into going along with his sadistic circuit of evil.

She's getting pretty freaking impressive at taking down men twice her size though, so I'm not going to fight him over her treatment.

North arrives at the door with Kieran in full Tac gear and three other TacTeam operatives the same time that Gryphon's phone starts blowing up. I hit the stop button on the treadmill and climb down, grabbing a towel to wipe off my face as I stalk over to the crowd. Sage glances over at me and comes up to my side, eyeing Kieran. It's still super freaking weird around them at the moment while they figure their shit out, but I also like him a lot after our time in the camps. I'm all for them figuring this shit out together.

I'm more for him than I'll ever be for Riley, even knowing he's been manipulated. I can't just forgive and forget, that shit isn't in me.

"There's been an attack at Draven and in the surrounding township," North says. Gryphon is cursing viciously under his breath as he stalks over to the changing rooms to get into his gear.

Sawyer shares a look with North and walks out

without a word, which seems weird to me, but I'm too worried about what is about to happen to ask about it right now. "Is it still happening or is this a cleanup? Let me grab a shirt. I'm going too."

North steps in my path with a look right as Gryphon walks back out of the changing room, fully dressed in record time as he adjusts the straps on his holsters by feel alone. Both of them are death glaring at me like I'm being an unruly child right now, and I'm not. I'm being totally reasonable.

"It's a cleanup, and only fully trained, active TacTeam operatives are going, which means Gryphon is the only one in our Bond Group going. We also don't want to be moving in large numbers at the moment unless there's a good reason for it, so you'll be staying here with me and everyone else."

Gabe grabs my towel off of me and uses the dry side to wipe his own face down, knocking my arm with his in his quiet show of solidarity, but it only itches at my skin today.

My bond is also *hungry* right now, which makes the irritation a million times worse. "I'm more help out there than I am in this stupid house!"

North shakes his head and Gryphon just turns on his heel and moves to stand with Kieran, the two of them disappearing with a *pop*.

I want to scream.

"We're all staying here for now, Oleander, but you can all come to my office and watch the reports come in until we decide what the plan of action will be."

I share a look with Sage and we both nod, following him out without another word. Everyone chooses to come as well and when we get there, Sawyer is already set up at North's desk with a laptop, tapping away furiously. North grabs one of his spare chairs to direct me into with a hand to my shoulder, giving it a squeeze as he gets his phone out and starts texting someone.

"What's happening? What are you doing?" I murmur, nosy and grumpy at being left behind in this freaking house, but he's good about it.

"I'm calling Bassinger down to watch with us. He has been very good about giving us information, and there might be something here that flags with him. I'll use every resource at our disposal if it will keep you safe."

My cheeks heat and Sage perches on her chair, holding a hand out to me for comfort. I take it, giving her fingers a little squeeze. When North finds an extra chair for himself, he pulls it up to my other side. Grey stands behind Sawyer and watches him work, while Gabe and Felix both grab chairs from the dining room to sit by the wall together, murmuring quietly about what this all means for us. I try not to think about it too much.

Atlas arrives after a few minutes, ignoring everyone and making a beeline for me. The office chairs aren't really big enough for the two of us to share one, but when I stand up to give him a hug, he just maneuvers us around until I'm perched in his lap.

North gives him a *very* unimpressed look. Atlas just shrugs it off, drawling, "You've kept her as far away from me as you can manage without it hurting her, you can get over it for now."

Sage bites her lip to stop herself from smirking and then Sawyer clears his throat. "I've got it. I'll get the streams on the big screen. Shore, Black, and Rockelle are all wearing cams, so we can see what they're seeing. They all have comms as well, so if you need them to backtrack on something, just tell me."

Atlas nods and North shoves his phone away to watch as the large flatscreen on the wall lights up and we can see the footage of three cameras up there.

The area hasn't just been raided…

It's a massacre.

We all sit there in silence as the three operatives walk around the area and we see the carnage. There are bodies everywhere. Top Tier Gifted and the lower families alike, there are corpses littering the streets for everyone to see. Kieran walks past a Non-Gifted reporter trying to get past the barriers and talking a whole lot of bullshit about the situation, not surprising, but the Tac guys there won't let her through.

After a few minutes of watching, North says to Atlas, his voice low, "Do you see anything?"

I feel Atlas shrug. "I can only guess for most of it… except the scorch marks. That's absolutely Peter, one of my sister's Bonded. The patterns? A dead giveaway for his gift. Wait! That, there. Sawyer, can you pull it back? Three seconds. Yeah, pause it. That injury? That's pretty specific. My father was definitely a part of this too. Fuck. Okay, that helps. He has a team of people he won't work without, so that narrows the list down greatly on where they'd be taking people. Dad only works with three camps. Oli took out one of them, and I can make an educated guess on which of the other two he'd pick."

I lean into him. "Has your mom told them? That you're in this Bond Group yet?"

He glances at me and shrugs. "The last I heard from her before I gave up my phone, she hadn't. Things could have changed. North would know more if she attempted to contact me about it."

We both glance at him, and he shakes his head. "She hasn't sent anything through. If we all go to the camp for a clean out, you'll have to be prepared for them to know."

"Can't we just… keep Atlas here? Won't they change things up if we go now?"

North shakes his head. "We're already about to change everything around, this raid has just sped that process up a few weeks. As long as Bassinger is sure he's given us all of the information we need, then it's a risk we're taking."

Atlas nods. "It's everything I had stashed away as important and everything else you've asked for. If I think of anything else or something comes up, I've already said I'll give it to you. Whatever keeps Oli safe, it's yours."

My heart spasms in my chest like I'm having some sort of episode over his words. He's so loyal to me, even before he met me, and I feel so unworthy.

North glances at me and shakes his head. "You withstood two years of torture without ever giving any of us up. No one deserves our loyalty more, Bonded."

I blanch and then groan under my breath, "Don't tell me you can see in my head now too. I can't take much more of this."

He sends one last text on his phone before he slides it into his pocket, loosening his tie as he prepares himself for the change into the Tac gear that's about to happen. "No. I'm just getting better at reading your facial expressions. You really don't see yourself the way we see you, not at all. We're going to have to change that."

I don't have anything to say back to that, so I turn back to the screen and keep watching the bloodbath. When Gryphon turns to the grassed area, all of the air leaks out of my lungs.

There's a white sheet covering some of the carnage, but the little row of legs sticking out are clearly small, grade school and under. The Resistance wiped them out as easily as they'd murdered the grown men and women who had chosen to stay behind.

"I'm going to be sick," Sage mutters, and Felix jumps

up to grab the wastepaper basket and shove it under her nose. She retches a little, and while my stomach cramps and roils as well, I choke down the bile creeping up my throat.

I already knew this sort of retaliation was coming, we all did, but to see it is something else. To know that... that I'm responsible for it in some way is truly horrifying.

The children.

Of course he's gone after the children. This is Davies' way of letting me know personally.

"How? How does this let you know?"

I didn't realize I'd said it out loud.

I glance up to find that not only are all of their eyes on me, but that Nox has snuck into the room as well while I was transfixed by the horror on the screen.

I try not to lash out at any of them because of how uncomfortable it's making me. "Towards the end... of my time with him, Davies figured out that the best way to get to me was through kids. I couldn't handle what he would do to them. My Bond took over without the pain it usually took because I would let it just so I didn't... have to watch."

The disgust on Nox's face has me wanting to curl

up and die. I get it entirely. I hid from the pain and the horror of what was happening and was no use at all to the children—

North snaps, "Stop it. You didn't do anything—"

"Yes, I'm aware, please don't rub it in."

He grabs my arm and jerks me around to face him, almost pulling me out of Atlas' lap in doing so. "Listen to me, Bonded. You were a child as well. You were fourteen when he took you and sixteen when you got out, no one here thinks you're responsible in any way for what that man did. No one."

My eyes flick to Nox because, well, he's the one who judges me as harshly as I judge myself. If anyone was going to tell the complete honest truth here about my responsibility, it'll be him.

He doesn't even bother to return my gaze.

"Well, Black caught wind of their Transporter's trail, right? Let's go kill the sadists and get this over with. They all need to die screaming, and I think we can do something about that," Nox says, turning his back on us all and walking out of the office.

North stands up and helps me to my feet with a warm hand on the base of my spine, murmuring quietly to me,

"I'd rather you stayed here but if you want to come and do your part, then we need to move now."

I glance up at him, but I already know what my answer is.

I'm going to let my bond kill as many of them as we can find.

Gryphon's voice pops into my head without warning. *That's my girl.*

I want to wear what I've already got on, but my Bonded are having none of it. I'm manhandled, coerced, snapped at, and forced into a full set of Tac gear by North, which I complain loudly about because I'm sure I look like a toddler in her dad's wardrobe.

It also doesn't help that when I step out of the changing room and into the foyer where everyone is waiting, Gabe cackles at the sight of me, slowly dissolving into full belly roaring laughter.

I shoot North a savage look, but he ignores me. Gryphon, who had returned with Kieran to transport us all in, smacks Gabe in the back of the head and snaps,

"Shut up, idiot, before she starts whining about it all over again."

"What are you talking about? She never stopped," North drawls, and I discover the advantages of the heavy-soled boots when I stomp on his foot and the surly Bonded actually winces.

I'm taking the win.

Atlas walks out in a modified Tac suit, mostly because there's less protective panels on it, and my heart skips a beat for a second until I realize that he's indestructible and there's no need for them.

"If you get shot, does the bullet just, like, bounce off, or do you just heal faster? How much am I going to have to worry about you?"

He grins at me and slings an arm around my shoulders. "It bounces off, which is another reason why I'm allowed to come today. I'm your human shield for the trip, your Gifted shadow following your every move."

I blink up at him for a second, trying to imagine bullets just bouncing off of his skin and then grin, grabbing his hand and tugging his body close to mine. "Perfect. Get ready to meet my bond. Try not to judge me too harshly when she starts torturing everyone in our general vicinity."

He smirks back at me, dropping his head down to murmur, "I told you before, I already know all about your bond. There's nothing that could happen that'll scare me away. You and I, nothing can come between us."

If there weren't a million other TacTeam operatives swarming around us in the tight space, I would kiss him, but it feels wrong to start making out with him around them all, so I take a little step back and a deep breath.

Gabe glances between us both and then steps up to flank my other side, making me feel tiny between them both. Gryphon finishes up his planning session with Kieran, barking out orders to each of the teams, and North is having a quiet discussion with Nox in the corner. They look as though they're both itching to go and, sure enough, there's a dark ring of smoke around North's wrist, one of the few signs he has of being close to the edge with his power. He feels just as responsible for the attack as I do, but from the other side.

He's the councilman who is being hamstrung at every turn, trying to get as many people out of this situation alive as he can, but the other Top Tier families want to hide in their money and do nothing. They want to waste their Gifts and Bonded power because they feel above this sort of work, no matter what he's said to them all.

Still, he feels like he hasn't done enough.

Get your head in the game, Bonded, or I'm leaving you behind.

I snap my attention back to Gryphon and raise an eyebrow in his direction. *I am. Nothing will make my bond angrier than Resistance scum upsetting my Bonded and my Bonds. It's very touchy about what belongs to us.*

His mouth quirks up just a little at that and then he's barking out more orders, reeling out jump times that have everyone preparing around us. We're going with Kieran, naturally, and jumping as the third wave. All of these terms I've never been taught before and am learning on the fly are kind of fun, and when both of the Dravens walk back over to our group so that we're all going together, I feel a little rush of adrenaline in my blood.

Look at me, getting worked up about being a monster for good.

No monster talk either, Gryphon says. I answer him out loud. "I'm harnessing the monster for good. Like I give a fuck what anyone else thinks of what my bond can do."

Kieran glances at me, then around the group, before murmuring, "That's the spirit! The more you take out, the less of them out there killing innocent little kids. Kill them all, Fallows."

I just might.

Then we're all being thrown into space by his gift, popping back into existence on the edges of a camp, the sun already set in this part of the world and visibility shitty.

Gryphon comes to my side and murmurs to both Atlas and me, "Stay where I can see you at all times. Black will take you home the second either of you step out of line."

I nod, trying to look as obedient and solemn as I can while Atlas just gives him a curt nod.

Harrison scoffs and snarks, "We all saw what she did to the last camp, Shore. She's the best defense we have. You should really ease back on her a little."

Gryphon gives him a look that I'm sure is shriveling his balls and North steps up to my side, pulling his own riot helmet over his perfect hair, and snaps, "Get your eyes and your opinions off of my Bonded before I set a nightmare on you, Rockelle."

He blanches a little, freaking out even more when

August bursts out of North and immediately turns to heel at my feet, his jaws opening so his tongue can loll out as he gives me a silent plea for pets.

I bend down to give them to him as I bring Brutus down from behind my ear at the same time, stroking them both and murmuring about all of the bloodshed and horror we'll be doing here together for the night.

There's a moment of dead silence around me and then Rockelle mutters, "That is fucking terrifying—"

Kieran cuts him off. "I told you! I told you to just stay away from her. You have to be the idiot that sticks his nose in where it doesn't belong. Shore will reach down your throat and rip your spleen out with his bare hands if you so much as look at her again, just keep out of her way. In fact, all of you should just treat Fallows as though she's a shadow creature as well, because if her bond decides to join the party, she might as well be a rabid, bloodthirsty shadow, because she'll kill you just as easily as they do. Keep. Fucking. Clear."

The group murmurs their compliance and then scatters obediently, moving into the formations that they've all been trained into by my Bonded. I watch them go and then straighten up, snapping my fingers to get the pups to follow me, which they do like the perfect boys they are.

"Tell me if you recognize anyone," I murmur to Atlas and he glances down at me, faltering just a little. He thinks I'm doubting him, and I immediately feel guilty as hell about it.

I rush to reassure him. "I just mean that if there's anyone worth keeping alive for North or Gryphon to question. Most of these people are worth more to us dead but... if there's someone who might know what's being planned, Gryphon should talk to them."

He nods and pulls his helmet off, throwing it to the ground. "I can't see as well with that thing on. Let's go burn this hellhole to the ground. Preferably, with my father still in it."

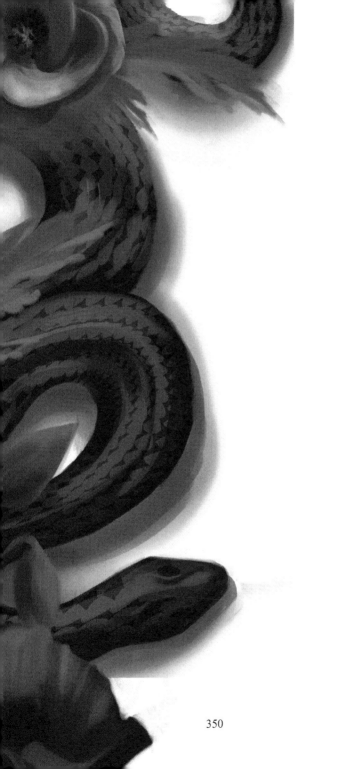

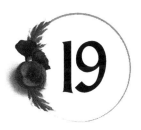

OLI

I've never been to this camp before which is both a blessing and a bit annoying. A blessing because there's no hidden memories about to jump out and paralyze me and annoying because how many of these stupid things does the Resistance have hiding around the place? How many innocent Gifted have they kidnapped, brainwashed, tortured, and murdered?

How many little girls have been hurt and assaulted here?

"Don't think about it; I don't want your bond triggered right now. We're going for stealth. We don't need an outright massacre here just yet," Gryphon murmurs, and I glance at him with a slow nod. He's right, but it's hard to shake those feelings. The ghosts walking around here with us are thick in the air, and the ominous feeling has my bond on high alert.

The camp either doesn't have Gifted-sorting people, or there's still so much chaos happening with the new arrivals that no one sounds the alarm that we've arrived. Gryphon uses mostly hand signals to move his teams through the small amount of swampy bush cover that's here, and I just follow his instructions that he gives me directly through our Bond connection.

Just let the Teams do what they're trained to do. We're here as support, not to do the heavy lifting.

I glance at North and nod, tucking into Atlas' side a little tighter to visibly show them all that I'm playing by the rules. Not because I've lost my spine or anything, I just don't want them getting hurt from being distracted by me running off for no good reason.

I trust Gryphon and his team. I trust Kieran because he's already proved himself to me, and I trust the rest of them because anyone trained and vetted by Gryphon is good enough for me.

He's sort of a hard-ass, and no one could skate through under his watchful eye.

There's a few minutes of quiet where only noises from the camp can be heard as we creep forward through the scrub as one, and then there's an explosion on the other side of the camp as one of the tents goes up in a giant ball of flames.

My bond takes the helm immediately, my panic at the unexpected fire show kicking its protective measures into action. I'm still in there enough to know what's going on and to argue with my bond if I need to, but it's definitely in control. The shadows both come to heel at my feet, ready to protect me from anything that might come my way.

The Everlasting One notices straight away but stays close, dipping his head at me respectfully. He's known about me for a long time, learned all of the ways to court a bond like me, and when I smile back at him, it's all teeth.

"We should kill them all now. The only good Resistance soldier is a dead one."

There's movement around us as the operatives all move into the camp, gunfire and shouts ringing in the air, but the Everlasting One ignores it all. He inclines his head to me as though he agrees but says, "Mostly yes, but information is key right now. Someone here might know where Davies is, or what they're planning next, and we want the man who dared to touch you gone."

A carrot on a stick, effective because it's true.

I want that man dead. I want to be fully Bonded and tear him apart slowly. I want to feed him piece by piece to the shadows at my feet.

A voice sounds in my ear through a small machine. "Bassinger, stop riling her up and keep clear of the rest of us until we've secured the area."

I don't like hearing them in my ear like that, but when I move to bat the earpiece out, the Everlasting One grabs my hand to stop me, gently moving me over to where there's cover for us to watch the operatives work.

They're efficient.

Outnumbered ten-to-one, they pick off the runners and what Transporters they can. I watch as they work and the Everlasting One takes out a gun of his own, checking the safety as he holds it at his side. He offers me one, but I shake my head. I'm a god, a gun means nothing to me.

We need to have a conversation about this 'god' stuff

sometime soon, Bond.

I ignore my Bonded and watch as he directs his people into the camps to flush out more of the enemy soldiers. There are stragglers everywhere, a few of them making it to the scrub before the operatives take them out. I don't think we're expecting much from it but when the Everlasting One curses viciously, I look up to find a blonde woman staring back at him, shell shocked.

When her face finally twists into a snarl, the girl inside of me whispers that it is his sister.

She takes a step towards him and I move in front of him, raising my own arm, only to have him press up close to my back, murmuring to me, "Don't kill her, Bond. We can take her in and deal with her however North decides, but just—"

His sister turns on her heel and runs, bullets hitting her body and bouncing off of her because her gift is the same as her brother's.

The girl tries to take control again, to force me into submission, but I keep the helm. "Agreed. The shadows will take care of this for us."

The Everlasting One looks over at me, but I snap my fingers until the shadow pup comes to my side. "I need her alive and as untouched as you can manage without being hurt yourself. Fetch her for me."

The shadow blinks at me and I know that the Dark One is seeing through his eyes, that's why he is pausing.

The girl inside speaks directly to him before I deal with it myself. *Atlas didn't attempt to hide her or talk her way out. He just asked to take her in instead of killing her, for now. I think we can give him that, right?*

There's a pause and then the shadow is off, moving faster than my eyes can properly track as he chases the enemy girl down. The Everlasting One takes a deep breath and watches but doesn't attempt to interfere. I feel a deep need to destroy his family once again, to hunt them all down and feast on their souls until they are nothing but ash and dirt beneath our feet.

The Dark One speaks directly to us again. *I'll have August bring her to Kieran for an immediate jump. I don't want her talking to Atlas and attempting to manipulate him. Let's keep it as clean as we can for now, Bonded.*

I look out at the carnage around us and say, "The Dark One is getting her out now, taking her back to be detained. She's alive and will stay that way."

The Everlasting One gives a curt shake of his head.

"I don't want to see her. I don't want to see any of them. Let's finish this and get the fuck out of this shithole."

There's another explosion of fire and he wraps his arms around me again, ready to cover my body with his own to protect the girl from the heat and damage. There's a Flame there controlling the fire, making sure to only burn the enemy and their camp without taking out our own. My Shifter is in full wolf form and tearing through the camp, snapping and tearing men apart with nothing but his powerful jaws. Pride swells within me at the magnificent sight of him.

I want to be involved but I also want to watch them work, to know what my Bonds are capable of and to know that they're worthy of the Bond Group they're in. It's good to see that they are.

Then I feel it.

One of my Bonds is hurt.

My eyes shift and it's game over on the whole night, the mission, these men and women. My bond just wipes the entire camp clean of them all as I cast out my web to find which one of them has been hurt and where *the fuck* they are. Tearing their souls out is easier than breathing and there's a satisfaction to the unanimous thump nose as they all fall to the dirt as one.

There's shouts and chaos around me from the TacTeams but I ignore them, single-mindedly stalking through the mess.

Gabe, the girl whispers, and my heart skips a beat. I mean, rationally I know that it has to be the Shifter or the damaged Dark One. If it was one of my Bonded, I'd know exactly who it was and how they were hurt, and the Everlasting One is bullet-proof.

Where is he? What happened? I send out to both of my Bonded, but neither of them have an answer for me. He's out there somewhere by himself.

My web finally finds him in one of the larger holding tents and I take off at a sprint in that direction. The bodies are thick here, most of them my kills, but there are a few with bullet holes and visible Gifted wounds. There's a Flame doing some serious damage around here and I quietly admire his work even as I move towards my Bond.

I can appreciate these people feeling some pain before their inevitable deaths.

The girl doesn't like me thinking like that, she doesn't like what that means for her morality, but such pettiness belongs to me. What use are morals to a God of Death?

Nothing. They are nothing to me or mine.

When I duck into the tent, there's rows of cages filled with haggard and terrified-looking prisoners and a large pile of dead men in front of the Shifter. He's been shot, a through-and-through wound on his arm that looks painful but not life-threatening. It still makes me furious to see him bleeding, and I stalk over to him with a scowl.

He looks very alarmed to see me, his eyebrows shooting up his forehead as he holds his good arm out as if to stop me. "I had two choices. I chose the one that had us all surviving. I'll heal just fine, Bond. Calm—"

I roll my eyes at him as my gift bursts out of me and into him as I cut him off. "No. No more being hurt. Not for anyone, do you understand? I will not tolerate it."

He stares at me, looking into the depths of my eyes before he nods slowly, pressing the fingers at the end of his freshly healed arm to the comms earpiece and muttering, "Oli is in full bond mode, are you all aware of this?"

I hear it in my own earpiece, and then the damaged Dark One says in a drawl, "The piles of dead bodies everywhere did give that away, yes."

My dark Bonded says, "Just keep her with you and

don't let her near the abducted Gifted. I'm not sure what she'll read off them, and I don't want her killing anyone who might be useful."

The Shifter watches me and when I cock my head at him, he mutters, "That's easier said than done. She is listening to us right now."

The damaged Dark One says, "Figure it out."

Then the Everlasting One says, "I'm coming to you both. I'll help get her out of there."

The Shifter stumbles on one of the bodies and mutters, "How many of them have you taken out? Jesus."

The Everlasting One scowls at him and moves as though he's going to strike the Shifter, then glances at me and changes his mind. "Don't talk like that. Her bond might be at the helm but Oli is still in there, and she doesn't need to hear you making fucking comments."

I ignore them both but the girl has a lot of feelings about the conversation. Feelings mean nothing to me.

We arrive at the clearing and find that the men and women wearing black and vests with lots of weapons are standing around taking stock of the damage here.

It's mostly my work.

The Shifter and the Everlasting One direct me over

to a group and begin talking to some of the men, all of whom are watching me from the corners of their eyes like they think I'll be taking them out next.

What fun that would be, but not right now.

As my bond finally leaves me with that last little delightful thought, slipping back into the inner recesses of my mind, I shake out my limbs until I feel more like myself again. There's some pain in my legs that I'll need to stretch out later but, otherwise, I'm okay.

We got through that experience *okay*.

"If you're about to lie down and take a nap, lemme know. I'll call Shore to come carry you around again," Kieran snarks at me and I shoot him a look, rolling my eyes.

"Thank you for your concern, but I'm fine. Look at us getting a camp cleaned out without having our asses handed to us first! Not a broken bone in sight. I'm proud of you, Black!"

The guys around him all snicker under their breaths, but they shut up quickly when he turns to give them all a death glare. They might not revere him the way they do my Bonded, but he's clearly still respected.

I can see why.

Atlas moves to stand a little closer to me as we wait everyone else out. I can see every last one of my Bonds, except North. I'm not worried, because I'd know if there was something wrong with him, but it still makes my skin itch a little.

Where are you?

He's quick to answer. *In the holding tents. Are you back now, or is this just another small moment of clarity?*

I roll my shoulders back and glance around. The holding tents are close, and I tell Atlas where I'm heading. He turns to watch me but stays behind easily enough, trusting me.

I duck into the space and find that while the cages have been opened, most of the healing and assessment is still happening inside them. Some of the Gifted who have been here for a long time are so frail that they'll need to be carried out, and some look too sick to be moved. My chest tightens at the sight of them. I walk over to where North is watching them all, his face giving away the sheer amount of disgust and loathing he has for the men and women responsible for this.

I clear my throat and murmur, "I'm back. Properly, I mean. Sorry for going off script."

He nods. "It was for the best. They had a lot more on their side than we originally accounted for. They always do, no matter how much extra we throw in."

That does seem to be one of the Resistance's many advantages. Because of their unscrupulous ways, they'll just kidnap and brainwash a whole new set of soldiers that they're willing to sacrifice to get through to us.

Silence falls between us as we watch one of the women in the cage break down and start screaming at the operatives who approach her. She's terrified, clawing at her own skin like she's trying to dig something out that we can't see. When the operatives switch so that it's a woman approaching her, she breaks down, sobbing uncontrollably in a heap.

I want to cry with her.

It takes me two attempts to get my voice to work. "What happens to them?"

North grimaces. "You don't really want the answer to that, Oleander. Those who can be taken home, are. Hold onto that instead of the alternative. It's what I do."

Looking at the crowd... I'm not sure any of them can really go home.

"Who does it? Who has to put them down if they can't

be saved?"

His eyes narrow at me. "No. Don't ask, and don't think like that. That's not what your gift is going to be used for."

"I'm already a monster, North. What's a few more souls when I've already taken thousands? Yep, there it is. It's in the thousands, thanks to my time in one of these camps. What does it matter?"

He tears the helmet off and shoves the gaiter down the column of his neck so that I can clearly see the blinding rage written all over his entire face, but he speaks quietly so that no one further inside the tent can hear us. "It matters because your voice is shaking, Oleander. Don't you hear it? It matters because you're writhing with guilt over it all."

I shake my head at him but he gets a hand up to grab my chin and stops me, leaning in close and snarling, "It matters because you're mine, and I'd never let you do it. Killing to protect yourself? Fine. Killing to wipe out the enemy who hurt you? Great, do it. Them? Never. Not you, not ever."

I want to scream at him, argue with him, because why shouldn't it be me? Why should I get to live untouched by all of this ugliness just because I have them as my Bonds, but he gets a hold of my arm and drags me back out of the tent and into the clearing where everyone else is waiting for us to get back home.

Kieran waits for a second and when my eyes stay their usual color, he holds out his arm for us all to grab.

When we *pop* back into existence again, my stomach roils rebelliously and I clap a hand over my mouth. Gryphon shoves Atlas out of the way just a little more forcefully than he probably had to as he reaches out to get a hand on my neck, the heat searing me as he manipulates my nervous system and stops me from puking everywhere.

The sweats and shaking stop immediately, and I almost profess my undying love to him out loud in front of all of his friends and subordinates.

Like I'd care if they heard, Bonded.

My cheeks heat and I knock his hand away from my skin as I duck my head. I listen to him chuckle at me and he pulls me in close to his chest for a quick hug before he's off barking orders at people again.

Atlas reaches out to give my hand a squeeze before he follows North out of the room. I assume he's going back to his solitary confinement because he's doing it without question.

I hate it, but I'm not going to call North out about it right now in front of all of these people.

I take a breath and let my shoulders slump down a little, checking in with my bond and my body, but I don't feel the usual impending three day nap coming. I'm tired, but only the same amount as if Gryphon had run me into the ground in the gym, so a good night's rest should cover me. When I open my eyes, my surroundings finally filter into me and my brows drop down. "Where are we? This isn't the mansion. North said to take us home."

Kieran gives me a lopsided grin and holds his arms out. "This *is* home now, Fallows. The raid got us here quicker than was planned, but the Sanctuary is home now."

I glance up at Gabe and he slings his arm around my shoulders to direct me over to the large set of doors, opening them and directing me out to look out over... the Sanctuary.

It's a whole-ass city.

Okay, it's more of a town or a village really, but there's dozens of houses and buildings here and people *everywhere*. The sun is barely setting, so I'm guessing we're back in the States, but there's mountains on every side of the clearing and a slight disturbance in the air around us that says we have Shields working overtime to keep this place off of the maps.

I stare around it all in wonder.

"What the hell is this place?"

Gabe kisses the side of my head and murmurs, "William and Nolan Draven started building it forty years ago. When North was old enough to take the seat on the Council, he started helping with it too. It's been the Draven family's mission for a lifetime. It wasn't due to be ready for another decade or so, but when North found out about you, he moved the deadlines up. He's poured literally hundreds of millions of dollars into it since he took over the build. He's been recruiting to get the best and strongest Gifted here, all of them vetted by Gryphon so we know that you'll be safe here. Except North refused to leave behind the Gifted communities who couldn't get out by themselves so that's why it's this... big. He brought everyone who would come and could pass the testing. The Resistance will never find us here. North has made sure of it."

I stare around at the people, the *children*, around us in wonder. They're all looking a little shell-shocked but moving their personal items into the houses and smiling at each other happily enough.

"How do you move that many people at once without leaving a trace?"

I feel a Bond walk up behind us and then Atlas says, "Transporters. A *lot* of fucking Transporters. This is the most impressive thing I've ever seen."

I spin around to face him. "I thought you were going back to your very comfortable and humane prison cell?"

He smiles at me but it's not his usual warm and open grin, the day has clearly worn him down. "I went with North to see about the actual cells here and make sure they'd be able to contain my sister. I'm back to being free. North believes that I want you more than I've ever given a shit about the family business."

He spits out the last few words like they're poison on his tongue, and I pull fully away from Gabe to go to him. It's hard to see him like this, hard to think about everything he's going through while he faces that his family aren't just the enemy, but they're *his* enemies as well.

They'd all kill us in a heartbeat to further their campaign, everyone except his mom.

And Lord knows what she's going to do now that Atlas has disappeared on her entirely.

Atlas tucks his face into my neck and breathes me in a little shakily, and I try to be strong for him. I try to be everything that he was for me when I first got here and I didn't know who I could trust. I know I'm falling short, but I try.

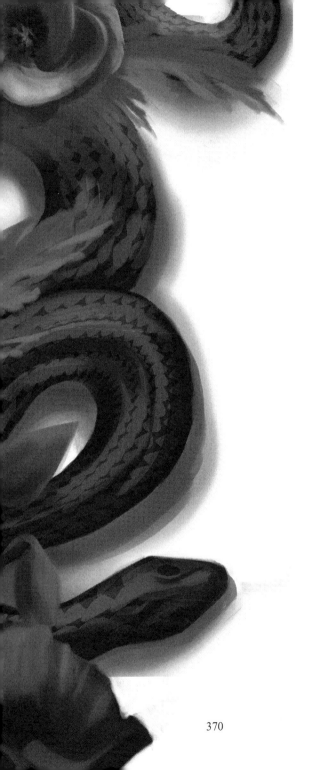

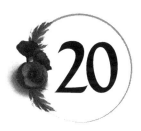

GRYPHON

After years of coming to the Sanctuary to test out the security measures, help with building the houses and setting up the facilities, stocking the stores and building an arsenal big enough to take out an attack from literally any of the world's biggest militaries, it's something else to finally be here and know that it's home.

With Oli here, it actually feels like it.

The house that North built for our Bond Group isn't ready yet, so we're in one of the smaller houses that was put aside for other council members' families, though only three have chosen to join us. There's only four bedrooms, so Gabe and Bassinger volunteer to share. Oli doesn't get one to herself, which she says she's fine with, but I know she's already getting frustrated at not having her own space on the very first day.

She doesn't breathe a word about it though, and I keep my mouth shut about what's going on in her head to the others. She already has no privacy, no need to make it worse by airing out what's going on in her head.

Two peaceful but busy days after we arrive here, I wake up with a very naked Bonded in my arms, still asleep and dreaming of nothing but warmth and comfort. She'd been reluctant to have sex in this house with us all sharing walls, and I'd only managed to persuade her by eating her out until my entire face was dripping with her cum. My shoulders were clawed up and her hand was bleeding from where she'd bitten it to stay quiet.

I don't have the heart to tell her that all of her Bonds could feel her last night. Her climax at such close proximity? Every last one of them was squirming over it, and Gabe had taken an hour-long cold shower when she'd finally passed out.

Except Nox, who left the house the second I peeled her panties off and got wasted in North's offices, where I assume he's still sleeping it off.

"Why do you look so smug?" she murmurs, her voice still rough with sleep, and I want to go for another round instantly, my dick already hard and rubbing against her pert ass.

"A man can't help it when he's made his Bonded come eight times on his tongue. I'm thinking about doing it again."

She blushes so prettily, but her eyes flick down to my mouth as she grins. "Don't you have a meeting to go to this morning? You told North you'd be leaving here at seven, it's already a quarter to. I don't think you can make me come that quickly and still get out the door in time."

I grab her chin and tilt her face up to meet my lips, kissing her deeply as my other hand slips down to her pussy and finds it still as wet as it was last night. "You're assuming that I'm going to shower, but I'm going to smell like you all fucking day, Bonded. I'm going to sit in that stupid fucking meeting with your pussy all over my face, and it'll be the only thing that gets me through the day."

She blushes again, her hips moving to grind on my hand as her breath stutters in her chest. She's so responsive, so ready to take what pleasure she wants from me and, fuck, if that isn't perfect.

She was made for me.

I have her shuddering out her release on my fingers in under a minute, whispering filth in her ear about everything I'm going to do to her when I get her next until she's writhing.

When she finally comes down from her high, I take her chin again, prying her mouth open and shoving my fingers into her mouth until she's licked them clean again. When I pull them back out, I kiss her, chasing the taste that's even better on her tongue.

I make it to the door with two minutes to spare, my boots laced up and my dick still hard as fucking nails at the sight of her spread out on my sheets. Her hair is a mess and there's still dark circles under her eyes that shouldn't be there.

I lean down before I leave to kiss her one last time, murmuring, "Go back to sleep. There's nothing you need to do until after lunch, so just get some more sleep."

She nods and lets her eyelids flutter shut, but her mind is already busy with shit to do today and I doubt she'll actually manage to do it. I send a text to Gabe to get him to leave her alone until she comes out and he cusses me out in the reply.

I can't help but feel even more smug about it.

North meets me at the front door, looking me over as his nostrils flare. He doesn't say anything until we're out of the house and pacing to his office in the next building over.

"You smell like her."

I look him dead in the eye and smirk. "Good."

He bristles, and I know that it's got nothing to do with cleanliness or decorum or jealousy over my night with our little Bonded. He doesn't want anyone else catching our Bonded's most intimate scents because he's a possessive bastard about her. He always has been, and while he's perfectly fine sharing her with the rest of her Bonds, the idea of anyone else so much as smelling her on me?

Unacceptable.

I already knew it. He's assuming I'll let anyone close enough to me to get a whiff of her. I already know what my scheduling looks like and if I put a savage enough scowl on my face, everyone will steer clear of me. I'll get to wallow in her all day, and that might just get me through until she's back in my bed, soaking my sheets and coming like a good girl for me.

When we arrive at the offices and one of the office workers approaches, North steps in front of me like a buffer. I snort at him, enjoying the fuck out of watching him have a little petty fit over this. The fact that Oli misses out on seeing this side of him half the time doesn't elude me, and I seriously consider sending her the image of it, except when I check in with her, I find that she has actually gone back to sleep. I'm not waking her for this.

I'll save it for later.

When the worker finally moves away, North snaps at me, "I'm glad you're enjoying this."

I shrug. "It's been too quiet around here. I need something to keep me amused."

"Well, go build something with Gabe. Lay some carpets. There's tiling in Oleander's bathroom that needs ripping up, that'll keep you busy."

The *tiling*. He's being a fusspot about the colors of tiles. It's going to drive us all mad. I swipe my card after he's done with his to get us both in the elevator and headed into his office. The security here is the best money can pay for. Aside from housing North's offices, there's also a bomb shelter panic room in the basement with concrete walls that are six feet thick on every side.

It could withstand Unser going off.

We know. We've tested it.

North waits until the elevator closes behind us before he starts his usual debrief, starting with the Bonded Group. "Bassinger is on his way over. He went for a run this morning and has already volunteered to help Gabe with the housing over in the third quarter. Obviously because Oleander will be there as well, but it's a good sign."

I nod and then broach my least favorite topic. "Is Nox still here? Do you need me to step in, or are we just going to… continue to let him spiral?"

North's eyes flash over to me. I'm his biggest, and only, ally when it comes to his brother and all of his issues. Our friendship had started the day North brought Nox home, and because of that, I know pretty much everything there is to know about the brothers. Every twisted, fucked-up thing.

And so long as it doesn't hurt my Bonded, I'll keep helping to manage the situation.

"He's back to drinking and training. The camp cleanup was good for him. We'll need to send him on some more missions with you to keep him level. I'm taking him leaving the house last night as a good sign. He's getting better at spotting his triggers and leaving before it becomes a problem. Just… leave him to me for now."

"If he goes after her again—"

He cuts me off, probably because he doesn't want to think about it either. "He won't. I've spoken to him."

I shake my head slowly as the doors open in front of us again and we find Nox passed out on the small couch in the corner of North's office. One of his shadows is resting over his chest and two more are lying on the floor in front of him, but they stay put as we walk over to North's desk. They watch us though, obsessively. They're waiting for the moment we dare to step towards their sleeping master.

The moment *anyone* dares.

"Did we bring a psych with us as well? Did you find the guy Sage was seeing?"

North cringes and starts his computer up, plugging in his laptop and getting all four of the screens on the desk set up. "I found him, and he's already left the country. His family decided on an extended stay in Singapore, not that I blame them."

The elevator dings again and then Bassinger steps out,

his cheeks still pink from the run, and his hands shoved into his pockets as he comes over to slump in the chair beside me.

North ignores us both for his emails for a second, scowling and muttering under his breath in a furious tone, and I take the moment to look Bassinger over. His leg is bouncing under the desk, a sign of agitation that he's struggling to hide.

I pitch my tone to be something friendly enough, which is something that he doesn't always take kindly to, and I ask, "How are you doing? The run doesn't seem to have helped."

He stares at me for a second and then says, "It's still hard for me to talk to you guys about it. I'm not used to... this sort of Bond Group dynamic. It messes with my head sometimes."

North nods from behind the desk but doesn't add anything, so I try instead. "This is the way that we keep Oli safe. Even when we don't like it, we talk about shit and we're honest. If something happens to her because we're acting like dickheads with each other, we only have ourselves to blame."

His jaw flexes a little but he nods. "I'm just still...

surprised that my father would be involved in the killing of children, but that's probably just me being naive. It's fucking with my head, but I'm dealing with it. It's not going to be a problem."

Truth.

Solid truth, and I'll respect the hell out of that sort of honesty any day of the week.

North's eyebrows inch up just a little at the admission but he nods again, taking a second before he murmurs, "It's hard to see people crossing lines that we assume would be unfathomable to ever consider, especially someone we think we know so well. Don't be too hard on yourself."

This feels like progress.

It has to be, right?

An hour later, Bassinger and I step into the elevator together, ready to be transported back to the council offices to finish up after the raid and dismantling of the Resistance camp we took out. We've already had an influx of intel thanks to the chatter in the aftermath, and Bassinger has been pivotal in recovering it. There's always the chance that he's a deep cell spy, someone sent in to us to sacrifice his own family just to get to Oli and take us all out, but I'm starting to really believe the kid.

There's something about his single-minded devotion to her at the expense of everything else in his life that is very convincing to everyone except Nox, but he's not exactly known for being reasonable about anything Bond related.

Bassinger is quiet for a moment while the elevator doors close, but once it starts moving, he clears his throat, his voice coming out steady enough. "I don't want to see my sister. I know you're probably going to try to convince me, and I get it, it makes sense to have me in there to get her talking and thinking shit but… that's my line. If it's not about Oli's safety, I'm not doing it."

I look at him and shrug. "It might come down to that. I'll talk to her and see what I can get, but if I need help with it—"

He cuts me off. "If you need it, I'll do it. If Oli needs it, I'll always do it, but not unless it comes to that."

I can respect that.

I can respect a lot of what he's said actually. If it weren't for his last name, his parents, his entire upbringing, he'd absolutely be climbing his way up to my inner circle of people I trust.

I can't do that though, not right now, and not with so much at stake.

I nod at him right as the doors open to reveal Black and Rockelle waiting there for us, both of them in full Tac gear. Heading out of the Sanctuary means needing at least three fully trained operatives per group, and there's no one I trust more than these two.

Even if they are the mouthiest assholes on my damn team.

"So we're not taking the harbinger of death this time?"

I already know Rockelle is attempting to stir shit about Oli, but I'm not going to let him. "North is dealing with the council bullshit as remotely as possible these days, so he'll be here. Or did you mean Nox? He's sleeping off a hangover."

He grins at me and shrugs it off, easy and friendly as always. "Sure, those two Death Dealers were the ones I was talking about. I've already been warned."

Bassinger stares him down. "Obviously it didn't sink in."

Black and I share a look. Bassinger is never going to make friends with the blunt and cutthroat treatment he gives everyone when Oli isn't with him, but I'm also starting to figure out that he doesn't really give a fuck either. He doesn't want friends. The weird companionship he's found himself in with Gabe seems like the only concession he's been willing to make… that and the truce he just declared with North.

Anyone outside of our Bond Group is fair game to his acid tongue.

I motion for him to step in closer to the other two so that we can get this job over and done with. Rockelle is grinning at him with an edge to it like he's itching for a fight. They're as bad as each other, and I'll need to remember to keep them apart in the future.

As we get within touching distance of each other, Black cocks his head at me before shaking it, clapping his hand onto my shoulder to transport me a little more forcefully than usual. "New cologne?"

My eyes narrow. "Don't breathe a word. I have enough shit on you to bury you."

He just smirks at me and motions like he's zipping his lips shut, which is the biggest fucking lie because the asshole just thinks everything he *would* say, which is just as effective.

He knows how to send me information, has for years, and it's been useful in our line of work, so I find him thinking in my direction. *I'd call you a degenerate but... I guess you're Bonded and it's to be expected.*

I answer out loud, "You shouldn't call me anything as your superior and definitely not in Councilman Draven's hearing."

He has been friends with North almost as long as I have been, and I don't have to say anything else for him to get what I'm saying, loud and clear. He snorts and shakes his head again. "They're both as jealous as each other, and yet neither of them have figured it out yet. Fucking hilarious."

Bassinger doesn't like any of this conversation, and the smirk he gives Black is all sorts of venomous. "How's your Bond Group treating you?"

Black has gone toe-to-toe with Nox for decades; Bassinger's shitty attitude is nothing to him. "Well, there isn't a Resistance snake in mine, so better than others for sure."

Bassinger just raises an eyebrow at him and snarks

back, "Are you so sure about that?"

No one here wants to think about the Riley and Giovanna mess we're still attempting to untangle for Sage, or what doing so is going to cost us.

Black grimaces and transports us without another word, the *pop* loud enough to ring in my eardrums and scramble my head for a second once our feet hit solid ground again. He's brought us to the underground parking space of the offices, right in front of the elevator to the basement. There's no one else around us, nothing to say that anything is happening here that we'd need to worry about, and a pit of unease starts in my gut.

It always does when things go smoothly.

I don't trust that shit at all.

As per protocol, no one else speaks or moves until I've cast my gift out to check for other Gifted around us. There's no one in the parking lot or the first three upper levels of the building. The raid has made sure of that, and when I push my gift to its limits, I only find the prisoners and other Gifted we have held down in the cells.

"We're clear. Let's get this over with."

Black nods and takes point, letting Rockelle fall behind and cover our backs. Bassigner watches their movements with keen eyes but keeps his mouth shut, following along with the rules and guidelines he's been told about coming along today.

Nox had railed hard about having him here, still so sure that he's a spy, but North and I had agreed. Whatever we need to do to get the upper hand on the Resistance, as long as it's not sacrificing innocents, then we're doing it.

Anything to get Oli clear of Silas fucking Davies.

When we make it to the lower levels and the doors of the elevator opens, Black and I both watch as Bassinger steps out and gets a good look at the cells. It feels a little like deja vu, like I'm back to a few weeks ago when Oli had been here for the first time and Carlin Meadows had gotten an eyeful of her.

Render.

Fuck, when I'd heard her spit that word at my Bonded, I didn't believe it. Not until Oli had immediately freaked the fuck out and run away like she was being chased by the devil. Every pore of her being was terrified.

Of me.

Me hearing it, me rejecting her, me telling the others and them all turning on her. My head had felt as though it was about to split from everything screaming out of my

Bonded, and every protective instinct in me kicked in. I wanted her safe and secure in my arms, a million miles away from this place, and I'd barely made it through watching the interrogations without dragging her out.

Bassigner walks slowly down the hallway, oblivious to the memories of Oli assaulting me. The Gifted inside the cells are all thin, haggard-looking men and women with blank sort of eyes. They are all fed and taken care of, but most go on hunger strikes to attempt to kill themselves.

I usually end up here forcing them to eat with my gift.

I get my head back into the game. "Any you recognize?"

Bassinger is slow and methodical as he checks them over slowly. He's taking this seriously, and I'll give him credit for that too.

He points between two of the cells. "Him. And that woman. They're both familiar, but that's it. I'd have to look through the footage to pinpoint it exactly. Well, them, and I know Carlin, but you already know that. You should kill her for what she did to Oli."

She does deserve it, she deserves a lot more than we've done to her so far, but she's still being processed for now.

One day she'll face North's nightmares, and I'll enjoy nothing more than watching her being consumed into nothingness.

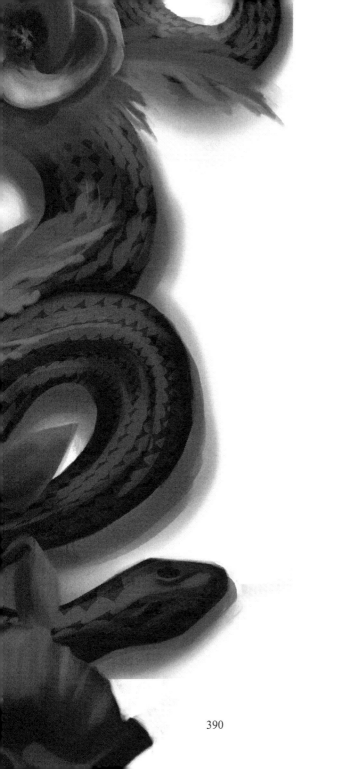

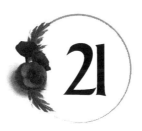

OLI

When I finally climb out of Gryphon's bed close to noon, I drag my ass into the shower and attempt to look as though I slept well and didn't have my brains eaten out by him last night. I was kind of under the impression that guys only really went down on girls to get their dicks sucked, but Gryphon just blew that theory out of the water.

I turn beet red when I think about him walking around right now, smelling like me and honestly being smug about it. Literally, my skin is glowing and hot as I brush my hair out, and the color of it looks even more bleached out, more white now than silver.

I need to do something about it before it sends me into a full spiral and my Bonded freak out about the mess my head is in.

Brutus sits by the door with me, but August is nowhere to be seen. Gryphon refuses to let them sleep on his bed, and while Brutus will sleep on the floor, under protest, to stay with me, August mostly goes back to North when he's not allowed to be all over me while I sleep. I miss him and need to go rescue him from North later.

When I leave Gryphon's room, I can feel one of my Bonds in the living room, and I find Gabe sitting there with the TV off and his phone in his hand as he scrolls aimlessly. He looks up at me and grins the moment I walk in, holding out a hand for me to take as he draws me into him.

"North had breakfast and lunch sent up for you if you're hungry. Everyone is working. I'm heading into the fifth zone to work on the houses there if you want to come with me."

I nod and give him a quick kiss, moving over to the small kitchenette to poke around in the fridge until I find the loaded steak sandwich wrapped up in there for me.

The chef and kitchen staff are all working in the huge communal food hall for now while the food supply chain starts working and people can go back to eating in their own homes. One of the many things that North is working on at all hours of the day and night. I still can barely believe that this is something he's been working on for literally ten years, and his uncle for decades before that, just to keep us all safe.

It makes me very proud to be his Bonded, and also a little guilty for not being the perfect Bond for him. I'm too much work, too hard, and too freaking emotional for the good councilman. But I can try to help out and, at the very least, not be a burden to him.

Thank God Gryphon is working this morning and not tripping over my thoughts, I'd never hear the end of it.

I grab the sandwich and take a bite as I walk back over to the couch, thanking all of my lucky stars again for the chef who was clearly blessed by the gods themselves, because this sandwich is orgasmic. Gabe smirks at the look on my face, moving a little so I can join him on the couch and then dragging the coffee table closer for me to put my plate down.

I clear my throat and attempt to look civil as I tear

into my food, murmuring around my mouthful, "How are the houses coming along down there? Are they close? I know we're struggling with occupancy."

He shrugs and shoves his phone away. "It's not so bad. The families are mostly bunked in double, but everyone has enough rooms to handle it. This place is about making do and keeping everyone safe, so mostly the lower families are just grateful to be here. The Top Tiers are giving North shit, but he's put Nox in charge of complaints, so they've all shut the fuck up for now. His attitude does come in handy for some situations."

I snort with laughter at the thought of Nox dealing with those spoiled assholes. "I'm sure he's loving the work too. Telling people how pathetic and useless they are is kind of his superpower."

Gabe pulls a face and takes the other half of the sandwich when I offer it to him. There's so many different fillings in it that I can only manage half, and what a beautiful thing that is.

"He's been worried about North, so he offered to help the best way he knows how. We all are. Atlas and Gryphon are working through the Resistance stuff, I'm helping with the buildings, and you're—"

I cut him off. "I'm sleeping in and being hand-delivered food by men who have better things to do. I might go crazy here, Gabe. I can't sit on my ass doing nothing just because my Bonds would prefer to keep me somewhere safe at all times. I can't be useless."

He scowls back at me. "You took out another camp and then came back here to recover from it. Now we're going to go build some shit. That's helping out, Bond. If you have anything else you want to do instead, just tell me and we'll go find North."

The problem is that I don't have anything else I can do because I'm a high school drop out who has only ever worked as a damn waitress. I guess I could go work in the kitchens and help feed people, that's important work. But then North would move security around so I have a TacTeam operative with me, and I don't want to move people away from other areas just to babysit me.

So building with Gabe it is.

I wash up my plate and grab a Coke out of the fridge to take over to the building sites. I'd love a coffee, but I feel like I've taken up too much of Gabe's morning already, so the Coke will have to do. Gabe pulls on a set of work boots and pulls out a brand new pair for me as well, grinning at me when I sputter out a thank you. It always catches me off-guard when my Bonds buy me things, even just basic necessities, and it takes me a minute to get them laced up properly. They feel like clown shoes on me, big and bulky, but I'd rather have the protection because there's nothing quite like the pain of a broken toe.

I'm already wearing jeans and one of Gabe's plaid work shirts over a tank top, like a dress-up doll of what a Builder Barbie would look like. It's funny, and when Gabe gets a proper look at my whole outfit, he cackles at me, taking a photo that I ham it up in.

When we leave the house on foot, he catches my hand in his and threads our fingers together, sliding on a pair of aviators that make his look unbearably cool. Ridiculously hot too, like almost too much to freaking look at.

How can I feel this way about more than one man? I do, and I don't feel guilty about it either. I just feel like maybe we need to head back into the house for a quick minute.

Fuck.

Right, distraction. I need one and quick. "I'm dying my hair again. I'm thinking hot pink. Or maybe some lime green streaks. Which do you like better?"

Gabe pulls a face at me. "I thought you were good with North now; who are you trying to piss off with that choice?"

I roll my eyes at him and make kissy noises at Brutus until he comes to walk behind me, butting into the backs of my thighs with his little comfort nudging that he does. He's always extra affectionate in the mornings, as though me sleeping and not being awake to love on him makes the nights unbearable. "No one. I hate the silver, and now it's almost freaking white. Black won't stay in, I've tried it before. The purple washed out fast, but at least it stuck around for a few days. I just... don't want to look at the white for a few days. Maybe I should just shave it off."

He looks incredibly alarmed and starts rummaging around in his pockets for his phone in a very obvious display of calling in backup. It's almost comical and, with extreme effort, I keep my face straight as I watch him fumble around for words.

"I don't think you need to do that—I mean, you can do whatever you want, obviously, it's your hair but—pink is good."

He gives me a shaky smile, tapping on his phone

without even looking at the screen, and I start counting, because he's about as obvious as a smack in the face. Honestly, if it wasn't so freaking funny, I'd be chewing him out for it.

Don't you dare shave your head. I don't care what color your hair is, but do not shave it.

I giggle at North's stern tone and shake my head at Gabe, who doesn't even attempt to look innocent.

"You're lucky you're hot, Ardern, because you're also a total freaking narc."

He shrugs. "I work with what I have, and you can't deny that North is the best person to convince you to do *anything*. If being an asshole is Nox's superpower, then this is his brother's."

It's true, and when Gryphon chimes in, he goes for a very different and effective tactic, one I'm not going to tell Gabe about because I don't need him setting Gryphon on me more regularly.

What am I going to wrap around my fist when I fuck you from behind if you so much as trim it? You'd look good with the pink, the purple was hot too. Just don't touch the length.

Well.

That sounds very reasonable.

Watching Gabe help with the construction is a great way to spend the afternoon, and I can see why this is where he's most useful. He's strong, smart as hell, and knows exactly what the builders need when they start with the framing on the new structure. There's six other houses on this street in various stages of being built at the moment, and I help with the one that is at the lock-up stage, carrying in supplies and holding up giant sheets of drywall for the guys working there.

At first they all eye me like I'm just there to get in their way, but after a couple of hours of good, honest work, they're including me in their stories and joking around. It's hard, but it clears my brain out to actually be helping out. By the time Gabe comes looking for me, I'm up on a ladder having a go at one of the nail guns and whooping with joy when I actually get a piece of the ceiling fixed in place without any new holes in my fingers or hands.

He grins at me like I'm the sun, warming him right down to his core.

I stare back at him the same way, both of us looking like sappy idiots in love. I know this for sure because Elliot, the foreman, tells me so with a hell of a lot of snark in his old, gravelly tone.

"I'm not sure if you noticed, but she's my Bond. There'd be something majorly fucking wrong if I wasn't a sappy shit over her. Besides, look at her with all that dirt over her and that big grin. Can't blame me," Gabe drawls. Elliot waves us both off for the night, demanding we show up on time tomorrow *morning*.

"No promises. I'm a delicate princess about my sleep," Gabe calls back, draping his arm over my shoulders. He's just as dirty and sweaty as I am, so I don't feel self-conscious of how bad I must smell.

We walk together through the almost empty streets, it's mostly dirt and loose gravel on this side of the town because the houses are not move-in ready yet. Eventually, there'll be cars and all sorts of vehicles here, but we're not quite at that point yet. The logistics of starting a whole new town and community makes my head hurt. I can't think about it too much without wanting to puke on North's behalf.

How is money going to work here?

Job allocation, education, what do we do about crime and neighborhood disputes? I'm fairly certain we're still in the States, but does the government know about this place? Taxes?

Too much for me right now.

So I focus on the small stuff, the questions I can ask and get simple answers for instead. "How did you learn how to build houses? Or are you just a natural at it?"

He scoffs at me. "I'm not sure there's any such thing as being a natural at framing, but my dad was a partner in the family construction company. My great-grandfather started it, and it was sort of a tradition that all of the family worked there during the summers. My dad took over the business side of it, but one of my uncles is still on the tools. He's finishing a job in Nevada and then heading over here, but his family is here. What's left of it, I mean."

I grimace, that seems to be a recurring theme with everyone here in the Sanctuary. Loss of family, loss of Bonds, loss of the people that matter most to us all.

He hesitates for a second and then asks, "What did your family do? Before the accident?"

It throws me for a second, but of course he'd ask

about my family. Of course he'd be interested. We're Bonds, and I've told him basically nothing about my life before the Resistance took me. Very, very little.

"We mostly moved a lot. I didn't understand why but now—now I'm pretty sure that Davies knew about me. I think my parents were on the run to keep him away from me. But my father, my biological father, he did something with the stock market. Andrew was an engineer; he ran a business remotely and always had his computer with him while he did consulting work. Vincenzo was once a chef, but gave it up to stay home with me and mom. He was a Neuro and spent a lot of time training me on how to manage my emotions and my bond. My mom… I don't actually know what she once did. I never asked."

My voice breaks a little as I say that and his arm tightens around me, bundling me into his warmth a little closer. "You were a kid. You didn't get the time to grow up and ask her all the shit you wanted to. Nothing to feel guilty about, Bond."

I nod, but it's there nonetheless. It always will be.

When we get back to the house, I duck into North's room to use his bathroom. No one else is home yet, and when Gabe offers to grab dinner for us both, I shake my head.

"I want to find North. It's Nox's night tonight, and I need to… make sure it's going to be okay. I always do."

Gabe scowls but nods, walking me over to North's offices without another word. He sees me all the way to the elevator before kissing me goodbye soundly. It's only been two days since I slept in his bed, but without being Bonded, it still feels like an age.

I'm not sure the ache will ever really go away. I'm doomed to feel incomplete forever.

I scan my card to get access to North's level and when the elevator doors open back up straight into North's office, he's on the phone, frowning and rustling papers in a very frustrated-looking way. He glances up at me and his frown eases a little. August comes out from behind him and bounds over to me joyfully.

I stoop down to give him scratches, cooing at him in a hushed tone so I don't interrupt the phone call, but North's tone gets snappier as it goes on, clearly trying to get it over with so he can speak with me.

I feel bad for interrupting, but not quite enough to leave. I've barely seen him since we got here, and I'm already missing those long days of being trapped in his bed in the post-Bonding haze.

"Councilman Rockelle, I'm done for the evening. We can get back to this tomorrow. I'm not having another late night. Even I have limits."

When I take a seat on the other side of his desk, August tucks his head into my lap as he sits on my feet, a weightless bundle of smoke that is still comforting as hell. North glances up at me again and scowls at the distance between us, pushing his seat back a little and then motioning to his lap like he really expects me to get up and climb onto him, no matter that he's on the phone doing important councilman things.

Well.

That's exactly what I do.

The frown melts right off of his face as my ass settles in his lap, his hand closing around my thigh to pull me right into his body. I almost make embarrassingly happy noises about being with him again.

I'm not sure Councilman Rockelle would like that.

I lean forward to bury my nose in his neck and North hangs up on the councilman, throwing his phone down onto the desk and leaning further back in his chair and winding his arms tightly around me until I can barely breathe.

"I'm quitting the council. I can't keep playing the docile role and being kept away from you."

I laugh into his neck, more breath than noise, kissing the skin behind his ear as I murmur, "We both know you'd be bored in under a minute… or I'd run away. I can't take the full force of all of your bossiness."

He huffs and then groans. "The Council should be about doing what's right for the community, not arguing about what to name things and how many lobster tails each family should be allocated each fucking week."

I pull back from him a little to make a face. "Seriously? That's what the Councilman is talking your ear off about? Tell him to come build houses with Gabe, Elliot, and I. We'll have him too busy to worry about stupid things. Can I get a nail gun? Is there room in the budget for that?"

He raises an eyebrow at me and then rubs a hand over his eyes. "Of course they gave you a high powered weapon to play with, because that's the latest nightmare I need to occupy myself with."

He genuinely looks like he's about to start yelling at people, so I attempt to distract him and save Elliot. "So you're working overtime on lobster tails and names?

Should I be leaving you alone more? Sleeping elsewhere so you're not distracted?"

He doesn't move his hand from his eyes as he drawls, "Wherever you sneak off to on my nights, I'll just come to get you. If you want me to fuck you on Atlas' sheets while he watches and sees exactly what he's missing out on, then go right ahead, Bonded."

My cheeks heat and he knows he's managed to embarrass me a little, his casual and filthy flirting is a little harder to wrap my head around than Gryphon's. I'm not sure why, but when he says *fuck,* my knees go a little weak.

His nostrils flare and he glances down at me, a dark ring circling the outer rim of his irises like he's desperately holding on to his control. "Do you want me to fuck you here instead? You smell like sex."

I take a deep breath, but all I smell is his very expensive cologne, the musky undertones of it like an aphrodisiac to me now that I know what his cock tastes like. I swipe my tongue over my bottom lip before I say, "Let's just say it's a good thing you can't read my mind like Gryphon can. You'd know way too many embarrassing things about me now."

His eyes drop down to my lips and he murmurs back, "If it were anyone else's night tonight, I'd spread you out on this desk and fuck you until you couldn't walk straight."

I swallow and nod. We both know that's not a good idea on Nox's nights. Not that I know exactly why, but I know enough about his careful lines with his brother to understand that he won't cross it. I'm not sure if it's for my safety or Nox's, but I'll play along.

I'm getting awfully good at it.

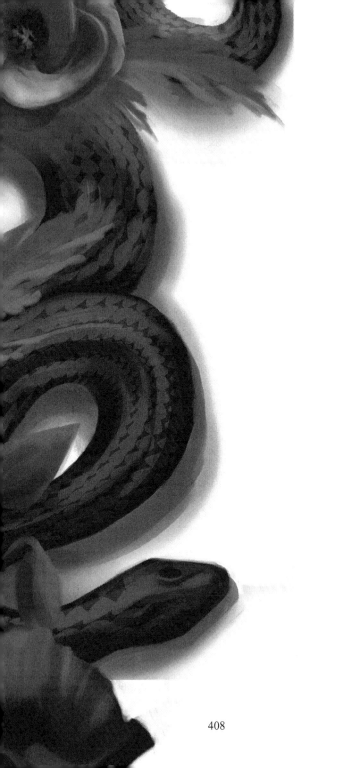

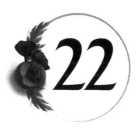

NOX

The bedroom is quiet as I slip in, trying not to bleed everywhere as I do. The late night training sessions that have taken over from my late night drinking sessions aren't any easier on my body, and blood is still pouring out of my nose from the lucky shot Black had gotten in.

My knuckles are a bloodied, raw mess from the beating he'd gotten in return.

He's going back to his rooms with access to the best Healer of our generation, so I don't feel an ounce of guilt. Azrael lifts his head from my bed, and I feel his relief in my presence. North's creature is there as well and when

I scowl at him and gesture to the door, I can feel my brother's frustration. I don't need a fucking babysitter. If he wants me to let the girl sleep here, then he'll have to just trust that she'll make it out alive.

The creature leaves, his legs being snapped at by Rahab, who is my most savage creature. I have to step between them to make sure they don't wake the girl up with their childish bickering.

I move slowly into the space, my eyes shifting so that I can see clearly. There's nothing out of place. There never is when she comes here. She just slips into the bed and sleeps on my pillow, burying into the scents of me as though they're the only thing keeping her heart beating.

It's strangely respectful, and more than I've ever offered her in return.

If I didn't know my brother better than he knows himself, I might guess that he'd told her. Even something small, just a tiny detail about the absolute mess that he calls a brother, but he wouldn't.

He never even told William, his closest blood relative after our father was put to death. No, I was the one to spill out the truth to him in one of my episodes. I'd feel a little more self-loathing about that moment but I was nine, and there's been enough therapy poured over my soul by now that I'm past that phase of my life.

Now I just try to forget it all, drink it out or fight until the pain replaces the memories.

Once I get out of the Tac gear I'd worn down to training, a shirt and utility pants, I find an old towel to wipe the blood away from myself. As I loosen my muscles and take some deep breaths, my creatures slowly pour out of me. Mephis stops at my feet and stays with me, even as the others all come out and spread out across the room. I shouldn't be surprised that more of them are adopting the form of puppies and other sweet creatures.

They all want her to love them.

It's sickening.

Literally, my gut turns at the sight of them all trying to fight their way onto the bed to be near her. They're fierce enough with it that she sighs and rolls in her sleep, her hair spilling out of the tie she had it in and falling out over my pillows in an enticing way.

I look away and get to pulling a pair of sweats on, digging through the small collection I'd brought with us until I find one of the soft tees to throw on with it. They're the only ones I like sleeping in and, sure enough, they've become the girl's favorite to steal from me as well.

I rub a hand over Mephis' head, ruffling his ears a little and enjoying the way he preens under my attention. Both Mephis and Rahab wait for me to decide where I'm going to sleep before they move, always staying close to my side. As much as they also want the girl, they would never leave me for her.

I *should* sleep on the couch a safe distance from her. It's comfortable enough. I should, but the bed is too tempting, and it's not like I haven't already slept in it with her before.

Always when I'm sure she's out cold and only on rare occasions.

It's easier to do now that I've spoken to her bond. Now that I know exactly what it wants from me and told it what it can't have, we've reached an agreement between the two of us and, sure enough, when I slide between the sheets, the girl's eyes are open.

But the bond is who stares back at me.

I stare back at it, not really in the mood to talk, and it doesn't move towards me. It knows better.

When Mephis crawls up to slip between us, the bond finally speaks. "Do you need the pain to sleep? I don't like it."

I reach up to press a finger against my nose and enjoy the throbbing pain of it. "I don't need it. It's cleared my head already. I'm fine now."

Her gift floods me instantly and the pain disappears all at once. There'll be questions tomorrow from Gryph and Black about where the injuries went, and with the girl having no recollection, it'll be harder to dodge them, so I'll need to find work away from them for a few days.

Avoiding them all has become a great skill for me, keenly honed.

As I roll onto my back and attempt to get comfortable now that I'm not babying sore points, the bond speaks again. "They're coming. They won't leave us alone."

I nod up at the ceiling. "Of course. They'd be stupid to leave someone like you behind enemy lines."

She is quiet for a moment and then says, "And you? When they find out about you, what do you think they'll do to get their hands on a dark god like you?"

Dark god.

It is obsessed with that line of thinking, but I've spent a long time trying to avoid the other being who shares my skin. North might be worried about the creatures, but I've always known it's the voice, the other soul, that's the real thing to be feared.

I know our bonds are not like the others.

"Let me speak to him. I miss him."

I side-eye the bond but it hasn't moved, it hasn't crossed any of my very carefully established boundaries.

It never does.

I'm the one who breaks things, not the bond trapped in the girl who looks as though she was dragged out of my deepest, darkest fantasies and splayed out over my pillows.

I don't trust either of them. "If you two Bond while she sleeps, they'll kill me, you know. They'll never believe that I didn't do it."

The bond smirks slowly, looking somehow older than the nineteen-year-old's face it's wearing. "I'll be on my best behavior. Let me have him for a little while. Just sleep and leave us to it."

I shouldn't, but my own bond wakes up from the darkest recesses of my mind to let me know that he wants to speak.

No fucking. North will kill us both.

My bond prickles at the ruling but answers, *No*

Bonding. I want my Bond for a night.

It's reckless, but I let go of my control and leave them to their reunion. I try to stick around enough to at least know what they're doing, but my bond blocks me out so they can be left alone.

I wake, hours later and only just before dawn, with the girl splayed out over my chest and her nose pressed against my neck, my heart thumping the second I come to and feel her there.

The only reason I don't throw her across the room to get her the fuck off of me is because I don't want to have to explain to any of them why I'm in the bed.

I manage to get her back onto her pillows and the bed straightened up before I lurch into the bathroom and get the shower running to cover the sounds of my retching. Once that part is over with, I climb under the hot spray still in my clothes. I can't stand the sight of myself right now, not the scars or the reaction to waking up with her on top of me that hasn't been deterred by the vomiting.

Rahab sits at the bottom of the shower, the water moving through his body as though he were a ghost, and Mephis keeps watch at the door. His head sticks through the solid wood every now and then to see what's happening in there.

Gryph comes to collect the girl while I'm scrubbing my hair. He scowls at the bathroom door and Mephis when she mentions needing the bathroom, but leads her out to use his before they train. I should feel bad. I should have some level of empathy for how my fucked-up brain ruins everything, but I can't.

I'm too busy trying to scrub her off of me before I completely lose my fucking mind.

"What happened to you? Wasn't Oleander supposed to be in with you last night? You look like shit."

I don't stop to speak to him on my way to the coffee pot, picking up the biggest cup in the collection and pouring out the black liquid until it hits the rim. The bonds obviously spent the entire night speaking to each other, and while my mind 'slept', my body did not.

North's new office looks exactly like his old one layout-wise, but with none of his usual decadent luxury. I'm sure if we're here for long enough, he'll find a way to get some marble installed in here.

"Nox? Do I need to go find my Bonded and check if she's okay?"

I send him a dark look. "Sleeping on a couch so that *your* Bonded can get what she needs isn't very restful. If you're so desperate to pant after her, then I'm not stopping you. Go be pathetic elsewhere."

His eyes flash black at me for a split second, a tiny slip of his control, and I smirk at him. I will never not enjoy watching him crumble over a little girl made of poison.

How the mighty fall. It really is pathetic.

"Stop taking your bad mood out on me. If you want the day off to hole up with your books, then just say it. No one is forcing you to be here."

Ah, but he's wrong about that. I'd had to open up all three of the windows in my room to attempt to air it out and get her sweet smell out of there. My bond refused to let me change the sheets, it threw a bitch fit over it if I'm being honest, so I was forced to just get rid of the rest of it as much as possible.

I'm going to have to drink tonight. The only way I'll get through sleeping in there is if I'm wasted, and for once, my bond agrees with me.

"The water supply has been compromised."

My eyes snap up from my cup of coffee to meet North's scowl. He nods at me and continues, "There are only two points of the line that aren't covered by security, it had to happen there. The filtration system picked up the foreign bacterias there and automatically shut down. Sawyer was woken by the alarms and called me at seven. He's already been through what footage we have, but it looks like there's someone living here that is a plant."

I curse under my breath. We'd always known it wasn't just possible, but probable that we'd be bringing a sympathizer with us.

"Any guesses on who it was?"

North rounds the table and slides a tablet towards me with a list of names on it. "These are the people who weren't in their beds at that time. Sawyer has been slowly tracing their movements, but it's a big job for one man, even a skilled Technokinetic. We are very lucky to have him. We need to recruit another."

Easier said than done. Technos are rare. Second only to Renders and Death Dealers, we've somehow managed to start this little community with a very special set of skills. A Shifter who can take any form and an insanely strong Neuro with the ability to sniff out lies also helps immensely.

Indestructible Boy can still disappear for all I care.

North takes a seat in his chair and opens up his laptop, frowning at the screen like he's just been assaulted by the onslaught of bullshit there. I have no doubt that he's being harassed by the remaining members of the Council and the other Top Tier families who want him to deal with their problems even though they refused to come here with the lower families.

Scum, the lot of them.

I memorize the list of names and say, "I'll look into it. I can set up creatures in the blind spots until we have them covered with cams."

North nods and clicks around on the keyboard without looking up at me. "We need to go on a supply run as well. Get bottled water to get us through until the clean out happens."

I nod, sipping at my coffee again.

The door swings open and Gryph stalks through, jerky in his movements, like he's frustrated. I would've thought a morning on the mats with the girl would've fixed that, but apparently not.

He takes one look at me and says, "Oli healed you."

It's not a question and I'm careful with my answer. "She was asleep when it happened, but yes, she healed me."

Gryph nods, hearing the truth in what I'd chosen to say, and it's only when he turns to the coffee pot that North shoots me a look. He doesn't need to be a Neuro to hear what I'm not saying. He's good about keeping Gryph out of it though, ever the loyal brother.

I don't really give a shit though.

"Her bond spoke to me. I said it could heal me if it needed to. That's it, brother. That's what happened. Your Bonded won't remember it, and I never attempted to touch either of them."

He doesn't look at Gryph, but when he doesn't interrupt to call out a lie, North nods and gets back to whatever he's doing on the computer.

"Who's going on the supply run? If there's a plant, then we can't all go."

North shrugs. "You and Gabe can stay. You can keep looking for the plant, and Gabe can keep going with the building. He's better than any of the rest of us at it, and he's a good backup for you."

Gryph nods and takes the list from me, looking it over. "Half of these names are lower families who are training with me in the mornings. I can give Sawyer some ideas on where to look for them to rule them out."

North nods and then pauses, letting out a slow breath. "Show them to Atlas. The list and then point out the people to him. See if anything rings a bell."

Over my dead body. "No. Absolutely not. I'm not going to give what little information we do have to someone we know is a part of the Resistance."

Gryph and North share a look, but I shake my head at both of them. I don't care what they say, I don't care if he's part of the Bond Group, he's a fucking Bassinger.

He was the first sign of the poison the girl is.

"I'll take care of it myself, so leave him out of it. I'll have the sympathizer by the end of the week."

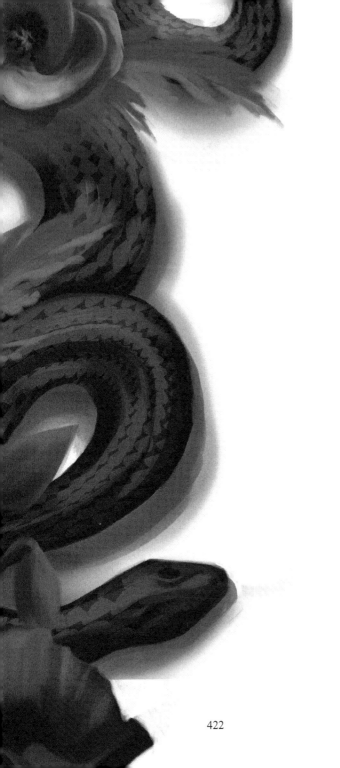

422

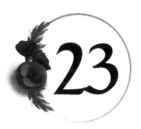

OLI

As much as building houses is actually fun and rewarding, going on a supply run with three of my Bonds is exactly what I need right about now.

I'd slept in Nox's room, and even though I'd gotten in a solid eight hours of sleep, I'd woken up feeling as though a truck had backed over my decaying corpse, so I chalk it up to an uncomfortable atmosphere and get to training with Gryphon when he comes for me.

An hour later, North arrives, not yet in his suit, to tell us about the water contamination issue. It's a little concerning because I'd showered and already drunk a coffee brewed with that water but as far as Sawyer can tell, the contamination happened between six and seven in the morning, so I should be safe.

North and Gryphon still drag me to Felix for a check up, just to be sure. I point out that Gryphon also drank the coffee, but neither of them give a shit about that. Felix, who was asleep when we showed up to the house he's sharing with his Bond Group, Sawyer, and Grey, slaps a very gentle but tired hand over mine for half a second before declaring me fine and stomps back to bed, still wearing nothing but a pair of haphazardly shoved on boxer shorts.

Sage pokes her head out of the room but when I tell her I'm fine, she stumbles back to bed without a word, still half asleep and not coherent enough yet to form words.

I chew North and Gryphon both out using our mind connection as we leave, but neither of them seem to care.

"Someone who knows our morning routines did it. They know that you're an early riser," North says, pulling his sweater off and shoving it over my head. It's still warm enough, even in my gym gear of a tank top and a pair of shorts, but Gryphon helps him to straighten it over

424

me until I'm covered to my knees.

I don't get why he's trying to cover me up until I see the hordes of workmen walking along in the opposite direction, all of them waving or tipping their heads respectfully at North, who I'm sure is absolutely thrilled to be wearing nothing but sweatpants right now.

Gryphon shakes his head slowly, grabbing my hand when I lose my balance a little on some loose gravel. "It was a test. The Resistance don't actually want Oli dead. They want to know how secure this place is and what we have in the way of failsafes. They'll be watching our reactions to things and how we pivot when they attack, even on smaller scales like this."

I scoff at them. "Well, they've learned that you both panic and find me a Healer, and if they want me alive, then they'll be extra pleased about that."

Gryphon shrugs again, refusing to let go of my hand as he directs me up the path to our house and says, "This is the one time I'm fine with doing exactly what those assholes want. Safety above ego, always."

I nod and wait for North to get the door open, stumbling over my feet into the house and trying not to get frustrated at the fact that Gabe leaves his shoes at the door. North doesn't give out the same courtesy and curses under his breath, striding off to snap at him and wake my poor Bond up.

Living in such close quarters is harder than any of us thought, and there are a lot of alpha males in one spot here.

"Stop worrying about it. It's not your problem to deal with, and they've had years to figure out a friendship that you have no responsibility over," Gryphon murmurs, directing me over to the breakfast bar in the kitchen and helping me up onto the stool.

I nod and tuck my arms around myself, taking a deep and calming breath of North's scent on the sweater before propping my chin up on my fist as I watch Gryphon move around the kitchen. He's still wearing his gym gear and I get to enjoy the flexing of his arms and shoulders in his harshly cut out tank top. I barely notice that he's getting out frying pans and all of the fixings for scrambled eggs and bacon. It's only when he slides the plate across to me, that I realize he's made us both breakfast.

I stare down at it for a second and then back up to where he's shaking his head at me. "I'm not the chef, but I can make eggs. I worked in the cafe with Kyrie for a few years during college, they'll be edible at the very least."

I blush a little and grab the knife and fork he's also slid across the counter to me. "I'm sure they're delicious. I was more shocked that we have the food. I thought we weren't at the rationing stage yet?"

He shrugs and digs in to his own plate. "We're not. I grabbed them when I had to go into the Council offices. There's occasionally perks to dealing with the Resistance assholes we bring back here."

I nod and eat along with him, impressed as hell that he not only cooked them to the perfect consistency but he seasoned them well too. They're freaking great eggs.

"I didn't think we got any prisoners? I thought my bond took the entire camp out."

He nods, his mouth full, and waits until he's swallowed before replying, "It did. These were those we'd grabbed and transported out before you joined the fight. We got a handful, a few higher ranking Gifted so that was helpful."

I nod and North stalks through the kitchen, his hair still a little sleep rumpled where he hasn't bothered fixing it too much, but his suit makes him look far more like himself. He nods at Gryphon and then swoops down to give me a kiss, snapping his fingers at August who appears at my side obediently. The change in their relationship has been dramatic since I spoke with his bond. I've noticed that even when August returns to him, North will mostly leave him out to guard whatever space he is in.

It makes me fall for him just a little more every time I see it.

"Stay with one of the Bonds at all times today until we get this under control."

I nod, because I was already planning on it, and let him kiss me again as his hand cradles the back of my head possessively. When he straightens, he shares one last look with Gryphon and then he's gone, out the door and dealing with the newest crisis here.

I get back to my plate of delicious eggs and to the conversation with Gryphon. There's too much I want to know about the happenings of the Resistance. "Have you gotten anything useful from the people you took back yet? Did Atlas know anyone?"

He nods and scrapes the last of his eggs onto his fork, still standing in the kitchen like he can't even take the time to sit down. Thanks to North crashing our training session, we're over an hour earlier than we usually are, but he's moving like he's halfway out the door already.

Before he answers my questions, he cocks his head as his eyes flash, his gift reaching out to check where Atlas is. When he finds him sleeping away, he murmurs to me, "Bassinger's sister is a mess. I've spent two days sifting through her memories, but the inside of her head is like looking in one of those mirrors at a sideshow. The world through her eyes is distorted and misshapen. Growing up in Resistance propaganda and then having four Bonds with the same opinions? She's... a mess. She's also being abused by most of her Bonded, physical and mental abuse. That isn't uncommon in the families from the East Coast Gifted community, but the fact that her parents both know about it and do nothing for her is fucking disgusting."

My heart breaks a little more for Atlas, the stuff he didn't want to have to tell me but that he was willing to if it meant I'd believe him. It feels a little bit wrong to be talking about it with Gryphon, but he's also my Bonded and I know this is weighing on him too. Everything he has to see and experience in his work as a TacTeam leader, it's a heavy load to carry.

Isn't it exactly my job to help lighten the load?

"I wouldn't ask you to, Bonded. I would never put too much of this shit on you, your own burdens are heavy enough. I'm heading into North's offices to sort out what we're doing about the water issue. You just get on with your day the same way you would normally. Just keep Bassinger and Gabe with you at all times, okay?"

I nod and grab his plate, hip bumping him out of the way as I load them and the other dishes into the dishwasher. He kisses me soundly and heads off to get dressed for the day, and I enjoy the view of his ass in those shorts the whole damn way.

I almost forget and climb into the shower when Gryphon leaves, but instead I text Sage and apologize about the rude early morning wake up. She gets back to me straight away, calling me to say that she's totally fine about it because she's the best and we spend a good hour on the phone.

Mostly gossiping about Bonds, which is annoyingly fun.

When we get to the fun shit, I break Sage's poor brain

with my own little updates, and it's the funniest freaking thing. "Both of them at the same time?! Oleander Fallows! That feels… scandalous. And they were just…fine with that?"

I snort and prop the phone up on my shoulder. "Well, it's not like I suggested it! I was more… convinced that it was a good idea. Listen, once the Bonded ones start having creative ideas, you're going to be swept up into crazy shit that no one warns you about. We might need other friends in Bonded Groups, just for, like, a heads up for this shit. It's not like we can just ask your parents—"

She makes a gagging noise and cuts me off with a squeal. "Shut your mouth right now! I do not want to think about my parents in an orgy. Fuck, I could vomit. Why would you even say that? They've only done it twice, just for me and Sawyer. That's it! Gross."

I hear Sawyer's dramatics in the background, cussing her out for so much as talking about something so gross, and I cackle at them both. They're such typical siblings in a really normal family dynamic, now that her family isn't being obnoxious to her about shit outside of her control, and it's nice to just experience it vicariously through them both for a minute.

Sage clears her throat. "Okay, so now that I need my entire brain dipped in bleach, what is the plan for today's incident? Are you going to help out with whatever they do about it?"

I flop back onto Gryphon's bed, tucking my nose into his pillow a little bit just to get one last whiff of him before I get on with my day. "No news yet. There's a meeting happening now about it, but I've just been told to stick with Gabe and Atlas today."

Sage hums down the line. "Kieran said the same to me. He wants me with someone in this house at all times."

I could make a joke about possessive, overprotective Bonds, but there's a knock at the door and then Atlas' head is poking through. "Shore called, we're heading out of the Sanctuary on a run. You're coming with… as long as you want to."

Hell yeah I do. "Gotta go, Sage. I'll call you when I get home."

I bounce off of the bed and straight into Atlas' arms. He looks tired, he has since we got back from the camps with his sister in our custody, but he grins down at me.

"I don't think your bond is going to be needed much today. I hope you're not bounding around because you think it's going to be… fed."

I snort at his teasing, because I already know he's not actually serious, and shrug. "You never know, one of the Tac personnel could piss me off and end up as lunch."

He chuckles at me as we get to the front door together, pulling on shoes and grabbing jackets. "I know which ones I'm voting for. Rockelle is a fucking dickhead and deserves his soul to be gobbled up."

I shrug with a smirk, but I already know that he's one of Gryphon's closest friends and trusted personnel, so even with his smart mouth and irreverent jokes, he's safe for now.

We don't have enough trusted people in our circle as it is. I can't take out the few we do have.

We make our way over to North's offices, but the crowds of Tac operatives are waiting outside, already dressed and fully armed. There's no way I'm going to be allowed to go out in the jeans and sweater I'm currently wearing, but I guess there's no way to get used to the gear unless you wear it.

I just feel like some sort of fraud when I'm in it, like a civilian pretending to be a superhero.

Kieran spots us both coming and snaps at the

stragglers of the group to get out of our way until we can make it into the building. There's only a handful of people waiting around in the foyer, all of them the higher-up operatives, and I get the feeling they're waiting on my Bonded so we can head out.

We stop when we get to Kieran, happy to wait with him for now. He's looking good, about a million times better than when we were rescued from the camps, and I have to fight to keep the smirk off of my face.

I can't help but comment about it, messing around a little with him because I feel like we're practically family now that he's watched me get carved up by the most terrifying man in the world. "Bonded life treating you well?"

He raises an eyebrow at me, his face completely straight as he says, "About as well as Gryphon's new cologne is faring for him, yes."

It takes me a second to get what he's saying, and then I want to die a little. Scratch that, I want to die a whole lot.

I groan and bury my face into my hands as though I can disappear if no one can make eye contact with me anymore. "I'm going to murder him, right after I find a nice hole to die in."

Kieran shrugs at me and eyes the murderous look that Atlas gives him for so much as mentioning something that embarrasses me, though he doesn't really have a clue as to why I'm dying. Thank God, because Kieran knowing is bad enough.

Freaking Bonded.

When the elevator chimes and opens up to reveal North and Gryphon, I turn my back on the asshole and cross my arms, in full shameful pout mode and giving zero fucks about it. August bounds over and sits at my feet, looking up at me with his perfect void eyes as though he can tell I'm ready to stab someone.

"You're in deep shit," Kieran drawls and Gryphon scowls back at him, striding over to me like he can fix this, but I'm already so freaking embarrassed that I don't want to discuss it anymore. It was hot as fuck at the time but now, standing around here thinking about it? No, thanks.

Kill me.

"Something about cologne," Atlas snarks, grabbing my hand tugging me away from them both, "Come on, Sweetness. We'll go get changed so that we can get out of here."

We turn our back on them as North snarls at Gryphon in a very non-Draven way. Nope, I glance back just to check that his bond hasn't burst out of him in the middle of the freaking foyer, but I just find both of my Bonded squaring off about me.

Atlas drags me into one of the gear rooms, joining me in the women's area once he's grabbed his own stuff, and then he flicks the lock so we won't get anyone walking in on us. I'm still too far in my own head to give a shit about changing together and when I pull my sweater and shirt off, he doesn't bat an eye, just gets to changing as well.

My scent, all over Gryphon while he went about his day.

I blink back into myself, coming face-to-bare-chest with Atlas and, man, is it a good sight. I'm not sure if his gift makes him extra cut or if he's kept up a brutal training regime without me knowing, but he is cut. Like, professional bodybuilder levels of cut, and the delicious looking V that draws my eyes down to the top of his jeans looks incredibly inviting.

I clear my throat, mostly to attempt to find my voice, but it gets his attention. Atlas mistakes my nervous actions for me stressing over Gryphon and shakes his head at me. "I know enough to make a guess about it, Sweetness. Don't try to explain it. I already want to tear his arms off and shove them up his ass for having everything I want. I don't need any more details."

I blush again and duck my head as I nod. "I don't think—I don't feel any stronger. I think maybe you were right."

His eyebrows shoot up and I bite at my lip, unbuttoning my jeans and watching as he swallows, his eyes dropping down to follow their path down my legs. I'm wearing a simple black thong, nothing flashy or anything, but it might as well be crotchless, lacy lingerie for how he reacts to the sight of me. His legs buckle a little and he takes a step forward, taking a deep breath and groaning softly like he's been wounded.

I could fuck him right here. Bond with him and take him for my own. Shit, is this really me thinking this?! Not my horny bond? Nope, it's me practically dripping for him in a very inopportune moment.

His eyes flare and flash white for a second, returning to the clear green in an instant as he reins himself in. "Don't tease, Sweetness. Not when there's a whole fucking horde of Tac operatives out there listening, because I'll do a helluva lot worse than Shore ever did. Fuck, the thought of them all out there listening to me Bond with you, it's too tempting."

My voice is barely more than a rasp as I reply, "I'm sorry. I'm not thinking straight. I just—I think North would kick the door in and murder you anyway."

He nods and steps back again, his movements jerkier, like he's really struggling to let this heated moment pass. I am too, no matter where we are or how many people are waiting on us to get ready.

I scramble around in the locker that was put aside for me, swiping my card to get through the security to open the damn thing. I grab my Tac gear and start pulling it on. The pants hang a little looser on me now that I'm back at training and spending less time eating creamy seafood sauces on my ass in North's bed.

Once I'm dressed and ready, I move to the door, only to have Atlas stop me, gently grabbing my upper arm to tug me back into his body. I go to him easily, lifting up onto my toes to kiss him back when he ducks down to meet my lips.

He kisses me like a vow of what's to come for us, a

branding promise that I can't wait to fulfill.

When we walk back out of the changing rooms together, I meet North's eye across the room and he gives me a nod before he speaks to all of the team leaders there, briefing them on what we're doing today.

"We're after water, mostly, and there have been some other requests that we said we'd look into. Mostly comfort items, but there's also some 'scripts we need to fill. Felix has been busy doing diagnostics and basic healing that a simple 'script could take off of his plate."

He continues through the protocol and I nod along, all of it the same stock-standard stuff we followed last time. I'm not surprised that we're going after things to help Felix out. Every time I've seen the Healer, other than this morning's early wake up, he's been run off of his feet and haggard looking. Sage has also been super worried about how much he's working, but the other Healers have refused to work without pay, even though they're being housed and fed for free, so everything is currently landing on his shoulders.

North is going to end up killing someone and making an example of them for sure. Well, actually, he wouldn't, but I for sure will because there's nothing quite like rich men being on their high horses about unimportant things while there's an actual crisis going on.

Typical Top Tier bullshit.

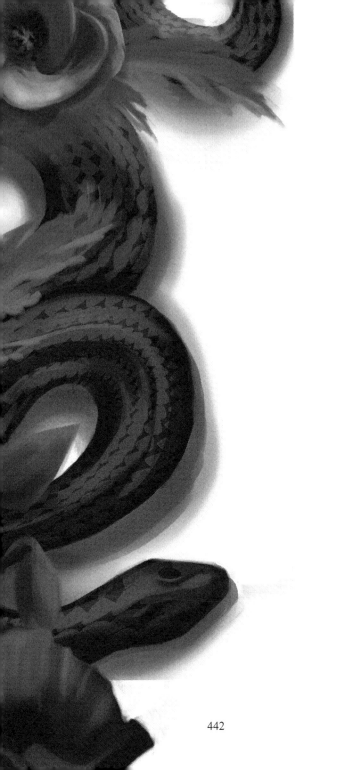

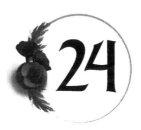

OLI

We're transported into a pickup area full of Tactical vehicles. I'm wedged between Atlas and North, with Gryphon, Kieran, and Rockelle closing the tight circle we make together. Gryphon's eyes flash as he checks out the area and, just to be extra sure, I cast out my own gift. North's eyebrows draw down a little as he watches me, not in a bad way though, just like I've taken him by surprise.

Gryphon mutters, "I'm not picking up on anyone. Oli?"

I shake my head. "Closest is half a mile away, in a

car driving in the opposite direction, so I think we're good. I didn't sense anything 'wrong' either. Like shit that shouldn't be here."

Kieran gives me a look. "How does that work? You can just tell if something is… what, *bad*?"

I wriggle out from between my Bonds, stepping around until I'm taking in the surroundings with my eyes and not my gift. I roll my shoulders back, poking around at the warehouse a little as the other teams start filtering in. "I don't know how it works, really, just that my bond can tell if things are there to hurt me."

Atlas stretches out his arms, like being transported has run through his muscles and left an ache behind. "That's how it knows who to take out when it's Rending. It just takes the souls of people there to harm you."

Rockelle nods along and then grins. "So we're safe so long as we wish you no harm? Noted. Shore better grovel before anything goes down."

I roll my eyes at him and then follow Atlas over to the vehicles. We're all going to be traveling together and we're going to be the third car in the convoy. I feel bad for whoever is lead car, the most dangerous spot, because if someone is contaminating our water supply, then there's every chance that this entire trip is happening on the Resistance's whim. They could be anywhere, at any time, and I need to stay sharp.

Gryphon has clearly learned that the best way to approach me is the one where no one will ever know it's happening and just talk to me through our mind connection. *I'm not groveling. Black was being a dick, but I'm not ashamed of my Bonded or what we do together, and you shouldn't be either.*

I duck down to check the undercarriage of the truck North points out for me, pushing at my gift just to be extra sure there's nothing under there. *Then why was North so pissed off about it? If it's all just a proud Bonded moment then that isn't at all embarrassing.*

If he had his way, North Draven would have you locked in a tower right now, completely unreachable to anyone who isn't in our Bond Group, and even then, he'd only give the rest of us access to you because it would hurt you not to. He's a jealous, possessive dickhead, and I'm not. I want everyone to see what's mine and know that they'll never get to have something as fucking perfect as my Bonded. I'm a smug asshole, but an asshole all the same.

Damn.

It's a very good explanation, even if I really want to stay pissed at him, I can't. I can't because I've known he was smug, and *proud*, about having me. I knew how much he loved being the first to Bond with me, no matter the circumstances, and it's always made me feel like maybe I could have this.

Maybe I could keep them all and not become a mindless killing machine.

Are you still pissed? I'll slit Black's throat and bleed him out right now.

I straighten up and give him a very sassy look. *No the hell you won't! That's not just your friend and colleague anymore, he's Sage's Bond. But fine, your soul can escape the next killing round. I'll let you live to make it up to me later.*

His eyes smolder back at me, fiery depths beneath the calm facade he's putting on for everyone else. I love those depths and the stream of filth that comes out of his dirty mouth when he leans into it.

If you two are done, can we get back to what we're supposed to be doing here?

I startle at North's haughty tone and duck my head,

climbing up into the backseat of the truck without another word.

"Are they giving you shit again? You'd think they could leave you be for a couple of hours while we work," Atlas grumbles as he slides in next to me, pulling on his seat belt before helping me with mine.

"Gryphon was just apologizing. He's not great at it, but it'll do," I tease, ignoring the way Rockelle overhears and cackles as he climbs into the back section. He's got a gun in his hands, and when he clips himself down to the floor and sets up like he's about to be shooting out of the back of the truck, I give North a look.

"Why does this feel like we're entering a war zone? It's a trip to Walmart for water," I sass, wiggling my ass a little to get settled.

North climbs in and takes up all of the remaining room in the backseat so that I feel as though I'm being crushed between him and Atlas again. Weirdly, it's more comforting than problematic.

Bonds are fucking weird about this stuff.

He doesn't bother with his own seat belt, just grabs the bar that runs above his door frame and holds on while Kieran gets us on the road. Gryphon's in the front seat, his eyes still white as he monitors everything around us.

North has to speak loudly so that I can hear him over the truck's engine, even with all of the windows sealed shut with bulletproof glass. "We have supply runs and incoming resident drop offs every day, and at least sixty percent of them have been attacked or raided in some way. Since this trip has been forced by the Resistance, I'm betting it's not going to be a smooth ride. There's a reason we're all coming along. Water is too important to hold off on, but with our gifts, we should be able to minimize the fallout."

Interesting.

"Is there any chance that you guys would let me be involved in the supply runs and incomings? I could be really useful here, more useful than learning how to build houses."

All three of my Bonds speak over each other in agreement.

"No."

"Absolutely not."

"I didn't want you coming today, these two insisted."

I glance at Atlas, surprised at his reply, but he just shrugs. "I'm a lot happier with you being in the Sanctuary.

I'm not going to lie and say this is all fine with me, but there was also no way that they were bringing you and leaving me behind."

I sputter over my words, "I—my bond is more than capable of handling shit if things go wrong!"

"Yeah, and yet you still spent two years being tortured by Silas Davies. I don't doubt you, but I also don't doubt that he's a fully Bonded Neuro with the ability to shut your brain *and* bond down."

I cross my arms. "He's powerful, but his range is shit. Gryphon's gift is better."

Atlas nods and shrugs again. "And yet, Silas is still our biggest threat. Maybe, and I really mean *maybe*, the Draven nightmares could deal with him. If North or Nox's ranges are as good as they seem to be, we *might* be able to use one to take him out."

I already know their range is phenomenal, Brutus came to the camp with me, and while Nox couldn't tell where we were, he could still see through his creatures' eyes. Gryphon had told me that and told me how worried they'd all been when I'd given him to Kyrie.

Still the best decision I'd made in that stupid camp.

I glance up at North, but he's still scowling at the road

like he's expecting trouble, so I take a small breath in and call on my bond.

Let me out.

I internally roll my eyes. *I just need to know if there's danger. I don't need you going full death god on this mission.*

I can feel the ripple of frustration and then it speaks again, *Let me out and I'll keep them safe. All of them, even the non-mine ones.*

Is it strange of me to be jealous about my bond being that possessive over my Bonds? Probably. Maybe I do need that therapy.

My eyes void out and the Everlasting One stiffens in his seat, his hand on my thigh tenses but doesn't move. He's not scared, just ready to move should he need to.

The Dark One doesn't react, just turns to speak to me. "Is there danger? Is she safe?"

Still very devoted to the girl.

I like that.

"Not yet. She's going to be fine, whatever that takes."

He nods and makes a hand motion at my Bonded. My *first* Bonded, the one I finally got to taste. The one who unlocked more of my power, more of the potential living inside the girl, until I could access more and keep her safe and alive.

I want *more*.

"No more of that thinking. You're not going to keep her safe like that," he says in a tight voice, and I smile back at him, all teeth and sharp edges.

"You're no fun. Give me my Bond instead."

The girl disagrees with me. She attempts to wrestle back some of the control as the driver curses under his breath, hitting the gas and getting the vehicle moving faster underneath us. I look out, but there's nothing there. Nothing but miles of farm land and livestock around us. This place we've been brought to is somewhere remote enough to barely exist on a map.

"How far away are we?" the Everlasting One says.

The driver snaps back, "Too far with her doing *that* back there. Can you get Oli back now?"

The Dark One cuts in. "No. If her bond is out, then she's taking this seriously. Just get us there and don't worry about her. You're on her safe list anyway. Rockelle is the only one who needs to be sweating."

There's quiet in the cab for a moment, only the roar of the engine to be heard, and then the Gifted in the back says, "How do I get on that safe list? Is there an application process, or do I just have to break my own leg? I'm not against it or anything, just not exactly my first choice."

I turn to look at him and smirk at the sheer terror that flits over his face before he regains control of himself, tightening his grip on the gun.

When I turn back to the front he mutters, "Fuck. It's so much worse when it looks at you."

The Everlasting One turns to snap, "Stop calling my fucking Bond an *it*. She's Oli, and she's trying to keep your worthless hide alive, so keep your mouth shut."

I don't feel the need to show affection or prove my connection to any of my Bonds, but I cover his hand with mine on my leg as a form of praise. His loyalty to me and our Bond has never been in question. It's not his fault he was born in a pit of snakes. He came home the moment I called to him. He came for the girl and offered her comfort when she needed it.

The Everlasting One leans down to kiss my cheek, murmuring to me, "You're glowing. It's cute as fuck, but Black is sweating in the front over it, so you might want to work on it."

I shake my head. "He can work to get over it. I'm perfect as I am."

The Walmart parking lot we pull into is in the middle of nowhere. Literally, there's fields full of cows surrounding us on all sides, and then a massive superstore just appears out of thin air.

When we park, Gryphon gets out first, doing the initial sweep. It takes a lot longer this time, mostly because he's vetting the hordes of people who are here shopping, and filtering through that many brains the way he does takes longer than searching out an empty warehouse or a road ahead of us.

When he meets my eye and jerks his head at me to join him, the Dark One gets out to open my door, his body shielding me as I work. There's no one here from the Resistance. There's no danger here at all, which I feel is more of a warning than a relief.

Where are they hiding, lying in wait for us?

Why won't they come out and play with me?

My Bonded looks down at me and when I nod at him

for an all clear, he starts barking out orders to the Gifted surrounding us. They move the moment they have their directives, but when he gets to me I shake my head.

"Oli will go—"

"No."

Both of my Bonded turn to look at me, but my eyes stay on the side of the building where there's a driveway to the back for the receiving area. There's a large truck already around there being unloaded, and while there's nothing there so far, that is a warning to me. I don't like it.

I don't like it at all.

"Okay. Oleander, Draven, and Bassinger will stay here and help with the perimeter patrol while we get the supplies. No one get in my Bonded's way or approach her, especially when she's working. You don't want to catch her bond's interest, trust me."

There's a murmur of agreement and then they all move out. I couldn't care less about them or what we're actually here for.

I want that truck.

There's no need to say that out loud or to discuss a plan, I just stride over there, secure in the knowledge that mine will follow me. Of course they will, where else would they need to be when I am in their presence?

So they follow me and we walk together over to the loading area at the back of the huge building where the truck has caught my attention. I can't focus on anything else, which is all that needs to be said because I am a god.

I am never wrong.

The communicator in my ear makes a noise and then my Bonded's voice comes through clearly to me. "Do not leave her side. Whatever ambush they're planning, she's feeling it. *Do not leave her*."

The Dark One answers, "We already had that figured out. No one is leaving her. Get the stock and get out of there. Keep your head in the mission."

I come to a stop in the center of the road about ten feet away from the truck. Both of my Bonds attempt to move me, but this is the spot. There is nowhere else to be right now and if any vehicle approaches, then that's an issue for them to deal with.

I cannot be moved.

We stand there and when either of my Bonds attempt to speak to me, I ignore them, waiting for the moment. I know it's coming. I know it as surely as I know that I must protect the girl. I will not be swayed from this spot until it comes. Whatever it is, whatever is coming for us, this is where I will deal with it.

I lose track of the passing of time.

I know that there's movement around me, a lot of Tac personnel approaching us and being redirected in their rounds as they patrol the area. I can feel their tension, the way that my *strangeness* and *otherness* is getting them all rattled. Even though they're all very well trained and aren't reacting to it, I can feel it.

I can taste it in the air.

My Bonded's voice comes down the comms again. "We're loaded and ready to go. I'll send the other two groups, ours can stay until Oli is done."

The driver speaks again, "I'm packed and ready to move, just give the word."

The Dark One replies, "She's fixated on the truck. We're not going to move until she's ready. We trust the bond above all else."

I almost preen at that, almost, but then there's a *pop* sound five feet in front of us and three men appear out of thin air. I don't recognize any of them, but I know who they are and what they're here for.

Me.

The girl *and* the being inside her.

My Bonds as well, if they can manage it.

"Little Render, you are proving to be quite the pain in the ass now, aren't you?" the older man in the middle says, his pockmarked skin stretching over his toothy grin a little too tautly.

I wave a hand and the souls of the other two men tear out without any real effort, their bodies falling to the ground with twin thuds.

The Dark One steps into my body a little closer, his shadows falling from his body like dark smoke on a lake in the clearest night. He looks like death immemorial and pride swells in my chest at the magnificent sight of him.

The Everlasting One is struggling to hold himself back, struggling not to throw himself over me because the urges to protect his most beloved Bond are so strong. I want to reach out to him, to comfort him and remind him that all of this is meaningless to me.

I just want to know what else the Transporter has to say because why else would they send us three men? Granted, the one still breathing is strong. Very strong, strong enough that I'm not just going to waste a good soul and tear it out.

No.

He's a delicacy, something worth taking and consuming slowly, piece by delicious piece.

"Well, well, not strong enough for me? You probably should have counted on us sending someone higher up than Franklin for you. He was the lowest of what we have. You're going to regret running. Oh, the things Silas is going to—"

"I'm done with this," I interrupt and reach out a hand, something to call the soul over to my body with. I don't need to do this when I cleave the souls out, when I'm just doing this to kill people. No, I let them disappear into nothing just like they deserve.

But this one looks yummy.

"What the fuck is she doing?" the Everlasting one mutters, but the Dark One doesn't answer. He's too busy watching me rend the soul away from the body and tuck it into my being for later.

As the last man's corpse lands on the ground, my Bonds both stand there for a second and then, when no one else *pops* into existence around us, the Dark One steps over to turn the body using his foot. His shadow walks around it with him, sniffing at the corpse as though he can get more information that way.

"That's Giles Andrews. He's one of Silas' favorites, a Transporter who has never been caught before. He doesn't have to touch you to move you, and his range is... *was* unmatched," the Everlasting One says, and the Dark One nods.

"He's been on our list for years. He was pivotal in the riots back in the seventies. He just removed half of the Resistance when things weren't going their way."

I step around the Everlasting One. "He's testing the girl and me. He's testing to see how much stronger we have gotten. Killing Franklin proved to him that we've Bonded and gotten stronger, but he's not going to come himself unless he's sure he's still stronger, so he's sending in the others. Sacrificing them for information, and they're following his orders like the good little brainwashed sheep they are."

The Dark One stops to look at me, his shadows still moving forward. "We need to talk about this."

The answer to that is simple, especially with the voice that shares my mind chiming in. "The girl says no, so I will not. She says not right now, and you will agree to that."

He blinks at me once and then nods slowly, and the Everlasting One looks between us in shock at the interaction.

I can feel the soul wriggling in my belly, waiting for me to take the time to properly consume it, but I will not take the risk while the girl is still out here in the open.

"Take us back to the safe place now. I'm hungry."

They do as I say without another word shared between us, flanking me as we walk back over to the truck that is already on and ready to leave. My Bonded stares over the hood at me like he's trying to pry everything out of my mind, but I just need the girl safe so that I can eat.

He nods and gets in the car, then we're off, back on the road at breakneck speeds, leaving the bodies of the Resistance men behind like the worthless trash they are. No one speaks on the trip back, not any of my Bonds or the other two, not even the mouthy one.

I stay focused on my prize, right until the driver parks the truck. We get out as one and he Transports us back to the safe place. I can finally leave the rest of this to the girl.

Dinner time.

My bond leaves me in a rush, like a balloon deflating, and I double over as I retch. It hasn't ever felt like this before, like the power of tearing that Transporter's soul out and... *consuming* it has messed my stomach right the hell up.

I feel strong hands sweep my hair up and hold it away from my face. Even though nothing is actually coming up, it's sweet of North to attempt to help out with this.

When I stand back up, he tugs me into his arms, his hand moving from my hair to the nape of my neck to hold me close. "Motion sickness? Or the bond?"

"The bond. I think I'm processing the soul, which is the most horrifying sentence of the week. I can—it's *in* me. I can feel it there while my bond is snacking on it. Gross. I'm officially a mon—"

"Don't. Don't even mutter that word around me, Oleander. You just took out another key player in the Resistance arsenal, another Gifted we no longer have to factor into our plans thanks to you and your bond. I hate that you're going through this, but it will *never* make you a monster."

I want to believe him, and my bond agrees with him completely, but as I feel the squirming in the pit of my gut, it's not exactly easy. There's a living soul in there.

Someone's essence, their life force, the thing that makes them a human, and my bond is chomping away at it like a kid with a hefty slice of chocolate cake.

I don't want to think about it anymore.

I don't want to think about anything.

North walks me back to the house and hands me one of the bottles of water we'd brought back, pressing it into the palm of my hand and then standing over me until I've drunk the entire lot. I have to threaten him to get him to leave me here alone and go back to his office, mostly because I don't want him hovering over me if I'm going to actually be sick.

Once he leaves, I climb into Gabe's bed and pull the blankets over my head, wallowing in his scents like a lovesick brat while I attempt to ignore the happy munching happening deep in my gut.

It's really disgusting.

Atlas finds me in there an hour later, huffing and rolling about like an idiot. When I glance up at him, just a little embarrassed about the state I'm in, he smiles at me, leaning against the door frame.

"How are you feeling? Are we about to take an epic nap?"

I sigh and pull myself up into a sitting position, shaking my head. "No, I'm trying not to have a freaking meltdown about this new and improved party trick my bond has pulled out. You can't even act like it's normal and fine, Atlas. I was still aware in there. I saw your face."

He grimaces a little and then takes a seat next to me, slinging an arm over my shoulder and pressing a kiss into my hair. "I was just shocked. It's not... something I've heard of before. I thought—I don't know what I thought it was doing, to be honest. What can I do, Sweetness? What can I do to make this better for you?"

I sigh and lean my head back to look at him properly. "I'm tired. I don't want to face everyone once North tells them all what happened, and they'll all want to talk about it. I'm also sick of living on top of each other. I'm irritable, and I know that none of this matters because we're safer here and protecting vulnerable people, but I'm so fucking sick of this shit."

He nods slowly and brushes the hair away from my

face gently, looking so deeply into my eyes that I almost feel shy about the intimacy of it. "Use your mind link and tell North we're going for a ride on the ATVs. Tell him you're safe and that we'll stay in the view of the cameras the whole time. I know where they are; we can drive in their path. I think we all know that your bond has you covered even if something happens to me."

I raise an eyebrow at him but when he doesn't say anything else, I do as he asks. North is good about it, only replying, *Tell me when you're on your way back so that I know you're safe. Don't do anything stupid, Bonded.*

Atlas shoos me out of the room and tells me he'll pack for us both and to go grab the ATV. I give him a curious look, but he just shoos me out of the house entirely.

I duck into the garage, looking for the keys I need, and find Gryphon already there with a helmet for me. When I roll my eyes at him, he just puts it onto my head for me and drawls, "As if I'd let you sneak off without saying goodbye. Bassinger is probably going to find a cave to hole up in for a month and I'll have to come looking."

Hmm.

I'd probably be okay with that. I let him buckle the strap before I reply, "You're not going to be mad at me for running away?"

He shrugs and adjusts the straps until the helmet is snugly in place. "Nope. I heard everything going on inside your head when it happened. You need a minute to figure that out, and you're going to get that minute, even if I have to use every trick in the book to keep North from coming out there after the two of you."

Well, shit. Now I want to break down and cry over his thoughtfulness. "I just need a break. I love you all, but I really need to breathe. And, like, a whole day of just dealing with one of you and not the whole bunch arguing about rationing and Tac bullshit."

His eyes are hot as he swoops down to kiss the life out of me, a blistering show of force that nearly sweeps me off of my feet. I have no idea of what prompted it but, hell, maybe I want Gryphon to come along for the ride too.

When he finally breaks away from my lips, he trails kisses from my shoulder up my neck to just under the strap until he can murmur into my ear, "I love you too, Bonded, but maybe you should have saved saying that to me for my night, because now I'm thinking about stealing you away and leaving Bassinger to himself."

I flush, realizing now what I said, but I snark back, "I don't want to sleep in the hut, that's the whole point. I feel like I'm... on show, twenty-four seven, and it's so freaking uncomfortable. I'm—it's—I need a break."

He nods and sucks on the skin under my ear. "We'll figure something else out. We're already doing what we can to get the big house done as soon as possible. Once you've Bonded with everyone, you'll feel less... exposed."

I scoff at him and snap, "Well, that's never going to freaking happen, because Nox would rather cut his own dick off than sleep in the same bed as me, let alone Bond. Shit. Forget I said that and don't you dare narc on me. I mean it, no Dravens."

He bites the inside of his cheek like he's stopping himself from speaking, but when I glare a little more, he nods. "Your secrets are safe with me. Even the ones in your head."

He glances up as though he's checking the door for anyone coming in to spy on us both, then leans down to whisper my deepest, darkest fantasies to me. "Like how much you want that orgy you've been dreaming of."

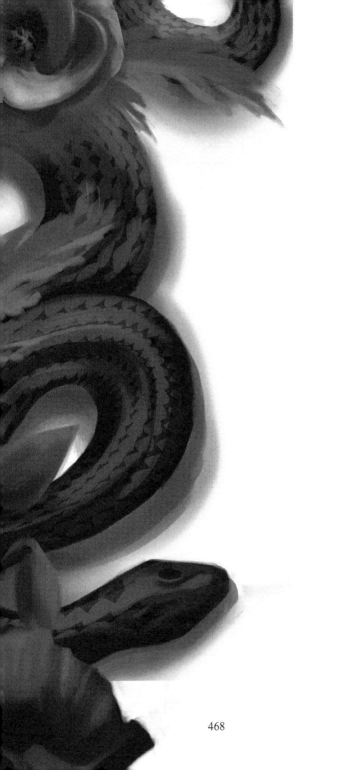

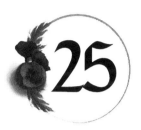

ATLAS

I watch as the tension leaks out of my Bond's body more and more the further we get from the town site of the Sanctuary.

I have no real idea of where the fuck we are, other than the fact that we're still in the States, but there's a sandy sort of desertscape on the edges of the town and a warren of caves out here that I spent a few days walking through after we'd found my sister. I've been struggling just as much as Oli has been with the close quarters, especially with not having any sort of alone time with her thanks to Ardern sleeping a foot away from us in his own bed.

Not that I'm pushing for anything with her.

Never, and especially not while she's still battling the bond living inside her that is nothing like mine. I'm nothing like the men in my family, and I'm definitely not a fucking Draven.

Not that North has turned out so bad, but his brother? I'd kill him in a heartbeat if Oli gave me the word. I've been watching him closely enough to know his weak points, and those nightmares of his? They can restrain me, sure, but they're never really going to do damage.

I'd have his fucking neck snapped in a second.

"What's wrong? You're breathing like you're trying not to kill someone," Oli murmurs, her voice pitched low and sweet.

I calm down the second she opens her mouth. Her voice is more than enough to break me out of my murderous thought spiral.

"It might seem like I'm doing something extra thoughtful for you, but it's also pretty selfish. I needed this as much as you did."

She nods and looks out over the mountains that surround us, their peaks casting shadows over the entire valley. "I get that. The others all grew up together and have had a whole lifetime to get used to living in each other's pockets. We're both sort of on the outside with that."

I catch her hand in mine and bring it up to my mouth to kiss the back of it. "It's worth it. All of it. Having you here safe is worth it all. As much as I loathe admitting it, Draven outdid himself with this place. It's like he knew that we'd need it for you, and he just did it. He just poured all of that Draven wealth into keeping our Bond safe… I can get behind that. I also didn't have to learn a new language just to keep you safe, which is handy because I barely passed Spanish at school. I'm really shit at pronunciation."

She giggles at me like I'm telling a joke, but I'm really not.

We get over the last of the small ridges to the opening of the first big cave, the one we'll be camping out in tonight that the cameras cover the opening of. It's clean and dry and secure, everything we need for a night out in the wild.

While also being completely safe at all times.

"How the hell did you ever find this? And are we taking bets on how long it takes someone to come find us, because I'm not sure we're going to make it the whole night." She giggles at her own joke, which is cute as hell, her eyes lighting up like she's already feeling giddy about our time alone.

That makes two of us.

I park the ATV and kill the engine, sitting back in the seat a little and letting the cool afternoon air wash over us both. "I took one of these things out when we brought Aurelia back from the camps. I just needed to clear my head, and then I found this place. I've been planning on bringing you out here since I found it, I just wasn't expecting you to be needing it so badly."

She looks over at me and grins, pulling off her helmet and getting out of the ATV to walk around the rocks. I point out the cameras to her so that she knows we're being watched and are safe enough here, and she waves to Sawyer.

And I'll bet North has a live feed of us directly into his office as well, but at least we have complete privacy inside the cave.

I grab the bags I'd packed from the back and follow her up to the opening. There's a small outlook there that is the perfect viewing point for the town lights and the giant, fortress-like concrete wall that North put up at either end of the valley to keep this place a secret from anyone who might stumble upon it.

I watch as the awe settles over Oli's face, and it's a fucking beautiful sight. Her eyes light up and she sort of backs her way up the path so that she doesn't have to look away from the view. The sun is already starting to fall into dusk, low over the trees, and the brilliant burst of orange over the sky warms her skin in a gorgeous glow.

I take a photo of her.

Then I make it my background on my phone like a complete sap, because she looks like a fucking model, absolutely breathtaking and *mine*.

She glances over to me and blinks a little like she forgot what we were doing here. "Did you happen to bring dinner? I forgot about food during my bond's weirdness, but now it's taking a nap and I'm starving. I should've thought of that."

I grin at her and brush past her to put the bags down a little further into the cave where I'm sure they can't be seen by the camera. They're my maker, my way to know if I've set our bed up too close to the opening and Sawyer is getting a free show of my Bond sleeping.

Or of us at the very least making out, which would cause me to kill the man. He should never know the way that her cheeks pink up or the fall of her chest when she's struggling for breath because she'd rather the taste of my lips than oxygen.

I pull out the sandwiches I'd thrown together for us both as I'd packed and take one to her, holding it out and watching her face light up all over again. She's sweet behind all of the sass she throws at everyone. I feel smug that I get to see it so often, a perk of being her safe place when the others were still up their own asses about her.

She giggles at the overloaded state of the sandwiches, the only way to eat them, and opens hers up right away, acting as though it's a big deal as she takes a bite. "My bond is having a field day right now. Two of my Bonds cooking me food in the same day? This is practically the dream."

Ah.

The old trick North had used to his advantage back when he was pretending to hate her. I'm still not convinced that any of his bad feelings were real because the way he treats her hasn't really changed, just the delivery and how it's received.

She's a lot better about doing what he says now they're Bonded.

"What are you thinking? You're frowning again," she mumbles with her mouth still full.

"You. I'm thinking about how to make things better for you here."

She walks over to the small ledge and sits down, hanging her legs over the edge and kicking them out. There's a small drop, only a couple of feet, but I park my ass next to her straight away in case she falls.

She'd probably barely scratch herself on the way down, but I'm not taking the risk.

She swallows her mouthful and says, "Things are fine. They're good, really. I'm not as scared anymore. I'm—okay. I mostly feel guilty now, but I keep telling myself that everyone is safe here, thanks to North pulling the trigger on the move. I don't think he would've if I wasn't in danger, so those kids running around that new school? They're safe, thanks to his need to protect me."

I scowl at her. "Why would you feel guilty?"

She groans and shoves the last of the sandwich half into her mouth like she wants to avoid the question. I wait her out, patient enough to plow through the rest of my own sandwich while she chews at the pace of a geriatric.

"I'm not an idiot. I know that Davies will have a list somewhere with my Bonds' names on it. Yours? Not so much, thanks to your family, but the rest of them? A Shifter who can become any living animal? A Neuro like Gryphon, whose range is better than his? The Dravens, who need nothing more said but their name to strike terror in the population? Yeah, he knows about them all, but he's never hunted them before. Not the way that he will now that he knows they're in my Bond Group. Andrews was the very first, easiest test. They're going to come, thick and fast, and I brought that on you all. I'm no real help around here because all of the work I'd be good at, North refuses to let me do because he's... overprotective of me. I'm a liability with a bond who *eats souls*."

I nod slowly, taking the last bite of my own sandwich and balling up the paper wrappings to pack away for recycling back in town. "Are you pissed at me as well then? Because I'm finding safety here too. My mom couldn't keep my being here a secret forever. I'm sure now that Aurelia is gone, my dad and Peter have figured out that I'm here too. They'd have found me and killed me if I weren't here. I know exactly nothing about building houses. I'm a security risk for joining a TacTeam, so I'm only allowed to go if I'm your protector. Other than my knowledge of the Resistance, I have nothing to offer this place, and even my knowledge is starting to run out. There's not a huge amount of intel left to tell North and Gryphon. I've gotten all of the important shit out already."

She frowns and bumps my shoulder. "There's a million things you can do here. The best I can do is wash dishes in the food hall, which is fine! That's work that needs to be done, but it also makes me feel like I'm letting everyone down. Gabe is literally building houses. He was tiling a bathroom while we were gone. We'll have more space for people soon."

I nod. I've been impressed with what he's been doing as well. I'm probably going to go over there to help out in the next few days as well, but my building knowledge is at a zero. I'm not great at taking instructions from surly, asshole men who think I'm an idiot, so I'm not expecting great things.

When I say this, Oli giggles and hands me the last of her sandwich. "Elliot is pretty great. He let me use a nail gun, and it's definitely the highlight of my building career so far. Is there a job where that's all I do? Just nail things?"

It's so cheesy, but I can't help it. "Yeah, nail me. That's literally the only job you really need to do here, Sweetness."

She snorts and rolls her eyes, the tiny dimples at the edge of her cheeks deepening beautifully, and I feel like I'm a fucking hero for getting them out of her like that.

"You're playing your cards right. If there's a comfortable bed in that bag of yours, I might even be tempted to second base."

Fuck second, I'm getting her naked and begging underneath me. Fuck, then I want to have her naked and begging *on top* of me. I want every variation of my Bond fucking me that I can get right now.

Her eyes flare and I know I'm doing a shit job of keeping my thoughts off of my face, but she's mine and it's impossible to not want her. Every part of her was made for me in a way that I've never really experienced before.

None of my family act like that.

My dad barely tolerates my mom's presence. Thomas is the same way. Three out of four of Aurelia's Bonded treat her like a power source and a pair of tits. It's why

I hated them all so much, even before I figured the Resistance shit out for myself and realized that my family are the bad guys in every superhero movie ever.

None of them act with the worship I feel when I look at my Bond.

I take her hand and help her off of the ledge and back over to the cave. I get her settled on one of the small boulders there with a bottle of water and get to work unpacking the bed rolls and pillows I've brought out. There are solar lamps in there as well, and I set a couple of them up to light up the space for us. I do a quick sweep of the place just to be sure that no animals or creepy-crawlies have set up camp since I was last here because I'm not sure how Oli would react to a furry friend creeping up on us.

She watches me with a little smile, glancing over her shoulder at the view and the cameras every now and then. "Are you sure we're not going to be giving Sawyer a free show? He's a little *too* interested in all of my Bond's dicks for my liking, and I don't really want him getting an eyeful."

I shoot her a grin over my shoulder and nod. "I'm sure. I made him go through all of the cameras to map this place out. Is he still talking about us like that? I'll kill him for you."

She scoffs and slides off of the rock. "No. He hasn't in months, but you never really forget that sort of thing. We also can't kill one of our most trusted friends over a small amount of voyeurism."

I could.

I would, but I let it drop.

"How do you know so much about camping? I thought the Bassingers were the type of filthy rich that comes with ski resorts and hotels on the water in the Bahamas."

"They are, but Jericho, Aurelia's one decent Bond, grew up on a farm. He took me camping a lot after they Bonded, mostly as an excuse to get away from my family. He's probably the only one of them who is actually missing her. I don't exactly feel sorry for her. She was at the camps and there's only a few things she'd be there to be doing, but she followed everything our parents told her to. Then she did everything her Bonds said. I guess... meeting you, knowing everything you've done, it's made me judge her a lot more harshly. You would never have let any of us talk you into joining the Resistance. You'd... break your own heart to do the right thing. I know it. We all do."

She ducks her head like she's trying not to cry, and I move to duck down and fuss with the pillows to give her a minute. Normally I'd be up in her space, pulling her into my chest and trying to fix everything for her, but we're here because she's feeling like she's under a fucking microscope, so I'll cool off for a day.

I can handle a day.

"That's an awful lot of pillows," she says as she slides off of the boulder to come over.

I nod. "My mattress wouldn't fit on the ATV, I've already measured it."

She scoffs as she steps over to me, checking for the camera, so I pull her another step closer to be sure that it can't see her. I try to keep my expectations low, but she bites her bottom lip and I almost haul her up into my arms to find a good cave wall to fuck her against.

Calm down, Bassinger. Don't ruin it now.

Except I don't need to keep going with that pep talk because she tugs my hand until I duck down to meet her lips, my hands moving to her ass to pull her back into my chest. She feels so tiny against me, so fucking fragile, and it's been years since I worried about losing control of my gift and crushing someone, but when I feel her bond come out and brush against me as well, calling out to mine, I almost snap and lose my shit on her.

She feels too fucking perfect.

I barely break away from her to speak, and the whimper she lets out is my new addiction. "Tell me I can get you naked now, Sweetness. Tell me that you want this as much as I do, because I'm going to have to take a walk otherwise."

She giggles against my lips and nods. "I want you. I want this. I want to Bond with you and keep you forever. Even if it's selfish—"

I cut her off with another kiss, no more of that shit, and my hands move to get her shirt over her head. Her hands fumble against my clothes as we scramble at each other desperately. There's nothing practiced or suave about us, just two idiots who need each other more than they need air.

I've already seen her mostly naked. I had her in my arms with our chests pressed against each other as she pulled power from me to recover, but that moment was all about getting her well again. I'd had to threaten my dick so that I wasn't getting hard over my unconscious and mostly lifeless Bond.

Seeing her naked with her consent and participation is about a billion times fucking better, especially when she grins at me as she steps back to shove her jeans and underwear off in one go, kicking them away.

She grimaces when they end up a little too close to the cave opening, but I smooth down the silvery locks of her hair as I try to distract her back into us again, to forget about cameras and discretion and Sawyer's monitoring, because none of that shit matters.

I'm definitely not going to let that asshole bother her about it.

I run a reverent hand down her chest, between the swell of her breasts, and watch as she shivers, her nipples tightening up like an invitation. Everything about her is inviting actually, every inch of her is open and here and wanting.

Wanting me and what I'm so fucking ready to give her.

I finish unbuckling my jeans and belt, getting them off and placed a little closer than hers are, just in case. Just in case some fucking idiot shows up here and thinks about getting anywhere near my Bond.

She bites her lip again and I break, using my thumb to swipe along it and get her to stop. If anyone is biting that plump, pink flesh, it's going to be me.

I'm already as hard as fucking stone and I reach down to give my base a squeeze, something to hold off the load that is already growing heavy in my balls at the mere sight of her.

Her eyes flick down to the movement and she grins at me. "Well, I already know how you like it."

I grin back at her, groaning when she reaches over to knock my hand away as she wraps her fingers around the base of me. Her grip tightens and twists just how I like it. Her hand is smaller and softer than mine, and it does all the right movements. She's seen how I like it, but my Bond actually doing it? I'm going to be lucky not to shame myself here.

"Turn around, Sweetness," I say, grabbing her wrist and moving her around until she's where I want her to be, braced with both of her hands flat against the rock wall behind us and her back arched perfectly.

Fuck, the sight of her smooth legs and pert ass pulls a groan out of my chest, bringing me to my knees behind her to finally get a taste of her. She makes a surprised sound and moves like she's going to pull away from my mouth, but I get a firm hold of her hips to keep her right there while I feast on her until her slickness coats my tongue.

I might hate myself for fucking around while she was in the camps, but knowing how to make her legs shake like this is a definite perk.

As I eat her out from behind, her arms collapse until her face is pressed against the smooth rock of the cave walls, her hips pushing back against my tongue as she rides my face. Next time, I'm going to lie back and have her sit on my face so that I can watch her expressions and play with her tits while she rocks and grinds on my tongue exactly how she wants to.

When I slap her ass with one hand, the other keeping her spread open, she groans and rocks back, her body begging for more. She doesn't have to beg, I'll give her whatever the fuck she wants.

When I move to roll her clit with my tongue, her thighs clenching around my shoulders like she's trying to pull me in closer, she starts begging, her words more moans than anything coherent. "Atlas, fuck, I can't—I need to come with you. I need to Bond with you, please,

please, fuck, *please*—"

I can go straight to hell right now as a complete man. Her words ring in my ears as I stand up, my hands staying on her hips, before I move her over to the blankets and pillows, her back tight against my chest even as I curve over her to kiss her again. She's not worried about her wetness all over my lips and chin. If anything, I think she likes it. When she tries to turn around in my arms, I stop her with a hand on her chest until I get us both kneeling on the bedroll amongst the pillows and blankets.

I hold her there with that hand on her chest as I use the other one to line my dick up with her dripping pussy, pushing in as easy as fucking pie because she's already shaking with her need to Bond. Her need to come with me, to come on my cock and seal us together for the rest of time.

One last kiss and then I push her down until she's on all fours, my hips picking up the pace until I'm pounding into her, the wet sounds of us echoing around the cave. Thank fuck the cameras don't have microphones because neither of us are even trying to keep it down, her moans like music to my ears.

I run my hand down her spine, enjoying the way that

she flexes up into it, and when I get to her head, I grab a fistful of her hair, jerking her head back to bend her back to my lips as I kiss her, my tongue fucking her mouth the same way my that cock is pounding her pussy.

She makes the best noises, like she's been surprised to be taking everything I'm giving her, but also terrified that it's going to stop before she comes.

Her bond is ready to burst inside of her.

I can feel it growing and swelling inside of her, racing to get out of her and take me over the moment we come together and Bond. My own bond is pushing at my skin, reaching out for hers and ready to be tied to her forever. I'm almost angry that it's happening so quickly, that they're both so desperate to be with each other that they're pushing us both right to our limits.

I don't want this to end.

Oli's arms wobble a little and then she ducks down to rest on her elbows, biting the pillow when I slap a pink patch on her ass again. The skin there is hot when I rub my hand back over it, but the rhythmic clenching of her pussy on my cock tells me everything I need to know about whether my Bond likes a little pain with her pleasure.

It also pushes me right over the edge, my hand slipping around her hips to brush over her clit and pull her right over with me, into the greatest orgasm of my life. Not only because it's with her, my Sweetness, but because the euphoria in my bond at finally connecting with our other half has me seeing stars.

I almost pass the fuck out.

That's embarrassing, but Oli just collapses underneath me into the blankets, my body following hers like she's the goddamn sun. Her body trembles as her breaths come out in sobs and her skin glows unnaturally as my bond washes over her and gives her *everything*. Fuck, she writhes there on my cock and I almost come again.

I didn't even know that was possible.

I wait until I can see again and then I pull out, taking her into my arms and bundling her into my chest, kissing her soundly on the lips even though she's still barely coherent. The haze settles over her eyes and, fuck, it's incredible to see. As much as it had grated on me to see on her after she'd Bonded with Gryphon... when it's my Bond she's settling into, it's fucking amazing. When it's my neck she's wrapping her arms around tightly so that I won't even let her go... I could die the happiest Bonded on Earth right now.

There's a moment right after our bonds settle and slip away from us that I see the panic rise a little in her, the terror of what might happen if she gets stronger, and I have to clamp down my own feelings about her bond in that moment. I have to shut down the frustration that it's scared her this badly with everything that it's done, because it was all to keep her alive and as safe as it could manage.

It's my family that I should hate.

She blinks rapidly, trying not to let the tears fall, and scrubbing at her cheeks when they do regardless. "You promise not to regret this, right? Even if—even now that my bond will get stronger and start something else new and gross?"

I stoop down a little so we're eye to eye, grabbing the back of her neck in one hand gently so that I'm sure I have all of her attention. "Oli, I need you to listen to me right now, because I've never been so fucking serious about anything in my life. You're my Bond. If you get stronger and burn the whole world to the ground, then I'll be there at your side, watching it burn. I'm not the good guy, Oli. I'm not one of the Dravens or Shores of the world. It's you and me, and *nothing* else matters to me."

She ducks her head back down into my chest and I can feel the tears there. She's had a long day, but it still rips me apart that she's feeling like this. "Don't cry, Sweetness. Don't cry, because it makes me feel violent, and this whole town is going to end up rubble around us if I lose my shit right now."

My lips chase the hot stream of tears down her cheeks and, fuck, I would do anything to take this fear and pain away from her. Anything to stop this world from hurting her any more than it has. Every time I shut my eyes, I can see her lying on that table with Silas fucking Davies standing over her with a knife, and I can't take it anymore.

"Oli, I want you more than I've ever wanted anything in my life… except for how badly I want you to be safe. I want you as strong as we can get you, even if that means your bond starts eating every soul it comes across. Does that make me as bad as my father and the rest of the Resistance? Maybe. Maybe, but that's the price I'll happily pay. The road to hell for me is paved with everything I would do for you, and that list never fucking ends."

I wake up just before dawn to pee. I hate to leave the comfort of the blankets and my Bonded, but when I get back to the cave entrance, the dawn sky brightening around us, Oli looks perfect lying there on her stomach amongst the blankets.

There's one thrown over her waist and ass like she was attempting to be modest as we fell asleep together but failed miserably at it. Her hair is fanned out and her cheeks are a little rosy from the warmth of the cave. It was the perfect night, one I don't want to leave behind any time soon.

I want to remember this moment forever.

I would take a picture of her there, but I'm monitored by the Dravens and Benson so much that they'd end up seeing it, and this moment isn't for them. This is for me and my beautiful Bonded, glorious and dangerous that she is, and I wouldn't share it with any of them even if my life depended on it.

I grab my phone out from my jeans where they lay forgotten on the cave floor after I kicked them off last night. There's a voicemail from an unknown phone number blinking there, and dread pools in my gut.

I have no loyalty to my father after everything the man has done. I have nothing for my mother's other Bonded either, but my mother... she tried. For the wrong reasons, but she's the same brainwashed human that my sister is too.

Aurelia.

I don't want it to be one of her Bonded on the line either. I've been chasing my own demons for so fucking long that it's almost impossible not to feel shitty over every little part of this.

There is a little bit of guilt too because I know I'm on the right side of history now, and I will always choose my Bonded. I will always choose my Bonded, no matter what happens here.

I glance over my shoulder at her again and enjoy the sight one last time without the bullshit waiting for me on my phone clouding the moment. She sighs in her sleep as though she can feel my eyes on her, rolling over onto her back, and the blanket slips away from her body until she's completely bared to me.

Fuck, she is magnificent.

I know that it's natural for a Bonded to think that way, but Oleander Fallows is the most gorgeous woman I've ever laid eyes on. Every inch of her was created to draw me in, and there was never a world in which I'd choose my family's suicidal ideology over her.

I turn back to my phone and step out of the cave, wearing nothing but my boxer shorts in the sticky night air.

"Son, you need to stop and think very carefully about what you're doing here. I get it now. I understand what you were so angry about, but we need the girl. You're thinking with your bond too much. Take a step back and look at the bigger picture here."

Useless fucking drivel.

How he ever thought he'd be able to convince me to sell out my own Bonded with this is unfathomable. Is this all it would take for him to sacrifice Mom? Cold fingers of dread creep down my spine. Thomas would never. I take a deep breath, secure in the knowledge that even if my father has fallen this far from what is right in the world, at least Mom's other Bonded wouldn't.

He's loyal to the Resistance, but not above her.

I can hear someone trying to get through to me while

I listen to Dad's voicemail one last time, hoping for some indicator of what he's got planned, but I let it go to voicemail as well.

The moment I play the newest recording, I wish I'd picked the damn thing up.

Mom's voice is strong down the line. "Call me. Your father is coming for you, and he's not thinking straight. Peter is with him. Neither of them are thinking straight, Atlas. Call me back and... keep the girl away from them. If they get her, they'll use you both."

Peter.

My sister's asshole Bonded that I once caught slapping her. When I confronted him about it, he laughed at me, told me she was indestructible and could take a hit.

I broke his skull in four places.

It took three Healers hours to stop his brain from being permanently damaged. Aurelia didn't speak to me for a month. She told me I'd understand when I found my Bonded, but the very idea of *anyone* raising their hand to Oli makes me sick.

There's no way they can find us, no way that they can actually make it through the Shields, but I hit dial on North's number anyway, my loyalties firmly with the beauty over there on the floor of the cave with me.

In the distance, with the sun rising slowly over the wall, I see the massive gates swing open right as Draven picks the line up. All the security measures in the world mean nothing when they have someone on the inside.

"They're here, and someone has just let them in."

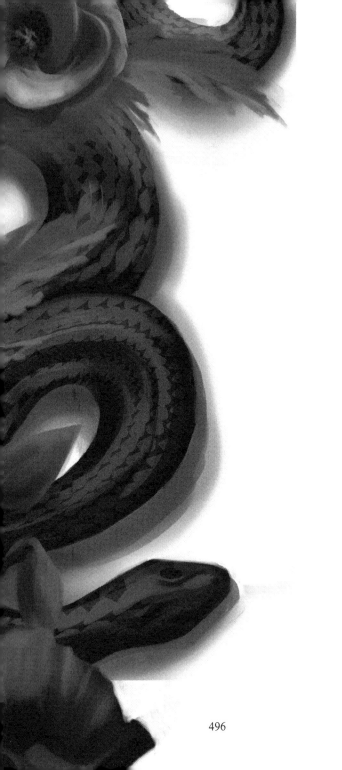

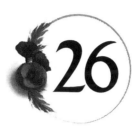

OLI

I wake to Atlas' stern voice, my brain taking a second to process exactly what he's saying.

"Oli, get up and get dressed. The gates are open, the Shield is out, and we need to get moving right now."

I jolt up out of bed as he hands me my clothes, his jeans on but still unbuttoned and his shirt tucked under one of his arms as he throws himself together.

Unfortunately, it's not the worst joke Atlas has ever told because North's voice floods my head in a demanding sweep. *Stay where you are, Bonded. Stay there until we have this taken care of. Stay safe with Bassinger.*

I wrench myself to my feet, stumbling a little on the blankets and stuttering over my words. "How? Someone had to let them in, have you called—"

He cuts me off, shoving his shirt over his head before he starts helping me with my clothes. "Sawyer and I both called North at the same time. The TacTeams are already mobilized. We just need to get dressed and be ready if we need to move out. You heard North, we're staying put."

It takes me a second to realize he's heard North talking to me, that he is also a part of the mind connection I share with the other two, which is both daunting and a relief.

I like the connections, but he's the most likely to argue with the other two about the things that they say to me using that form of silent communication.

The moment I'm completely covered, I follow Atlas back to the mouth of the cave to look back over at the town. If I had any doubt about what Atlas was saying to me before, I certainly can't deny what's happening right there in front of my eyes. We watch in horror as the Resistance pour through the open gates, dozens of trucks and more than a hundred armed and lethal Gifted soldiers here to kill, abduct, and maim.

Our Shield has betrayed us... or someone has taken

them out. Either way, hundreds of enemy Gifted are here and the entire town are sitting ducks, sleeping in the early morning in the so-called safety of their new homes.

There's children in the town.

A lot of the lower families who had come along were mostly Bond Groups with kids who were rattled after the last raids, none of them are prepared for this sort of thing.

"We can't just… sit here and wait. *I* can't do that."

Atlas turns to me, but my eyes have already shifted to the black voids. My bond hasn't fully taken over and it won't unless I am in pain, but I'm not going to run away from this fight. No matter how much my Bonds would like me to.

Good girl, my bond purrs to me, and I feel all three of my Bonded have very strong reactions to that.

"Oli, if we go back to the town, you're only going to be a distraction to your Bonds and Bonded. We need them all focusing on taking out the Resistance—"

"No. They can watch me do it," my bond says, and I shake my head a little to clear it, my eyes shifting back so I can speak for myself.

"Sorry, I'm not going to wait around here while people die. If there's one thing you should know for sure about me by now, Atlas, it's that I'm not going to sit around and wait to be rescued."

He doesn't like that answer one bit, but he walks over to the bags that he'd brought out with us and pulls out the same guns that he'd been assigned when we were on the supply run. I have absolutely no interest or use for a gun, so when he tries to talk me into one, I just scowl at him and lift my hand up as though he can see the soul-sucking gift writhing under my skin at the prospect of the carnage we're about to walk into. He nods without another word and climbs into the ATV, buckling me into it before he takes off.

"Can you do the net thing you do? Just to be sure they haven't started scouting for us yet? My dad was the one who called this morning, there's a good chance he's here looking for me."

Shit. Is now the time to talk about the fact that I might have agreed to keep his sister breathing... but his dad? Dead and gone the second I can get within gift usage distance, which is relatively far away these days.

When I mention this to him, he rolls his eyes and snaps, "Well, obviously, Bonded. Anyone who came here today is fair game, even my mom if she tagged along to work her diversion bullshit."

With that shit out of the way, we get to work, him driving like a maniac and me scouting. North feels it the second I cast it out, thanks to his creatures and shadows already being spread out throughout the town, taking down Resistance soldiers like the good babies they are.

Tell Bassinger I will make his death a painful and messy affair.

I press my lips together to keep the giggle in. *He can hear you. Also, he's just doing what my bond told him to, can't blame the man. It's persuasive.*

He doesn't find that funny at all. When we get within a mile of the town's edge, I motion for Atlas to park. Good thing I've been training with Gryphon for all of these months, because I can run an eight minute mile without completely dying, so we're going to get into this town and deal with anyone and everyone we come across.

Stay with me, Oli. We're doing this, but we're doing it together.

I turn to look at him and hold out my pinkie finger, something stupid to break the tension out of the air. I feel calm about this for once. I'm not a liability or the one doing the harm here.

I'm going to *save* people.

He scoffs at me but links his pinkie with mine all the same, using it to tug me into his body to kiss me one last possessive time, and my body has a little flashback to the earth-shattering orgasm from last night.

I was hoping for at least two more this morning, and that disappointment is enough to kill a whole army of Resistance soldiers.

Atlas keeps pace with me, and we make it three minutes into the run before we come across the first soldier. My gift net is still out and even without it, my bond flags the guy wearing black with blood on both of his arms as the enemy.

He moves to lift his hand, but before my bond can deal with him, a black mass the size of a bear appears suddenly out of the shrub and devours him, its jaws opening to the size of a small car and just swallowing the guy whole.

Atlas gets an arm around my waist and yanks me behind him, lifting me clean off of my feet, but I'm too busy trying to fight off a nervous giggle to be really worried.

The black mass turns to look at us, the form shimmering

and folding in on itself until August is left standing there, his tail wagging behind him and a mysterious green liquid dripping from his jaws.

"*Baby!*" I whisper as I drop down to greet him, Brutus coming down from behind my ear to sniff at his brother while I give them both pets and scratches. Atlas pokes around the area like he's expecting to find pieces of the guy left behind.

I already know there's not anything to find.

Not there, anyway. But the group of four more soldiers coming our way need to be dealt with.

I straighten back up and step over to his side, murmuring quietly, "There's more coming. I'm just going to deal with them and anyone else that comes our way."

He straightens up and comes over to stand with me, just a little in front of me before he nods. "Do it. Leave no one behind, but let me know when you're starting to tap out."

I swallow roughly, his words rattling me, but not for the reasons that he would guess.

I don't tap out. My gift *never* taps out.

The souls I take just give me more power.

I swallow again and reach out to kill the men, taking

their souls without another thought, and my bond doesn't attempt to eat these ones, thank God. The moment their bodies hit the ground, I tug on Atlas' hand to get us moving.

We're close enough now to hear the chaos and screaming coming from the town.

"Stay at my side, Oli, *please*," Atlas says with the low-level demand that I'm starting to read a little more clearly from them all.

They've figured out that I'm a do-it-my-own-way kind of girl, and they're all alpha men who don't really want to have to play along nicely with that sort of attitude.

In the mix of the gifts flying around, it's hard to clearly pick out who is Resistance and who are the Tac personnel, especially since most of them are wearing civilian clothes, thanks to the dawn ambush. I duck behind an overturned car to dodge a giant ball of electricity that is thrown my way, and Atlas moves with me to cover, zigging at the last second to avoid being burnt by the retaliating stream of fire a Flame sends back. We're separated, but only by a couple of feet.

It's not so bad.

When another car goes flying, right towards a group

of Gifted who are huddled behind a half-destroyed wall, he lurches up and catches it mid-air, as easily as you'd catch a tennis ball.

It's fucking incredible.

I've got them, just focus on the net. Take them out, Sweetness. The faster you do it, the safer we all are.

I squeeze my eyes shut and try to focus, asking my bond to kick in just a little and help out with this, and even through the deafening sounds of the fighting, I hear the click of a hammer pulling back on a handgun a few feet away from myself.

I turn, but then there's a hot spray of blood over my face as a bullet hits the woman directly between the eyes, instant lights out for her. It's a little bit traumatizing, just a smidge, but only because the death I would've given her was less messy.

Harrison grabs my arm and jerks me out of the way. "If you're not going to go full death demon on us, then you might want to go wait somewhere safe. Where's Bulletproof Boy gone?"

Brutus stares up at him, waiting for my command to kill the operative for touching me, but August is a little more trigger-happy and snaps at his ankles savagely. I try not to giggle at the sound Harrison makes. He stays standing, apparently catching a bullet to his own head is preferable to crouching down closer to the pups.

I duck at the sounds. "My bond is very pro 'death to everyone' and I'm trying to make sure we don't lose anyone to friendly fire. Where the fuck are the rest of my Bonds?"

I could just ask them with our mind connection, but I really don't want to distract any of them and get them hurt. Plus, that would only get me my Bonded.

I'm also itching to know that Gabe and even Nox are okay and have backup in this freaking mess.

Atlas uses the hood of one of the destroyed trucks to barricade the Gifted into one of the houses, securing them the only way we can here, while I pick off the Resistance in this area of the town methodically. I'm careful, and with my bond's help, I'm sure of my choices.

Harrison's murmur of praise at my work as he watches over the truck reinforces my choices.

"Good work, kid. If only you were Bonded to someone other than Draven, you'd be a fucking massive asset."

Atlas stalks over and helps me back onto my feet. "Draven doesn't decide what Oli does. If she really wants to, then we're here cleaning up. Now, where the fuck is Ardern? We're going after him next."

I like his choice, and I let them talk through town routes while I extend my nets, slowly reaching out and cleaning up more of the soldiers on the edges of where we are.

I feel Sawyer in the security room at the base of North's office, the elevator going down to the basement there, and there's no question that I need to get a look at those screens.

Could I use them and clear everything out? Maybe. It's definitely worth a try.

We find Sawyer in an absolute mess in front of his computers in his underwear, blood still dripping from a gash on his forehead. He doesn't look up as we walk into the room. He's the one who opened up the security door for us, so he knew we were coming.

The moment we step into the room, my mouth drops open at the sight of the screens in front of us.

The town has been blown apart.

Either there's been explosives used, or the Resistance has sent in someone with a truly destructive gift, because there are entire buildings with holes in the side of them and paths with giant craters in them, as if a bomb had gone off.

"Holy shit," I whisper, and Sawyer doesn't look up from his keyboard to answer me.

"North is clearing out the first five zones, his creatures have it under control. I've never seen someone last this long but every time it looks as though he's flagging, something happens and he gets a kick back."

Atlas glances at me and I raise a finger to my lips.

I already knew it was happening, I could feel it. The more souls I take, the more power there is for me to send his way.

"Gryphon and his TacTeam are moving through six to ten. Nox is with them, but he's in full Draven nightmare mode and torturing everyone he comes across."

I nod and step forward to stand right behind him. "And Gabe? Where's he holed up?"

"The schoolhouse. He got out of the house early, grabbed everyone he could, and got them over there. He's protecting at least a third of the town population there. North and the others have been finding people and sending them over to him, escorting when they can or just getting them to make a run for it. We've had casualties in the civilians, but it could have been a hell of a lot worse. Kieran found Sage early on and has her holed up in one of the trucks, and Felix is barricaded in the medical rooms."

I take a breath, a deep one, and then he finally looks at me. "Oli, I need you to find Grey. Everyone else is accounted for. I can't see him, but he was in the kitchens helping out with the changes with the water supply, please just find him—"

That I can do. Sawyer has been here the whole time keeping my men safe, there's no way I'm leaving family behind. "I'll get him here, don't worry about it, Sawyer! You keep my Bonds safe, and I'll get your man here safe, I swear it."

He looks at me for a second longer and then nods, turning back to the computers and putting on his earpiece again to listen in to the Tac chatter there. I know he'll keep everyone as safe as he can, but I also know that he's going to prioritize our family.

Our family, because that's what we do.

So now I have to get Grey back here safely. I already

know he can hold his own, but the Resistance only ever sends in their biggest and best fighters, so he needs some goddamned backup.

Atlas, who is standing at the door, cursing under his breath, mutters desperately, "Oli, please stay here with Sawyer and let me go. This place is a fort and you can just guide me—"

Absolutely not. "No. I'm the biggest weapon we've got. I'm not running scared anymore."

Atlas scoffs and lets his head drop back against the wall behind him, muttering under his breath, "You never did. You never fucking did, Sweetness."

Atlas grabs another gun from the cabinet next to Sawyer, and throws the holsters over his shoulders. There's a full Tac uniform in there but it'll be too small for him, and I refuse to change now. I don't need the superhero outfit, I need the range for my arms, but I do take an earpiece. Sawyer does too, shoving an extra one in his pocket, and then we get our asses out of there.

I keep the net out and kill every Resistance soldier that I come across the second I hit them. Word that I'm here and that I'm hunting seems to spread quickly, and through the comms I hear comments of Transporters making speedy exits. They haven't taken anyone with them so far, but we're on guard nonetheless.

We get through the debris and corpse-filled streets easily enough and find Grey in the kitchens, exactly where Sawyer had last seen him, holed up in one of the walk-in fridges along with the chef and half a dozen other kitchen staff. Atlas gives him the spare comms and then we all regret it when Sawyer cusses him out very openly and unabashedly for daring to be somewhere that wasn't covered by the cameras.

I have no doubt that North will be finding room in the budget for more in the very near future.

We make the choice that Grey is safer here than us trying to move him, and with a way to get intel from Sawyer and a gun from Atlas, he'll be able to protect himself and those with him.

He's also Telekinetic and could for sure kill a man if he needed to, we have no doubts.

I take the risk and open up to call out to my Bonded, praying that I'm not going to get either of them killed.

We're going to find Gabe now. Do either of you need anything?

Gryphon answers first, *Come grab Sage and get her*

over to the schoolhouse. She's a distraction for Black, and he's useless to me with her here.

Easily done, I definitely want her out of the firing line anyway. *On my way.*

North takes a second longer to reply and I feel the tendrils of guilt in my stomach at his words. *Should I expect my power to go on forever? Or just until the Soul Rending is done? Exactly how strong are you, Bonded?*

Atlas glances at me again and shakes his head, more than happy for there to be secrets for only us to keep. I already know we can't live like that.

There is no limit. Or at least, I've never found one.

Atlas curses under his breath again, but I move forward, taking all of the right turns towards zone six. I might be freaking horrendous at directions, but my bond is good, and it can follow the invisible strings that connect me to my Bonded easier than breathing.

It almost becomes soothing, the sounds of the bodies dropping to the freshly poured pavement. I become completely numb to the meaning of it, my bond quietly pleased as we take the energy and funnel it to our Bonded. Atlas' skin begins to glow softly next to me, but he's too focused on protecting me to notice it.

The moment we get to where the last of the fight is, I let my eyes flash to the voids and trust my bond to take out the last of the Resistance soldiers there. I can see the relief on half of the TacTeam there, all of them looking a little haggard and worn out.

Except, of course, for Nox, who looks up from the corpse he's now holding in place of the man he was *creatively questioning* and sneers at me.

Great.

He stands up in a rush, beating Gryphon to me, and Atlas pulls me back into his arms like he's trying to get me away from the Bond.

"Why the fuck are you risking yourself out here? Do you want the Bond Group to fucking implode just because you're bored and don't want to sit somewhere safely for an hour while we sort it out?" he snarls at me, shoving his gaiter down his throat so that all I see on his face is the significant rage thrumming so clearly through him.

"Because it's my fucking fault! Do you think I'm going to let them take other people just because I escaped? They were killing *children* the last time."

Nox snorts and my eyes snap up to meet his. There's a ring of black around them, his bond sitting just below the surface, and the smirk on his face is savage and mocking. "You think this is the first time they've killed children? Well, I suppose usually they just grab them. Half the Resistance is made up of stolen and brainwashed kids. Davies started taking them thirty years ago. Those Gifted you killed today *are* those kids... they're just old enough now that you didn't think twice."

My stomach drops so quickly that I think I'm going to puke all over Atlas' shoes, my head spinning and my moral compass once again taking a hit.

Gryphon's temper snaps and he gets right up in Nox's face, crossing the invisible lines that they usually leave securely in place. "Don't fucking say that shit to her! If you're worried about what's happening, then deal with it. She is not your fucking punching bag. North won't save you this time."

Atlas' arms tighten around me, and I realize I'm shaking. I killed all of those men and women. I killed them. Without thought, I just ripped all of their souls out of their bodies. They could have been anyone.

Children and parents, siblings, every last one of them have family somewhere, and I just... didn't fucking care.

I really am the monster they all called me.

I'm the fucking monster.

Gryphon pulls me around again and cups my chin. "Go find Gabe. We'll finish off here and get the gates secured again. We have another Shield on the way. You go to Gabe. Ignore all of this shit, Bonded. It's all just bullshit that doesn't matter anyway. They came here to kill us all, you've done nothing wrong."

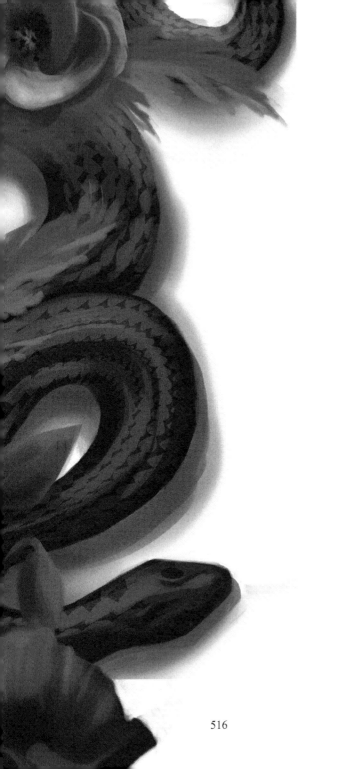

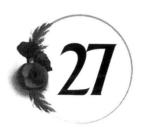

GABE

I can't see Oli from where I am in my shifted form, but Gryphon's reassurance filtering into my brain that he's heard from her, that she's alive and ripping people's souls out left and right, is the only thing keeping me from abandoning the people here and running to her. The impulse to find and covet her is strong, but I have a job to do and I need to trust the rest of the Bond Group.

It's a good thing too, because there's a lot of Healers and low-level Neuro types running towards me for safety that would be decimated by the gifts being thrown around.

There's a Charge around here somewhere, blowing

holes in the sides of buildings, and I'm feeling particularly shitty about it after a week of working on the damn things.

I have to shift back into human form to call out to the terrified crowd and direct them to safety. They blink at me like rabbits caught in headlights, a giant naked guy will do that to a person, but I open the doors up to the school to usher the newcomers in and they go quickly enough. I send them down to the storm cellar underneath the building with the rest of the Gifted that I've found and stashed under there. It's mostly women and children and Top Tier idiots who are too scared to fight for our town and our community.

There are going to be a lot of changes around here once we've dealt with this nightmare.

The moment I get the door shut and barricaded behind them, dragging a slab of concrete from the debris in front of the door for extra protection, I shift back into my largest panther form and jump down from the small porch to join the other shifters, sniffing at the air as the next wave rolls in.

North and the others are doing a great job of keeping most of the fighting away from us, but there's a group of Transporters here bringing in wave after wave of soldiers, and there are too many slipping through to us for me to leave and join the fight.

In my fully shifted form, I can tear through three men at a time, which is helping keep the crowd at bay. Ezra shifting behind me into the tiger form he has and being able to take out one at a time also helps. Elliot stoops down to place his palm on the ground, sending a sheet of ice that grows out of his fingers to cover the ground and freeze the approaching soldiers, making them easy game for me to rip in half.

It's messier than the other deaths, but there's something very satisfying about doing it.

There's a quiet moment, a lull in the hordes of insurgents around us, and then I turn towards the footsteps coming up quickly from behind. Kyrie has a scrape down one of her cheeks, a split lip, and a child she's found somewhere tucked under one of her arms, but her eyes are clear and she's still sharp as she looks around the side of the school building, spotting me and deflating a little in relief.

She helps the kid onto the porch and then winces a little as she pulls herself up. "Tell me you have guns here as well? I only had three in my room, and I'm already out of ammo."

I jump up to lead her over to the pile of clothing I'd torn off to shift, and she stoops down to grab two of the guns and some clips that I'd grabbed and brought with me when North had called.

She sweeps her hair back into a ponytail, all business and looking so much like her brother with the no-bullshit look on her face. "There's some houses on the edge of zone three, just over there, and there's people trapped in there. They have kids, and they're too scared to move them without an escort. I'll go now. I have an earpiece, and that Benson kid has been directing me."

I drop my head down in a nod, because I'm not going to shift back and have this conversation butt-ass naked with her. My bond ripples in my chest at the idea and the seething sort of jealousy that Oli's bond had shown around us makes it a non-option.

If her bond is out here tearing souls out, I'm not going to provoke it into hurting Kyrie.

There's a boom as the Charge takes out another building, one of the trucks they'd rolled in here lifting into the air and landing a few feet away in a charred and smoking mess. I jerk my head at Kyrie to get her moving and jump back down to where the others are waiting.

The next wave of Resistance arrives in front of us, guns and hands raised as they begin firing at us but the bullets bounce off of an invisible barrier. We might not have a Shield hiding in the school strong enough to protect the entire Sanctuary, but there are three mothers and a father in there doing everything they can for their kids, and I would protect them over the Top Tier Flame bureaucrat shitting himself next to them any day of the fucking week.

The barrier isn't enough to keep them away from us though, but we've been at this for over an hour, so we know how it works. I focus on the bulk of the soldiers while the other two grab whoever I miss. It's bloody work, but it's also cathartic, taking out every last ounce of my frustration on these fucking pieces of shit who came here after our most defenseless population.

When I've taken out the six men who crossed the barrier, I look up to find the Charge there, hand out as if he's about to blow a fucking crater into the ground where I'm standing.

Except then Oli strides around the corner with her hand up and her eyes voided out. There's nothing here that my Bond can't handle. Dozens of the Resistance fall as one until there's no one left for me to deal with. I watch Ezra and Elliot both drop back, moving away from her with a look of fear in them so strong that even shifted, you can tell they're shitting themselves.

I think she just looks hot as fuck.

"Ugh, what was that? That guy there, what was his power?"

I glance down and then shift back to my human form, enjoying the little squeak she lets out at the sight of me. I glance around but there's only the building workers still out here, and I don't think she'll give a shit about them. "He was a Charge. A living bomb. He's the one doing all of the damage. He flipped a truck over on a few of Gryphon's guys early on, and North has been working at pushing him back this whole time. He had a Shield working with him but... well, that's the other guy you just took out."

Oli looks around, very scandalized about my dick still being out, and says, "Shift back! There's cameras everywhere, and I don't want Sawyer talking about how fantastic your ass is."

Bassinger snorts and shakes his head, drawling, "I

don't think it'll be his ass—"

"Don't even suggest his dick right now! I'm doing what I can to distract my bond, and talking about it isn't helping, Atlas!" she snaps, and I shift back, easy as breathing, to butt my head against her legs. I'd shifted to talk to her, sure, but also because I wanted to take a second to just hold my goddamned Bond.

Alive and massacring the enemy like they deserve. We're all fucking *blessed*.

She crouches down to wrap her arms around my neck, burying her face there. "Sorry. I want to talk to you but... you're also mine and I'm not sharing."

It's a good thing too because right as she sighs with relief at having me back, Kyrie pops back up with a couple of families, at least a dozen kids between them, and starts moving them back towards the school. Brutus jumps over to sniff at them as they walk and a couple of the kids squeal and burst into tears at the sight of him, their parents scooping them up in fear.

Kyrie nips that in the bud. "The beast is back again? Shit. It's okay, kids. He's a friendly pup. That's his mama over there. She wouldn't let him misbehave. He won't hurt you; he's here for the bad guys."

Everyone who has an earpiece turns to stone for a second, hearing something from Sawyer, but my feline hearing can only pick up the high frequency noise of the technology.

Oli lets out a sigh and tucks her face back into my neck. "I got the last of the Transporters. North just took out the last of the soldiers in his zones, and Gryphon has the gates back in place."

Atlas nods and takes a step towards the corpse of the Charge. "They got the new Shields in. We have three backups now, instead of one. That should help."

Oli's stomach makes a noise and I move back a little so that I can look at her, ready to go hunt for something to feed her if she needs it after all of the power she's used, but she looks sick.

"Ignore it. My bond... is eating the Charge's soul in there. He was the strongest Gifted here, and even stronger than Andrews. I guess we just passed the next strength test."

Well, fuck.

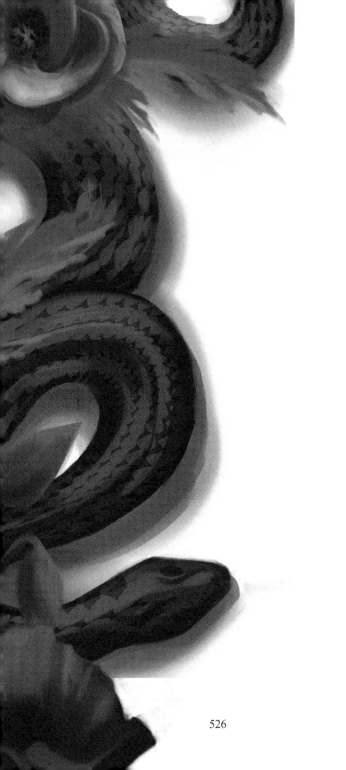

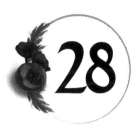

OLI

We wait in front of the school with Gabe and the other Shifters until the Shields have the Sanctuary completely covered. Sawyer gives us the all clear before we let the families out of the school and start moving people to the medical center.

Gabe, who is once again dressed in his sleep sweatpants and one of Atlas' sweaters that he'd grabbed in his rush to get down here, has a kid on each of his shoulders as he helps to move people who are injured or low mobility. Atlas has a man draped over his own shoulders who has been shot in the leg and very crudely patched up by one of the useless Healers in the storm shelter. He is still doing his best not to groan at every little movement.

None of the families want to touch me.

I'm okay with that, but both of my Bonds take it a little personally on my behalf.

Kyrie snorts at them and jiggles a little to adjust the toddler on her hip. "The Dravens get the same treatment. It's just fear. Even knowing you were the pivotal piece of our victory, they can still sense that something *else* is walking with them."

I shrug and pet down August's back, ruffling his ears a little, exactly how he likes it. "I know. That's survival instinct for you, I would stay away from me too."

I don't tell her that I'm fine with it because Nox verbally tore me a new asshole less than an hour ago and that shit is still stinging like a bitch, because then Atlas will drop the guy he's holding and just go full kamikaze on him for my honor.

I don't need that.

So I put a smile on my face and keep the puppies close to my legs. There's no point in scaring people more by letting them roam freely.

When we get to the medical center, which is in the main area of town and across the way from North's offices, we find the TacTeams mostly congregating there, and I can duck off to find my Bonded.

I need to find North and see him alive and well for myself, thank you very much.

He's easy to spot, being the most highly sought after person in the town while also being terrifying enough to require a two foot personal bubble from everyone while the memories of what nightmares he was inflicting on the enemy are still strong. I'm not exactly kind or tactful in the way that I use the puppies to get people the hell out of my way as I make a beeline to him.

The relief on his face at the sight of my dust-covered, sweaty, gross face is exactly what's on my face as well. I don't need to see it to know it.

I'm not sure if he's really into PDA, but I throw myself in his direction and he catches me without hesitation, his arms tight around me as he pulls me in as closely as the laws of physics will let him.

"You really couldn't stay somewhere safe, just to stop me from having a heart attack?"

I scoff at him, but his arms stay tight around me so I

can't move. "Kyrie just called me pivotal to our win here. Pretty sure you guys needed my help. Besides, we both know the Charge was sent for me."

There's murmuring behind us, and I feel my Bonds approaching. All of them, even Nox, surprisingly.

I get tugged out of his arms gently, even though he doesn't want to let me go, and Gryphon snarks at him, "Stop hogging her, you possessive shit. You have people to speak to and important councilman shit to do."

North glares in the general direction of Foggarty and the other two Healers gossiping amongst themselves just a few feet away, staring at him like they're vultures.

I tuck myself up back into his side to murmur, "Which one do you want me to scare the shit out of? I can totally kill one of them if you want me to."

When he shoots me a look, I grin at him innocently with a little shrug, teasing, "For the greater good, I can do what's necessary."

"Liar. You wouldn't, but your bond would. Maybe you should let her out for a bit longer, thin the overfed and over-important crowd a little for us."

Gabe scoffs and kicks his sneaker into the dirt a little, but he's caked in it already from the fight, so it doesn't make a difference. "Just throw them out. You owe them nothing, not safety or comfort. If they're not going to help, then get rid of them."

North rolls his eyes and rubs a hand over his face, smearing more of the blood and dirt around. "It's not that easy. Nothing is ever that easy."

I pull a face but nod, because that's a big part of growing up. Learning that everything comes with consequences, some of them too devastating to contemplate.

So I change tactics. "Where did Kieran end up stashing Sage? I need to keep doing my rounds and check over the whole family."

Gryphon huffs, still pissed as hell at his second, and says, "They're in with Felix."

North gives him a look and then nods like they've come to an agreement. "You can head right over there and be checked by Davenport as well. Gabe and Bassinger too. I have this to deal with, and Gryphon can go through the security processes one last time, then we can regroup. Don't go anywhere alone."

Where are you?

I roll my eyes at the sound of North's voice in my head because he was the one to tell me not to leave this room without backup, so naturally I'm right where he put me.

The man should trust me a little more.

Oli, who is with you right now? Don't say anything out loud or react, you need to be discreet.

I fight to keep a scowl off of my face at Gryphon chiming in. I still don't fully understand how this mind-talking thing works, and the fact that they both talk over each other makes me sure that they're both hearing each other.

Atlas glances over to me and that confirms it, they're all in my head right now, talking to me, but at each other as well.

I glance up to where Kieran is holding Sage, petting at her hair and murmuring to her quietly about the blood he's covered in. She doesn't actually seem fazed by it at all, she's more worried about getting as close to him as she can get, and my heart does a little tug at my own Bonded.

I'm in the medical center, exactly where North told

me to be. I have Gabe and Atlas with me. Kieran, Sage, and Felix are too. I'm safe.

There's a pause and my stomach begins to churn. It's only Gryphon's warning to stay discreet that keeps me in my seat. If I'm being watched somehow, like a hacker in the security system, then I can't just run out of here like my ass is on fire.

But what if one of my Bonds has been hurt?

Would I know? I'd have to, right?!

Tell me now. Whatever it is, tell me now.

I send it to both of them and I attempt to sound firm, but I'm not sure how well that translates to them when I'm met with silence.

I could scream.

"What's wrong? Your heart rate just hit the roof," Felix murmurs, obviously trying not to startle me in my entirely freaked out state.

I swallow roughly as I try to figure out how to warn him that something is going on without speaking about it, in case the room is bugged. It's impossible. There's no way without Gryphon's Neuro ability to do it. So I just sit there and wait, trying not to lose my shit.

Then Gryphon sends me through a perfect image.

I don't know how the hell he does it, it almost killed me to send North the image of the shadow pups, and yet Gryphon is sending me through a series of images that play in my head like a film reel.

My palms break out in a sweat.

I can handle a lot of things.

So I already know how much bullshit I can survive.

Seeing Sage slit our first Shield, Dara's, throat and then opening the gates to the Resistance, might not be one of them.

Also by J Bree

The Mounts Bay Saga

The Butcher Duet
The Butcher of the Bay: Part I
The Butcher of the Bay: Part II

Hannaford Prep
Just Drop Out: Hannaford Prep Year One
Make Your Move: Hannaford Prep Year Two
Play the Game: Hannaford Prep Year Three
To the End: Hannaford Prep Year Four

The Queen Crow Trilogy
All Hail
The Ruthless
Queen Crow

The Unseen MC
Angel Unseen

The Bonds That Tie
Broken Bonds
Savage Bonds
Blood Bonds
Forced Bonds

About J Bree

J Bree is a dreamer, writer, mother, farmer, and cat-wrangler. The order of priorities changes daily.

She lives on a small farm in a tiny rural town in Australia that no one has ever heard of. She spends her days dreaming about all of her book boyfriends, listening to her partner moan about how the wine grapes are growing, and being a snack bitch to her two kids. For updates about upcoming releases, please visit her website at http://www.jbreeauthor.com, and sign up for the newsletter or join her group on Facebook at #mountygirlforlife: A J Bree Reading Group

Printed in Great Britain
by Amazon